Defining Excellence in Simulation Programs

EDITED BY

Janice C. Palaganas, PhD, RN, NP

Director, Institute for Medical Simulation
Principal Faculty, Center for Medical Simulation
Massachusetts General Hospital
Department of Anesthesia, Critical Care, & Pain Medicine
Harvard Medical School
Boston, Massachusetts

Juli C. Maxworthy, DNP, MSN, MBA, RN, CNL, CPHQ, CPPS, CHSE

Assistant Professor, Director of Traditional DNP Program and Chair of Simulation Committee
School of Nursing and Health Professions
University of San Francisco
San Francisco, California
CEO, WithMax Consulting Inc.
Orinda, California

Chad A. Epps, MD

Associate Professor and Director of Simulation
School of Health Professions, Department of Clinical and Diagnostic Sciences
School of Medicine, Department of Anesthesiology
School of Nursing, Department of Adult/Acute Health, Chronic Care, and Foundations
School of Engineering, Department of Mechanical Engineering
University of Alabama at Birmingham
Birmingham, Alabama

Mary Elizabeth (Beth) Mancini, RN, PhD, NE-BC, FAHA, ANEF, FAAN

Professor
Associate Dean and Chair, Undergraduate Nursing Programs
Baylor Professor for Healthcare Research
The University of Texas at Arlington College of Nursing
Past President, The Society for Simulation in Healthcare
Arlington, Texas

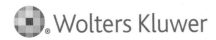 Wolters Kluwer

Philadelphia • Baltimore • New York • London
Buenos Aires • Hong Kong • Sydney • Tokyo

Acquisitions Editor: Shannon W. Magee
Product Development Editors: Ashley Fischer and Maria M. McAvey
Developmental Editor: Louise Bierig
Senior Marketing Manager: Mark Wiragh
Editorial Assistant: Zachary Shapiro
Senior Production Project Manager: Cynthia Rudy
Design Coordinator: Holly Reid McLaughlin
Manufacturing Coordinator: Kathleen Brown
Prepress Vendor: S4Carlisle

9 8 7 6 5 4 3 2 1

Printed in China

Library of Congress Cataloging-in-Publication Data
Defining excellence in simulation programs / edited by Janice C. Palaganas, Juli C. Maxworthy,
Chad A. Epps, Mary Elizabeth (Beth) Mancini.—First edition.
  p. ; cm.
 Includes bibliographical references and index.
 ISBN 978-1-4511-8879-0 (alk. paper)
 I. Palaganas, Janice C., editor. II. Maxworthy, Juli C., editor. III. Epps, Chad A., editor. IV. Mancini, Mary E., editor.
 [DNLM: 1. Patient Simulation. 2. Competency—Based Education–methods. 3. Education, Nursing—methods.
4. Evidence—Based Nursing—methods. WY 105]

 RT51
 610.73—dc23

                                                                                          2014021575

DEDICATION

This is dedicated to the field of simulation: current users of simulation, members of the Society and affiliating groups, and future simulationists.

Janice C. Palaganas, PhD, RN, NP
Juli C. Maxworthy, DNP, MSN, MBA, RN, CNL, CPHQ, CPPS, CHSE
Chad A. Epps, MD
Mary Elizabeth (Beth) Mancini, RN, PhD, NE-BC, FAHA, ANEF, FAAN

CONTRIBUTORS

Guillaume Alinier, PhD, MPhys, PgCert, SFHEA, CPhys, MInstP, MIPEM
Professor of Simulation in Healthcare Education
School of Health and Social Work
University of Hertfordshire
Hatfield, United Kingdom
National Teaching Fellow, Higher Education
  Academy, UK
Simulation Training and Research Manager
Ambulance Service
Hamad Medical Corporation
Doha, Qatar
Visiting Fellow, Department of Public
  Health and Wellbeing, Northumbria
  University, Newcastle, UK

Aditee Ambardekar, MD
Assistant Professor
Department of Anesthesiology and Pain Management
University of Texas Southwestern Medical Center

Pamela B. Andreatta, EdD, MFA, MA
Assistant Professor, Department of Medical Education
Director, Clinical Simulation Center
Executive Director, American Heart Association
  Training Center
University of Michigan Medical School
Ann Arbor, Michigan

Wendy Anson, PhD, CHSE
Educational Psychology & Technology
Research Analyst
Certified Healthcare Simulation Educator
Simulation and Training Education Lab,
  MedStar Health
Washington, District of Columbia

Soledad Armijo, R MD, EdD
Associate Professor
Director Centro de Simulación Clínica
Centro de Simulación Clínica
Facultad de Medicina
Universidad Diego Portales
Santiago, Chile

Jennifer L. Arnold, MD, MSc, FAAP
Assistant Professor
Department of Pediatrics
Baylor
Medical Director, Simulation
Simulation Center
Texas Children's Hospital
Houston, Texas

Marc Auerbach, MD, MSc, FAAP
Assistant Professor
Department of Pediatrics
Section of Emergency Medicine
Yale University School of Medicine
Attending Physician
Associate Director Pediatric Simulation
Associate Pediatric Trauma Medical Director
Yale New Haven Children's Hospital
New Haven, Connecticut

Jeanette L. Augustson, MA
Senior Director, Education Administration
HealthPartners Institute for Education
  and Research
HealthPartners
Bloomington, Minnesota

Eric B. Bauman, PhD, RN
Affiliate
Games+Learning+Society
University of Wisconsin–Madison
Founding and Managing Member
Clinical Playground, LLC
Madison, Wisconsin

Fernando Bello, PhD
Reader in Surgical Graphics and Computing
Department of Surgery and Cancer
Imperial College London
St. Mary's Hospital
London, United Kingdom

David J. Birnbach, MD, MPH
Vice Provost for Faculty Affairs
University of Miami
Professor of Anesthesiology and Obstetrics
  and Gynecology
Miller School of Medicine
Associate Dean and Director
UM/Jackson Memorial Hospital
  Center for Patient Safety
Coral Gables, Florida

Teri Boese, RN, MSN
Associate Professor (Clinical)
Director
Center for Simulation Innovation
University of Texas Health Science
  Center at San Antonio
San Antonio, Texas

Brian C. Brost, MD
Operations Director, Mayo Clinic Multidisciplinary
    Simulation Center
Maternal Fetal Medicine Fellowship Director
Maternal Fetal Medicine Division Director
Professor, Mayo Clinic College of Medicine
Rochester, Minnesota

Eric A. Brown, MD, FACEP
Physician Executive
Palmetto Health Richland
Executive Director
Palmetto Health—USC School of Medicine Simulation
    Center
Faculty
Department of Emergency Medicine
Palmetto Health
Columbia, South Carolina

Janine A. Buis, RN, BSN, BSHCA, MBA
Manager Education and Simulation
Education Service/Community Health Education and
    Simulation Center
Northwest Hospital & Medical Center/UW Medicine
Seattle, Washington

Jennifer A. Calzada, MA
Director
Tulane Center for Advanced Medical Simulation and
    Team Training
Tulane School of Medicine
New Orleans, Louisiana

**Dylan Campher, Cert AT, Adv Dip Perf., Dip PM, Dip
Buss. Management, Grad. Cert. Healthcare Simulation**
Director of Simulation
Director of Graduate Certificate in Healthcare Simulation
Clinical Skills Development Service
Queensland Health
Brisbane, Australia

Cecilia Canales, MPH
Director of Operations
Medical Education Simulation Center
University of California, Irvine
Irvine, California
Director of Clinical Research
Department of Anesthesiology and Perioperative Care
UC Irvine Medical Center
Orange, California

Adam Cheng, MD, FRCPC, FAAP
Associate Professor
Department of Pediatrics
University of Calgary
Director
KidSIM-ASPIRE Simulation
    Research Program
Alberta Children's Hospital
Calgary, Alberta, Canada

Don Combs, PhD
Vice President, Dean of the School of
    Health Professions
Eastern Virginia Medical School
Norfolk, Virginia

Leslie Coonfare, MBA, BSN, RN-BC
Senior Director of Strategic Partnerships
Ohio University
Dublin, Ohio

Jeffrey B. Cooper, PhD
Professor of Anesthesia
Harvard Medical School
Executive Director
Center for Medical Simulation
Senior Biomedical Engineer
Department of Anesthesia
Critical Care and Pain Medicine
Massachusetts General Hospital
Boston, Massachusetts

**Ian Curran, BSc, AKC, MBBS, FRCA, PgDig MedEd
(distinction)**
Reader (Assistant Professor)
Innovation and Excellence in
    Healthcare Education
Centre for Medical Education
Queen Mary University of London
Consultant Anesthetist in Pain Medicine
Boyle's Department of Anesthesiology
St. Bartholomew's Hospital
London, United Kingdom

Rebekah Damazo, RN, CPNP, CHSE-A, MSN
Rural SimCenter Director
Professor of Public Health Nursing
California State University, Chico
Chico, California

**Rita F. D'Aoust, PhD, ACNP, ANP-BC, CNE,
FAANP, FNAP**
Associate Dean for Academic Affairs
Director for Interprofessional Initiatives
University of South Florida College of Nursing
Tampa, Florida

Cathy Deckers, RN, MSN, EdD
Clinical Instructor
School of Nursing
California State University, Long Beach
Clinical Instructor
Clinical Workforce Development
Long Beach Memorial Medical Center
Long Beach, California
Hospital Services Account Manager & Simulation
    Consultant
CAE Healthcare
Sarasota, Florida

Shad Deering, MD
Assistant Dean for Simulation Education
Department of Obstetrics and Gynecology
Uniforms Services University of
 the Health Sciences
Maternal Fetal Medicine Staff
Department of Obstetrics and Gynecology
Walter Reed National Military Medical Center
Bethesda, Maryland

Ignacio del Moral, MD, PhD
Executive Director
Hospital Virtual Valdecilla
Santander, Spain

Ellen S. Deutsch, MD, FACS, FAAP
Director, Peri-Operative Simulation
Center for Simulation, Advance Education and
 Innovation
Department of Anesthesiology and
 Critical Care Medicine
The Children's Hospital of Pennsylvania
Philadelphia, Pennsylvania

Peter Dieckmann, PhD, Dipl.-Psych
Director of Research
Danish Institute for
 Medical Simulation (DIMS)
Capital Region of Denmark
Herlev Hospital, Denmark

Yue Dong, MD
Assistant Professor of Medicine
Multidisciplinary Simulation Center
Mayo Clinic
Rochester, Minnesota

Thomas A. Dongilli, AT
Director of Operations
WISER
University of Pittsburgh
Pittsburgh, Pennsylvania

Bonnie J. Driggers, RN, MS, MPA
Professor Emerita
School of Nursing
Oregon Health & Sciences University
Portland, Oregon

William F. Dunn, MD
Associate Professor of Medicine
Mayo Clinic College of Medicine
Consultant
Department of Medicine
Division of Pulmonary and Critical Care Medicine
Mayo Clinic
Rochester, Minnesota

Chad A. Epps, MD
Associate Professor and Director of Simulation
School of Health Professions, Department
 of Clinical & Diagnostic Sciences
School of Medicine, Department of Anesthesiology
School of Nursing, Department of Adult/Acute Health,
 Chronic Care, and Foundations
School of Engineering, Department of Mechanical
 Engineering
University of Alabama at Birmingham
Birmingham, Alabama

Sandra J. Feaster, RN, MS, MBA
Assistant Dean
Center for Immersion and Simulation-Based Learning
Stanford University School of Medicine
Stanford, California

Diane M. Ferguson, BSN, RN
Director
HEB Clinical Skills Center
Department of the Medical Dean
The University of Texas Health Science Center at
 San Antonio
San Antonio, Texas

Sherry D. Fox, RN, PhD, CHSE
Professor Emerita
Department of Nursing
California State University, Chico
Chico, California

David M. Gaba, MD
Associate Dean for Immersive and Simulation-Based
 Learning
Stanford School of Medicine
Stanford, California
Staff Physician and Co-Director, Simulation Center
VA Palo Alto Health Care System
Palo Alto, California

Kathleen Gallo, PhD, MBA, RN, FAAN
Associate Professor
Science Education
Hofstra-North Shore-LIJ School of Medicine
Hempstead, New York
Senior Vice President and Chief Learning Officer
The Center for Learning and Innovation
North Shore-LIJ Health System
Lake Success, New York

Wendy L. Gammon, MA, MEd
Assistant Professor of Medicine
Director, Standardized Patient Program
Interprofessional Center for Experiential Learning
 and Simulation (iCELS)
University of Massachusetts Medical School
Worcester, Massachusetts

Susan J. Garbutt, DNP, RN, CIC, CNE
Simulation Coordinator
Lecturer
Department of Nursing
The University of Tampa
Tampa, Florida

Jesika S. Gavilanes, MA
OHSU Simulation Operations
Chair Oregon Simulation Alliance
Member of Simulated Code Interdisciplinary Team
 Training (SCITT)
Oregon Health & Science University Simulation
Portland, Oregon

Gayle Gliva-McConvey, BA
Director, Professional Skills Teaching & Assessment
Sentara Center for Simulation and Immersive Learning
Eastern Virginia Medical School
Norfolk, Virginia

Jean Claude Granry, MD
Professor
Department of Anesthesia and Intensive Care
University of Angers
Chief
Department of Anesthesia and Intensive Care
University Hospital
Angers, France

Debra Hagler, PhD, RN, ACNS-BC, CNE, CHSE, ANEF, FAAN
Clinical Professor
College of Nursing and Health Innovation
Arizona State University
Phoenix, Arizona

Roberta L. Hales, MHA, RRT-NPS, RN
Lead Simulation Educator
Center for Simulation, Advanced Education and Innovation
The Children's Hospital of Philadelphia
Philadelphia, Pennsylvania
Adjunct Associate Faculty
Master of Science in Medical and Healthcare
 Simulation Program
Drexel University College of Medicine,
 Department of Emergency Medicine
Philadelphia, Pennsylvania

Daniel A. Hashimoto, MD, MS
General Surgery Resident
Department of Surgery
Massachusetts General Hospital
Boston, Massachusetts

Nancy Heine, RN, CANP, MSEd
Assistant Professor of Medicine and Medical Education
Director, Clinical Skills Education Center
Loma Linda University
Loma Linda, California

Danyel L. Helgeson, MS, RN
Interim Associate Dean of Allied Health
Chief Nursing Officer
Academic Affairs
Riverland Community Center
Austin, Minnesota

Wendy Hewitt, BSEE
Operations Manager
Department of Medical Education
Hannaford Center for Safety, Innovation,
 and Simulation
TUSM, Maine Track Program
Maine Medical Center
Portland, Maine

Margaret Hinrichs, M.Ed.
Coordinator and Trainer, Family Meeting
 Project Volunteers
Beth Israel Deaconess Medical Center
Boston, Massachusett

Valerie M. Howard, EdD, MSN, RN
Dean and Professor
School of Nursing and Health Sciences
Director
Regional RISE Center
Robert Morris University
Past President
International Nursing Association for Clinical
 Simulation and Learning (INACSL)
Moon Township, Pennsylvania

Ismaël Hssain, MD, MSc (MEd)
Attending Physician in Emergency
 and Disaster Medicine
Center for EMS Education and Simulation in
 Healthcare Unit
Department of Emergency Medicine, Prehospital
 Care and HEMS
Mulhouse General Hospital
Mulhouse, France

Yue Ming Huang, EdD, MHS
Associate Adjunct Professor
Department of Anesthesiology
David Geffen School of Medicine at UCLA
Education/Operations Director,
 UCLA Simulation Center
Los Angeles, California

Joshua Hui, MD, MSCR, FACEP
Assistant Professor
Department of Emergency Medicine
David Geffen School of Medicine at UCLA
Los Angeles, California
Director of Simulation
Department of Emergency Medicine
Olive View–University of California Los Angeles
 Medical Center
Sylmar, California

Aisha Jamal, CPA
Senior Project Manager
Strategic Planning and Business Development
Texas Children's Hospital
Houston, Texas

Pamela R. Jeffries, PhD, RN, ANEF, FAAN
Professor
Vice Provost for Digital Initiatives
Johns Hopkins School of Nursing
Baltimore, Maryland

Gail Johnson, MS, RN, CCRN, CPHQ, CHSE
Director
Clinical Simulation
Health Partners Institute for Education and Research
St. Paul, Minnesota

Ashwin A. Kalbag, MBBS, DA, MD, FFARCSI, FRCA
Consultant
Department of Anesthesia and Pain Medicine
Imperial College NHS Trust
London, United Kingdom

Suzan E. Kardong-Edgren, PhD, RN, ANEF, CHSE
Jody DeMeyer Endowed Chair
Research Associate Professor
Department of Nursing
Boise State University
Boise, Idaho

Sara Kim, PhD
Research Professor, Director of Educational
Innovations and Strategic Programs
Department of Surgery
Institute for Simulation and Interprofessional
    Studies (ISIS)
University of Washington
Seattle, Washington

Roger L. Kneebone, PhD, FRCS, FRCGP
Professor
Division of Surgery
Department of Surgery and Cancer
Faculty of Medicine
Imperial College London
Clinical Skills Centre
St. Mary's Hospital
London, United Kingdom

Sabrina Koh, RN, MHS(Edu), PGDip(CC), CHSE
Assistant Director, Nursing
Nursing Administration
Sengkang Health, SingHealth
Singapore

Jared M. Kutzin, DNP, MS (MMEL), MPH, RN, CPPS
Director
Simulation Center
Winthrop University Hospital
Mineola, New York

Richard R. Kyle Jr., MS
Instructor
Department of Anatomy, Physiology, and Genetics
Uniformed Services University of the Health Sciences
Bethesda, Maryland

David M. LaCombe, BSM, CPLP
Emergency Care Portfolio Director–Americas
Laerdal Medical
Wappingers Falls, New York

Stephen E. Lammers, PhD
Professor Emeritus
Lafayette College
Easton, Pennsylvania
Ethics Program Consultant
Division of Education
Lehigh Valley Health Network
Allentown, Pennsylvania

Samsun Lampotang, PhD
Professor
Department of Anesthesiology
University of Florida
Director
Center for Safety, Simulation & Advanced Learning
    Technologies
University of Florida
Gainesville, Florida

Michael C. Lauber, FAIA
President
Ellenzweig
Architecture Planning
Cambridge, Massachusetts

Farrah F. Leland, JD
Assistant Director
The Institute for Simulation and Interprofessional
    Studies (ISIS)
University of Washington
Seattle, Washington

Tom Lemaster, RN, MSN, MEd, Paramedic
Program Director
Center for Simulation and Research
Cincinnati Children's Hospital
Cincinnati, Ohio

Adam I. Levine, MD
Professor
Department of Anesthesiology, Otolaryngology, and
    Structural and Chemical Biology
Icahn School of Medicine at Mount Sinai
Program Director and Vice Chair for Education
Department of Anesthesiology
Mount Sinai Hospital
New York, New York

Keith E. Littlewood, MD
Assistant Dean, School of Medicine
Vice-Chair, Department of Anesthesiology
Medical Director, UVA Medical Simulation Center
Director, Clinical Performance Education Center
University of Virginia Health System
Charlottesville, Virginia

Justin L. Lockman, MD
Director, Pediatric Anesthesiology Fellowship Program at
    The Children's Hospital of Philadelphia
Assistant Professor of Anesthesiology, Pediatrics,
    and Critical Care
Perelman School of Medicine at the University
    of Pennsylvania
Philadelphia, Pennsylvania

Connie M. Lopez, MSN, CNS, RNC-OB, CPHRM
National Leader, Patient Safety & Risk Management
National Risk Management
Kaiser Permanente
Oakland, California

John W. Lutz, BS
Director of Information Technology
WISER
University of Pittsburgh
Pittsburgh, Pennsylvania

Leslie A. Lynch
Administrative Director
Continuing Medical Education
OhioHealth Learning
Columbus, Ohio

José M. Maestre, MD, PhD
Education Director
Hospital Virtual Valdecilla
Department of Anesthesiology and Critical Care
Hospital Universitario Marqués de Valdecilla
Santander, Spain

Mary Elizabeth (Beth) Mancini, RN, PhD, NE-BC, FAHA, ANEF, FAAN
Professor
Associate Dean and Chair, Undergraduate Nursing
    Programs
Baylor Professor for Healthcare Research
The University of Texas at Arlington College of Nursing
Past President, The Society for Simulation in Healthcare
Arlington, Texas

Juli C. Maxworthy, DNP, MSN, MBA, RN, CNL, CPHQ, CPPS, CHSE
Assistant Professor, Director of Traditional DNP Program
    and Chair of Simulation Committee
School of Nursing and Health Professions
University of San Francisco
Vice-Chair, Accreditation Council, Society for Simulation
    in Healthcare
San Francisco, California

Catherine A. McIntosh, MBBS, FANZCA
Director
Hunter New England Simulation Centre
Hunter New England Health
Conjoint Senior Lecturer
School of Medicine and Public Health
University of Newcastle
Australia

Anne Marie Monachino, MSN, RN, CPN
Clinical Educator
Center for Stimulation, Advanced Education, and
    Innovation
Children's Hospital of Philadelphia
Philadelphia, Pennsylvania

Brian Moores
Vice President
Drake Systems Group, Incorporated
Yorba Linda, California

J. Bradley Morrison, PhD
Associate Professor of Management
International Business School
Brandeis University
Waltham, Massachusetts

Deborah D. Navedo, PhD, CPNP, CNE
Director
Health Professions Education Program
MGH Institute of Health Professions
Educational Specialist
MGH Learning Laboratory
Massachusetts General Hospital
Boston, Massachusetts

Debra Nestel, PhD, FAcadMEd, CHSE-A
Professor of Simulation Education in Healthcare
School of Rural Health/Health PEER
Faculty of Medicine, Nursing & Health Sciences
Monash University
Clayton, Victoria, Australia

Cate F. Nicholas, EdD, MS, PA
Director, Simulation Education and Operations
Clinical Simulation Laboratory
University of Vermont
Assistant Professor, Family Medicine and Ob/Gyn
Fletcher Allen Health Care
Burlington, Vermont

Nichole Oocumma, PhD (ABD), BSDH, MA, CHES, CHSE
Director, CareConnect Training
OhioHealth
Dublin, Ohio

Tamara L. Owens, MEd
Director, Clinical Skills and Simulation Centers
Instructor, Department Community and Family Medicine
Howard University
Washington, District of Columbia

Janice C. Palaganas, PhD, RN, NP
Director, Institute for Medical Simulation
Principal Faculty, Center for Medical Simulation
Massachusetts General Hospital
Department of Anesthesia, Critical Care, and Pain Medicine
Harvard Medical School
Boston, Massachusetts

Christine S. Park, MD
Director, Simulation Technology and Immersive Learning
Center for Education in Medicine
Associate Professor
Department of Anesthesiology
Northwestern University, Feinberg School of Medicine
Chicago, Illinois

Amar P. Patel, MS, NREMT-P, CFC
Adjunct Instructor
School of Medicine
Department of Emergency Medicine
University of North Carolina at Chapel Hill
Chapel Hill, North Carolina
Director
Center for Innovative Learning
WakeMed Health & Hospitals
Raleigh, North Carolina

Mary D. Patterson, MD, MEd
Professor
Department of Pediatrics
Northeast Ohio Medical University
Rootstown, Ohio
Director
Simulation Center for Safety and Reliability
Akron Children's Hospital
Akron, Ohio

Dawn Taylor Peterson, PhD
Director of Simulation Education and Research
University of Alabama at Birmingham, Department of
    Pediatrics
Pediatric Simulation Center, Children's of Alabama
Birmingham, Alabama

James C. Phero, DMD
Professor Emeritus Anesthesiology,
College of Medicine, University of Cincinnati Academic
    Health Center
Anesthesia Attending,
UC Physicians, UC Medical Center,
Cincinnati, Ohio

Roy Phitayakorn, MD, MHPE (MEd), FACS
Assistant Professor of Surgery
Harvard Medical School
Director of Surgical Education Research
Department of Surgery
Surgical Lead, Strategic Initiatives and Operations
MGH Learning Laboratory
The Massachusetts General Hospital
Boston, Massachusetts

Paul E. Phrampus, MD, FACEP
Associate Professor
Departments of Emergency Medicine and Anesthesiology
University of Pittsburgh School of Medicine
Director, Peter M. Winter Institute for Simulation,
    Education, and Research (WISER)
University of Pittsburgh and University of Pittsburgh
    Medical Center
Pittsburgh, Pennsylvania

Paul J. Pribaz, MS
Executive Director, Jump Innovation
Jump Trading Simulation & Education Center
OSF Healthcare System
Peoria, Illinois

Daniel B. Raemer, PhD
Founding President, Society for Simulation in Healthcare
Director of Clinical Programs, Center for Medical
    Simulation, Boston, MA
Associate Professor of Anaesthesiology
Harvard Medical School, Boston, MA

Penny Ralston-Berg, MS
Senior Instructional Designer
World Campus Learning Design
The Pennsylvania State University
University Park, Pennsylvania

Patricia A. Reidy, DNP, FNP-BC
Clinical Associate Professor
School of Nursing
MGH Institute of Health Professions
Boston, Massachusetts
Family Nurse Practitioner
Family Health Center of Worcester
Worcester, Massachusetts

Troy E. Reihsen
Director of Operations
SimPORTAL Medical School
University of Minnesota
Minneapolis, Minnesota

John Rice, PhD
Chairman of Technology and Standards Committee
Society for Simulation in Healthcare (SSH)
Virginia Beach, Virginia

Mary Anne Rizzolo, EdD, RN, FAAN, ANEF
Consultant
National League for Nursing
Washington, District of Columbia

Laura K. Rock, MD
Instructor
Harvard Medical School
Pulmonary and Critical Care Medicine
Beth Israel Deaconess Medical Center
Boston, Massachusetts

Brian K. Ross, PhD, MD
Executive Director
Institute for Simulation and Interprofessional
  Studies (ISIS)
University of Washington
Professor
Department of Anesthesiology and Pain Management
University of Washington
Seattle, Washington

Alicia Gill Rossiter, MSN, ARNP, FNP, PNP-BC, FAANP
Instructor
Coordinator of Graduate Nursing Simulation
College of Nursing Military Liaison
University of South Florida College of Nursing
Tampa, Florida

Jenny W. Rudolph, PhD
Assistant Clinical Professor of Anaesthesia
Harvard Medical School and
Massachusetts General Hospital
Director, Graduate Programs
Institute for Medical Simulation
Center for Medical Simulation
Boston, Massachusetts

Jill S. Sanko, MS, ARNP, CHSE-A, PhD(c)
Research and Simulation Education Specialist
Department of Anesthesia
University of Miami School of Nursing and Health
  Studies
University of Miami
Miami, Florida

Taylor L. Sawyer, DO, MEd
Assistant Professor
Department of Pediatrics
University of Washington
Neonatologist
Department of Pediatrics
Seattle Children's Hospital
Seattle, Washington

Augusto Scalabrini-Neto, MD, PhD
Associate Professor
Emergency Department
University of Sao Paulo Medical School
Teaching Coordinator
Emergency Department
Hospital das Clinicas da FMUSP
Sao Paulo, Brazil

Kathryn A. Schaivone, MHA
Clinical Instructor and Director
Clinical Education and Evaluation
University of Maryland
Baltimore, Maryland

Morgan A. Scherwitz, MSN, RN
Instructor and Manager of the Nursing Skills
  Laboratories and Simulation Center
Center for Clinical Simulation & Competency
Tarleton State University*
Stephenville, Texas
*Member of the Texas A&M University System

Dawn M. Schocken, MPH, PhD(c), CHSE-A
Director
Center for Advanced Clinical Learning
USF Health Morsani College of Medicine
Tampa, Florida

Michael A. Seropian, MD, FRCPC
Professor
Department of Anesthesiology
Director of Anesthesia Simulation Services
Oregon Health & Science University
Past President, Society for Simulation
  in Healthcare
President, The SimHealth Group
Portland, Oregon

John H. Shatzer, PhD
Associate Professor
Medical Education and Administration
Vanderbilt University School of Medicine
Nashville, Tennessee

Ilya Shekhter, MS, MBA, CHSE
Director of Simulation Operations
Center for Patient Safety
University of Miami
Jackson Memorial Hospital
Miami, Florida

Robert Simon, EdD
Education Director, Center for Medical Simulation
Instructor, Harvard Medical School and
Massachusetts General Hospital
Boston, Massachusetts

Frederick L. Slone, MD
Medical Director
Center for Advanced Clinical Learning
University of South Florida College of Medicine
Tampa, Florida

Amy B. Smith, PhD
Associate Professor
Educational Affairs
University of South Florida Morsani College of Medicine
Tampa, Florida
Medical Educator
Division of Education
Lehigh Valley Health Network
Allentown, Pennsylvania

Andrew E. Spain, MA, NCEE, EMT-P
Director of Accreditation and Certification
Society for Simulation in Healthcare
Wheaton, Illinois

Demian Szyld, MD, EdM
Associate Medical Director
New York Simulation Center for the Health Sciences
  (NYSIM)
New York University Langone Medical Center and City
  University of New York
Assistant Professor
Department of Emergency Medicine
New York University School of Medicine
New York, New York

Brent Thorkelson, BSc, EMT-P
Senior Staff Development Officer
Clinical Compliance, Training and Standards
Patient Care Simulation Program
Albert Health Services, Emergency Medical Services
Calgary, Alberta, Canada

Stephanie A. Tuttle, MS, MBA
Administrative Director
Center for Simulation, Advanced Education, and
  Innovation
The Children's Hospital of Philadelphia
Philadelphia, Pennsylvania

Sandrijn M. van Schaik, MD, PhD
Associate Professor of Clinical Pediatrics
Fellowship Program Director
Pediatric Critical Care Medicine
Education Director, Kanbar Center for Simulation,
  Clinical Skills and Telemedicine Education
University of California San Francisco
San Francisco, California

Angie Wade, MPH, CCRC
Sr. Measurement and Assessment Consultant
OhioHealth Learning
OhioHealth
Columbus, Ohio

Katie Walker, RN, MBA
Director, Assistant Vice President
New York City Health and Hospitals Corporation
  Healthcare Simulation Center
The Institute of Medical Simulation and
  Advanced Learning
New York, New York

Kelly D. Wallin, MS, RN
Assistant Director
Simulation Center
Texas Children's Hospital
Houston, Texas

Marcus Watson, BSc Hon, Grad Dip CS, MS, PhD
Associate Professor
School of Medicine
University of Queensland
Executive Director
Clinical Skills Development Service
Queensland Health
Brisbane, Australia

Penni I. Watts, MSN, RN, CHSE
Instructor and Director of Clinical Simulation and
  Training
School of Nursing, Department of Adult/Acute Health,
  Chronic Care, and Foundations
The University of Alabama at Birmingham
Birmingham, Alabama

KT Waxman, DNP, MBA, RN, CNL, CENP
Assistant Professor
School of Nursing & Health Professions
University of San Francisco
San Francisco, California
Director
California Simulation Alliance
California Institute for Nursing & Health Care
Oakland, California

Marjorie Lee White, MD, MPPM, MA
Associate Professor
Department of Pediatrics
University of Alabama at Birmingham
Director of Medical Student Simulation
University of Alabama School of Medicine
Medical Co-Director
Pediatric Simulation Center
Children's of Alabama
Birmingham, Alabama

Graham Whiteside, BSc (Hons) Nur Sci,
DipHE MHN, RMN, RGN
Chief Operating Officer
Limbs and Things, Incorporated
Savannah, Georgia

M. Scott Williams, PhD, MBA
Associate Superintendent of Instruction and Student
  Services
Chief Instruction and Student Services Officer
Tulsa Technology Center
Tulsa, Oklahoma

Rebecca Wilson, PhD, RN, CHSE
Director of Interprofessional Education
Health Sciences
University of Utah
Salt Lake City, Utah

H. Michael Young, BBS, MDiv
Simulation Technology Specialist
Center for Instructional Innovation
Tarleton State University*
Stephenville, Texas
*Member of the Texas A&M University System

Jason Zigmont, PhD, CHSE-A
System Director of Learning Innovation
OhioHealth Learning
OhioHealth
Columbus, Ohio

FOREWORD

When the modern era of simulation in healthcare started, in the early 1990s or so, a few brave souls ventured forth in resurrecting an old idea while thinking it was new. This emerging educational technique was the product of individuals discovering, inventing, and reinventing methods for teaching in healthcare that were outside of the paradigms that had developed in nursing, medicine, and allied health during the 20th century. The prevailing methods for teaching at that time, providing didactic material through writing or lecturing combined with extensive bedside instruction, mirrored the trends in healthcare itself. That century saw steady growth of the scientific knowledge about disease and its treatment and the development of the modern hospital. The educational paradigm was characterized by the specialized learning and apprenticeship model. The teaching methods and the healthcare learners' needs were a fine marriage until, toward the end of the century, the rate of growth of science showed itself to be exponential and overwhelming and the singular model of the inpatient hospital began to crumble. Thus, as healthcare has evolved into the 21st century, the educational paradigm is again necessarily changing. While the simulation pioneer's motivation was originally technologically driven, it is now becoming clear that the field of simulation is growing because it is meeting the new needs of the learner. The impetus for procedural and problem-solving skill development in a distinctly interprofessional healthcare environment is well matched with simulation's application-based teaching, which is well suited to different professions and specialties even at the same time. What appeared to be a revolutionary and innovative educational technique in the early 1990s is rapidly becoming a mainstream component of healthcare teaching and learning.

At the beginning of this century, the Society for Simulation in Healthcare (SSH) emerged. As one of the founders of that organization, I had a selfish motive. I was asked to manage a simulation program and wanted a forum to share ideas so that I did not have to reinvent everything *de novo*. Also, my foundation in management sciences and formal education was weak. I envisioned a gathering place where like-minded risk-taking educators and simulation managers could exchange their fresh experience, growing expertise, and mistakes to be avoided. I imagined that it would be interprofessional, as I was learning from people with whom I had no prior interactions and realized they faced many of the same problems and had created novel solutions. This book, *Defining Excellence in Simulation Programs*, is an embodiment of those dreams. There is no longer a reason to start from scratch or reinvent, as the experience, knowledge, and wisdom of SSH are captured within. No matter what profession, specialty, or background you come from, the contents of this book will surely be valuable. There are three things that the relationship between this book and SSH represents. First is the unique perspective of the editors and many of the authors who have played a central role in SSH's efforts to examine, learn, and define best practices for simulation and simulation program management through its accreditation, certification, and affiliation efforts. Second, the book is accessible, practical, and timely. While it is well referenced and scholarly, the authors have recognized the value of offering guidance from practices and ideas that have not been proven or sanctified. It is important to recognize that in any young field, the evidence base may be shallow, but the need to share experience remains. Finally, the interprofessional nature of the author list and their diverse perspectives is a refreshing reminder of the power of simulation itself. The editors and authors, all simulationists, come from nursing, medicine, and allied health, with a plethora of specialties represented, as well as many nonclinical arenas such as organizational behavior, psychology, statistics, business, and engineering. They have worked together as a team, a healthcare education team, to provide guidance for everyone interested in simulation education regardless of their affiliations or persuasions. How inspiring is that in a healthcare world that is rapidly becoming a truly team-based domain?

Daniel B. Raemer, PhD
Founding President, Society for Simulation
in Healthcare
Director of Clinical Programs, Center for Medical
Simulation, Boston, MA
Associate Professor of Anaesthesiology
Harvard Medical School, Boston, MA
April 2014

ACKNOWLEDGMENTS

The editors thank the Society for Simulation in Healthcare, whose collective members and efforts have guided the creation and development of this textbook. The Society has supported this production, encouraging the editors and consistently asking for ways to further support this large endeavor.

The editors thank the team at Wolters Kluwer for the assistance, support, and motivation provided throughout the process of editing and writing. Louise Bierig, our Developmental Editor; Ashley Fischer and Maria McAvey, our Product Development Editors; and Shannon Magee, our Acquisitions Editor, were key in facilitating our needs and timelines. Thank you.

The editors would like to acknowledge guest editors who have helped us in the process of reviewing the material in this book to ensure expert peer review, as well as review for clarity. We'd like to specifically acknowledge Dr. Maria Rudolph for reviewing a number of chapters to provide clarity from the perspective of someone new to healthcare simulation.

Dr. Palaganas wishes to thank …

…this editorial team for all of the hard work and time poured into the writing, editing, revising, and decision making for this textbook. Thank you to all of the authors for your contributions. Specific thanks to the team at Wolters Kluwer for all of your guidance and commitment.

I'd like to thank my strongest supporters: my parents, Gerry and Cora; my life partner, Alex; and our children, Jayden and Jianna, who have found ways to encourage and help me make time for this project. I would like to thank my simulation mentors, who happen to be my work family at the Center for Medical Simulation, specifically Robert Simon, Jenny Rudolph, Dan Raemer, and Jeff Cooper, as well as my interprofessional and simulation friends and colleagues around the world.

Dr. Maxworthy wishes to thank …

…my coeditors and the many authors whom through this process I have had the opportunity to get to know as peers but more importantly as friends. This process has been one of great learning for me professionally and personally.

I'd like to thank my best friend and husband, Gary Witherell, who has always been my strongest supporter. My children, Becka, Trevor, and Kaiti, during the writing of this book have blossomed into amazing young adults, and I couldn't be prouder of them. I would like to thank KT Waxman who, while we were in our doctoral program together many years ago, introduced me to the world of healthcare simulation.

Dr. Epps wishes to thank …

…the pioneers of healthcare simulation who led the way for utilizing simulation to improve patient care. We are fortunate that many of these pioneers contributed to this textbook. In addition, thanks to the many contributors for their expertise and commitment and to the editorial and production teams.

Above all, I'd like to deeply thank my wife, Deborah, and two daughters, Evelyn and Ellis, for their patience and support through the many nights and weekends required to edit this book.

Dr. Mancini wishes to thank ….

All of the remarkable individuals in the Society who are committed to enhancing patient safety and outcomes through healthcare simulation.

In addition, I wish to thank David, Carla, Laura, and Jake…. I couldn't do what I do without your love and support.

INTRODUCTION

This book is intended to assist in defining excellence in healthcare simulation. It has a specific focus on management and the development of quality simulation programs. The book was conceived and supported by the Society for Simulation in Healthcare (SSH) and is written for several audiences. Whether you have limited management experience and have been selected to operate a simulation center or you have significant management experience and recently been awarded a grant to develop a new simulation program or you have just been hired as a new simulation educator or researcher, this book serves as a resource for you. In addition, this book can serve as foundational reading for undergraduate or graduate students in a program that focuses on healthcare simulation.

It is our hope that the text makes a contribution by exposing readers to the operational aspects of a simulation program, particularly simulation standards. We describe a variety of simulation methodologies, simulators, simulation program types, program funding mechanisms, program management strategies, center designs, educational development opportunities, strategies of faculty development, research in simulation, and resources in our field.

HOW THIS TEXTBOOK CAME ABOUT

The idea of this textbook stemmed from the SSH Accreditation Program. After reviewing a number of simulation programs seeking accreditation, the Accreditation Council recognized that there were common needs and areas for improvement among surveyed programs. This need for a shared pool of knowledge resulted in the development of this textbook as a resource for programs as well as a guide for improvement and systems development.

WHY THE NAME?

While "excellence" in simulation is yet to be defined, our interactions with simulation colleagues, observations, interviews, and visits to simulation programs around the globe support the notion that there are common practices that lead to success. There is a well-known book by Thomas Peters and Robert Waterman, Jr. (1982) entitled *In Search of Excellence*. Peters and Waterman studied 43 of America's best-run companies, looking at a variety of business sectors. After reviews, observations, interviews, and visits, they identified practices that they felt made these organizations successful. In our attempt to define standards of excellence for simulation programs, we essentially were in search of excellence, visiting many programs that demonstrated what we felt were successful and sustainable practices. Like Peters and Waterman, we are continuing to uncover practices that we feel make simulation programs successful. This textbook is a compilation of successful practices we have uncovered thus far.

A TAXONOMY OF HEALTHCARE SIMULATION

Simulation propagates new technology, methodology, purposes, and areas of study. The variety of simulation use is not only ponderous but also procurable—making healthcare simulation an exciting, alluring, and promising field. While the opportunities for simulation are endless, current healthcare simulation is fraught with limitations that can be resolved by matching purpose with combinations of methods and modalities. There are common purposes, methods, and modalities in healthcare simulation. Understanding these taxonomies (classifications) and types can provide simulationists with tools that can be leveraged to engineer simulations that provide rich learning experiences.

As SSH developed its Accreditation and Certification Programs, it was challenged to deal with the vast array of simulation programs. The SSH Accreditation Board of Review remains impressed by the differences as well as the similarities they see in the programs reviewed every quarter. There are, however, some general perspectives of simulation that are consistent. These perspectives provide categories that can be used to describe the science of simulation. This taxonomy has been used in this book and can serve as a base to examine areas in need of further study. It also provides a fundamental infrastructure for the activities of societies, standard-setting groups, researchers, scientists, inventors, educators, and healthcare providers.

In healthcare, simulation can be categorized by purpose, modality, and methods.

Purpose. The *purpose* of a simulation is to achieve the expressed learning objectives. There are many types of learning objectives identified in a healthcare provider's training and continuing education. Generally, simulation is used for education (teaching, training, and practice). Simulation can also be used for assessment, research, systems integration, and patient safety.

Modality. The term *modality*, as used in this textbook, refers to the simulator. A modality also has multiple dimensions, including the patient and/or anatomical simulator, embedded actor/facilitator roles, clinical setting, patient care equipment, and other physical equipment or technology. The fidelity and interactive ability of each modality dimension is vital to the simulation's achievement of the learning objectives.

Each simulator has advantages and limitations to its use. In order to best meet the needs of the learners, these advantages and limitations should be explored before choosing a simulator. Often, simulation staff will choose the one with which they are most comfortable without realizing that another available simulator has capabilities that are more appropriate for the simulation's learning objectives. In this book we review various modalities and how their use can be facilitated and amplified.

Methods. *Methods* describe the teaching, learning, assessment, or research methods used during the simulation. Different methods are used in simulation, particularly in how feedback is provided. The teaching method should be determined and planned on the basis of the objectives and the modality used. The selected teaching method should be facilitated during the simulation and debriefing based on the formative feedback or learner interactions that demonstrate learning needs. The repercussions of using an inappropriate method could cause adverse learning, assessment, or research experiences. For example, using a mannequin-based immersive patient care simulation presenting unstable vital signs with a new medical student who is learning how to perform a proper preoperative introduction and history assessment may derail the learning objectives, impede any learning around the objectives, and create an anxiety that may negatively affect future performance with an actual patient. Because of this, it is imperative that the instructional and facilitative methods used in simulation be appropriate to the learning objectives and the modalities selected.

Awareness of the limitations of existing modalities and methods encourages programs to focus more on developing faculty on how to use simulation and technology to support the purpose rather than letting the technology drive the teaching. With the variety of simulation purposes, methods, and modalities, simulation managers and educators have the responsibility to know the limitations of their simulators and use them to their best capability to match learning objectives. By covering concepts discovered in the field and attempting to define perspectives within this taxonomy that are recognized to support successful programs, this textbook seeks to provide educators, managers, and students with a foundation in simulation-based healthcare education.

OVERALL STRUCTURE OF THE BOOK

Based on common issues in the field, we have organized this book around 10 key themes:

1. Simulation Standards
2. Types of Simulation Programs
3. Simulators
4. Funding
5. Management
6. Environmental Design
7. Educational Development
8. Faculty Development
9. Research
10. Resources

There are 54 chapters from 137 authors with experience in simulation programs that vary in type, geography, and purpose. There are eight "Consider This" boxes within chapters that provide information on related topics for consideration. Additionally, identified experts and founding fathers and mothers in the field of healthcare simulation have provided open commentary in 26 "Expert's Corner" boxes scattered throughout the textbook, revealing current thinking and areas for future research.

TERMS OF REFERENCE

Yue Ming Huang, John Rice, Andrew Spain, and Janice C. Palaganas representing the SSH Lexicography Committee

ABOUT THE AUTHORS

Dr. Yue Ming Huang is Adjunct Associate Professor of Anesthesiology and Education and Operations Director at the UCLA Simulation Center. After serving as the first Education Chair for the Society for Simulation in Healthcare, Dr. Huang chaired the Simulation Alliance Task Force for several years, bringing together stakeholders from different organizations to initiate a simulation taxonomy project, led the submission of a grant, and conducted focus groups at the International Meeting for Simulation in Healthcare.

Dr. John Rice is retired from the Department of the Navy, where he had over 40 years of experience in many aspects of modeling and simulation for military training and research. Dr. Rice has completed all but dissertations for doctors in philosophy of Instructional System Technology and in Special Education both with emphasis in M&S application research. Upon retirement, he worked as a Standardized Patient at EVMS and affiliated with the Society for Simulation in Healthcare, where he has chaired the Technology and Standards Committee, bringing extensive knowledge of the M&S body of knowledge that has existed long before its application to healthcare training.

Mr. Andrew E. Spain is the Director of Accreditation and Certification for the Society for Simulation in Healthcare. Part of his work for SSH includes the collaborative development of terminology to support healthcare simulation. This work is being done with lexicographic principles and processes being key to the development. He has an MA in Political Science and is currently working on a PhD in Education at the University of Missouri (emphasis in Educational Leadership and Policy Analysis).

Dr. Janice C. Palaganas was the implementing Director of Accreditation and Certification, leading the development and vetting of the Society for Simulation in Healthcare's first working glossary. Dr. Palaganas continues this work as a member of the SSH Terminology & Concepts Committee.

PREFACE TO THE TERMS OF REFERENCE

This introductory section is an attempt to consolidate what is currently known about simulation terminology and taxonomy, to serve as a basis and guide for those new to simulation, and a reference to those who have observed its many changes. We accept the fact that this is an evolving area for discussion, and the short glossary presented here is by no means definitive. We are basing our definitions on best practice cross-checked with other domains. We discuss here the need for common language and, while some chapters may provide definitions for that chapter, we suggest terms for simulation reference that have been identified and vetted by focused committees and groups within the society.

WHY DO WE NEED THIS?

Everything we know needs to be given names with a defined meaning for human communication to take place. A rose is a rose even if you decide to call it something else, but someone would correct you if you label it incorrectly. On the other hand, one would not call a daffodil a rose, so the concept of defined terms interjecting meaning to otherwise nameless objects is very important and must be adhered to by everyone in order to maintain a common understanding. The future of simulation requires an unambiguous manner to coherently express research, data, techniques, and assessment. The verbiage must represent concepts, and the definitions of words and classification of meanings associated with words and phrases must be clear.

Simulation is not a new concept. One can imagine that thousands of years ago, people likely threw rocks and sticks at stationary and moving targets in preparation for using them for hunting or defense from wild animals. Hunters likely "simulated" attacks on woolly mammoths long before there was a word for simulation. "Simulation" is used in complex and high-risk domains such as civil aviation, military preparation, and the nuclear industry for both engineering design and training to rehearse for potential real-life events. Yet many formally stated definitions can be found for simulation, and current articles continue to contain the phrase "For the purpose of this study, 'simulation' is defined as ABC" (with a new definition distinct from how others have defined it).

Indeed, the very term "simulation" in healthcare seems to generate a lot of confusion. Part of this confusing conceptual ambiguity stems from an exponentially increased jump in simulation usage in the last decade. During the early years, emphasis was on the technique and usability of relatively simplistic representation of human bodies or body parts for use in simulations. The apparent training benefits from these models led to the design and development of increasingly sophisticated and expensive simulators. Technology was and still is trying to catch up to create more "realistic" replicas of the human body on which to practice medical procedures while avoiding risk to living bodies. Early pioneers of healthcare simulation had to improvise greatly, thus relying on imagination and impromptu cues from instructors and actors. Simulation today still relies greatly on and often uses the variously defined concept of "suspension of disbelief" and, more recently, the "fiction contract" (Dieckmann et al., 2007). The problem with imagination is that each person has different perspectives, and therefore our imaginations are slightly different, creating many variations of what we may call the same thing. With technology moving forward to provide "realistic" physical and computer/computational "models," it has become imperative that we also evolve our simulation "techniques" and taxonomic "classes" of simulators and simulations to propel both learning and technological advances in a way that will leave room for imagination, but still be understood by all who read about it.

Without doubt, the use of simulation in healthcare training and education will continue to grow at a rapid pace, providing an ideal time to harness this energy to make Healthcare Simulation an officially recognized Professional Community of Practice with defined systems, methods, guidelines, and standards. Paradoxically, the growth will nevertheless be hindered and confused by the lack of a consistent and coherent way of expressing projects, research, assessments, techniques, and data. Indeed, even the term "simulation industry" is controversial, as it refers to different "fields" of simulation. Unless cross-disciplinary taxonomies and language are clarified, efforts by the National Training and Simulation Association and other organizations to apply for Simulation to be recognized and coded by the Department of Labor as an industry will have little likelihood of success.

Everyone recognizes that there is a lot of ambiguous language that is "sacred" to those who have created their own definitions. The only way to overcome this is to engage the entire community to evolve and then promote a common lexicon. If we do not engage in this endeavor now, we may never have the opportunity to overcome our current disjointed means of describing the same thing. Research interpretations will be inconsistent and unable to be compared, and quality guidelines would be difficult if not impossible to establish. The growth of the field is in fact being hindered by this exact problem. Without a common nomenclature and taxonomy for classification, progress in the field of healthcare simulation will be stymied.

Although there are many similar examples, consider the example of three articles that seemingly study the same thing, yet use different terminologies.

1. In the article "Simulation-based training is superior to problem-based learning for the acquisition of critical assessment and management skills" (Steadman et al., 2006), "full-scale simulation" (SIM) was compared with "interactive" "problem-based learning" (PBL).

2. In the article "A randomized comparison trial of case-based learning versus human patient simulation in medical student education" (Schwartz et al., 2007), the authors used the terms Human Patient Simulator (HPS; a term that one simulator manufacturer claims as their own via a trademark symbol) and "case-based learning" (CBL) for small group discussions using a written case vignette.

3. In "Simulation-based medical education is no better than problem-based discussions and induces misjudgment in self-assessment" (Wenk et al., 2008), the terms "simulation-based teaching" (SBT) and "problem-based discussions" (PBD) were used.

The terms and abbreviations in these examples point out that there is great variance in defining words to describe simulation-based education. While we tend to accept synonyms in our language, the converse is generally not acceptable: studies that use the same terms but mean different things.

One would hope that each of the terms we place in quotations is a label for a well-described concept such that in any group 8 out of 10 independent observers would recognize exactly what kind of event it was. Though the same technologies and techniques may be used (in this case, full-body computerized mannequins and paper cases in small group settings), the terms are different and require further description in the methods section for comparison. Moreover, a lack of classification of the different types and levels or "fidelity" of simulation tools adds to the difficulty when making comparisons. Because there is no standard taxonomy for classification, nor nomenclature for a glossary of terms for "simulation-based" education, authors, and very often readers, are left to their own to define things to meet their immediate need as they deem appropriate.

It is time that we recognized that a growing field such as healthcare simulation will not reach its optimal potential if we do not have a reasonably standard language with which to communicate. Healthcare professionals communicate via technical terms and a classification schema of differentials to identify and describe a patient syndrome or condition. Relatively independent care and treatment can occur because medical terminology and adherence to a common language and taxonomy is a significant part of healthcare professionals' training. Simulation users and developers need to do the same.

Why not directly adopt aviation and other industries' definition of simulation into the healthcare domain? First, even this seemingly simple approach would require a consensus conference to adopt or transfer nomenclature from other applications of simulation. Second, the healthcare simulation community is in some ways unique with regard to the taxonomic base and language associated with simulation as a potentially valuable technology and instructional medium. Indeed, instead of using a computerized mannequin or a noncomputerized model or a computer-based program as the simulation medium, one may use humans with or without disease to simulate a variety of circumstances that caregivers may encounter. At some high and as yet unrecognized level, we appreciate that there may be an impetus for language that applies to simulation across all domains of use. While there should, and will, be many concepts and attributes related to simulation in any domain that we must be prepared to use, there are also many unique areas specific to healthcare. A broad-based stakeholder initiative is required to lay this fundamental foundation for growth.

EXPERT OPINIONS

A number of individuals have addressed this lack of a common language in the simulation community. Heinrichs et al. (2004) described a structured vocabulary for designing surgical curricula and simulators. This, however, was very specific to technical procedural skills used in surgery and represents a very narrow scope of simulation. Definitions of what constitutes a "low-," "mid-," and "high-fidelity" simulator (Brydges et al., 2010) as well as discussions regarding "realism" in simulation applications (Dieckmann et al., 2007) have emerged within the simulation literature. Others have attempted to create a classification schema or review the different types of available simulators (Alinier, 2007; Huwendiek et al., 2009; Meller, 1997; Mihalas et al., 1995; Norman, 1985). Alinier noted that "even if two institutions reported their intention to use the same simulation technology in their project, they were adopting very different teaching approaches." He also stated that "misuse of terminology can give false impressions to trainees, making them believe that they are fully prepared to confront reality" and proposed that "a set of nationally [we would add "internationally"] recognized standards should be developed for the use of educational simulation techniques at different levels to enable trainers and trainees to compare learning experiences."

A report from the Association of American Medical Colleges, "Toward Hypothesis-Driven Medical Education Research: Task Force Report from the Millennium Conference 2007 on Educational Research" (Fincher et al., 2010) ranked simulation-based educational research as their top priority for future efforts. Edler and Fanning (2007) note that a common terminology is needed to avoid misinterpretations of data and results. The need to have standard guidelines for communication and research is apparent in two Best Evidence in Medical Education meta-analyses conducted by Issenberg and McGaghie, which determined that methodologies and terminologies reduced the number of applicable studies to compare (Issenberg et al., 2005; McGaghie et al., 2010). Before more funds are used to produce results that are difficult to compare, we need to reach a consensus on the language for reporting and discussions.

At the 2010 International Liaison Committee on Resuscitation, sponsored by the American Heart Association (AHA), delegates voiced the need for a common lexicon to support the AHA's goals of improving training for cardiac arrest using simulation techniques. The American College of Surgeons and the Association of American Medical Colleges each have reached the same conclusion. Furthermore, the American Society of Anesthesiologists and the American College of Surgeons have had to define terms and criteria for their respective accreditation and simulation endorsement programs (Sachdeva et al., 2008; Steadman, 2008). The Department of Defense (DOD, 2011) has funded a project at the University of Central Florida to update their Modeling and Simulation glossary. Rather than each addressing this problem on their own, a broader meeting to convene like minds will achieve this common goal in a more collaborative manner.

Loftin (2009) proposes a need to create an undergraduate degree, because students become acculturated to a field and speak the technical terms from that field during their undergraduate studies. Currently, a few universities, such as the University of Arizona/Arizona State University, the Naval Postgraduate School, Old Dominion University, and the University of Central Florida, offer master's and/or doctoral degrees in Modeling and Simulation. Yet more and more doctoral students in the health sciences are seeking to focus their studies in medical education, and as interest grows, universities will have to respond. The product of this project, a standard language and taxonomy, could serve as an educational foundation for both an undergraduate degree for simulation and for master's and doctoral-level professionals.

PRELIMINARY EFFORTS

Two reports from simulation conferences serve as preliminary studies (Huang et al., 2008; Sinz, 2006) of efforts to tackle the simulation language problem. At the 2006 meeting, the definition of the term simulation was discussed, as were current uses for simulation (testing, evaluation, credentialing, teaching, research, product safety assessment), types of simulation (full mannequin patient simulation, task trainers, standardized patients, case reports/PBL, virtual environments, flat screen computers), and controversial and provocative statements were voted upon. The conclusions formed from this meeting were that there were common ground first-tier themes of interest, which included research and standards and guidelines for simulation. Furthermore, the group expressed the desire to create collaborative forums to share and exchange information.

As a follow-up to the 2006 Summit, the second Summit in 2007 convened delegates from various organizations to discuss the criteria needed for various training and assessment applications using simulation. A preliminary framework for standards in simulation-based education was drafted. There were many additional areas identified as needing further discussion, including the need to agree on common definitions and taxonomy. Unifying themes emerged; however, much more work and discussion was clearly needed for true consensus. It appeared premature to establish a process for approving simulation standards, as there was much confusion and controversy among the topics discussed, including the language for simulation. The group concluded that SSH should help set up a Simulation Alliance, as an organized consortium of representatives from the different organizations, to be the "think tank" for simulation initiatives. This group would work on establishing a unified set of standards for simulation-based education and training.

In 2012, a Simulation Terminology and Concepts Committee was created within SSH in an effort to create a dictionary by collating existing terms, definitions, and concepts. The work continues. There may be terminology and concepts new to you within each chapter. Terms are defined within each chapter. We provide a list of terms with definitions related to the content in this book that we feel are critical to healthcare simulation, and indicate with a preceding asterisk ("*") terms that are currently controversial or in development and require additional consideration prior to use.

TERMS OF REFERENCE

* Denotes terms in development or variable in the field that require additional considerations.

Term	Definition(s)
Accreditation	A process whereby a professional organization grants recognition to a simulation program for demonstrated ability to meet predetermined criteria for established standards (Society for Simulation in Healthcare [SSH] Accreditation, 2014).
*Actor(s)	See **Embedded Simulated Person**.
Advocacy and Inquiry	A communication method within debriefing that pairs a statement of observation and point of view (advocacy) with a question directed at understanding an action through a participant's cognitive construct or frame (inquiry). Used in debriefing with good judgment (Rudolph et al., 2006).
Assessor	A person who assesses human performance by a set of standards. Assessors should have specific and substantial training, expertise, and demonstrated competency in the art and science of human assessment (SSH Accreditation, 2014).
Assessment	**Formative Assessment** is assessment for learning and usually includes both observation of a learner's actions and feedback. Formative assessment informs the educator about the degree to which the learner's needs are being met. **Summative Assessment** is the measurement of knowledge, skills, or abilities at a discrete moment of time, usually for a high-stakes evaluation. Data is often used to determine a learner's proficiency or competency.
Augmented Reality	A type of virtual reality in which synthetic stimuli are registered with and superimposed on real-world objects, often used to make perceptible information otherwise imperceptible to human senses. An example of augmented reality in healthcare simulation is the use of simulated equipment (stethoscope with built-in sounds) and a standardized patient (Department of Defense, 2011).
Avatar	A participant's graphic representation in a virtual reality simulation or game (Health Workforce Australia [HWA], 2012).
*Briefing	See **Prebriefing**.
Clinical Scenario	Also referred to as **Simulation Scenario, Simulated Case**. A plan of an expected and potential course of events for a simulated clinical experience. The clinical scenario provides the context for the simulation and can vary in length and complexity, depending on the objective. A clinical scenario may include the following components: • Participant preparation • Prebriefing: objectives, questions, and/or material • Patient information describing the situation to be managed

Term	Definition(s)
	• Learning objectives • Environmental conditions, including mannequin, patient, embedded simulated person preparation • Related equipment, props, and tools and/or resources for assessing and managing the simulated experience, e.g. pathology results, defibrillator • Expectations, limitations, and potential roles of participant • A progression outline including a beginning and an ending • Debriefing process • Evaluation criteria (HWA, 2012)
Clinical Skills Examination (CSE)	Also referred to as **Clinical Skills Assessment (CSA), Clinical Practice Examination (CPX)**. A clinical skills or clinical practice examination is a station or series of stations designed to assess the key clinical competencies of history-taking, physical examination, communication, and interpersonal and professional skills. Learners are expected to structure the history, physical examination, and other tasks necessary (e.g., counseling, education) based on the presenting complaint. Documentation of findings, differential diagnosis, diagnosis, diagnostic workup, and/or therapeutic workup may be included. Learners are evaluated via direct observation, checklists, learner presentation or written follow-up exercises. The examinations can be either formative or summative and may involve feedback. The length of time at each station is typically 10–20 minutes (Association of Standardized Patient Educators [ASPE], 2009).
Coding	Indicating or marking chunks of data with symbols, descriptions, or categories. Video recordings or other data used in simulation or research can be coded for review or study.
Computer-based simulation	Also referred to as **Computer Simulation**. Simulation activities that are performed via a computer program; a dynamic representation of a model, often involving some combination of executing code, control/display interface hardware, and interfaces to real-world equipment (Hancock et al., 2009; SSH Certification, 2014).
*Confederate	See **Embedded Simulated Person**.
Continuing Education (CE)	For medical providers, also referred to as **Continuing Medical Education (CME)**. The process within a scope of practice that provides activities designed to maintain and improve the ability of the practitioner to provide healthcare.
Confidentiality	A set of rules, agreement, or a promise that limits access or places restrictions on certain types of information. In simulation, it primarily applies to the agreement and maintenance of privacy as it relates to one's performance during the simulation.
Conflict of Interest (COI)	When an individual or organization is involved in multiple interests, one of which could possibly corrupt the motivation for an act in another.
Contingency Plan	A plan for when things do not go as expected, i.e., when a contingent event or condition occurs during a simulation such as technological glitches.
Continuous Quality Improvement (CQI)	A system that works to improve processes with an emphasis on future results, often using a set of statistical tools to understand subsystems and uncover problems, with emphasis on maintaining quality in the future, not just controlling a process.
Continuum of Care Simulation	Simulated patient care that develops over time, contexts, or emerging issues, and involves sequential settings, series of communications, and multiple clinicians that must communicate effectively to provide optimal care (e.g., simulation in a home environment that moves to emergency department to operating room to recovery to medical-surgical to home care).
*Crisis Resource Management (CRM)	An approach to managing critical situations in a healthcare setting. CRM training emphasizes communication skills. Originally developed in aviation and, as a result, also called **crew resource management**, CRM emphasizes the role of "human factors"—the effects of fatigue and perceptual errors, as well as the effects of different management styles and organizational cultures in high-stress, high-risk environments.

Term	Definition(s)
Critical Incident Stress Debriefing (CISD)	Seven-step structured debriefing process for emergency services professions, including healthcare, police, military, airlines, railroads to mitigate or prevent the onset of posttraumatic stress disorder (PTSD) after (real) traumatic situations.
Debriefer	An individual or individuals who guides or facilitates a **debriefing** activity.
Debriefing	A formal, reflective stage in the simulation learning process; a process whereby educators/instructors and learners reexamine the simulation experience and foster the development of clinical judgment and critical thinking skills designed to guide learners through a reflective process about their learning (SSH Accreditation).
Debriefing with Good Judgment	A debriefing method with three key components: (1) understanding actions within the frames of participants, (2) a stance of supportive and genuine inquiry, and (3) the investigative method of advocacy-inquiry (Rudolph et al., 2006).
Deliberate Practice	A highly structured activity explicitly directed at improvement of performance in a particular domain.
Discrete Event Simulation (DES)	A common systems engineering tool for process analysis and system optimization by many industries, including those high-reliability industries (aviation, nuclear power stations, etc.); a computer simulation of system operations that is presented as a chronological sequence of events. Each event occurs at an instant in time and marks a change of state in the system. DES provides the user with a "test bed" to perform experiments via computer modeling and test the likely effectiveness of different solutions before their implementation. In healthcare simulation, different "what if" scenarios can then be carried out in a "prototype" testing environment.
Disruptive Innovation	Also referred to as **disruptive technology**. The introduction of new technologies, products, or services promoting change and gaining advantage over the competition.
Distributed Simulation (DS)	The concept of high-fidelity immersive simulation on-demand, made widely available wherever and whenever it is required, usually structured as an easily transportable, self-contained "set" for creating simulated environments within an enclosure (e.g., disaster simulations are often inflatable enclosures; Kneebone, 2009).
***Embedded Simulated Person**	Also referred to as **Confederate, Actor, Embedded Actor, Embedded Simulated Participant, Standardized Patient**. When a person portrays a patient (**simulated patient**), family member (**simulated family**), or healthcare provider (**simulation healthcare provider**) in order to facilitate or meet the objectives of the simulation. A simulated person may also be called a **Standardized Patient/Family/Healthcare Provider** if they have been trained to act as a real patient to simulate a set of symptoms or problems used for healthcare education, evaluation, and research. There is continuing debate around the use of the word "actor" because standardized patients often engage in assessment as an educator by providing feedback to the learner.
Experiential Learning	The use of concrete experiences (real or simulated) to gain knowledge. Simulation is a type of experiential learning. In contrast, didactic learning is often used synonymously with unidirectional learning, implying teaching content focused on cognitive knowledge in a sitting or lecture style, as opposed to hands-on training.
Experiential Learning Cycle	A theoretical model developed by David A. Kolb presenting a cycle required for effective learning, and includes four stages: experience, reflection, conceptualization, and experimentation.
Faculty Development	A systematic process of preparing educators to provide educational content of experience and improve their skills.
Failure modes effect analyses (FMEA)	An inductive analysis used in product development, systems engineering, reliability engineering, and operations management for analysis of failure modes within a system for classification by the severity and likelihood of the failures; a proactive approach to assist with mitigating issues prior to implementation.

Term	Definition(s)
Feedback	Information given or dialogue between participants, facilitator, simulator, or peer with the intention of improving the understanding of concepts or aspects of performance (van de Ridder et al., 2008).
*Fidelity	Also referred to as **Realism**. The believability or the degree to which a simulated experience approaches reality. The level of fidelity can involve a variety of dimensions, including (a) physical factors such as environment, equipment, and related tools; (b) psychological factors such as emotions, beliefs, and self-awareness of participants; (c) social factors such as participant and instructor motivation and goals; (d) culture of the group; and (e) degree of openness and trust, as well as participants' modes of thinking (Dieckmann et al., 2007; National League for Nursing Simulation Innovation Resource Center [NLN-SIRC], 2013).
Formative Assessment	See **Assessment**.
Game-Based Environment	Created digital environment where game-based learning can take place.
Gamification	The use of game elements in nongame contexts.
GAS Debriefing	A debriefing method with the phases of Gathering data, Analysis, and Summary that has been developed for use by the American Heart Association.
Guided Reflection	Process used by the facilitator during debriefing that reinforces the critical aspects of the experience and encourages insightful learning, allowing the participant to assimilate theory, practice, and research in order to influence future actions (NLN-SIRC, 2013).
Haptic	The use of devices that provide tactile feedback or touch technology and that interact with a user's motions or applications during a simulation (Robles-de la Torre, 2008).
Healthcare Simulation	A technique that uses a situation or environment created to allow persons to experience a representation of a real healthcare event for the purpose of practice, learning, evaluation, testing, or to gain understanding of systems or human actions; the application of a simulator to training, assessment, research, or systems integration toward patient safety (SSH Accreditation, 2014).
*High-fidelity Healthcare Simulation	See **High-technology Healthcare Simulation** when describing the use of simulation modalities or mechanisms to create a realistic patient model or healthcare situation. See **Mannequin-based Simulation** when describing the use of mannequin simulators. High-fidelity simulation is a term that is often used to imply the use of mannequin simulators in a realistic setting. The term is argued to be ill defined and frequently misapplied. While high-fidelity simulation has been used synonymously in the literature for mannequin-based simulation, low-technology modalities may have more fidelity than a mannequin depending on learning objectives (e.g., laparoscopic procedural training).
High-reliability Team	A group of individuals who operate in a setting with an inherent high risk of errors (and high consequence for each error) and who successfully decrease the incidence of these errors by the use of teamwork training, communication skills, and cultural change in order to improve outcomes (e.g., the aviation industry, the nuclear power industry, and, more recently, the healthcare industry).
*High-technology Healthcare Simulation	See **Mannequin-based Simulation** when describing the use of mannequin simulators. The use of computerized simulation modalities that are controlled or programmed by a person external to the learner, including mannequin-based simulation, where functions may be altered by a simulation facilitator/technician/educator as an interactive result of learner actions. This term is often confusing since the use of audio/visual equipment can also be considered high-technology and any use of A/V could be described under this term.
Human Factors	The discipline or science of studying human–machine relationships and interactions (DOD, 2011). Note: the term covers all biomedical and psychological considerations; it includes, but is not limited to, principles and applications in the areas of human engineering, personnel selection, training, life support, job performance aids, and human performance evaluation.
*Hybrid Simulation	The integration of multiple modalities of simulation (e.g., simulators and standardized patients to achieve learning objectives in a simulation); a simulation that combines constructive, live, and/or virtual simulation, typically in a distributed environment (SSH Accreditation, 2014).

Term	Definition(s)
*Immersive Simulation	Also referred to as **High-technology Simulation**. Simulation education or experiences that encourage participants to become immersed in a task or setting as they would if it were the real situation. It involves the participant suspending disbelief and making decisions as they would in a real-life situation. The ability to create an immersive simulation depends on the participant characteristics, the fidelity of the simulation in terms of context (scenario), equipment, and role-plays (HWA, 2012). This term is often confusing since the realism of simulation is influenced by a variety of factors, experiential learning may be associated with "immersive," and "immersive" is used in psychotherapy as a specialized method for purposes that differ from healthcare education.
Informed Consent	The process by which an investigator communicates the purpose, procedures, risks, benefits, and confidentiality related to a proposed research study in such a way that the participant understands and can actively agree to participate in the study.
In Silico	An activity that is performed in a location absent from actual clinical care (e.g., computer, simulation center).
In Situ	An educational activity that takes place in the actual patient care area, professional practice areas, or clinical setting in which the healthcare providers would normally function; this does not include a setting that is made to look like a work area (SSH Certification).
Interdisciplinary Learning	The integration of the perspective of professionals from two or more professions, by organizing the education around a specific discipline, where each discipline examines the basis of their knowledge (Howkins & Bray, 2008).
*Interprofessional Education	When students from two or more professions learn about, from, and with each other to enable effective collaboration and improve health outcomes (World Health Organization, 2010). "Informal" (or "serendipitous") interprofessional education is unplanned learning between professional practitioners, or between students on uniprofessional or multiprofessional programs, which improves interprofessional practice. At its inception, it lacks the intention of interprofessional education. At any point in time after that it may be acknowledged that learning with, from, and about each other is happening between participants. However, in many such initiatives, this remains unacknowledged or is only recognized on reflection in and on the learning practice. Formal interprofessional education aims to promote collaboration and enhance the quality of care; therefore, it is an educational or practice development initiative that brings people from different professions together to engage in activities that promote interprofessional learning. The intention for formal interprofessional education is for curricula to achieve this aim.
Interprofessional Learning	Learning arising from interaction between members (or students) of two or more professions. This may be a product of *interprofessional education* or happen spontaneously in the workplace or in education settings (e.g., from *serendipitous interprofessional education*; Freeth et al., 2005).
Intraprofessional	Involves activity between or among individuals within the same profession with similar or different specialties or levels of practice (e.g. Surgeon and Emergency Physician; Clinical Nurse and Nurse Practitioner, Resident and Physician).
Just In Time Education (JIT)	Training conducted directly prior to a potential intervention. JIT is derived from the manufacturing field where just in time is a production strategy that strives to improve a business return on investment by reducing in-process inventory and associated carrying costs. "Just in place" refers to training that is at or near the site of the potential intervention.
*Low Fidelity	See **Low-technology Simulations**. Used to describe experiences such as case studies, role-playing, using partial task trainers or static mannequins to immerse students or professionals in a clinical situation or practice of a specific skill (NLN-SIRC, 2013). There is disagreement in the field around this term since low-fidelity simulations may be simulations that do have a high degree of realism to the actual event or anatomy (e.g., laparoscopic procedure).
*Low-Technology Simulation	The use of simulation modalities that are not computerized or electronic and may not be controlled or programmed by a person external to the learner.

Term	Definition(s)
*Mannequin	Also referred to as **manikin;** see **Mannequin-based Simulation.** A human-like simulator used for healthcare simulation. A mannequin (French origin) is "a form representing the human figure, whereas a manikin (Dutch origin) is a life-sized anatomical human model used in education" (National League for Nursing Simulation; Merriam-Webster Dictionary, 2012). Both terms have been used interchangeably for human-like simulators with a majority of simulation literature using "mannequin" and a majority of resuscitation literature using "manikin." After much debate and research, in the summer of 2006, "mannequin" was the term recommended by Simulation in Healthcare, the journal for the Society for Simulation in Healthcare (Gaba, 2006). Some authors have also used the term human patient simulator; however, Human Patient Simulator is the trade name of a METI (CAE) product, and appending "human" to patient is thought to be a pleonasm.
*Mannequin-based Simulation	The use of human-like mannequins to create a patient case/scenario/situation via heart and lung sounds, palpable pulses, voice interaction, vital signs monitor, movement (e.g., seizures, eye blinking), bleeding, blood flashback with intravenous insertion, and other human capabilities that may be controlled by a simulation specialist using computers and paralleled software.
Massed Learning	Training periods very close together with very short rest intervals in between (e.g., 1-week course, undergraduate semester, or quarter course).
Mastery Learning	An instructional methodology that states that nearly all learners can achieve subject or skill mastery when provided adequate time, individualized feedback to address learning needs based on formative assessments, and progress through the subject in an organized manner, typically in smaller units that permit a stepwise approach to mastery level.
Mixed Reality Human (MRH)	In simulation, this would represent the head (and perhaps the body) of a virtual human portrayed on a monitor screen with physical legs (e.g., stuffed trousers, jeans, or scrubs pants) hanging below the monitor to represent the legs. The mixed reality human is programmed to have verbal interactions with the learners or real humans around it.
*Mixed Simulation	Also referred to as **Multimodality Simulation, Mixed Methods Simulation, Hybrid Simulation.** The use of a variety of different types of simulation simultaneously; differentiated from Hybrid Simulation in that it is not characterized by the use of one type of simulation to enhance another, but rather the use of multiple types of simulation as part of the overall educational activity (SSH Certification, 2014).
Modality	A type of simulation being used as part of the educational activity; the simulator (e.g., Task Trainers, Mannequin-Based, Embedded Simulated Person, Computer-Based, Virtual Reality; SSH Certification, 2014).
Modeling and Simulation (M&S)	The use of models (e.g., emulators, prototypes, simulators, and stimulators) either statically or over time to develop data as a basis for making managerial or technical decisions (Hancock et al., 2009).
Monte Carlo Simulation	A commonly used method for modeling complex systems having recursive processes and events that are impractical and time-consuming to test in the physical world, generating numerous output scenarios by repeatedly picking random samples from an uncertain variable based on probability distribution (Hancock et al., 2009).
Moore's Strategic Triangle	A concept that describes how to create public value with three points of a triangle: creating value, building political legitimacy, and nurturing operations.
Moulage	Techniques used to simulate injury, disease, aging, and other physical characteristics specific to a scenario, supporting the sensory perceptions of participants and the fidelity of the simulation scenario through the use of makeup, attachable artifacts (e.g., penetrating objects), and smells (Mercia, 2011; Smith-Stoner, 2011).
Multidisciplinary	When professionals with different perspectives are brought together to provide a wider understanding of a particular problem (Howkins & Bray, 2008).
Multimodality simulation	See **Mixed Modality Simulation.**
Multiprofessional Education	When members (or students) of two or more professions learn alongside one another: in other words, parallel rather than interactive learning (Freeth et al., 2005).

Term	Definition(s)
Needs Assessment	A systematic exploration to collect and analyze information, including the needs of the institution and the present state of skills, knowledge, and abilities of the current and/or future learners.
*Nontechnical Skills	Also known as behavioral skills or **teamwork skills**. See **Teamwork Skills**.
Novice to Expert	Describes the Dreyfus model of skill acquisition, in which learners proceed through sequential stages as their skills increase: Novice, Advanced Beginner, Competent, Proficient, Expert.
Objective Structured Clinical Examination (OSCE)	A station or series of stations designed to assess performance competency in individual clinical or other professional skills (ASPE, 2009). Stations are carefully structured and designed to be easily reproducible. Learners are evaluated via direct observation, checklists, learner presentation, or written follow-up exercises. The examinations are generally summative but may involve feedback. Stations tend to be short, typically 5–10 minutes, but can be longer.
Observation Room	A room that allows additional learners access to the scenario and freedom to discuss the behaviors without disrupting the students with the simulated patient.
Observing Participant/Learner	In Healthcare Simulation, there are frequently Observing and Active Participants owing to limited resources and because a typical clinical event has fewer providers than the number of students. Observing participants learn by observing the simulation with active participants actively undergoing the scenario. The debriefings typically involve both observing and active participants.
*Orientation	Any activity that occurs prior to an educational activity in order to prepare the faculty/instructors or learners; often a formatted, structured set of instructions, rather than an informal or ad hoc event (SSH Certification, 2014). A **Prebriefing** may be part of the orientation.
*Part-task Trainers	See **Task Trainer**.
Participant	One who is a learner in a simulation-based learning activity created for the purpose of gaining or demonstrating knowledge, skills, and attitudes of professional practice (e.g., learner, student).
Physiologic Modeling	During the operation of a simulator, when a parameter is changed, other variables are automatically adjusted on the basis of mathematical models of physiology. Also known as mathematical modeling to simulate physiologic principles.
Plus/Delta Debriefing	A debriefing method in which actions are considered for successful strategies ("plus") and those that might be improved upon in future applicable circumstances ("delta").
Pocket Simulation Center	Also known as **Satellite Center**. Locally operated simulation areas within the clinical environment or as built facilities with administrative, technical, and equipment support from a larger center; an area that is physically distanced but is an extension of a larger simulation center.
Policies	A principle or protocol to guide decisions and achieve rational outcomes; a statement of intent implemented as a procedure or protocol. Most simulation centers create policies pertaining to use of the facility, development of scenarios and content, and code of conduct.
Practice Analysis	A systematic collection of data describing the knowledge, skills, and/or competencies required to competently practice a profession.
*Prebriefing	Also referred to as **Briefing**. An information or orientation session held prior to the start of a simulation-based learning experience in which instructions or preparatory information is given to the participants (International Nursing Association for Clinical Simulation and Learning [INACSL], 2011). The purpose of the prebriefing is to set the stage for a scenario and assist participants in achieving scenario objectives. Suggested activities in a prebriefing include an orientation to the equipment, environment, mannequin, roles, time allotment, objectives, and patient situation.
*Procedural simulation	A training method that utilizes simulation to teach the technical skills and cognitive knowledge required for the safe execution of a clinical procedure, spanning a range of techniques ranging from individual skill training to group and multidisciplinary training.

Term	Definition(s)
Psychological Fidelity	The extent to which the simulated environment evokes the underlying psychological processes that are necessary in the real-world setting; this includes the degree of perceived **realism** or **fidelity**, including psychological factors such as emotions, beliefs, and self-awareness of participants in simulation scenarios (Dieckmann et al., 2007; Edmondson, 1999).
Psychological Safety	A feeling (explicit or implicit) where in a simulation-based learning activity, participants can speak up, share thoughts, perceptions, and opinions without risk of retribution or embarrassment.
*Realism	Also referred to as **Fidelity**. The ability to impart the suspension of disbelief to the learner by creating an environment that mimics that of the learner's work environment and includes the environment, simulated patient, and activities of the educators, assessors, and/or facilitators (INACSL, 2011; Rudolph et al., 2006; SSH Accreditation, 2014).
Reflective Thinking, Reflective Practice	The engagement of self-monitoring that occurs during or after a simulation experience; considered an essential component of experiential learning since it promotes the discovery of new knowledge with the intent of applying this knowledge to future situations (Decker et al., 2013, Decker & Litke, 2007; Dewey, 1933; Kolb, 1984; Schon, 1984, 1990). Reflective thinking is necessary for metacognitive skill acquisition and clinical judgment and has the potential to decrease the gap between theory and practice. Reflection requires the creativity and conscious self-evaluation to deal with unique patient situations.
Remediation	The act or process of correcting a performance gap (INACSL, 2011).
Root cause analysis (RCA)	A reactive approach to explore an event; a structured approach to identifying the factors that resulted in the nature, the magnitude, the location, and the timing of the harmful outcomes (consequences) of one or more past events in order to identify what behaviors, actions, inactions, or conditions need to be changed to prevent recurrence of similar harmful outcomes and to identify the lessons to be learned to promote the achievement of better consequences.
Scenario	See **Clinical Scenario**; also referred to as **Simulation Scenario, Simulated Case**.
Serious Gaming	A game designed for a primary purpose of solving a problem (versus pure entertainment; Australian Defence Simulation Office, 2013). In the military defense context, serious games are used to rehearse, train, or explore military options in a simulation of real-world events or processes.
Shared mental model	Also known as shared frame, shared schema. A shared understanding of the task that is to be performed and of the involved team work.
*Simulated Patient	See **Embedded Simulated Person**.
Simulation-based Education	See **Healthcare Simulation**.
Simulated/ Synthetic Learning Environment (SLE)	An area or service that reproduces components or aspects of the real-world environment, for the purpose of learning and related activities, and/or research.
Simulation	A technique that uses a situation or environment created to allow persons to experience a representation of a real event for the purpose of practice, learning, evaluation, testing, or to gain understanding of systems or human actions (SSH Accreditation, 2014). Simulation is the application of a simulator to training and/or assessment.
Simulation Fidelity	See **Fidelity**.
Simulation Guideline	A recommendation of the qualities for simulation fidelity, simulation validity, simulation program, or for formative or summative evaluation (versus **simulation standard**).
Simulation Program in Healthcare	An organization or group with dedicated resources whose mission is specifically targeted toward improving patient safety and outcomes through assessment, research, advocacy, and/or education using simulation technologies and methodologies including formal workshops, courses, classes, or other activity that uses a substantial component of simulation as a technique (SSH Accreditation, 2014).
Simulation Standard	A statement of the minimum requirements for simulation fidelity, simulation validity, simulation program, or for formative or summative evaluation (SSH Accreditation, 2014).

Term	Definition(s)
Simulation Time	(a) a simulation's internal representation of time. (b) the reference time (e.g., Universal Coordinated Time) within a simulation exercise. This time is established by the simulation management function before the start of the simulation and is common to all participants in a particular exercise.
Simulation Validity	The quality of a simulation or simulation program that demonstrates that the relationship between the process and its intended purpose is specific, sensitive, reliable, and reproducible (Dieckmann et al., 2007; SSH Accreditation, 2014).
Simulation-enhanced Interprofessional Education	The use of healthcare simulation modalities for interprofessional education. Simulation-based Interprofessional Education (SimBIE) describes simulations that were created using interprofessional learning objectives and students from two or more professions learn with, from, and about each other during the simulation; whereas Interprofessional simulations (IPsim) describe simulations that were created using clinical, diagnosis-centered, or task-focused learning objectives and students from two or more professions participate in the simulation (Palaganas, 2012).
Simulationist	A simulationist is a person who is involved, full-time or part-time, with at least one of the following activities: collects and/or specifies data to be used for/by simulation models (in analysis problems, by designing experiments, by performing instrumentation, calibration … In design problems, by providing explicit assumptions, by allowing implicit assumptions, and by formulating and certifying specifications); develops models to be used for simulation purposes; engages in validation, verification, and accreditation studies; performs simulation studies, [that is], specifies simulation problems, causes generation of model behavior and performs analysis/interpretation of the generated model behavior; formulates (specific or policy) solutions to problems based on simulation; develops simulation software, simulation software generators, or simulation tools; manages simulation projects (engineering or administrative management); advertises and/or markets simulation products and/or services; maintains simulation products and/or services; advises other simulationists; promotes simulation-based solutions to important problems; advances simulation technology; and advances simulation methodology and/or theory (Ören, 2000).
Simulator	Any object or representation used during training or assessment that behaves or operates like a given system and responds to the user's actions (SSH Accreditation, 2014).
Situated Learning	A theory by Lave and Wenger (1991) that posit that learning is situated in a way that learning occurs as it normally occurs and is embedded within activity, context, and culture. This is in contrast to most classroom learning activities that involve abstract knowledge not within the context of the activity.

Situational Awareness	Also referred to as situation monitoring.
	    The degree to which one's perception of a situation matches reality; in the context of crisis management, where the phrase is most often used, situational awareness includes awareness of fatigue and stress among team members (including oneself), environmental threats to safety, appropriate immediate goals, and the deteriorating status of the crisis (or patient).
	    Failure to maintain situational awareness can result in various problems that compound the crisis. In a simulation, maintaining situational awareness might be seen as equivalent to keeping the big picture in mind.

*Standardized Patient (SP)	See **Embedded Simulated Person**. Individuals who are trained to portray a patient with a specific condition in a realistic, standardized, and repeatable way (where portrayal/presentation varies based only on learner performance); used for teaching and assessment of learners including, but not limited to, history/consultation, physical examination, and other clinical skills in simulated clinical environments; SPs can also be used to give feedback and evaluate student performance (ASPE, 2009).
Summative Assessment	See **Assessment**.
SWOT analysis	An identification of *s*trengths, *w*eaknesses, *o*pportunities, and *t*hreats (SWOT), where strengths and weaknesses typically reflect attributes within the program, and opportunities and threats are external to the program.

Term	Definition(s)
Systems Integration	Programs that demonstrate consistent, planned, collaborative, integrated, and iterative application of simulation-based assessment, research, and teaching activities with systems engineering and risk management principles to achieve excellent bedside clinical care, enhanced patient safety, and improved outcome metrics across the healthcare system(s) (SSH Accreditation, 2014).
Task Trainer	Models, part-mannequins, or other jigs and working simulations used to reproduce components of a task, usually by imitating patients' anatomy generally used to support procedural skills training and may be used in conjunction with other learning technologies to create integrated clinical situations.
Team-based Learning	A teaching approach with small groups of students with diverse skill sets learning together after preliminary individual accountability and with incentive to work together through an activity and experiential exercises (Michaelsen et al., 2008).
Teamwork Skills	Cognitive functioning and observable behaviors that underpin safe and effective clinical practice, including communication (patient–doctor, team) leadership, teamwork, situation awareness and decision making, resource management, safe practice, adverse event minimization/mitigation and professionalism.
*Technical Skills Training	See **Procedural Training**. Domain-specific components of clinical practice directly required, including patient assessment and clinical diagnostic reasoning, judgment and decision making regarding therapy, procedural knowledge and technical skills relevant to execution of procedures.
Unannounced Standardized Patients	Standardized patients who are trained to portray a patient, family member, or healthcare provider and enter the clinical environment unannounced to assess the provider's interaction with patients or the system. Also referred to in the literature as unannounced standardized patients (USPs), incognito standardized patients (ISPs), invisible patients, fake patients, secret shoppers, and mystery shoppers.
Uniprofessional Education	When members (or students) of a single profession learn together.
Video Retention	The proper labeling, storing, accessibility, and securing of video or photography. When video is recorded at a simulation center, center management will need to determine the retention time, archival rules, data formats, and the permissible means of storage, access, and encryption.
Virtual Patient	A computer program that simulates real-life clinical scenarios in which the learner acts as a healthcare provider obtaining a history and physical exam and making diagnostic and therapeutic decisions (HWA, 2012).
Virtual Reality Simulation	Simulations that use a variety of enhanced technology to enhance reality in order to replicate real-life situations and/or healthcare procedures (SSH Certification, 2014). Note: This is distinguished from Computer-Based Simulation in that it generally incorporates physical or other interfaces (such as surgical instrumentation) that more readily replicate the actions required in a given situation or setting.
Virtual Reality Simulations	A wide variety of computer-based simulation applications conducted in a Virtual Reality Environment (e.g., participants may engage with other persons via Avatars; HWA, 2012). Note: The Human Machine Interface may be by the computer keyboard, mouse, speech, motion sensors, or haptic devices.
Virtual Simulations	Re-creations of reality depicted on a computer screen (e.g., avatars, surgical simulators used for on-screen procedural training and usually integrated with haptic devices); a simulation involving real people operating simulated systems injecting human-in-the-loop in a central role by exercising motor control skills (e.g., flying an airplane), decision skills (e.g., committing fire control resources to action), or communication skills (e.g., as members of an air traffic control team; McGovern, 1994; Robles-de la Torre, 2011).

REFERENCES

Alinier, G. (2007). A typology of educationally focused medical simulation tools. *Medical Teacher, 29*(8), e243–e250.

Association of Standardized Patient Educators. (2009). *Terminology standards*. Retrieved from http://www.aspeducators.org/node/102

Australian Defence Simulation Office. (2013). *Australian defense simulation glossary* (Version 2.2). Canberra, Australia: Department of Defense.

Brydges, R., Carnahan, H., Rose, D., Rose, L., & Dubrowski, A. (2010). Coordinating progressive levels of simulation fidelity to maximize educational benefit. *Academic Medicine, 85*(5), 806–812.

Decker, S., Fey, M., Sideras, S., Caballer, S., Rockstraw, L., Boese, T., ... Borum, J. C. (2013). Standards of best practice: Simulation standard VI: The debriefing process. *Clinical Simulation in Nursing, 9*(6), S26–S29.

Decker, S., & Litke, I. (2007). *Simulation as an educational strategy in the development of critical and reflective thinking: A qualitative exploration.* Denton: Texas Woman's University.

Department of Defense. (2011). *Modeling and simulation (M&S) glossary.* Washington, DC: Modeling and Simulation Coordination Office.

Dewey, J. (1933). *How We Think. New York*: D. C. Heath.

Dieckmann, P., Gaba, D., & Rall, M. (2007). Deepening the theoretical foundations of patient simulation as social practice. *Simulation in Healthcare, 2*(3), 183–193.

Edler, A. A., & Fanning, R. M. (2007). "A rose by any other name"? Toward a common terminology in simulation education and assessment. *Critical Care Medicine, 35*(9), 2237–2238; author reply 2238.

Edmondson, A. (1999). Psychological safety and learning behavior in work teams. *Administrative Science Quarterly, 44*(2), 350.

Fincher, R. M., White, C. B., Huang, G., & Schwartzstein, R. (2010). Toward hypothesis-driven medical education research: Task force report from the Millennium Conference 2007 on Educational Research. *Academic Medicine, 85*(5), 821–828.

Freeth, D., Hammick, M., Reeves, S., Koppel, I., & Barr, H. (2005). *Effective interprofessional education: Development, delivery, and evaluation.* London, UK: Blackwell.

Gaba, D. (2006). What's in a name? A mannequin by any other name would work as well. *Simulation in Healthcare, 1*, 64–65.

Hancock, P. A., Vincenzi, D. A., Wise, J. A., & Mouloua, M. (Eds.). (2009). *Human factors in simulation and training.* Boca Raton, FL: CRC Press.

Health Workforce Australia. (2012). *Australian Society for Simulation in Healthcare simulation directory data dictionary.* Retrieved from www.simnet.net.au/get/1863.pdf

Heinrichs, W. L., Srivastava, S., Montgomery, K., & Dev, P. (2004). The fundamental manipulations of surgery: a structured vocabulary for designing surgical curricula and simulators. *Journal of the American Association of Gynecological Laparoscopy, 11*(4), 450–456.

Howkins, E., & Bray, J. (2008). *Preparing for interprofessional teaching: Theory and practice.* London, England: Radcliffe.

Huang, Y. M., Pliego, J. F., Henrichs, B., Bowyer, M. W., Siddall, V. J., McGaghie, W. C., & Raemer, D. B. (2008). In collaboration with the 2007 Summit Consortium. 2007 Simulation Education Summit. *Simulation in Healthcare, 3*(3), 186–191.

Huwendiek, S., De leng, B. A., Zary, N., Fischer, M. R., Ruiz, J. G., & Ellaway, R. (2009). Towards a typology of virtual patients. *Medical Teacher, 31*(8), 743–748.

International Nursing Association for Clinical Simulation and Learning. (2011). *Standard I: Terminology.* Retrieved from http://www.nursing-simulation.org/issue/S1876-1399%2811%29X0005-1

Issenberg, S., McGaghie, W., Petrusa, E., Lee Gordon, D., & Scalese, R. (2005). Features and uses of high-fidelity medical simulations that lead to effective learning: a BEME systematic review. *Medical Teacher, 27*(1), 10–28.

Kneebone, R. L. (2009). Practice, rehearsal, and performance an approach for simulation based surgical and procedure training. *Journal of the American Medical Association, 302*(12), 1336–1338. doi:10.1001/jama.2009.1392

Kolb, D. (1984). *Experiential learning: Experience as the source of learning and development.* Englewood Cliffs, NJ: Prentice-Hall.

Lave, J., & Wenger, E. (1991). *Situated learning: Legitimate peripheral participation.* Cambridge, England: Cambridge University Press.

Loftin, R. B. (2009). The future of simulation. In J. A. Sololowski & C. M. Banks (Eds.), *Principles of modeling and simulation: A multidisciplinary approach.* Hoboken, NJ: Wiley.

McGaghie, W., Issenberg, S., Petrusa, E., & Scalese, R. (2010). A critical review of simulation-based medical education research: 2003–2009. *Medical Education, 1*, 50–63.

McGovern, K. T. (1994). Applications of virtual reality to surgery. *BMJ, 12*(308), 1054–1055.

Meller, G. (1997). A typology of simulators for medical education. *Journal of Digital Imaging, 10*(3, Suppl. 1), 194–196.

Mercia, B. (2011). *Medical moulage: How to make your simulations come alive.* Philadelphia, PA: F.A. Davis.

Michaelsen, L., Parmelee, D., McMahon, K., & Levine, R. (2008). *Team-based learning for health professions education.* Sterling, VA: Stylus.

Mihalas, G. I., Lungeanu, D., Kigyosi, A., & Vernic, C. (1995). Classification criteria for simulation programs used in medical education. *Medinfo, 8*(Pt. 2), 1209–1213.

National League for Nursing Simulation Innovation Resource Center. (2013). Retrieved from http://sirc.nln.org/

National League for Nursing Simulation Merriam-Webster Dictionary. (2012). *The Merriam Webster dictionary.* Retrieved from http://www.merriam-webster.com/dictionary/

Norman, G. R. (1985). Simulation in health sciences education. *Journal of Instructional Development, 8*(1), 11–17.

Ören, T. (2000). Responsibility, ethics, and simulation. *The Society for Computer Simulation International, 17*, 165–170.

Palaganas, J. (2012). *Healthcare simulation as a platform for interprofessional education* (Doctoral dissertation). Ann Arbor, MI: Proquest.

Robles-de la Torre, G. (2008). Principles of haptic perception in virtual environments. In M. Grunwald (Ed.), *Human haptic perception* (pp. 363–379). Berlin, Germany: Birkhauser Verlag.

Rudolph, J. W., Simon, R., Dufresne, R. L., & Raemer, D. B. (2006). There's no such thing as "nonjudgmental" debriefing: A theory and method for debriefing with good judgment. *Simulation in Healthcare, 1*(1), 49–55.

Sachdeva, A. K., Pellegrini, C. A., & Johnson, K. A. (2008). Support for simulation-based surgical education through American College of Surgeons—accredited education institutes. *World Journal of Surgery, 32*(2), 196–207.

Schon, D. (1984). *The reflective practitioner: How professionals think in action.* Boston, MA: MIT Press.

Schon, D. (1990). *Educating the reflective practitioner.* Boston, MA: MIT Press.

Schwartz, L. R., Fernandez, R., Kouyoumjian, S. R., Jones, K. A., & Compton, S. (2007). A Randomized comparison trial of case-based learning versus human patient simulation in medical student education. *Academic Emergency Medicine, 14*(2), 130–137.

Sinz, E. (2006). Simulation summit. *Simulation in Healthcare, 2*(1), 33–38.

Smith-Stoner, M. (2011). Using moulage to enhance educational and instruction. *Nurse Educator, 36*, 21–24.

Society for Simulation in Healthcare Accreditation. (2014). *SSH accreditation informational guide.* Retrieved from http://www.ssih.org/Accreditation/Full-Accreditation

Society for Simulation in Healthcare Certification. (2014). *CHSE handbook.* Retrieved from http://www.ssih.org/Certification/CHSE/Handbook

Steadman, R. H. (2008). The American Society of Anesthesiologists' national endorsement program for simulation centers. *Journal of Critical Care, 23*(2), 203–206.

Steadman, R. H., Coates, W. C., Huang, Y. M., Matevosian, R., Larmon, B. R., McCullough, L., & Ariel, D. (2006). Simulation-based training is superior to problem-based learning for the acquisition of critical assessment and management skills. *Critical Care Medicine, 34*(1), 151–157.

Van de Ridder, J. M., Stokking, K. M., McGaghie, W. C., & ten Cate, O. T. J. (2008). What is feedback in clinical education? *Medical Education, 42*(2), 189–197.

Wenk, M., Waurick, R., Schotes, D., Wenk, M., Gerdes, C., Van Aken, H. K., & Popping, D. M. (2008). Simulation-based medical education is no better than problem-based discussions and induces misjudgment in self-assessment. *Advances in Health Science Education Theory and Practice, 14*(2), 159–171.

World Health Organization. (2010). *Framework for action on interprofessional education & collaborative practice: a health professions networks, nursing & midwifery, human resources for health.* Geneva, Switzerland: World Health Organization.

CONTENTS

SECTION 1

Simulation Standards

CHAPTER 1.1

SSH Accreditation Standards

Ellen S. Deutsch, MD, FACS, FAAP, and Janice C. Palaganas, PhD, RN, NP

ABOUT THE AUTHORS

ELLEN S. DEUTSCH was Chair of the Council on Accreditation from 2010 to 2012. She led the Council through the implementation of the formal Accreditation process, and the initial development of Preliminary Accreditation and Re-Accreditation. She has an interest in using simulation as a powerful tool to improve the safety and quality of healthcare, including individual, team, and systems applications, while seeking to optimize patient and provider satisfaction.

JANICE C. PALAGANAS was the implementing Director for the SSH Accreditation Program and led the development of the standards, processes, quality improvement, and launching of the program from 2008 to 2010. In this role, she trained the first cadre of SSH Reviewers, reviewed all applicants in the pilot phase, and assisted in the program's transition and growth from committee to Council for the Accreditation of Healthcare Simulation Programs.

Acknowledgments: The authors would like to acknowledge SSH leadership and those individuals who have contributed to the development of this Program and reviewers and applicants who continue to improve the Program (see Appendix). Among the many individuals who have contributed their time and expertise, to create and improve exemplary standards, Mary Elizabeth ("Beth") Mancini has provided invaluable vision, and Jenn Manos has provided unwavering support. The authors and the Council for Accreditation of Healthcare Simulation Programs would also like to thank Dr. Mark Haviland, who assisted and guided the Committee with the psychometric analysis of the accreditation tool.

ABSTRACT

This chapter discusses the accreditation standards as set by the Accreditation Program of the Society for Simulation in Healthcare, providing some history, significance, and benefits. This chapter describes the formatting structure of the standards that can assist applicants with a better understanding of the measurement criteria. Each area of accreditation (i.e., Core, Assessment, Research, Teaching/Education, and Systems Integration/Patient Safety) is described, providing more details to the intended exploration of each standard and measurement criteria. Sites who have already been granted accreditation explain their post-accreditation activities, as well as the results of their experience with SSH accreditation.

CASE EXAMPLE

You attended the Accreditation Program presentation at the International Meeting for Simulation in Healthcare. You realize that your program is now eligible to apply for accreditation. You feel that this would support the goals of your program's Steering Committee: to provide quality healthcare education and to gain recognition for creative education. You downloaded the standards from the Society for Simulation in Healthcare's Web site. Most of the standards make sense. Now what?

INTRODUCTION AND BACKGROUND

As advances and knowledge of simulation were collected and shared within the Society for Simulation in Healthcare (SSH), an incredible variety of simulation methods, philosophies, frameworks, and modalities became apparent. In addition to the variety in simulation technology, content, and programs came the recognition that the simulation programs around the globe were seeking ways to develop, measure, and improve the quality of their efforts, educators, and technology.

In response, in 2007, the executive leadership of SSH charged a small group of leading simulationists to initiate processes for developing certification, accreditation, and technology standards, earning the acronym "CATS." Early in the process, the group acknowledged a significant dilemma: given that a large variety of simulation programs, educators, and technology existed, developing a set of standards to embrace this variety would be difficult. With executive guidance, the members of the CATS Committee determined a process for the creation of these three related efforts and decided that the efforts would be staggered. Development of the Council on Accreditation to design accreditation standards for simulation programs would be the first effort launched. This would be followed by the creation of programs to address certification and then technology standards. This chapter outlines the work of the SSH Council on Accreditation.

STRUCTURING THE ACCREDITATION STANDARDS

Challenged by the great diversity in the types of simulation along with the varied settings for implementation of simulation programs, the Council on Accreditation developed and tested accreditation criteria that incorporated both structure and flexibility, thus contributing to the development of common terminology and definitions necessary to advance this nascent field. The Council appreciated that while effective simulation programs might focus in one or more areas of assessment, research, or teaching and education, there is a stable core infrastructure that should be demonstrated by all Programs. In addition, some Programs would impact systems improvement within a larger healthcare delivery system, and this specialized endeavor would warrant a unique area of accreditation. The accreditation categories became known as Core plus ART-S (Figure 1.1.1). The required elements for accreditation are shown in Figure 1.1.2.

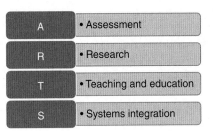

FIGURE 1.1.1 These categories of simulation activity became known as Core plus ART-S.

Developing the standards involved methodical, iterative consultations with experts in various forms of simulation, including standardized patients, accreditation, education, assessment, research, systems processes, and psychometrics. More than a dozen Programs with diverse simulation modalities and programmatic structures generously participated as beta-test programs and, as pilot programs, their feedback was invaluable in improving and clarifying the standards. The development process has been transparent, and vetted in public forums.

While opportunities for accreditation have been available to qualified applicants since 2009, the Council continues to solicit feedback and methodically improve the Accreditation process on an ongoing basis.

The following sections address these five areas of accreditation:

- Core
- Assessment
- Research
- Teaching and Education
- Systems Integration

Each section presents the standards, intent, development, and significance of the respective area of focus.

SECTION 1 • Simulation Standards

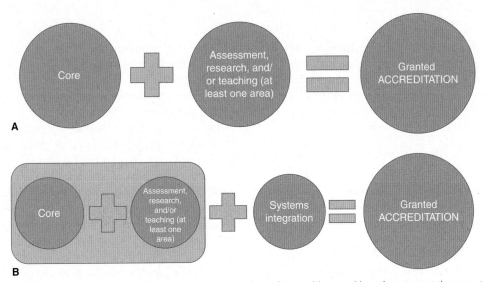

FIGURE 1.1.2 In option **(A),** an applicant can apply for assessment, research, and/or teaching area(s), and must meet the core standards in addition to the standards of one of these areas to be granted accreditation. Option **(B)** is for those Programs opting to apply for systems integration. In order to be granted accreditation in systems integration, a Program would need to meet core standards, the standards of at least one area of assessment, research, or teaching, as well as the standards of systems integration.

SIMULATION: MORE THAN ANOTHER TOOL IN THE TOOLBOX

Kathleen Gallo, PhD, MBA, RN, FAAN
Senior Vice President and Chief Learning Officer, North Shore-LIJ System
Former Examiner for the Malcolm Baldrige Quality Award Program

Simulation as a tool focusing on patient safety has evolved over the past 15 years. Historically, simulation in healthcare owes much of its creditability to the aviation industry. Flight simulation for pilots began in the early 20th century. The principles of Crew Resource Management (CRM) developed in the late 1970s owing to what has been infamously known as the "deadliest accident in aviation history": a reference to the collision between two 747 jumbo jets (KLM and Pan AM) that occurred at Tenerife Airport in 1977 resulting in 583 fatalities. Subsequent to this disaster, there was a clear and compelling "call to action" by the aviation industry to significantly improve its safety record.

Fast-forward to 1999. The Institute of Medicine's landmark report "To Err is Human: Building a Safer Health System" is released and startles all healthcare stakeholders with its findings: between 44,000 and 98,000 people die each year as a result of preventable medical errors—analogous to 75 to 170 Tenerife disasters. Thus, the call to action to improve patient safety begins to gain momentum.

Today, the patient safety movement, among other things, strongly embraces an interprofessional model of teamwork to improve communication and advocates the systematic use of simulation. Using Rouse's (2000) definition of healthcare as an exemplar of a complex adaptive system (CAS), the following characteristics are noted: complex adaptive system is nonlinear and dynamic, composed of independent intelligent agents where adaptation and learning tend to result in self-organization whereby behavior patterns emerge rather than being designed into the system. Emergent behaviors may range from valuable innovations to unfortunate accidents. Simulation combined with an interprofessional learning model has emerged as a disruptive innovation not only in education and assessment but also in systems integration.

SSH developed both standards and criteria for accreditation for simulation programs in 2007. This process has not only brought about a common language within this area, but has facilitated self-study, quality improvement, and internal and external validation of the resources necessary for a quality simulation program. SSH has been a steady force in the adoption of simulation as a new paradigm for healthcare education and overall system improvement related to patient safety.

While simulation is an effective tool for assessment, education/teaching, and research, its fourth domain—systems integration—can have an overarching influence on organizational outcomes. As such, simulation used within a systems approach offers the best opportunities for improving patient safety and achieving business goals. The diffusion of using simulation within a complex adaptive system such as healthcare will take time. Diffusion is a process through which innovation spreads through communication channels over time among members of a social system. Simulation, highly recognized for its benefits in assessment, training/education, and research, and its capacity for influencing organizational behaviors, processes, and outcomes, will need to be encouraged and fortified by the current simulation innovators and early adopters.

As leaders of healthcare organizations pursue the goal of building a safer healthcare system, it is incumbent upon them (and us) to recognize that a systems approach using simulation is an effective and powerful tool when used strategically.

As the adoption rate of simulation as a tool for assessment, education/training, and research approaches a tipping point, I suspect that the diffusion of systems integration as defined by SSH:

". . . those simulation programs which demonstrate consistent, planned, collaborative, integrated and iterative application of simulation-based teaching and assessment activities with systems engineering and risk management principles to achieve excellence in clinical care, enhanced patient safety, and improved metrics across the health system . . ." will follow the path of other disruptive innovations.

Whether using these standards as an applicant, for development, or for ongoing quality improvement, it is important to understand the structure of the published standards. Figure 1.1.3 illustrates how the standards and criteria are presented so that the overarching theme of the standard helps to clarify the intent of the specific criteria.

Core Standards

A successful simulation program requires a foundation that provides resources and stability. The Core Standards have been developed to articulate the basic attributes that should be present in all simulation programs so that they can provide quality simulation opportunities in a sustainable manner. The additional attributes essential for Programs providing simulation in support of teaching and education, research, assessment, and systems improvements are described later in this chapter.

Clearly articulating the Program's purpose is a cornerstone of the Core Standards. This exercise may seem trivial, but a carefully honed statement of the intent and function of the Program provides direction and may help when prioritizing resources and investment. The statement of purpose could be a mission or vision statement, or a variant, and may address stakeholders, participants, general goals, and philosophy (see chapter 5.4 for writing a mission and vision statement). In most cases, a simulation program is a component of a larger organization, and it is similarly important to articulate the governance of the simulation program by the larger organization, the reporting structure from the program to the larger organization, and the funding relationships between the Program and the larger organization.

The Program's organizing framework should provide adequate resources to support the mission of the program, including fiscal, human, and material resources (see chapter 2.1 for developing a simulation program

**Core Standards and Criteria
(Required of All Applicants)**

Core Standards are the fundamental operational standards that underpin the success of a program. There are standards associated with seven (7) elements that all programs must meet regardless of the specific area in which they are applying for accreditation.

The 7 Core Standards are related to: (1) Mission & Governance, (2) Organization & Management, (3) Facilities, Application, & Technology, (4) Evaluation & Improvement, (5) Integrity, (6) Security, and (7) Expanding the Field.

CORE STANDARDS FOR ALL APPLICATIONS

TO BE ACCREDITED, **CRITERIA IN BOLD FONT ARE REQUIRED**. HOWEVER, ALL CRITERIA CONTRIBUTE TO THE ACCREDITATION PROCESS. APPROVED OR WRITTEN DOCUMENTS ARE PREFERRED

1. MISSION AND GOVERNANCE: *There is a clear and publicly stated mission that specifically addresses the intent and functions of the simulation program, and how the program is linked to the larger organization, if one exists*

a. Provide a brief summary of how the simulation program meets the mission and governance standards described within Section 1 (not more than 250 words)

b. *There is clear and publicly stated mission that specifically addresses the intent and functions of the simulation program*
    i. Provide a copy of the program's mission and/or vision.

c. *The simulation program is linked to the larger organization, if one exists*
    i. Describe how the simulation program is linked to the larger organization, if one exist

d. *Describe the process used to review and approve the activities/functions of the program by its designated governing or oversight body (e.g. the body to which the simulation program reports)*
    i. The program's organizational chart or structure (at least up to the level of the governing body to which the program reports)
    ii. A letter of support from the senior administrative officer to whom the program reports

2. ORGANIZATION AND MANAGEMENT: *There is an organizing framework that provides adequate resources (fiscal, human, and material) to support the mission of the program. There is a strategic plan designed to accomplish the mission of the Program.*

FIGURE 1.1.3 Step 1. In the dark (title) box, the text underneath the title indicates program requirements and the overall intent of the accreditation area. Step 2. Within the blue box, the bold text describes the topic, and the italic text describes the conceptual components of the standards and the general intent of the criteria that follow. Step 3. Applicants are asked to demonstrate specific criteria under each standard. Clarification of the intent of the criteria can often be obtained by referring back to the information reviewed in Steps 1 and 2. Criteria presented in bold font are required, but the degree of fulfillment of all criteria is a consideration during review of the application.

SECTION 1 • Simulation Standards

infrastructure). Periodically developing a strategic plan provides an opportunity for reevaluation of current and desired resources, as well as a blueprint for structured growth (see chapter 5.4 for writing and implementing a strategic plan). Within this framework, written policies and procedures will help the Program meet its obligations and support the provision of high-quality services. Some of these policies will be unique to the Program; some can be borrowed from, and all should align with, the policies of the larger organization (see chapter 5.3 for writing policies and procedures). Program leadership may be based on academic, professional, and/or experiential qualifications; SSH has recently developed a certification program for simulation educators. Because of the large number and wide variety of backgrounds and experiences typically present in simulation program members, a thoughtful and effective orientation is essential.

The modern field of simulation is relatively young and is rapidly evolving, particularly with respect to technologic advances. The Program should have an appropriate variety and level of simulation modalities, as well as an appropriate physical and psychological environment, to achieve the Program's goals. Simulation modalities typically include, but are not limited to, standardized patients, high-technology mannequins, task trainers, virtual reality simulators, and biologic material (see Introduction for types of simulation). Sufficient human resources are essential to develop and implement simulations using appropriate simulators, and to manage equipment and programs.

Consistent with the theme of education and learning that is woven into most simulations, Programs should engage in continued self-improvement, including collecting and evaluating feedback (see chapter 5.5 for implementing a systematic evaluation plan). Opportunities for ongoing professional development for program staff and associates may be based within the simulation program or sought externally (see chapter 8.1 for faculty development).

All activities, communications, and relationships should demonstrate a commitment to the highest ethical standards, and policies and protocols should be in place to ensure that data security and learner confidentiality are maintained. Finally, as a core function, Programs should contribute to developing and improving the field of simulation (Table 1.1.1).

TABLE 1.1.1

Core Standards

Core Standards and Criteria
(Required of All Applicants)
Core Standards are the fundamental operational standards that underpin the success of a Program. There are standards associated with seven elements that all Programs must meet regardless of the specific area in which they are applying for accreditation.

The seven Core Standards are related to: (1) Mission and Governance, (2) Organization and Management, (3) Facilities, Application, and Technology, (4) Evaluation and Improvement, (5) Integrity, (6) Security, and (7) Expanding the Field.

1. **MISSION AND GOVERNANCE:** *There is a clear and publicly stated mission that specifically addresses the intent and functions of the Simulation Program, and how the Program is linked to the larger organization, if one exists.*
   a. ***Provide a brief summary of how the Simulation Program meets the Mission and Governance standards described within Section 1 (not more than 250 words).***
   b. *There is a clear and publicly stated mission that specifically addresses the intent and functions of the Simulation Program.*
      i. **Provide a copy of the Program's mission and/orvision.**
   c. *The Simulation Program is linked to the larger organization, if one exists.*
      i. **Describe how the Simulation Program is linked to the larger organization, if one exists.**
   d. *Describe the process used to review and approve the activities/functions of the Program by its designated governing or oversight body (e.g., the body to which the Simulation Program reports).*
      i. **The Program's organizational chart or structure (at least up to the level of the governing body to which the Program reports)**
      ii. **A letter of support from the senior administrative officer to whom the Program reports**

2. **ORGANIZATION AND MANAGEMENT:** *There is an organizing framework that provides adequate resources (fiscal, human, and material) to support the mission of the Program. There is a strategic plan designed to accomplish the mission of the Program. There are written policies and procedures to assure that the Program provides high-quality services and meets its obligations and commitments.*
   a. ***Provide a brief summary of how the Simulation Program meets the Organization and Management standards described within Section 2 (not more than 250 words).***
   b. *There is an organizing framework that provides adequate resources (fiscal, human, and material) to support the mission of the Program.*
      i. **Provide a norganization chart(s)for the Programthat:(1) reflects its position within the organization (if different than governance structure as described in Section1.d.i) and (2) outline sprogrammatic lines of responsibility and authority within the Program, including a director or equivalent for the Program.**
      ii. **Describe the Program's budget process, and identify the individual(s) responsible for fiscal affairs.**
   c. *The Program is managed by an individual(s) who is/are:*
      i. **Academically and/or experientially qualified; submit curriculum vitae/resume/biosketch of the Program leadership as demonstrated in the organizational chart.**
      ii. **Responsible for, and has authority for, the operations of the Program; submit job description(s) of the above individual(s) that demonstrate(s) job function and responsibility.**
      iii. **Assigned sufficient time in the role(s) to achieve the goals of the Program; describe the amount or proportion of time dedicated to the Simulation Program (e.g.,letter from supervisor and/or job description).**
   d. *There is a process in place to provide oversight of simulation activities in the Program.*
      i. **Describe the process for oversight of simulation activities in the Program.**
   e. *There is a plan designed to accomplish the mission of the Program.*
      i. **Describe the goals for the future of your Program and how they will be achieved (e.g.,business plan/strategic plan/operational plan).**
   f. *There are written policies and procedures to assure that the Program provides quality services and meets its obligations and commitments.*
      i. **Provide a complete copy of your Policy and Procedure Manual (or equivalent operations manual) for the Simulation Program. At a minimum, this must include a Table of Contents and policies/procedures that address the criteria described in numerals *ii–vi*.**
      ii. **Quality Improvement Process**
      iii. **Confidentiality Procedures (including, but not limited to, learner confidentiality)**
      iv. **Mechanisms to protect and address physical and psychological safety of individuals involved in simulation**
      v. **Appropriate separation of simulation and actual patient care materials (e.g., equipment, supplies, and patient information)**
      vi. **Storage and maintenance of equipment and supplies**
   g. *There are processes in place to orient and support Simulation Program members (e.g., administrators, educators, operators, assessors, facilitators, standardized patients, and technicians).*
      i. **Demonstrate how Simulation Program members are oriented and supported in their roles within the Program.**
      ii. Document or demonstrate that Staff meetings are conducted at least twice a year.
      iii. Document or describe how ongoing professional development opportunities are provided and/or supported for Program members.
   h. *There are processes in place to manage and prioritize the use of simulation resources.*
      i. Describe the process(es) and/or provide copies of related policies/procedures.
      ii. Provide up to three examples that demonstrate how simulation resources are prioritized.

3. **FACILITIES, TECHNOLOGY, SIMULATION MODALITIES, AND HUMAN RESOURCES:** *There is an appropriate variety and level of simulation modalities (e.g., standardized patients, mannequins, virtual reality, task trainers, etc.) and human resources to support/achieve the goals of the Program. The environment is conducive to accomplish the Program's teaching, assessment, research, and/or systems integration activities.*
   a. ***Provide a brief summary of how the Program meets the Facilities, Technology, and Simulation Modalities standards described within Section 3 (not more than 250 words).***
   b. *The Program has a process for determining what simulation modalities and relevant technologies are selected for use in various educational, assessment, research, and/or systems improvement activities.*
      i. **Document or describe how the Program accesses expertise regarding thea ppropriateness of technology devices, applications, and integration thereof within the Program.**
      ii. **Document or describe the Program's process to identify the optimum simulation modality and equipment to achieve the intended objectives.**
      iii. Document or describe the Program's process to identify and recruit individuals to design and deliver the courses/programs (with appropriate content and/or simulation expertise).

TABLE 1.1.1 *(continued)*

Core Standards

  c. *The Program has technology resources that support its functions consistent with its mission and vision. The Program has the ability to obtain, maintain, and support simulation modalities and relevant technologies to achieve its educational, assessment, research, and/or systems improvement activities.*
    i. Provide a list of simulation equipment.
    ii. Document or describe the mechanism(s) for maintenance of simulation equipment.
    iii. Describe resources or processes to continue ongoing facility, technology, and application improvements.
  d. *The Program has appropriate physical areas for activities such as education, technology storage, and debriefing, in keeping with the mission of the Program.*
    i. Provide narrative description of the facility, detailing the environment for education, functionality, and intended use of the rooms.
    ii. Provide floor plan/blueprints and/or photographs of facility associated with the Program as appropriate (i.e., in situ simulation setup).
  e. *The Program provides an adequate number and a variety of simulation offerings to develop and maintain expertise.*
    i. **Provide a list of simulation courses offered, including targeted learners.**
    ii. **Provide a list of educators (e.g., content experts, instructors, facilitators, trainers).**
    iii. Provide a list of Certified Healthcare Simulation Educators (CHSE).
    iv. Provide the number of participants this year.
    v. Describe the types and/or groups of learners this year.
    vi. Provide total numbers of Learner Contact Hours this year.
    vii. Describe the anticipated trends of simulation use for the forthcoming year (e.g., areas of expansion or change).

4. **EVALUATION AND IMPROVEMENT**: *The Program has a method to evaluate its overall program and services areas, as well as the individual educational, assessment, and/or research activities in a manner that provides feedback for continued improvements.*
  a. **Provide a brief summary of how the Simulation Program meets the Evaluation and Improvement standards described within Section 4 (not more than 250 words).**
  b. *The Program has a plan for systematic quality improvement (QI) performance improvement (PI) that includes but is not limited to assessment of learner outcomes and achievement and course evaluation by course participants, at least annually.*
    i. **Document or describe quality or performance improvement processes.**
    ii. **Document or describe quality or performance improvement activities identified in last 2 years. A minimum of three improvements is required.**

5. **INTEGRITY**: *All activities, communications, and relationships demonstrate a commitment to the highest ethical standards.*
  a. **Provide a brief summary of how the Simulation Program demonstrates its commitment to high ethical standards (not more than 250 words).**

6. **SECURITY**: *There is appropriate documentation and organizational policies and mechanisms in place to assure that data/test security and learner confidentiality are maintained.*
  a. **Provide a brief summary of how the Simulation Program meets the Security standards described within Section 5 (not more than 250 words).**
  b. *The Program is compliant with accepted standards for data security and participant confidentiality.*
    i. **Document or describe the process to maintain confidentiality about participant performance.**
    ii. **Document or describe the process to maintain data confidentiality.**
    iii. **Describe the process of maintaining the confidentiality of records, including videos.**

7. **EXPANDING THE FIELD**: *The Program demonstrates commitment to advocate for healthcare simulation and contributes to the field of simulation.*
  a. **Provide a brief summary of how the Simulation Program meets the Expanding the Field requirements standards described within Section 6 (not more than 250 words).**
  b. *Activities of the Program and its staff extend beyond the Program (reaching an institutional, community, regional, national, and/or international audience) and contribute to the body of knowledge in the simulation community.*
    i. **Provide documentation that at least one individual active in the Program is a member of a local, national, and/or international simulation society.**
    ii. Provide a list (up to 10) of activities, published articles, research, and/or book chapters that contribute to knowledge within or about the simulation community (locally, regionally, nationally, and/or internationally).
    iii. Provide a list (up to 10) of presentations at local, regional, national, and/or international meetings and conferences that are based on its simulation activities.

Assessment Standards

Assessment activities may include simulations for the purposes of grading a student, determining competencies in an individual or team, certifying a set of skills, or as a final exam known as "high-stakes testing." Some assessees may be learners, while others may be applicants or candidates; for simplicity, the word "learner" will be used in this section.

Assessment activities utilize a structured modality to measure performance, and hence the modality must be administered and measured in the same way for each learner. To achieve this, an assessment activity must be standardized. Healthcare simulations are extremely difficult to standardize given the variety of potential variables (e.g., modality used, equipment glitches, variation among simulationists controlling or participating in the simulation, interactions prompted by candidate actions, timing of transitions, etc.). Simulations used for assessment must be rigorously structured at all the levels, including the testing or assessment conditions, the assessors, and the assessment tool. Administrative and personnel resources are needed to support such activities (see chapter 7.3 for use of simulation in assessment activities).

Faculty who are developing the assessment should match and select the most appropriate and realistic simulation modality with the aim of accurate assessment, despite the temptation to select a modality based on availability, convenience, or comfort. In addition, there should be strict controls for potential confounding variables. Resource availability of a modality often depends on the focus, mission, and vision of the simulation program, where the likelihood of resource availability increases as the assessment activities align with the goals of the Program.

Any assessment activity must have validity, the ability to fairly measure what it is intended to measure. An assessment activity must also be reliable in that repeated assessments of the same learner or assessments by different judges should yield approximately the same scores.

A fair assessment activity must include a standard orientation process for each candidate. The strength of an assessment Program relies on the assessment Program leadership and faculty. The Program should have access to faculty experienced in the art and science of human performance assessment as they are usually attuned to these concerns around orientation, validity, and reliability that are critical to fair and accurate assessment activities.

Validity and reliability in simulation assessments depend not only on the equipment and technology being used, but also on the people or "assessors" measuring and judging the learner(s). Assessors must be qualified by virtue of their education and experience, understand the advantages and limitations of assessment, be familiar with the simulation activity, and be adequately trained to assess a learner in the simulation. Training for assessors should include practice using the relevant simulation modality as well as a learner from the population they will likely be assessing. Assessor group training is often an effective venue for clarifying and calibrating assessment processes, and addressing areas of confusion including purpose, measurement, degrees of measurement, or the structure of the simulation.

A thoughtful process for the selection, adaptation, or development of assessment tools is essential to the quality of the assessment Program. Assessment Programs often use published assessment tools for which validity and reliability have already been established in peer-reviewed literature. Establishing the validity and reliability of a measurement tool often takes years of dedicated research and analysis. Because of this, Programs are encouraged to evaluate existing valid and reliable measurement tools that align with the aim and objectives of their assessment. At times, an appropriate tool may be difficult to find, and a Program may decide to adapt an existing tool or develop a new instrument or measurement tool. During the development of a tool, the validity and reliability of the tool will depend heavily on the expertise in assessment available to the Program. Human factors, psychometric and/or statistical expertise can be invaluable.

The data generated by assessment activities can be extensive. This data must be analyzed appropriately and managed confidentially. Assessment Programs require qualified analysis and adequate administrative support. As with instrument development, expertise in human factors, psychometrics, or statistics should be applied in an ongoing manner so as to ensure proper analytic processes, maintain the quality of analyses, and provide support for the overall simulation-based assessment Program (see chapter 7.3 for use of simulation in assessment activities) (Table 1.1.2).

Research Standards

The goal of research is to discover new knowledge and explore understandings in the field. Therefore, dissemination of knowledge is key to advancing the science of healthcare simulation. Findings from rigorous simulation research Programs are extremely valuable to the growth of the field of simulation, and existing research Programs should find ways to share their findings through meeting presentations, internal and external forums, gray literature, and, ultimately, peer-reviewed publications (see chapter 9.1 for simulation research).

Simulations used for research face the same challenges as simulations used for assessment: the need for rigor (including validity and reliability), expertise, oversight, and programmatic support (see chapter 9.2 for simulation research considerations). Research activities require extensive resources for development, implementation, data gathering, analysis, and dissemination of knowledge. Successful Programs require adequate organizational and financial support, and a commitment to research in the larger Program's overall mission, strategic and operational.

Developing rigorous research activities requires a strong research Program, which includes resources, relationships, researchers, and mentorship. A robust research Program depends heavily on dedicated expertise among the educators and researchers involved as principal (or lead) investigators and coinvestigators. Dedicated time for a Director of Research should be formalized in his/her job description. Mature research Programs often have an organized, systematic approach to optimizing research proposals, selection, ethical review, assignment, development, recruitment, implementation, data storage, confidentiality, analysis, evaluation, and publication, as well as an effective training program for newer researchers, or experienced researchers seeking to expand their expertise. These are often described in programmatic policies and procedures and must be in compliance with the standards of the institution, region, and country (see chapter 9.3 for institutional review boards).

Because of the large variety of methods that could be used in research, it is important for the Program to have diverse expertise, either within the Program or by access to a network of experts that can be consulted at different stages of various projects. Statisticians, psychometricians, human factors specialists, qualitative researchers, and data managers or Program consultants may all be valuable resources. Just like any Program, to ensure quality, the effectiveness of simulation within the Program must be continuously assessed (Table 1.1.3).

TABLE 1.1.2

Assessment Standards

Assessment Standards and Measurement

Application for accreditation in *Assessment* will be limited to those organizations conducting simulation assessments characterized by trained raters, valid and reliable tools, and consistent testing conditions. Assessment leadership and assessors must be competent in the art and science of human performance assessment. Assessment tools may be (1) obtained from a peer-reviewed journal (2) defined by professional societies, licensing bodies, or certification organizations, or (3) modified or created *de novo* if justified via expert panel review process.

1. **Resources and Technology: Facilities, technology, and simulation modalities such as standardized patients and equipment are appropriate for the summative assessment of individual and team knowledge and/or skills.**
   a. **Provide a brief summary of how the Simulation Program meets the Applications and Technology standards described within Section 1 (not more than 250 words).**
   b. **Facilities, simulation modalities (e.g., standardized patients), and availableassessment technology are appropriate for assessment of individual and team knowledge and/or skills.**
      i. **Document or describe the process in place to link the assessment activities to the Program goals.**
      ii. **Provide a list of the Simulation Program's assessment activities and the associatedassessors for the past 2 years.**
      iii. **On-site, the Program provides documentation of three assessment activities (selected by reviewers on-site).**
      iv. **Document or describe how the facilities are appropriate for theindividuals/teams being assessed and level of assessment being undertaken.**
      v. **Document or describe how simulation modalities are selected for assessment activities; provide three examples.**
2. **Assessors and Staff: There are qualified assessors and staff to conduct the assessment activities.**
   a. **Provide a brief summary of how the Simulation Program meets the Assessors and Staff standards described within Section 2 (not more than 250 words).**
   b. **Assessors are qualified by virtue of their education and/or experience to conduct valid and reliable assessments.**
      i. **Document or describe the process used to match the assessor to the type of assessment activity.**
      ii. **On-site, the Program provides documentation that threeassessors (selected by reviewers on-site) follow the described process.**
      iii. **Provide curriculum vitae, biosketch, or resumes for all core assessors (maximum of five).**
   c. **Assessor performance is evaluated, at least annually, to assure ongoing professional development and competence.**
      i. **Describe or document the process to evaluate assessors.**
      ii. **Provide evaluation of all assessors for the past 2 years (maximum of five).**
      iii. **Provide curriculum vitae, biosketch, or resumes of the two most active individuals who evaluate the assessors.**
3. **Assessment Tools: There is a systematic process to select appropriate assessment tools.**
   a. **Provide a brief summary of how the Simulation Program meets the Assessment Tools standards described within Section 3 (not more than 250 words).**
   b. **Assessment methods and tools are consistent, reliable, and valid.**
      i. **Provide examples of three to five tools used for assessment.**
      ii. **Document or describe how assessment tools are aligned with learner objectives.**
      iii. **Document or describe how students are oriented to the environment and the assessment process.**
      iv. **Document or describe the process for assuring that assessment tools are reliable and valid.**
      v. **Document or describe the process to develop or select assessment tools.**
      vi. **Document or describe the process to ensure inter-rater reliability.**
4. **Assessment Support: There is adequate support for analysis of data.**
   a. **Provide a brief summary of how the Simulation Program meets the Assessment Support standards described within Section 4 (not more than 250 words).**
   b. **The Program can demonstrate that it has access to qualified assessment analysis support (e.g., human factors, psychometrics, and/or statistical support).**
      i. **Document or describe access to appropriate qualified assessment analysis support.**
      ii. **Provide documentation from all individuals or services providing assessment analysis support acknowledging their involvement with the Program (maximum of five).**
      iii. **Document or describe resources available to develop assessment tools.**

Teaching and Education Standards

The vast majority of simulation programs accredited by SSH have sought, and achieved, accreditation for Teaching and Education. Teaching and Education are almost always essential components of a simulation program's mission, and the mainstay of a Program's activities. This section of the accreditation standards was developed to ensure that Programs provide simulation-based learning activities that are based on sound educational principles, are designed and delivered by qualified individuals, and take advantage of the rich diversity of available simulation modalities.

Educational activities should be related to the overarching Program goals, and should include specific educational activities that take place on a regular, recurring basis. It is important to have a system to track Programs and courses as well as learner and faculty contact hours. The individual overseeing the Program's educational activities should have simulation education expertise. Simulation-based learning must be integral to the Program's learning activities, and having access to a broad range of simulation capabilities and modalities will enrich the learning opportunities. Non-simulation learning modalities may also be incorporated in a Program's portfolio as supplementary resources.

TABLE 1.1.3

Research Standards

Research Standards and Measurement

Application for Accreditation in Research will be limited to those programs actively involved in data gathering, analysis, and dissemination of knowledge for advancing the science of simulation.

RESEARCH STANDARDS

TO BE ACCREDITED, **CRITERIA IN BOLD FONT ARE REQUIRED**. HOWEVER, ALL CRITERIA CONTRIBUTE TO THE ACCREDITATION PROCESS. APPROVED OR WRITTEN DOCUMENTS ARE PREFERRED.

1. **MISSION:** *The mission statement includes a specific and credible commitment to research activities.*
   a. ***Provide a brief summary of how the Simulation Program meets the Mission standards described in Section 1 (not more than 250 words).***
   b. *Research activities are linked to the Program goals.*
      i. *Document or describe the process that links the research activities to the Program goals.*
      ii. *Provide a list of all research activities related to simulation and the associated researchers for the past 3 years (maximum of 20).*
      iii. *On-site: Document or describe how three research activities (selected by reviewers on-site) are consistent with the strategic and/or operational plan.*
      iv. *Provide a list of all funded and unfunded research within the past 3 years (maximum of 20).*
   c. *The Program has an established record of organizational and/or financial support for simulation research.*
      i. **Document or describe the Program's organizational and/or financial commitment to simulation research.**
2. **RESEARCH EXPERTISE:** *Instructors/educators/researchers demonstrate a capability to perform research.*
   a. ***Provide a brief summary of how the Simulation Program meets the Research Expertise standards described in Section 2 (not more than 250 words).***
   b. *Basic elements of Program assessment are present.*
      i. **Document or describe an organized, systematic program of research.**
      ii. **Provide a policy and/or procedure related to research program assessment.**
      iii. **Document or describe the process utilized for research program assessment.**
   c. *There is evidence of publication and/or presentation of research findings in peer-reviewed forums.*
      i. *Provide a list of presentations involving simulation research within the past 3 years at local, regional, national, and/or international meetings or conferences (maximum of 12).*
      ii. *Provide a list of peer-reviewed publications involving simulation research within the past 3 years (maximum of 12).*
   d. *The Program has qualified individuals involved in data gathering, analysis, and dissemination of knowledge for advancing simulation research.*
      i. **Provide a biosketch for the two most active researchers.**
3. **RESEARCH OVERSIGHT:** *There is a designated individual(s) who is responsible for administering the research programs.*
   a. ***Provide a brief summary of how the Simulation Program meets the Director of Research standards described in Section 3 (not more than 250 words).***
   b. *The role and functions of a Director of Research are provided for within the organizational structure.*
      i. **Document or describe a Director of Research who is responsible for research related to simulation.**
      ii. *Provide a job description that reflects designated, dedicated time, recommended 20% minimum, for administration of simulation research (e.g., letter from supervisor and/or job description).*
      iii. **Provide a biosketch, curriculum vitae, or resume of Director of Research.**
4. **RESEARCH ACTIVITIES:** *The Program emphasizes and supports the application of scholarly approaches to evaluate teaching, assessment, and/or systems integration programs and to conduct studies of validation of simulation systems, approaches, or modules.*
   a. ***Provide a brief summary of how the Simulation Program meets the Research Activities standards described in Section 4 (not more than 250 words).***
   b. *Activities of staff promote collaborative relationships and research communications internal and external to the Program.*
      i. *Provide a list of at least two collaborative and cooperative research relationships within the last 3 years external to the Program (collaboration can be within or beyond the institution).*
      ii. *Demonstrate or describe the research used to assess simulation effectiveness within the Program's environment.*
      iii. *Demonstrate or describe appropriate research support (e.g., access to statistical, human factors, and/or psychometric expertise).*
   c. *There are instructors/educators with specific research training and internal/external documentation of collaboration.*
      i. *Document or describe specific research training and collaboration of instructors and educators.*
      ii. *Document or describe periodic, at least quarterly, conferences related to simulation (e.g., research forum, grand rounds, visiting professors, journal club).*
   d. *There is mentoring of simulation research.*
      i. *Provide a list of all mentoring and/or coaching pairs (mentors and mentees) in the last 3 years who have participated in the mentoring process with a brief description of their involvement with the Program (maximum of 10 pairs).*
5. **COMPLIANCE:** *Research protocols are in accordance with accepted research standards.*
   a. ***Provide a brief summary of how the Simulation Program meets the Compliance standards described in Section 5 (not more than 250 words).***
   b. *There is access to and documentation of compliance with national research standards processes.*
      i. **Document or describe research policies and procedures, including data storage policies and procedures.**
      ii. **Document or describe compliance with your national, regional, and/or institutional research standards (IRB; e.g., letter of approval from IRB and/or a statement of compliance in a peer-reviewed publication).**

Individuals from a variety of backgrounds may function as educators, faculty, or facilitators. The current lack of consensus on terminology for this role reflects the diverse backgrounds and functions of various individuals who actively participate in teaching; in general, they may be qualified by virtue of expertise in simulation or expertise in a specific subject or content area. Some individuals may have skills and knowledge in both areas; others will require orientation to the complementary components and principles of the material being taught. Educators should be able develop and deliver material appropriate to the learner group's level of study. Educator development (e.g., the development of the educators themselves) should address orientation for new individuals, and ongoing professional development for all educators. Regular evaluations of educators will help the Program maintain and improve quality (see chapter 8.1 for faculty development and evaluation).

In preparing the learning opportunities, course and curricular development can be based on needs or gap analysis, expert assessment, learner request, or regulatory requirements. Simulation design and development, and simulator selection, should occur in an organized, rational manner based on currently understood educational theory (see chapter 7.2 for common educational theories used in simulation) and the principle of finding the best fit between resources and educational needs. A template or protocol can be useful in ensuring that the Program meets the needs of both the organization and the learners.

After the learning events have concluded, courses should be evaluated in a systematic and routine manner using expert review, peer review, internal feedback, or other appropriate processes. Typically, evaluations of courses by learners include a formal component (e.g., a feedback questionnaire or survey) and may also include a debriefing. Course evaluations by educators and course faculty are also essential and should be documented, although the process to obtain feedback and the debriefing is often less formal (see chapter 5.5 for implementing a systematic evaluation plan).

While simulation for the purpose of assessment inevitably includes some threshold of success, simulation for the purpose of teaching should be as supportive, nonjudgmental, and respectful as possible (see chapter 7.3 for assessment using simulation). This does not preclude constructive feedback, but does allow exploration without penalty. Learners, particularly those participating in group simulations, should be reminded that participant performance during simulation does not always reflect the full capabilities of individuals during actual patient care. "What happens in sim, stays in sim" is a common refrain (see chapter 8.5 for psychological safety) (Table 1.1.4).

Systems Integration and Patient Safety Standards

Simulation is a tool that can have a powerful impact when it is used to improve the systems within which we work, whether it is patient flow, transfer of care from provider to provider or unit to unit, policies in an organization, or organizational culture. These system-based improvements may address quality, safety, risk management, enterprise improvement, resilience, or other system-wide desired attributes. Simulated events allow exploration of the functionality of equipment, teams, protocols, processes, team structures, and even healthcare delivery settings of various scales. Simulation can be used in an intentional manner, as a probe or "ping," to evaluate new or renovated patient care spaces and to ensure that essential components have been addressed and incorporated, as well as to allow individuals and teams to practice in a new environment. Even earlier, during the design process, simulation can be used to develop the layout and details of healthcare delivery spaces; or, conversely, to identify essential

TABLE 1.1.4

Teaching and Education Standards

Teaching/Education Standards and Measurement

Application for Accreditation in the area of Teaching/Education will be limited to those Programs that demonstrate regular, recurring activities with defined curricula and ongoing validation that employs simulation methodologies appropriate for learning objectives to instruct, teach, or train participants for formative integration of cognitive, procedural, and attitudinal goals. The Program will be able to demonstrate the effectiveness of their curriculum.

1. **LEARNING ACTIVITIES:** *The Program offers comprehensive learning activities using simulation. The Program provides expert orientation to simulation education for instructors/educators and learners. Educational methods are reliable, valid, engaging, effective, and, where possible, evidence-based. Appropriate simulation modalities are used to support learning objectives and design.*
    a. **Provide a brief summary of how the Simulation Program meets the Learning Activities standards described within Section 1 (not more than 250 words).**
    b. *Educational activities are linked to the Program goals.*
        i. **Document or describe the process that links the educational activities to the Program goals.**
    c. *Educational activities using simulation occur on a regular, recurring basis.*
        i. **List all simulation-based educational programs, and the associated educators, offered over the past 2 years (see definition of educators in Section 2).**
        ii. Document or demonstrate that at least two courses occur on a regular and recurring basis.
        iii. Provide the number of learner contact hours for the Program each year for the past 2 years.
    d. *An expert in simulation education oversees the Program's educational activities.*
        i. Document or demonstrate the qualifications of a simulation expert who oversees programs and educational activities.
    e. *Simulation education curricula and education materials are reviewed and updated at least annually, using expert review, peer review, internal feedback, or other appropriate processes.*
        i. **Document or demonstrate how simulation education materials are reviewed and updated.**
        ii. Document or demonstrate the process to develop or utilize curricular compo nents on the basis of needs or gap analysis, expert assessment, learner request, and/or curricular or regulatory requirements.
    f. *Simulation modalities are appropriate for the learning objectives.*
        i. **Describe how simulation modalities are selected for specific educational activities.**

(continued)

TABLE 1.1.4 *(continued)*

Teaching and Education Standards

2. **QUALIFIED EDUCATORS:** *There is access to qualified educators for the educational offerings provided. For the purposes of this section, an educator is an individual who may be an expert in simulation or an expert in a specific subject or content area who participates in providing an educational experience for the learner(s). Instructors, facilitators, content experts, and simulationists may all be considered educators in the appropriate circumstances.*
   a. *Provide a brief summary of how the Simulation Program meets the Qualified Educators standards described within Section 2 (not more than 250 words).*
   b. *The Program has access to qualified educators.*
      i. **Provide a list of key educators (maximum of five) with biosketch specific to simulation (e.g., orientation, professional development, years of experience).**
   c. *Simulation educators and/or content experts are selected to match the learner group's level of study.*
      i. **Describe the process to match the qualifications of the educator to the characteristics of the learning activities.**
   d. *Simulation educators are evaluated at least annually to assure ongoing development and competence.*
      i. **Describe the process to evaluate educators.**
      ii. On-site, the Program provides documentation that three educators (selected by reviewers on-site) follow the described process.
   e. *Simulation-based courses involve personnel with expertise in simulation in the development and/or delivery of the courses.*
      i. Describe how personnel with expertise in simulation are involved in the development and/or delivery of courses.
      ii. Provide curriculum vitae, resumes, or biosketch of the individuals (maximum of five) involved in the development and/or delivery of courses.
   f. *Simulation educators receive initial orientation and engage in ongoing professional development.*
      i. **Document or demonstrate the process for initial orientation including: (1) feedback/debriefing techniques and (2) appropriatedocumentation and evaluation tools.**
      ii. **Document or describe how content experts who may not be simulation experts are oriented to the environment, including appropriate documentation and evaluation tools.**
      iii. **Document or demonstrate the evaluation and feedback processes for educators, including feedback from participants and changes implemented; provide three examples.**
      iv. **Document or describe how educators engage in ongoing professional development to improve their simulation skills, such as attending meetings, performing simulation education research activities, and so on.**
3. **CURRICULUM DESIGN:** *Curriculum design follows a rational process based on currently understood education theory.*
   a. *Provide a brief summary of how the Simulation Program meets the Curriculum Design standards described within Section 3 (not more than 250 words).*
   b. *The Program uses a curriculum design process that involves appropriate learning theories.*
      i. **Describe the curricular design process, and provide tools used in the simulation curricular design process.**
      ii. **On-site, the Program provides documentation of three teaching activities (selected by reviewers on-site).**
   c. *There is a logical approach for simulation design, development, and selection.*
      i. **Document or demonstrate that educational principles are used in the design anddevelopment ofcourses.**
4. **LEARNING ENVIRONMENT:** *Simulation event is conducted in an environment to optimize the achievement of learning objectives.*
   a. *Provide a brief summary of how the Simulation Program meets the Learning Environment standards described within Section 4 (not more than 250 words).*
   b. *The learning environment of a simulation event is conducted in a manner to optimize the achievement of learning objectives.*
      i. **On-site: Provide videos of actual learning activities for reviewers to select on-site for review.**
5. **ONGOING CURRICULUM FEEDBACK AND IMPROVEMENT:** *The Program continually updates and improves its courses.*
   a. *Provide a brief summary of how the Simulation Program meets the Ongoing Curriculum Feedback and Improvement standards described within Section 5 (not more than 250 words).*
   b. *The Program has mechanisms in place to obtain feedback from course participants and course educators.*
      i. **Document or demonstrate that course evaluations are conducted in a systematic and routine manner.**
      ii. **Provide evaluations, completed by either course participants or course educators, from three to five courses offered within the last year.**
   c. *The Program has a mechanism for incorporating feedback into future offerings and record keeping supports evaluation, validation, and research of curriculum:*
      i. **Document or demonstrate how evaluations have been used to prompt course or program changes.**
   d. *Records of all learner, instructor, and coordinator activities are maintained.*
      i. **Evaluations describe whether courses met the educational objectives.**
      ii. **Document or demonstrate how learner, educator, and administrative records are maintained.**
6. **EDUCATIONAL CREDIT:** *The Program has a mechanism to offer formal credit for educational activities in the form of continuing education credits as appropriate for various disciplines.*
   a. *Provide a brief summary of how the Simulation Program meets the Educational Credit standards described within Section 6 (not more than 250 words). If no educational credit is provided, please provide a brief explanation.*
   b. *The Program has a demonstrated ability to offer continuing education credit.*
      i. **List all continuing education (CE) courses within the last year (maximum of five).**

system components that must be maintained despite space, resource, or other limitations. Simulation can be used in an iterative fashion to evaluate processes and protocols during their development so as to help bridge the gap between design based on "work as imagined" versus design based on "work as done." Creatively designed simulations can be used to intentionally explore almost any aspect of the healthcare delivery environment, or to optimize system-wide capabilities (see chapter 2.8 for systems integration and patient safety using simulation).

Simulation can also be used for system improvement by identifying opportunities in a serendipitous manner.

During debriefing of a simulation designed to improve individual and team skills, discussion may lead to the identification of local or pervasive conditions, latent hazards, or other information that impact healthcare delivery at a system level. This information can be used to mitigate potential problems in a proactive manner, for example, to remedy a condition that has been identified in simulation as posing an apparent risk, before that problem contributes to a serious safety event, or even a near miss. The more realistic the team composition, setting, and equipment, the more likely serendipitous opportunities to identify latent hazards will occur and be identified.

Bidirectional information and impact are hallmarks of simulation designed at the system level. For example, an organization may use simulation to address specific safety concerns. In response to a serious safety event, or a near miss, simulation could be used to "replay" the event, in order to probe the causes, or simulation could be used to practice specific skills, to mitigate system-wide deficiencies.

Some organizations may accomplish this process in a formal manner, using a specific production or engineering methodology; others may use an informal or organic approach. What is important is that the feedback is looped throughout those involved in the process studied and is bidirectional; for example, the simulation program also provides information back to the organization, either about the results of simulation intervention initiated in response to a system concern or, proactively, about problems or opportunities identified during simulation, which deserve organizational attention. For example, if a few people are identified who lack specific skills or knowledge during a simulation, further education for those individuals may be appropriate. If simulations in diverse units throughout an organization demonstrate that the lack of skill or knowledge is pervasive, then the mitigation should be system-wide education. Because this process often includes multiple parties, it is important that information and guidance flows both to and from all parties involved. This integration of simulation into the larger healthcare organization is most effective when it is carefully planned, collaborative, and iterative (Table 1.1.5).

TABLE 1.1.5

Systems Integration and Patient Safety Standards

Systems Integration: Facilitating Patient Safety Outcomes

Application for accreditation in the area of Systems Integration: Facilitating Patient Safety Outcomes will be available to those Programs that demonstrate consistent, planned, collaborative, integrated, and iterative application of simulation-based assessment; Quality and Safety; and teaching activities with Systems Engineering and Risk Management principles to achieve excellent bedside clinical care, enhanced Patient safety, and improved outcome metrics across a healthcare system.

1. **MISSION AND SCOPE:** *The Program functions as an integrated institutional Safety, Quality, and Risk Management resource that uses Systems Engineering, Human Factors, Quality, Safety, and/or Risk Management principles and engages in bidirectional feedback to achieve enterprise-level goals and improve quality of care.*
   a. ***Provide a brief summary of how the Simulation Program meets the Mission and Scope standards described in Section 1 (not more than 250 words).***
   b. *Simulation activities are clearly driven by the strategic needs of the involved clinical facility or healthcare system(s).*
      i. **The Mission or Vision statement(s) of the Program specifically addresses the intent and functions of the Simulation Program including: (1) impacting integrated system improvement within a complex healthcare environment, (2) enhancement of the performance of individuals, team, and organizations, and (3) creating a safer patient environment and improving outcomes.**
      ii. **Document or describe how the Simulation Program has been used as a resource by Risk Management, Quality/Safety, and/or similar organizational structure for enterprise improvement with bidirectional feedback during the past 2 years.**
      iii. **Provide a letter (twopages maximum) from organizational Risk Management, Enterprise Improvement, Safety, and/or Quality Improvement leadership supporting the Program's role in achieving Organizational Risk, Quality, Value, and/or Safety goals.**
   c. *The Program has a demonstrated history of participation in organizational process improvement including measurement of outcomes for purposes of improvement.*
      i. *Document or demonstrate three examples of simulation used by the Program in an integrated fashion to facilitate Patient Safety, Risk Management, Enterprise Improvement, and/or Quality Outcomes projects/activities. Optimum supporting documentation for each project/activity would include items ii–v below.*
      ii. *Document or describe Systems Engineering, Human Factors, or other systematic approach used to solve or mitigate an enterprise-defined safety, quality, or value concern(s), including bidirectional accountability for the activity/project (e.g., charter, A3, process improvement map, root cause analysis, cycles of improvement, etc.).*
      iii. *Report of findings to organizational leadership, including minutes demonstrating review and feedback.*
      iv. *Provide documentation of sustained assessment of associated relevant outcomes.*
      v. *Provide evidence that demonstrates organizational leadership's ongoing assessment of outcome metrics.*
2. **INTEGRATION WITH QUALITY AND SAFETY ACTIVITIES:** *The Program has an established and committed role in institutional Quality Assessment and Safety processes.*
   a. *Provide a brief summary of how the Simulation Program meets the Integration with Quality and Safety activities standards described in Section 2 (not more than 250 words).*
   b. *There is clear evidence of participation by Simulation leadership in the design and process of performance improvement activities at the organizational level.*
      i. *The Program provides Performance Improvement Committee rosters and minutes from at least two meetings during the past 2 years that demonstrate involvement/contributions of personnel associated with the Simulation Program.*
   c. *There is access to appropriate qualified human factors, psychometrics, systems engineering, and/or other appropriate support or resources.*
      i. *Demonstrate or describe access to appropriate qualified Human Factors, Psychometrics, Systems Engineering, and/or other appropriate support or resources.*

BEEN THERE, DONE THAT

Many applicants report that the process of self-study using the standards as a guide has stimulated invaluable enhancements in their Programs. Programs have developed or improved their existing processes or shaped new areas of focus using accreditation standards. Some Programs use these standards with the intent to apply for accreditation in the future, while other Programs use these standards purely for their own development.

Programs report that the benefits of using these accreditation standards and principles continue to accrue, even after receiving accreditation. They report that SSH accreditation helps in obtaining external and internal support, and in providing an external recognition of quality, as well as validating their resource needs. The process of external review and feedback allows Programs to understand their strengths and areas for improvement, guiding efforts toward maintenance and growth. Many Programs have reported that they developed many new methods and activities during the application process and continue to benefit in self-assessment as they work to sustain and improve their processes and activities. Many Programs are using the standards as a map to develop a new area of accomplishment within their Program (e.g., a Program accredited in assessment and teaching is now working toward developing their Program in the area of research using the research standards). Programs have also reported the value of performing an annual self-assessment using the standards. Examples of how accredited Programs have made changes as a result of accreditation are presented in Boxes 1.1.1 to 1.1.5.

BOX 1.1.1

During its first year, the Carolinas Simulation Center focused on the things most urgent for a new center: determining and meeting users' needs, mastering the technology, finding places to store everything, and convincing prospective users of the value of simulation. As the Center grew and staff proficiency increased, the number of users exploded. And as the number of users exploded, guess what happened. The staff focus intensified on meeting users' needs, mastering the technology, finding storage, and so on. The Center was busy, bustling, and doing urgent work. Had we not set our sights on accreditation, we'd have remained very busy, doing all those urgent things. But to meet our goals, the staff did the impossible: they carved out time for the not so urgent, but highly important, work of becoming an accredited site. Priorities didn't change, they simply doubled! But what a difference it has made. The new priorities were the ones that elevated the Center from very good to excellent. The accreditation quest led to vital new policies, to research that has enriched the body of simulation knowledge, to a stronger alignment with our users' goals. Thanks to the accreditation journey, Carolinas Simulation Center went from using simulation to improve healthcare education, to transforming healthcare through education. Along the way, the staff became simulation professionals; the users became partners in work that far transcended daily skill goals. When we celebrated the Center's first grant of accreditation, we also celebrated our emergence as professional partners in improving healthcare delivery.

Ellen Sheppard, EdD
President, Carolinas College of Health Sciences
SSH Accreditation Recipient 2010

BOX 1.1.2

The NorthShore Center for Simulation and Innovation (NCSI), Evanston, IL, participated in the SSH Simulation Center accreditation process in 2012. We have reaped several benefits from attaining accreditation. The first was recognized value from our Health System. Accreditation from SSH validated our simulation programs and demonstrated to our hospital administration that our simulationists have developed a level of expertise that met an international standard. Since our accreditation, our administrators have been more proactive in promoting our department, both internally and externally. It has helped with increasing collaboration with our Quality and Risk Departments, and our hospital now touts our Center as an integral piece of our HealthSystem's Mission.

The second benefit was internal. The process helped us to better organize our internal structure (from an organizational structure, policies and procedures, etc.), to focus on our Mission, to critique and reflect on our current programs in a way that made us reevaluate how we deliver the educational content to provide the best educational product from a learner and educator perspective.

The third was in the area of evaluation. Prior to the accreditation process, we focused primarily on collecting evaluation/feedback from the learners regarding our courses. The SSH accreditation self-study and site visit motivated us to develop an instructor evaluation process to improve the skills of our faculty and to ensure that all our instructors are delivering simulation-based debriefing in a standardized fashion.

Ernest Wang, MD, FACEP
Pam Aitchison, RN
Alvin H. Baum Family Fund Chair of Simulation and Innovation
NorthShore University HealthSystem, Evanston, Illinois
SSH Accreditation Recipient 2012

BOX 1.1.3

SSH Accreditation of the Virtual Hospital at Metropolitan Community College–Penn Valley Health Science Institute (MCC-PV-HSI) provides a standardized formal process for ongoing evaluation, quality improvement of our simulation program, along with high-stakes accountability. Participation in the accreditation process not only assists in identifying areas of concern, but also validates areas of excellence. The accreditation process requires a self-reflective, holistic, in-depth analysis and evaluation of policies, procedures, and operations in conjunction with peer reviews conducted by respected content experts from across the country. Access and engagement with these experts bring exposure to a broadened vision of simulation best practice, direction, and need for continuous quality improvement. National accreditation sends a message to both our students and external users that MCC-PV-HSI is committed to quality and excellence in simulation through participation in the rigor of external analysis and evaluation and meeting the high quality standards set by SSIH. SSIH accreditation is a stamp of quality that we display proudly.

Liz Santander RN, MSN
Sandy McIlnay
Lester Hardegree
Metropolitan Community College–Penn Valley
Health Science Institute: Virtual Hospital
SSH Accreditation Recipient 2011

BOX 1.1.4

Our teaching hospital was recently granted accreditation in simulation. The educational benefits are immense and have far-reaching broad implications. The advantages extend beyond improvements in individual knowledge base; we've had a noticeable increase in physician comfort, confidence, and proficiency with procedures and topics where simulation was used as the primary teaching modality.

The SSH Accreditation legitimizes our simulation program and commitment to simulation training. As a result, we've successfully secured funding to advance and improve our program. We are administratively centralized for planning, purchasing, and facilitator training, resulting in reduced redundant spending by individual departments. Challenges faced after securing accreditation include long-term budget considerations to keep the simulation program active and involved within its organization and the community. Such considerations include sufficient staffing, renewal fees, and faculty development.

Joshua Fenderson, MD
Jefferson Roberts, MD
Tripler Army Medical Center
Honolulu, HI
SSH Accreditation Recipient 2011

BOX 1.1.5

For the Simulation, Teaching and Academic Research (STAR) Center, the value of undergoing accreditation was twofold, beginning with the application process and carrying on after accreditation was granted as we continue to comply with the standards.

Applying for teaching accreditation required our team to procure documents and evaluate our policies. It was a great effort where all team members played an important role. The regular meetings that happened and the e-mail exchanges that circulated not only garnished a wonderful portfolio of paper, it also brought our team closer in the process. We learned about each other, about our center, and bonded over our toils in collectively working toward a goal.

When our center was granted accreditation, the bonding continued as we shared each other's joy, celebrating this momentous achievement. As we proudly added the SSH accreditation logo to our website and other forms of literature, people noticed, and our center gained instant credibility. Since we have been accredited, our center has developed more courses, all designed to meet the unique and diverse needs of our internal and external users, using the SSH standards as a guide. By following these standards, we ensure our users the most effective and efficient means of simulation education.

Being an accredited institution has broadened our perspective, and we continually reach for national and international opportunities to present and publish research and ideas. The value of being recognized by society is so high that we have the goal of applying for accreditation in the other areas also.

Laura Daniel, PhD
Simulation, Teaching, and Academic Research (STAR) Center in Allegheny, Pennsylvania
SSH Accreditation Recipient 2011

SUMMARY

The Council for Accreditation of Healthcare Simulation Programs has developed standards designed to support Programs providing teaching, assessment, research, or systems integration and improvement activities using simulation. Using the standards as guidelines facilitates the development of excellent simulation programs. Programs that have achieved accreditation have recognized the value of the accreditation process and many continue to use the standards for sustainability and improvement. The accreditation standards can be used as guidance for internal development and self-assessment; many simulation programs have risen to the challenge of fulfilling all of the criteria, thus achieving accreditation and public recognition of the quality of their Programs.

SECTION 1 • Simulation Standards

APPENDIX

Individual Members

2008 CATS Members
- Bill Dunn
- Beth Mancini
- Lisa Sinz
- Tamara Owens
- Gerry Moses
- Robert Simon
- Vinay Nadkarni
- Janice Palaganas
- Mary Patterson
- Bill McGaghie
- Beverlee Anderson
- Sally Rudy
- Katie Walker
- William Rutherford
- William Hamman

2008 Accreditation Subcommittee Members
- Bill Dunn
- Beth Mancini
- Lisa Sinz
- Tamara Owens
- Gerry Moses

- Vinay Nadkarni
- Janice Palaganas
- Mary Patterson

2009 Inaugural Accreditation Council
- Beth Mancini (Chair)
- Janice Palaganas (Director)
- Vinay Nadkarni
- Kathy Gallo
- Ellen Deutsch
- Jose Pliego
- Emily Hinchey
- Jennifer Manos
- Stephanie Tuttle
- Leo Kobayashi
- Tamara Owens
- Karen Reynolds
- Bill Riley
- Tom LeMaster
- Mary Patterson
- Bill Dunn
- Cate McIntosh
- Gerry Moses

CHAPTER 1.2

The INACSL Standards of Best Practice

Suzan E. Kardong-Edgren, PhD, RN, ANEF, CHSE, Teri Boese, RN, MSN, and Valerie M. Howard, EdD, MSN, RN

ABOUT THE AUTHORS

SUZAN (SUZIE) E. KARDONG-EDGREN is an Educational Researcher, Consultant, and the Editor-in-Chief of *Clinical Simulation in Nursing*. She is an active member of both the Society for Simulation in Healthcare and International Nursing Association for Clinical Simulation and Learning. She holds the Jodie DeMeyer Endowed Chair in Nursing at Boise State University in Boise, Idaho.

VALERIE M. HOWARD serves as Dean, Professor of Nursing, and the Director of the Regional Research and Innovation in Simulation Education (RISE) Center at Robert Morris University in Pittsburgh, PA. She is past president of the International Nursing Association for Clinical Simulation and Learning and an active member of the Society for Simulation in Healthcare.

TERI BOESE is an Associate Professor at the University of Texas Health Science Center at San Antonio and serves as the director of their Center for Simulation Innovation. She is the cofounding president of the International Nursing Association for Clinical Simulation and Learning, and has been an active member of the Standards Committee since their work began; she is also a member of the Society for Simulation in Healthcare.

ABSTRACT

Standards are created by experts within a discipline and reflect best practice. The International Association for Clinical Simulation and Learning (INACSL) developed the first set of published Standards for Best Practice: Simulation in 2011, and added guidelines in 2013. The INACSL Standards serve as a framework for providing simulation-based educational experiences within healthcare, and can be applied to multiple professions and settings. This chapter provides an overview of the comprehensive development process and summary of the seven INACSL Standards, with examples for their use within healthcare education and training. Utilizing the INACSL Standards in any setting creates a standardized foundation on which to build simulation-based educational experiences and demonstrates adherence to best practices for internal and external stakeholders.

CASE EXAMPLE

You are tasked with training new faculty at your program to run and debrief scenarios. You wonder what others have done in this situation and whether there are resources to help you save time and adopt best practices. After a Google search for nursing and simulation, you discover the International Association for Clinical Simulation and Learning (INACSL). INACSL provides a set of standards of best simulation practice that are evidence-based and updated every 2 years. They provide a useful planning and training road map for using simulation effectively with accompanying rationale.

INTRODUCTION AND BACKGROUND

Standards provide a road map for successful simulation program development within a hospital or academic setting. They provide an authoritative reference for program administrators seeking additional resources to properly run and manage a simulation center. When standards are adopted, they provide a stamp of approval for both standardization and quality for participants and stakeholders. Those charged with making a case for a simulation center will have the ability to say that they adhere to a set of standards engendering confidence that resources are being used in the best manner possible. Following internationally recognized standards prepares a simulation center for the next logical step: certification of its faculty (see chapter 1.4) and accreditation of the center (see chapter 1.1).

The pedagogy of simulation has continued to develop over the last decade. This growth has led to the need for the development of simulation practice standards. The Board of Directors (BOD) of INACSL began a multipart process for developing simulation standards in 2009. After determining an appropriate format, a list was developed to identify simulation concepts that should be contained in standards.

The INACSL surveyed members regarding their priorities for simulation standards development. The INACSL BOD (2011a) collated those responses into the 20 major concepts that emerged, and then regrouped the concepts into themes, forming 7 major standards. Work groups composed of board members further developed each of the seven standards. In 2010, a first draft of these standards was sent to both the INACSL membership and simulation experts for critique and comment. A Standards Committee task force was appointed to oversee the revision of the standards, on the basis of this feedback. The first publication of the standards appeared in *Clinical Simulation in Nursing*, in the August 2011 supplement.

After the Standards of Best Practice were published in 2011, the INACSL BOD Standards Committee immediately began the work of developing guidelines to accompany Standards II through VII, to provide further clarity using evidence-based guidelines. The distinction between standards and guidelines was discussed at length initially and clarified. The INACSL BOD chose to define standards as "policies" describing shared values, principles, and guidelines. The INACSL Standards set the criteria for decisions and actions and provide a definition of what is considered competent. Standards seek to identify what level of performance must be achieved, not the detailing of how to achieve that performance. Guidelines were viewed as the actions that assist in meeting standards. Guidelines are not necessarily comprehensive, but provide the framework for developing policies and procedures. The Standards Committee chair appointed experts to update the first Standards of Best Practice to meet the ongoing knowledge development related to simulation and develop practice guidelines to accompany each standard, for the next round of publication. These simulation experts were invited on the basis of their experiences with writing the standards and simulation expertise; they in turn solicited subcommittee members to work on guideline development. Each subcommittee reviewed the current literature related to the assigned standard and drafted practice guidelines for each criterion included in the standard. The first drafts were reviewed by the INACSL BOD and were sent back to the subcommittees for further revisions. After the revisions were made, the guidelines were reviewed by a solicited panel of external experts, with their edits incorporated before publishing (Table 1.2.1).

TABLE 1.2.1

Standard Title and Standard Statement Changes from 2011 to 2013

Standards of Best Practice: Simulation 2011	Standard's Statement (2011)	Standards of Best Practice: Simulation 2013	Standard's Statement (2013)
Standard I: Terminology	Consistent terminology provides guidance and clear communication and reflects shared values in simulation experiences, research, and publications.	Standard I: Terminology	Consistent terminology provides guidance and clear communication and reflects shared values in simulation experiences, research, and publications. Knowledge and ideas are clearly communicated with consistent terminology to advance the science of simulation.
Standard II: Professional Integrity of Participant	The simulation learning and testing environment will be one of clear expectations for the attitudes and behavior of each participant and an area where mutual respect is supported. Professional integrity related to confidentiality of the performances, scenario content, and participant experience is expected to be upheld during a simulation experience. These performances in simulation experiences may be live, recorded, and/or virtual.	Standard II: Professional Integrity of Participant(s)	The simulation learning, assessment, and evaluation environments will be areas where mutual respect among participants and facilitator(s) is expected and supported. As such, it is essential to provide clear expectations for the attitudes and behaviors of simulation participants. Professional integrity related to confidentiality of the performances, scenario content, and participant experience is required during and after any simulation. Confidentiality is expected in live, recorded, and/or virtual simulation experiences.
Standard III: Participant Objectives	The simulation experience should focus on the participant objectives and experience level.	Standard III: Participant Objectives	All simulation-based learning experiences begin with development of clearly written participant objectives, which are available prior to the experience.

Standards of Best Practice: Simulation 2011	Standard's Statement (2011)	Standards of Best Practice: Simulation 2013	Standard's Statement (2013)
Standard IV: Facilitation Methods	Multiple methods of facilitation are available, and use of a specific method is dependent on the learning needs of the participant(s) and the expected outcomes.	Standard IV: Facilitation	Multiple methods of facilitation are available, and use of a specific method is dependent on the learning needs of the participant(s) and the expected outcomes.
Standard V: Simulation Facilitator	A proficient facilitator is required to manage the complexity of all aspects of simulation.	Standard V: Facilitator	A proficient facilitator is required to manage the complexity of all aspects of simulation. The facilitator has specific simulation education provided by formal coursework, continuing education offering(s), and/or targeted work with an experienced mentor.
Standard VI: The Debriefing Process	All simulated experiences should include a planned debriefing session aimed toward promoting reflective thinking.	Standard VI: The Debriefing Process	All simulation-based learning experiences should include a planned debriefing session aimed toward promoting reflective thinking.
Standard VII: Evaluation of Expected Outcomes	This standard addresses summative evaluation as opposed to formative assessment.	Standard VII: Participant Assessment or Evaluation	In a simulation-based experience, formative assessment or summative evaluation can be used.

STANDARD I: TERMINOLOGY

The INACSL BOD and Standards Committee supported the use of standard definitions or a common language to be used when communicating about concepts related to simulation. Therefore, the Standards Committee developed nearly 50 definitions of simulation-related terms: for example, simulation, scenario, simulation learning environment, and debriefing. These terms were defined using current literature, reviewed by experts, revised, and published. The use of a standardized terminology enables communication among those involved in simulation and provides consistency when developing, implementing, evaluating, and publishing simulation-related activities, and will serve to advance the science of simulation-related efforts. Standardization of terms in research studies also allows easier aggregation of small-study findings for meta-analyses, for future use (INACSL BOD, 2011b). During the process of standards revision and guideline development, the Standards Committee identified the need for revision of certain terms already, on the basis of evidence and usage. This updated standard will be published with Standards II to VII in the summer of 2013. Nearly 70 terms are now defined within this INACSL Standard. Many of the international simulation societies, including the Society for Simulation in Healthcare, are now joining forces to work on a joint lexicography for all simulationists (see chapter 3.2).

STANDARD II: PROFESSIONAL INTEGRITY OF STUDENT

Simulated learning experiences should be conducted in an environment that fosters professionalism, confidentiality, and mutual respect. The simulated learning environment provides unique challenges and anxieties for the participant, often related to being recorded, evaluated by peers, and judgment (Blazeck, 2011; Clapper, 2010; Howard et al., 2011). Failure of the participants, and/or the facilitator, to maintain a mutually respectful environment can undermine the benefits of simulation and debriefing. In addition, participants are asked to keep the events related to the simulated learning experience confidential so that future participants can benefit from similar learning experiences. Maintaining professional integrity and confidentiality of all participants provides the same standardized experience for all participants (INACSL BOD, 2011c).

STANDARD III: PARTICIPANT OBJECTIVES

Simulation is an experiential teaching and learning methodology that should be guided by sound educational principles. Prior to any educational activity, the facilitator should develop specific learning objectives. This educational planning activity takes time and resources, but is integral to the proper development of the learning experience (Howard, et al., 2011; Jeffries, 2007). The objectives should be clear, measurable, and reflect the purpose and outcomes of the simulated learning experience. In addition, the objectives should reflect the experience and prior learning of the participant, and be rooted in the most current clinical evidence. Participants should be able to meet these objectives during the time frame provided during the simulation-based learning experience. The participant objectives should directly correlate with the evaluation methods discussed in Standard VII and should address the cognitive, psychomotor, and/or affective domains of learning (INACSL BOD, 2011d).

STANDARD IV: FACILITATION

Facilitation at some level is needed and expected, from before the scenario starts through the debriefing. This helps move a simulation forward and assists participants in gaining the maximum learning possible from the experience, long before the scenario ever starts. Facilitation begins with the alignment of participant objectives with coursework or learning outcomes and continues with sharing those objectives with the participants before the scenario (Waxman, 2010), orienting participants to the mannequins and simulation space (Posmontier et al., 2012), and planning evaluation methodologies. Partial facilitator prompting of a simulation can be done by cueing as the voice of the patient, or with a helpful charge nurse, or by an embedded participant family member in the room, or resident dropping by, or by the "voice from out of nowhere" approach, over the loudspeaker providing cues. The latter is the least desirable form of cueing as it breaks the participants' concentration and might lead participants to expect this to occur in the practice setting also. It is also the most directive form of facilitation: the facilitator virtually talks the participants through a scenario. No facilitator prompting during simulation suggests that the facilitator interjects only if a simulation is heading away from the stated participant objectives. Comments are held for debriefing (INACSL BOD, 2011e). Ultimately, the determination of what facilitation methodology to use in any given situation is based on the participant objectives and the expected outcomes of the simulation. Research is needed in this area to determine the best kinds of facilitation for differing levels of participants and practitioners.

STANDARD V: SIMULATION FACILITATOR

This standard describes who the facilitator is and what the facilitator does. The facilitator is defined in Standard I. A *facilitator* (INACSL BOD, 2011f) is an individual who guides and supports participants toward understanding and achieving scenario objectives. When the original standards were conceived, the decision was made to differentiate between what facilitation is and what the facilitator does; Standard IV addresses the process of facilitation and describes different facilitation methods, while Standard V describes the characteristics of the facilitator.

The facilitator should be able to clearly communicate the goals and expectations of the simulation. In addition, the facilitator creates an environment in which the participants can make mistakes without fear of reproach and in which the participants experience active learning (Ackermann et al., 2009; Kuznar, 2007; Waxman & Telles, 2009). If participants are to think critically, the learning environment must be psychologically safe. Stress during the simulation should not inhibit the participants' ability to learn and grow from the experience (INACSL BOD, 2011f).

It is important for the facilitator to acknowledge that the simulation will not be exactly like real life, but an effort is made to ensure that the simulation setting is as true to the real experience as possible. While preparing the participants for the simulation, the facilitator explains what is real, what is not real, and how elements are made real for the participants. The participants should understand that there will be ambiguity, and they are asked to maintain a suspension of disbelief during the simulation (Dieckmann et al., 2007). The facilitator must be knowledgeable about teaching and learning principles in order to design the experience to meet the level of the participant and the desired outcomes. The facilitator must also demonstrate ethical and professional behavior throughout the simulation experience. An atmosphere of mutual trust and respect is maintained with the participants, and the facilitator maintains their commitment to adhering to the Standards of Best Practice in simulation.

Methods of evaluation, of the participants and of the simulation, are established by the facilitator who provides guidance during the review of the relevant, significant elements of the experience. The facilitator also assists the participants in understanding how concepts learned or practiced in the simulation can be adapted to the clinical practice (Simon et al., 2009).

STANDARD VI: DEBRIEFING

Debriefing is an integral part of the simulation experience; simulations should not be conducted without time for debriefing built into the experience (see chapter 8.2). Debriefing should be done by a facilitator who observed the simulation scenario and who is competent in the process, by virtue of training, certification, or experience. Debriefing allows participants to reflect on the events and interventions, their own performance and the performance of others, and how they interacted as a team. Debriefing is an area of increasing interest and study (Beyer, 2012; Chronister & Brown, 2012; Dieckmann et al., 2009; Mariani et al., 2013; Neill & Wotton, 2011; Reed, 2012; Rudolph et al., 2006; Shinnick et al., 2011). The most effective practices in debriefing are only now beginning to emerge and vary with the level of the participant and complexity of the scenario (INACSL BOD, 2011g).

Accurate self-reflection during the debriefing process for both individual and team performance is essential. Research consistently demonstrates that high-performing scenario participants will more accurately rate their own performances than poor performers. Poor performers consistently overrate their performances, even with video evidence (Paul, 2010; Sadosty et al., 2011). Reasons for these findings remain unclear but are consistent across all disciplines. This is an area ripe for further research.

STANDARD VII: PARTICIPANT ASSESSMENT OR EVALUATION

Standard VII was renamed in the updated 2013 Standards from "evaluation of expected learning outcomes" to "participant assessment or evaluation." The 2013 Standard VII includes criteria for formative and summative evaluation and high-stakes testing. Benner et al. (2010) and others (Berkow et al., 2008; Howard et al., 2010; Hunt et al., 2012; Kolb & Shugart, 1984; Yanhua & Watson, 2011) suggested increased rigor in the evaluation preparation for professional practice, beyond the currently used methodologies. Simulation is effective for evaluating learning in the psychomotor, cognitive, and affective domains and could be used for rigorous summative evaluation. Kirkpatrick (1994) suggests that how one acts in a simulation may not reflect actual behavior in a real situation; however, recent research suggests that simulation scores do correlate with subjective educational rankings by faculty (Mudumbai et al., 2012). Even though medicine has embraced objective structured clinical examinations (OSCEs) for many years as part of the licensure process, nurses remain ambivalent about summative evaluations using simulation (Kardong-Edgren et al., 2011). Standard VII outlines very specific criteria to follow for establishing a reliable and valid summative simulation environment (INACSL BOD, 2011h).

As research in using simulation for summative outcomes testing continues, new considerations arise (Boulet et al., 2011; see chapter 7.3). The number of scenarios required to obtain an accurate assessment of a student's overall performance remains in question (Mudumbai et al., 2012), and the use of an evaluator who is familiar with the student is a significant source of bias affecting scoring outcomes (Stroud et al., 2011). New questions will continue to emerge as new answers are found, as the standards for best practices continue to be refined and published.

The INACSL Standards presented the best evidence to date when they were first presented in 2011. With the simulation field changing rapidly and more research studies reported, the work of updating the standards to reflect evolving best practices will be ongoing. Revisions to the initial standards with the addition of guidelines were published in 2013. During the development of guidelines and the updating of the standards, three additional standards were identified for the next revision cycle. These standards will be related to simulation design, simulation research, and interprofessional simulation.

BEEN THERE, DONE THAT: HOW CAN I CONTINUE TO IMPROVE OR SUSTAIN WHAT I HAVE ACHIEVED?

The INACSL Standards can be used as the basic building blocks of simulation instructor courses and simulation center orientations for all participants and facilitators. They reflect current evidence-based practices in simulation pedagogy; thus they apply to all levels and types of simulation and simulators, from novice to expert, center type, and profession. The Standards were used to build the simulation faculty development ladder at Boise State University (Rosemary Macy, personal communication). For example, new simulation faculty are initially oriented to the terminology used in simulation by reviewing INACSL Standard I. Standards II through VII provide a thorough orientation (each standard with the evidence-based rationale) to guiding and debriefing a simulation scenario. The faculty are required to observe multiple simulations with an experienced simulationist. Then, the faculty are apprenticed with a faculty member and observed and debriefed as the new faculty member gains experience with facilitating and debriefing simulations. As proficiency increases, the faculty move from a Simulation I to Simulation II level. Once faculty members are speaking at simulation and educational conferences and publishing articles, they achieve Simulation III status.

Many schools have chosen to adopt the INACSL Standards as the framework for their simulation programs. The faculty at the Robert Morris University School of Nursing and Health Sciences chose to adopt the Standards within the regional Research and Innovation in Simulation Education (RISE) Center. This means that all simulation experiences within the RISE Center align with the INACSL Standards. For example, the standardized lesson plan/programming form in the RISE Center addresses standard terminology, clear measurable objectives, facilitation methods, debriefing questions with evidence-based rationales, and methods of evaluation, which are all in alignment with the INACSL Standards. This information was placed into a simulation policy that has been communicated to all faculty and students using the RISE Center. The RISE Center Confidentiality Policy describes the importance of professional behavior and maintaining the academic integrity of the simulations, which aligns with Standard II: Professional Integrity of Student (Figures 1.2.1 and 1.2.2). Simulation educators can reference the Standards when making the case for funding requests for simulation experiences. For example, demonstrating how your simulation activities align with national Standards of Best Practice provides evidence that your simulation center is conducting high-quality simulation learning experiences. The RMU Regional RISE Center received several grants, and with each one, the funding agency reacted positively to the simulation approach that was guided by national standards. At the University of Texas Health Science Center at San Antonio, the Standards have been adopted as the authority to guide the development of the policies and procedures for the Center for Simulation Innovation. The use of the Standards demonstrates that a simulation facility is utilizing the best evidence available when developing, implementing, and evaluating simulation experiences. New opportunities for center accreditation (see chapter 1.1) and individual certification (see chapter 1.4) all support and build on criteria such as the INACSL Standards for simulation.

College of Health Sciences
Simulation Center
Facilitator Development Guide

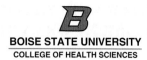

Facilities INACSL Standard I	Level #1	Level #2	Level #3
Tour College of Health Sciences Simulation Center	✓	✓	✓
Tour Practice Labs	✓	✓	✓
Tour Learning Resource center (LRC)	✓	✓	✓
Simulation Center General Use **INAC SL Standard I, II**			
Orientation to scheduling	✓	✓	✓
Orientation to policies/procedures	✓	✓	✓
Orientation to roles and responsibilities	✓	✓	✓

Simulation Scenario Development Process INAC SL Standard I, II, III, IV, V, VI, VII			
Complete the level 100 (4) online free simulation modules from the University of Washington's Center for Health Science Interprofessional Education, Research and Practice website.	✓	✓	✓
Complete simulation stipend requirements		✓	✓
		✓	✓

Facilitating a Simulation Scenario INAC SL Standard I, II, III, IV, V, VI			
Participate/observe facilitation/debriefing of simulations with an experienced facilitator.	✓ (2)	✓ (2 more)	✓ (2 more)
Independently facilitate/debrief a minimum of three simulations per ser		✓	✓
			✓

Professional/Dissemination Activities INAC SL Standard I, II, III, IV, V, VI			
Member of the SON and/or COHS Simulation Team			✓
Submit a minimum of one simulation related Journal article/conference abstract or demonstrate participation in a minimum of one simulation related research project every two years			✓
			✓

Level Achieved (circle appropriate) – Level #1   Level #2   Level #3

Signature: _____

Date: _____

FIGURE 1.2.1   Sample faculty simulation facilitator development path (Courtesy Boise State University).

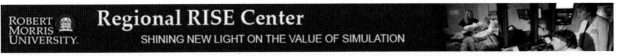

RISE Center INACSL Standards of Practice

Policy:

Simulation offers the ability to provide standardized applied learning opportunities for students within the safe environment of the RISE Center, thus reducing the risk of harm to our patients. The RMU Nursing department supports the substitution of simulation for a minimum of 10% of the total number of clinical hours designated for a clinical course, as long as each activity is guided by the International Nursing Association for Clinical Simulation and Learning (INACSL) Standards of Best Practice: Simulation (INACSL Board of Directors, 2011).

> Standard I: Terminology
> Standard II: Professional Integrity of Participant
> Standard III: Participant Objectives
> Standard IV: Facilitation Methods
> Standard V: Simulation Facilitator
> Standard VI: The Debriefing Process
> Standard VII: Evaluation of Expected Outcomes

Procedure:

- Each 1 hour of simulation equals 2 hours of clinical time, for a 1:2 ratio. The course faculty member should designate the allotted equivalent on their syllabus and inform the students accordingly.
- The RISE High Fidelity Center will assist faculty members in designing, implementing, and evaluating simulation experiences for their students according to the INACSL Standards of Best Practice: Simulation (2011).
- Each RISE High Fidelity Center simulation experience will be followed by an evaluation of the learner's experience.
- To schedule high fidelity simulation experiences, contact the RISE Center at least two weeks prior to the experience.
- Experiences are scheduled based upon the date of request.
- The schedule of RISE Center high fidelity simulation experiences can be viewed on the RISE Center calendar at risecenter.rmu.edu.
- Concerns related to RISE Center activities should be addressed with the RISE Center Director.

Approved 9/2012
RISE Center Administration, Faculty and Staff
and SNHS Faculty

FIGURE 1.2.2 Sample simulation policy (Courtesy Robert Morris University).

SECTION 1 • Simulation Standards

SUMMARY

This chapter presents a synopsis on the development and use of the current INACSL Standards of Best Practice in Simulation. Standards are outlined for terminology, professional integrity of participants, participant objectives, facilitation, facilitator, the debriefing process, and participant assessment and evaluation. Standards are updated and published every 2 years by the INACSL organization.

REFERENCES

Ackermann, A. D., Kenny, G., & Walker, C. (2009). Simulator programs for new nurses' orientation. *Journal for Nurses in Staff Development, 23*(3), 136–139.

Benner, B., Sutphen, M., Leonard, V., & Day, L. (2010). *Educating nurses.* San Francisco, CA: Jossey-Bass.

Berkow, S., Virkstis, K., Stewart, J., & Conway, L. (2008). Assessing new graduate nurse performance. *Nurse Educator, 34*(1), 17–22.

Beyer, D. A. (2012). Enhancing critical reflection on simulation through wikis. *Clinical Simulation in Nursing, 8*(2), e67–e70. doi:10.1016/j.ecns.2010.12.003

Blazeck, A. (2011). Simulation anxiety syndrome: Presentation and treatment. *Clinical Simulation in Nursing, 7*, e57–e60. doi:10.1016/j.ecns.2010.05.002

Boulet, J. R., Jeffries, P. R., Hatala, R. A., Korndorffer, J. R., Feinstein, D. M., & Roche, J. P. (2011). Research regarding methods of assessing learning outcomes. *Simulation in Healthcare, 6*, s48–s51. doi:10.1097/SIH.0b013e318222237d0

Chronister, C., & Brown, D. (2012). Comparison of simulation debriefing methods. *Clinical Simulation in Nursing, 8*(7), e281–e288. doi:10.1016/j.ecns.2010.12.005

Clapper, T. C. (2010). Beyond Knowles: What those conducting simulation need to know about adult learning theory. *Clinical Simulation in Nursing, 6*(1), e7–e14. doi:10.1016/j.ecns.2009.07.003

Dieckmann, P., Gaba, D., & Rall, M. (2007). Deepening the theoretical foundations of patient simulation as social practice. *Simulation in Healthcare: The Journal of the Society for Simulation in Healthcare, 2*(3), 183–193. doi:10.1097/SIH.0b013e3180f637f5

Dieckmann, P., Molin Friis, S., Lippert, A., & Ostergaard, D. (2009). The art and science of debriefing in simulation: Ideal and practice. *Medical Teacher, 31*, e287–e294. doi:10.1016/j.ecns.2009.10.004

Howard, V., Englert, N., Kameg, K., & Perozzi, K. (2011). Integration of simulation across the curriculum: Student and faculty perspectives. *Clinical Simulation in Nursing, 7*(1), e1–e10.

Howard, V., Ross, C., Mitchell, A. M., & Nelson, G. (2010). Human patient simulators and interactive case studies—A comparative analysis of learning outcomes and student perceptions. *Computers, Informatics, and Nursing (CIN), 28*(1), 42–48.

Hunt, L. A., McGee, P., Gutteridge, R., & Hughes, M. (2012). Assessment of student nurses in practice: A comparison of theoretical and practical assessment results in England. *Nurse Education Today, 32*(4), 351–355.

INACSL Board of Directors. (2011a). Standards of best practice: Simulation. *Clinical Simulation in Nursing, 7*(4S), s1–s2.

INACSL Board of Directors. (2011b). Standard I: Terminology. *Clinical Simulation in Nursing, 7*(4S), s3–s7. doi:10.1016/j.ecns.2011.05.005

INACSL Board of Directors. (2011c). Standard II: Professional integrity of participants. *Clinical Simulation in Nursing, 7*(4S), s8–s9. doi:10.1016/j.ecns.2011.05.006

INACSL Board of Directors. (2011d). Standard III: Participant objectives. *Clinical Simulation in Nursing, 7*(4S), s10–s11. doi:10.1016/jecns.2011.05.007

INACSL Board of Directors. (2011e). Standard IV: Facilitation methods. *Clinical Simulation in Nursing, 7*(4S), s12–s13. doi:10.1016/j.ecns.2011.05.008

INACSL Board of Directors. (2011f). Standard V: Simulation facilitator. *Clinical Simulation in Nursing, 7*(4S), s14–s15. doi:10.1016/j.ecns.2011.05.009

INACSL Board of Directors. (2011g). Standard VI: The debriefing process. *Clinical Simulation in Nursing, 7*(4S), s16–s17. doi:10.1016/j.ecns.2011.05.010

INACSL Board of Directors. (2011h). Standard VII: Evaluation of expected outcomes. *Clinical Simulation in Nursing, 7*(4S), s18–s19. doi:10.1016/j.ecns.2011.05.011

Jeffries, P. R. (2007). *Simulation in nursing education: From conceptualization to evaluation.* New York, NY: National League for Nursing.

Kardong-Edgren, S., Hanberg, A. D., Keenan, C., Ackerman, A., & Chambers, K. C. (2011). A discussion of high-stakes testing: An extension of a 2009 INACSL conference roundtable. *Clinical Simulation in Nursing, 7*(1), e19–e24. doi:10.1016/j.ecns.2010.02.002

Kirkpatrick, D. (1994). *Evaluating training programs: The four levels.* San Francisco, CA: Berrett-Koehler. doi:10.1097/SIH.0b013e31823d018a

Kolb, S., & Shugart, E. (1984). Evaluation: Is simulation the answer? *Journal of Nursing Education, 23*(2), 84–86.

Kuznar, K. A. (2007). Associate degree nursing students' perception of learning using a high-fidelity human patient simulator. *Teaching and Learning in Nursing, 2*(2), 46–52. doi:10.1016/j.teln.2007.01.009

Mariani, B., Cantrell, M. A., Meakim, C., Prieto, P., & Dreifuerst, K. T. (2013). Structured debriefing and students' clinical judgment abilities in simulation. *Clinical Simulation in Nursing, 9*(5), e147–e155. doi:10.1016/j.ecns.2011.11.009

Mudumbai, S. C., Gaba, D. M., Boulet, J. R., Howard, S. K., & Davies, M. F. (2012). External validation of simulation-based assessments with other performance measures of third-year anesthesiology residents. *Simulation in Healthcare, 7*(2), 73–80.

Neill, M. A., & Wotton, K. (2011). High-fidelity simulation debriefing in nursing education: A literature review. *Clinical Simulation in Nursing, 7*(5), e161–e168. doi:10.1016/j.ecns.2011.02.001

Paul, F. (2010). An exploration of student nurses' thoughts and experiences of using a video-recording to assess their performance or CPR during a mock objective OSCE. *Nurse Education in Practice, 10*, 285–290.

Posmontier, B., Montgomery, K., Smith Glasgow, M. E., Montgomery, O. C., & Morse, K. (2012). Transdisciplinary teamwork simulation in obstetrics-gynecology health care education. *Journal of Nursing Education, 51*(3), 176–179. doi:10.3928/01484834-20120127-02

Reed, S. J. (2012). Debriefing experience scale: Development of a tool to evaluate the student learning experience in debriefing. *Clinical Simulation in Nursing, 8*(6), e211–e217. doi:10.1016/j.ecns.2011.11.002

Rudolph, J. W., Simon, R., Dufresne, R. L., & Raemer, D. B. (2006). There's no such thing as "nonjudgmental" debriefing: A theory and method for debriefing with good judgment. *Simulation in Healthcare, 1*(1), 49–56.

Sadosty, A. T., Fernanda Bellolio, M., Laack, T. A., Luke, A., Weaver, A., & Goyal, D. G. (2011). Simulation-based emergency medicine resident self-assessment. *The Journal of Emergency Medicine, 41*(6), 679–685. doi:10.1016/j.jemermed.2011.05.041

Shinnick, M. A., Woo, M., Horwich, T. B., & Steadman, R. (2011). Debriefing: The most important component in simulation? *Clinical Simulation in Nursing, 7*(3), e105–e111. doi:10.1016/j.ecns.2010.11.005

Simon, R., Rudolph, J. W., & Raemer, D. B. (2009). *Debriefing assessment for simulation in healthcare—Rater version.* Cambridge, MA: Center for Medical Simulation. Retrieved from http://www.harvardmedsim.org/debriefing-assesment-simulation-healthcare.php

Stroud, L., Herold, J., Tomlinson, G., & Cavalcanti, R. B. (2011). Who you know or what you know? Effects of examiner familiarity with residents on OSCE scores. *Academic Medicine, 86*, S8–S11.

Waxman, K. T. (2010). The development of evidence-based clinical simulation scenarios: Guidelines for nurse educators. *Journal of Nursing Education, 49*(1), 29–35. doi:10.3982/01484834-20090916-07

Waxman, K. T., & Telles, C. (2009). The use of Benner's framework in high-fidelity simulation faculty development: The Bay Area Simulation Collaborative Model. *Clinical Simulation in Nursing, 5*(6), e231–e235. doi:10.1016/j.ecns.2009.06.001

Yanhua, C., & Watson, R. (2011). A review of clinical competence assessment in nursing. *Nurse Education Today, 31*(8), 832–836.

CHAPTER 1.3

Simulation Center Program Metrics

*Sandra J. Feaster, RN, MS, MBA, John W. Lutz, BS, Troy E. Reihsen,
Farrah F. Leland, JD, and John H. Shatzer, PhD*

ABOUT THE AUTHORS

SANDRA J. FEASTER is the Assistant Dean for Immersive and Simulation-based Learning at Stanford University School of Medicine. Over the past 8 years, she has opened and managed two key simulation centers at Stanford, the 1,500 square feet (139.4 m^2) Goodman Surgical Simulation Center (which is an ACS AEI level 1 accredited center) and the 28,000 square feet (2601.2 m^2) Goodman Immersive Learning Center. She is active in the Society for Simulation in Healthcare and the American College of Surgery Accredited Education Institutes.

JOHN W. LUTZ is the Director of Information Technology and Co-Director of Research at the Peter M. Winter Institute for Simulation, Education, and Research (WISER) at the University of Pittsburgh and the University of Pittsburgh Medical Center (UPMC). He provides management and guidance for all software development projects as well as new hardware implementation and information technology support. He is the architect of the Simulation Information Management System (SIMS), which WISER uses to manage the facility.

TROY REIHSEN is the Administrator of the SimPORTAL and CREST labs. He is also the Director of the Anaplastology Lab, which creates patient-specific models with novel organosilicate-based artificial tissues benchmarked from our Human Tissue Database. He has over 8 years in Anesthesiology (clinical and animal) and Urologic Surgery (education) research. He also has over 22 years of military service as a 68W combat medic with combat zone experience.

FARRAH F. LELAND is the Assistant Director of The Institute for Simulation and Interprofessional Studies (ISIS) at the University of Washington. She serves as Vice Chair of the Administration and Management Committee for the American College of Surgery Accredited Education Institutes. Ms. Leland earned a Juris Doctorate from Gonzaga University and was admitted to the Washington State Bar Association in 2007. She holds an undergraduate degree in Cell and Molecular Biology from the University of Washington.

JOHN H. SHATZER received his PhD from the University of Illinois in 1991 and is an Associate Professor of Medical Education and Administration at Vanderbilt University School of Medicine. He is the founding Director of the Center for Experiential Learning and Assessment there, and has worked in simulation since the mid-80s, contributing articles, workshops, and presentations to further our understanding of simulation education, focusing on the best practices from the learning and assessment sciences.

ABSTRACT

This chapter discusses the importance of collecting data to enable simulation leadership to document the activities in the center, provide data necessary for obtaining accreditation by various accrediting bodies, and to provide justification for programs and activities. This chapter also demonstrates various methods and terms used for data collection and analysis. The use of Excel spreadsheets and pivot tables will be demonstrated in various examples.

CASE EXAMPLE: DEVELOPING A WORKSHOP FOR IMSH ON METRICS, WHAT TO CALL THINGS, HOW TO COMPARE PROGRAMS, AND MORE

Five centers were participating in data collection to present a workshop on Data Metrics at a recent International Meeting on Simulation in Healthcare (IMSH). The presenters thought it would be interesting to demonstrate how each center compared with the others. As they began to gather data, they quickly realized that everyone had a different name for similar data, or collected data in different ways.

The five programs collected data for one month using a specific template. Data was collected from every class run at the centers and included the course name, start/stop time, date, number of learners, number of rooms, and number of simulators. Additional data was collected on the **course, class, session,** learners, **simulators, simulator type, clinical domain, learner type, training type,** and **department** (see Glossary for definitions).

Formulas were developed to describe, analyze, and compare activities individually and between centers. These included learner hours, **educational hours, room hours,** contact hours, and duration. Table 1.3.1 provides comparison data on the five centers using the following formulas:

TABLE 1.3.1

Five-Center, 1-Month Analysis

	No. of Participants	Participant Hours	No. of Classes	Room Hours
PORTAL	339	820	28	193
Stanford	1,455	5,701	95	869
WISER	1,035	3,873	217	1,070
STP	310	927	57	334
ISIS	1,403	6,211	167	852

- **No. of Learners:** The number of students that have participated in simulation classes. The same person can be counted multiple times if they attended multiple classes during the time frame reported on.
- **Learner Hours:** 1 learner hour = 1 class hour × 1 learner. If a class lasted 4 hours and there were 10 learners, there would be 40 learner hours.
- **No. of Classes:** Each class is defined as a set number of hours during a day where a specific number of learners are involved in one or more structured learning activities.
- **Room Hours:** Multiply the number of rooms by the class time. If there were 4 rooms used for a 4-hour class, there would be 16 room hours.

From this exercise, a passion for describing and standardizing terminology used for developing and discussing simulation centers was born. This passion was founded upon our struggles to come to an agreement on a common language and a desire to help colleagues effectively and efficiently communicate with one another.

INTRODUCTION

Over the past several years of collaboration and presentations on metrics, it has become clear to many in the simulation community that there is a huge gap in understanding, developing, and collecting metrics that accurately and consistently describe the activities of healthcare simulation programs. The unfortunate old adage "if you have seen and measured one program, you have seen and measured one program" holds true, even today. By collecting and measuring data, program managers can understand and analyze activities that have occurred and use that data to try to project activities into the future. This data can be used to create and report information to administration, develop and publish reports, highlight activities to funding sources, and demonstrate productivity and utilization to accrediting bodies and others.

Many accrediting bodies are beginning to request data about simulation: for example, the Society for Simulation in Healthcare (SSH) (http://ssih.org/committees/accreditation) and the American College of Surgeons–Accredited Education Institutes (ACS-AEI) (http://www.facs.org/education/accreditationprogram/). In addition, specialty organizations that provide program endorsements are also starting to look at data. For example, the American Society of Anesthesiology (ASA) (https://simapps.asahq.org/) and the American College of Obstetrics and Gynecology (ACOG) (http://www.acog.org) are developing programs that are specific to simulation.

The Accreditation Council for Graduate Medical Education (ACGME) (http://www.acgme.org/acgmeweb/GraduateMedicalEducation/AccreditedProgramsandSponsorSearch.aspx) is also suggesting that simulation play a part in **training**. With this will come further demand for data that should be reported in a standard comparable format.

The ability to track various activities and report those activities to accrediting bodies is on the rise (Box 1.3.1). Data requirements and reporting related to simulation

BOX 1.3.1

EXAMPLE OF ACCREDITATION REQUIREMENTS

SSH has data reporting requirements that are required for accreditation (see accreditations standards here: https://ssih.org/accreditation/how-to-apply).

In the seven Core Standards, Standard 3 is a key standard that can benefit from data collection and analysis.

3. Facilities, Technology, Simulation Modalities, and Human Resources

There is an appropriate variety and level of simulation modalities (e.g., standardized patients, mannequins, virtual reality, task trainers, etc.) and human resources to support/achieve the goals of the Program. The environment is conducive to accomplish the Program's teaching, **assessment, research,** and/or systems integration activities.

Section e. The Program provides an adequate number and variety of simulation offerings to develop and maintain expertise:

   i. Provide a list of simulation courses offered, including targeted learners.

   ii. Provide a list of educators (e.g., content experts, instructors, facilitators, trainers).

   iii. Provide a list of Certified Healthcare Simulation Educators (CHSE).

   iv. **Provide the number of participants this year.**

   v. **Describe the types and/or groups of learners this year.**

   vi. **Provide total numbers of Learner Contact Hours this year.**

   vii. Describe the anticipated trends of simulation use for the forthcoming year (e.g., areas of expansion or change).

ACS-AEI

The ACS-AEI has various data that must be reported both at the time of initial application and again for reaccreditation. The information required includes, but is not limited to, items listed below:

   1. The specific learner group (s) and the percentage of time each group participates in center activities.

   2. The learning domains that activities address (cognitive, psychomotor, affective, and team training).

   3. Assessment of learning, performance and outcome, faculty, and continuous improvement in the education and training programs.

In these requirements, one can see that learner attendance is required. In the case of the ACS-AEI, learner groups are identified as surgeons in practice, physicians from other disciplines, residents from any discipline, medical students, **allied health** professionals, nurses, and others. You need to know not only the number of attendees, but also their discipline, besides being clear about what constitutes "attendance."

In the ACS-AEI criterion that addresses administrative and support staff requirements, it specifically states that "staff will create an annual report and utilization data for the Education Institute." Sites are also required to pursue research and scholarly activities, which again require data that support assessment of learners, technologies, and so on.

---

can often intersect with other data requirements for other accreditation and reporting purposes. Reviewing accreditation requirements prior to seeking accreditation is prudent in helping determine the data needs and perhaps guide the data format and collection methodology used.

Going one step further, administration, accrediting bodies, and others are asking how programs compare. By comparing metrics, programs can benchmark activity, collaborate to help develop best practices, and ultimately perform collaborative research. However, before this can happen, programs must speak the same language.

Understanding how one program did "X" with "Y" resource can lead to improved program efficiencies. In the past, and even continuing today, simulation in healthcare develops and grows in a very organic and ad hoc manner, with simulation programs creating their own processes for program development and execution. There continues to be very little standardization and even less collaboration between programs. As healthcare simulation evolves, standardization of procedures and measurement of the effectiveness of the activities and procedures will require collection of standardized data and a standardized taxonomy.

Because healthcare simulation is a rapidly developing field, the following discussions about definitions, metrics, and structures are not absolute. As simulation activity grows, the methods and terminology used to measure activity and discuss functionality will change as well. This chapter will discuss measuring activities from several different aspects and applications. In addition, there will be demonstrations provided in how to calculate metrics with the use of some simple Excel techniques.

Stakeholders in Simulation

Every stakeholder (e.g., student, simulation leadership, administration, institution,) may, and likely will, have a different perspective on what is important and what reflects their investments made in simulation. An honest and transparent needs assessment will be required with all stakeholders to understand their unique perspective, as well as the common ground upon which there is agreement. These conversations must then be translated into the data collected to report simulation utilization.

TAXONOMY

Taxonomy, as defined by the Merriam-Webster dictionary, is the "classification" according to presumed natural relationships, or being clear and consistent with "what things are called." Having a defined ttaxonomy helps develop and organize methods of classifying simulation activities, and it can help programs relate in new ways (see Introduction).

Although no one method is perfect for every center, the goal is to create a base of descriptors or "taxonomy" that allows a common language for centers to use to classify and quantify activities and engage in conversation. As noted in the case example above, without a baseline common language, it is difficult to have such discussions and develop a model for comparison.

This chapter is not intended to be a primer on taxonomy, but merely hopes to highlight the importance of a common language.

METRICS AND MEANING OF METRICS

The importance of collecting and reporting program metrics has been described above. The road to achieving a shared lexicon that brings common meanings to metrics, however, can be perilous. Regardless, if a common "language" of simulation is to be achieved, programs will need to agree to common meanings. It is a somewhat arbitrary decision to make for each term, but a necessary one.

Consider, for example, agreeing on the term "encounter." The meaning of encounter within the standardized patient (SP) world has typically meant the interaction event between the SP and the learner. Initially, it likely grew out of the "clinical encounter" terminology with a one-on-one interaction between physician and patient, but it becomes more complicated in the learning environment if there is more than one SP or learner in that event.

Vanderbilt's Center for **Experiential** Learning and Assessment considers an "encounter" to be an interaction with:

1. a high-technology mannequin,
2. or a hybrid patient,
3. or a SP,
4. or watching a live feed of the same and then participating in a debriefing of that scenario by an instructor.

At Vanderbilt, a student would be considered to have had two encounters if the student had one encounter with a high-technology mannequin simulator including a debriefing and another one with an SP including a debriefing. With three simulations, each student would have three encounters, consisting of three hands-on or live-feed interactions and a debriefing with each one. For Vanderbilt, a "session" would reference a class event of students.

To contrast, the Peter M. Winter Institute for Simulation Education and Research (WISER) center at the University of Pittsburgh considers the entire time that someone spent engaged at their simulation center in a contiguous time period defined as an "encounter." In one educational encounter, a student may come to WISER at 9:00 a.m., take a prequiz, listen to a brief lecture, go through a scenario using a high-fidelity simulator, have a session with a SP, be debriefed on both encounters, take a postquiz, and complete a course survey, and leave at noon. In the WISER program metric system, that is considered one educational encounter, with many (up to seven) separate activities within that "encounter." Some of those activities (simulator and SP) are called "sessions."

These examples illustrate how the terminology developed at various programs will impact the conversation about a common lexicon, and perhaps make agreement more difficult. However, if programs are ever to move beyond local metrics to gain a greater insight into the entire enterprise and the impact on learners, clients, and patients, programs will have to decide on a standardized taxonomy, or at least understand the taxonomy of various programs, and where they differ, so effective comparisons may be made.

PROGRAMMATIC ASSESSMENT

More and more, programs are being asked to provide very specific details of programs or learner groups. These requests come with different purposes. For example, they may be financially driven (who should pay for center use) or to determine the true costs of activities for budget purposes.

Given below are case studies that will present data requests from or about programs.

CASE STUDY: Data Request for Determining Graduate Medical Education Program Volume

At Stanford School of Medicine, the Immersive Learning Center (cisl.stanford.edu) was charged with providing Graduate Medical Education (GME) program statistics. The purpose of this exercise was to engage the hospitals in a discussion on finances and the value that the simulation center provides to the hospital and residency program by running a variety of GME activities for various departments in the School of Medicine's Immersive Learning Center. These activities include mostly mannequin-based simulation, but more requests for SP exercises (difficult conversations) and the use of task trainers (airway, lumbar puncture, central line insertion, etc.), particularly for new interns, are being made. The goal of this analysis was to identify the time and resources required for planning, preparing, and running these GME activities so the School of Medicine could dialogue with the hospital about funding.

There were several challenges in responding to this request.

1. **Data Accuracy**—Ensuring that the data downloaded from a scheduling system accurately reflected the following: correct rooms, times of activities, staff and resources, setup and takedown time, and learner population. Given below is an example of the initial data pull that is obtained from a scheduling system, R25 (an enterprise-level

scheduling system used by the University and other universities—http://corp.collegenet.com/products/Series25_overview.html). The screenshot is only a portion of the data pull, which is then placed in a spreadsheet for data manipulation (Table 1.3.2).

TABLE 1.3.2

Initial Data Pull from Resource 25 Scheduling System

Rsrv	Month & Date	Start Time	End Time	Setup Start Time	Pre-event Start Time	Event Start Time	Event End Time	Post-event End Time	Takedown End Time	Room No
5964307	4/2/12	10:30:00 AM	12:29:00 PM	10:30:00 AM	10:30:00 AM	10:30:00 AM	12:29:00 PM	12:29:00 PM	12:29:00 PM	LK033
5964307	4/2/12	10:30:00 AM	12:29:00 PM	10:30:00 AM	10:30:00 AM	10:30:00 AM	12:29:00 PM	12:29:00 PM	12:29:00 PM	LK037
5964307	4/2/12	10:30:00 AM	12:29:00 PM	10:30:00 AM	10:30:00 AM	10:30:00 AM	12:29:00 PM	12:29:00 PM	12:29:00 PM	LK040
5964307	4/2/12	10:30:00 AM	12:29:00 PM	10:30:00 AM	10:30:00 AM	10:30:00 AM	12:29:00 PM	12:29:00 PM	12:29:00 PM	LK043
5964307	4/2/12	10:30:00 AM	12:29:00 PM	10:30:00 AM	10:30:00 AM	10:30:00 AM	12:29:00 PM	12:29:00 PM	12:29:00 PM	LK047

2. **Understanding the Data**—After the data is downloaded, the activity, hours, setup, resource, and so forth must be either sorted or calculated. Note in the example above that the same exercise used several rooms for 2 hours only.

3. **Manipulating the Data**—Identifying the learner population is done by developing an Excel lookup table that matches the activity with the learner population. From there, pivot tables could be used to manipulate the data. This was not an easy process because:

   a. The data pull collected is extremely large and in an enterprise system that is not particularly user-friendly.
   b. Data must be downloaded into a spreadsheet and additional calculations and lookup tables need to be developed.
   c. Course activities are often entered under different names as the person that enters them does not necessarily know the courses, so just enters what is provided. For example, an Emergency Medicine Crisis Resource Management course may be entered as EMCRM, EMCRM-A, EMCRM R1, Emergency Medicine CRM, and so forth. As one can imagine, not calling the exercise the same name when it is entered can cause various issues when trying to perform data analysis, pivot tables, and so forth. This was a new learning for the authors who are working on common tables for identifying activities.
   d. The data must be reported and collected accurately to really define the activity exercise times, setup time, learners, and so forth. If not, additional time-consuming manipulation is necessary. A standardized setup time for key exercises is essential to developing consistent reporting and analysis activities.
   e. Because of the enormous amount of data (resources, rooms, setup, takedown, etc.), it can become daunting and difficult to manage without expertise in analytical skills.

Center Utilization

Identifying who is utilizing the center globally is important to determine capacity, staffing requirements, learners, and so forth. The case studies discussed below will explore how comparing the center year to year provides insight into various key variables. This information can be presented in annual reports, to funders (such as administration, donors, etc.). It can also help in identifying capacity and when new staffing is necessary to increase courses or activities. There may also be a system in place whereby programs or departments are allowed a certain amount of time or percentage use of the center. Having this data can assist in arbitrating those discussions and allocations.

CASE STUDY: Annual Report Data

WISER (wiser.pitt.edu) identifies six key metrics for their annual report. These metrics also provide a means of assessing the success of their program (Table 1.3.3).

TABLE 1.3.3

WISER Annual Report Metrics

Academic Year Ending	2005	2006	2007	2008	2009	2010	2011	2012
Number of classes	1,002	1,159	1,329	1,307	1,369	1,366	1,357	1,317
Educational encounters	7,928	9,537	11,079	11,997	10,938	11,542	11,168	12,362
Unique learners	2,082	2,706	3,307	3,383	3,590	3,112	3,519	3,260
Facilitators	143	164	222	270	250	261	312	314
Learner hours	33,059	39,539	46,021	47,845	41,461	42,363	43,906	51,083
Room hours	9,017	11,480	13,225	14,136	13,947	14,223	12,556	13,770

Trends, from the 2005 to 2012 academic years (July to June), from these numbers include the following:
- Number of classes increased by 31%.
- **Educational encounters** increased by 56%.
- Unique learners increased by 57%.
- The number of facilitators increased by 120%.
- Learner hours increased by 55%.
- Room hours increased by 53% (Box 1.3.2).

BOX 1.3.2

CALCULATING THE PERCENT CHANGE (ROOMS, PARTICIPANTS, EXERCISES, ETC.)

% Change—Subtract the old value from the new value, then divide the result by the old value. That will show as a percentage.
Step 1: Calculate the change (subtract old value from the new value).
Step 2: Divide that change by the old value (results in a decimal number).

Step 3: Convert that to a percentage (by multiplying by 1,000 and adding a % sign).
Note: if the new value is greater than the old value, it is a percentage increase, otherwise it is a decrease.
The Formula: [(New Value − Old Value)/Old Value] × 100%

These trends identified the following issues for WISER to address:
- Room hours increased more than the number of classes. Does this mean classes are taking more space, or are they are running longer?
- There are significantly more instructors teaching at WISER per class. Is this good?
- Room hours are increasing. If there is not a significant increase in the average number of classes that each student is taking, are there more rooms being used per class?

CASE STUDY: Tracking Model

The SimPORTAL (www.simportal.umn.edu) supports training for third-year medical students and beyond. The SimPORTAL primarily focuses on the perioperative surgical subspecialities, including all surgical domains, anesthesia, critical care, emergency medicine, and trauma, as well as image-guided and microvascular skills.

The SimPORTAL created a tracking model to analyze learners as well as utilization of equipment and supplies in the center. Details are listed below. Some of the data collected included medical devices (anesthesia gas machine, syringe pumps, warmers, etc.), instruments, disposables, simulator use, room use, repair/downtime, orientation to simulators, **tours, meetings,** conferences, and personnel.

To date, 100% of funding comes from the medical school. This made sense at the inception of the new center, but as more hospital staff began to be trained, the time has come to revisit the funding model and explore sustainability options.

Data was captured and analyzed surrounding the following domains:
1. Services
   a. Facility use
   b. Mannequins, virtual reality (VR) simulators, costly task trainers
   c. Less expensive task trainers
   d. Disposables
   e. Testing—OSATS/OSCE
   f. Video services—recording, editing, 3D video, streaming
   g. Software/hardware creation
2. Operations
   a. Administrative operations
      - General
      - Scheduling
      - Depreciation of office equipment
      - Meetings/planning
   b. Technical operations
      - Medical devices
      - Simulators
      - Computers/audio visual (AV)
   c. Design operations
      - Simulator design and development
   d. Grants/travel/publications

Tracking gave SimPORTAL the ability to project the monetary utilization by each domain, and further analysis determined domains that were the highest consumers of financial resources. Analysis of time was not included during the development phase of tracking, owing to the unbalanced allocation of resources on complex templates, one-time occurrence workshops, and research data collection. Personnel were not included in these calculations, because the salary of a technician was defined for the entire year, and spread across all activities equally. Space charge is also a constant rate determined by the University. These numbers were used to establish Independent Service Organization (ISO) rates. These rates include time, personnel, and space as staples of the charges. The unknown cost categories below are representative of unknown flexible expenses that were used to establish *a la carte* rates for these domains. After 1 year of tracking, the percentage cost of each category relative to the sum of all categories is shown (Table 1.3.4).

On the basis of these percentages and usage of the program, a funding model can be built. Begin by collecting metrics around use of the center (by course and department), associated costs with each course and each learner—MS1 through PP+ year (practicing physician). This funding model resulted in a percentage "tree" for allocation of resources.

Below is the proposed funding tree model:

- Courses required to fulfill medical school requirements—100% funded by medical school (trunk).
- Courses to fulfill residency requirements *and* are multidisciplinary—75% funded by medical school (large branch).
- Courses that either fulfill residency requirements *or* are multidisciplinary—50% funded by medical school (medium branch).
- Courses that are not required but are multidisciplinary—25% funded by medical school (small branch).
- Courses that are not required and not multidisciplinary—No funding from the medical school.

The SimPORTAL team is in the process of evaluating the fairness of the model, implementation strategies, and vote by their Advisory Board.

TABLE 1.3.4

Allocation of Resources

Facility/general	35.24%
Mannequins	26.57%
Task trainers	4.93%
Disposables	3.41%
A/V—computers	6.68%
Design/development	3.21%
Travel and publications	5.42%
Depreciation	14.54%
TOTAL	100.00%

Data Collection for Research, Grants, Quality Improvement, and Safe Patient Care

Often, data collection is required for research, but it is being used more and more to determine whether an activity can demonstrate quality improvement and safe patient care. It has been well documented that practicing skills and techniques can lead to proficiency and ultimately improved patient care. The simulation center has a key role in deliberate practice (or skill acquisition), as described by Dutta and Proctor (1992).

Also, if data collection is part of a research study and/or grants, data requirements are even more stringent. Data collection and metrics required for research and grant work involves congregating evidence that allows for analyzing the information that will best answer the proposed questions. This data must be honest, accurate, consistent, and repeatable.

There are many consequences to poor or inaccurately collected data. Repeatability, distortion in findings, misleading, and compromising the decisions that result from this data can negatively impact the nature of the research. Therefore, asking the right questions and accurately collecting and reporting the data is crucial.

The case presented below looks at how a central line simulation program can improve patient care and reduces associated costs due to central lines. Much like a research project, specific data must be collected to get the true cost and true outcome.

CASE STUDY: Central Venous Catheter Implementation

The primary goal of the Institute for Simulation and Interprofessional Studies (ISIS) (isis.washington.edu) at the University of Washington (UW) is to provide leadership in the use of simulation technologies to improve the quality of healthcare education and improve patient safety and outcomes (Figure 1.3.1). In 2008, the Center for Medicare and Medicaid Services (CMS) declared that it will no longer pay for care related to central line–associated bloodstream infections (CLABSIs). The average cost of care for a CLABSI is around $45,000. This change in reimbursement got the attention of the UW Medicine leadership. As described by Figueredo et al. (2012), a team of content experts were formed to gather information and devise a plan on how to reduce the rate of catheter-related complications. An internal review revealed variation in care due to several issues, including (1) lack of compliance with maximal barrier precautions, (2) lack of training in ultrasound-guided placement, and (3) lack of standard technique and equipment.

After much discussion between specialties on standardized education and training for central line placement, it became clear that simulation would add value to this training. UW Medicine system committed to change the culture

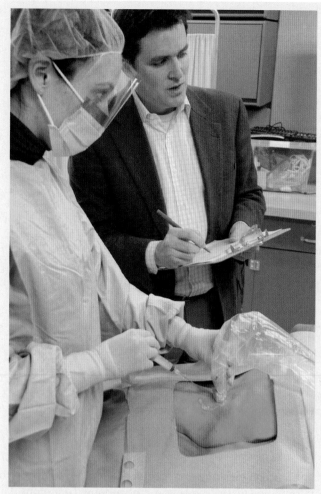

FIGURE 1.3.1 Faculty member using the standardized CVC checklist for completion of the simulation-based education.

and practice through an approach of intensive simulation-based education combined with a system-wide quality improvement process. The education components included the following:

1. Complete the CVC e-Learning Module
2. Simulation testing on Central Line Man Simulator (http://www.simulab.com)
3. Supervised line placement on patients documented

ISIS then considered what data points/information would need to be collected on the basis of the activities that required the following resources:

- Space and time: one room, 8:00–4:30, one learner, 30 minutes for training, setup, and takedown.
- Center staffing and supplies: CVC kit, task trainer, ultrasound machine, disposables, and one technician.

The data points chosen for collection by ISIS include the following:

- Room usage, learner hours, staff time (including setup and takedown), supply costs, cost/learner, pass/fail rate.

Initially, most of the data collection done was around completion of the training and infection rates/patient outcomes. The data was compelling, with an improved compliance with documentation from 0% in January 2008 to nearly 100% at the time of the study. The rate of CLABSI progressively declined, and since 2008 the rate is consistently below 0.9 CLABSI/1,000 catheter-days. Additionally, it was estimated that 25 central line–related complications were prevented, saving $30,000 per complication for a total savings of $1,050,000 annually. This certainly provides strong support for such a program.

Analyzing the cost of the program was equally important. Analysis followed to document the cost of the training program (both development and implementation). Some points to consider when developing and/or implementing any program are as follows:

- Development of training modules/curriculum. If unable to use existing curriculum or need to customize a curriculum, the cost of that development must be considered. Both content experts and technologist/developer should be included.
- Maintenance and updating of modules curriculum, taking into account, again, the time of both the content experts and the technologist/developer.
- Supplies, materials, and equipment are a bit easier to retrospectively include, but it is always useful to collect them from the onset. One may want to look at the retail cost of such supplies and equipment to get the "real" cost for future reference. Often, a center is able to reuse, get donated, damaged, or other materials or supplies that do not have a cost associated at that time. However, if the true cost of the program is to be recognized, the retail costs of the materials should be calculated. In this example, because ISIS is able to reuse simulated tissue and use outdated and donated CVC kits, the real costs are estimated to be $66.48 per person, but the actual costs are $22.48 per person.

CASE STUDY: Personnel Justification Based on Equipment Use and Repair

Simulator purchase, use, and repair rank high as a costly item for SimPORTAL's expenditures, second only to personnel. The justification for a $150,000 simulator goes all the way to the Regents of the University of Minnesota. The justification for a new employee goes only as far as the local Human Resources department.

As simulators advance in capabilities, and increase in operation costs, one needs to determine at what point to hire a technician to maintain the simulators versus purchase the extended warranty for each. SimPORTAL reviewed the out of warranty (OOW) costs, and it was noted that the purchase of an extended warranty for these simulators did not always increase their ability to perform. The following categories were tracked: computer software, simulator hardware, computer hardware, connectivity, simulator software, medical device, scenario, fluids, battery, and disposables as items that affected the use and acceptability of simulators as teaching tools. These items were captured by incident reports and by customer satisfaction surveys. A Pareto chart to evaluate these findings given frequency and cost issues was explored (see Figure 1.3.2).

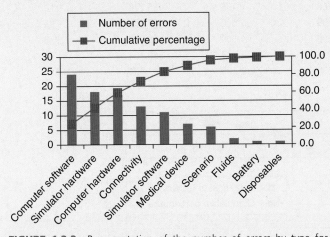

FIGURE 1.3.2 Representation of the number of errors by type for simulators.

Evaluation of the costs of OOW errors indicated that simulator hardware made up over 80% of the costs. Furthermore, the number of errors (24) was higher for simulator hardware, as well as the cost per error ($2,935.00) (Figure 1.3.3).

The next step is to compare the actual manufacturer warranty costs. This is illustrated in Table 1.3.5, and was accurate at the time of analysis. Note that these costs are not a current reflection of the manufacturers' warranty costs and coverage timelines.

Evaluation of the percentage of manufacturer warranty costs that each simulator contributes is displayed in Figure 1.3.4. As one might assume, these are in line with the specific fidelity and capabilities of the simulators. The more complex the model, the more it costs to operate and maintain.

The total cost for SimPORTAL (with the Center's specific use) was simulator "errors" ($112,015) and warranty

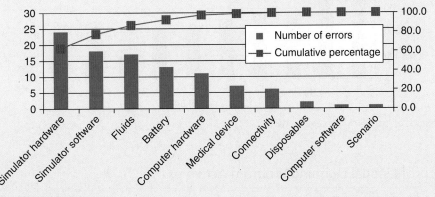

FIGURE 1.3.3 Error costs of OOW repairs.

cost ($61,304), totalling $173,319. This does not include the business loss estimates relative to simulators' downtime for repair, and does not include customer satisfaction survey data indicating a use of lower-fidelity simulators to get the job done due to reliability issues.

In conclusion, the costs for warranty issues were $173,319. The cost for a technician at SimPORTAL is approximately $75,000 per year, including fringe and benefits. By hiring a technician, the Center was able to increase customer satisfaction, spent less time on simulator repair, and there was less simulator downtime.

TABLE 1.3.5

Manufacturer Warranty Costs

Simulator/ Equipment	Warranty Cost—Total ($)	No. of Years— Warranty	Cost per Year ($)	Total Cost of Repairs per Year ($)	Cumulative Costs ($)	Cumulative %
A	16,958	2	8,479	16,958	16,958	27.6
B	32,995	5	6,599	13,198	30,156	49.1
C	117	1	117	5,850	36,006	58.7
D	13,995	5	2,799	5,598	41,604	67.8
E	7,500	3	2,500	5,000	46,604	76
F	4,500	1	4,500	4,500	51,104	83.3
G	12,500	3	4,166	4,166	55,270	90.1
H	6,000	3	2,000	2,000	57,270	93.4
I	1,500	1	1,500	1,500	58,770	95.8
J	4,000	3	1,333	1,333	60,104	98
K	1,200	1	1,200	1,200	61,304	100

FIGURE 1.3.4   Percentage of manufacturer warranty costs.

CASE STUDY: Interprofessional Learning Program Activities

The Vanderbilt Program in Interprofessional Learning (VPIL) (https://medschool.vanderbilt.edu/vpil/) was created as a collaboration between the Vanderbilt University Schools of Medicine and Nursing, Belmont University College of Pharmacy, Lipscomb University College of Pharmacy, and Tennessee State University Master of Social Work Program. As a part of VPIL, performance-based formative assessment experiences were created using SPs from the Program in Human Simulation of the Center for Experiential Learning and Assessment (CELA). As the plan has been developed, student teams from each profession work in groups of four at CELA, to interview an SP. During a session at CELA, every student in each team takes a turn interviewing the SP (10 minutes), who presents with multiple medical issues, as well as social issues surrounding the illnesses. The learner gathers information appropriate to their respective discipline, and then the SP sees the next student in the interprofessional team. During their downtime, post interview, each student writes up their finding and recommendations using one of the conference rooms in CELA. When the entire team has interviewed the patient, the team discusses their impressions and comes up with a collective plan for the SP. Then the SP returns to the full team, and they present their care plan (30 minutes). Their faculty observes both the individual and team interactions with the SP and provides feedback after the session. There are typically 10 to 12 interprofessional teams in VPIL each year. Each team visits CELA on three occasions (September, December, and April) and interviews the same SP to construct a longitudinal experience for the interprofessional teams.

There are several perspectives from which to count the center utilization. The first perspective might be that of the VPIL program that is the primary responsible party in these exercises. What is an encounter or a session? As has been emphasized, commonly agreed-upon terms are critical for a shared language and equivalent comparisons. How are sessions or encounters counted (definitions may differ between the SP program perspectives vs. the technical simulation perspective)? Another perspective might be from the individual schools that send their respective students and faculty as mentors to this exercise. These statistics could be useful in supporting the program within the school administration. These statistics likely need to reflect aggregated individual metrics for each program. And of course, from a simple utilization perspective for CELA, statistics that reflect the overall staff effort, room use, and direct costs are necessary aspects of annual reports and center justification.

Center Utilization as It Relates to Staffing Requirement

The activities and offerings of the center will drive the staffing requirements. Technology-heavy centers require more technically savvy staff, while teaching-heavy centers would benefit from an educator focus. The "CASE STUDY: Personnel Justification Based on Equipment Use and Repair" focuses on justifying a technician to offset the cost of expensive equipment. Knowing your maintenance fees, equipment downtime, and other specifics of running your activities can help justify your decisions.

Assessing Interprofessional Education Program Activities

The challenges with room and learner population programs having multiple learners are often challenging to capture metrics. Not only the room usage issues and how they are allocated, but also the individual learners and how they are logged and analyzed are challenging. The CASE STUDY: Interprofessional Learning Program Activities explores the complexity of the interprofessional education (IPE) activity.

DATA ANALYSIS: SPREADSHEETS AND PIVOT TABLES

Spreadsheets that feature the capability to have pivot tables (Microsoft Excel and Google Spreadsheet) provide the ability to quickly enter basic data in column format and derive complex reports in tabular format to make trends and anomalies readily apparent.

A basic example follows: Start by entering class data into specific columns in the spreadsheet: date, start time, end time, course name, number of learners, number of rooms used, and number of simulators used (Table 1.3.6). Then, formulas can be created to automatically calculate various metrics on the basis of the simple data that was filled in above. For example, the end time can be subtracted from the start time to get the class time. Multiplying this by the number of rooms will calculate the room hours for that particular class. This can be used for utilization calculations.

CALCULATIONS

Class time = end time − start time

Room hours = class time × number of rooms

TABLE 1.3.6

Excel Basic Table Example

Date	Start Time	End Time	COURSE Name	No of Participants	No of Rooms	No of Simulator Type
09/01/11	9:00	11:00	4TH YR EM	9	1	1
09/01/11	13:30	15:30	CCM FELL ORIENT	2	2	1
09/01/11	8:00	17:00	CEM Paramedic Lab	50	6	5
09/01/11	7:30	12:30	CTT	9	2	2
09/01/11	13:00	15:00	Patient Management EM Res	2	1	1
09/02/11	8:00	11:00	3RD YR CCM	14	1	1
09/02/11	11:00	13:00	4TH YR CCM	8	1	1
09/02/11	13:00	17:00	DAM ANES RES	4	3	2
09/02/11	17:30	19:00	Med Anatomy MS1: US	3	2	1
09/06/11	11:00	13:00	4TH YR CCM	8	1	1
09/06/11	9:00	11:00	4TH YR EM	9	2	2
09/06/11	12:00	14:00	ACLS HC	1	1	1
09/06/11	13:00	15:30	ANES CLERK DAY 3-EMR SURG	9	3	3

TABLE 1.3.7

Excel Basic Table Example with Automatic Fill-Ins

Date	Start Time	End Time	COURSE Name	No of Participants	No of Rooms	No of Simulator Type	Department	Room Hours	Participant Hours	Month	Year	Academic Year
01/02/13	7:30	9:00	ANES ELECT A/W GET	3	1	1	SOM	1.5	4.5	Jan-13	2013	FY13
01/02/13	10:00	12:00	ANES CLERK DAY 1-A/W GET	7	2	1	SOM	4	14	Jan-13	2013	FY13
01/02/13	10:00	11:30	Peds CA2 CHP	10	1	1	PEDS	1.5	15	Jan-13	2013	FY13
01/02/13	11:00	12:30	Peds CA2 CHP	4	1	1	PEDS	1.5	6	Jan-13	2013	FY13
01/02/13	11:00	13:00	4TH YR CCM	12	1	1	SOM	2	24	Jan-13	2013	FY13
01/02/13	14:00	17:00	RAUL	3	2	1	Anesthesia	6	9	Jan-13	2013	FY13
01/03/13	8:00	12:00	ALT	2	2	1	Anesthesia	8	8	Jan-13	2013	FY13
01/03/13	9:00	11:00	4TH YR EM	5	1	1	SOM	2	10	Jan-13	2013	FY13
01/03/13	11:00	13:00	4TH YR CCM	12	1	1	SOM	2	24	Jan-13	2013	FY13
01/04/13	8:00	11:00	3RD YR CCM	13	1	1	SOM	3	39	Jan-13	2013	FY13
01/04/13	11:00	13:00	4TH YR CCM	12	1	1	SOM	2	24	Jan-13	2013	FY13
01/04/13	13:00	15:30	ANES CLERK DAY 2-IND GET	7	1	1	SOM	2.5	17.5	Jan-13	2013	FY13
01/07/13	8:00	13:00	ERT - MKS	3	2	1	Health System	10	15	Jan-13	2013	FY13

Spreadsheets can use lookup functionality to automatically populate cells on the basis of the data that was entered into other cells. If date entry is consistent (using the worksheets data validation feature, for instance), cells can be automatically filled with useful information. In the example above, by consistently naming courses, data can be entered specific to the type of activity or responsible departments (Table 1.3.7).

Pivot tables take data that is in the columns and combine them, by, for example, summing the data, into tabular format. The rows and columns of the pivot table are defined by selecting the two (or more) columns of data. A third column of data populates the data fields themselves. Note that the original data set could be thousands of rows long, but is expressed into a simple 4 × 4 table (Table 1.3.8).

For the interested simulation program manager, pivot tables allow for fairly sophisticated reports using the simple data collected above. For example, total room hours can be shown, grouped by department, for whatever month range has been specified. Totals can be generated for both rows and columns (Table 1.3.9).

TABLE 1.3.8

Pivot Table Example

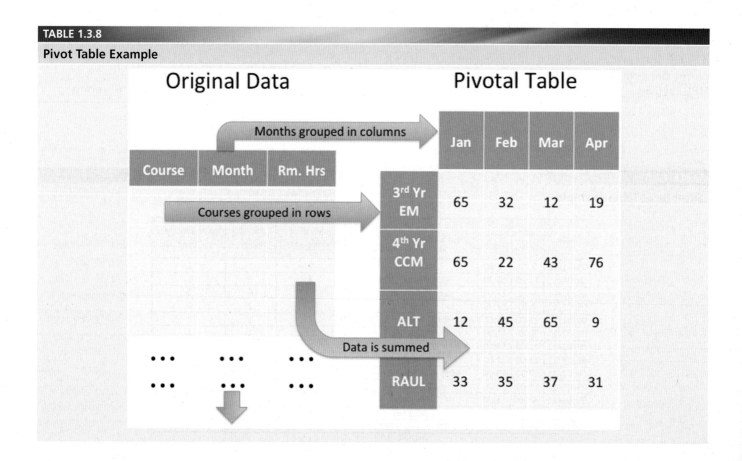

TABLE 1.3.9

Pivot Table Example

Sum of Room Hours	Column Labels			
Row Labels	Jan-13	Feb-13	Mar-13	Grand Total
▼ Anesthesia	18	122	272	412
ALT	8	8	8	24
RAUL	6	6	2	14
FOB ANES RES	4	24	12	40
MOCA		60	75	135
DAM ANES CRNA		24	168	192
ACLS ANES RES			5	5
RSCH ANES Project			2	2
▶ CCM		9.5		9.5
▶ Health System	92.5	108.5	104.5	305.5
▶ EM	21	88.5	31	140.5
▶ PEDS	17.5	63.5	50.5	131.5
▶ SOM	238	432	180.5	850.5

Pivot tables allow for quick creation of reports on a wide variety of metrics given a fairly straightforward set of data. For example, with three clicks of the mouse, the report above can be changed to tabulate the number of students by course by department.

BEEN THERE, DONE THAT: HOW CAN I CONTINUE TO IMPROVE OR SUSTAIN WHAT I HAVE ACHIEVED?

Other Data Capture Options: Why Databases Are Good

While spreadsheets provide a quick and easy way to record activities at your simulation program, they have limitations in terms of accurately depicting those activities.

In the previous example(s) using spreadsheets, all activity for a given class was represented on one row of the spreadsheet. This would be fine if all the collected metrics could be reduced to a single number, but this is often not the case. For example, what if, instead of simply the number of students in the class, a list of student names is desired? There is no easy way for a spreadsheet to represent this. This is where a database would be more effective.

Databases in this sense usually refer to relational databases. This means that the items in the database relate to each other on the basis of the relationships that they represent in the real world. These relationships can be on a one-to-one basis or a one-to-many basis, or many-to-many basis. For example, each class has a one-to-one relationship with the length of the class in hours. There is a one-to-many relationship with the names of each of the students (Figure 1.3.5).

The ability to have one-to-one and one-to-many relationships allows databases to accurately model the real world. While the ability to accurately model what happens in real life is a definite plus, it does not come without a

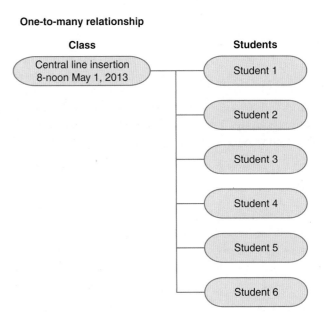

FIGURE 1.3.5 One-to-one and one-to-many relationships database example.

price. Databases are significantly harder to set up, maintain, and enter data into than simple spreadsheets. First, tables need to be created by the database that will group together similar data (e.g., classes, student names, rooms) and then specify the relationships between those datasets. Then an interface to input data needs to be built. There are a number of databases that could be used. Databases that can be used with standard desktop computers include Microsoft Access (PC) and FileMaker (Mac). Enterprise-level databases that require more computational horsepower, setup, and maintenance include Microsoft SQL Server, Oracle, and MySQL.

In the end, a decision needs to be made as to whether the extra cost (both in financial and human resource terms) is worthwhile to the needs of the program. The authors recommend starting with a spreadsheet to understand its benefits and limitations, and then moving toward a database solution as a more sophisticated understanding and needs are developed.

SUMMARY

Data metrics have various components, and the requirements vary for each center. It cannot be stressed enough how important the collection of metrics is. Hopefully, the examples provided will pique interest and inspire programs to collect and analyze data. Simulation programs should always strive to "do it right versus doing it over";

however, in the rush to ramp up a simulation center, get activities booked, and entice faculty to enter the world of simulation, programs often forget to collect data that are useful for demonstrating and justifying resources necessary for future work. Having and using a common taxonomy so you are being able to articulate and compare data with others is key.

Programs that are just starting out and have limited time to collect data may begin by logging courses, start and end time, and number of rooms. For programs developing or revising a business plan, it may be helpful to gather the stakeholders to determine what information is and will be important to them; a good brainstorming session is always helpful. It is also vital to think about what will be necessary to justify resources (e.g., staff, space, faculty) in the future. As long as a record of the information

is kept somewhere, even if it is handwritten to start, programs are able to at least retrieve and work backward (although this is not recommended). One of the key elements in making the analysis easier is developing a common language for courses—as demonstrated by the case studies provided in this chapter. In the words of Peter F. Drucker, "What's measured improves."

REFERENCES

Dutta, A., & Proctor, R. W. (1992). Persistence of stimulus-response compatibility effects with extended practice. *Journal of Experimental Psychology: Learning, Memory, and Cognition, 18*(4), 801–809.

Figueredo, E. J., Sinanan, M. N., Makarewicz, V., Kim, S., & Wright, A. S. (2012). Improving patient safety and reducing hospital costs: The University of Washington Central Venous Catheter Project. *MedSim Magazine,* (4), 14–18.

CHAPTER 1.4

Development of the SSH Certified Healthcare Simulation Educator Program: Design of a Valid, Defensible, and Cost-Effective Program

Cate F. Nicholas, EdD, MS, PA, Andrew E. Spain, MA, NCEE, EMT-P, Connie M. Lopez, MSN, CNS, RNC-OB, CPHRM, and Katie Walker, RN, MBA

> Professional accountability requires a self-regulating profession to set and maintain credible, useful standards for its members. Voluntary certification and recertification—evaluation by peers—serves the responsibility of the profession to establish and enforce its own standards.
>
> —*Benson (1991)*

ABOUT THE AUTHORS

CATE F. NICHOLAS, Director of Simulation Education at FAHC/University of Vermont Clinical Simulation Laboratory, sits on the Society for Simulation in Healthcare (SSH) Certification Committee and is an SSH Accreditation Site Reviewer. She is Chair of Grants and Research for the Association of Standardized Patient Educators (ASPE) and 2011 ASPE Outstanding Educator of the Year. She is associate editor of Standardized Patient cases for MedEd Portal and sits on the Editorial Board for the International Nursing Association for Simulation and Clinical Learning (INASCL) Journal.

ANDREW E. SPAIN is the Director of Accreditation and Certification with the Society for Simulation in Healthcare and has been with SSH for over 3 years. He has a clinical background as a Paramedic for over 20 years, and is currently a PhD student at the University of Missouri in Education, with an emphasis in Educational Leadership and Policy Analysis.

CONNIE M. LOPEZ leads Kaiser Permanente's National Risk Education and Healthcare Simulation Programs. Ms. Lopez has 10 years' experience researching and implementing simulation in the clinical setting, and has focused her in situ simulations on improving teamwork and communication of practicing clinicians. Connie has been asked to present simulation-related topics nationally and internationally over the past 7 years. Connie is a member of the SSH Certification Committee and Co-Chair for the 2014 International Meeting on Simulation in Healthcare (IMSH) and National Patient Safety Foundation (NPSF) conferences.

KATIE WALKER is the Director of the New York Health and Hospital's Corporation Simulation Program. Prior to this appointment in December 2011, she was the Program Manager of a national simulation program being established in Australia through the peak Government agency, Health Workforce Australia. She has Co-Chaired the 2010 IMSH in Phoenix, Arizona, and the first Asia-Pacific meeting on Simulation in Healthcare in Hong Kong in May 2011.

ABSTRACT

Certification in healthcare simulation is an important component in ensuring professional development and verification of knowledge, skills, and abilities. This chapter discusses the origination, development, rigor, and collaborative nature of the certifications that have been or are being developed for healthcare simulation by the Society for Simulation in Healthcare (SSH), and the simulation community as a whole. Through this collaboration, and in partnership with industry experts, the certifications for healthcare simulation educators can be seen to have the rigorous process and standards necessary to demonstrate their value and validity, and to support the healthcare simulation industry educators and operations specialists.

CASE EXAMPLE

The budget deadline is coming up, and part of your plan for this year includes certification for your educators and **operations specialists**. While this is a small part of your budget, you know that the money gurus are going to challenge you on this as well as all parts of your budget. You sit back, reflecting on how to make the argument for certification. You instinctively know that certification is a good idea for your staff, and you want to support this part of their professional development. How do you demonstrate the value of the certifications they will achieve, and show how this will improve your simulation program?

INTRODUCTION AND BACKGROUND

The role of the Healthcare Simulation Educator has emerged as a new role within the healthcare simulation profession. But with over 100 definitions of simulation, and as many paths to becoming a simulation education expert, how is the Healthcare Simulation Educator defined? The Society for Simulation in Healthcare (SSH) recognized a need to establish a level of standards and core competencies and has developed a process for providing a globally recognized certification program for healthcare simulation educators. The goal of the SSH Certification Program is to enhance healthcare education and have a positive impact on patient safety by recognizing, developing, and promoting excellence in the role of the Healthcare Simulation Educator. As defined by SSH, an individual who has become certified has the knowledge, skills, behaviors, and accomplishments needed to create, deliver, and evaluate effective healthcare simulation experiences. It validates and provides a formal professional recognition essential for educators in the field, and adds value to not only the individual but also their organization and the community by regulating the providers of healthcare simulation education and thereby promoting best practices. What began as a committee agenda item in 2006 ended with the development and successful launch of the SSH Healthcare Simulation Educator Certification Program in 2012 and 235 new certified healthcare simulation educators (CHSEs) in 2013. The process of designing a valid, defensible, and cost-effective program for Healthcare Simulation Educator certification has been completed, but the story is still unfolding.

BENEFITS OF THE SSH CERTIFICATION PROGRAM

The SSH was established in January 2004, to lead in facilitating excellence in (multispecialty) healthcare education, practice, and research through simulation modalities. The Society is made up of educators, researchers, technicians, clinicians, and administrators who see the benefit from using an array of simulation techniques in a variety of settings with learners across the continuum of healthcare education. Proponents of simulation see its potential to improve individual and team performance with the ultimate goal of improving clinical outcomes and patient safety.

In addition to other goals, SSH was created to (SSH, n.d.):

- Develop and foster standards for simulation education and applications that affect healthcare practices.
- Stimulate and promote the professional development of those individuals and institutions interested in simulation modalities and their applications.
- Partner with professional societies having common goals for the benefit of patient safety and the Society.
- Provide for continuing professional development of individuals who serve the patient through simulation-based education, research, and development.

Over the years, the simulation educators and researchers began to take on more important roles within healthcare education. Most healthcare simulation educators learned on the job, through taking courses or through apprenticeship models. With no formal educational path for these individuals, the development of a certification program was a way to provide a benchmark for simulation educators to meet to demonstrate that they had acquired the requisite knowledge and experience for the expanding roles in the field. In addition, certification would demonstrate their potential to contribute toward assuring the quality of the simulation educational experiences and promote the professional development of the educators.

SSH took on the task of developing a certification process for educators focused on simulation in healthcare. Consistent with its mission and goals, SSH's Certification Program was developed with inputs from other international simulation societies, healthcare organizations, and individuals representing a wide variety of disciplines, professions, simulation modalities, and experience in healthcare simulation.

From its inception, the benefits of SSH's Certification Program to the profession, the public, and the individual were identified as:

- Meeting the needs of employers, practitioners, and the public by identifying educators with specialized knowledge and skills in healthcare simulation education.
- Strengthening organizational, community, and learner confidence in the quality of education.
- Providing formal professional recognition of specialized knowledge, skills, abilities (KSAs), and accomplishments in simulation education.
- Encouraging performance improvement and knowledge expansion of the individual educator.
- Assuring a commitment to continued professional development and lifelong learning.

REACHING OUT TO THE STAKEHOLDERS AND TARGET AUDIENCES

Working with both stakeholders (those individuals who have a vested interest in ensuring that the standards are set appropriately and the results are reliable) and the target audience (those who have an interest in being certified) was deemed equally important. At the start of the process, a commitment was made to work collaboratively with international and national simulation societies, and leaders in the field to further understand the needs and hear the opinions of educators who would be seeking certification.

Stakeholders

Discussion within SSH began with the Board of Directors, followed by the Education Committee, and ultimately the Committee on Certification, Accreditation and Technology (CATS). In 2008, a Subcommittee on Certification was formed within CATS, and invited members from international and national simulation societies (see Table 1.4.1) and thought leaders in simulation to participate. These members and leaders were selected to ensure that as many simulation modalities and disciplines were represented as possible to be inclusive of the breadth of healthcare simulation. In 2009, the Certification Committee was established. The committee was charged with establishing a certification program for simulation educators focused on this mission statement: "*The SSH Simulation Certification Educator Program is to promote and recognize excellence in the specialty role of Healthcare Simulation Educator, advancing the*

TABLE 1.4.1

Simulation Society Abbreviations

ASPE: Association of Standardized Patient Educators

ASSH: The Australian Society for Simulation in Health Care

INACSL: International Nursing Association for Clinical Simulation and Learning, London Deanery

NLN: National League of Nursing

SESAM: Society in Europe for Simulation Applied To Medicine

EXPERT'S CORNER

FACULTY DEVELOPMENT

Ignacio del Moral, MD, PhD
Founder and First President Elect of the Spanish Society for Simulation in Healthcare

Bertha is a cardiologist who loves simulation and wants to become a simulation instructor. She became involved with simulation observing a program designed to train a cardiovascular team to become a cardiac transplantation high-performance team. Debriefing her experience after the program, she was confused. She thought it was going to be different, more teaching-oriented, less interactive, and more planned. Her initial reaction was to abandon her idea of being an instructor because of how different it was from her routine job as a cardiologist.

Healthcare and allied health professionals face a challenge once we enter into simulation-based education (SBE). We have been trained for years to take care of patients. Over time, we have developed the knowledge, skills, and attitudes to deliver of care in a variety of situations, from routine to high-stakes ones. When we run an SBE program, we are no longer clinicians taking care of patients; we are educators designing learning experiences to facilitate learning and support change. Traditionally, it has been assumed that an expert clinician is automatically an expert teacher. However, effective teaching requires a new set of knowledge, skills, and attitudes that come from disciplines outside of healthcare: education, pedagogy, psychology, and organizational behavior domains. Working with professionals from these

domains will foster our programs and ultimately enrich our working environment.

In my experience, the best investment that can be made in a simulation endeavor is the investment in educator training. It requires considerable motivation, investment of time, effort, and resources to deeply understand the foundations and theories of adult learning, and to identify and apply best practices in order to improve the quality of education.

Becoming an educator demands mentorship to advance in the field. Eventually, with practice and reflection, excellent healthcare professionals can become excellent healthcare educators. Having excellent educators makes a difference in each program and for each participant.

Because we are in simulation to make a difference, we should invest the resources needed to become well-qualified educators; it is a fascinating path that will change our mental models as nurses or physicians. Furthermore, simulation is a very contemporary methodology in education. There is a considerable amount of evidence of what works and what should be different. But that's not enough. There are new areas to explore, new methods to try, and ideas to research.

The faculty development process is a never-ending process as it is for healthcare. The more we learn, the more we realize we have to practice.

field of simulation and improving patient safety." A decision was made to work within the framework laid out by the National Commission for Certifying Agencies (NCCA) with the goal of becoming an accredited certification program in the future.

Thought leaders from the Association of Standardized Patient Educators (ASPE), Australian Society for Simulation in Healthcare (ASSH), International Nursing Association for Clinical Simulation and Learning (INASCL), the London Deanery, National League for Nursing (NLN), Society in Europe for Simulation Applied to Medicine (SESAM), and other subject matter experts (SMEs) spanning the full spectrum of simulation modalities joined the committee in London for a face-to-face meeting to discuss two key questions:

1. What knowledge, skills, and attitudes would a CHSE possess?
2. What are the standards that a certified simulation educator would need to meet?

The goal was to develop a set of competencies in specific domains in terms of knowledge, skills, and behaviors. The simulation educator would be assessed against these standards to demonstrate competency.

This meeting resulted in the first draft of standards that would be used as a development tool in the certification process. Table 1.4.2 displays the final version of the standards that were adopted.

Target Audience

The target audience of the CHSE Program consists of professionals from various disciplines; however, they are all required to have the same set of knowledge, skills, and behaviors in certain areas (SSH, n.d.). Once the standards were drafted, they were presented and vetted at several different venues to potential target audiences.

TABLE 1.4.2

Standards: Final Version

Standard	Measurement Criteria
Knowledge	Simulation
	Education
Skills	Debriefing
	Simulation
	Education
	Course design
Environment	Technology
	Resources
Assessment	Self
	Students
Communication	Supervisors
	Students
	Organizations
	Society

TABLE 1.4.3

Demographics

Field	%	Instructor Skills Level	%	Interest in Certification	%
Nursing	39	Advanced	34	Yes	73
Medical	25	Beginner	23	No	10
Administration	18	Novice	3	Not sure	17
Biomedical	14				

TABLE 1.4.4

Method of Training

Method	%
Self-taught	54
Coursework	35
Apprenticeship-trained	12

The first was at the 2010 International Meeting for Simulation in Healthcare (IMSH) during a town hall–style meeting. The demographics of this group are presented in Table 1.4.3.

The standards document was sent to the leadership of SSH, ASPE, ASSH, INACSL, the London Deanery, NLN, and SESAM for their membership to review along with other subject matter and provide feedback to the committee. This pattern of program development with stakeholders and then feedback from the target audience would become the standard operating procedure for the committee.

The demographics obtained from the IMSH town hall meeting in 2010 were from a small cross section of the simulation community. Later, the committee sent out a Simulation Educator Demographic and Needs Assessment Survey to the membership of ASPE, ASSH, INACSL, NLN, SESAM, and SSH. Approximately 9,000 surveys were sent out, with a 51% return rate. Seventy-one percent of respondents indicated they would be interested in applying for certification. The question asking the respondents to indicate how they were trained to become simulation educators further supported the need for a certification exam (see Table 1.4.4).

PROGRAM ELEMENTS

Once there was agreement to proceed with the development of the CHSE Program from stakeholders in the professional societies, educational institutions, and thought leaders in the field, the next step was to develop the specific elements of the program. Some members of the target audiences also indicated an interest in becoming certified, which was encouraging for the developers. Typical elements required for certification fall into the following categories:

- Education, training, or development: what kind, for how long?
- Tests: what kind; what knowledge, skills, and or attitudes should be assessed? Who should administer them, how often, and who will score them? What criteria will be used?
- Experience: how much? For how long and how recently should it be? What type and under what circumstances?
- Work samples: should they be required? What format? Who will review them?
- Endorsement: who will endorse? What will they endorse?
- Fees: what will the charges be for the certification process?

Heuristic issues then arose regarding what combination of the six elements above would serve the purpose of the SSH Certification Program. The SSH Board of Directors, in reviewing the workload that would ensue for this program, suggested to SSH staff that it might be beneficial to hire a project manager to oversee the project and assist the Chair of the Committee. To consider these questions, the Curriculum Committee hosted a face-to-face meeting in Washington DC under the facilitation of the Chair and a new project manager. The results of that meeting were as follows:

- The transformation of the certification standards into competency domains (criteria):
  - Professional Values and Capabilities
  - Knowledge of Educational Principles, Practice, and Methodology in Simulation
  - Implementing, Assessing, and Managing Simulation-based Educational Activities
  - Scholarship—Spirit of Inquiry and Teaching
- The delineation of two different levels of certification that would initially include an entry level and, later, an advanced level (see Table 1.4.5). The advanced level would include the submission of a portfolio. The advanced level was to be known as CHSE-A.

Once the decision was made to use a portfolio review for the CHSE-A, the discussion turned to how to evaluate competency at the CHSE level. The decision was made to

---

TABLE 1.4.5

Eligibility Requirements

Certified Healthcare Simulation Educator-Advanced (CHSE-A)—A master's degree or equivalent. At least 5 years of simulation experience. Has used simulation for healthcare learners. Has used simulation continuously for 5 years.

Certified Healthcare Simulation Educator (CHSE)—A bachelor's degree or equivalent. At least 2 years of simulation experience. Has used simulation for healthcare learners. Has used simulation continuously for 2 years.

---

use commonly accepted methods of competency assessment. These included the following:

- Assessment of knowledge with a multiple-choice exam;
- Assessment of skills and attitudes to be assessed through reference reports and targeted questions;
- Review of the application and three reference reports by two Certification Committee members.

It was determined that the certification would be valid for 3 years.

PRACTICE ANALYSIS

As the development of the program progressed, it was determined that a practice analysis would be required to fully understand the scope of simulation educators' positions and the work that they do—a process called a practice (or job or task) analysis. The analysis was developed through a series of steps, including a review of the literature and other source documents, consulting stakeholders, and sending a structured survey to as many of those in the field as possible for comment.

In January of 2011, The Board of Directors issued a request for proposal (RFP) for the services of a practice analysis and test development company. In June 2011, Schroeder Measurement Technologies (SMT) was chosen to perform the practice analysis. A literature search, Web site, job description, and published research were reviewed and the results used to develop an exhaustive list of tasks and KSAs required of competent practice. The Certification Committee and SMT convened a panel of 14 expert stakeholders who represented a full spectrum of simulation modalities, disciplines, professions, and geographic regions. Prior to the meeting, an outline of KSAs was developed by SMT. The outline was compiled from articles and job descriptions. The SMEs reviewed, edited, modified, and approved the final list. During the meeting, the outline was reviewed for task importance and frequency of practice. This outline was transformed into the practice analysis survey that included a demographic survey to provide data regarding geographic location, discipline, profession, and simulation modality to assure adequate cross representation of the target audience.

The online survey was then sent to 10,900 potential respondents who were members of SSH, ASPE, ASSH, SESAM, INASCL, and NLN. The survey was available for 4 weeks. Approximately 1,100 individuals responded to the survey, with a return rate of 10.1%. The survey showed reliability coefficients above 0.9 for frequency and importance for the 70 tasks and KSAs. Over 99% of those surveyed said they agreed with the tasks as described. The results were presented via Webinar and conference call to either remove any nonessential tasks based on the survey results or add any tasks based on the comments written

TABLE 1.4.6

Domain Weights

Domain	Weight (%)
1. Display Professional Values and Capabilities	4
2. Demonstrate Knowledge of Simulation Principles, Practice, and Methodology	34
3. Educate and Assess Learners Using Simulation	52
4. Manage Overall Simulation Resources and Environments	6
5. Engage in Scholarly Activities	4

by the respondents. No tasks were removed, and five tasks were added to the knowledge competency (SSH, n.d.). Further discussion was held to determine the complexity of the tasks, importance, and time spent in each of these domains. The results were to establish domain weights for the content outline for the examination blueprint (Table 1.4.6).

EXAMINATION BLUEPRINT

Once the practice analysis was complete and the domain weight established, the next step was to create the examination blueprint upon which the content of the CHSE examination is based. The blueprint was completed in the fall of 2011 (see Table 1.4.7 for the final test blueprint).

DEVELOPMENT OF THE CHSE CERTIFICATION EXAMINATION

The CHSE certification test questions were developed to accurately reflect the knowledge and problem-solving skills used by the CHSE in diverse simulation educational settings and ever-evolving practice environments. The test taker should be confident that the examination accurately assesses their knowledge and skill. In this section, we will describe how the Certification Committee

TABLE 1.4.7

Certified Healthcare Simulation Educator Detailed Examination Blueprint

Display Professional Values and Capabilities

a. Demonstrate leadership capabilities (e.g., assume a leadership role in activity, serve as a mentor for a novice simulation educator)
b. Advocate for simulation in local healthcare community
c. Demonstrate awareness of diversity issues (e.g., cultural, gender, age)

Demonstrate Knowledge of Simulation Principles, Practice, and Methodology

a. Understand the relationship between learner engagement and the learning and assessment environment
b. Understand the legal implications of simulation
c. Understand the ethical implications of simulation
d. Understand regulatory requirements (e.g., student confidentiality, drug and device, research)
e. Understand the principles of utilizing simulation as an educational tool (e.g., learning taxonomies, assessment, learning theories)
f. Understand the theories of utilizing simulation as an educational tool (e.g., experiential learning, reflection)
g. Understand the principles of integrating simulation into a curriculum
h. Understand the theories of feedback
i. Understand the theories of debriefing
j. Understand the various modalities of simulation training (e.g., mannequins, standardized patients, virtual environments)
k. Understand the variety of content areas to which simulation can be applied (e.g., basic science, crisis management, basic assessment)
l. Understand the impact of location on simulation (e.g., in situ, center-based, mobile)
m. Understand the scope of application of simulation (e.g., individual, team, systems)
n. Understand when to use simulation-based training/education
　i. Advantages
　ii. Limitations
　iii. Risks
o. Understand the capabilities of simulator technologies/modalities
p. Understand the need to be able to operate or direct the operation of simulation resources in your program (e.g., money, people, space)

q. Utilize resources effectively and efficiently (e.g., money, people, space)
r. Understand concepts
　i. Realism
　ii. Reliability (e.g., assessment tools, implementation process)
　iii. Validity (e.g., content, construct)
　iv. Feasibility (e.g., efficient, effective, achievable)
　v. Learner-centered education
　vi. Interprofessional education
　vii. Teamwork (e.g., leadership, role delegation)
　viii. Human factors
　ix. Patient safety
　x. Risk management

Educate and Assess Learners Using Simulation

a. Plan training and educational simulation activities
　i. Perform needs assessment (e.g., technical, behavioral, cognitive)
　ii. Define goals
　iii. Create measurable learning objectives
　iv. Select evaluation type (i.e., formative or summative)
　v. Select evaluation methods (e.g., debriefing, feedback)
　vi. Select and implement evaluation tools (e.g., instruments, metrics, checklists)
　vii. Design simulation activity (e.g., course, class, session)
　viii. Select simulation modality
　ix. Identify resources (e.g., content experts, location, technicians)
　x. Organize simulation team (e.g., patients, technicians, educators/content experts)
　　a. Recruit
　　b. Orient
　　c. Train
　xi. Prepare materials for learners and simulation team
　　a. Instructions
　　b. Equipment
　　c. Environment
　xii. Conduct pilot activity for new simulations (e.g., dress rehearsal, field test, run-through)

b. Implement simulation activity
  i. Briefing/orientation
    a. Determine the information to provide to simulation participants
    b. Communicate potential physical and psychological risks
    c. Create a psychologically safe environment
    d. Orient (e.g., equipment, environment, expectations)
  ii. Conduct simulation
    a. Manage personnel and equipment
    b. Adapt to evolving simulation and learner needs
    c. Problem-solve issues that arise during the simulation (e.g., equipment failure, unexpected behaviors or events)
    d. Manage physical and psychological risks related to the simulation
    e. Assess performance gaps
  iii. Conduct learner evaluation
    a. Manage physical and psychological risks during the evaluation process
    b. Address performance gaps
    c. Facilitate debriefing
      1. Specific to the learning objectives
      2. Consistent with the simulation modality
    d. Provide feedback
      1. Specific to the learning objectives
      2. Consistent with the simulation modality (e.g., standardized patients, virtual reality)

c. Evaluate simulation activities
  i. Self-evaluation
  ii. Peer evaluation
  iii. Learner evaluation
d. Modify simulation activities in response to feedback from learners and team members
e. Communicate opportunities for practice and curricular improvement to responsible parties

Manage Overall Simulation Resources and Environments

a. Understand the basic operational principles associated with delivering simulation activities
b. Assess and modify the physical environment to maximize simulation-based learning
c. Follow policies, procedures, and practices of the simulation program
d. Understand and respond to technical and material issues (e.g., video capture, simulator failures, material supplies)

Engage in Scholarly Activities

a. Participate in professional development (e.g., conferences, courses)
b. Identify and use credible resources in simulation education (e.g., Web sites, listservs, literature)
c. Understand the role of qualitative and quantitative research

controlled for three sources of bias that can negatively affect the validity of an examination: sampling error, design error, and administrative error (Institute for Credentialing Excellence, n.d.).

Sampling Process

To avoid sampling error, the committee designed a test that accurately reflected the knowledge required of a simulation educator on the basis of the results of a two-step process. A consensus conference of representatives from all major disciplines and international organizations representing the full spectrum of simulation methods agreed on the basic competencies required of a Healthcare Simulation Educator. On the basis of those competency domains, simulation educators were surveyed to systematically gather information that described job behaviors and activities. They were asked to rank these with regard to importance and frequency. The test design was based on the results of the practice analysis. The domains and examination weights are shown in Table 1.4.8.

Design Process

Inappropriate or poorly constructed test items, or inadequate sampling of all domains, can result in design error. To minimize this error, the CHSE examination was designed to test knowledge across all domains at three levels of difficulty: recall, application, and evaluation. Two test forms were developed, each consisting of 115 multiple-choice questions (MCQs), of which 100 are counted toward determination of achieving a passing score. The remaining 15 questions were more recently developed and are

TABLE 1.4.8

Domain Weights Comparison

Domain	Weights (%)		
	Respondent	Empirical	SME
Display Professional Values and Capabilities	16	4	5
Demonstrate Knowledge of Simulation Principles, Practice, and Methodology	26	34	46
Educate and Assess Learners Using Simulation	29	52	31
Manage Overall Simulation Resources and Environments	17	6	14
Engage in Scholarly Activities	12	4	4

included in the examination to statistically validate these test items prior to their becoming an accepted item for scoring. Mapping questions to an examination blueprint confirms that both test forms cover the same content in the same way. The exam was developed collaboratively with SMT, examination development experts, and healthcare simulation experts across disciplines, methods, and geographic locations.

MCQs were chosen because they are frequently used to test knowledge, test takers are familiar with MCQs, and they are a valid method to measure knowledge across levels of difficulty (Institute for Credentialing Excellence, n.d.). The key is to have MCQs that are without technical flaws: testwiseness and irrelevant difficulty (*Certified Healthcare Simulation Educator Job Analysis Report*, 2011). Table 1.4.9 lists these elements.

SECTION 1 • Simulation Standards

TABLE 1.4.9

Item Writing Rules and Guidelines

Testwiseness	Irrelevant Difficulty
• Grammatical cues: one or more distractors doesn't follow from the stem	• Options long or complicated
• Absolute terms: "always" or "never" in some options	• Numeric data not stated consistently
• Long answer is correct	• Terms are vague like "rarely "or "usually"
• Word repeats in the stem and the correct answer	• Language in options not parallel—requires editing
• Convergence strategy—correct answer includes most elements in common with the other options	• Options in nonlogical order
	• None of the above is an option
	• Stems are "tricky"
	• Answer to item hinged to answer of a related item

The probability that the test taker will answer the question correctly should be related to their knowledge and not to their test-taking strategy.

CHSE exam writers attended an in-person workshop on item writing and review conducted by SMT, where over 200 exam items were generated. Following this face-to-face workshop, item writing was moved to a Webinar-based format, which allowed for asynchronous writing and where additional items could be written and reviewed. SMT conducted online examination item reviews, with healthcare simulation experts, and items were accepted, rejected, improved, or sent back to the author. The exams were created with an approximately 50% overlap between the two forms. Review included specific filters as well. The first filter was related to making the examinations international and removing any terms or idioms that might be country-centric. The second filter was to ensure that any use of a specific modality was neither overly extensive nor mandating a need for in-depth knowledge of any specific simulation modality, but rather focused on the principles of healthcare simulation, no matter which modality was used.

Healthcare simulation experts reviewed each form and continued item improvement. This occurred iteratively for all questions, meaning that each item was reviewed and improved multiple times by many individuals. Finally, the full forms were reviewed individually, then compared with each other, and approved for the pilot phase. The final reviews were done by six to eight SMEs.

Standard Setting

The pilot phase was launched with the goal of having 200 examinations completed to ensure statistical validation of the overall form and allow for individual item analysis. The pilot phase was open for 4 months. The split between the two forms was approximately 50–50, and the number completed for each form met the requirements for statistical analysis. Standard setting used a group of SMEs and the Modified Angoff process. The Modified Angoff process is described below.

Determining the Passing Score

The *pass point* is the minimum score required to pass the certification examination or the point where a candidate's knowledge, skills, and behaviors equal the certification threshold. There are several different methods commonly used to set passing scores for certification examinations. SSH chose the Modified Angoff Method. Pass points for the certification exam vary with each test, but usually they fall between 65% and 75% of all test items answered correctly. A Modified *Angoff Method* is used to determine the pass point for each version of each test. The Modified Angoff Method uses expert judgments from SMEs to determine the difficulty level of the test. The easier the test, the higher the pass point; the more difficult the test, the lower the pass point.

The following is a basic outline of the Modified Angoff Method. A group of SMEs independently rate each test question within a given test. The ratings are defined as the probability, or likelihood, that an acceptably (minimally) competent person with the requisite education and experience will answer the question correctly. An acceptably (minimally) competent person is defined as someone who adequately performs all job functions safely and requires no further training to do so.

1. The SMEs review each test question as group. A consensus is reached for the rating of each test question. During this time, the SMEs review comments submitted in writing by test takers. Any test question that is judged to be ambiguous, has more than one correct answer, or has no correct answers is eliminated from the scoring process for that test. These test questions are then revised for future use, reclassified, or deleted from the test item bank.
2. After the data are refined, the final step is to calculate the mean, or average, of all the test question ratings. This becomes the overall pass point estimation.

Why Use Modified Angoff?—Each version of a given certification test pulls questions from a test item bank. Each of these questions varies in difficulty. Because a different mix of questions is used in each test, the overall difficulty level is not fixed. Thus, it is important to make sure that the varying difficulty level is reflected in the pass point of each test to ensure that test results are reliable. Test reliability is concerned with the reproducibility of results for each version of a given test. In other words, for a test to be reliable it must yield the same result (pass or fail) for the same individual under very similar circumstances. By taking into consideration the difficulty level of the test, the Modified Angoff Method significantly increases the reliability of the tests. Also, because each test is adjusted for difficulty level, each test version has the same standard for passing. Thus, test takers are treated equitably and fairly even if they take different versions of the test.

Item Analysis: Poor-Performing Item—Each item on the test is reviewed statistically, and if it is found to be performing poorly, it may be removed, or rewritten. A poorly performing item is identified when it is unable to discriminate between a competent and incompetent test taker or all test takers are writing the wrong answer to the item.

Administration and Governance of the Program

To provide quality assurance for the program, administrative and governance practices need to be carefully determined.

Administration: To avoid administrative error, the Certification Committee standardized how information about the examination is given to all interested and eligible examinees. The Society's Certified Healthcare Simulation Educator Handbook provides information to help the individual prepare their application and describes the certification program. The handbook can be found at ssih.org/certification.

Preparation: While many fields can rely on formal education programs to help prepare examinees for certification exams, healthcare simulation educators have diverse educational and training backgrounds, and one formal preparation program is not warranted. Most opportunities for training in simulation-based education methods have come from on-the-job experience, workshops, preconferences, courses, and other simulation-based educational opportunities. The SSH Certification Committee developed a series of recommendations to applicants on how to prepare for the examination:

1. Review the literature and survey the latest research.
2. Access various networking tools and review conversation and information shared to gain insight into the latest trends and techniques.
3. Consider taking a course on simulation and educational techniques.
4. Review the list of references provided by the SSH Certification Committee (https://ssih.org/certification/chse-examination). It is a collection of articles related to simulation, education, and research that should help the candidate review information. Further, many of the articles listed were used as source material for the questions on the examination. The list is targeted toward helping the candidate prepare for the examination. It is not to be considered a comprehensive list of seminal articles in simulation.

Rather, the list should be used as a tool to help prepare for the examination. *NOTE:* The candidate need not read each of these items, nor is this expected. The list is made up of articles from which the candidate can select what is needed to gain knowledge in areas where knowledge may be lacking, or to allow the candidate to refresh knowledge.

Remediation: If the candidate is unsuccessful on the CHSE exam, they may retake the examination once every 90 days, and no more than four times in a calendar year. Information from the previous examination may be used to determine where further study is needed.

Governance: What began as a subcommittee has now grown into a large committee with a subcommittee structure and a full-time Director of Certification (Figure 1.4.1).

Results: By December 2012, 264 individuals had applied for certification, 231 applications were approved, and 185 applicants had taken the examination. On the basis of that number and using the Modified Angoff Method, cut scores were set and 150 applicants had passed the examination. These results demonstrated that by using a process that was methodical and evidence-based, SSH had designed and was set to deliver a valid and defensible cost-effective program. At the IMSH 2013 Conference in Orlando, new CHSEs were honored with a reception and recognition.

BEEN THERE, DONE THAT: HOW CAN I CONTINUE TO IMPROVE OR SUSTAIN WHAT I HAVE ACHIEVED?

Future Plans

The pilot phase for the CHSE-A certification process was launched in October 2013. This advanced certification should be available in 2014 after the pilot study has been completed and the processes for application, evaluation, and approval have been reviewed, approved, and disseminated. Key to this will be to assure that applicants receive a fair and equitable review no matter who is assigned to review the application. To achieve this goal, the processes to ensure inter-rater reliability will be robust and transparent to all.

The SSH Certification Director and committee are in the process of developing a certification for the individuals who fulfill another key role in the healthcare simulation. The Certified Healthcare Simulation Operations Specialist (CHSOS) certification is intended for those individuals

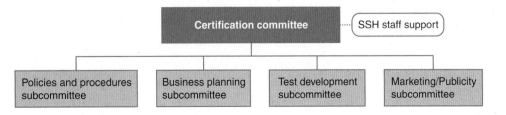

FIGURE 1.4.1 Initial Certification Committee organization chart.

SECTION 1 • Simulation Standards

who are key to the infrastructure and delivery of simulation. They go by many different titles—simulation technicians, technologists, information technology (IT) support, operators, coordinators, and many more. This group of individuals has been identified as having a unique set of KSAs that complement and support those of the CHSE, as well as having some common knowledge. Shared ground includes things like simulation principles and the ability to speak the same language of education and healthcare, ensuring good communication and teamwork. The development of this certification is following the same path and rigor of the development of the CHSE. A pilot phase is planned in early to mid-2014.

In order to continue to provide SSH stakeholders and the SSH target audience with the confidence that the SSH Certification Program will continue to serve their needs, SSH will be applying for Accreditation through the NCCA. The SSH Certification Program will thus evolve into an independent commission—the next key step in the maturation of the program.

SUMMARY

The development of any certification program is a challenging process, particularly when developing a formal certification for a profession that is new and growing. The Healthcare Simulation Educator profession has responded to the need to develop the standards and define the KSAs that are required to be a successful professional in healthcare simulation. As we move forward and the field changes, repeat analysis of practice will help keep the certification requirements up-to-date and supportive of what each healthcare simulationist does, every day.

REFERENCES

Benson, J. A. (1991). Certification and recertification: one approach to professional accountability. *Annals of Internal Medicine, 114*(3), 238–242. Retrieved from http://www.ukpmc.ac.uk

Certified healthcare simulation educator job analysis report. (2011, pp. 7–8). Parsons, TN: SMT Inc.

Society for Simulation in Healthcare. (n.d.). Retrieved from http://www.ssih.org

Institute for Credentialing Excellence. (n.d.). *NCCA accreditation.* Retrieved from http://www.credentialingexcellence.org/ncca

SELECTED READINGS

Case, S. M., & Swanson, D. B. (2002). *Constructing written test questions for the basic and clinical sciences* (3rd ed.). Philadelphia, PA: National Board of Medical Examiners.

Hale, J. (2000). *Performance based certification.* San Francisco, CA: Jossey Bass Pfeiffer.

CHAPTER 1.5

Quality Improvement

Juli C. Maxworthy, DNP, MSN, MBA, RN, CNL, CPHQ, CPPS, CHSE and
Jared M. Kutzin, DNP, MS (MMEL), MPH, RN, CPPS

ABOUT THE AUTHORS

JULI C. MAXWORTHY is the former Director of the Simulation Center at Holy Names University and currently serves as the Chair of the Simulation Committee at the University of San Francisco. Prior to entering full time into academia, her last "clinical" role was that of Vice President of Quality and Risk. Dr. Maxworthy has advanced degrees in nursing administration, business, quality, and patient safety. She is currently the Vice Chair for the Society for Simulation in Healthcare (SSH) Accreditation Council and has been a surveyor of simulation programs since 2010.

JARED M. KUTZIN is the Director of Simulation at Winthrop University Hospital and sits on the institution's patient safety committee. A registered nurse with advanced degrees in health policy and management, public health, leadership, and medical education, Dr. Kutzin completed the clinical quality fellowship program (CQFP) offered by the Greater New York Hospital Association and the United Hospital Fund. Dr. Kutzin is active in SSH and the National Patient Safety Foundation (NPSF).

ABSTRACT

As simulation as a modality has been evolving, evaluation and determination of areas for improvement has also been evolving. This chapter provides a brief historical perspective on quality improvement and the role simulation can play in these quality improvement efforts. Tools, tips, and methods are provided using case studies from both the simulation center and the acute care perspectives. The ideal situation is when there is a **bidirectional relationship** between the simulation center and the clinical sites that enable both to assess, implement, and evaluate activities for the betterment of patient care and outcomes.

CASE EXAMPLE

Throughout the chapter there are two cases portrayed, both are about the aftermath of a fall, one occurs in a simulation center and the other in an acute care setting. These areas are being highlighted due to the content of this textbook and to demonstrate what quality and patient safety efforts can be applied.

INTRODUCTION

Those involved in simulation are commonly invested in building, innovating, and collaborating. Simulation provides an intersection where education, clinical practice, theatrical performance, and healthcare quality and safety meet. Simulation-based curricula are often implemented to affect a particular area of concern, regardless of whether that concern is national (central line infection rates) or local (disaster preparedness). These uses of simulation require simulation educators and administrators to be knowledgeable not only about clinical practice and curriculum design but also about the methods of process improvement.

Simulation can be used to investigate errors in healthcare, as part of a **failure modes and effects analysis** (FMEA) before a sentinel event occurs and as part of a **root cause analysis** (RCA) after an error or mistake occurs. In either use of simulation, simulation administrators and educators must be keenly aware that quality and patient safety is the primary focus of the effort. A broad understanding of the theories of patient quality and patient safety as well as the knowledge of specific tools can allow the simulation experts to become a more integral part of the healthcare safety team.

To demonstrate how quality tools can assist in assuring students and patients receive optimal experiences, two scenarios are presented. One takes place in a simulation center and one in a hospital. These scenarios present a challenge to management and staff and force them to be involved in addressing the problems that arise. It is essential in both instances that concepts from the field of **continuous quality improvement** (CQI) be applied in an organized, evidence-based manner to reach solutions that address the root causes of the events.

The first example provided below is one that could happen at any simulation center in the world (see Box 1.5.1). The next situation is unfortunately a common one in the inpatient setting (see Box 1.5.2).

A POINT OF REFERENCE

To set the stage for the review of these cases, it helps to know some of the history related to total quality management (TQM) and CQI, as they relate to healthcare. In 1910, Dr. Ernest Codman, a physician at Massachusetts General Hospital, proposed the "end result system of hospital standardization" (Neuhauser, 2002). Codman left Massachusetts General Hospital and opened his own hospital, where he recorded each patient discharged and the end result. Between 1911 and 1916, there were 337 patients discharged from his hospital, and 123 errors were caught and measured during this time. He grouped each error by type:

1. Lack of knowledge or skill
2. Surgical judgment
3. Lack of care or equipment
4. Lack of diagnostic skill

In addition, he noted, there were four "calamities of surgery or those accidents and complications over which we have no known control. These should be acknowledged

---

BOX 1.5.1

SIMULATION CENTER EXAMPLE

It's Thursday, 3:00 p.m. local time, and your simulation center is preparing for a final team training simulation for the day. The simulation center has been utilized every day this past week for 12 hours a day. The simulation support staff has been working hard to meet the needs of course faculty and learners throughout the week. Their job hasn't been made any easier, because one simulation technician is away on vacation. The final scenario for the day requires the simulated patient (mannequin) to be moulaged. The simulation technician fills the fluid reservoirs (blood and sweat) with fluid, places simulated injuries on the patient, lubricates any necessary mannequin components, and sets the room with the necessary equipment. As they finish, the faculty member checks with the simulation technician to inquire whether the room is ready for the next group. The simulation technician finishes a few last-minute items and returns to the control room to control the mannequin. Within a few moments, the learners enter the room to assess the patient. As they enter the room and approach the foot of the bed, a learner steps in a puddle of fluid spilled when filling the reservoirs, slips, and falls to the floor. The other learners, unsure whether this is part of the scenario, continue to treat the simulated mannequin. As this is not part of the scenario, the simulation technician and faculty observer wait to see whether the learner gets up or whether they are injured and need assistance. When the learner doesn't get up, the scenario is stopped, and the learner assessed. The learner complains of back and wrist pain from the fall. The learner, now patient, is subsequently seen in the emergency room and diagnosed with a wrist fracture.

The quality and safety components to discuss are immense, but include the following:
1. Production pressure
2. Workload
3. Policies (filling the mannequin in the room)

BOX 1.5.2

HOSPITAL EXAMPLE

On 4 West, a busy 32-bed orthopedic floor, Mr. Smith, a 2-day postoperative hip replacement patient, has been pushing his nurse call bell frequently during the evening because he needs to urinate and has been unsuccessful in using the urinal while lying in his bed. Mr. Smith decides to get out of bed on his own to use the urinal. He is able to get to the side of the bed, stand up, and successfully uses the urinal by moving a few steps away from the bed and holding on to the side rail of his bed. While using the urinal, he accidentally spills some of the urine on the floor. Mr. Smith keeps the room dark so his roommate can sleep, and while returning to bed, slips on urine he spilled on the floor. Mr. Smith lands on his surgical site causing damage to the incision, requiring additional tests and ultimately more surgery to repair the incision and prosthetic device. Mr. Smith is the third patient on 4 West in the past 3 months to fall and sustain an injury while toileting. The manager is concerned that there is lack of patient education and collaboration occurring on her unit and requests to meet with the quality, safety, process improvement, and risk management personnel. The team decides to approach the manager of the simulation center that is affiliated with the hospital and share their concerns. The risk manager advises the group that she has been contacted by nurse managers throughout the organization with similar concerns. The risk manager advises the Chief Nursing Officer (CNO) of the increased number of incidents and shares the concerns that have been brought to her. The CNO along with the nursing leadership team requests a Root Cause Analysis (RCA) of these recent events to determine any linkages. They will then work to develop scenarios in which nurses can be assessed for their competency of certain activities that could prevent a patient fall. Together with the nurse managers and the environmental services group, the risk manager develops a scenario and brings in the staff for assessment.

to ourselves and to the public and study directed to their prevention." Codman was the first to publicly report his measures. In his annual report, he admitted the mistakes both publicly and in print and sent a copy to major hospitals around the country, asking them to do the same (Neuhauser, 2002).

Shewhart, Juran, and Deming are considered the three key founders of the quality improvement movement (Best & Neuhauser, 2006). W. Edwards Deming, who worked during the summer months in 1925 and 1926 with Juran and Shewhart at the Western Hawthorne Electric Plant, later developed his philosophy of quality. Deming's philosophy requires simultaneously seeing an organization as a set of interrelated processes with a common aim, understanding that processes have common cause and special cause variations, understanding how new knowledge is generated within an organization, and understanding how people are motivated and work in groups or teams within the organization (Best & Neuhauser, 2005).

Deming also contributed his "fourteen points of management" to the field. His 14 points have at their core leadership, organizational learning, cooperation, and systems thinking. His 14 points include the following:

1. Create a constancy of purpose
2. Adopt the new philosophy
3. Cease dependence on inspection
4. Do not award business on the basis of price tag alone
5. Improve constantly the system of production and service
6. Institute training
7. Adopt and institute leadership
8. Drive out fear
9. Break barriers among staff areas
10. Eliminate slogans, exhortations, and targets
11. Eliminate numerical quotas
12. Remove barriers
13. Institute a program of education and self-improvement
14. Take action to accomplish the transformation (Best & Neuhauser, 2005).

After being a patient in a hospital, Deming realized that his philosophies applied to the healthcare system, just like they applied to the industrial setting. Deming stated that management's job was to optimize the whole system. Additionally, he recognized that nurses were working as hard as they could (Best & Neuhauser, 2005). They were well educated, but discouraged and defeated by the broken system in which they worked. While recognizing that the healthcare system had flaws, Deming did not blame the people working in it. Rather, he noted that only leadership could redesign the system to reduce unwanted variation in care (Best & Neuhauser, 2005).

In 1954, following World War II, Joseph Juran and W. Edwards Deming were invited to Japan where they helped restructure the Japanese production methods. In less than 5 years, Japanese products gained the market edge, whereas previously they were thought to be inferior (Best & Neuhauser, 2006). Juran stated that what was known as Pareto's principle, 80% of the wealth of Italy in the 19th century was held by approximately 20% of the population, also applied to defects (Best & Neuhauser, 2006). In essence, 80% of problems are caused by 20% of the defects. Juran also developed his quality trilogy, providing a frame to link finance and management to **quality improvement**. The three components are as follows:

1. Quality Planning—define customers and how to meet their needs
2. Quality Control—keep the process working well
3. Quality Improvement—learn, optimize, refine, and adapt (Best & Neuhauser, 2006)

Moving forward approximately 30 years, the **Institute for Healthcare Improvement** (IHI) was founded in the mid-1980s by Dr. Donald Berwick, a pediatrician, along with a group who were committed to making significant changes to healthcare. They realized that healthcare needed to make major changes to reduce harm and waste. They had seen what the airline industry had done in the previous decade to make substantial strides in improving the safety of the industry and began to translate those lessons into healthcare. Those lessons include "flattening the hierarchy" in healthcare, between physicians, nurses, and other staff, much like the way the airlines flattened the hierarchy in the cockpit, allowing copilots and first officers to "speak up" to the captain. Other lessons include the importance of teamwork and communication between professionals to ensure safe operating conditions for both staff and patients.

In 2000, the **Institute of Medicine** (IOM) published a critical report, "To Err Is Human" (Kohn et al., 2000). This report described the harm that was affecting patients across the United States. It was estimated that at least 44,000 and as many as 98,000 people were dying annually because of preventable medical errors (Kohn et al., 2000). This information sent shock waves throughout healthcare, and after a decade the industry is still trying to improve patient outcomes. The failure to resolve this situation is evidenced by recent reports that identify as many as 187,000 deaths that occur each year in hospitals owing to preventable medical mistakes (Goodman et al., 2011). The major types of errors being found to cause unnecessary deaths are listed in Table 1.5.1.

There are several key areas where simulation can mitigate harm, and their foundations lie in IOM's *Crossing the Quality Chasm: A New Health System for the 21st Century*. This monumental report concluded that merely making incremental improvements in current systems of care would not suffice (IOM, 2001). To be able to provide appropriate care would require a major redesign of the current system at every level. The mantra was described "to continually

SECTION 1 • Simulation Standards

TABLE 1.5.1

Types of Errors

Diagnostic

Error or delay in diagnosis

Failure to employ indicated tests

Use of outmoded tests or therapy

Failure to act on results of monitoring or testing

Treatment

Error in the performance of an operation, procedure, or test

Error in administering the treatment

Error in the dose or method of using a drug

Avoidable delay in treatment or in responding to an abnormal test

Inappropriate (not indicated) care

Preventive

Failure to provide prophylactic treatment

Inadequate monitoring or follow-up of treatment

Other

Failure of communication

Equipment failure

Other system failure

Source: Leape, L. L., Lawthers, A. G., Brennan, T. A., & Johnson, W. G. (1993). Preventing medical injury. *QRB. Quality Review Bulletin, 19*(5), 144–149.

reduce the burden of illness, injury, and disability, and to improve the health and functioning of the people" (IOM, 2001). The document proposed six specific aims for improvement. These aims are built around the core need for healthcare to be:

- *Safe*: avoiding injuries to patients from the care that is intended to help them.
- *Effective*: providing services on the basis of scientific knowledge to all who could benefit, and refraining from providing services to those not likely to benefit.
- *Patient-centered*: providing care that is respectful of and responsive to individual patient preferences, needs, and values, and ensuring that patient values guide all clinical decisions.
- *Timely*: reducing waits and sometimes harmful delays for both those who receive and those who give care.
- *Efficient*: avoiding waste, including waste of equipment, supplies, ideas, and energy.
- *Equitable*: providing care that does not vary in quality because of personal characteristics such as gender, ethnicity, geographic location, and socioeconomic status (IOM, 2001).

In January 2005, the IHI launched the 100,000 Lives Campaign that helped spread best practice changes throughout healthcare. It was the first time in the history of US healthcare that competitors were working together to help save lives. IHI followed up the successful campaign with the 5 Million Lives campaign that continued the building of networks for improvement, working on reducing needless deaths and preventing harm from care (IHI.org).

The opportunity for simulation to be an integral part of the solution to healthcare improvement is quite evident. As the studies suggest, there are many areas for improvement within healthcare. There is an expectation that simulation staff, and in particular their leadership, be knowledgeable in the area of quality improvement techniques and be advocates for how simulation can serve as a tool to achieve the goals of enhancing safety and improving care.

TOOLS OF THE TRADE

As you can see, quality in healthcare is not a new topic. Healthcare professionals and healthcare leaders are involved in the continuing dialogue on quality and patient safety. These individuals and many others throughout healthcare are working to motivate and build the will for change; identify and test new models of care in partnership with both patients and healthcare professionals; and ensure the broadest possible adoption of best practices and effective innovations. These strategies require an understanding of CQI tools. When an adverse event occurs, there are basic steps that should occur in a systematic order to ensure that proper investigation and process changes are implemented. These steps include the following:

1. Identification of the issue
2. Investigation of the issue
   a. Determination of who was involved
   b. Determine policy/procedures involved
3. Perform an RCA
   a. Utilize the "five whys"
   b. Flowchart event
   c. Break down elements utilizing a fishbone diagram
4. Utilize a Plan-Do-Study-Act (PDSA) process to institute proposed changes to processes identified during RCA

In addition, other performance improvement systems such as **Lean**, the Toyota Production System (TPS) (Ohno, 1988), and Motorola's **Six Sigma** methodology (Tennant, 2001) can be utilized. For quality improvement efforts to be successful and sustained over time, senior leadership needs to provide the necessary support. It is also critical that the organization is one in which a "*Just Culture*" exists (Marx, 2001). In his testimony before Congress, Dr. Lucian Leape noted, "Approaches that focus on punishing individuals instead of changing systems provide strong incentives for people to report only those errors they cannot hide (Leape, 2000). Thus, a punitive approach shuts off the information that is needed to identify faulty systems and create safer ones. In a punitive system, no one learns from their mistakes" (Leape et al., 1993). As an alternative to a punitive system, application of the *Just Culture* model, which has been widely used in the aviation industry, seeks to create an environment that encourages individuals to

EXPERT'S CORNER

KAISER PERMANENTE'S APPROACH TO PATIENT SAFETY

Connie Lopez, MSN, CNS, RNC-OB, CPHRM
National Leader, Simulation and Risk Education, Kaiser Permanente

As a risk manager, my primary responsibilities are to identify potential sources of loss or risk for my organization, to develop programs to reduce adverse events, and to improve patient safety. At Kaiser Permanente, we significantly stepped up our efforts to create an effective patient safety program shortly after the November 1999 publication of the Institute of Medicine's report, "To Err is Human: Building a Safer Health System." The report outlined the far-reaching effects of medical errors:

> "Errors are costly in terms of loss of trust in the health care system by patients and diminished satisfaction by both patients and health professionals. Patients who experience a long hospital stay or disability as a result of errors pay with physical and psychological discomfort. Health professionals pay with loss of morale and frustration at not being able to provide the best care possible."

In early 2000, a team of Kaiser Permanente risk and quality leaders came together to determine how we could develop a successful patient safety program that would proactively prevent medical errors and promote a culture of safety. The team outlined three fundamental success factors:

1. Leadership commitment and ongoing support: Obtaining early buy-in was essential to the successful launch of Kaiser Permanente's patient safety program and to sustaining the program.
2. Focus on real outcomes supported by reliable data: Examples of outcomes we have focused on include decreased infection rates, improved response times to emergencies, and decreased patient injuries in the OR. To establish baselines and monitor program effectiveness, we have reviewed data from patient satisfaction scores, Safety Attitudes Questionnaires, and closed malpractice claims.
3. Simulation-based training: Providing opportunities for teams to practice real events and deal with emergency situations has been a key element in the success of our patient safety program.

One of my responsibilities as the national leader for simulation and risk education has been to develop a simulation-based training program and to roll it out to the Kaiser Permanente's seven regions, with the support of regional leadership and staff. In developing simulation activities, we first evaluated our organization's risk data to determine key areas in need of improvement. We decided to begin by focusing on perinatal patient safety. One perinatal claim might cost millions of dollars, but the emotional effect on patients, their family members, and our health care personnel, along with the reputational loss to our organization when errors occur, is immeasurable. This emotional piece is a primary force in driving risk managers to find ways to improve patient care and safety.

Our perinatal patient safety program focuses on training in human factors and provides simulation-based scenarios in which all perinatal team members participate in briefings, debriefings, time-outs, hand-offs, and closed-loop communication in real OR settings. In developing this first safety program, we felt that having clinical and executive leaders sign what we refer to as a "memorandum of understanding" would help formalize their agreement and fortify their commitment. The memorandum for the perinatal patient safety program outlined the goals of the program, the role of leaders, the support needed, improvements on which team efforts would be focused, and what success would look like. Since its inception, our perinatal program has contributed to a significant decrease (i.e., greater than 50%) in birth injuries and claims. We are now transferring our learning to simulation-based training in our surgical units and other areas and are hoping to see the same improvements in patient care and safety as we have seen in our perinatal patient safety program.

Most recently, we have included Patient Advisors in our *in situ* simulations. By involving patients and family members who have real-life experience with the care provided in our hospitals and medical centers, we gain valuable information and insights. One example is a woman whose husband had an acute *Clostridium difficile* infection. Her husband died despite all our efforts to save him. Following his hospitalization, we enlisted his wife to become a Patient Advisor. She later participated in a simulation in which she posed as a patient being treated for *C. difficile*. She provided vivid feedback in the debriefing sessions on her reactions, impressions, and emotions based on her experience in the simulation and her husband's illness. Staff who participated in the simulation were tremendously moved and motivated to enact improvements.

Simulation training gives our teams an opportunity to practice dealing with a broad range of critical safety issues and has greatly contributed to the success of our patient safety programs. From the data-supported results we have attained to date, and the highly favorable feedback we have received from medical personnel and leaders in our regions, we have demonstrated that our simulation program is an important way to help sustain a culture of patient safety across our organization.

report mistakes so that the precursors to errors can be better understood in order to fix the system issues. The term "*Just Culture*" was first used in a 2001 report by David Marx (2001), who popularized it in the patient safety field (Agency for Healthcare Research and Quality, n.d.).

Traditionally, healthcare's culture has held individuals accountable for all errors or mishaps that befall patients under their care. By contrast, a *Just Culture* recognizes that individual practitioners should not be held accountable for system failings over which they have no control. A *Just Culture* also recognizes many individual or "active" errors represent predictable interactions between human operators and the systems in which they work. However, in contrast to a culture that touts "no blame" as its governing principle, a *Just Culture* does not tolerate conscious disregard of clear risks to patients or gross misconduct (e.g., falsifying a record, performing professional duties while intoxicated).

RCA and FMEA are means by which an incident (or potential incident) can be reviewed in an intentional, meaningful way for all those involved. There are many tools consistently utilized to assist in the review of an incident, and they are provided in alphabetical order after a basic overview of the RCA and FMEA.

Root Cause Analysis

An RCA is a reactive yet structured approach to analyzing an event. An RCA is aimed at identifying the factors that resulted in the nature, the magnitude, the location, and the timing of the harmful outcomes (consequences) of one or more past events in order to identify what behaviors, actions, inactions, or conditions need to be changed to prevent recurrence of similar harmful outcomes and to identify the lessons to be learned to promote the achievement of better consequences. The most effective RCAs occur when those involved believe in the process and are committed to making improvement.

Failure Modes and Effects Analysis

Unlike the reactive approach of RCAs, FMEAs are an inductive failure analysis used in product development, systems engineering/reliability engineering, and operations management for analysis of failure modes within a system for classification by the severity and likelihood of the failures. It is a proactive approach to assist with mitigating issues prior to their occurrence. A successful FMEA activity helps a team to identify potential failure modes on the basis of past experience with similar products or processes or on the basis of common failure mechanism logic, enabling the team to design those failures out of the system with the minimum of effort and resource expenditure, thereby reducing development time and costs. It serves as a form of design review to erase weakness out of the design or process. It is widely used in development and manufacturing industries in various phases of the product's life cycle. *Effects analysis* refers to studying the consequences of those failures on different system levels.

Flowcharts

Creating a flowchart is often the first step in determining the root cause of a particular event. A flowchart is created to identify the flow of activities in a process and is used to map the process, identify where errors may occur, and review the process(es) that occurred. **Flowcharts** use standard symbols, identified in Figure 1.5.1. These symbols identify beginning and end points, decision points, standardized processes, and the direction of flow. To begin with, all **stakeholders** or involved individuals should be together in an area conducive for creating a flowchart. Whiteboard space or adhesive notes are helpful in creating the flowchart, as are computer programs such as Microsoft Visio or Internet programs such as Webspiration. After gathering stakeholders, the main activities or tasks should be identified and recorded. Often, it may be beneficial to work backward, listing the end point first. The activities or tasks should be rearranged until a representation of the actual process is reflected. Reviewing the hospital example above, the nurse manager, nursing staff, nursing assistants, unit secretaries, environmental service staff, biomedical engineering, and other hospital staff should be convened. This group should also include an identified team leader or project manager, a recorder/scribe, process improvement specialist, and quality and safety personnel.

Standard flowchart symbols

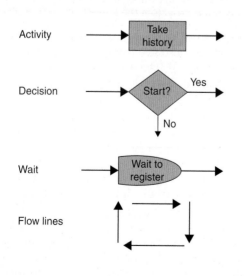
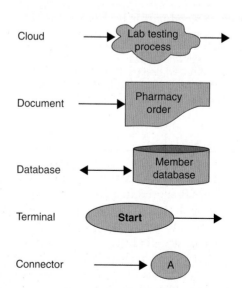

FIGURE 1.5.1   Standard flowchart symbols.

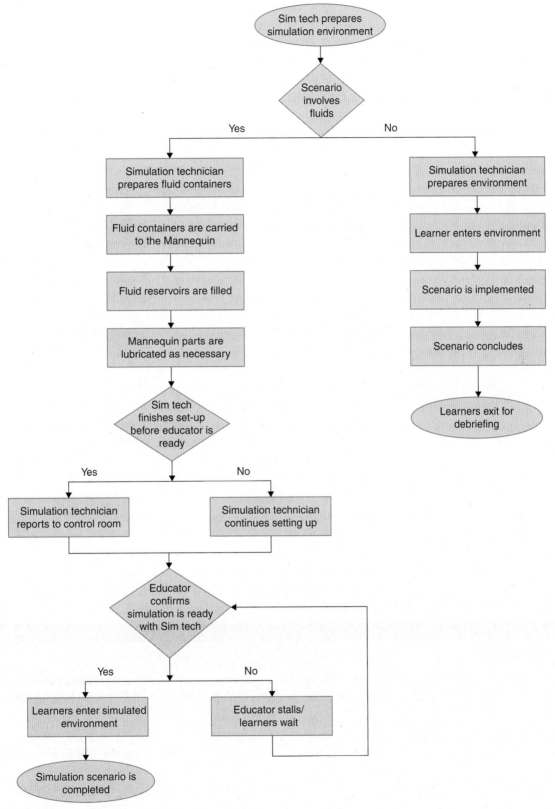

FIGURE 1.5.2   Flowchart: Learner fall in simulation center example.

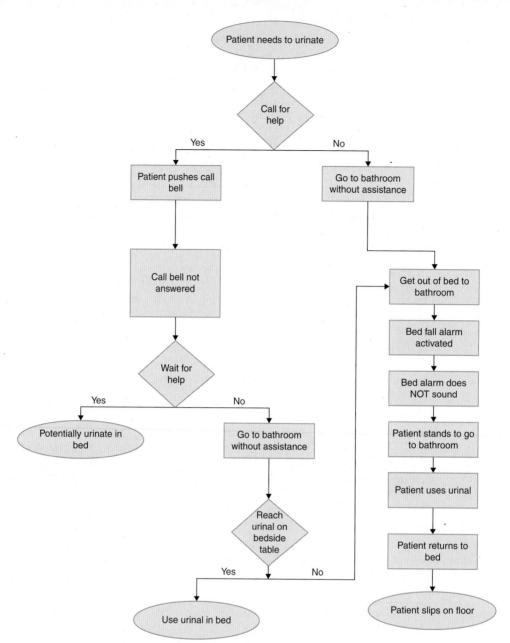

FIGURE 1.5.3 Flowchart: Patient fall in hospital example.

HOSPITAL EXAMPLE

The flowchart in Figure 1.5.3 identifies the starting point as the patient identifying their need to urinate. The flowchart then reaches a decision point—whether the patient calls for help or attempts to urinate on their own. This is important to list, as the barriers to calling for help (location of call bell, responsiveness of staff, etc.) may be an important factor in determining the patient outcome. This is the first branch point of the flowchart. The flowchart then follows the separate branches. Assuming the patient attempts to call for help and the call bell goes unanswered for a period of time, the second decision point is reached—whether to continue to wait for help. If the patient continues to wait, the end of the branch concludes with the patient potentially soiling themselves, in bed. The other branch point at this point leads to the patient attempting to go to the bathroom without assistance. This brings the flowchart to the third decision point—whether the urinal could be easily reached. If it is easily reached, then the patient may be able to use it while remaining in bed or could use it by sitting on the edge of the bed. If the urinal cannot be reached, then the flowchart moves to another branch, where the patient attempts to use the bathroom without assistance. This section of the flowchart leads to a series of actions, including getting out of bed, the failure of the bed alarm to sound, the patient using the bathroom, and ultimately slipping on the wet floor while returning to bed. It is important to list out each action and process in the flowchart to attempt to identify each area that leads to the outcome under investigation.

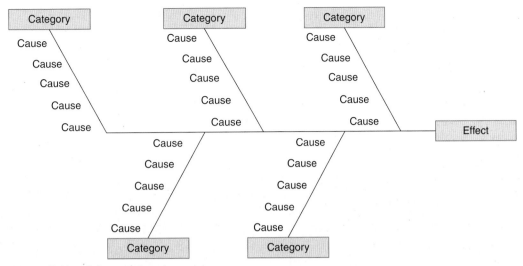

FIGURE 1.5.4   Ishikawa (fishbone) diagram: Generic example.

Fishbone (Ishikawa) Diagrams

A **cause-and-effect diagram** identifies the relationship between the problem and its associated causes (Figure 1.5.4). The tool uses a systematic approach for listing the causes and effects after a brainstorming session is held among participants. After identifying possible **causative factors**, the most likely ones can be addressed.

There are two methods for creating the cause-and-effect diagram. One method begins with listing the effect on the right side of the diagram and listing groups of causes on the "bones" of the diagram. These common groupings include people, environment, materials, methods, and equipment. The stakeholders then identify all possible causes under each group. The other method does not begin with these common groups but instead asks the participants to list all potential causes. These causes are listed as they are generated and then grouped into categories once they are all identified. Either method leads to the same end point: a diagram listing all the causes under separate groups that contribute to an effect (Figure 1.5.5). In the diagram in Figure 1.5.5, people are identified as part of a group. In Figure 1.5.6, under People, each profession is listed

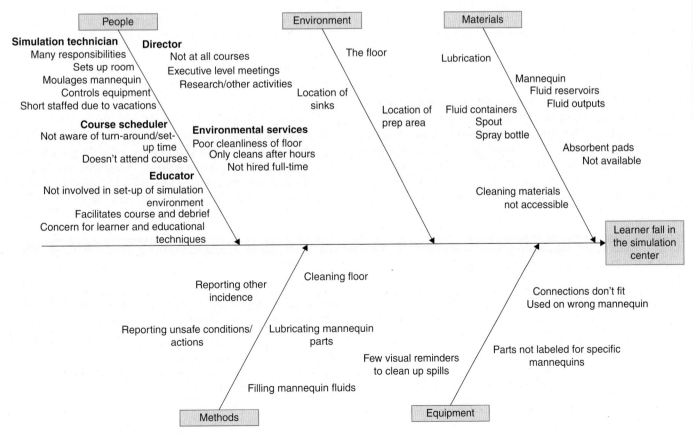

FIGURE 1.5.5   Ishikawa (fishbone) diagram: Simulation center example.

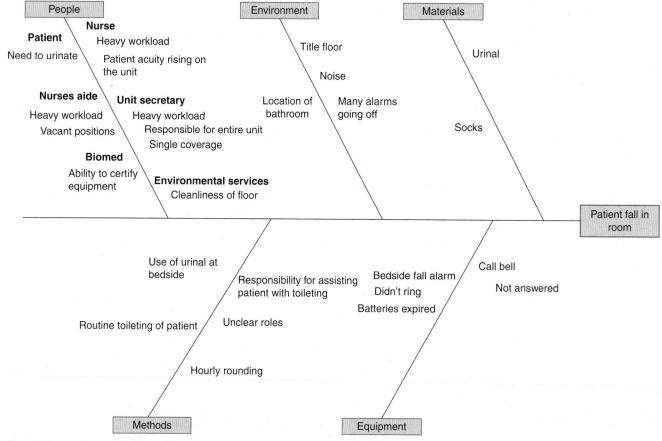

FIGURE 1.5.6 Ishikawa (fishbone) diagram: Hospital example.

separately, and further causative factors are listed under each profession. Boxes 1.5.4 and 1.5.5 describe the implications for the hospital and simulation center incidents.

The Five Whys Method

The "five whys" method of identifying the root cause is a relatively simple method to uncover the reason why an event occurred. The five whys method begins with the result and continually asks "why" until the root cause becomes apparent. It is generally well accepted that asking "why" five times will get to the root cause (or at least close). It is important to remember, when asking the five whys, to remain focused on the process and not on the person or people. Asking "Why did the process fail?" may help keep the RCA on track. The process may require more than five whys being asked to reach the root cause, as seen in Boxes 1.5.6 and 1.5.7.

Lean

Lean is both a strategy and a set of techniques. The strategy of Lean is simple yet compelling: minimize waste and maximize customer satisfaction. Translated to healthcare, Lean continuously seeks to drive out waste in healthcare processes so that patient needs are more effectively

---

BOX 1.5.4

SIMULATION CENTER EXAMPLE

A learner fall in the simulation center may have many causative factors. The Ishikawa diagram can help simulation center staff identify the root causes. On the basis of the scenario described above, multiple people are involved in simulation center operations. These include the simulation technician, the course scheduler, the educator, the director, and the environmental staff. Each staff member has specific roles and responsibilities, but both extrinsic and intrinsic factors may affect their performance. For example, the simulation technician has many responsibilities, including room setup, mannequin moulage, and controlling the equipment; however, they are short-staffed because of an employee being on vacation. The materials include the fluid containers, types of lubrication, as well as cleaning materials that may all contribute to the slippery surface encountered by the learner. The methods, including cleaning the simulation environment and filling the mannequins, combined with the materials, environment, and equipment all lead to the dangerous situation that in turn caused the learner to fall.

BOX 1.5.5

HOSPITAL EXAMPLE

The lack of an available nursing assistant to help the patient was identified as a potential cause. The nursing assistant was not available because they were busy in another room (heavy workload). They had a heavy workload because of vacant nursing assistant positions that have not been filled. Looking at another branch, such as equipment, the bedside

fall alarm is listed. The bedside alarm is a causative factor because it did not ring. The bedside alarm failed to ring because the batteries were expired. The cause-and-effect diagram identifies each cause and allows the stakeholders to narrow down the areas that could be changed to affect the outcome.

BOX 1.5.6

SIMULATION CENTER EXAMPLE

Why did the learner fall? Because they slipped on the wet floor.
Why was the floor wet? Because staff filled the mannequin reservoirs in the simulation room.
Why were the mannequin reservoirs filled in the simulation room? Because the prep area was too far away and there was little time between scenarios.
Why was there limited time between scenarios? Because courses were scheduled back-to-back.

Why were courses scheduled so close together? Because the course scheduler was unaware of the vacation schedule of the simulation technicians.
Why was the courses scheduler not aware of the vacations schedule?
Continuing would require further questioning and uncovering additional causes.

BOX 1.5.7

HOSPITAL EXAMPLE

Why did the patient fall? Because he got out of bed without assistance.
Why did the patient get out of bed without assistance? Because staff didn't respond to the call bell.
Why did the staff not respond to the call bell? Because the call bell wasn't heard.
Why wasn't the call bell heard? Because no staff were at the nursing station.

Why were there no staff at the nursing station? Because the unit coordinator was on break and the patient care assistants were busy in other rooms.
Why were all staff busy with other activities? Because acuity level on the floor was high and the staffing was suboptimal.
Why was the staffing suboptimal? Because staff were on vacation and not enough per-diem staff were on the roster to be contacted.

and efficiently met. Lean focuses on waste elimination, and in healthcare we perceive that to be anything other than the minimum amount of supplies, equipment, personnel, space, and time that is absolutely essential to delivering a quality level of clinically accepted patient treatment. Lean emphasizes the continuous movement toward a best process and is constantly reevaluating to ensure that waste is continually being removed from the equation. This attitude of striving for continuous improvement must be embraced by the entire organization and become part of the cultural DNA if it is to be truly successful.

A **Pareto chart** is a useful representation of the data (Figure 1.5.7). It shows the frequency of the reasons for the occurrence and the percentage of the frequency. This principle is known as the **Pareto principle** or the 80–20 rule, and can be applied throughout healthcare. In Figure 1.5.7, a red line has been added to identify the 80% mark, and the green line identifies the cumulative

percentage of the causes. The data shows that three reasons caused 80% of the falls on this unit:

1. The call bell not being answered.
2. Staff not available to assist the patient.
3. The bed alarm failing to work.

These areas should be targeted first as they will have the largest impact on the overall fall rate by potentially reducing falls by 80%.

After examining incident reports and talking to participants and simulation staff, a list of causes of falls can be generated. After the frequency and cumulative percent are input into a database, graphical representations can be made. The graph in Figure 1.5.7 identifies five causes of patient falls. The green line is the cumulative percentage of falls, while the red line marks the 80% region. Figure 1.5.8 identifies that electrical wires (mannequin wires, equipment wires, etc.) were the primary reason for participants tripping and falling in the simulation center.

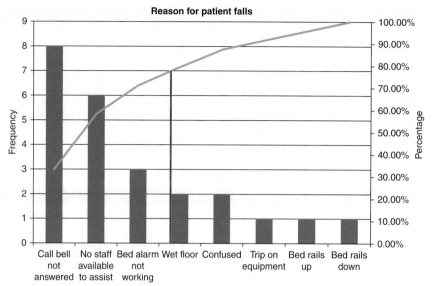

FIGURE 1.5.7   Pareto charts: Reason for patient falls.

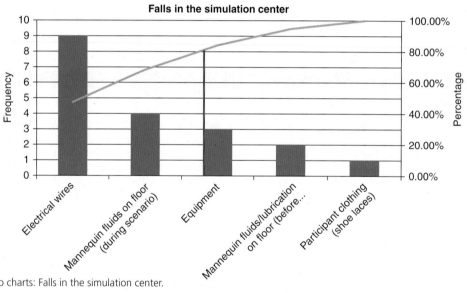

FIGURE 1.5.8   Pareto charts: Falls in the simulation center.

The fluids that come out of the mannequin (blood, sweat, etc.) during a scenario added to the number of falls, but not to the same extent as the wires. Therefore, directing efforts toward this minor cause of participant falls may not significantly impact the overall number of falls. However, the ultimate goal is zero falls and all causes should be addressed as time allows.

The Pareto chart allows staff to prioritize their actions on the basis of data. However, consideration must also be made regarding the severity of the injury. If the nine individuals who tripped on electrical wires in the simulation center suffered no injury but one of the participants who slipped on fluids before the scenario suffered significant injury, then attention may be directed to the cause of this more serious injury to prevent it from occurring in the future.

The Perfect Storm

Another method of identifying potential root causes of incidents is to create the "**perfect storm.**" The perfect storm begins with the scenario that we want to avoid. In our example, that would be a patient or participant fall. A diagram like the one used in Figures 1.5.9 and 1.5.10 can be used to record all the actions that would be taken to cause the event to happen.

As this technique causes us to think through the elements necessary to cause an untoward event, we start by listing the outcome we want to achieve—in this case, a patient fall. Next, we list everything we would do to make sure that the event occurs, such as making sure the patient is out of bed, the patient doesn't have socks on, the floor is wet, and so forth. After brainstorming all the possibilities, they are

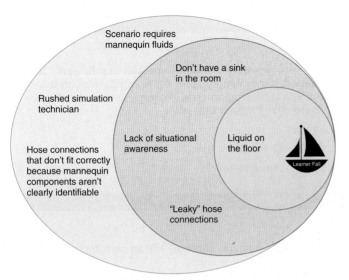

FIGURE 1.5.9 The perfect storm method: Patient fall example.

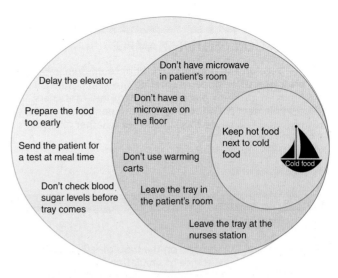

FIGURE 1.5.10 The perfect storm method: Cold food example.

grouped and arranged according to their proximity to the cause in a wave of events that lead to the outcome. With the diagram complete, potential issues can be addressed. This method is especially useful when an incident hasn't occurred or hasn't occurred with much frequency but still needs to be addressed.

Plan-Do-Check-Act/Plan-Do-Study-Act

Walter A. Shewhart first discussed the concept of **Plan-Do-Check-Act** (PDCA) in his 1939 book, *Statistical Method from the Viewpoint of Quality Control*. However, it was Shewart's protégé Deming who encouraged a systematic approach to problem solving and promoted the now widely recognized four-step process for continual improvement (Best & Neuhauser, 2006). Deming refers to it as the PDSA Cycle or the Shewhart Cycle. The Japanese call it the Deming Cycle. Others call it the PDCA Cycle or the Deming Wheel. Whatever the title, the purpose of the method is to continually assess and improve the system. The model can be used for the ongoing improvement of almost anything, and it contains the following four continuous steps:

Plan	Develop a plan for improving quality at a process
Do	Execute the plan, first on a small scale
Study/Check	Evaluate feedback to confirm or to adjust the plan
Act	Make the plan permanent or study the adjustments

The IHI has a PDSA template that can be downloaded from their Web site (IHI.org). This template provides a simple, straightforward way to address an issue. Utilizing one patient and one staff on one day to test whatever the small test of change may be can provide valuable information that can build to become a system-wide improvement.

Simulation is an important piece of the process improvement strategies to improve patient outcomes. Figure 1.5.11 shows how the PDSA process can be adapted to incorporate

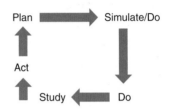

FIGURE 1.5.11 PDSA worksheet: Simulation center example.

simulation. Boxes 1.5.8 and 1.5.9 describe how this adaptation could be part of the improvement activities.

Six Sigma

Whereas the strength of Lean lies in providing a set of proven techniques for eliminating waste, Six Sigma provides a structured methodology on the basis of quantitative analysis for carrying out and sustaining initiatives. Lean and Six Sigma complement each other in driving process improvement and are often used together by quality programs. The standard Six Sigma methodology for process improvement is called the **DMAIC** process, an acronym that stands for the following steps:

Define the most important problem to resolve as determined by the "voice of the customer" (i.e., what the patient values most).

Measure the current performance of the process that is failing to meet objectives as determined by the voice of the customer.

Analyze the process to find cause-and-effect relationships (i.e., how independent or decision variables affect dependent or performance variables).

Improve the process by finding the solutions that best achieve the desired performance and then implement these solutions (this is where Lean solutions come into play).

Control the implemented process improvements through monitoring and feedback mechanisms.

BOX 1.5.8

SIMULATION CENTER EXAMPLE

Plan—Develop and update checklist of room preparation prior to staff or students entering site, and ensure that fluids are properly placed in the identified containers.

Do—Implement checklist for a 1-month period.

Study/Check—Analyze checklists to see whether all elements are being completed.

Act—Make necessary changes to checklist or process if needed. If completion rate is 100% and staff found the document helpful, consider making it permanent, thereby "hardwiring" it into the system.

BOX 1.5.9

HOSPITAL EXAMPLE

Plan—Develop fall scenario on the basis of fall prevention protocols with assistance of simulation staff, and have staff from the affected unit participate and test for competencies of fall protocol.

Do—Implement fall protocol scenario in the simulation center. Have all staff participate in simulation.

Study/Check—Analyze outcomes of staff performance and evaluate knowledge gaps.

Act—Reeducate staff on areas that were found deficient utilizing simulation and then retest. If significant deficiencies exist, should consider educating and testing all staff.

The DMAIC process is intended to be repeated as a cycle of continuous improvement as a means to objectively and quantitatively evaluate solutions.

Just as more complex systems restrict the number of different options the human mind is capable of considering, it also restricts the ability to quantitatively evaluate the impact of proposed solutions. This makes the selection difficult and forces one to resort to make a best-guess estimate of performance or allows strong-willed people to sway decisions.

Instead of relying on subjective opinions, simulation gives objective and accurate estimates of performance improvements. For example, when a new piece of equipment is being proposed, simulation can provide the vehicle by which the use (and misuse) can be determined, and potential errors can be mitigated before it ever touches a patient (Figure 1.5.12).

WHAT DO I NEED TO DO TO IMPROVE

Incorporating these tools into the simulation vocabulary is an important step in ensuring high-quality, safe learning opportunities. Taking a cue from healthcare, simulation administrators and educators should be reporting their quality and safety data to their administration. Adopting CQI can assist in assuring that processes are being utilized consistently throughout the facility. When issues arise, the performance improvement tools can be utilized to identify opportunities for improvement. Publicly reporting quality data that is not standardized provides little benefit or means of comparison; therefore, a standardized evaluation of learner's perception of the simulation center and education should be developed so that learner evaluations can be publicly reported and compared between simulation centers.

Variability between assessment mechanisms does not allow for comparison, and therefore a benchmark of acceptability cannot be defined. Certainly, within a simulation center, consistent use of an assessment tool allows for investigation of variability between sessions and over time, but little can be said about the simulation center as compared with other simulation programs.

Berwick has been quoted as saying, "Every system is perfectly designed to get the results it achieves" (Berwick, 1996), meaning that if four learners slip and fall per year in the simulation center, then the system currently in place

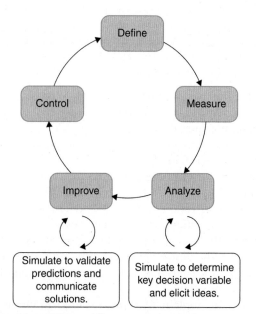

FIGURE 1.5.12   PDSA worksheet: Hospital example.

is designed for that to happen. Only by restructuring the system will different outcomes occur.

Restructuring the system requires investigating the incident and leading a team to implement a new system. If we look at the example from the simulation center, an RCA investigation may reveal multiple reasons that the learner fell during the scenario. These reasons include work production pressures (many classes for multiple days in a row), staffing availability (limited resources due to vacation), policy and procedures (filling of the equipment in the simulation space as opposed to another location), communication (between educator and technician), time pressure (limited time between scenarios and between moulage and simulation), environment (no drains in floor or poor choice of flooring), and inappropriate footwear by learner. These are only some of the potential causes of the participant's injury.

BEEN THERE, DONE THAT: HOW CAN I CONTINUE TO IMPROVE OR SUSTAIN WHAT I HAVE ACHIEVED?

It is essential that quality improvement activities have a lasting effect. Many staff will state that these initiatives are just the "flavor of the month" for the institution and with changes in the corporate leadership, so go the initiatives that are expected to be done by staff. This in turn with the daily challenges in both the simulation center and the inpatient environment makes changes incredibly difficult. However, with proper stewardship when launching new CQI initiates, staff will be able to interpret these initiatives and find ways to make them "stick" in their particular environment. It is essential that leadership ensures that staff are not overwhelmed and that their unique needs are met in light of the initiatives. In healthcare, we often do not stop long enough to notice the improvements that have been made. It is essential to celebrate the successes as it keeps people motivated and focused on the desired outcome. A simple "thank you" can go a long way.

Becoming an accredited simulation program by the Society for Simulation in Healthcare (SSH) is a goal for many centers. There are many standards that pertain to being a quality-based center of excellence. Throughout the core standards, there are expectations that sites have written plans for quality monitoring and improvement activities and have a demonstrated history of systematic, comprehensive, and ongoing quality improvement and performance improvement. The Systems Integration certification standards state that those simulation programs wishing to be recognized for their efforts must "function as an integrated institutional safety, quality, and risk management resource that uses systems engineering principles and engages in bi-directional feedback to achieve enterprise-level goals and improve quality of care" (Society

for Simulation in Healthcare, 2012). It is critical for the success of the center to be diligent in their documentation of their work as they progress through the various steps in the process of obtaining accreditation.

The inpatient scenario provided earlier provides a good example of how a simulation center could/should work with the organization in assisting with improvement in processes. It is essential that simulation centers work collaboratively with their inpatient partners to provide a vehicle by which continuous improvements will occur. Simulation center directors need to be part of the performance improvement committees as well as participants in RCAs. Quality and continual performance improvement is a cornerstone of a successful simulation program.

SUMMARY

CQI activities can improve the operations of the simulation center, allow the staff to respond to adverse events that take place in the simulation center, and potentially prevent dangerous situations. Being familiar with CQI concepts presented also allows the simulation staff to be integrated into the healthcare system. Simulation centers can be used to identify the root causes of actual adverse clinical events, identify potential system or equipment failures if used proactively, and develop corrective action plans to prevent adverse events in the future. The utility of simulation extends beyond clinical and interpersonal skills, and includes identifying and responding to system failures in an effort to improve the quality and safety of care.

The importance of healthcare providers—especially those involved in simulation—understanding the basic principles of quality and risk cannot be stressed enough. By understanding ways to analyze and improve quality, we can all help to make healthcare safer for the patients under our care.

REFERENCES

Agency for Healthcare Research and Quality. (n.d.). *Patient safety network glossary.* Retrieved from http://www.psnet.ahrq.gov/glossary.aspx#J

Berwick, D. (1996). A primer on leading the improvement of systems. *BMJ (Clinical research ed.), 312,* 619–622.

Best, M., & Neuhauser, D. (2005). W Edwards Deming: Father of quality management, patient and composer. *Quality and Safety in Health Care, 14*(4), 310–312. doi:10.1136/qshc.2005.015289

Best, M., & Neuhauser, D. (2006). Joseph Juran: Overcoming resistance to organizational change. *Quality and Safety in Health Care, 15*(5), 380–382. doi:10.1136/qshc.2006.020016

Goodman, J. C., Villarreal, P., & Jones, B. (2011). The social cost of adverse medical events, and what we can do about it. *Health Affairs, 30*(4), 590–595. doi:10.1377/hlthaff.2010.1256

Institute of Medicine. (2001). *Crossing the quality chasm: A new health system for the 21st century.* Washington, DC: National Academy Press.

Kohn, L. T., Corrigan, J., & Donaldson, M. S. (2000). *To err is human: Building a safer health system.* Washington, DC: National Academy Press.

Leape, L. (2000, January 25). *Testimony, United States Congress, United States Senate Subcommittee on Labor, Health and Human Services, and Education.*

Leape, L. L., Lawthers, A. G., Brennan, T. A., & Johnson, W. G. (1993). Preventing medical injury. *QRB. Quality Review Bulletin, 19*(5), 144–149.

Marx, D. (2001, April 17). *Patient safety and the "Just Culture": A primer for health care executives.* New York, NY: Columbia University and University of Texas Southwestern Medical Center in Dallas.

Neuhauser, D. (2002). Heroes and martyrs of quality and safety: Ernest Amory Codman MD. *Quality and Safety in Health Care, 11*(1), 104–105. doi:10.1136/qhc.11.1.104.

Ohno, T. (1988). *Toyota production system* (p. 58). New York, NY: Productivity Press.

Society for Simulation in Healthcare. (2012). *Accreditation standards.* Retreived from http://ssih.org/uploads/committees/2012%20Accreditation%20Standards39.pdf

Tennant, G. (2001). *Six sigma: SPC and TQM in manufacturing and services* (p. 6). Hampshire, England: Gower.

SECTION 2

Types of Simulation Programs

CHAPTER 2.1

Creating the Infrastructure for a Successful Simulation Program

Sara Kim, PhD, Wendy Hewitt, BSEE, Janine A. Buis, RN, BSN, BSHCA, MBA, and Brian K. Ross, MD, PhD

ABOUT THE AUTHORS

SARA KIM is the Director of Educational Innovations and Strategic Programs at the Institute for Simulation and Interprofessional Studies (ISIS), School of Medicine, University of Washington. She leads multiple initiatives to strengthen ISIS operational, training, and research capacity as well as implement local, regional, and national outreach programs for creating and sustaining a rich network of partners in simulation education and research. An active researcher, she focuses on improving interprofessional team communication skills.

WENDY HEWITT is the Operations Manager for the Hannaford Center for Safety, Innovation and Simulation, Department of Medical Education at Maine Medical Center. Since its opening in 2010, she has led the strategic and operational efforts of the Hannaford Simulation Center, which includes a leadership role on the Simulation Governance Committee and an active member of the Society for Simulation in Healthcare Director's SIG. She led the Hannaford Simulation Center through two successful organizational restructuring efforts.

JANINE A. BUIS manages the Community Health Education and Simulation Center, Education Service for Nursing, and the system-wide Learning Management system. She manages and teaches a variety of programs and enterprises in both the hospital system and the community setting. Janine facilitates the collaboration between a variety of healthcare entities to provide educational opportunities for educators, healthcare providers, and community members. She also assists educators and clinical staff in their professional development.

BRIAN K. ROSS is the Executive Director of the Institute for Simulation and Interprofessional Studies (ISIS), School of Medicine, University of Washington. In 1994, Ross established the first medical simulation center in the University of Washington School of Medicine (SOM) housed in the Department of Anesthesiology. Since then, he has been a champion and leader in the SOM for all the major simulation initiatives.

Acknowledgments: Peter M. Wiser Institute for Simulation Education and Research, University of Pittsburgh, Pittsburgh, PA.

ABSTRACT

The main goal of this chapter is to illustrate how both mission and vision statements of simulation programs can be used to guide an organizational structure, governance, and staffing model to support the mission and vision of the program or institution. A simulation infrastructure that is consistently aligned with the strategic direction of a simulation program contributes to advancing the organizational mission and vision. Conversely, when the infrastructure is misaligned, the mission and vision can lose their core focus, leading to missed opportunities for innovations, inefficiencies in resource and personnel deployment, and low staff morale. In this chapter, three examples of basic organizational models of simulation programs all requiring very different infrastructures to meet their mission and vision are provided: (1) A program focused on resident/fellow, clinical professionals, and medical student training; (2) A program focused on patient safety, quality, training, and research initiatives; and (3) A program focused on community outreach, including nurse training programs and K-12. A description of roles and responsibilities are provided in each model section. The conclusion provides a set of recommendations for simulation program leaders to consider when they may be involved with creating a new entity; reviewing and/or structuring a currently existing entity; or serving as advisors or consultants to other internal and external organizations.

CASE EXAMPLE

Kay arrived at her first day on the job as operations manager for a brand-new simulation center. She had just finished meeting her team of four new employees for the first time. What was to follow included several meetings with senior leadership and multiple internal stakeholder groups. Her head was filled with the following questions:

1. What is the purpose of the new simulation center?
2. Who are the stakeholders that are concerned with the center's activities?
3. What are the short- and long-term goals?
4. Who are our customers?
5. What assets are at my disposal such as staff, finances (capital dollars, operational funding), and facilities/space?
6. What underlying infrastructure could I depend on from the hospital, such as marketing, payroll, HR, benefits?

These are fundamental questions that every new business needs to ask of itself. A simulation center is no different. Quite frankly, in Kay's mind this was a start-up business, and all of these questions needed to be answered. Fortunately for Kay, her leadership had already developed an excellent business plan and strategic plan (see chapters 4.4 and 5.3). In many situations, this is not the case, and many new operational managers find themselves handed the reins of a center without a clear blueprint. When that happens, a set of foundation plans must be written before the work of making the center operational can begin.

In the process of writing plans for this center, Kay's leadership took the time to research several simulation centers nationally and internationally, realizing that this process might identify some basic fundamental principles, but that each center will be driven by very contextualized forces and requirements. The review was comprised of interviews with the respective leadership and collecting significant benchmark data pertaining to the questions posed above. One key question they tried to address was how to appropriately configure the operational components of the center. This included settling on the governance of the organization, designing the organizational chart, and developing the respective roles, responsibilities, and job descriptions of the employees.

Since Kay's team was hired prior her arrival, her first challenge was getting to know each of the employees personally, assessing their strengths and weaknesses, and performing a gap analysis with respect to the job descriptions and the current organizational chart. She then reviewed the overall description/purpose of the center, as defined in the mission and vision, particularly in reference to the depth and breadth of skills available in the team. She had to answer the following questions: "Do I have the right mix of talent?" "Is everyone in the right role for the center to be successful?" "If not, what changes need to be made and how quickly?" As the leader of the center, it will be Kay's responsibility to determine the gaps in the organization and make decisions on the best way to bridge those gaps over time.

INTRODUCTION, BACKGROUND, AND SIGNIFICANCE

There are many factors that contribute to a successful operation of a simulation program. These factors support the educational, research, patient safety and quality mission of a simulation entity and include both human and technical infrastructure, for example, leadership buy-in, organizational governance, stable funding source, and adequate administrative and technical staffing (Kim et al., 2011). A common definition of "infrastructure" typically includes the enabling components that are necessary for a program to be successful. The cornerstone of a simulation program's infrastructure is a talented team that brings the program to life. Fostering a successful team requires that due diligence is applied up-front to clearly map out the needs of the program and critical resources to meet the goals and objectives.

A simulation infrastructure that is consistently aligned with the strategic direction of a simulation program contributes to advancing the organizational mission and vision. Conversely, when the infrastructure is misaligned, the mission and vision can lose their core focus, leading to missed opportunities for innovations, inefficiencies in resource, personnel deployment, and low staff morale. This chapter illustrates how different mission and vision statements of simulation programs are used to guide the development of an organizational structure as well as the governance and staffing model to support the mission and vision.

A review of key elements that facilitate a simulation program's infrastructure plan provides a stage for understanding the need for a mission- and vision-guided organizational structure. A strategic plan—the overall plan that both defines the end goals and identifies how one intends to meet the goals—is an "ends" and "means"

SECTION 2 • Types of Simulation Programs

summary. Within the strategic plan, one will typically see both the mission and vision statements for the organization (see chapter 5.3). In comparison, the business plan is a living and breathing document that should be flexible enough to change with market and economic pressures as well as business fluctuations. The business plan outlines in greater detail more of the daily operations (see chapter 4.4), and the best means of achieving the goals outlined in the *Strategic Plan*.

It is important not to confuse vision and mission statements. Sometimes, they are used interchangeably, but they are, in fact, very different. The vision statement summarizes "where one wants to be" once the goals and objectives have been met. For example, a group might self-describe their vision as wanting to "End World Hunger."

The mission statement succinctly describes how one will accomplish the vision. It answers the question "Why do we exist?" In the example above, the mission needs to reflect "how" the vision will be accomplished—such as "give a man bread and feed him for a day, but teach him to farm and feed him for life".

What flows into an infrastructure plan is derived from the *Strategic Plan* in combination with the institution's mission and vision statements. As a leader designing the infrastructure for the program, he/she needs to identify the key elements that are essential to success. One has to be realistic and identify the most critical pieces of the infrastructure, without which the program will fall short of fulfilling its core mandate.

Every institution has both a reporting structure and a governance model. A simulation program will reside within an organization's reporting structure on the basis of the business model of the organization. The responsibility of managing the simulation program's operating budgets, strategic plans, and capital investments needs to be reported up through this organizational structure. However, there is the need for a secondary level of governance that is aligned with the simulation program's internal organization. Part of the governance comes from within the structure mentioned above, but there needs to be a way for the "influencers" and "stakeholders" of the simulation program to get their voices heard. Furthermore, it is important to pull together senior leadership within the organization to provide strategic guidance as the program matures. The leadership can serve as the rudder and compass as the program navigates its way through a sea of overwhelming requests for services. They are the program's allies as policies and procedures are built to filter requests, manage tough budgetary issues, and prioritize business opportunities for the program.

To help bring some clarity to this process, three specific examples are presented here that demonstrate how different types of organizations have applied this model. The institutions are first described briefly, identifying their setting, customers, and then mission and vision statements. Details follow on how each institution aligned their mission statements with the design of their respective organizational charts.

METHODS

As an illustration of the critical importance of aligning a simulation program's mission and vision with an appropriate infrastructure and personnel mix, three simulation programs were selected to illustrate unique and varied organizational models. The first model represents a simulation program in a large community hospital and tertiary care center, whose mission supports medical research along with the education of residents/fellows, clinical professionals, and medical students. The second model represents a simulation institute that is integral to the patient safety, quality, training, and research mission of an academic medical center with the main constituents including residents, practicing physicians, and interprofessional providers. The third model is a simulation program in a community-based medical center with a primary mandate for community outreach, including nurse training programs, K-12, and supporting the hospital education with simulation opportunities. These models stem from the authors' current organizations that richly reflect diversity and synergistic organizational structures to illustrate the key points highlighted in this chapter.

The descriptive profile of each of the simulation models provided below has a specific focus on how the evolving mission and vision impact the organizational structure and staffing needs. The analyses are grouped into three distinct sections to illustrate how each of the models compares and contrasts. The first section describes a high-level overview of each program's facility, the second section contains the current vision and mission statements of each program, and the third section describes and discusses both the governance models and organizational structures that support these programs.

EXAMPLE 1

Hannaford Center for Safety, Innovation and Simulation—Education-Centered Mission and Vision

A. **Setting:** Large hospital (600+ bed facility, 6,000+ employees), premier referral and tertiary care hospital in the state of Maine. The Hannaford Simulation Center occupies the entire third floor of a rehabilitation hospital, located 1.8 miles (approximately 3 km) from the main hospital campus, and has a dedicated Simulation Van to support **in situ** (off-site) events.

B. **Customers:** Undergraduate Medical Education (UME) Program, Graduate Medical Education (GME) Program, Continuing Medical Education (CME), nursing department, attending physicians and ancillary clinical staff, affiliate hospitals, and other outside entities throughout the state.

C. **Major Funding Source:** The majority of funding comes directly from the hospital. The Hannaford Simulation Center is looking for alternate funding sources, including donations, grants, and possibly charging for courses delivered to nonhospital entities.

D. **Vision Statement:** "The Hannaford Center for Safety, Innovation and Simulation, at Maine Medical Center, will strive to become a highly regarded, nationally accredited, multidisciplinary learning environment. Using sophisticated simulation technologies and educational practices, we will enhance the quality of care and patient safety at our hospital and throughout the state of Maine. Providing a safe, learner-focused, and patient-oriented environment, the center will promote the inclusion of simulation into the training of all healthcare providers. By active engagement in simulation-based research, the center will become a laboratory that discovers and disseminates the highest standards of medical education and clinical care. We will serve as a unique resource to other healthcare providers and educators in the region."

E. **Mission Statement:** "Our Mission is to research and advance the delivery of high quality, safe, and effective patient care throughout the institution and the region by integrating cutting-edge simulation technologies and educational practices into the training of all learners in a safe, interactive, and transformative environment."

F. **Organizational Governance:** The hospital has 11 specialty departments that support the education of 240 residents and fellows across 19 Accreditation Council for Graduate Medical Education (**ACGME**) accredited programs. In addition, in 2009, Maine Medical Center (MMC) formed a medical education partnership with Tufts University School of Medicine (TUSM), creating an education track called the "TUSM-MMC Maine Track Program." The program includes 36 students per year and provides a unique curriculum, focused on rural education. The students spend the majority of their first 2 years on the Boston campus and complete the remainder of their education at both MMC and in other hospitals and communities around the state of Maine.

Organizationally, it was decided that the best position for the new Hannaford Simulation Center was that it be embedded in the Department of Medical Education and reporting up through the Division of Medical and Academic Affairs (Figure 2.1.1).

It was recognized that the simulation center had a unique vision and mission and that the potential positive impact of such a facility would have far-reaching implications, not only within the walls of the hospital, but to the community, the region, and throughout the state.

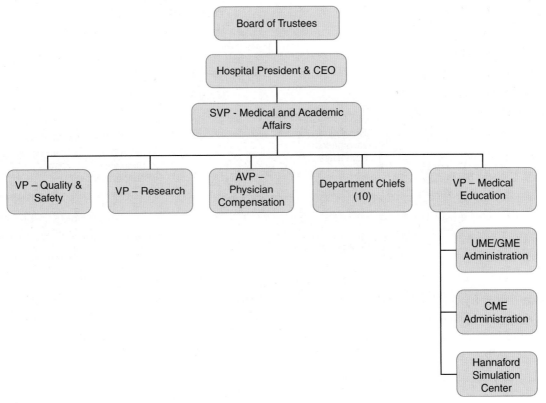

FIGURE 2.1.1 Organizational reporting structure for the Hannaford Simulation Center.

Figure 2.1.2 represents a combination of the priority initiatives within MMC along with major committees that were formed within the first year to help guide the center through its start-up challenges.

- The **Simulation Governance Committee.** This committee is responsible for reviewing and overseeing ongoing simulation-related operational goals, costs, and planning and development activities as well as prioritizing spending (of operational and capital budgets) for all Hannaford Simulation Center activities and projects. This committee ensures that the needs of the primary key audiences as well as of the hospital and community at large are being evaluated and addressed within the operational capabilities of the simulation center.

- The **Simulation Education and Research Committee**. This committee is comprised of the simulation faculty champions within the hospital, representing each department and discipline. This committee is charged with:
  - Development of department-specific simulation curriculum.
  - Development of common curriculum that can be leveraged across all the departments.
  - Evaluation and recommendations regarding lab-related training devices and equipment.
  - Development of clinical/educational research protocols relevant to the simulation environment.
- The **Undergraduate Medical Education Committee**. This committee is comprised of course directors (clerkship, 4th year, foundational courses),

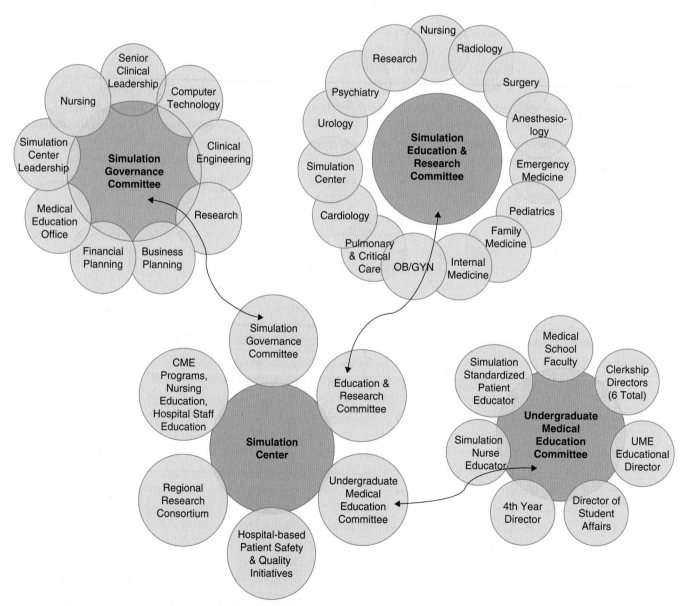

FIGURE 2.1.2   Primary stakeholders, customers, and programs developed within the first 2 years of the Hannaford Simulation Center's existence.

including senior faculty from the TUSM, clinical directors from our partner sites around the state of Maine, GME program directors, nursing, administration, and educators (nurse educator and standardized patient educator) from within the Hannaford Simulation Center. This committee is charged with reviewing and vetting innovative ideas and proposed changes to the TUSM-MMC curriculum to ensure the program is meeting all the required curricular elements of the Tufts curriculum.

- **Regional Research Consortium**. In 2011, the Hannaford Simulation Center spearheaded the creation of a regional research consortium with other simulation centers in the northeast. The Northern New England Simulation Education and Research Consortium (**NNESERC**) is a group of clinicians and educators from regional centers of excellence in healthcare education who have joined together voluntarily in a joint effort to advance the quality and effectiveness of simulation-based medical education for all healthcare professionals and to further the cause of high-quality health education outcomes research. The NNESERC's mission is to provide quality and safety in healthcare by fostering cooperation, dissemination of information, collaborative research, educational program sharing, and the development of standardized methods of training and measurement across participating consortium simulation centers. The consortium's ultimate goal is to link state-of-the-art techniques in healthcare education with improved patient outcomes and safer patient care in a cost-effective manner. (For more information on the NNESERC, please visit www.nneserc.org.)

G. **Department Staffing Model**: In 2010, the Hannaford Simulation Center's original organizational chart consisted of the following roles to support the day-to-day operations of the facility: Simulation medical director (0.5 FTE), operations manager (1.0 FTE), nurse educator (1.0 FTE), simulation administrative coordinator (1.0 FTE), chief simulation specialist (1.0 FTE), simulation specialists (2.0 FTEs), IT analyst (1.0 FTE), standardized patient educator (1.0 FTE), for a total of 8.5 FTEs. A brief job description of the core roles is as follows:

- **Simulation Medical Director** (0.5 FTE)—He/she needed to be a clinical professional, preferably an MD. Needed to not only demonstrate a passion for simulation, but also have first-hand experience in the industry. Be a visionary and evangelist for simulation-based education and research, with the ability to navigate the political dark alleys as well as the bright lights of the Board Room.
- **Nurse Educator** (1.0 FTE)—This role was critical to the development and delivery of the clinically sound high-fidelity scenarios and skills events.

The nurse educator would be responsible for working with each of the department program directors and faculty, and guiding them through the process of developing their simulation cases. This individual would also be the focal point for coordinating and scheduling the high-fidelity and skills activities for the center, working closely with the simulation team members to ensure resources were secured (people, equipment, and space). A registered nurse (RN) was the starting point, then we searched for someone with the passion for raising the education and clinical expertise within the hospital, and someone who knew the ropes of the organization politically. It would be ideal if this person were already a basic and advanced life support instructor and possibly a unit-based educator in the hospital. The individual also needed to have a passion for learning new technology and an open mind for new and inventive ways to teach clinical learning objectives.

- **Information Technology (IT) Analyst** (1.0 FTE)—To say that this position initially received significant pushback is a gross understatement. Many stakeholders in the process voiced strong opposition to this role, insisting that all IT support should be part of the hospital's enterprise IT organization. The team knew that this start-up business was going to push the envelope with new technology and the infrastructure would not look anything like the enterprise system deployed throughout the hospital. The simulation center was unique by design, and would require instantaneous support for a wide range of technology issues. Consensus was finally reached that the level of support and attention the simulation center required could not be guaranteed by the hospital's IT department. In the end, placing this position within the center's organizational structure was one of the best decisions made.

The IT analyst had several responsibilities: maintenance and support of all hardware/software in the center, which included the video-conferencing system, audio/visual/recording and scheduling system, the IT server room, built-in overhead projector systems, and supporting all computer-related equipment (laptops, Windows and Macintosh operating system [OS] desktops), i-Pads, all-in-one devices, mannequin laptops, just to name a few. It was believed that this person should be an internal hire because to be successful right out of the gate, he/she needed a strong professional relationship with the hospital's IT group. A huge component of the job would rely on getting real-time support in areas that touched the hospital's enterprise environment (i.e., wifi system, failover system, etc.). He/she would also need to have keen troubleshooting and debugging skills. A lot of what was initially installed in the center would need to be modified or built upon over time. This person would also be relied upon to create and maintain databases, work with vendors (obtain quotes, create functional objective specifications, request for quotes, develop/execute/verify test plans, etc., then supervise the work once a bid was accepted), and would be our technical expert supporting our external and internal Web presences (Intranet and Internet). He/she needed strong project management skills because many of the challenges would require bringing a team together to get the job done (internal and external technology-specific resources).

• **Chief Simulation Specialist** (1.0 FTE)—Ideally, this would be someone who had several years of hands-on experience as a simulation specialist, working with a wide range of mannequins, task trainers, and the like. The chief simulation specialist would have several years running high-fidelity events and be well-versed in the overall process of developing/delivering a clinical scenario, and the ability to work well with physicians and other clinical professionals. In addition, the individual would need to possess expertise with the control rooms, be familiar with multiple versions of computers and software, and very familiar with the audio/visual world. It would be ideal if this person was an RN or a respiratory therapist, but at a minimum, he/she needed to have experience as an emergency medical technician (EMT).

The overall strategy in hiring this person was for the individual to mentor the two simulation specialists and quickly get them prepared to work in the high-fidelity and skills arenas. The goal was to introduce learners to the high-fidelity simulation in a way that helped them suspend reality and make the learning experiences come to life. The chief simulation specialist would be the cornerstone in building an expert simulation staff to run all high-fidelity events and support all skills-related training. The role also included managing the preventive maintenance (PM) schedules for all the simulation equipment, building a comprehensive inventory management system, and preparing annual operation budgets to support high-fidelity and skills events. It was critical to have the means to forecast when the simulation equipment needed OS upgrades and firmware/hardware upgrades, to track equipment usage and forecast when components would need to be repaired or replaced. (E.g., rubber materials degrade over time even if they are not used. What is the expected life of a material? Task trainers that are frequently stuck with needles will eventually reach the end of their useful life based on the

number of needle sticks. At what point are they beyond repair?) This person would be responsible for tracking the useful life of all the equipment in the labs, for building an annual operation budget forecast that incorporates the replacement/repair costs of all equipment, track and manage all service contracts and warranties, and build an internal tracking system for maintaining levels of disposable medical supplies.

• **Simulation Specialists (2.0 FTEs)**—Initially, the simulation specialists would be hired for their expert knowledge in the clinical arenas, and we envisioned hiring them from within the hospital. They needed to be experts in operating room and intensive care unit spaces of the hospital, instinctually knowing how a specific clinical setting should look, what typical medical supplies were needed in these spaces and why, how to operate all the clinical equipment with ease, and have a well-established network within the hospital. Once on board, an aggressive cross-training plan would be developed and executed by the chief simulation specialist, and in turn the chief simulation specialist would receive training on the inner workings of the clinical environments from the simulation specialists.

The simulation specialists would be responsible for the setup and teardown of high-fidelity and skills rooms, care and maintenance of all equipment (mannequins, trainers, virtual trainers), programming the complete family of mannequins, moulage techniques, how to set up and teach faculty how to use the wide array of virtual trainers, assist in the development of policies and procedures for all events that take place in the high-fidelity and skills areas, ensure all medical supplies are tracked during each event and reordered as needed, perform frequent preventive maintenance on all mannequins and trainers, and become intimately familiar with all the technology in the control rooms (including the specialized software used to schedule and record all the events).

• **Standardized Patient Educator** (1.0 FTE)—At the Hannaford Simulation Center, an entire wing was initially built to support the UME program in the form of a standardized patient lab. Very much like the nurse educator, this person needed to develop a close relationship with the Tufts Medical School faculty and help them develop Objective Structured Clinical Examination (OSCE) cases to enrich the learning of the medical school students and Objective Structured Teaching Events (OSTE) for the faculty. The standardized patient (SP) educator would be charged with operationalizing the SP Lab, which included managing an entire pool of SPs (ongoing recruiting, hiring, firing,

SIMULATION PROGRAM SCHEDULING

Chad A. Epps, MD, and Penni I. Watts, MSN, RN, CHSE

Effective scheduling in a busy simulation program is essential for efficient operation. This includes scheduling of program resources (educators, technicians, equipment), courses, learners, and even visitors. Designing a scheduling framework may be time-consuming, but if done well will save the program time, aggravation, and even money. When developing a scheduling framework, programs should consider factors such as course load, capacity for learners, space, equipment, and staff requirements (educators, technicians, etc.). Close attention should be given to ensure that the scheduling framework is appropriate for the program's hours of operations and provides flexibility (if desired) to meet needs outside of the normal operating schedule.

Simulation programs often underestimate the amount of time and resources (staff) necessary for course setup and breakdown. Careful consideration needs to be given to ensure that these essential activities are appropriately included in the scheduling framework. In addition, successful simulation programs often reserve days (or weeks) where no activity is occurring to ensure proper time for center maintenance, team huddles, professional development, and so on. Once a framework for scheduling has been designed, the schedules should be published and updated, regulated, and monitored for any feedback that would indicate the need to revise the framework.

Many scheduling solutions are available to meet the needs of simulation programs. Smaller programs sometimes find a simple Outlook or Google calendar to suffice for their scheduling needs. Inevitably, however, as the program grows, the demands outpace the capabilities of simpler solutions, so taking time to investigate scalable solutions is a wise choice. There are scheduling systems designed specifically for simulation programs, while others are more generic in their application. Simulation programs that are linked to a larger organization may benefit greatly by using a scheduling system that is already in use even if it is not specifically designed for a simulation program. These systems are sometimes limited in their ability to specifically track simulation resources, but may be modified to meet basic needs. The cost savings associated with using a system in place within the larger organization may outweigh any limitations.

Advanced enterprise solutions built specifically for simulation programs vary greatly in their sophistication and specificity to simulation. Factors that should be considered include the following:

1. What type of simulation program are you? Some scheduling systems are better suited for standardized patient programs, while others are better for programs using mannequin-based or team simulations.
2. How will learners and educators access your system? In the event learners and educators will be accessing the scheduling system, programs should consider how they will be registered. Some systems allow self-registration, requiring users to remember an additional log-in and password, while others offer a form of LDAP integration where users are authenticated using an already-assigned log-in and password from the institution.
3. What is your process for scheduling an event? Ease of scheduling an event can be a factor, especially when resources are scheduled with the event (simulators, staff, equipment, etc.). Some scheduling systems, particularly those with Web- or cloud-based interfaces, can be simple to use. Some interfaces require a laborious series of "clicks" to schedule an event with multiple resources. A feature to look for in a scheduling system is ease of assigning recurrent courses or ease of copying and pasting courses.

4. Do you want your schedule to be available publicly? Some scheduling systems allow for a public-facing interface and calendar, while others do not. If programs have multiple sites with different calendars, consideration should be given to the ability of the scheduling system to merge multiple schedules and resource utilization into an overarching organizational calendar.
5. How are learners assigned to courses? Assuming a program is using its scheduling solution for more than just scheduling space, some consideration should be given to the process for learners to be added to a course. Some systems allow learners to self-register for courses, while others require learners to be "dropped in" the course by an administrator. The latter option will require greater administrative support. In the event learners will be relied on for self-registration into courses, you need to ensure that there is an easy way to point learners to the appropriate course or, at the very least, that searching the calendar can be done with ease.
6. What is the pricing structure? Some scheduling systems require an up-front investment, while others are on annual terms. Programs should consider whether the system adjusts pricing depending on the number of users and whether there is a maintenance cost in addition to the license purchase.
7. What resources can be tracked and how? Some programs are only interested in scheduling space/rooms, while others would like to track usage of simulators, task trainers, technicians, educators, learners, and so on. Also, additional functionality may be required if a program wishes to track resource utilization at a higher level (by client or department, for instance).
8. What types of notifications are needed for your program? Scheduling solutions often include a system of notifying the learners and instructors of assignments, locations, changes, and so on. It is important to investigate the level of notification required for the program's users and either develop a process for internal notifications or ensure the scheduling solution's notification capabilities are adequate.
9. What staff effort is required for managing the system? Some systems require a great deal of effort by system administrators, while other systems rely on users (learners and educators) to manage content and scheduling.
10. Do you want to be part of an "early-adopter" club? Many of the currently available enterprise solutions for simulation scheduling and program management are in their infancy. A great deal of patience may be required in dealing with these vendors. It is wise in this situation to consider avoiding a long-term agreement in the event the vendor is unable to deliver a product that meets the program's needs.
11. Are there management needs beyond scheduling? There are multiple enterprise solutions available that have capacity well beyond scheduling; these capabilities may be included but most often are modules that can be added for an additional price. Programs that desire additional functionality in course/program evaluation, learner assessment, simulation content management, and/or digital recording should investigate the options available.
12. What reports can be generated? Do you depend on your scheduling system to calculate your utilization rates by learners? Learner experiences? Faculty? Learning programs? How accurate does this need to be? Do you depend on these reports to determine bills for your funding sources? Some scheduling systems are very detailed—offer options for generating different reports—while some allow estimates.

training, and scheduling). It would be ideal to hire an RN, but not critical. More important was that this person was detail-oriented, organized, and with a strong educational background in the development and delivery of teaching curriculum.

- **Simulation Administrative Coordinator** (1.0 FTE)—This person would have the primary responsibility for supporting the needs of the simulation medical director and operations manager. The coordinator would work closely with the nurse educator and assist with the scheduling of events on the center's event calendar, ensuring there were no double bookings, and help minimize conflicts. This individual needed to be an expert in Microsoft Office applications, extremely well organized, and possess superior skills in multitasking.
- **Operations Manager** (1.0 FTE)—The center had filled the position of simulation medical director first. He was an anesthesiologist for half a week and simulation medical director for the other half. This meant that the operations manager would be required to represent the simulation medical director when he was absent. Unlike a few of the roles for the simulation center, this position did not absolutely require a clinical background. Instead, the center needed someone with a strong propensity for finances, someone who was extremely detail-oriented, possessed strong project management skills, and was very organized. This individual would have a business background, possess excellent team-building and people skills, and be politically savvy. The operations manager needed to be adept at creating policies and procedures, and business case development (including budgetary design and justification). In addition, this

position would be responsible for managing the department staff, budgets (capital and operations), developing/refining the business plan over time, and ensuring that the simulation center met its strategic goals. This meant opening the search beyond the walls of the hospital and reaching out to those with a background in business, technology, and even engineering disciplines (Figure 2.1.3).

In the first 3 years since its grand opening, the Hannaford Simulation Center has made several enhancements. These changes were necessary for several reasons:

- The initial gap analysis was completed within the first year. We analyzed the skills of the team and the demands placed on the center, and two roles were completely rewritten in order to align with the needs of the center.
  - Redesigned the role of **IT analyst**, changed the title to a **projectmanager** (1.0 FTE), and wrote a new job description.
  - Redesigned the role of **chief simulation specialist**. The position title was changed to **simulation lab supervisor** (1.0 FTE), and a new job description was written. After 2 years of developing and delivering high-fidelity and skills events, we realized it would be ideal for this role to include the requirement for RN background with several years of both clinical and managerial experience, and preferably hire someone from within the hospital that had already developed a strong professional network.
- Upon review of the first 2 years of activity and the mix of courses and attendees, models were created to help forecast the volume and type of activity that would come to the center over the next few years. In the end, the hiring of two additional

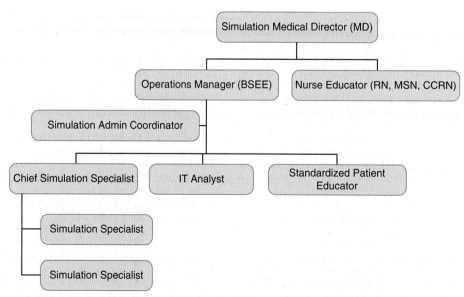

FIGURE 2.1.3   The 2010 organizational chart for the Hannaford Simulation Center.

full-time staff was justified. These included the following:

- Another **simulation specialist** (1.0 FTE), who was added to the team to bring the overall total to 3.0 FTEs.
- A new position called **standardized patient program coordinator** (1.0 FTE) was created requiring a new job description. This person would take ownership of the SP scheduling system, maintain the SP database, be responsible for scheduling the recruitment, orientation, and training of the SPs, and serve as the SP educator's right hand in operationalizing the standardized patient lab.

The organizational chart for the Hannaford Simulation Center currently looks like the one shown in Figure 2.1.4.

EXAMPLE 2

Institute for Simulation and Interprofessional Studies (**ISIS**)—Patient Safety, Quality, Research-Centered Mission and Vision

A. **Setting**: The simulation institute is located in an academic medical center that consists of four hospitals, including community-based hospitals and a Level I adult and pediatric trauma and burn center, serving a five-state region. The medical school is situated in a unique regional context, as it is the only school in the five-state region, therefore serving the healthcare needs of the citizens across a vast geographic distribution.

B. **Customers**: The simulation institute serves a diverse range of constituents, including health science students (medical, nursing, pharmacy, physician assistant, social work), residents from multiple specialties, nursing staff, and faculty across the academic medical center. The institute annually hosts large-scale interprofessional student training programs in team care. In addition, the institute provides leadership in developing patient safety and quality e-learning modules in areas of the clinical enterprise priorities. Lastly, the institute is a national **TeamSTEPPS** training center (Team Strategies and Tools to Enhance Performance and Patient Safety), providing training to over 300 national trainers from hospitals, clinics, and healthcare programs. (See teamstepps.ahrq.gov.)

C. **Major Funding Source**: Three major funding sources support the operation of the simulation institute: the medical school and two hospitals. The simulation institute also receives a significant amount of extramural grant funding to support its research and development efforts.

D. **Vision Statement**: "To provide leadership in the use of simulation techniques, technologies and resources to advance the quality of healthcare education and improve patient safety and outcomes via innovations and research."

E. **Mission Statement**: "To train healthcare providers and trainees to be effective, efficient clinicians in their medical and technical knowledge, adept communicators within teams and competent in their interprofessional team-based care."

F. **Organizational Governance and Chart**: The simulation institute was established in response to a need

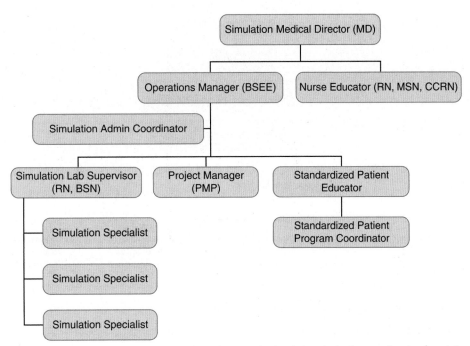

FIGURE 2.1.4 Hannaford Simulation Center—how the organizational chart looks 3 years after the Grand Opening.

SECTION 2 • Types of Simulation Programs

for a centralized multidisciplinary center of simulation expertise at the organization. Over 30 departments in SOM, programs, and their faculty became affiliated to the simulation institute, thus fulfilling a unique vision of a central governance model at our institution. Figure 2.1.5 illustrates the initial governance structure of the simulation institute. The institute created a Board that consists of multiple stakeholders from the medical school (vice dean of academic affairs, vice dean of graduate medical education, associate deans, and department chairs) and from the clinical enterprise. The Chair of the Department of Surgery that administratively houses the simulation institute serves as the Board Chair, who is supported by an executive committee that consists of the following: the executive director of the institute, senior executive advisor, chief executive officers, chief medical officers, chief nursing officers, and the chairs of Curriculum Development Committee, Research and Development Committee, and Patient Safety and Quality Committee. These last three committees were established to develop the critical educational, research, patient safety, and quality infrastructure for the new simulation institution.

The key mandate of the *Curriculum Committee* was to create simulation-based curriculum materials in collaboration with clinician-educator faculty whose roles largely involve teaching. These curriculum materials were submitted to a national peer-review system, such as the Association of American Medical Colleges' (**AAMC**) MedEdPORTAL, in order that the faculty members who author curricula receive scholarly credits for their promotion in an academic medical center. (See www.mededportal.org for more information.)

The *Research and Development (R&D) Committee* was created to develop an infrastructure for building a research capacity, such as identifying projects, writing grants, recruiting subjects, collecting research data, and so on. The committee hosts a monthly forum to showcase ongoing simulation-based research projects, to brainstorm on grant proposals, and to invite guest speakers from the wider university community to foster collaborations.

The *Patient Safety and Quality Committee* was established to position the simulation institute as an operational arm of the clinical enterprise and identify the hospital's priority patient safety and quality targets that can be addressed via simulation-based interventions. The chair of this committee participated as a member on the clinical enterprise quality committee as a way to facilitate this synergy. The initial administrative support at the simulation institute included a full-time administrator, a program coordinator, a technician, and a scientific instructional technician.

After 3 years of operation, the institute faced a turning point in its need to revise the mission to explicitly embrace the growing trends in integrating simulation into interprofessional team training. Thus, the institute shifted its governance and strategic focus away from being medicine-centric to being interprofessionally oriented in its scope. Figure 2.1.6 illustrates how a modified governance structure reflects this change in the renewed

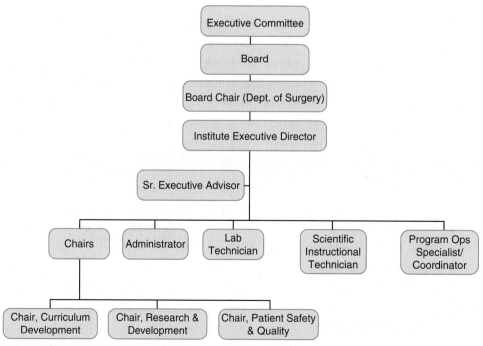

FIGURE 2.1.5 Initial Simulation Institute governance structure.

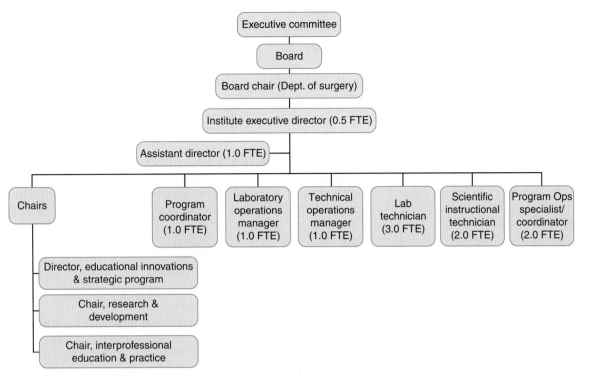

FIGURE 2.1.6 Modified Simulation Institute governance structure.

mission. Compared with the initial governance structure, the major change included creating a new committee, *Interprofessional Education and Practice Committee*, headed by a nationally renowned interprofessional education expert with a mandate to create a network of colleagues to advance interprofessional teamwork both at the health sciences students' level and at the practice level.

While the commitment to developing simulation-based curriculum remains strong, the institute created a full-time position staffed by an education faculty member to help advance the educational efforts of the institute at the larger organizational level and engage in ongoing strategic initiatives that sustain the value of the institute in both the educational and clinical enterprises.

The purposeful emphasis of the institute's mission on interprofessional teamwork and team communication led to institutionally visible initiatives as follows:

• Serving as the TeamSTEPPS training center for master trainer certification
• Implementing in situ, point-of-care simulation-based mock code blue response and emergency medicine training
• Developing and implementing large-scale simulation-based team training involving health sciences students

The ongoing research efforts have also resulted in productive outcomes such as securing funding from the Department of Defense and Internal Patient Safety Innovations Project that have enabled

the institute to pursue cutting-edge simulation-based educational practices and research.

G. **Staffing Model:** The institute currently has the following staff dedicated to the day-to-day operations: Executive Director (0.5 FTE), Associate Director (0.25 FTE), Assistant Director (1.0 FTE), Director of Educational Innovations and Strategic Programs (1.0 FTE), Program Operations Specialists (2.0 FTEs), Laboratory Operations Manager (1.0 FTE), Technical Operations Manager (1.0 FTE), Laboratory Technicians (3.0 FTEs), Scientific Instructional Technician (2.0 FTEs), and Program Coordinator (1.0 FTE) for a total of 11.5 FTEs.

A brief job description of the core roles follows.

• **Program Operations Specialist** (2.0 FTEs): The Program Operations Specialist is responsible for the programmatic and operational support and reports to the Administrator for ISIS with a matrix-designed reporting relationship to the Executive Director of ISIS. The individual in this position organizes the operations of the Program and manages and coordinates its activities with responsibilities to include oversight of educational proposal and events, creation of materials for publication, and management of ISIS expenditures in particular areas.

The major aspects of this position fall into the following four categories:

• Development of educational program, events, and governance operations (approximately 60%)
• Management of ISIS research and development operations (approximately 20%)

- Management of ISIS publications (approximately 15%)
- Grants, contracts, and financial operational duties (approximately 5%)

  A portion of this position's time is applying appropriate financial policies and procedures and appropriately expending ISIS funds within the scope of the position.
- **Lab Operations Manager** (1.0 FTE): The Lab Operations Manager is responsible for the operational coordination and reports to the Administrator for ISIS with a matrixed reporting relationship to the Executive Director of ISIS. The individual organizes and oversees the operations of the ISIS simulation labs and provides support to ISIS research projects. The individual supervises lab technicians and is involved in hiring, training, and supervision on a day-to-day basis. The Lab Operations Manager is responsible for seeing that the labs are appropriately staffed at all times and for ensuring that all lab tasks are completed by the lab technicians in a timely and accurate manner. The individual also provides assistance and support to ISIS research activities.

  The major aspects of this position fall into two categories:
  - Management of ISIS Simulation Lab and Operations = 70%
  - Operation of Research Studies = 30%
- **Technical Operations Manager** (1.0 FTE): The Technical Operations Manager is the technical professional responsible for designing and implementing computing and simulation infrastructure solutions for ISIS. This position reports to the Administrator for ISIS with a matrixed reporting relationship to the Executive Director and IT Director of ISIS. The individual in this position receives direction regarding ISIS strategic goals and general deliverables and receives direction from the IT Director of Surgery/ISIS IT Director for specific projects and for direction regarding compliance issues and ISIS compatibility with Surgery IT infrastructure. Working closely with ISIS Leadership and the department of Surgery IT Services, this position will perform advanced-level coordination, analysis, programming, and design tasks for existing and new simulation, Web, and e-learning content delivery systems. The position requires someone with the requisite technical skills, a self-starter, expert time manager, and an individual comfortable with a range of projects.

  The major aspects of this position fall into four categories:
  - ISIS Technology Planning and IT Support (approximately 65%)
  - ISIS Web Resource Management (approximately 25%)

- ISIS Backup Lab Technician (approximately 10%)
- **Laboratory Technician** (3.0 FTEs): These individuals perform laboratory and related work under general supervision in support of ISIS and other areas of the Department of Surgery. Major duties include the following:
  - General maintenance and operation of laboratory equipment
  - Setup and calibration of laboratory apparatus and instruments
  - Data collection (read and record data and keep laboratory records)
  - Set up human patient simulator and run scenarios
  - Setup and cleanup of courses, including human cadaver labs
  - Take down equipment
  - Prepare labs for classes
  - Perform minor maintenance and repair of laboratory apparatus and instruments
  - Wash, clean, and arrange laboratory areas and equipment
  - Assist instructors with laboratory operations
  - Within scope of position, participate in laboratory research
  - Perform inventories of supplies and equipment
  - Stock laboratory areas as required
- **Scientific Instructional Technician** (2.0 FTEs): The scientific instructional technicians are responsible for performing laboratory-related work under general supervision. This position performs key simulation lab duties, including assisting with curriculum development, maintenance and repair of simulators, and running simulation exercises. In addition, the individual directs the work of other, more junior personnel in the simulation lab before, during, and after simulation exercises. This position also participates in various simulation-related research projects by collecting, reducing, and tabulating data, and reviews the equipment and supply needs for both simulations and assigned research projects, and arranges for their purchase/procurement.

  The major aspects of this position fall into three categories:
  - Operating/assisting with ISIS simulations, including cadaveric courses
  - Class Scheduling, Curriculum Development, and Data Management
  - Outreach and Event
- **Program Coordinator** (1.0 FTE): The program coordinator is responsible for the coordination of specified operational aspects of ISIS. The individual exercises judgment in interpreting and applying rules and regulations and will advise students, staff, program participants, and/or the public

regarding program content, policies, procedures, and activities. He/she has extensive involvement with students, staff, the public, and/or agencies and coordinates, schedules, and monitors selected program activities.

The major responsibilities of this position fall into three categories:

- Schedule and Coordination of ISIS Educational activities (approximately 50%)
- Coordination of ISIS Committees and events (approximately 35%)
- Financial Operational duties (approximately 15%)

EXAMPLE 3

Community Health Education and Simulation Center (**CHESC**)—Community Outreach–Centered Mission and Vision

A. **Setting**: A 250-bed community hospital–based simulation center with two hospital rooms, a city street environment, and a van for off-site courses.
B. **Customers**: Participants include clinical and nonclinical hospital staff, university and college healthcare provider students, community healthcare providers, and community nonhealthcare providers.
C. **Major Funding Source:** Originally funded by a Health Resources and Services Administration (**HRSA**) grant and donations, the center is now supported by funding from the community hospital, the larger medicine system, fees, donations, and small grants.
D. **Vision Statement:** Original Vision: The original directive from administration was to fulfill the goals listed in the HRSA grant application and maintain the community focus. The center's vision was strongly influenced by a partnership with Peter M. Wiser Institute for Simulation Education and Research (WISER), University of Pittsburgh, PA, and the program goals proposed in the original HRSA application. The vision was patterned after the hospital's vision and included goals from the HRSA program application:
- The hospital as a caring community of healthcare professionals will actively engage in learning opportunities with a curriculum of detection, prevention, intervention, new clinical practices, and competency.
- The hospital patients and clients will engage in learning opportunities to enhance their health and lifestyle.
E. **Mission Statement**: "Raise the long-term health status of our community by providing educational opportunities using low- and high-fidelity technology for our practitioners and staff in creating a safe

and evidence-based care environment for our patients. Provide a safe environment of learning to our patients and clients so they may actively participate and raise their own personal health care status.

We support a culture of safety and learning using:
- Team-oriented communication across disciplines.
- Standardization, competency, problem-based error forgiving, supervised scenarios.
- A virtual hospital with medical technology which facilities acquisition of knowledge, skills and clinical decision-making.
- Curriculum tailored to staff needs for addressing simple to complex patient needs.
- Leadership management for a delivery team that is culturally sensitive, friendly, and respectful.
- Affiliation agreements with colleges, universities, health programs, community responders."

In the first 2 years of the center's operation, it became evident for cost and efficiency considerations that the CHESC would be unable to provide individual patient/client education. The center would provide a more successful model of raising the health and lifestyle of the community by providing education to diverse groups of community healthcare providers.

F. **Organizational Governance and Chart**: The organizational chart shown in Figure 2.1.7 reflects the reporting lines from the President to Education. The Manager of Education Service and CHESC reported to the Director of Clinical Services for the majority of education responsibilities. For the duration of the HRSA grant, the Manager reported additionally to the Director of Clinical Support Services. This reflected his/her responsibility for managing the budget, communicating with the state delegates, and completing the required HRSA documentation. The manager made a request to administration for a governance committee; it was decided that the CHESC team could set the departments' organizational priorities. If an issue remained difficult to resolve, the Chief Nursing Officer would make a determination on the basis of organizational priorities.

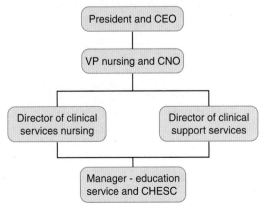

FIGURE 2.1.7 2009 organizational chart.

At this point in time, the only support requested was for administrative staff to complete requested project timelines. Hospital administrators, managers, and coordinators support initiatives and work within the priority setting of the CHESC team. The CHESC team remains cognizant of organizational priorities (Figure 2.1.8).

The original staffing chart for the center was created from recommendations from the WISER consulting team. On the basis of their experience, it was recommended that 2.5 FTE staff members be added for simulation operation. The department continued with the present 2.5 FTEs for Education Services, which remained focused on the present hospital programs.

- The **Unit Manager** (1.0 FTE) has the primary responsibility to hire staff, develop workflows and protocols for the CHESC, market and grow simulation programs both internally and externally. There were many requirements for the HRSA grant that had to be fulfilled, including reporting and inventory creation. The manager promoted the use of simulation technology throughout the organization, designed new curriculum, and ordered equipment that would be needed for future programs. She managed the department staff, budget, developed the business plan and Program to reach the strategic goals.

- The **Staff Development Coordinator** (1.0 FTE) integrates simulation methodology into present programs such as residency and orientation and develops new programs or classes, assists with policy and procedure development, and reviews equipment needs and placement. The coordinator is responsible for the unit when the manager is not present. The coordinator became the champion for simulation throughout the organization and mentored many of the clinical nurses to integrate simulation when appropriate. She participated in the monthly all-day nursing meeting to assist in developing practices and education for

the division. This position required an RN with a strong clinical background in medical-surgical nursing. This was the initial target audience for the hospital simulation development.

- The **Clinical Coordinator/Educator** (1.0 FTE) assumes responsibility for the Education Service programs. She manages the Basic Life Support (BLS) program, orientation, continuing nursing education programs, and develops an on-campus Advanced Cardiac Life Support (ACLS) program. The clinical coordinator/educator is expected to integrate simulation teaching methodology into the present classes offered where appropriate. In addition, she began to colead the formal Continuing Nursing Education credentialing team. The background for this role was a very experienced critical care nurse, who would introduce simulation to the monitored units. This was a secondary priority as it soon became clear that these staff members were the most resistant. She was then encouraged to support the nursing staff caring for the medical-surgical population with mock codes and introduce simulation into ACLS.

- A **Simulation Specialist** (1.0 FTE) was hired in June 2009. This person needed to be a digital native with no reluctance to work with a variety of new and unusual technological systems and equipment. The specialist must have the technical ability to provide physical repairs to a variety of equipment. The center opened in May 2009. In retrospect, the simulation specialist should have been hired as the equipment was delivered and connected. This delay negatively impacted the workflow of the CHESC operations and created great stress for the nursing educators who are technical immigrants. The specialist is responsible for programming and running all the simulation equipment, inventory of all equipment, installing updates to software, performing maintenance, and integrating systems to function seamlessly. Also included in the job description is the requirement to catalog all scenarios, provide scenario setups, breakdowns, and moulage.

- **BLS/ACLS Instructors** are reserve staff who teach courses to staff as needed. They are members of the Education Service department and support simulation in ACLS courses.

- The **Training Coordinator** (0.5 FTE) is responsible for the support of the two departments, including clerical support, classroom setups, and act the role of confederate when requested. This role eventually proved to be inadequate to support the center as the person was supporting two different departments and torn by competing responsibilities.

- The **Medical Director** was not supported with salary from the center for this role. The center

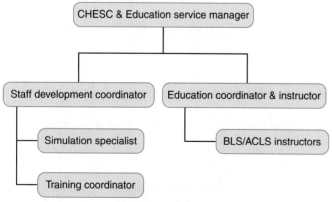

FIGURE 2.1.8 Education Service and Community Health Education and Simulation Center organizational chart 2009.

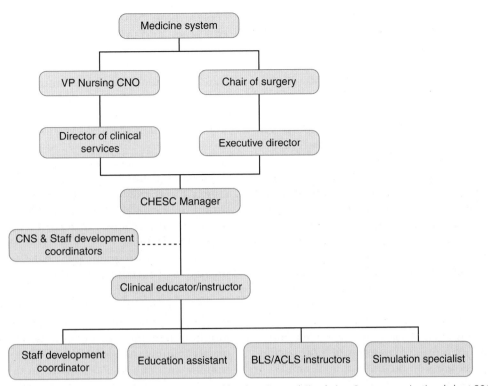

FIGURE 2.1.9 Education Service and Community Health Education and Simulation Center organizational chart 2013.

was extremely fortunate to have the medical director of the Emergency Room take on this role voluntarily. He facilitated mock codes, promoted our services, and became an ACLS instructor for physician classes. A hospitalist also volunteered to support our endeavor and has taken turns with the ED doctor in supporting in situ mock codes (Figure 2.1.9).

G. **Staffing Model**: It was identified within a year of operations that the Clinical Educator, Staff Development staff, the Clinical Nurse Specialist (CNS) team and other healthcare providers would need to be trained to fully integrate simulation education into present and future hospital programs. Several of these instructors continued to support the CHESC community outreach programs. These educators were utilized for their expertise in their specialty areas and openness to learn simulation methodology. Not all educators were open to this concept or identified it as a priority with their present work requirements. While the CNS/Educators are not under the leadership of the CHESC manager, they are part of the simulation team and relied on the center team's expertise in developing programs. The center was ready to create a third organizational chart as the customer mix and funding sources changed.

In 2009, a local academic medical center integrated the community hospital simulation center into their simulation program. The Education Service department continues to function at its present level and remains under the community hospital

administration. In reality, the small department's staff and team overlap continually. A contract was written and signed in 2013 to clearly identify lines of certain responsibilities between the larger medical system, the CHESC, and hospital-based Education Service. The following reflects changes in staff's roles and responsibilities.

• The **Unit Manager** (1.0 FTE) relinquished more of the teaching responsibilities and took on the role of marketing, billing, grant writing, interagency collaborations, and administrative functions. The unit manager serves as the liaison between the medical system and hospital with the adoption, integration, and ongoing use of the online learning system.

• The **Staff Development** (1.0 FTE) role has transitioned to education services and assumed responsibility for orientation, residency, and preceptor programs. The nurse is now the second lead support person for the new hospital-wide online learning management system. The community hospital adopted the system-wide learning system. This has created a new program with many requirements to learn and maintain.

• The **Clinical Educator/Instructor** (1.0 FTE) transitioned into the school nurse program, BLS/ACLS, support for cardiac classes, took on secondary lead for the community-based record system, and maintained continuing nursing education responsibilities. She is the primary support for the community education courses and facilitates communications between the university/college and hospital clinical opportunities. She is now the second leader on the team.

- The **Simulation Specialist** (1.0 FTE) added responsibilities for the community-based record system for students and course registration. In addition, the online learning system has a software program for creating courses, which the specialist supports. The addition of the two software programs has greatly added to time requirements for this position.
- The **Education Assistant** (1.0 FTE) replaced the training coordinator position and continues with clerical support but is the primary resource for the hospital-wide online learning system and resource to the larger medicine system. The education assistant participates as a confederate in simulation and has begun to learn the use of mannequin equipment. Involving the nonclinical staff in simulations creates a positive team environment and sense of belonging to the simulation team.
- Everyone in the department provides marketing on site and mentoring to a variety of internal and external customers on the utilization of simulation methodology.
- There is a need to add a 0.6 FTE simulation specialist owing to increased requirements, especially with the addition of the Learning Management System (LMS) and the desire for increasing the amount of data that is needed. Owing to time and staffing constraints, there is currently no ability to increase customer and simulation programs.

THEMES

The day-to-day operations of all simulation programs have many similar themes. There is a need for a strategic plan that clearly identifies overall goals. The business plan reflects the approach to meeting the strategic plan, and outcome measurements are used to assess meeting those goals. The program should be an active reflection of the organization's mission and vision. The program must have an identified branch on the organizational chart and a governance body of a formal or informal nature that advocates the utilization and growth of the program. The program can be a physical building or a mobile unit. Marketing and recruiting, high-quality education programs, financial stability, and possible profits (including a measurable return on investment) allow the program to continue to be a desirable investment and asset in the changing healthcare environment. Job descriptions, roles, facilities, and equipment should align with the organization's processes and overall goals and objectives. Policies and procedures should reflect the latest evidence and clearly guide the education and workflow in the program.

In the first model, Hannaford Simulation Center is situated in a large community hospital and tertiary care center whose focus includes undergraduate and graduate education, and interprofessional training at the hospital. Medical schools, resident and fellowship programs have a structured curriculum in order to maintain and enforce standardization across the continuum. The hospital uses an evidence-based curriculum and an interprofessional teaching approach that incorporates the unit culture, patient population, staff experience, and medical case mix. We also observe that the level of adult learning theory being successfully adopted within the hospital environment is dependent upon the hospital staffs' experience, how closely the curriculum correlates with clinical challenges within the hospital, and the overall level of support from within the unit groups, the departments, and the hospital's senior leadership.

The second program, ISIS, has several focuses, which include medical education and interprofessional training. A focus on research requires strict guidelines with quality measures and reportable data. The research is piloted in the simulation environment and then transitioned and monitored in the live environment. As a TeamSTEPPS master training site, simulation is integrated into the team-training curriculum. Participants in this program include diverse population in a variety of healthcare organizations from around the nation. The last focus is satellite simulation opportunities being developed for utilization in five states. Standard curriculum is integrated into simulation vignettes using remote communication and prepackaged short programs for teaching.

The last model, CHESC, highlights a community simulation program with three primary focuses. Housed in a hospital setting, the facility provides an opportunity to focus on the education efforts of the clinical and nonclinical staff, including orientation, in-services, formal courses, competencies, and mock codes. Having facilities, staff, and equipment on site promotes easy access for staff classes, in situ training, and as a resource for requests. The second focus is on the university and college students, including medicine, therapies, and nursing. All clinical instructors are provided one opportunity without a fee to utilize the lab for a scenario during the clinical rotation. The scenario promotes review of didactic theory. The program has also contracted with a local college to provide their nursing school the services as the simulation center. The third focus is on clinical and nonclinical community members. There is support to school nurses, chronic care facilities, opportunities for first responders, and sharing clinical approaches with visiting students from around the world. The nonclinical community members include a variety of school-age children and young adults who participate in scenarios that are age-appropriate. The program uses standard curricula for the schools and the variable approach for hospital staff. The community outreach program utilizes a variety of educational approaches based on the participants. An example would be the Boy Scouts exposure to a trauma module on triage. The school-age boys were assigned a variety of roles such as EMT, police, and photographer, with the more senior boys as chiefs. None of the victims who were unconscious were parents. Awareness of their age, growth, and development phase and need to physically move after being in school all day were taken into consideration.

THE "HOW TO . . ."

". . . Start with Only a Mission and Vision in Hand and Jumpstart the Program!"

In the third example, the CHESC did not have a formal strategic or business plan, but by applying business acumen and focusing on the program goals, an overall plan evolved. Funded initially from grants and donations, the parallel strategic plan was to incorporate and develop simulation into present and new programs, while developing programs and relationships with partners who would provide future funding sources.

The first order of business was to start at a very high level and evaluate the present education programs and decide which would benefit from the addition of simulation teaching methods and, secondly, to identify future education needs within the organization. After these two steps were completed, it was time to start promoting the simulation center at the two targets: internal and external customers.

Internal Awareness

- An Open House was provided to all staff, and the first in situ class, called *Code Readiness,* was held. Marketing within the hospital was continual to introduce high-fidelity mannequins to all the clinical staff. Working with the Unit Base educators, the mannequins were scheduled to visit the units for a variety of short learning opportunities. To add to the realism, the mannequins were always dressed in street clothes and made to appear as lifelike as possible. An example is the Women in Red Campaign (AHA), where the mannequin was dressed totally in red and heart sounds were the emphasis for the day. For Halloween, all rooms were decorated, and mannequins were in costumes or hospital clothes. The entire hospital staff was invited to participate in a safety assessment with prizes to those staff that could identify the most hospital safety issues in the lab.
- Targeting the Early Adopters: Mentoring of hospital educators, outreach to managers, and being identified as the education solution for the organization were reinforced. Clinical management identified the center staff as problem solvers for their education needs. Selected nonclinical management has begun to use the center, and others shy away owing to the costs. The hope is to provide examples of opportunity in which the simulation experts can support the nonclinical team's education needs.

External Awareness

- Community customers are gained from referrals from staff such as Boy Scout troops of staff children, and free marketing to schools and businesses. Schools with clinical experiences are provided one free simulation event each quarter. Workforce grants support Instructor Courses and students in nonclinical coursework. Collaboration with one school system has led to an annual school nurse conference.
- Statewide Collaborative: It was important to be one of the primary catalysts for the creation of a Simulation Collaborative in the western Washington state. The collaborative endorsed exposure and networking with 35 institutions in various phases of Simulation Center development. Reaching out to potential customers with the offering of a free class engaged several prospective groups. Previous work with a Training Fund led to a collaborative grant between colleges and industry partners. It yielded 36 simulation scenarios, which will be available for all nursing instructors in the state.

The organizational chart will be changing in the future as ISIS and the CHESC begin to integrate and collaborate owing to a business merger. The organizations are at a precipice to align and develop strategically while merging the individual mission and values into the greater system. At present, participating in the larger system simulation activities provides credibility and networking. The hope is to continue to expand staff and programs, and begin to engage in research while maintaining increasing financial contributions to the budget.

". . . Start with a Mission and Vision, and Strategic Plan, and Ultimately Arrive at a Business Plan and an Organizational Chart"

Assume the center has a strategic plan, and both a mission and vision statement. How do they connect the dots and arrive at a business plan that includes an organizational structure?

This is a process that has several steps and provides a good overall structure for any simulation program, no matter what your mission and vision:

1. You MUST start with the most basic "needs assessment":
   a. What is the history of simulation training at your institution?
   b. Who have been the players regionally?
   c. What are the political and economic challenges that need to be addressed?
   d. Who is charged with training? Residents, staff, medical students, RNs, paraprofessionals?
   e. What is the "expected" return on investment?

2. Perform an initial assessment, called an "Is Map," a detail analysis of how training is being done today, by whom, along with the tools/facilities used, the trainees, and training costs. Identify current and future simulation-enhanced training and teaching tools at the facility.

3. Then develop a "To-Be Map" that outlines the plan to introduce or extend simulation-based training into the organization over the next 1 to 5 years and what changes accompany that transition. You will need to collect the same information in both scenarios to arrive at a reasonable forecast involving the facility's size, equipment needs, staffing profile, and costs (operational and capital).

4. Develop thorough a Strengths, Weaknesses, Opportunities, and Threats analysis (SWOT).

5. Define those who are key stakeholders and involve relevant staff (clinical and administrative) in the discussions from the outset. Be sure to examine both internal and external stakeholders. Identify and empower departmental leaders in the development of department-based simulation teams.

6. Learn from other simulation programs that have similar goals or have a similar model. There is the good, the bad, and the ugly out there. Not every simulation program has done a perfect job in configuring the facility, the staff, and the budget. If a program is willing to share their knowledge, learn from them.

At the end of this analysis, you will have identified who needs to be trained, why, what numbers, the frequency, and the equipment needed to support the training. This analysis can take as little as 6 months if the institution is supportive, and it will directly drive the ultimate request for space, equipment, staff, and funding.

The most common error most institutions make is to build first without any clear understanding of the current needs and growth potential. This has been a very expensive mistake made by most simulation programs. Most programs have either focused on building a program quickly just to get something in place and then it ends up not being used, or the program is built without doing the analysis and it quickly becomes either too small or incapable of meeting the needs of the organization. If all target users are not initially surveyed, the program may observe a subsequent surge in requests from these groups, and the site will not be capable of delivering on its promises.

Here is an example of how the Hannaford Simulation Center followed these guidelines and arrived at their first pass of a comprehensive organizational structure. To start off, this program had already established a mission, vision, and a strategic plan. What came next was the process to create the business plan that will include these elements:

a. Restated strategic plan
b. Benefits of simulation-based medical education
c. Emerging support for simulation in healthcare
d. Current state of the institution
e. Potential users
f. Overview of the proposed simulation program (with visual examples and explanations)
g. Proposed location and concept plans
h. Governance and staffing
i. Project schedule
j. Financial analysis: proposed capital budget and operations budget

The very first step in the process was to perform a comprehensive *Needs Analysis*, and it took this group approximately 6 months to complete. The guidelines (outlined above) were followed, and in the end each department (customer) in the model contributed their best guess assessment of how their educational curriculum would morph over the next 1 to 5 years as it began to include simulation tools and techniques. Some groups were very aggressive in their adoption of high-fidelity simulation, task training, and SP events into their portfolio, while a small percentage of departments were slow adopters and contributed little to the process. In the event a department was slow to contribute, the simulation center made an educated guess and forecasted the usage ramp rate and equipment needs on the basis of other programs and centers evaluated around the nation.

Each department also included a plan to ramp the training of their faculty on how to develop/deliver/debrief simulation events. They built in the need to send at least one faculty member from each department to a simulation instructor course every year. This would help build the intellectual foundation inside the institution for creating their library of simulation scenarios, cases, and courses, and build expertise with their faculty who were charged with delivering the course curriculum.

In parallel, the simulation center had its own plan to develop its staff's expertise. They began by sending those simulation staff members directly involved with creating and delivering scenarios to at least one simulation instructor course (if not two) within the first year. Over the next year, the center then created their own simulation instructor course that would incorporate the custom scenario templates, cases, use the mannequins in their inventory, and implement the software tools of their A/V recording system. This strategy has several benefits:

1. Faculty are taught how to create cases/scenarios from the ground up.
2. Faculty would be immersed in the simulation program's methods and processes for the development and delivery of a course, and learn the debrief techniques and adult theory teaching style adopted by the center.
3. The simulation team would educate the faculty on the use of the center's A/V recording system.
4. Faculty would become familiar with the center's mannequins and trainers because they would be incorporated into the training course.

While information gathering took place to support a needs analysis, a special team was formed within the organization whose charter was to physically visit several simulation programs throughout the country and learn what these programs did well, and not so well, and gather their candid recommendations for this new simulation program. All of the team members were given dedicated time to work on this project.

The team consisted of:

- Simulation medical director
- Senior IT project manager
- Director of medical education
- Nursing director
- Finance director
- Director of planning

Before embarking on the site visits, they created a basic set of questions to ask each program. They also carefully handpicked a number of simulation programs that were a close match to their institutional profile and had a similar mission and vision.

Some lessons learned from these trips were as follows:

- Do not become a babysitter service. In other words, the education of the learners needs to be owned by the departments, not the simulation program. Departments may try to just send their people to the program to get their training. That is not how it works. The creation of the educational curriculum, the delivery of the courses, and the debrief closeout all need to be owned and managed by the departments. In addition, the departmental faculty need to become certified simulation instructors.
- Build a big enough classroom—one that will hold at least 40 people.
- Storage—you will never have enough. Plan on having at least 20% of your facility reserved for storage.
- Develop a pay-for-service fee for users. It may be decided that some users are not charged, but it is important to communicate what the fee would be if they were charged. Using the simulation center is never free. Someone has to pay the bills.
- Make sure there are specific, dedicated rooms for task training or settings.
  - Task Training: airway trainers, central line training, training on computer systems and workflows, code training
  - Settings: build rooms that are identical to spaces on a typical hospital floor: ICU, ER, OR
  - Skills room: a place to practice laparoscopy, for example
- When building the high-fidelity rooms, make sure you have separate control rooms for each one. Some programs try to conserve space by building just one control room that will serve dual purpose and support two high-fidelity rooms. While it may sound like a good idea and may be a way to make the most use

of the floor plan, in the end it is very counterproductive. Trying to run two sessions at the same time, sharing one control room has many drawbacks:
- Not enough room for simulation staff and faculty. Some people will have to stand outside the control room and just observe the scenario, others left in the room are fighting to sit or stand and orchestrate the event.
- The noise may become unmanageable, and to try and compensate for this, everyone may be forced to wear headsets, leading to frustration and the inability to concentrate on the events.
- The communication between the control room and the confederates in the scenario has a high likelihood of being compromised because walkie-talkies are the means to send in instructions. The control room is a very busy space when a scenario is running at full speed, and it is important to address noise and physical crowding concerns early.
- Staff: at a minimum four to six infrastructure staff will prove to be critical to your success. They include simulation medical director, operations director, administrative support, IT engineer (project manager), and audio/visual expert.
- Involve biomedical-purchasing personnel in the process of outfitting your spaces with clinical equipment, task trainers, and simulators. Leverage the buying power of the institution and the knowledge of the clinical engineering (and purchasing) departments to ensure that the warranties and service agreements are written to the institution's standards.
- Having a mobile simulation unit helps buy-in when the time comes to get support for the program. This means having the capability of taking a training event on the road to other parts of the institution, other hospitals, or other teaching venues.
- Develop policies and procedures for the program as soon as possible. It will not be long before there is a long list of inquiries to use the space. You need to quickly establish rules of conduct, and clearly spell out consequences if the guidelines and rules are not followed. In turn, clearly explain what services the program offers and how to request the services.
- Faculty must receive competency training in designing, developing, delivering simulation events and conducting a proper debrief. One cannot simply walk into a simulation program and just "wing it."
- Faculty teaching time must be protected. Teaching time cannot be simply added on to a faculty member's workload. It is important to formally incorporate it into their roles and responsibilities. If they are expected to teach 20% of their time, they need to be provided protected time to teach, and learn how to teach, in a simulation lab.

SECTION 2 • Types of Simulation Programs

From Needs Analysis to an Organizational Chart

This section will focus on just one aspect, and that is how the Hannaford Simulation Center arrived at their initial staffing model.

To be honest, it was mostly an organic process for them. They started with their mission statement, which was heavily weighted toward medical education. They paired that with the results of their multiple site visits, took into consideration the type of curriculum their customers (departments) planned on delivering, along with the volume of simulation-specific equipment they would need to support. The details on how they went about mapping out the roles, responsibilities, and framing the team was discussed in great detail at the beginning of this chapter, so the analysis and job descriptions will not be repeated here.

At the conclusion of the analysis, the total number of dedicated simulation staff came to 8.5 FTEs. The high-level strategy was to build a team of individuals that possessed extremely strong skills in specific areas of expertise. Once the individuals were on board, a comprehensive plan would be developed to cross-train several members of the team.

This strategy worked very well for the Hannaford Simulation Center. It has been just over 3 years since they initially formed their team, and they have revised/rewritten a total of two job descriptions and hired two additional personnel: one simulation specialist and a standardized patient program coordinator. In hindsight, this team did a great job in understanding the needs of their customers, and as a result "right-sized" the organization pretty well.

It is important to remember that no matter how well you do your research and analyze your results, you will not get your organizational chart *perfect* the first time, but you will get very close if you pay attention, follow the process, do the legwork, ask the tough questions, and really understand the potential demands on the program.

BEEN THERE, DONE THAT: HOW CAN I CONTINUE TO IMPROVE OR SUSTAIN WHAT I HAVE ACHIEVED?

Simulation programs operate within an evolving organizational context and culture. The fast-paced changes in healthcare as well as in simulation as a field compel simulation programs to develop an organizational readiness to create solutions to complex and novel organizational challenges.

As a mature program with a process to continuously evaluate the mission, vision, and operational priorities through strategic planning, your program may be well positioned to envision a new organizational mandate that can not only advance your mission and vision but also lead cutting-edge simulation-based innovations.

As a well-established simulation infrastructure, you may have the capacity to design, test, and implement a large-scale simulation event in your organization such as staff orientation in a new care facility, disaster preparedness training, or training innovations associated with priority patient safety and qualities initiatives. If your program already possesses rich expertise in developing curriculum, creating scenarios, training faculty, deploying suitable technologies to support targeted learning goals, and tracking data, you can scale up your existing capacity to deliver visible institution-wide simulation-based events.

Another opportunity for a mature program is to engage in developing a formal professional development model for simulation program staff members. Simulation is such a relatively young field that it is without an established career path that is consistently used. At ISIS, we now have 11 staff members including technical, administrative, and special project staff. Apart from technical and administrative professional positions that have preexisting organizational job pathways for professional mobility, other positions in the simulation field do not necessarily have professional pathways to follow. This is where leaders of the simulation program may need to work closely with the Human Resources (HR) department to create new professional roles and positions to retain a competent simulation workforce.

As more and more simulation programs move from a novice state to a more mature state, it does not take a leap of faith to imagine that job descriptions specific to simulation programs will start to become standardized. Work has already begun in several programs to network with their counterparts and share organizational charts and job descriptions. In order to recruit, hire, and retain talented personnel, it is important that job descriptions be enriched and standardized as much as possible. It is also important to meet with your HR department representatives and help them understand that simulation is a new industry that requires a specialized set of skills in some roles. You can help by doing the legwork for your HR department and bring back comprehensive job descriptions that will enable HR to perform their benchmark analysis and help you justify not only the position, but the respective salaries.

Lastly, another evolving role for your program may be in the "operational simulation" domain that tests hospital workflow. At ISIS, this is emerging as a growing need as the clinical enterprise is slated to become an Accountable Care Organization. As an example of workflow simulation (see chapter 2.8), Environmental Services (EVS) was having difficulty with their patient survey scores. The team was brought in, six staff members at a time, provided with scripting for greeting and leaving the room with a review of the room-cleaning process. The mannequin interacted with staff in the room. Most EVS staff speak English as a second language and tend to be quiet in patient rooms, and patients did not even realize their rooms were being cleaned. This simulation intervention resulted in improved scores. Another example involved the call center in the Food and Nutrition department. On the basis of a script, an SP called into the control room, and the staff member took the call. The patient could be difficult and

MAKING A CAREER IN SIMULATION

Jeffrey B. Cooper, PhD
Founder and Executive Director, Center for Medical Simulation

You can choose from many philosophies about planning your life and your career. I'll just tell you mine. Don't plan. Follow your instincts and take opportunities; if one doesn't work out, try another. Do what will make you feel good about yourself. I'm not sure the axiom "Do what you love and you'll never work a day in your life" is quite true, but it's in the right direction. Do things that make going into work something to look forward to every day. Everything else follows, including your career. It's an easy philosophy to have when you are closer to the end of your career than to the beginning as I am. Maybe I just got lucky. I'm just one data point. Take what you want from it.

I was fortunate to have a cooperative work experience education in engineering. I learned early that I wanted to do something that involved doing things that made a positive difference in people's lives. By chance I landed in a bioengineering lab in my undergraduate college; one thing led to another and I ended up in the Anesthesia Department at the Massachusetts General Hospital right out of graduate school. I didn't really know what I was doing there. I had more good fortune to land in a place with colleagues who were all smarter than I, and also collaborative and generative. Through an immersion in the world of the operating room and with the freedom to explore, I stumbled into the study of human error. It was itself something of an accident, born out of curiosity about why people made mistakes fairly regularly and how their technology was more hindrance than help to prevent errors. My interests extended beyond the technology into the relationships between people. And that's where simulation came in.

I stumbled into simulation in my quest to find a way to change the culture, to help people get better in working together, to prevent the use of patients as objects to learn on.

After over 20 years in patient safety, I've spent the next 20 using simulation to effect change. It doesn't matter so much what I did at every step of the way. What matters is that I had a general idea of what I wanted to make happen. Every time an opportunity popped up that seemed to draw me in that direction, I took it. Some worked; some didn't. But the overall process did work. I don't think I bring any special intelligence or skills. What I have done is always push myself beyond what I thought I could do—just what we want our students to do in simulation. It's how mastery is developed. It really works. I had no life objective to create a new organization, to be a leader, or to get promoted academically. All of those things came as a result of following the path of doing things that made a difference in the lives of other people. It's my neurosis you might say. Not a bad one to have, I suppose.

I'd say the most critical aspect of developing your simulation career is to find good mentors, more than one. They can help you figure out what risks are worth taking and how to navigate the minefields of whatever culture you are in. Being deliberate about mentors isn't something I did, but I had them and used them. They taught me, they opened doors, and propped me up when things weren't going well.

What's it mean for you? Your choice. Take the normal path (create a life plan and intermediate goals, take the path that others have mapped out), or try to carve out your own. Stretch yourself. You can't find a better place to do that than in the simulation community, a place where people want to make a difference, are collegial, collaborative, and eager to help their colleagues succeed. And I can't think of a better tool than simulation to enable you to make that difference, especially in making healthcare safer. So if that gives you fulfillment, just do it. The career will likely follow.

confusing to the staff member, which deliberately targets the skills that we would like staff members to demonstrate in terms of their patient-centeredness.

SUMMARY

What have we learned about the organization and governance of the three very different simulation program models that have been presented in this chapter? The organizational infrastructure as well as the governance and reporting structure of each of these programs is quite different, unique to their own institution or enterprise. After careful consideration, one can see that the programs are all currently organized to meet their mission and vision. How and why did this happen? Did it happen at the moment of the programs' formation and opening, or was there a more organic iterative process at play? Most importantly, how might the mission and vision statements have played a role in the evolution of these programs as the organizations developed and matured?

A mission statement, when thoughtfully created, defines the purpose and primary objectives of the organization. It is a document that should be used primarily for internal purposes whose primary audience is the leadership team and stockholders. It should, in its body, define the key metrics by which the success of an organization can be measured. This document should be used as a compass to guide the decisions and actions of the organization as well as a framework or context around which strategic decisions are formulated.

The vision statement, on the other hand, should also define the organization's purpose, but this time in terms of the organization's values—guiding beliefs, how things should be done—rather than hard metrics. It provides both direction to employees on expected behaviors while inspiring them to a common shared mental model of "destination postcard" for the organization, but should also shape the "customers'" understanding of why they should work with and for the organization.

We have found that mission and vision statements should not be crafted by single individuals or the immediate simulation program leadership but are best crafted by a wide representation of simulation program personnel, stakeholders, and potential customers. Every hour spent on thoughtfully crafting these documents has huge benefits in avoiding wasted time, resources, as well as minimizing conflict or disappointment of faculty, department, or industrial partners.

Lessons Learned—Mission and Vision Statements

Are Essential to the Successful Birth and Evolution of a Simulation Initiative

The leadership of these three programs have all learned that the mission and vision statements are not just static documents that are crafted early in a program's life (or unfortunately and commonly not so early) and end up languishing at the entrance of their program, serving as marketing tools or tag lines in its advertising materials. Often times, the creation of mission and vision statements is seen as a necessary "hoop" through which start-up organizations must jump. In reality, however, our experience has taught us that these two documents are much more than that. They, in actuality, play a vital role in the birth, life, and evolution of an organization. It is also important to realize that both the mission and vision statements become living breathing documents, which undergo revision, evolution, and maturation.

Can Help Minimize Scope Creep

These two documents should serve as the compass or GPS for the organization. We have found that early in a simulation program's life, as simulation initiatives gain traction, the pace of activities, decisions, funding, development activities, the donation, and entrepreneurial opportunities becomes more and more hectic—frenetic at times—and with that there is a significant risk of distraction or scope creep. There is a tendency to want to become everything to everybody. From experience we can tell you that scope creep has to be guarded against, and focusing on the mission and vision statements often brings clarity to many of these distractions.

During the start-up phase of a simulation program, frequently measured in months to several years, we have found that it is helpful to commit to regularly and formally reading aloud both the mission and vision statements, particularly when leadership groups gather to make important strategic or organizational decisions. After all, a compass is simply a tool that functions well only when the crew actually looks at it to verify they are on the proper heading.

Aid in Mundane to Complicated Decisions

It might not be inherently obvious, but the mission and vision statements should actually guide decisions—from what might appear to be the most mundane decisions such as the naming of the program to the most complex organizational, governance, and strategic planning decisions.

One of the first decisions the mission and vision statements can guide is the naming of the program or simulation enterprise. This may sound trivial, but, in fact, the name of the simulation program is the first introduction potential trainees, faculty, stakeholders, and development/donors see. Their early impressions, which frequently make or break the willingness to partner, can be based on their impressions of what the program provides as advertised by their name. Unavoidably, the program becomes what their name implies. If the program is named after a donor, for example, the message is uninformative and neutral; however, if the program's name has in it the words "patient safety," this may send a clearer message of the mission and vision. Equally telling are words such as surgical, anesthesia, interprofessional, and so on. Words in program names are powerful beyond their first impressions. Thus, the first introduction to the world by the program must align with its mission.

As an example of the impact of a name, one of the programs in this document initially was named "Institute for Surgical and Interventional Simulation." After several years, the leadership realized that the name both did not align with their mission and vision, and the program was not attracting the depth and breadth of partners the institution had wished to touch. It subsequently changed its name to "Institute for Simulation and Interprofessional Studies," and the nature and numbers of potential clients diversified significantly.

At the other end of the spectrum of decision-making are the important and often-complex decisions that must initially be made concerning day-to-day operations, staff reporting structure, and low- and high-level governance. Mission and vision statements should play a central role in identifying the need for specific committees and leadership positions that will ensure a successful launch of the initiative. The statements will also help in making strategic decisions concerning the governance structure of the organization so that the power leaders of the organization are in place to provide the necessary support and guidance for this start-up program. From reviewing the three organizational models presented in this chapter, it is clear that the organizations had very different 3- and 5-year end points, and thus their initial organizational infrastructures look markedly different.

Aid in Sorting Evolution from Confusion

Mission and vision statements provide a view of what many of us term the "destination postcard" or the shared mental model of what the simulation initiative will look like in 3, 4, or 5 years. There is no reason to believe that the organizational structure (i.e., operational committees or subcommittees), reporting, and governance of a simulation initiative should remain static. These documents should give direction as to how the organizational and governance structures must evolve with time to meet the 3- and 5-year goals. From the outside it might appear that there is confusion and lack of direction as committees, reporting structures, and stakeholder leadership form up and are then replaced. One must recognize that the first several years of a simulation initiative are the formative years as the organization is in start-up mode. The needs and resources change, often more quickly than might be expected. If crafted appropriately, the mission and vision statements will serve as a vital compass to the organization, particularly when they are reviewed regularly. They will clearly point out the necessary changes that are on a predictable trajectory on the road map that is contained within these documents. It is also clear from the three simulation program models that significant changes occurred within their organizations, committees came and went, and new ones emerged. This is a healthy sign of good planning and thoughtful missioning and visioning.

REFERENCES

Kim, S., Ross, B., Wright, A., Wu, M., Benedetti, T., Leland, F., & Pellegrini, C. (2011). Halting the revolving door of faculty turnover: Recruiting and retaining clinician educators in an academic medical simulation center. *Simulation in Healthcare, 6*(3), 168–175.

CHAPTER 2.2

Optimizing Education with In Situ Simulation

Justin L. Lockman, MD, Aditee Ambardekar, MD, and Ellen S. Deutsch, MD, FACS, FAAP

ABOUT THE AUTHORS

JUSTIN L. LOCKMAN is Assistant Professor of Anesthesiology, Pediatrics, and Critical Care, Attending Physician in Pediatric Anesthesiology and Pediatric Critical Care, and Director of the Pediatric Anesthesiology Fellowship Program at The Children's Hospital of Philadelphia. Justin has utilized his experience as a leader in simulation for both Anesthesiology and Critical Care Fellowships to develop and refine comprehensive in situ curricula for trainees in both specialties. His particular interests include multidisciplinary simulation, patient safety, and team building/crisis resource management activities.

ADITEE P. AMBARDEKAR is Assistant Professor of Clinical Anesthesiology and Critical Care, Attending Physician in Pediatric Anesthesiology, and Associate Program Director for the Pediatric Anesthesiology Fellowship at The Children's Hospital of Philadelphia. Dr. Ambardekar is an active simulation faculty member in the Center for Simulation, Advanced Education, and Innovation, and specializes in in situ simulation in the operating room for anesthesia trainees and faculty. She has developed a comprehensive simulation-based curriculum for anesthesiology residents and fellows.

ELLEN S. DEUTSCH is Director of Perioperative Simulation at The Children's Hospital of Philadelphia, Immediate Past Chair of the Society for Simulation in Healthcare's Council for Accreditation of Healthcare Simulation Programs, and Chair of the American Academy of Otolaryngology's Surgical Simulation Task Force. Her interests include emerging educational strategies and technologies, including simulation, and she is particularly interested in synergies between human factors principles, simulation, healthcare quality, and patient and provider safety.

Acknowledgments: The authors wish to thank all of the team members of the Center for Simulation, Advanced Education, and Innovation at The Children's Hospital of Philadelphia, whose unrelenting quest to improve education for the entire medical center staff and to advance patient safety and quality have created the foundation on which this chapter is written.

ABSTRACT

This chapter focuses on the use of in situ simulation for both routine and just-in-time training. Advantages (including realism, timeliness, convenience, and systems-based improvement) are contrasted with challenges (such as poor control of time, space, equipment, and personnel availability in the actual clinical setting). Finally, a value analysis is included to promote discussion between simulation faculty and hospital administration about possibilities for utilizing in situ simulation.

CASE EXAMPLE

It is 2:00 in the morning, and your emergency department team has had a busy night. You receive a call that there is a child with a severe traumatic brain injury who will arrive at your facility via helicopter in 30 to 45 minutes. After notifying the trauma team, the neurosurgery service, and the ICU team of the impending arrival, you open the door to examination room 10, which houses a high-technology, in situ simulator. You quickly start the preprogrammed simulation scenario for pediatric traumatic brain injury, and then call overhead for help from the emergency department team. The two nurses, pediatric resident, medical student, and pharmacist who respond to your call for help have never worked together before today. Additionally, several of the team members have never cared for a patient with severe traumatic brain injury before participating in this 10-minute scenario. In the remaining 20 minutes before the patient arrives, your debriefing and high-fidelity **"just-in-time"** education ensure that the entire team understands the goals of airway protection, adequate ventilation, circulatory stability, and diagnosis and treatment of intracranial hypertension. Several minutes later, the patient arrives at your resuscitation room, and the team is able to replay the scenario, this time with a real patient but with more understanding of the goals and necessary tasks.

INTRODUCTION AND BACKGROUND

In situ simulation, in its simplest form, may be conceptualized as actual care of a simulated patient. In contrast to the controlled, often remote location of a dedicated simulation center, in situ simulation utilizes a functional clinical environment, along with staff, equipment, and systems to provide rehearsal and ultimately mastery among team members, with minimal need for creation of an artificial experience or removal of team members from their clinical duties. This can optimize both the fidelity and the convenience of the simulation.

Interestingly, the recent emergence of in situ simulation as a cost-effective strategy for medical education and teamwork building represents a return to the earliest days of medical simulation. Long before dedicated simulation centers with full-time staff were conceived, a few dedicated pioneers who saw great potential for this relatively new realm of education utilized mobile simulation. Since the invention of the mannequin cardiopulmonary resuscitation (CPR) trainer in 1960 by Asmund Laerdal and colleagues, point-of-care simulation, typically using low-technology simulators, has become a mainstay of CPR training courses, some of which travel to schools, community centers, and medical facilities to train both medical professionals and laypersons (Cooper & Taqueti, 2004; Perkins, 2007). Decades prior to that, in the 1920s, Chevalier Jackson demonstrated the technique of emergency tracheotomy on a doll in the backseat of his limousine (American Bronchoesophagological Association, n.d.).

With the embrace of healthcare simulation in the last decade by many healthcare facilities and medical training programs, the advantages of dedicated space, staff, time, and equipment have resulted in the creation of "simulation centers," which are sometimes in locations remote from clinical care areas. These centers, which may be large and expensive, may be ideal for training large groups of individuals when dedicated time is available (McKeon et al., 2009). Examples include specific groups of students (such as medical or nursing students) and specific mandatory training courses (such as advanced life support training courses). However, there are distinct disadvantages to this method. Most notably, complex clinical environments, including current equipment, such as operating rooms and critical care units, may be very expensive and even impossible to fully replicate in a simulation center. Additional challenges include multidisciplinary team member unavailability (physicians, nurses, respiratory therapists, and pharmacists are unlikely to be free to leave the clinical area simultaneously for a team simulation), and the inability to study and improve interdisciplinary communication and systems-based problems in a large healthcare facility. These are just a few of the challenges that may be easily overcome by in situ programs; indeed, these issues have led to a reemergence in recent years of in situ simulation as an innovative "leading edge" in team dynamics, communication training, patient safety, and systems-based improvements (Davis et al., 2008; Hamman et al., 2010; Hohenhaus et al., 2008; Miller et al., 2008). The remainder of this chapter will focus on the benefits and challenges of implementing an in situ simulation program.

ADVANTAGES OF IN SITU SIMULATION

Realistic/Believable Setting

A readily apparent advantage to in situ simulation is the lack of need for investment of time, space, and money to create an artificial environment for simulation. This benefit is amplified by considering the number of different potential spaces that may be needed for high-fidelity simulation. For example, one may wish to simulate a trauma bay, an outpatient clinic, an inpatient hospital room, an operating room, a cardiac catheterization lab, and a critical care facility; even the cafeteria may be helpful for simulating bystander/visitor events. Indeed, the ideal simulation center would create an entire "simulated hospital" to rehearse mass casualty incidents, multidisciplinary patient handoffs, and other complex events. In situ simulation eliminates the need to create any of these specialty locations, because they already exist in the real clinical setting of the hospital (Volk et al., 2011).

The inherent **realism** of the in situ environment is also a significant benefit. It may be difficult to replicate in a dedicated simulation center, at any cost, the equipment and resources available in and around the clinical settings in which the learners work. The realism of this situation enhances the **experiential learning** opportunities.

Notably, the **fidelity** and "believability" of in situ simulation does not end at the physical location. Instead, it includes many unexpected benefits. For example, the use of actual clinical equipment and supplies allows for troubleshooting and discovery of safety concerns that may affect real patients (Geis et al., 2011; Guise et al., 2010; Hamman et al., 2010). Rather than having participants role-play as various members of the team, the bona fide team members work together in a simulation to develop rapport with each other, to understand each other's roles and challenges better, and to anticipate support that other team members will need to perform as expected.

The actual clinical milieu may also be explored using the in situ environment. For example, staff may know that they can use a fire extinguisher to contain a small fire, but may not realize where the actual fire extinguisher is located in their own work area until they practice fire safety simulations in situ. Nursing staff may be surprised to learn how long it takes for the "code team" to arrive in a clinical setting when called; physician staff may not understand what goes into accurate medication dilution by the pharmacist or administration by a nurse; or child life specialists may not appreciate the steps of a rarely performed procedure and thus may not be able to adequately prepare a child for it. All of these obstacles may be overcome by having the team function in their native environment as though caring for actual patients.

Timely Education

Another major benefit of in situ simulation is temporal proximity. As described in the scenario above, in situ simulation may represent the optimal in "just-in-time" education, whereby the team members may simulate unusual events immediately prior to the occurrence of these events (see chapter 2.6). This may occur either in an ad hoc fashion, as in the case above, or in a planned fashion such as the simulation of a complex, multistep surgical procedure as a "dress rehearsal" for all involved team members on the day prior to a scheduled procedure. In other instances, spontaneous teaching may occur during team downtime. For example, a recent study by Sutton et al. (2010) demonstrated that high-frequency episodes of brief bedside CPR training with a task-training simulator resulted in improved CPR skill retention among hospital-based providers (Figure 2.2.1). Utilizing very brief episodes of spontaneous teaching when team members have even a few moments free results in improved retention of critical skills. The ease of in situ delivery supports this concept of "refresher" training.

Alternatively, in situ simulation may be used after rare or unexpected events as a method of reenactment to improve systems. Some centers include in situ event simulation as part of their root cause analysis or failure modes and effects analysis processes, uncovering previously unrecognized hazards or patient safety risks (Davis et al., 2008). This may result in changes to hospital safety protocols to prevent future serious events and enhance patient safety.

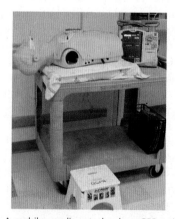

FIGURE 2.2.1 A mobile, medium-technology CPR trainer, consisting of a CPR mannequin (Laerdal, Wappinger Falls, NY) and a monitor defibrillator, which provides qualitative assessment of CPR performance (Royal Philips Electronics, Amsterdam, The Netherlands) used for frequent exposure training in our intensive care unit. Use of this relatively inexpensive system has been proven to improve CPR skill retention among hospital-based providers.

Systems-Based Benefits

The same process described above for the *post hoc* reenactment of serious safety events may be effectively utilized for prospective evaluation of existing or novel systems for potential improvements. The principles of actual team and protocol utilization allow for probing of existing systems with intentional exploration for improvements (Davis et al., 2008; Hamman et al., 2010). For example, the quality and efficacy of patient transport from the operating room to the intensive care unit has been studied in our institution using in situ simulation both to understand the circumstances that may hinder or enhance safety and efficiency and to develop processes targeting improved safety. Alternatively, the use of in situ simulation for educational or other purposes may (and often does) result in serendipitous discovery of opportunities for systems-based improvements in efficiency, patient safety, or resource use (Kobayashi et al., 2010; LaVelle & McLaughlin, 2008).

Some centers have also prospectively used in situ simulation to troubleshoot new or renovated systems prior to implementation. Isolated systems have been tested, such as trial of new clinical equipment or information technology systems prior to implementation to test functionality in the actual clinical environment (Kushniruk et al., 2011). Other centers have implemented broader use of simulation, such as in situ simulation of clinical care prior to opening a new hospital wing to ensure optimal teamwork and integration of systems (Bender, 2011). In situ simulation may also be used during policy and procedure development as well as for training for staff during updated protocol implementation. In situ simulation can be used in an iterative fashion, as an ongoing cyclical process to identify opportunities for improvement, design system changes, test the effects of changes, and then identify further opportunities for refinement.

Technical Benefits

Some of the technical benefits of in situ simulation are self-evident. For example, the use of mobile carts for simulation (as described below) allows for great flexibility in determining where or how the simulation may occur. For example, simulations are not restricted even to patient care areas of the hospital. Indeed, even the walls of the hospital and the boundaries of the medical center need not limit simulation activities. Scenarios may be designed in administrative areas, outpatient centers, and even remote facilities. Simulation can be used for community disaster drills in public areas like parks. Additionally, simulation has become common for community outreach and education, such as for dental clinics practicing sedation; mobile in situ is a prerequisite for such activities (Brooks-Buza et al., 2011).

Finally, a fundamental tenet of adult educational activities is that they must be readily accessible for busy adults. While off-site simulation centers may provide dedicated time and space, they impose inherent inconvenience on the learner by forcing the learner to find both time and means to travel to the location of the center. This may not be a problem for medical students or even residents, who may be assigned to simulation activities during protected educational time. However, for other healthcare professionals, such as attending physicians, registered nurses, or clinical pharmacists, off-site simulation may interfere with clinical staffing needs or may require an investment in administrative costs to provide paid nonclinical time for the activity. In situ simulation decreases the magnitude of these problems by increasing the convenience of the simulation activities.

CHALLENGES OF IN SITU SIMULATION

Patient Safety Risks

Despite the many benefits of in situ simulation, there are also significant challenges. Although these can likely be mediated if properly anticipated (see discussion below), this is an area for future research as there are few data on this topic.

The spirit of in situ simulation requires some flexibility in planning. To achieve the maximal benefit from being in an in situ environment, both the educators and the trainees must be willing to accept certain realities: there will be unexpected times when patient or team acuity exceeds the usual expected level, and last-minute cancellation of simulation training may be required. Educators should work within the framework of the existing local practice to attempt to decrease or eliminate cancellations and lessen interruptions, and may provide some protection by using strategies such as temporary forwarding of telecommunication devices to other providers, or notifying the care team that a training activity is ongoing, and asking staff members to temporarily limit interruptions except for urgent or emergent issues. Particularly in the setting of teaching hospitals, there is established precedent for such "protected educational time," which may be extended to include in situ activities (Lasko et al., 2009; Parikh et al., 2008). In situ education should be treated with the same commitment as traditional educational modalities, such as Grand Rounds, with disruptions for patient care occurring only when essential.

There are also supply and equipment-related concerns with in situ simulation. Unlike the physical separation of training equipment that typically occurs in an off-site simulation center, in situ training necessarily runs the risk of confusing training equipment for patient-use equipment. This risk must be anticipated and should be mitigated or eliminated by the careful and thorough labeling of simulation equipment and supplies. Similarly, care should be taken to ensure that at the conclusion of each training activity, all training-related equipment and supplies are completely removed from the patient unit and stored safely in a separate location. This is particularly true of medications; "simulated" or expired pharmacologic medications used for training must be clearly labeled and removed from care areas to minimize the risk of inadvertent administration to a patient.

On a related note, there is a potential concern for damage to critical patient-use equipment if it is utilized for training purposes. For example, during an in situ scenario, the actual bedside monitor may be used, a patient-use defibrillator may be used, or a patient bed may be used. While the per-use risk of damage to each of these items is negligible, if employed on a widespread basis for many trainees across a large healthcare system, there is a potential risk of equipment damage and related costs caused by use for simulation. This risk can be reduced by establishing completely separate simulation training equipment, as noted above, but this is not always possible because of budget constraints, and would be counterproductive in simulations designed to probe patient care areas for latent hazards. The alternative is a thoughtful combination of the careful use of both real and simulated patient care equipment and supplies and consideration of including the costs of repairs to actual patient care equipment in the simulation program budget.

Psychological Safety

While attempting to improve teamwork, communication, patient safety, and team morale through simulation, it is important to be aware of the potential for unanticipated negative psychological effects of any training activities. As with all simulation activity, in situ simulation requires appropriate debriefing to optimize education and minimize trauma or negative feelings about actions or participants, but debriefing may be more challenging in the in situ environment. Additionally, the routine presimulation discussion of the fiction contract and the basic assumption that all learners have the best interests of their patients in mind is at times excluded from in situ sessions by the nature of "code call" events, which are not announced in advance.

In addition, there is a risk of untoward psychological effects on the patients and family members who may observe simulation training activities on the ward or elsewhere in a medical facility. It is beneficial to provide advance notice of a training event so that family members are not concerned about an actual patient emergency when they witness the crowd of staff working at a bedside.

Operational Challenges

Aside from the patient safety and equipment-related risks noted above, there are other challenges to developing an in situ simulation program. As previously alluded to, perhaps the most significant of these is the inability to control the environment surrounding the simulation. Even with the best of preparation, last-minute cancellations or mid-simulation interruptions may occur as a consequence

SECTION 2 • Types of Simulation Programs

of the nature of human health and the unpredictability of patient care responsibilities. While these risks may be decreased by creating an educational culture at the training site in conjunction with administrative leadership, they can never be completely eliminated, and flexibility is important.

Space in a medical facility is both limited and expensive; "extra" space is a luxury. Consequently, when working to develop an in situ program, it becomes necessary to acknowledge and deal with the problem of space limitation. Significant advance planning and workflow analysis may be required to optimize simulation opportunities, taking advantage of patterns of ebbs and flows in space utilization and personnel workloads while minimizing disruptions to normal activities. Truly in situ activities, such as simulation in an ICU room, always include the potential for last-minute space or participant limitations, requiring flexibility on behalf of educators. When in situ simulation is not possible, near-situ training (see text below) may be an option, trading an increase in available space for a decrease in realism.

In a dedicated simulation center, equipment is often used repeatedly for training multiple target audiences/trainees with little or no setup and takedown effort. For in situ activities, equipment and supplies must be completely removed for both equipment security and patient safety after each session, and then reset for the next session. Written equipment and supply checklists and, if possible, dedicated staff can be used to ensure the complete and consistent setup and thorough removal of training equipment after each session (Berenholtz et al., 2004; Hales & Pronovost, 2006).

One challenge that commonly arises is the limitation of audiovisual support in the in situ environment. As described elsewhere in this book, an entire industry has arisen around the audio and video recording of medical simulation sessions. These recordings are often utilized for the immediate feedback or "replay" of activities during educational debriefing, and increasingly have been used for both quality control and medical education research purposes as well.

Well-funded simulation centers often include multiple cameras installed with varying angles, as well as numerous microphones to capture audio (Seropian & Lavey, 2010). Centers seeking to optimize realism may also support dedicated control booths from which the educators may manage the scenario and potentially discuss "on-the-fly" changes as well without affecting the realism of the simulation room. Although realism may be compromised by the presence of the simulation operator in the room with participants, this is balanced by the benefits of improved realism conferred by the in situ environment.

Even if a separate control area is not feasible, audiovisual recording is still possible; a mobile cart for in situ simulation may include video and audio recording equipment (Paige et al., 2008). If in situ activities are repeatedly performed in specific locations, such as the emergency department, one patient room may be outfitted with audiovisual equipment for the above purposes. If this strategy is employed, care must be taken to avoid the audiovisual recording of patient care activities without consent or appropriate organizational protocols; in addition to the risk of healthcare privacy law violation, local and state laws vary regarding audio and video recording without consent for laypeople.

For those wishing to develop or participate in medical education research with simulation, there is an added difficulty that arises from the inability to completely standardize the in situ environment to the degree possible in a dedicated space. However, multiple authors have overcome this obstacle with the use of standardized scenarios with templates for simulation setup; consequently, a wealth of in situ–based research has recently been published (Allan et al., 2010; Hamman et al., 2009; Mondrup et al., 2011; Riley, David et al., 2011).

Debriefing, as discussed elsewhere in this book, is an essential element of any simulation program. This is no less true for in situ programs. There are additional challenges presented by in situ settings, as there may be no dedicated "debriefing room" on a busy clinical ward, but nearby conference space or even a bedside debriefing will often suffice.

VARIATIONS OF IN SITU SIMULATION

Until this point, the term "in situ simulation" has been used primarily as a single entity. This is not entirely accurate; in truth, the term "in situ simulation" encompasses several related but distinct types of simulation that will be defined further in this section. Countless variations and combination of in situ venues exist, including an increasing number of novel methods of achieving similar results. Table 2.2.1 includes common variations of in situ described in the healthcare literature and describes the various, often overlapping, concepts of in situ simulation.

Modified/Temporary In Situ Simulation Space

Likely the first thing that comes to mind after mention of the term "in situ simulation" is the temporary use of bona fide patient care areas for simulation. This is probably the most common application of in situ simulation,

TABLE 2.2.1

Variations of In Situ Simulation

Description	Cost	Realism	Setup Ease
Modified/temporary in situ space	Variable	High	Moderate
Permanent/dedicated in situ space	High	High	Easy
Near-situ simulation space	Variable	Variable	Variable
Mobile (self-contained) cart	Low	Variable	Easy

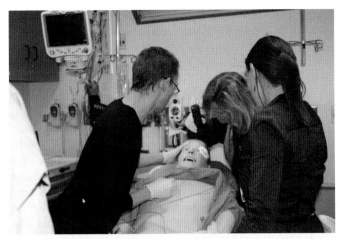

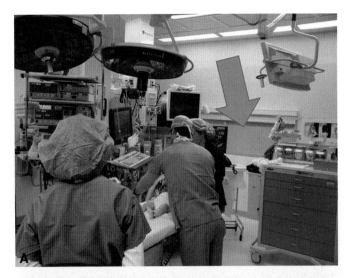

FIGURE 2.2.2 This patient care area is utilized for in situ simulation activities during a low patient census interval. The added cost in this case is minimal, as the room would be completely unused in the absence of this educational activity.

and involves the transient use of functional patient facilities for simulation. Figure 2.2.2 demonstrates educational activities utilizing this technique. An acute care setting is utilized for a simulation session at a time of day when patient load is predictably low. The benefit of this use of space is clear: this is the gold standard for realism of the simulation space. This can work quite well with planning and flexibility and allows limitless opportunities for creating simulations with local relevance.

Permanent In Situ Simulation Space

Actual patient care spaces that are used for simulation on a consistent basis can be considered permanent in situ locations. Patient care activities and simulation activities must be coordinated, but this consistency and commitment may justify the installation of enhanced audiovisual capabilities as well as appropriate cables, outlets, and conduits, which will then be helpful in decreasing the effort required to import, set up, take down, and remove simulation equipment for each educational session. This may be particularly feasible by utilizing a rarely used room in areas such as the Emergency Department or the Post-Anesthesia Care Unit, where there are large swings in patient census patterns with reasonable predictability.

Taking this a step further, a simulation control or observation room can be built immediately adjacent to a patient care room, allowing the simulator operator and observers to be out of the participants' sight during the simulations. This may be planned in advance, as during new construction or renovations, or it may take advantage of the fortuitous location of suitable space, such as a closet adjacent to a patient care room, that can be converted to a control area. An example of this technique is shown in Figure 2.2.3; this facility was constructed during an operating room construction project. The operating room is fully functional and is used on a daily basis by the perioperative care team. Note the arrow in Figure 2.2.3A indicating

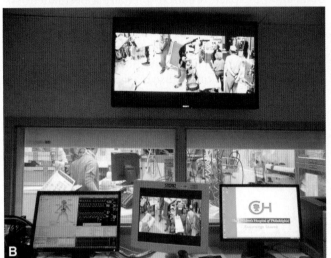

FIGURE 2.2.3 **A.** In this fully functional operating room, a simulation is taking place before the start of the daily surgical schedule when the space would be otherwise unused. Note the *arrow* indicating the location of the control booth window in this image. **B.** This is the operating room seen in Figure 2.2.3A, as viewed from within the simulation control room. Note the presence of several different cameras in the simulation space, which are useful for both scenario control as well as for playback of video and audio during participant debriefing.

the location of the control booth window at one end of the room. Figure 2.2.3B shows the view of the same room from within the simulation control room. If available, this approach combines some of the benefits of a permanent simulation facility with the realism of in situ simulation.

Near-Situ Simulation Space

One solution to the challenges of temporary and dedicated in situ simulation is the creation of a so-called "near-situ" simulation area. For example, an underutilized staff lounge, a redundant conference room, or perhaps even extra call-room space on or near the patient care area may be used to create a permanent simulation space. This combines many of the benefits of in situ simulation, such as the ability to maintain equipment in one place and ease of access for staff, with a lessened investment by the hospital administration that will not have to surrender a potential patient care area. While some realism may be lost, this does provide the advantage of relative convenience; not surprisingly, this is a popular program design for many centers.

Mobile Self-Contained Simulation Cart

Finally, a lower-cost and more flexible option for simulation across a healthcare system is the creation of a mobile, self-contained simulation cart. The concept behind this program design is a "permanent" simulation system built on wheels. This allows for use in quite variable locations, including both inpatient and outpatient settings, with reasonably high fidelity because the simulation happens in the actual patient care area, but without the dedication of space required to create a permanent system in any one patient care area, and without the need to gather equipment before the simulation and return individual items to storage after the simulation. Mobile in situ simulation is clearly the most flexible and potentially the lowest cost of the discussed options; it may range from simple, inexpensive systems as shown in Figure 2.2.1 through more high-technology systems. Depending on complexity, these carts may require a dedicated team to maintain, schedule, and manage the simulation equipment prior to and during each session (Weinstock et al., 2009; Yager et al., 2011).

VALUE ANALYSIS

In situ simulation is a relatively economical way to provide simulation-based education. Expenses involved in the creation of a simulation program include the purchase, upgrade, and maintenance of equipment; salary support for simulation staff; and the indirect costs of protected educational time for learners. Simulation has been demonstrated to improve the safety and quality of healthcare (Draycott et al., 2008) and is increasingly incorporated into medical and nursing education (Cohen et al., 2010; Harlow & Sportsman, 2007; Hunt et al., 2006; Langhan et al., 2009; Lasater, 2007; Lindquist et al., 2008; Nestel et al., 2011; Ziv et al., 2000); in fact, Ziv has suggested that simulation-based education is an ethical imperative (Ziv et al., 2003). In situ simulation decreases the additional potential cost of developing, outfitting, and maintaining dedicated space usable only for simulation, as well as the cost and disruption of transporting participants when simulation centers are located off-site (Calhoun et al., 2011; Edler et al., 2010; Kushniruk et al., 2011, Weinstock et al., 2009). Long events, and events with multiple participants, can be organized in an opportunistic fashion, adding value by taking advantage of the typical ebb and flow of patient care activity in spaces with intermittent use, such as treatment rooms, sleep laboratories, perianesthesia care units and operating rooms, and, less predictably, treatment rooms

and rooms equipped for trauma. Brief simulation events, such as "just-in-time" refreshers of specific skills, can be integrated with negligible adverse impact on patient care activities. For team training and systems evaluations, the added value of improved situational fidelity is difficult to accomplish in a simulation center. It may be difficult to ascertain the financial benefits of improved patient safety that will arise from the creation of an effective simulation program. Emerging data suggest that deficits in communication and team dynamics are significant contributors to adverse patient events (Pruitt & Liebelt, 2010). Healthcare is a complex system involving rare, high-risk events, and teams that are ever changing. Indeed, in a teaching facility it is unlikely that an identical team will ever encounter the same situation twice (Riley, Lownik et al., 2011). Unlike many **high-reliability teams** that benefit from knowledge of each member's strengths and weaknesses, constant leadership, and established feedback patterns, healthcare teams depend heavily on communication and team dynamics to allow for adaptive responses to a wide spectrum of situations (Cheng et al., 2012; Jankouskas et al., 2007; Sutton, 2009). We suggest that there is no better method of "practicing" these skills than by the regular use of in situ simulation to improve critical communication skills and teamwork (Allan et al., 2010). Only by maintaining proficiency in these skills in all staff can an impromptu team work effectively during rare, complex events.

THE "HOW TO ..."

Developing an in situ simulation program should include significant planning and preparation before the first piece of equipment is purchased. The first step is the identification of a "champion" for creation of the in situ program who will see the project through from start to finish (see Expert's Corner of chapter 4.5). A needs assessment should be performed to identify which areas of the medical center will benefit the most from the addition of simulation activities (see chapter 5.1). Next, the type of simulation design (see text above) should be selected, weighing factors including learner time availability, space availability (unit capacity and average census), financial constraints, and diversity of scenarios planned. Once a simulation design is planned, equipment should be researched and prices obtained. Generally, while there are several companies that manufacture mannequins and software for simulation as well as many high-end bells and whistles, a value analysis for a beginning simulation program will show that expensive technology may not be necessary to achieve stated goals.

With a budget planned, the hospital administration should be approached for funding. In some cases, the patient safety benefits of simulation have resulted in funding from hospital endowments; however, fundraising may be necessary to first create a small, effective but low-cost simulation program and demonstrate efficacy for the medical center (Edler et al., 2010; Weinstock et al., 2009). Depending on regional conditions, there may be a benefit to collaborating with nearby centers to purchase equipment and staff a simulation program jointly (Waxman et al., 2011). Starter grants may also be available to select entities, and should be fully researched prior to purchase of materials.

Once the equipment has been purchased, in situ scenarios may be written and staff education time scheduled as with any other simulation program. As noted above, a major concern is the separation of simulation equipment from actual patient care equipment, and this should be kept in mind during all stages of planning and execution of activities.

BEEN THERE, DONE THAT: HOW CAN I CONTINUE TO IMPROVE OR SUSTAIN WHAT I HAVE ACHIEVED?

In situ simulation provides for an ever-increasing number of potential scenarios. Indeed, the possibilities are endless when the simulator is mobile and can travel to locations as remote as the hospital parking garage, the helicopter landing pad, or the computed tomography gantry. There is truly no upper limit of benefit that may be obtained from continued rehearsal in teamwork, communication, and systems issues; thus, even when the medical knowledge has been mastered, in situ simulation is a useful tool for pushing the envelope and escalating teamwork to an increased level of proficiency (Riley, Lownik et al., 2011). This may include isolated teamwork training or continuum of care scenarios as discussed elsewhere in this text.

SUMMARY

In situ simulation is a broad term encompassing a myriad of differing techniques, unified in their application of simulation in locations where healthcare providers actually work. In situ simulation provides realism, flexibility, and convenience, with less expense and fewer space requirements than center-based simulation. In situ simulation also supports systems improvements at a level of detail and relevance not possible with off-site simulation. Although there are challenges in creating an in situ simulation program, there are countless benefits. Indeed, whether developed as a relatively inexpensive way to start a hospital-based simulation program or added to expand the capabilities of an existing simulation program, in situ simulation is an essential component of any comprehensive simulation curriculum.

REFERENCES

American Bronchoesophagological Association. (n.d.). *History: Jackson tracheotomy.* Retrieved from http://abea.net/about/historical/jacksontracheotomy/index.html

Allan, C. K., Thiagarajan, R. R., Beke, D., Imprescia, A., Kappus, L. J., Garden, A., … Weinstock, P. H. (2010). Simulation-based training delivered directly to the pediatric cardiac intensive care unit engenders preparedness, comfort, and decreased anxiety among multidisciplinary resuscitation teams. *The Journal of Thoracic and Cardiovascular Surgery, 140,* 646–652.

Bender, G. J. (2011). In situ simulation for systems testing in newly constructed perinatal facilities. *Seminars in Perinatology, 35,* 80–83.

Berenholtz, S. M., Pronovost, P. J., Lipsett, P. A., Hobson, D., Earsing, K., Farley, J. E., … Perl, T. M. (2004). Eliminating catheter-related bloodstream infections in the intensive care unit. *Critical Care Medicine, 32,* 2014–2020.

Brooks-Buza, H., Fernandez, R., & Stenger, J. P. (2011). The use of in situ simulation to evaluate teamwork and system organization during a pediatric dental clinic emergency. *Simulation in Healthcare, 6,* 101–108.

Calhoun, A. W., Boone, M. C., Peterson, E. B., Boland, K. A., & Montgomery, V. L. (2011). Integrated in situ simulation using redirected faculty educational time to minimize costs: A feasibility study. *Simulation in Healthcare, 6,* 337–344.

Cheng, A., Donoghue, A., Gilfoyle, E., & Eppich, W. (2012). Simulation-based crisis resource management training for pediatric critical care medicine: A review for instructors. *Pediatric Critical Care Medicine, 13,* 197–203.

Cohen, E. R., Feinglass, J., Barsuk, J. H., Barnard, C., O'Donnell, A., McGaghie, W. C., & Wayne, D. B. (2010). Cost savings from reduced catheter-related bloodstream infection after simulation-based education for residents in a medical intensive care unit. *Simulation in Healthcare, 5,* 98–102.

Cooper, J. B., & Taqueti, V. R. (2004). A brief history of the development of mannequin simulators for clinical education and training. *Quality & Safety in Health Care, 13,* i11–i18.

Davis, S., Riley, W., Gurses, A. P., Miller, K., & Hansen, H. (2008). Failure modes and effects analysis based on in situ simulations: A methodology to improve understanding of risks and failures. In K. Henriksen, J. B. Battles, M. A. Keyes, & M. L. Grady (Eds.), *Advances in patient safety: New directions and alternative approaches: Performance and tools.* (Vol. 3) Rockville, MD: Agency for Healthcare Research and Quality.

Draycott, T. J., Crofts, J. F., Ash, J. P., Wilson, L. V., Yard, E., Sibanda, T., & Whitelaw, A. (2008). Improving neonatal outcome through practical shoulder dystocia training. *Obstetrics & Gynecology, 112,* 14–20.

Edler, A. A., Chen, M., Honkanen, A., Hackel, A., & Golianu, B. (2010). Affordable simulation for small-scale training and assessment. *Simulation in Healthcare, 5,* 112–115.

Geis, G. L., Pio, B., Pendergrass, T. L., Moyer, M. R., & Patterson, M. D. (2011). Simulation to assess the safety of new healthcare teams and new facilities. *Simulation in Healthcare, 6,* 125–133.

Guise, J. M., Lowe, N. K., Deering, S., Lewis, P. O., O'Haire, C., Irwin, L. K., … Kanki, B. G. (2010). Mobile in situ obstetric emergency simulation and teamwork training to improve maternal-fetal safety in hospitals. *Joint Commission Journal on Quality and Patient Safety, 36,* 443–453.

Hales, B. M., & Pronovost, P. J. (2006). The checklist—A tool for error management and performance improvement. *Journal of Critical Care, 21,* 231–235.

Hamman, W. R., Beaudin-Seiler, B. M., Beaubien, J. M., Gullickson, A. M., Orizondo-Korotko, K., Gross, A. C., … Lammers, R. (2009). Using in situ simulation to identify and resolve latent environmental threats to patient safety: Case study involving a labor and delivery ward. *Journal of Patient Safety, 5,* 184–187.

Hamman, W. R., Beaudin-Seiler, B. M., Beaubien, J. M., Gullickson, A. M., Orizondo-Korotko, K., Gross, A. C., … Lammers, R. L. (2010). Using simulation to identify and resolve threats to patient safety. *The American Journal of Managed Care, 16,* e145–e150.

Harlow, K. C., & Sportsman, S. (2007). An economic analysis of patient simulators clinical training in nursing education. *Nursing Economic$, 25,* 24–29, 3.

Hohenhaus, S. M., Hohenhaus, J., Saunders, M., Vandergrift, J., Kohler, T. A., Manikowski, M. E., … Holleran, S. (2008). Emergency response: Lessons learned during a community hospital's in situ fire simulation. *Journal of Emergency Nursing, 34,* 352–354.

Hunt, E. A., Nelson, K. L., & Shilkofski, N. A. (2006). Simulation in medicine: Addressing patient safety and improving the interface between healthcare providers and medical technology. *Biomedical Instrumentation & Technology, 40,* 399–404.

SECTION 2 • Types of Simulation Programs

Jankouskas, T., Bush, M. C., Murray, B., Rudy, S., Henry, J., Dyer, A. M., … Sinz, E. (2007). Crisis resource management: Evaluating outcomes of a multidisciplinary team. *Simulation in Healthcare, 2,* 96–101.

Kobayashi, L., Dunbar-Viveiros, J. A., Sheahan, B. A., Rezendes, M. H., Devine, J., Cooper M. R., … Jay, G. D. (2010). In situ simulation comparing in-hospital first responder sudden cardiac arrest resuscitation using semiautomated defibrillators and automated external defibrillators. *Simulation in Healthcare, 5,* 82–90.

Kushniruk, A. W., Borycki, E. M., Kuwata, S., & Kannry, J. (2011). Emerging approaches to usability evaluation of health information systems: Towards in situ analysis of complex healthcare systems and environments. *Studies in Health Technology and Informatics, 169,* 915–919.

Langhan, T. S., Rigby, I. J., Walker, I. W., Howes, D., Donnon, T., & Lord, J. A. (2009). Simulation-based training in critical resuscitation procedures improves residents' competence. *Canadian Journal of Emergency Medical Care, 11,* 535–539.

Lasater, K. (2007). High-fidelity simulation and the development of clinical judgment: Students' experiences. *The Journal of Nursing Education, 46,* 269–276.

Lasko, D., Zamakhshary, M., & Gerstle, J. T. (2009). Perception and use of minimal access surgery simulators in pediatric surgery training programs. *Journal of Pediatric Surgery, 44,* 1009–1012.

LaVelle, B. A., & McLaughlin, J. J. (2008). Simulation-based education improves patient safety in ambulatory care. In K. Henriksen, J. B. Battles, M. A. Keyes, & M. L. Grady (Eds.), *Advances in patient safety: New directions and alternative approaches: Performance and tools.* (Vol. 3) Rockville, MD: Agency for Healthcare Research and Quality.

Lindquist, L. A., Gleason, K. M., McDaniel, M. R., Doeksen, A., & Liss, D. (2008). Teaching medication reconciliation through simulation: A patient safety initiative for second year medical students. *Journal of General Internal Medicine, 23,* 998–1001.

McKeon, L. M., Norris, T., Cardell, B., & Britt, T. (2009). Developing patient-centered care competencies among prelicensure nursing students using simulation. *The Journal of Nursing Education, 48,* 711–715.

Miller, K. K., Riley, W., Davis, S., & Hansen, H. E. (2008). In situ simulation: a method of experiential learning to promote safety and team behavior. *The Journal of Perinatal & Neonatal Nursing, 22,* 105–113.

Mondrup, F., Brabrand, M., Folkestad, L., Oxlund, J., Wiborg, K. R., Sand, N. P., & Knudsen, T. (2011). In-hospital resuscitation evaluated by in situ simulation: A prospective simulation study. *Scandinavian Journal of Trauma, Resuscitation and Emergency Medicine, 19,* 55.

Nestel, D., Groom, J., Eikeland-Husebø, S., & O'Donnell, J. M. (2011). Simulation for learning and teaching procedural skills: The state of the science. *Simulation in Healthcare, 6,* S10–S13.

Paige, J. T., Kozmenko, V., Yang, T., Gururaja, R. P., Cohn, I., Hilton, C., & Chauvin, S. (2008). The mobile mock operating room: Bringing team training to the point of care. In K. Henriksen, J. B. Battles, M. A. Keyes, & M. L. Grady (Eds.), *Advances in patient safety: New directions and alternative approaches: Performance and tools.* (Vol. 3) Rockville, MD: Agency for Healthcare Research and Quality.

Parikh, J. A., McGory, M. L., Ko, C. Y., Hines, O. J., Tillou, A., & Hiatt, J. R. (2008). A structured conference program improves competency-based surgical education. *American Journal of Surgery, 196,* 273–279.

Perkins, G. D. (2007). Simulation in resuscitation training. *Resuscitation, 73,* 202–211.

Pruitt, C. M., & Liebelt, E. L. (2010). Enhancing patient safety in the pediatric emergency department: Teams, communication, and lessons from crew resource management. *Pediatric Emergency Care, 26,* 942–948.

Riley, W., Davis, S., Miller, K., Hansen, H., Sainfort, F., & Sweet, R. (2011). Didactic and simulation nontechnical skills team training to improve perinatal patient outcomes in a community hospital. *Joint Commission Journal on Quality and Patient Safety, 37,* 357–364.

Riley, W., Lownik, E., Parrotta, C., Miller, K., & Davis, S. (2011). Creating high reliability teams in healthcare through in situ simulation training. *Administrative Sciences, 1,* 14–31.

Seropian, M., & Lavey, R. (2010). Design considerations for healthcare simulation facilities. *Simulation in Healthcare, 5,* 338–345.

Sutton, G. (2009). Evaluating multidisciplinary health care teams: Taking the crisis out of CRM. *Australian Health Review, 33,* 445–452.

Sutton, R. M., Niles, D., Meaney, P. A., Aplenc, R., French, B., Abella, B. S., … Sweet, R. M. (2010). Detecting breaches in defensive barriers using in situ simulation for obstetric emergencies. *Quality & Safety in Health Care, 19,* i53–i56.

Volk, M. S., Ward, J., Irias, N., Navedo, A., Pollart, J., & Weinstock, P. H. (2011). Using medical simulation to teach crisis resource management and decision-making skills to otolaryngology housestaff. *Otolaryngology—Head and Neck Surgery, 145,* 35–42.

Waxman, K. T., Nichols, A. A., O'Leary-Kelley, C., & Miller, M. (2011). The evolution of a statewide network: The bay area simulation collaborative. *Simulation in Healthcare, 6,* 345–351.

Weinstock, P. H., Kappus, L. J., Garden, A., & Burns, J. P. (2009). Simulation at the point of care: Reduced-cost, in situ training via a mobile cart. *Pediatric Critical Care Medicine, 10,* 176–181.

Yager, P. H., Lok, J., & Klig, J. E. (2011). Advances in simulation for pediatric critical care and emergency medicine. *Current Opinion in Pediatrics, 23,* 293–297.

Ziv, A., Small, S. D., & Wolpe, P. R. (2000). Patient safety and simulation-based medical education. *Medical Teacher, 22,* 489–495.

Ziv, A., Wolpe, P. R., Small, S. D., & Glick, S. (2003). Simulation-based medical education: An ethical imperative. *Academic Medicine, 78,* 783–788.

CHAPTER 2.3

Mobile Simulations

Brent Thorkelson, BSc, EMT-P

ABOUT THE AUTHORS

BRENT THORKELSON has been a registered Advanced Care Paramedic for 22 years. For the past 6 years, he has held the position of lead Senior Staff Development Officer in Clinical Compliance Training and Standards for Alberta Health Services Emergency Medical Services Patient Care Simulation. Brent's work with mobile simulation for the Emergency Medical Services workforce has been published in numerous media articles. When not coordinating the provincial simulation program, Brent raises funds for Kids Cancer Research.

ABSTRACT

You have been tasked to build an Medical Simulation Training Unit (MSTU). As available hospital space shrinks and the need to deliver experiential learning to a dynamic workforce grows, many hospitals and Emergency Medical Services are moving toward this method of delivering experiential education. There are several "pearls of wisdom" involved in building an MSTU. First, an environment that accurately portrays the area of service in which practitioners actually work in must be created. Second, if the MSTU is to travel long distances—as it should if it is being utilized to its fullest potential—it will need a chassis that is built for such a task, is easily maneuvered, and can ideally be operated without special licenses. Third, to maximize the return on investment for what will be an expensive vehicle, it should be active in all four seasons. Fourth, due to the public's growing awareness of reducing greenhouse gases, the MSTU should operate with minimal environmental impact. Fifth, special consideration must be given to the design of the audio/video system, as few systems are appropriate for mounting in a moving vehicle. Finally, interprofessional collaboration in designing the layout of the MSTU will be needed to facilitate the entire continuum of patient care, from the first responder to the Emergency Medical Services team, and finally to the emergency department staff.

CASE EXAMPLE

A patient safety division has been trending treatment rendered to patients suffering from myocardial ischemia for the past 3 years. Results have shown a need for additional practitioner education in the area of assessment and treatment of myocardial ischemic chest pain. This training is to be provided to all Emergency Department and Emergency Medical Services practitioners in an area that covers over 80,000 square miles (207,184 km²) and encompasses two main hospitals and three urgent care centers.

The Senior Leadership Team has agreed to fund four full-time Clinical Educator positions and the construction of a simulation lab. The two main caveats to funding this new simulation program are: simulation training is to occur with on-duty staff to prevent overtime costs, and training is not to interfere with ongoing patient care.

With funding for only one lab and training to occur while in close proximity to the practitioners' work location (so as to not interfere with ongoing patient care), there is only one cost-effective tool that can fit the program's needs: development of a mobile Medical Simulation Training Unit program.

INTRODUCTION

As health care simulation evolves and gains acceptance in the medical field, it is increasingly difficult to support all the practitioners who need this form of education. It is challenging to find available space in medical centers to house static simulation labs. As workloads grow and call volumes increase, moving staff off-site or out of their service areas to participate in scheduled simulations produces logistical challenges. As enhancing patient care through education is the key objective in any simulation program, pulling hospital staff or Emergency Medical Services (EMS) ambulance units from their areas, either in a large metropolis or in a rural area, is not conducive to good patient care. Further, the sheer cost of building multiple static labs across a province or state to serve what is a mobile workforce or hospital-based staff is simply not economically viable. The province of Alberta, for example, spans over 255,500 square miles (661,693.9 km^2) ("Alberta," 2007) and has approximately 3,000 EMS practitioners employed by Alberta Health Services (AHS) ("Employee Data Base," 2009). The main delivery model used by the AHS EMS Patient Care Simulation (PCS) program is a mobile **Medical Simulation Training Unit**(MSTU). This chapter will include the major elements to consider when building an MSTU, as seen through the lens of the AHS EMS PCS program.

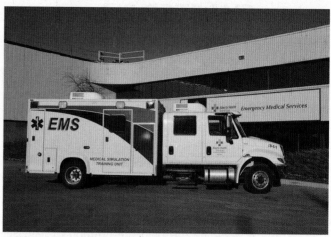

FIGURE 2.3.1 Photo of one of three mobile MSTUs operated by the Learning and Development division of the AHS EMS.

The Truck for the Job

The most important aspect of any project is the foundation that supports it. In the case of an MSTU, the project foundation is the **chassis** on which the vehicle will be built on.

The number of people intended to operate the MSTU along with its designated purpose will govern the selection of chassis size. The criteria of the AHS EMS PCS program includes the following:

- The truck must be easy to drive.
- There must be no need for any special federal driving endorsement.
- It must be capable of traveling long distances over a 10- to 15-year life cycle.
- There must be a network of service centers in the unit's general operating area.

The first two points are important, especially if there are going to be a variety of people taking turns at the wheel. An MSTU can be as small as an ambulance or large van, or as large as a converted full-sized diesel passenger bus. If there are only two or three consistent operators, the latter may be appropriate; however, if a greater number of operators will sporadically drive the vehicle, then a smaller simulation unit that still fits your needs may be best.

On the basis of the needs of the AHS EMS, a medium-duty truck chassis was decided upon (Figure 2.3.1). This size of chassis fits comfortably in the middle between a standard ambulance (or large van) and a full-size passenger bus. One of the key differences between a smaller chassis such (or light-duty chassis as in a van) and a medium-duty chassis is the options that are available to customize the chassis to best fit the program's needs. Here are the key elements to be discussed when choosing the MSTU's chassis.

Payload—Make sure that you take into account the full weight the vehicle will be carrying, including equipment, passengers, and a full fuel tank. These figures always need to be added up to determine your **gross vehicle weight rating**(GVWR) (Lyden, 2007), which is critical to prevent overloading and, by law, limits the maximum vehicle weight ("Gross Vehicle Weight Rating," 2013).

Truck Choice—A medium-duty truck is larger than a light-duty, typical pickup truck. Prices for a medium-duty truck start at around $60,000 for a new cab, chassis, and body (Brown, 2006). The good news is that the life of a medium-duty truck is much longer than that of a light-duty truck. Old age for a medium-duty diesel truck starts at 500,000 miles (804,650 km), and many last much longer if driven appropriately. Given this, the life expectancy of your simulation unit should be set at a minimum of 15 years, depending of course on the annual mileage (Brown, 2006).

Towing—If your simulation program includes towing a trailer with the mobile simulator chassis, perhaps to use as a classroom with task trainers, make sure to discuss the **gross combination vehicle weight rating** (GCVWR) with the vendor chosen ("Gross combined weight rating," 2013). Essentially, this is the maximum allowable weight determined by the manufacturer as the GCVWR, plus the weight of the trailer at maximum load (Lyden, 2007).

Rear Suspension—MSTUs typically traveling distances; not only is passenger comfort important, but also the safety and well-being of electronics and patient simulators. Choose a suspension that best suits the program's needs. If the MSTU's back bumper needs to lower or "kneel," as in the case of AHS EMS's MSTUs, then it is important to choose an air system (Figure 2.3.2A, B). This system provides a good compromise between comfort and lowering capabilities. If kneeling is not essential but a smooth ride is paramount, then a tapered-leaf setup will probably suffice (Lyden, 2007). Passenger comfort is easily accomplished by ensuring that the passenger cab is equipped with its own dampening system, something that is very common on today's modern medium-duty chassis.

Engine and Gearing—Unlike a regular passenger car, a medium-duty truck will have many types of engine and

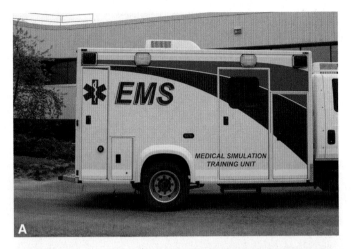

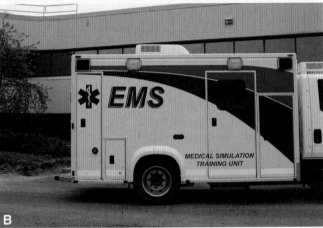

FIGURE 2.3.2 **A.** The AHS MSTU with air ride suspension in the transportation level. Note the placement of the "Medical Simulation Training Unit" decal placed at window height to advertise to the public that this unit is training their practitioners! **B.** Air suspension in the loading level to allow for easier loading and unloading of stretcher.

gearing configurations available. Due diligence in discussing options with the truck vendor is a necessity. When in doubt, go large; contrary to popular belief, a larger engine does not necessarily use more fuel. If a larger engine does not have to work as hard, it will burn less fuel than a smaller engine that works hard all the time (B. VanGastel, personal communication, May 7, 2013). The bottom line is that the vehicle needs to be comfortable with what it is carrying. This will decrease not only driver fatigue, but also long-term maintenance costs from having to repair an overstressed drive train.

As with any vehicle, an MSTU will need both scheduled and unscheduled maintenance. It is the unscheduled maintenance needs that necessitate choosing a chassis and engine configuration that can be serviced in the majority of locations it will be visiting. AHS EMS's MSTUs are all built on International chassis. At present there are 14 International Service Centers across the province of Alberta; if something goes wrong, it is highly likely that repairs can be made promptly. In this way we can avoid canceling a mobile simulation event, especially if we are a full day's travel from our home base.

Mobile Audio/Visual Considerations

When planning the audio/video system for a mobile simulation unit, special care must be taken to choose the correct vendor for the job: one who is willing to work through the idiosyncrasies that occur when electronics are put into a vehicle that will travel across the countryside, often on less-than-ideal roads. It is not necessary that the vendor has previously set equipment on a mobile platform; it is more important to ensure the vendor is in good standing and is willing to work closely with the project manager. The following guidelines suggest what you might bring to the table at the first planning meeting with the vendor. Focus on providing clear expectations and as much detail as possible.

- Plan on installing at least one computer to run the patient simulator as well as your audio/visual system. Through experience it has been learned that desktop tower computers and travel simply do not mix. If possible, use either a laptop or compact computer. Laptops, due to their internal packaging, withstand traveling far better. Another option is the Mac Mini that is both compact and very durable. An added bonus is that a laptop, at moderate operating speed, will draw far less power than a full-sized desktop computer (Williams, 2013).
- Running cable from one end of a mobile simulation vehicle to the other can present challenges, but these can be easily overcome by some simple preplanning. For both network and audio/video wiring, it is necessary to use stranded cabling rather than solid core. When subjected to the vibrations of a moving vehicle, stranded cable is much more reliable; solid core is likely to fatigue and break.
- Cable pathways should be run through the chassis of the vehicle so that network and microphone cables are each provided a separate path; these should be at least one foot away from any alternating current power cables. This helps prevent any electromagnetic interference from affecting these sensitive signals. If network and/or microphone cables have to cross alternating current power cables, make sure they do so at 90 degrees to one another.
- When planning out the cable pathways, make sure to allow for cycling out audio and video equipment. Designing conduits into the schematics through which to run cables will allow for easy change of equipment when needed.
- Be cognizant of the processing delay that occurs when computers are used to capture audio and video. Fortunately, newer computer systems are faster, so this delay is limited. Although a slight delay in the video feed is a minor inconvenience, it is not acceptable to have even a minor delay in the audio. Operators must hear—in real time—what is said in the simulation area. For example, a practitioner might ask, "Sir, are you having any chest discomfort?"

Even a one-second delay from the asking of the question to it being heard by the operator can cause confusion. The practitioner might think, for that moment, that the simulated patient is unresponsive, and the entire simulation exercise could begin to unravel. The use of an auxiliary audio microphone placed in the simulation area will ensure that all audio is heard in real time (R. Judd, personal communication, May 13, 2013).

- When laying out the audio and video plans, the patient simulation team must determine how the facilitator in the simulation area will communicate with the operator, who is usually in another area. Texting is a possible option to consider, but does depend on the speed of the person sending the text. Ideally, a wireless microphone system, complete with headset and boom microphone, should be installed. This will allow clear, concise communications between the operator and the facilitator.

- The type of **audio mixer** used depends on the layout. An audio mixer will allow the user to adjust the sensitivity of the microphones and speakers in both the simulation area and the operator's room. Ask the vendor to supply one that is simple to operate, with preset levels that can be locked in. When choosing the mixer, a good option is to ensure that it has acoustic echo cancellation. This allows both microphones and speakers to be on at the same time; it filters out the audio that has already been sent to the simulation area speakers so that the microphones do not pick it up and send it back to the operator. Without this feature, the microphones and speakers will have to be switched in such a way that the operator's speakers turn off when his/her microphone is turned on.

- In the event of a power outage (and this can happen), the use of appropriate **uninterrupted power supply** (UPS) units should be used. These will ensure that the sensitive electronics are protected against voltage spikes when the MSTU switches from **inverter** to shoreline (R. Judd, personal communication, May 13, 2013).

- The placement of the vital sign monitor is an important one. Initially, the AHS EMS PCS team had a regular computer monitor situated in close proximity to the defibrillator/monitor, allowing it to be easily seen by the practitioners. A refinement was made by one of our clinical educators, who replaced the computer monitor with a small mini screen attached to the front of the defibrillator/monitor (Figure 2.3.3). The layout of the screen is adjusted to match what the practitioners would normally see. This reduces the confusion of choosing which screen to observe at any given moment. If the simulation requires pacing or defibrillation, the small screen is popped off so the practitioners can view the regular screen.

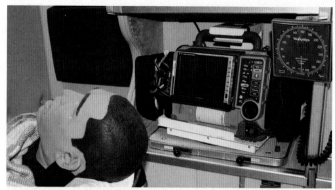

FIGURE 2.3.3 Inexpensive, small "mini screen" so that learners view the defibrillator as opposed to having to look elsewhere to get the patient simulator's information.

A MOBILE SIMULATOR FOR ALL SEASONS

The area serviced by the MSTU will dictate how to set up the mobile simulator for all seasons. Generally, spring and fall do not present major issues; however, summer and winter can each pose challenges to controlling the climate inside the mobile simulation unit.

If the simulator is built on a medium-duty truck chassis, then the options to park the unit indoors to conduct simulations will be limited, at best. Having the mobile simulation unit parked and idling outside an EMS/fire station or in front of a hospital is not ideal. Here are a couple of options that have been found to work well.

Heating—When considering heating, convenience and safety are important elements. A solution that has been very well received by our teams is the installation of small diesel-fed Webasto heaters. These units take up little space and draw a small amount of current. Convenience is enhanced as they are plumbed directly into the large diesel saddle tanks. AHS EMS MSTUs have found the heaters particularly useful for mobile simulations held in the winter. One heater is placed in the cab and another in the simulation area. We turn on the small diesel-fed heater in the simulation area the minute we leave base headquarters; it will remain on for the duration of the trip, which can last up to 7 days. The other unit in the cab area, or control room, is turned on while simulations are running, or when freezing temperatures are forecast and the unit is parked outdoors. The current draw is so minimal—between 1.25 and 2.40 A—that even with both heaters running overnight to keep the cab electronics and the patient simulator and medications warm, there is no risk of draining the chassis batteries when operating without the unit's engine running, even at $-22°$ F. Each heater also comes with a thermostat, and so temperatures can be easily regulated (Figure 2.3.4).

Air Conditioning (AC)—Providing cool air in both control and simulation areas on a hot summer day poses challenges when it comes to power demands. When an

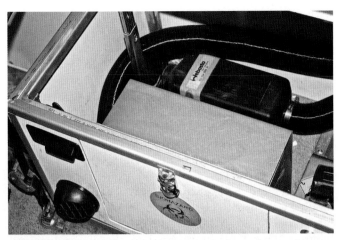

FIGURE 2.3.4 Small Webasto heater can be located in small spaces when room is at a premium. In this case, it is located under the bench seat in the simulation area.

the units off during the actual simulation. For small volume areas, such as the operator's area and the simulation room, this works very well, as the simulations last 20 to 30 minutes at most.

Another possible solution is to install an air diverter plate (Figure 2.3.6). This simple plate has worked well for the Simulation in Motion–South Dakota (SIM-SD) mobile program. It not only directs the air away from the tops of practitioners' heads, but it also decreases the amount of ambient noise so that communication between learners can be heard clearly through the microphones (T. Spier, personal communication, May 20, 2013).

Often overlooked, setting up a comfortable place where medical practitioners can learn is important. The term "turning up the heat" in simulation is not to be taken literally! The last thing learners want is to leave a simulation exercise needing showers and change of uniforms.

air conditioning unit is started, the general rule is that the hotter the ambient temperature, the greater the power draw needed to start the compressor. The way around this is to design a "soft start" for the compressors (Figure 2.3.5). Noise from the AC units can also be troublesome. To date, AHS EMS's PCS team have run the AC units presimulation to cool the area and then shut

DELIVERING AN ENERGY-EFFICIENT SIMULATION

When designing the MSTU, put thought and effort into lessening its impact on the environment. Plan to use a shoreline as the default power source for the mobile

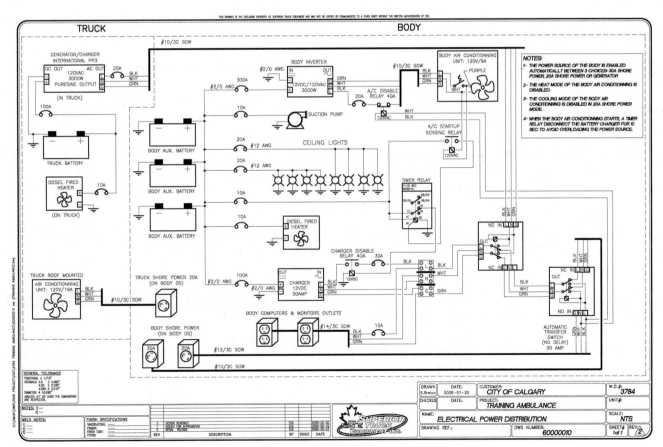

FIGURE 2.3.5 Engineering electrical schematic of wiring in the AHS EMS PCS mobile MSTU#2. Diagram illustrates the timer system that serves as the "soft start" for the AC units. Having diagrams accessible when traveling can be important if repairs are needed.

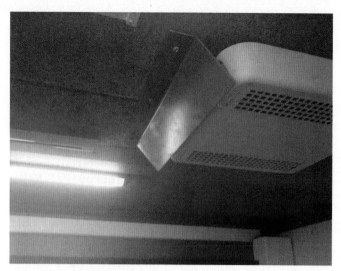

FIGURE 2.3.6 Air conditioning diverter plate on South Dakota's mobile simulation lab keeps noise down to a minimum during a simulation.

unit, rather than running a large diesel engine; or worse, a two- or four-stroke generator. Depending on the unit's size, operating completely on shoreline is an obtainable objective.

Using electrical power provides obvious environmental benefits, but has other advantages as well. Noise from a diesel engine or generator can disturb not only the learners in the simulation, but also residents, businesses, and services in the surrounding area. A generator large enough to run the air conditioning units or heaters as well as all electronics and lights will easily need to deliver 3,500 W. Though today's generators are quieter and much more efficient than they were even 5 years ago, they can still be very disruptive. Imagine sitting at a campsite enjoying a coffee by the morning fire, when a camper three sites down fires up a generator. The effect is similar to running the MSTU on diesel power.

When the program's MSTU arrives on-site to provide a full day of experiential learning, it is important to minimize the impact of noise and exhaust fumes, even if using a combustion engine. AHS EMS PCS's first MSTU could not operate strictly on shore power when air conditioning was needed. It did not take long for complaints from the adjacent hospital to be voiced, as it had inadvertently

parked near the fresh air intake to the facility. Take care to situate the mobile simulation unit appropriately, in order to avoid a similar situation.

Through the use of energy-efficient AC units, LED lights, Webasto heaters, large deep-cycle batteries, and switch timers, it is possible to run our mobile simulators on shore power alone (Figure 2.3.5). The use of LED lights, for example, works very well for two reasons. First, there is far less amperage draw than from incandescent bulbs; and second, far less heat is generated. When AHS EMS PCS initially set up its MSTUs, the actual incandescent lights that had been fitted to the decommissioned ambulance patient module were used. The lights, when on for extended periods of time, grew so hot that the plastic lens covers began melting. When LEDs were installed, the power draw and heat issues were resolved.

For the electrical supply on the side of the simulation unit, it is wise to choose 30-A receptacles, as these allow 30-A power to be plugged in, if available. If not, a 30- to 15-A "pig tail" cord can be used to adapt the side plugs to 15 A. On the AHS EMS PCS unit, there is one 30-A plug and one 20-A plug. The 30-A plug supplies all the electronics, the simulation area air conditioning, and also charges the deep-cycle batteries. The 20-A plug provides the operator's area AC only. This configuration allows for more flexibility (Table 2.3.1) (S. Breton, personal communication, May 9, 2013).

To run off shoreline power only, it is necessary to plan ahead. When traveling to a location, call ahead to the facility's security and building engineering or maintenance department, and specify that you require the use of two minimum 15-A receptacles that are on separate breakers. In our experience, this is almost always available. As well, the departments contacted appreciate the "heads up" regarding arrival. Often security will have placed traffic cones to cordon off the area in which to park the unit.

THE COST OF DOING BUSINESS

Is providing simulation an expensive way to educate medical professionals? The simple answer is "Yes." Factor in the cost of the MSTU and maintenance over its lifetime, the wages of the clinical educators, and the

TABLE 2.3.1

Possible Combinations of Power Supply and Accessories*

Ambient Outside Temperature	One 15-A Shoreline	Two 15-A Shoreline Power	Webasto Diesel Heaters	AC Unit for Simulation Area	AC Unit for Operators Area	Truck Engine Running Vanner 6000 Inverter
−22° F (−30° C)	YES	N/A	ON	OFF	OFF	OFF
	NO	N/A	ON	OFF	OFF	ON
+85° F (+30° C)	NO	YES	OFF	ON	ON	OFF
	YES	NO	OFF	ON	OFF	OFF
	NO	NO	OFF	ON	ON (using truck AC)	ON

*Audio and video are assumed to be ON regardless of power supply.

EXPERT'S CORNER

MOBILE SIMULATION AND THE DEVELOPMENT OF *SIMCOACH*
Eric A. Brown, MD, FACEP
Executive Director, Palmetto Health–University of South Carolina, School of Medicine Simulation Center

A mobile simulation component can add significant value to your simulation program. If you are considering a mobile component, you should begin with a thoughtful and targeted needs assessment of your client base. A few key questions that should be asked include:
- Do mobile capabilities serve your mission and vision?
- Is access to your fixed center or home base a barrier to serving your target client base?
- If you do not have a fixed center, can a mobile unit provide enough capacity to fulfill your mission?

It became clear to us several years ago at the Palmetto Health–University of South Carolina School of Medicine Simulation Center in Columbia, South Carolina, that our client's needs were on track to rapidly outpace our simulation infrastructure in a short period of time. It was then that we began a thorough expansion-planning process. The increase in our internal client base, comprised of multidisciplinary provider teams from partner institutions, clearly necessitated a plan for a larger fixed facility in the near term. However, we also recognized that a significant number of our learners were "externals" coming from across the state and region. Informal discussions with several of these clients revealed common themes about what led them to our simulation program. These themes included: (1) a belief that simulation-based education was the new standard, and (2) a lack of access to simulation resources in their local geographic area.

We formalized our needs assessment by surveying providers within a 50-mile (80.465 km) radius of our institution. We asked them to define their training needs, sources of funding for simulation training, and challenges to obtaining ongoing simulation training in their field of practice. The most common barriers cited were: (1) lack of simulation-training opportunities near their place of work, (2) inability to take a day off work to travel to an alternate site, and (3) concerns around cost of courses. These common themes led us to conclude that to meet our goal of being a regional resource in simulation-based training, we needed to provide a cost-efficient mobile simulation component to providers in our region.

Through the process of developing our mobile component, multiple advantages became apparent, including:
- The mobile unit would be a fully featured simulation space, available on demand and in proximity to any hospital, clinic, or community setting.
- The mobile unit would maintain the same level of control over the learning environment afforded by a fixed facility, including the appearance of the simulated clinical space, audio/visual capture capabilities, and so on.
- The mobile unit would serve as surge capacity for our fixed simulation center. When the unit is not deployed, the addition of two fully functional encounter rooms allows us to simultaneously serve multiple learner groups who would otherwise have to be scheduled during separate time slots.
- The mobile unit would serve as a sophisticated and efficient staging platform for both in situ and field-training exercises. The dedicated moulage and preparatory space can be critical to delivering a quality experience at an unfamiliar site.
- The mobile unit would engage a much larger and broader learner group for research purposes.
- The mobile unit would serve as an exceptional marketing tool, promoting our partner institutions as well as health care simulation in general.

We started our fundraising effort by immediately branding the mobile component so that our internal champions and funders could identify with the concept and mission. Our program moniker became Simulation in Medicine Collaborative Outreach and Community Health or SimCOACH. We designed a fully functional, mobile simulation unit, capable of delivering our full library of simulation courses to providers across the Midlands of South Carolina and the surrounding region. By telling our story and effectively articulating the potential impact of a mobile simulation component, we captured the attention of a donor who offered to fund the construction of our custom unit. SimCOACH is now a 38-ft long vehicle with double slide-outs, providing two encounter rooms, a control room, and ample storage for full capability deployment. We opted to base our design on a truck platform so that it remains within the weight limit required for a commercial driver's license. All of our employees are trained to operate the coach.

As medical simulation becomes an increasingly valuable and integrated set of methodologies bridging all domains in health care education, there is an increasing demand for simulation capacity. The right combination of fixed facilities, simulation equipment, and expert staff may meet your current local demands, but may be woefully inadequate as time goes on. Perhaps most importantly, the rising visibility of simulation over the past decade makes it clear that the ability to access simulation resources is transitioning from luxury to necessity, and will further incentivize those who have been waiting on the sidelines to get in the game. A mobile simulation component can be a high-impact mechanism to deliver simulation across multiple domains and serve your goals and mission.

purchase of fuel, accommodations, and patient simulator warranties, the costs of 1 hour of simulation can add up fast. The setup of the program's business model and the vastness of the area the team plans to cover will determine whether mobile simulation is the most practical solution. In many cases, it *is* the most cost-effective alternative (LeBlanc, 2008).

This chapter will use the AHS EMS PCS program's MSTUs.

MEDICAL SIMULATION TRAINING UNIT

In the province of Alberta, we serve approximately 3,000 EMS practitioners across 255,500 square miles (661,693 square kilometers). With the addition of a third MSTU, the AHS EMS PCS program's goal is to deliver 1500 simulations across the province in 12 months.

TABLE 2.3.2

Cost of Rural and Urban Simulations When Travel Times, Food, Fuel, and Accommodation Costs Are Factored in

Area	Hourly Cost of MSTU Based on 10-yr Life Cycle and Forecasted Repairs ($)	Average Cost of Consumables/1-hr Simulation Session ($)	Approximate Hourly Rate for Two Clinical Educators ($)	Costs for 1 hr/Practitioner and Two Practitioners/ Simulation ($)
Urban	75.00	26.00	100.00	100.00
Rural	75.00	26.00	100.00	211.00

The hourly cost of the MSTU is based on the expected maintenance cost of the unit over a 10-year life span, with a predicted recovery cost of zero at the end. Wages are based on two senior clinical educators. Rural trips include food and accommodations charges; these, however, would not be applicable in an urban setting. Equipment costs are also included as consumables. The AHS EMS PCS program also presently uses expired medications at no cost to the program (Table 2.3.2).

There is a way to bring the cost per practitioner down when dealing with a mobile workforce as well as training practitioners who are on active duty: organize relief practitioners through operational buy-in. If staffing and operations believe in the value of education through PCS, and extra staff are brought on to cover for the staff participating in the simulations, the rate of completing more simulations will increase. Inclusion into the program model of a relief staffing policy or understanding is essential; then the expectations from both areas will be understood upfront. This will not only improve the morale of your clinical educators, who will no longer be constantly waiting for people to become free to participate, but it will also decrease the cost per practitioner, especially when overnight trips are planned.

BEEN THERE, DONE THAT

Simulations are often restricted to focus on specific disciplines. This may involve designing and delivering simulations for an Emergency Department or perhaps an Operating Room. Once a mobile program is comfortable delivering discipline specific simulation, one may consider expanding the offering to include the care of patients across the entire continuum of care.

This has proved true with the AHS EMS PCS program. The program almost exclusively applies its mobile simulations to scenarios set in an ambulance. It is important, to expand the simulation environment outside of the MSTU when possible. Logistically, this takes more planning and is not always practical; however, on occasions it needs to be worked in. One interprofessional practice simulation designed by the AHS EMS PCS team had the attending crew take over care from a citizen, complete the simulation in the back of the MSTU, and transfer the pediatric patient simulator into the Alberta Children's Hospital. Care is then handed over to the Emergency Department, whose team continues to treat the patient (Luigi Savoia, 2010).

Utilizing an MSTU to include different health care disciplines or departments (or both) can be invaluable. Not only can it improve communication skills and help perfect the handoff between departments, it also builds interprofessional collaboration that may not normally be present (Berkenstadt et al., 2008).

When designing an MSTU, take into account this concept: If the mobile simulation is for EMS-specific practitioners (for example), build into it the ability to load and unload the wireless patient simulator from the unit. In this way, local first responders as well as the emergency room clinicians can be involved in the simulation.

This ability can be used to your advantage when raising funds for the project. For instance, run a simulation at a local area industrial plant where the first responders employed by the plant can get involved. The next time funding is needed, it is highly likely that the plant's senior management will remember their involvement and will enthusiastically contribute to the fundraising efforts.

SUMMARY

The "pearls of wisdom" offered in this chapter will undoubtedly inspire further questions that are unique to designing and building an MSTU. It is always preferable, and often less expensive, to solve a potential problem in the design stage rather than after the build has started.

Because mobile simulation has become more popular, there are many examples currently operating in the field. Give the project the time and funds to allow for a needs analysis of the unit that will be built. Take this information and travel to view some current, active MSTUs. It makes no sense to "reinvent the wheel" when someone out there has already made the mistakes and has found the ideal solutions. In the past 5 years, the AHS EMS PCS program has been approached by three different services. By viewing firsthand what may or may not work for their models of delivery, they can more efficiently design their own programs. This is a practical and commendable approach.

There are many MSTUs currently in operation. They range from units built "in-house" to those that are built by a manufacturer that specializes in unique applications. The budget for funding a unit can dictate what the model for construction will look like. AHS EMS PCS program acted as the general contractor when constructing the three current MSTUs active in Alberta. With each unit built, new and improved techniques have come to light. It is the AHS EMS PCS program's goal that every subsequent mobile unit built will be better than those that came before.

Once the keys to the new MSTU are picked up, what's next? It's time for a road trip! Get the unit out to as many hospitals and services to introduce this innovative and exciting model of delivering education. Make sure as many practitioners as possible get a chance to see the new unit; educate them as to how it will be used. The interest and enthusiasm generated will pay big dividends when the new MSTU arrives to offer them their first simulation-training experience.

REFERENCES

Alberta. (2007, March 7). Retrieved May 5, 2013, from https://en.wikipedia.org/wiki/Alberta

Berkenstadt, H., Haviv, Y., Tuval, A., Shemesh, Y., Megrill, A., Perry, A., … Ziv, A. (2008). Improving handoff communications in critical care: Utilizing simulation-based training toward process improvement in managing patient risk. *Chest Journal, 34*(1), 1–5.

Brown, C. (2006, January). First time's guide to the medium-duty truck. Retrieved from http://www.businessfleet.com/article/story/2006/01/first-timers-guide-to-the-medium-duty-truck.aspx?prestitial=1

Employee data base. (2009, April 1). Retrieved May 10, 2013, from AHSEMS.com

Gross combined weight rating. (2013, July 10). Retrieved July 25, 2013, from http://en.wikipedia.org/wiki/Gross_combined_weight_rating

Gross vehicle weight rating. (2013, March 31). Retrieved July 25, 2013, from http://en.wikipedia.org/wiki/Gross_vehicle_weight_rating

LeBlanc, D. J. (2008). Situated simulation: Taking simulation to the clinicians. In W. B. Murray & R. R. Kyle (Eds.), *Clinical simulation: Operations, engineering and management* (pp. 556, 557). Burlington, VT: Academic Press.

Luigi Savoia, P. C. (Director). (2010). *Calgary EMS bringing simulation to the streets* [Motion picture].

Lyden, S. (2007, September). Medium-duty chassis & suspension fundamentals. Retrieved from http://www.government-fleet.com/channel/equipment/article/story/2008/09/medium-duty-chassis-suspension-fundamentals/page/2.aspx

Williams, M. (2013, January 1). Green living: demand media. Retrieved from http://greenliving.nationalgeographic.com/laptops-save-electricity-bills-2998.html

CHAPTER 2.4

Simulation-Enhanced Interprofessional Education: A Framework for Development

Janice C. Palaganas, PhD, RN, NP, and Laura K. Rock, MD

ABOUT THE AUTHORS

JANICE C. PALAGANAS received her PhD, exploring healthcare simulation as a platform for interprofessional education (IPE). Dr. Palaganas has clinical and administrative emergency and trauma experience. Dr. Palaganas has held faculty positions in schools of medicine, nursing, management, and emergency medicine, and developed IPE programs. She is past Chair of the Society for Simulation in Healthcare IPE Special Interest Group. Dr. Palaganas has been an invited keynote speaker nationally and internationally to discuss simulation, IPE, and patient safety.

LAURA K. ROCK is a Pulmonologist and Critical Care Physician at Beth Israel Deaconess Medical Center (BIDMC) in Boston, Massachusetts; Instructor at Harvard Medical School; faculty at the Center for Medical Simulation; and Director of Simulation for the BIDMC Department of Medicine. Dr. Rock has designed and taught simulation courses involving nurses, pharmacists, physicians, and respiratory therapists in cardiac arrest and rapid response team training, procedural training, and effective and empathic communication skills.

Acknowledgments: The authors would like to acknowledge the Center for Medical Simulation, Drs. Betty Winslow, Mark Haviland, and Pat Jones for their assistance in the development of this work.

ABSTRACT

Using simulation as a platform for high-quality interprofessional education (IPE) presents many challenges that can impact interprofessional learning. When recognized and addressed, some of these may be explored, eliminated, or controlled. To do so requires significant planning, forethought, and dry runs to identify ways to create an effective simulation-enhanced IPE course. This chapter presents a framework that can be used as a guiding model to help educators identify and address these challenges. Recommendations from the 2012 Interprofessional Education and Healthcare Simulation Symposium on how to begin implementing simulation-enhanced IPE, as well as strategies to overcome challenges are provided.

CASE EXAMPLE

In a faculty meeting, the Dean of the School of Medicine shared a new vision for increasing interprofessional education, driven by accreditation reports. Dr. Robles proposes adding participants from other professions to the medical intern simulations she runs weekly at the Simulation Center as a starting point. She arranges to contact the Schools of Nursing, Pharmacy, and Allied Health.

INTRODUCTION AND BACKGROUND

Simulation-Enhanced Interprofessional Education

The critical need for interprofessional education (IPE) has been identified on the basis of medical error rates, root cause analyses, and patient outcome research, indicating that breaches in healthcare quality most often stem from poor communication within healthcare professional teams (Joint Commission, 2008). As healthcare disciplines have become increasingly specialized and focused in their training, the provision of quality healthcare has been recognized as requiring team practice—training that is rarely incorporated into traditional healthcare professional education. Communication skill training that does exist is largely focused on communicating with patients rather than with other professionals. Students are ultimately expected to know how to work effectively in diverse teams, though these essential teamwork skills are rarely incorporated into their education.

Review of examples of compromised patient care illustrates that professions often have difficulty figuring out how to work together as a team (Hean et al., 2012). As such, the patient safety community advocates IPE as a mechanism to achieve the competencies required for effective interprofessional collaborative practice. The need for IPE is increasingly recognized and promoted by professional, accrediting, and certifying bodies (Commission on Collegiate Nursing Education, 2009; Institute of Medicine, 2006, 2010; Interprofessional Education and Healthcare Simulation Collaborative, 2012; National League for Nursing Accreditation Commission, 2011) (Figure 2.4.1).

As IPE programs have developed over the past decade, healthcare simulation (HCS) has been evolving as a natural educational platform (see Figure 2.4.1). Still, many simulation programs lack the resources or knowledge to maximize the use of simulation as a methodology to enhance interprofessional practice and patient care. A review of the literature (Palaganas, 2012) showed that if an educator is not well prepared to deliver IPE course content, manage an interprofessional group, or adapt the teaching methods to achieve appropriate objectives for the diverse group of learners, the teaching event would not enhance student learning (Cooper et al., 2001; Freeth et al., 2005). The use of a simulator without a skilled educator to develop the experience and help the learners reflect on their behaviors and interactions and gain new perspective and skills is not going to be an effective learning experience. Unfortunately, the existing published literature to guide educators on how to successfully structure and implement simulation-based IPE is lacking (McGaghie et al., 2010; Palaganas, 2012; Reeves et al., 2012; Zhang et al., 2011). This chapter seeks to guide educators in understanding HCS as a platform for IPE by describing variables in simulation-enhanced IPE through a framework that assists in overcoming the implementation and practice challenges in this science.

In 2012, the Society for Simulation in Healthcare (SSH) and the National League for Nursing (NLN) convened the Symposium on Interprofessional Education and Healthcare Simulation to explore the use of simulation as an instrument for advancing interprofessional education and practice. Commonly reported barriers to effective simulation-enhanced IPE included the following:

- The lack of substantive and specific accreditation mandates
- Insufficient infrastructure and resources
- A paucity of research support mechanisms that demonstrate the impact of simulation-enhanced IPE on quality and safety
- Logistical challenges (e.g., scheduling and coordination)
- Cultural differences

On the basis of the identified need for IPE as well as the barriers to implementation, 10 consensus recommendations were developed.

1. Examine personal assumptions, knowledge, and skills related to healthcare simulation, IPE, and simulation-enhanced IPE.
2. Identify and engage local spheres of influence and share information about the IPEC competencies.
3. Conduct formal and informal educational offerings.
4. Promote IPE and simulation-enhanced IPE through the use of social media.
5. Participate in regional, state, and national conferences to showcase and improve understanding of simulation-enhanced IPE.
6. Publish simulation-enhanced IPE course descriptions and research outcomes.
7. Review and enhance current simulation scenarios to ensure that they align with the IPEC competencies.
8. Use research reports to provide evidence that links simulation-enhanced IPE to quality and safe patient outcomes.
9. Employ IPE-focused evaluation instruments.
10. Access and add simulation-enhanced IPE resources through the MedEdPortal or I-collaborative.

Educators and institutions can use these 10 recommendations to prepare and implement simulation-enhanced IPE.

A FRAMEWORK FOR SIMULATION-ENHANCED IPE

The experiential nature of HCS is highly engaging and forces learners to interact in a way that traditional learning does not. However, introducing HCS into curricula raises new challenges that must be appreciated in order to design effective IPE programs. Anticipating these important factors will enhance the quality and success of any simulation, especially those involving multiple disciplines.

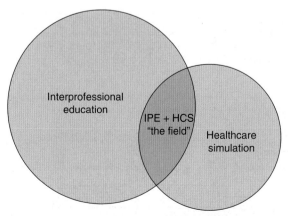

FIGURE 2.4.1 The overlapping sciences of Interprofessional Education and Healthcare Simulation (From Palaganas, J. [2012]. *Exploring healthcare simulation as a platform for interprofessional education [Doctoral dissertation].* Retrieved from ProQuest Dissertations and Theses database.)

EXPERT'S CORNER

TEAMWORK FOR SIMULATION TEAMS?

Jeffrey B. Cooper, PhD
Founder and Executive Director, Center for Medical Simulation

One of the great applications of simulation of various types is to improve the performance of healthcare teams. It's engaging, motivating, and there's reasonably good evidence that it's effective. Throughout healthcare, simulation is being used for teams to learn and practice to work together more effectively. So what about the teams that create the programs and conduct the simulations? How much team training goes on for simulation teams?

The question is simple and one that every team of simulation professionals needs to ask itself. If it's good enough for your students, shouldn't you be doing it for yourselves too? The "it" is any kind of training together to improve your group's teamwork and performance as a team. It doesn't have to be high-realism simulation. There are myriad experiential exercises for examining and

developing various aspects of your team's performance. We've looked at how we bring each other into conversations, allow and encourage each other to speak up, how good we are at setting limits on what we ask each other to do. Just as for teams of clinicians, good teamwork requires serious work, practice, and routine reinforcement. I think it's made us better, although of course that's hard to measure.

So if you are in a team of simulation professionals and haven't been working deliberately on your team's teamwork, it's time to do that. If you just do it as a one-off, then make a more regular event. Pick issues that you need to work on. Bring in a facilitator to lead you so you can all be equally involved. Do to yourselves what you would do unto others. You and your students will be better for it.

In IPE, content validity must be considered from the perspective of each of the professions involved in the event. Scenario reliability addresses learning objectives—that is, does the simulation meet the learning objectives for each group of target learners? Being mindful of these concepts while developing IPE scenarios will augment the versatility and usefulness of the courses.

Educators and researchers may benefit from considering an established framework that can assist in focusing on and screening for issues with the variables that influence the effectiveness of a simulation. Figure 2.4.2 illustrates the Simulation-based Interprofessional Education Reliability-Validity-Assessment (SimBIE RVA) Framework (Palaganas, 2012). Discussions in this section reflect the difficulty in

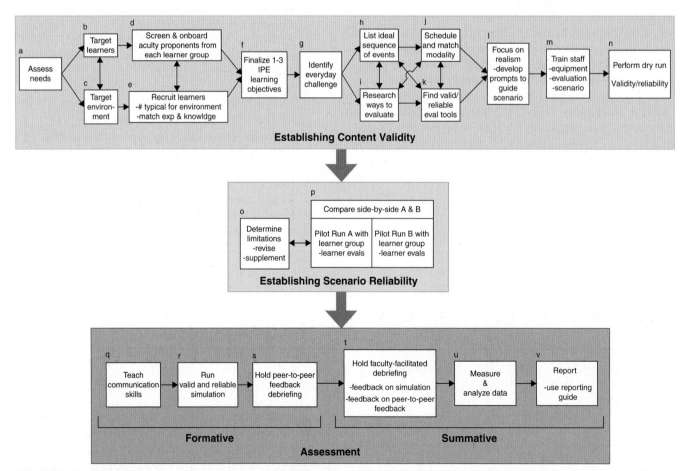

FIGURE 2.4.2 SimBIE RVA framework. (From Palaganas, J. [2012]. *Exploring healthcare simulation as a platform for interprofessional education [Doctoral dissertation]*. Retrieved from ProQuest Dissertations and Theses database.)

establishing validity and reliability due to the complexity of variables and uncertainties within the field. Complexity and uncertainty cause difficulties in establishing effective learning. The SimBIE RVA Framework may help educators and researchers further understand their simulation and IPE practice, clarify complex areas already studied, and build their own curricula for interprofessional learning (IPL) using existing data as a foundation. Assessment, as seen in Figure 2.4.2, is discussed in the "Been there, done that" section of this chapter (pp. 116).

The SimBIE RVA Framework offers a process for creating a high-quality simulation-enhanced IPE. It is best used as a general guide rather than stringently, using some steps and eliminating others as appropriate, on the basis of feasibility or processes, performing steps sequentially or nonsequentially. Most importantly, understanding the variables and challenges in each step fosters high-quality simulation-enhanced IPE.

Although this chapter uses the SimBIE RVA Framework to describe variables and challenges in the field, one effective way to implement simulation-enhanced IPE is to implement simulation-enhanced IPE. In other words, just do it. While educators may "reinvent the wheel" using a "do it" approach, this process has benefits. It is the social process of collaborating to understand and uncover new ways of doing things that generates new capabilities in a healthcare team rather than the specific techniques or methods that are developed. It is not the "wheel" but rather the social and relational work itself that may be the most productive goal.

Needs Assessment (See a in Figure 2.4.2)

Successful IPE programs address the needs of the organization and the learner. The organization's needs can be delineated from both external (e.g., national efforts or accreditation bodies) and internal sources (e.g., high-risk events, educator and learner feedback). Learner needs should be assessed from the perspective of each profession that will be included in the IPE course. Sustaining an IPE program is challenging and leadership support is more likely to occur when the impact of a program addresses well-established needs. (See chapter 5.1 for performing a needs assessment and chapter 7.1 for performing a learner needs assessment.)

GOING BACK TO THE CASE EXAMPLE

While it is common for educators making beginning efforts toward IPE to bring other professions into an already existing simulation that was developed for one profession, Dr. Robles should perform a needs assessment on the organization and across the professions she plans to involve in the IPE program.

Many of the driving forces for IPE flow from the leaders of multiple professional organizations. These leaders identified common core competencies for interprofessional collaborative practice. In 2010, an Interprofessional Education Collaborative Expert Panel (IPECEP) came together to establish interprofessional competencies applicable to all healthcare professions and teams (Canadian Interprofessional Health Collaborative IPECEP, 2011b). This group clustered the competencies under four major domains:

1. Values and Ethics of Interprofessional Practice
2. Roles and Responsibilities
3. Interprofessional Communication
4. Teams and Teamwork (IPECEP, 2011b)

In 2011, the IPECEP met again to develop competencies under each of these four domains. The competencies (listed in Table 2.4.1) may be used by educators as globally identified needs and as objectives for a simulation-enhanced IPE.

Target Learners and Environment (See b and c in Figure 2.4.2)

An effective needs assessment will indicate the target learners and environment. If the needs assessment identifies a clinical situation as an objective but does not specify the learners and environment, these may be determined using the following questions:

- Which professions are typically involved in this situation?
- When and where do these needs occur?
- What level of each profession is involved?
- What does the involvement of each profession look like?
- In which areas of the clinical environment do these needs most frequently occur?

Exploring the target learners will provide an idea of the type of scenario that should be developed to best address the need.

GOING BACK TO THE CASE EXAMPLE

The learners that Dr. Robles invites or involves in the IPE session may impact the nature and progression of the event. For example, if nursing students are involved in a simulation with emergency interns, the educators may consider beginning the simulation in triage or the emergency department lobby where a nurse would first interact with a patient.

Screen and Onboard Faculty (See d in Figure 2.4.2)

Once the target learners and environment are established, faculty with expertise in the focus area should be identified. There are myriad factors that influence learning effectiveness. A longstanding variable in education is the

TABLE 2.4.1

Interprofessional Collaborative Practice Competencies

Domain 1: Values/Ethics for Interprofessional Practice

VE1. Place the interests of patients and populations at the center of interprofessional healthcare delivery.

VE2. Respect the dignity and privacy of patients while maintaining confidentiality in the delivery of team-based care.

VE3. Embrace the cultural diversity and individual differences that characterize patients, populations, and the healthcare team.

VE4. Respect the unique cultures, values, roles/responsibilities, and expertise of other health professions.

VE5. Work in cooperation with those who receive care, those who provide care, and others who contribute to or support the delivery of prevention and health services.

VE6. Develop a trusting relationship with patients, families, and other team members (CIHC, 2010).

VE7. Demonstrate high standards of ethical conduct and quality of care in one's contributions to team-based care.

VE8. Manage ethical dilemmas specific to interprofessional patient-/population-centered care situations.

VE9. Act with honesty and integrity in relationships with patients, families, and other team members.

VE10. Maintain competence in one's own profession appropriate to scope of practice.

Domain 2: Roles/Responsibilities

RR1. Communicate one's roles and responsibilities clearly to patients, families, and other professionals.

RR2. Recognize one's limitations in skills, knowledge, and abilities.

RR3. Engage diverse healthcare professionals who complement one's own professional expertise, as well as associated resources, to develop strategies to meet specific patient care needs.

RR4. Explain the roles and responsibilities of other care providers and how the team works together to provide care.

RR5. Use the full scope of knowledge, skills, and abilities of available health professionals and healthcare workers to provide care that is safe, timely, efficient, effective, and equitable.

RR6. Communicate with team members to clarify each member's responsibility in executing components of a treatment plan or public health intervention.

RR7. Forge interdependent relationships with other professions to improve care and advance learning.

RR8. Engage in continuous professional and interprofessional development to enhance team performance.

RR9. Use unique and complementary abilities of all members of the team to optimize patient care.

Domain 3: Interprofessional Communication

CC1. Choose effective communication tools and techniques, including information systems and communication technologies, to facilitate discussions and interactions that enhance team function.

CC2. Organize and communicate information with patients, families, and healthcare team members in a form that is understandable, avoiding discipline-specific terminology when possible.

CC3. Express one's knowledge and opinions to team members involved in patient care with confidence, clarity, and respect, working to ensure common understanding of information and treatment and care decisions.

CC4. Listen actively, and encourage ideas and opinions of other team members.

CC5. Give timely, sensitive, instructive feedback to others about their performance on the team, responding respectfully as a team member to feedback from others.

CC6. Use respectful language appropriate for a given difficult situation, crucial conversation, or interprofessional conflict.

CC7. Recognize how one's own uniqueness, including experience level, expertise, culture, power, and hierarchy within the healthcare team, contributes to effective communication, conflict resolution, and positive interprofessional working relationships (University of Toronto, 2008).

CC8. Communicate consistently the importance of teamwork in patient-centered and community-focused care.

Domain 4: Teams and Teamwork

TT1. Describe the process of team development and the roles and practices of effective teams.

TT2. Develop consensus on the ethical principles to guide all aspects of patient care and team work.

TT3. Engage other health professionals—appropriate to the specific care situation—in shared patient-centered problem solving.

TT4. Integrate the knowledge and experience of other professions—appropriate to the specific care situation—to inform care decisions, while respecting patient and community values and priorities/preferences for care.

TT5. Apply leadership practices that support collaborative practice and team effectiveness.

TT6. Engage self and others to constructively manage disagreements about values, roles, goals, and actions that arise among healthcare professionals and with patients and families.

TT7. Share accountability with other professions, patients, and communities for outcomes relevant to prevention and healthcare.

TT8. Reflect on individual and team performance for individual, as well as team, performance improvement.

TT9. Use process improvement strategies to increase the effectiveness of interprofessional teamwork and team-based care.

TT10. Use available evidence to inform effective teamwork and team-based practices.

TT11. Perform effectively on teams and in different team roles in a variety of settings.

Source: From Interprofessional Education Collaborative Expert Panel. (2011). *Core competencies for interprofessional collaborative practice: Report of an expert panel.* Washington, DC: Interprofessional Education Collaborative.

expertise, quality, and "likeability" of educators by learners, colleagues, and superiors alike. IPE requires additional knowledge in the following areas:

- Interprofessional practice as applicable to the learner groups
- IPE competencies, as well as the newest research and recommendations for IPE
- IPE planning, design, implementation, and formulation of design and evaluation teams
- Spheres of influence and change theory
- Translational research
- Assessment of learners in IPE, including existing validated and reliable evaluation instruments (Hammick et al., 2008; Howkins & Bray, 2008)

Furthermore, educators using simulation benefit from additional knowledge in the following:

- Experiential teaching and learning theory
- Simulation equipment
- Simulation principles, practice, equipment, and methodology
- Assessment of learners using simulation
- Management of simulation resources and environments (IEHSC, 2012)

The level of an educator's knowledge in these areas, along with teaching talent, professional values, and capabilities, can greatly influence a learner group's outcomes. Once appropriate faculty members from each profession are identified, invitation, recruitment, and development activities can begin.

Challenge: Schedule conflicts preclude participation of faculty or content experts from all involved disciplines during scenario development.
Strategy: Implement an interprofessional curricula cross-matching committee whose responsibility is to represent the individual program needs, determine faculty, and IPE activities.

GOING BACK TO THE CASE EXAMPLE

Dr. Robles can establish an Interprofessional Education Committee with faculty members from each discipline. This committee can review existing curricula and professional competencies while developing a list of potential IPE activities. The group can highlight curricular and content overlap and find ways where courses or labs can be scheduled together.

Recruit Learners (See e in Figure 2.4.2)

Recruiting learners is a common challenge. Curricular and clinical scheduling, differences in calendars between schools and departments, and overloaded class and clinical schedules all contribute to the difficulty in scheduling learners for new learning programs. There are also important learner variables that should be considered during selection and recruitment of learners. These include the dynamics of IPE, group familiarity, and participatory role during simulation.

IPE Dynamics: Definition of IPE

By definition, in IPE, students are learning with, from, and about each other (IPECEP, 2011a). Each student possesses unique knowledge, experiences, energy, attitudes, perspectives, personality, mental frames, and communication skills. Together, these unique factors determine the cocreation of knowledge and greatly influence the IPL. Depending on the unique characteristics that each learner

brings and the composition of the group, the learning will differ.

Group Familiarity

Group familiarity with one or more members also influences learning outcomes. Generally, the within-profession learners are familiar with each other and not with the learners from other groups. Familiarity with team members may facilitate team comfort or, on the contrary, create subgroup fragmentation if only a few members among the group are familiar with each other. Whether IPL benefits from working teams versus ad hoc teams has not yet been studied in simulation-enhanced IPE, but may be a significant group characteristic affecting outcomes. This is an important question as courses may not match actual learning environments if they do not factor in the ongoing working relationship or ad hoc nature of the team.

Observing Versus Active

Owing to large group sizes and limitations on simulation resources, simulation often involves both observing and active participants. Observing learners often passively observe their peers in a simulation. While the observing participants often participate in reflection during team debriefings, they frequently become disengaged and distracted. Observing participants may become more engaged through the use of structured observational tools. Some simulation-enhanced IPE have individuals from various professions change roles and participate in the simulation as an alternative profession (i.e., doctor acting in the role of a nurse) to gain a sense of perspectives, role differences, and similarities. While this may be a valuable experience, it must be reserved for activities appropriate to objectives, such as promoting role clarity. If the course focus is communication and a nurse is acting in the role of a physician, the realism of the simulation is compromised, the nurse may not communicate the way a physician does, but rather the way he or she believes a physician communicates (often around his or her stereotype of this role). This dilemma is also present when using cross-profession evaluations or observations. Healthcare professionals are beginning to realize that each profession has a specialized language and culture that another profession may not understand, and therefore if one profession is evaluating another, there may be gaps in the observations, and the exercise may inadvertently lead to alienation or division among learners.

Challenge: Learners have varying needs and varying levels of experience.
Strategies: Stagger start time to allow for training and discussion of specialized skills, thereby maximizing the experience for diverse groups of participants and allowing sufficient technical preparation so the group can emphasize team training when they are all together.

GOING BACK TO THE CASE EXAMPLE

Dr. Robles and the IPE Committee have brainstormed two simulations that could be used for both students and practicing providers or a mixture of pre- and postlicensure students:

Simulation 1. Develop a scenario to involve a continuum of care from setting to setting or stage to stage to allow the case to be relevant to all learners. Didactic or practice simulations can be run prior to the scenario for learners who are not familiar with the content.

Simulation 2. Develop an extracorporeal membrane oxygenation (ECMO) scenario for managing massive pulmonary embolism and severe right ventricular failure. Begin the session with technical training on ECMO circuits and hands-on management of ports, tubing, and pumps for ECMO technicians and ECMO nurses only. Then, when the group is joined by critical care physicians and nurses, they will emphasize team communication and management while still practicing the technical skills they learned.

Logistical Factors for Course Implementation and Success

Logistical factors strongly influence the successful implementation and effectiveness of the course. Questions regarding simulation design include the following:

- What effect do required courses versus elective courses have on IPL?
- What is the most effective number of members and disciplines comprising a team for simulation-enhanced IPE?
- For prelicensure students, is it more effective for students to engage in simulation-enhanced IPE in their current role as students or in their postlicensure role?
- How do I minimize barriers to successful implementation such as absences and lateness?
- How do I improve attendance in the elective course?

Challenge: Students arrive consistently late.
Strategies: Procure department funding to provide lunch for a midday course, and inform participants they will get lunch at the start of the course. Use the time while they are eating to introduce the session, develop some rapport with participants, and review key concepts from didactic training, if relevant. Begin the course on time, if possible, rather than waiting for latecomers.

Challenge: Course poorly attended by one discipline, for example, nurses.
Strategies: Meet with nursing leadership to explain the course and obtain support. E-mail nurse educators and managers prior to each course to invite participants. Survey all participants at the end of each course to provide data regarding participant experience when soliciting support from department leaders.

Finalize IPE Objectives (See f in Figure 2.4.2)

Interprofessional education has been distinguished in the literature as different from multiprofessional education (MPE). MPE occurs when members (or students) of two or more professions learn alongside one another: in other words, parallel rather than interactive learning (Freeth et al., 2005). There is evidence in the literature that learning is better achieved through IPE as compared with MPE (CIHC, 2010).

The distinction between IPE and MPE can be clarified by illustrating two approaches to course design. These are Simulation-based Interprofessional Education (SimBIE) and Interprofessional Simulation (IPsim). SimBIE refers to a simulation that was designed according to IPE objectives in which two or more professionals learn with, from, and about each other to improve collaboration and the quality of care. IPsim corresponds with MPE and involves learners from two or more professions learning alongside one another in a simulated case where each profession has profession-specific objectives (Palaganas, 2012).

To avoid a uniprofessional focus, the course or simulation development team should have members from each profession involved in the IPE activity who can ensure the simulation is relevant to their profession. SimBIE often involves team behaviors and skills, and thus one to two objectives are adequate for a 20-minute simulation. IPsims often incorporate multiple skills and knowledge-based objectives specific to one or each profession. Most simulation-enhanced IPE proceeds with a simulation followed by a debriefing to allow team and individual reflection. IPsims that are built on uniprofessional objectives often lead to uniprofessional debriefing that the other professions may or may not find valuable to their learning.

Challenge: The debriefing appeared uniprofessional.
Strategy: Revisit the objectives of the simulation and ensure that they are relevant to all learners and revise the scenario as needed. Practice the session with a group of interprofessional volunteer learners who reflect the composition of the target group.

GOING BACK TO THE CASE EXAMPLE

Prior to exploring how to run IPE simulations, Dr. Robles was able to find nursing and pharmacy students to join the simulation she developed for her medical interns. She did not change the simulation or her debriefing focus and received mixed evaluations from the nursing and pharmacy students. Dr. Robles realized that to achieve IPL with all of the students, she would need to involve nursing and pharmacy faculty to revise the scenario objectives so that more nursing and pharmacy activities are embedded into the scenario.

Identify Everyday Challenge (See g in Figure 2.4.2)

An everyday challenge may be identified for the creation of a simulation—whether it is a clinical event, hospital policy implementation, leadership-to-staff communications, or team behaviors. This everyday challenge should be appropriate for the learners. Practice challenges may be identified through patient safety reviews or risk management analyses and would allow opportunity for collaboration between Patient Safety and Risk Management departments and the Simulation Program.

Challenge: The simulation allowed opportunities to meet the everyday challenge of the ICU intern, which was a focus during the debriefing. The nurses felt like they learned something new; however, these were procedures that nurses were not allowed to perform.
Strategy: Explore overlapping everyday challenges, or determine an everyday challenge and ask involved professions to identify common challenges relevant to them in that situation.

GOING BACK TO THE CASE EXAMPLE

Each member of the IPE simulation development group individually created a list of the top five things they wish students could learn prior to starting their clinical rotation in the medical-surgical unit. They found familiarity with the defibrillator was a common challenge that they then sought to integrate into the simulation lab.

List Ideal and Potential Sequence of Events (See h in Figure 2.4.2)

The ideal sequence of events for the chosen case describes the progression of the scenario. This sequence can be revisited and revised for alternative progressions on the basis of potential learner actions. As continued learner engagement relies on the interactive nature of the experience, progression of the simulation should be as realistic as the clinical environment. Owing to the wide range of potential learner actions, all possible choices must be anticipated, explored, and developed to be prepared for all possible simulator reactions.

GOING BACK TO THE CASE EXAMPLE

The IPE Simulation Lab Development group did a tabletop simulation (verbally simulated the scenario through discussion and sequence of events) and highlighted possible actions of learners—ideal and not so ideal. They then developed a table of "Ifs and Thens" (if the team does X, then Y will occur).

Modality Matching (See j in Figure 2.4.2)

Simulation may involve a wide variety of platforms and modalities. Selection of simulation modality should be based on the learning objectives of the IPE course, a concept referred to as "modality matching." Highly realistic and complex simulations are not always necessary or appropriate (Jeffries et al., 2009). All simulators have strengths and limitations. Simulation educators must be aware of the capabilities, strengths, and limitations of available simulation equipment, the learning objectives of a course, and the educational needs of the learners. As simulation-enhanced IPE courses usually aim to promote effective teamwork, communication, and resource management, realistic interactions and communication opportunities must be prioritized in simulation selection and scenario design.

GOING BACK TO THE CASE EXAMPLE

The IPE faculty decided to develop a simulation around breaking bad news to a patient regarding a medical error. Even though a standardized patient would be best for their objectives, some of the faculty members new to simulation were excited about the new high-technology mannequin that the simulation staff showed them. They thought the mannequin was so impressive that it would surely engage their students.

Dr. Robles was able to redirect the excitement of the group to the objectives of the simulation experience and explored the most appropriate use of existing resources. The group decided to create two simulations: one with breaking bad news to a patient using a standardized patient and another with breaking bad news to a family member with a standardized family member and the mannequin as adjunct to the simulation.

Research Evaluation Methods and Valid and Reliable Tools (See i and k in Figure 2.4.2)

Although evaluation methods and tools fall into course or program assessment, it is included in the initial development of scenario content in preparation to answer the following question. How will we know that what we created and implemented was effective for student learning? Addressing this question during program development will help validate the content of the simulation, help achieve the intent of the activity, and maximize student learning. Creating, validating, and testing reliability in an evaluation tool is an extensive process that requires expert psychometric guidance. With this in mind, identifying existing, valid, and reliable tools (or instruments) should be considered. If an established tool is chosen, the group might need to consider whether their objectives need to be edited to link more closely with the tool.

Challenge: Difficulty with assessing team performance.
Strategies: Faculty development in assessment, research existing assessment tools in team performance, contact programs that have performed team assessment.

GOING BACK TO THE CASE EXAMPLE

Dr. Robles and the development team ran the simulation for over 400 students. The Dean's Council was eager to hear how the lab was running and asked Dr. Robles to present evaluations from the simulation. Dr. Robles and the development team did not consider evaluations and did not have any to present. As they researched tools that they could start using, they could not find one that fit what they were doing. At a conference, one of the faculty heard of a group that has been doing team training using simulation for years. Dr. Robles called this group, and they sent them a list of evaluation tools they have been using, suggested one in particular, and shared their experience using each.

Focus on Realism (See l in Figure 2.4.2)

Team engagement depends heavily on the realism portrayed and facilitated through the simulation experience. Intrinsically, a team should agree on a "fiction contract"—a disclosure by faculty that it is not real, that the faculty tried their best to make it as real as feasibly possible, and to ask the students to agree to interact as best they could as though it is real (see chapter 8.3 Expert's Corner: Helping Learners "Buy in" to Simulation). This intrinsic motivation affects the experience of the other team members, as described above: each student affects the learning in IPE. Realism in healthcare simulation occurs at three levels of fidelity: physical fidelity (how real the environment and people appear), conceptual fidelity (the degree of each person's engagement with the fiction contract), and emotional/experiential fidelity (the interactive inputs that create the emotions and experience) (see chapter 8.3 Expert's Corner: Helping Learners "Buy in" to Simulation). Thus, the learning created during a simulation course relies on the realism engineered for the learning to occur with each individual's experience affecting other team members and the collective learning of the team.

Challenge: Students new to simulation giggle during the simulation, and the other students on the team get distracted.
Strategies: Faculty development in simulation moulaging and simulation facilitation methods explore ways to make the simulation more realistic in creating a team performance.

Train Simulation Educators (See m in Figure 2.4.2)

Given the unforeseen complexities of facilitating learning through HCS and IPE, simulation may be intimidating for faculty new to this field. Although many educators learn

through trial and error and have contributed to the field through this venue, there are also many activities that can help develop simulation educators, some of which are listed below:

- Faculty development in simulation (e.g., Simulation Instructor Training)
- Faculty development in IPE (e.g., IPE conferences)
- Faculty development in how to operate simulation equipment (e.g., vendor in-services)
- Faculty development in creative ways to overcome simulation equipment glitches (e.g., Program Training)
- Hiring experts in each of the above areas (e.g., On-site Consultants)
- Developing new roles responsible for each of these areas where expertise can be developed (e.g., Fellowships or Apprenticeship Programs)
- Developing technology (e.g., utilize organizational IT department or find faculty or students who are technologically inclined)

Challenge: Lack of faculty expertise in debriefing, specifically with interprofessional groups.
Strategies: Personal reflection on assumptions of other professions, involvement of interprofessional content experts (e.g., one skilled debriefer who facilitates the conversation with content experts from each profession available to discuss content-related issues), interview and observe other professions in their practice, faculty development (e.g., Debriefing Assessment for Simulation in Healthcare [DASH] training), separate debriefings, or uniprofessional debriefings followed by interprofessional debriefing (or vice versa).

Psychological Safety

A fundamental characteristic of simulation-based learning is the establishment of psychological safety (Council for the Accreditation of Healthcare Simulation Programs, 2012). For interprofessional students to fully engage in a team-based simulation and allow themselves to identify and explore errors, the educator must take the time to establish an environment of support, curiosity, and respect. An individual's contribution to the learning affects other team member's learning, as well as the collective learning of the group. Occasionally, a scenario may trigger memories of a prior bad experience that influences the discussion and learning of the entire group. Educators must be able to address such a breach in psychological safety, especially if the breach is regarding working in teams, should it arise.

Psychological safety is particularly critical with learners who work together on a day-to-day basis. If mistakes are made during the scenario, fear, embarrassment, and judgments may carry over to the day-to-day setting, creating discomfort and mistrust among the clinical team, which may contribute to ineffective patient care. Thus, safety must be established and team issues must be addressed and held as a priority during the debriefing.

Dry Run the Scenario (See n in Figure 2.4.2)

Equal Opportunity for Professions

Educators may seek students from other professions to add a more realistic experience to a simulation designed for one profession. This creates a uniprofessional design that may benefit one group of students more than other professional groups, inadvertently contributing to the very biases and misunderstandings that IPE strives to alleviate. When asking other professions to participate in simulation courses, educators should involve faculty (as content experts) from the added profession to dry run the scenario in order to create equal learning opportunities. During debriefing, assumptions and stereotypes arise from students and educators. Educators are role models and must be aware of their own personal assumptions around the professions involved and work consciously to avoid modeling disrespect or views that may be adverse to the intended learning goals.

GOING BACK TO THE CASE EXAMPLE

Dr. Robles asked her friend, a School of Nursing Professor, to bring her senior-level BSN students to an IPE event. The nursing students participated as learners alongside the interns during the simulation. The faculty debriefs the interns as he normally debriefs this course and then asks the nursing students to share their experience and perspectives developed from the simulation. While the nursing students were grateful to participate in a simulation with interns and learned about a procedure they are not allowed to perform, there were no specific objectives developed for them. The participation of the nursing students, however, helped the interns meet their learning objectives. This simulation may have had equal opportunity if objectives were developed for the nursing students to meet their specific learning needs and the Residents also helped them meet their learning objectives.

BEEN THERE, DONE THAT: HOW CAN I CONTINUE TO IMPROVE OR SUSTAIN WHAT I HAVE ACHIEVED?

Determine Limitations of the Scenario (See o in Figure 2.4.2)

Dry running a scenario often reveals many limitations that require creative engineering, revision of the scenario, or supplementation of equipment.

Challenge: Inadequate time.
Strategies: Prioritize and narrow simulation learning objectives and debriefing points.

GOING BACK TO THE CASE EXAMPLE

After two dry runs, the interprofessional lab development group realized that there was too little time and too many objectives. They limited their objectives to two, focusing on team skills.

Compare Pilot Runs (See p in Figure 2.4.2)

Learned from the standardization processes of Standardize Patients, a rigorous way to establish scenario reliability is to record two dry runs (or pilot runs) and play them side by side on a screen simultaneously. This allows visualization of variability. Because each learner should have an opportunity for the best learning possible, it is important to standardize the simulation as much as feasible. Evaluations may also be compared between groups. Many factors may influence variability, including faculty, debriefer, faculty knowledge and experience, the learners, and the simulation staff running the equipment and facilitating the simulation.

Teach Communication Skills (See q in Figure 2.4.2)

A study by Palaganas (2012) suggests that the simulation modality may not be significant to building teamwork and collaboration skills. In the debriefing sessions, the simulation serves as a common experience to allow discussion that fertilizes the learning during the debriefing experience. If debriefing becomes the actual learning platform for IPE, the debriefing may be enriched by some teaching of communication skills—specifically, how to effectively communicate with and provide feedback to team members of the same and different professions. This can prepare learners to engage in teamwork and collaboration skills during debriefing.

GOING BACK TO THE CASE EXAMPLE

The IPE Lab Development Group decided to engage in a semistructured debriefing, where they would facilitate the perspectives of each learner and encourage performance feedback to the team or specific individuals. In preparation for creating a healthy feedback debriefing, Dr. Robles gave a short lecture on the use of a structured way to communicate feedback.

Run Valid and Reliable Simulation (See v in Figure 2.4.2)

Although IPE simulations may be run without validation and reliability testing, validation and reliability increase the likelihood of a rich and relevant experience for the learners. Once all of the planning has occurred, the learners have been recruited, and the simulation has been scheduled, the simulation is ready to be run.

Hold Peer-to-Peer Feedback Debriefing (See s in Figure 2.4.2)

In debriefing, especially if a safe space has been created and sustained by the educator(s), learners are given the opportunity and are encouraged to share their individual perspectives and discuss team behaviors. It is at this moment that learners are able to learn the skills of talking to other professions and providing feedback to other team members—a skill most relevant to their everyday clinical practice and also most important for patient safety.

GOING BACK TO THE CASE EXAMPLE

Sara, a Pharmacy Student, has never been in class with a nursing student, a medical student, a physician's assistant student, and a social work student. She was surprised to learn the differences in how they are taught and the similarities they have in not knowing each other's professions, as well as roles in the care of a trauma patient. She has never interacted with different professions so candidly before. In her next clinical shift, she was eager to interact with other professions and did not feel awkward talking with them.

Hold Faculty-Facilitated Debriefing (See t in Figure 2.4.2)

Debriefing Facilitation Skills

Fanning and Gaba (2007) posit that debriefing, more so than the active simulation, is where learning takes place. It is thought that guided reflection or facilitator-led discussions create prolonged learning through reconstruction of the events, self-reflection, and cognitive assimilations. Whether IPL occurs primarily during the simulation (by working together) or during the debriefing (reflecting on team skills using a common experience) is unclear. In debriefing, students also learn how to provide peer-to-peer and profession-to-profession feedback and, in this process, learn how to communicate their thoughts to a team of other professions. This skill is relevant to clinical practice and often lacking in the clinical setting. A focus on developing this skill of feedback and communication may be key in teaching healthcare providers how to work together effectively. Educators should therefore have the debriefing skills to facilitate peer-to-peer feedback, as well as feedback on their feedback during the debriefing.

Challenge: Debriefings following in situ simulation-enhanced IPE are often held in a public area (e.g., staff break room or standing at the bedside of the mannequin) in a short time (e.g., 5–15 minutes).
Strategy to overcome challenge: It is critical for learners to feel a sense of support and safety to allow themselves to share their thoughts about one another's actions and professions. A public area and insufficient time become significant barriers to creating this comfort and opportunity

for deep reflection and feedback. Hence, the debriefer must possess effective facilitation skills that can be sensitive to these barriers and be effective within the limitations presented.

Preventing Adverse Learning

While creating and implementing simulation-enhanced IPE, educators have an obligation to recognize and be mindful that there is a possibility that negative perspectives may develop around interprofessional practice. Although adverse learning experiences may occur randomly, the likelihood of positive outcomes may depend on factors of faculty knowledge, including substantial planning using an anticipatory design, awareness and support of possible characteristics that lead to positive outcomes, as well as recognition of and purposeful muting of characteristics that may lead to negative outcomes.

GOING BACK TO THE CASE EXAMPLE

An Attending Obstetrician who was previously an L&D Nurse was leading a debriefing with the interprofessional students, the interns with whom she had mentored previously, and new nursing staff. Before the debriefing began, an Intern joked, "At least I wasn't the nurse." The Attending chuckled, remembering her days as a nurse. Throughout the debriefing, the nurses were very upset at the Intern's joke and were not engaging in the debriefing and gave the IPE low evaluation scores. The Attending was not aware of her light laughter, was not transparent in her thought in the moment, and was not aware of the negative impact it caused for other learners who did not know her background as a nurse.

Measure and Analyze Data and Report Findings (See u and v in Figure 2.4.2)

If evaluation tools were used in the course, these data can be measured and analyzed to improve the course, improve student learning, and improve the impact that this IPE activity has on patient care. Careful selection and description of methods and reporting will promote scientific excellence in this field as researchers and educators begin to establish methodology, equipment, and techniques. At this stage of the science, reporting of limitations is crucial to the field's evolution and success. However, current reporting mechanisms may limit the details necessary for replication (e.g., word limits, journal requirements for methods used). Finding additional venues (e.g., MedEd Portal, Web addendums to journals) to report details is necessary to addressing gaps in this science. Recognizing the limitations in reporting—whether it is journal editing or word limitations—when using a model that has been published, a more thorough report may be available through direct inquiry with the authors or researchers. Chances are many educators or organizations have already developed a similar simulation-enhanced IPE.

Seeking these resources may provide road maps that can assist in the development of new programs or improvement of existing programs.

SUMMARY

The Challenge of a New Science

Research on optimal simulation-based IPE strategies to inform course and research design is not available, and educators are frequently "reinventing the wheel." However, this process has benefits. It is the social process of working together to understand and find new ways of doing things that generates new capabilities in a healthcare team rather than the specific techniques or methods that are developed or used. In other words, it is not the "wheel" but rather the social and relational work itself that becomes the goal.

GOING BACK TO THE CASE EXAMPLE

In her continuing efforts, Dr. Robles has been asked to work with the simulation center to develop IPE for the schools of nursing, pharmacy, and medicine. In search of a model, she found a journal article that sounds like what she wants to implement and shows significant outcomes in learning teamwork. The article has only a paragraph on the simulation scenario, and she realizes that she needs to fill in details. She assembles a team of faculty from each of the schools to develop the scenario and the objectives of the IPE. The team spent three long meetings coming to agreement on the objectives alone. While Dr. Robles may have imposed the objectives and scenario from another model to facilitate the development, the process itself made substantial progress in furthering interprofessional goals. In this case, the group process included understanding the desires of the different faculty and schools, learning the gaps in the literature agreeing on objectives, and discovering ways to work effectively as a team. This process actually established a committed team and increased knowledge and ownership essential to the IPE they will develop, implement, measure, and report.

Because the field of HCS and IPE has entered a discovery and exploratory stage, thoughtful reporting will be crucial to future developments. This chapter has provided information on HCS and IPE from the literature, national discussions, and efforts and reflection of terminology and characteristics. It contributes to the growing findings around factors in IPE methods that influence positive and negative outcomes. This chapter also reveals many questions foundational for this science. Use of the information and tools presented in this chapter may assist in thoughtful planning for future simulation-enhanced IPE and research.

REFERENCES

Canadian Interprofessional Health Collaborative. (2010). *A national interprofessional competency framework*. Retrieved from http://www.cihc.ca/resources/publications

Commission on Collegiate Nursing Education. (2009). *Standards for accreditation of baccalaureate and graduate degree nursing programs*. Washington, DC: Author.

Cooper, H., Carlisle, C., Gibbs, T., & Watkins, C. (2001). Developing an evidence base for interdisciplinary learning: a systematic review. *Journal of Advanced Nursing, 35,* 228–237.

Council for the Accreditation of Healthcare Simulation Programs. (2012). *Informational guide for the 2011 Society for Simulation in Healthcare Accreditation Program*. Wheaton, IL: Society for Simulation in Healthcare.

Fanning, R., & Gaba, D. (2007). The role of debriefing in simulation based education. *Simulation in Healthcare, 2,* 115–126.

Freeth, D., Hammick, M., Reeves, S., Koppel, I., & Barr, H. (2005). *Effective interprofessional education: Development, delivery & evaluation.* Oxford, UK: Blackwell.

Hammick, M., Freeth, D., Koppel, I., Reeves, S., & Barr, H. (2008). A best evidence systematic review of interprofessional education. *Medical Teacher, 29,* 735–751.

Hean, S., Craddock, D., & Hammick, M. (2012). Theoretical insights into interprofessional education: AMEE guide No. 62. *Medical Teacher, 43(2),* 78–101.

Howkins, E., & Bray, J. (2008). *Preparing for interprofessional teaching.* Oxon, UK: Radcliffe.

Institute of Medicine. (2006). *Preventing medication errors: Quality chasm series.* Washington, DC: National Academies Press.

Institute of Medicine. (2010). *The future of nursing: Leading change, advancing health.* Washington, DC: National Academies Press.

Interprofessional Education and Healthcare Simulation Collaborative. (2012). *A consensus report from the 2012 interprofessional education and healthcare simulation collaborative.* Wheaton, IL: Society for Simulation in Healthcare.

Interprofessional Education Collaborative Expert Panel. (2011a). *Team-based competencies: Building a shared foundation for education and clinical practice.* Washington, DC: Interprofessional Education Collaborative.

Interprofessional Education Collaborative Expert Panel. (2011b). *Core competencies for interprofessional collaborative practice: Report of an expert panel.* Washington, DC: Interprofessional Education Collaborative.

Jeffries, P. R., Clochesy, J. M., & Hovancsek, M. T. (2009). Designing, implementing, and evaluating simulations in nursing education. In D. M. Billings & J. A. Halstead (Eds.), *Teaching in nursing: A guide for faculty.* St. Louis, MO: Saunders Elsevier.

Joint Commission. (2008). *Health care at the crossroads: Strategies for improving the medical liability system and preventing patient injury.* Retrieved from http://search.jointcommission.org/search?q=simulation&site=EntireSite&client=jcaho_frontend&output=xml_no_dtd&proxystylesheet=jcaho_frontend

McGaghie, W., Issenberg, S. B., Petrusa, E., & Scalese, R. (2010). A critical review of simulation-based medical education research: 2003–2009. *Medical Education, 44,* 50–63.

National League for Nursing Accreditation Commission. (2011). *NLNAC accreditation manual.* Atlanta, GA: NLNAC.

Palaganas, J. (2012). *Exploring healthcare simulation as a platform for interprofessional education (Doctoral dissertation).* Retrieved from ProQuest Dissertations and Theses database.

Reeves, S., Abramovich, I., Rice, K., & Goldman, J. (2012). *An environmental scan and literature review on interprofessional collaborative practice settings: Final report for Health Canada.* Li Ka Shing Knowledge Institute of St Michael's Hospital, University of Toronto.

Zhang, C., Thompson, S., & Miller, C. (2011). A review of simulation-based interprofessional education. *Clinical Simulation in Nursing, 7,* 117–126.

CHAPTER 2.5

Continuum of Care

Deborah D. Navedo, PhD, CPNP, CNE, and Patricia A. Reidy, DNP, FNP-BC

ABOUT THE AUTHORS

DEBORAH D. NAVEDO directs the Massachusetts General Hospital (MGH) Institute's masters program, which offers a concentration in simulation-based education, and works broadly across professions in her role as education specialist in the MGH Learning Lab. She also created the home healthcare simulation setting at the MGH Institute.

PATRICIA A. REIDY secured funding for and championed the use of standardized patients and actors in the Family Nurse Practitioner Program, implementing some of the scenarios described in this chapter. She also created the home healthcare simulation setting at the MGH Institute.

Acknowledgments: Special thanks to our colleagues at the MGH Institute and Partners Home Care who helped to design, implement, and evaluate the innovative continuum of care cases described in this chapter. To our mentors and colleagues at the Center for Medical Simulation, thank you for the inspiration.

ABSTRACT

Effective and safe patient care should occur across the continuum of care: from the initial complaint evaluation, through the acute care phase including any complications, and into optimized chronic care. As such, clinician competence must extend seamlessly beyond the management of resuscitations. Simulation-based learning is suitably robust to effectively facilitate learning in contexts beyond the standard rapid response cases. This chapter discusses the creation of meaningful learning experiences for learners that include sequential scenarios, which weave together patient encounters, professional communication, and management activities. These scenarios would realistically unfold over a span of time and settings as a continuum of care. Developing simulation centers will find a description of these complex cases, which may assist in defining faculty development plans for future implementation. Established simulation centers will find detailed discussions of learner-centered aspects that facilitate and impede the effective use of sequential scenarios, which become the continuum of care cases.

CASE EXAMPLE

Mrs. P, a 68-year-old retired teacher, is complaining of pain in her right knee, stating she can no longer walk to do her grocery shopping. A nurse practitioner performs an initial assessment in the primary care office and communicates her findings with the physician in the orthopedic clinic. A week later, the fearful patient is seen preoperatively in the surgeon's office and is scheduled for the knee replacement. During the operation, Mrs. P develops an allergic reaction to the antibiotic, and the anesthesiologist communicates the information with the postanesthetic care unit (PACU) team and the family. While in the PACU, the patient vomits and is confused, and the nurse updates her status changes with the family. Within a few days of being discharged from the hospital to her home, Mrs. P develops significant constipation, confusion about medications, and vertigo from her continued pain medication. She falls while attempting to get to the bathroom, requiring the visiting nurse to communicate the incident with the nurse in the orthopedic clinic. In the following weeks, the now very fearful Mrs. P arrives in the physical therapy clinic, where she experiences an episode of shortness of breath during treatment, and an ambulance is called.

Any one of these moments in the continuum of Mrs. P's care could be developed into a simulation scenario as brief encounters with rapidly changing patient conditions over minutes. In reality, patient status changes, responses to therapy, and even electronic communication can span hours to days. How can simulation-based learning be effectively implemented to consider the multifaceted and longitudinal care needed to effectively care for this very common case? This chapter offers a way to create meaningful learning experiences for learners that include sequential scenarios weaving together patient encounters, professional communication, and management activities as well as documentation that would realistically unfold over a span of time and settings, or a continuum of care.

INTRODUCTION, BACKGROUND, AND SIGNIFICANCE

In other chapters in this text, many best practices have been described in great detail. Attention has been given to the creation of realism and engagement through physical fidelity, conceptual fidelity, and emotional fidelity, resulting in meaningful learning (Dieckmann et al., 2007; Rudolph et al., 2007). Even so, many of these scenarios are bound by time and setting. Many healthcare simulations are designed to achieve learning in the recognition and management of quickly decompensating patients and to implement a rapid response. Simulation-based learning is significantly robust, and can be used to recreate other patient care contexts that might evolve over hours or days and across settings, including the home environment. Consider the case of Mrs. P, who progresses for total knee replacement from the primary care office, through orthopedic clinic, hospital setting, rehabilitative program, and finally into home care. As seen in the case of Mrs. P, care does not occur in isolated snippets or single offices, but rather is a continuum throughout the course of disease or even the life span. Yet it has been difficult to efficiently navigate the time gap, within a simulation experience, from one clinical situation or encounter to the next to recreate a realistic continuum of care as a coherent simulation experience.

To achieve the goal of augmenting conceptual fidelity and improving realism while including the passage of time, it is possible to create meaningful learning experiences that create sequential activities, which weave together

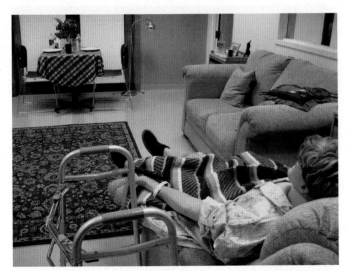

FIGURE 2.5.1 Continuum of care scenario that extends beyond the acute care setting: Mannequin in a home-setting recliner within the simulation lab.

patient encounters, professional communication, and management activities that would realistically unfold over a continuum of time (Figure 2.5.1).

Historically, learning about the patient's hospital course, or longitudinal care within the hospital, occurred at the bedside over hours and days. However, long work hours, especially for trainees, have fallen under increased scrutiny. Calls for educational reform in both medicine (Cooke et al., 2010) and nursing (Benner et al., 2010) seek to shift novice learner education from the bedside apprenticeship model to more intentional learning experiences, which can be facilitated through simulation-based learning. As such, there should be thoughtful consideration of integrating **continuum of care** cases into simulation-based learning.

The pedagogical precedents that support the use of **continuum of care** cases can be found across the health professions with origins in role-playing, case studies, and problem-based learning (PBL) (Dannefer & Prayson, 2013). More recently, **unfolding case studies** (Glendon & Ulrich, 2000), which provide sequential clinical updates and additional information within a case study, have been used to increase the realism of clinical problem solving (Day, 2012; West et al., 2012). These approaches are being increasingly utilized in the classroom (Svinicki & McKeachie, 2013, p. 210), and intersperse new events and/or information to an ongoing case study with pauses to consider how the change would affect the case in terms of pathology, assessment, and management options.

In the context of simulation-based learning, a continuum of care case would be offered to the same learner(s) in the form of multiple smaller scenarios. Although such integrated approaches are increasingly valued for learning effectiveness, few successful applications of such unfolding cases across the continuum of care in simulation can be found in the literature, demonstrating a field that is ripe for study.

FACULTY DEVELOPMENT, SCHEDULING, AND MAINTENANCE OF REALISM

There are three major challenges to the successful implementation of continuum of care cases in simulation: faculty preparation to teach effectively, scheduling the sequence of scenarios to optimize learning, and maintenance of realism.

The first and perhaps most significant challenge is related to faculty preparation. Formal education of faculty in pedagogy, meaningful learning, and effective assessment are the exception rather than the rule in healthcare settings. Current educators were largely trained in siloed educational structures with little exposure to simulation as a learning modality. Interprofessional practice and communication as explicit competencies have been recognized only in the past 5 to 10 years. As the desired learning outcomes for continuum of cases are often related to team-based care, the educators, but more importantly those individuals who conduct debriefing sessions, must be competent themselves in practicing and in teaching these skills. Additionally, faculty and staff development should include techniques for maintenance of realism, discussed later in this chapter.

Inattention to this area can contribute to the false sense of security that expertise in one professional clinical practice or specific content knowledge is sufficient to teach clinical care effectively. Clinicians rarely practice in isolation, and the continuum of care case includes patient encounters with multiple professionals with various roles. Faculty development that begins with the thoughtful communal study of effective pedagogy across the health professions and across settings, as seen in the continuum of care for the patient, should be the standard.

The second challenge relates to scheduling. Continuum of care cases involve a series of scenarios for the same learner(s), and are often longer sessions than the single scenario. Care must be taken to design cases that are reasonable in length to accommodate learner availability and to reduce learner fatigue. Most centers report scheduling problems, both in coordination of schedules and in securing release time from clinical demands, as significant barriers to effectively collaborative learning in these complex simulation cases. Institutional commitment to creating, coordinating, and protecting scheduled simulation time for both preprofessional and postlicensure or graduate learners is critical.

The third challenge appears to be the loss of realism and engagement when the participant is asked to move within the case from one scenario to the next. Following a patient status in real time is not feasible, as many results of interventions or new complications require significant time to manifest. Often, learners are verbally instructed that there has been a time lapse or that there has been a sudden progression in the case, such as "the patient in the holding area is now moved to the operating room" or "the patient has been successfully treated with drug *x* and is now. . . ." Referred to anecdotally as "time warps" within a case, learners describe such transitions as very disorienting, requiring reorientation within the new context.

Faculty and staff inexperience in managing the transitions within the continuum of care cases may be the most significant challenge facing simulation centers. Creating a believable remedy that minimally disrupts the realism, fiction contract, or the suspension of disbelief will become the focus of the remainder of this chapter (Table 2.5.1).

THE "HOW TO . . ."

There are specific planning needs that require attention in the continuum of care cases: (1) working with multiple learners, (2) the expanded simulation space, scheduling, and equipment needed, (3) the realism as it relates to the logical progression of learner experiences through the scenario transitions, and (4) the optimal method of debriefing to maximize the learning outcomes.

Working with Multiple Learners

As with any complex simulation case, preplanning of the simulation would benefit from consultation with an education specialist. This is particularly true when diverse learners are involved. Planning for effective learning should include the following:

TABLE 2.5.1

Comparison of Single-Scenario Case and Continuum of Care Case

	Single-Scenario Case	Continuum of Care Case
Number of scenarios	One	Multiple, at least one antecedent and one subsequent scenario
Transitions within the case	None	At least one
Time frame of case	Progresses in real time	Includes a transition between scenarios in which the time may have progressed quickly ("time warp")
Patient care setting	Single set or location	Includes a transition from one to the next such as operating room to recovery, or hospital to home
Resources	For single scenario	May occupy multiple rooms and simulators for a single learner
Faculty and staff	A developing center with new faculty and staff can manage with appropriate support and training	Should be sufficiently experienced to improvise effectively and follow the evolving case from one scenario into the next while protecting the realism for the learner
Desired learning outcomes	Understanding and management of a brief clinical encounter	Understanding and management across time or settings
	Communication in the moment	Communication across settings and time
Learners	One or many complete the scenario	The continuum of care learner will complete a sequence of scenarios
Debriefing considerations	Standard approach to debriefing immediately following the case	In addition to standard debriefing following any individual scenarios, overarching learning goals are debriefed at the end

- Identification of learners and their current learning levels
- Definition of appropriate learning outcomes for all learners and for each individual learner
- Decisions about what will be scripted and what will not

Being clear about who is participating as the learner and who is participating as part of the scenario as an **embedded simulated person (ESP)** is critical. In continuum of care cases, there are often many people involved in the team-based care of the patient. Learners will have learning objectives, while ESPs will have scripts to follow to create an experience that will benefit the learner. As an example, staff nurses may be invited to join a resident physician's resuscitation scenario with good intentions of creating an interprofessional experience and to improve the realism for the resident reviewing Advanced Cardiac Life Support (ACLS) protocols. The nurse is told to "be yourself" and to "do what you normally do." At the same time, the nurse may be asked not to help and to let the resident "do the scenario," when in reality, if a resident begins to struggle, the nurse would offer additional assistance and/or call for help. As described in the chapter on interprofessional simulation (see chapter 2.4), this creates a no-win situation for the participant who was invited to "join" but was ambushed without warning or consent and was restricted and used as a prop. Being clear about the specific roles of the many participants from the beginning will improve the success of continuum of care cases.

Clearly articulating the intended learning outcomes or objectives for each learner level from the beginning is essential in creating effective learning experiences. Particular consideration for the level of the learner, such as advanced beginner student versus competent staff, and matching the complexity of the case to accommodate the learner level should be part of all scenario-planning activities.

The continuum of care case is ideally situated for team-based care and communication as learning outcomes. However, regardless of the focus, these should be defined for each of the learners, and this will likely include objectives such as:

- Recognize and analyze changes in patient status over time or across contexts.
- Accurately report the status with changes in the handoff or consultation.
- Identify roles and responsibilities of the healthcare team.
- Demonstrate effective oral, written, and/or technology-assisted communication among the team members to provide safe, effective, patient-centered care.

Careful scripting of the scenarios within the continuum of care case will facilitate meeting the defined learning outcomes and protect the logical progression and transitions as the individual learners progress through the

sequence of scenarios (see section "Additional Realism and Relevance" below). Educators are encouraged to consult an education specialist early in the process to assure maximization of the case design, to clarify the intended learning outcomes, and to plan for the debriefings.

Another important but different use of sequential or progressive scenarios should be mentioned here. A simulation center may choose to have a single case or patient that progresses over a semester, which multiple learners encounter at various points, but a single learner would not experience the full sequence. For example, consider the care Mrs. P receives postoperatively. She may first be assessed and attended to by the nursing student, who writes a note. Subsequently, the physical therapy student might visit Mrs. P and read the previous nurse's note before treating Mrs. P, when she becomes short of breath. Each scenario would have discrete learners with separate learning outcomes identified. Each scenario should be carefully scripted for each learner's needs. Careful monitoring of previous student's work such as notes in the electronic health record (EHR) is essential to avoid introduction of elements that might become distracting if not controlled carefully, such as an error in the nursing note left by a previous learner. The same learner must be threaded through all of the **constituent scenarios** for a simulation to be called a continuum of care case as described here (Figure 2.5.2).

Expanded Space, Scheduling, and Equipment

When a simulation case contains multiple scenarios, as with continuum of care cases, multiple setups are needed, requiring additional space, staff, and equipment. Learners will transition between the progressive scenarios, which is discussed in more detail later in this chapter. However, there are setup implications that must be anticipated.

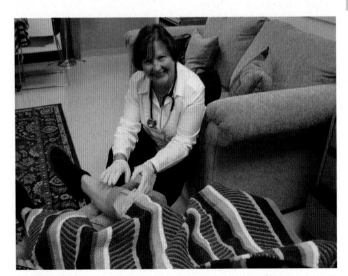

FIGURE 2.5.2 Continuum of care: A visiting nurse performs a comprehensive assessment of the home, including medication usage.

- Multiple rooms and setups may be required if a case transitions from one setting to another, such as the operating room to the recovery room.
- Multiple mannequins and other equipment may be needed at differing preset conditions.
- Additional staff may be required to run the scenario in the separate locations or with additional mannequins.
- Faculty and learners will need to be scheduled for an extended time or for several sessions to complete the multiple-scenario continuum of care case. If the same faculty/debriefer is to follow a learner, then coordinated scheduling becomes essential.
- Consideration for learner fatigue should be incorporated into the scheduling of multiple transitioning scenarios into a single session.

Continuum of care cases can be resource-intensive. As such, piloting these cases to work out the logistical coordination is highly encouraged.

Realism of Logical Progression and Scenario Transitions

In addition to the general best-practice strategies for simulation-based learning described in chapter 1.1, there are several unique learner considerations when designing continuum of care cases. Because there are patient developments across settings and/or time periods being portrayed, the realism of the progression and transitions should be considered beyond the mannequin settings and to the environment and communication to avoid disorientation.

When a continuum of care case is being planned, there will be at least two events or contexts involved. Learners will be expected to engage in the first scenario and then move to the next scenario and make appropriate connections in assessment, management, and communication on the basis of the patient status changes or situational differences presented to them.

It is possible that a learner will make a choice within an antecedent scenario, which will have implications for following scenarios. An "in-the-moment" decision will need to be made by faculty to pause between scenarios to debrief and adjust versus going ahead with a new status with consequences in the following scenario. This introduces an added level of complexity, which should be engaged cautiously by any simulation center. As such, centers are encouraged to carefully pilot these cases to understand the general range of learner behaviors prior to any high-stakes implementation.

Realism beyond the mannequin should be considered in conjunction with the defined learning outcomes. Dieckmann et al. (2007) relate physical, semantic (or conceptual), and phenomenal (or emotional) fidelity to realism within simulation-based learning. The physical fidelity across the transition might be the use of the same wig or the same equipment from one scenario to the next to create recognition and continuity from one scenario to the

next. Maintaining conceptual fidelity might mean assuring that if a drug was given in the **antecedent scenario**, the expected effects of this can be seen in the following scenario. Emotional fidelity might be reproduced within the learner across scenarios if there is consistency in ESPs in same character roles, as variability from one scenario to the next will be distracting from identified learning outcomes. Consider the effect on the learner if a mother of a patient is portrayed by one actor in an antecedent scenario and is suddenly portrayed by a different actor in a **subsequent scenario**. The initial disorientation is not insignificant and requires the learner to reestablish the context and realism of the case. All three forms of fidelity should be considered when creating a logical progression and promoting realism for the learner within the continuum of care cases.

Reality across **scenario transitions** should be considered through handoffs and consultations. For example, if effective use of communication skills was an expected learning outcome, then consideration should be given to the use of additional ESPs who serve as clinicians or family members outside the room, such as by phone or overhead consult. Additional forms of communication may include handoffs and likely various forms of documentation involved.

EXAMPLE

(Scripted Scenario): The nurse practitioner (NP) student examines Mrs. P in the primary care office and steps out of the exam room to make a consulting phone call with the orthopedist regarding her findings and to determine the next steps of care.

NP Student:	Mrs. P is a 68-year-old woman with a history of osteoarthritis and reports excruciating right knee pain that has progressively worsened over the past 6 months. She denies any trauma. Her pain is unrelieved with high doses of NSAIDS, and she reports she is unable to adequately walk or climb stairs. On physical exam, her right knee has a mild effusion, tenderness along the joint line, and crepitus with range of motion.
Dr. S:	What are her X-ray findings?
NP Student:	An X-ray performed 3 months ago reveals sclerotic changes and narrowing of the joint space.
Dr. S:	Obtain an MRI and schedule an appointment for her in the clinic. We will evaluate her and discuss her treatment options.

And finally, disorienting transitions that create a distraction from the learning goals should be avoided. These unnecessarily increase learner cognitive load while the learner sorts out what is "part of the scenario" and what can be ignored as part of the fiction contract. These may include even simple differences such as bedding, clothing, ESPs, or vital signs and displays. Such disorganized transitions may be perceived as frustrating for the expert learner as unrealistically increasing the signal-to-noise ratio, while the novice learner can become completely disoriented and lost. It is helpful for the planning team to explicitly create a list defining what will be consistent and not changing over the transition and what will be allowed to evolve. Some helpful suggestions for smoothing a transition and protecting fidelity and realism are offered:

- Be certain that a new orienting statement is given to the learner at the beginning of the new scenario. It should include elements of who the learner is (which should not change while within the continuum of care case), who the people in the room are (including the mannequin), what is going on, and what the new context and time is, especially if a "time warp" is used. This orienting statement about the new setting may need to be repeated if the learner remains frozen or stuck.
- If the vital signs on the monitor in the following scenario are not intended to be different than the first, have the confederate in the next scenario verbalize this. An example of such a statement would be, "I have been with Mrs. P for 15 minutes, and her vital signs have not changed."
- Do not expect the learner to read much unless this is part of the learning outcome. There is general consensus that clinicians will not read signs on walls during a 15- to 20-minute scenario. Detailed notes in medical records are also not likely to be reviewed in a short scenario.
- Debrief the learner about the transitions to identify any distractions that they experienced that may need to be adjusted.

Careful attention by the entire planning team to the continuity and alignment of the scenario is paramount for the learner to retain the fiction contract and to feel the realism sufficiently to stay engaged and to avoid being distracted unnecessarily by unintended discrepancies in the scenario transitions.

Debriefing

Continuum of care cases may require debriefing after each scenario to facilitate learning and explore the learner's knowledge, clinical judgment, and emotion as the case unfolds (Overstreet, 2010; Reese, 2011). Ideally, a single learner participates in all the continuum of care scenarios and may be interacting with various learners in individual scenarios. Debriefing strategies may vary throughout the course of the case according to the learning objectives for the specific scenarios and overall case. For example, the continuous learner in the case of Mrs. P may be the clinician in the orthopedic clinic who engages in all the scenarios from the initial referral through hospitalization and home care. After debriefing with the multiple learners for each scenario, the continuous learner may be asked to complete a reflection assignment to explore knowledge

and emotions. One innovative method (Reese, 2011, p. 345) is to ask learners to "finish the story" by projecting the patient's life over a span of time.

The developing simulation center should consider the use of continuum of care cases cautiously until they are implementing individual scenarios consistently and effectively. With appropriate attention to the intended learning outcomes, operational details, realism of transitions, and debriefing, established centers are encouraged to explore continuum of care cases.

BEEN THERE, DONE THAT: HOW CAN I CONTINUE TO IMPROVE OR SUSTAIN WHAT I HAVE ACHIEVED?

Expert educators can augment existing single scenarios by adding a follow-up scenario that serves the identified learning needs. This results in a continuum of care case. There are several approaches for taking the continuum of care case to the next level of realism and for assuring continued improvement.

Additional Realism and Relevance

As communication is often a central element in these cases, especially when they span time and settings, attention to these details should not be overlooked. Some examples of communication details within a continuum of care context follow.

One such addition could be the integration of the EHR to reproduce the reality of today's clinical environment, which is increasingly dependent on electronic communication. The EHR has become the basis for not only archival information or reports, but also for real time communication among caregivers of the same patient in the same moment. A variation of this might be the implementation of an EHR to facilitate interprofessional sequential care or visits by consultants. If labs are to be drawn as a result of an exam by one learner who participated in the scenario through that moment, then another learner may be sent in to share the lab results and to take any corrective action needed (such as a high coagulation time and adjusted anticoagulation therapy). The communication between the learners may occur only by EHR.

As the continuum of care is increasingly extended into the home, integration of home care into the scenario can be a challenging but rewarding addition. Mrs. P's problems at home are not unusual, and there is a significant need to think earnestly about implementing simulation-base education for the home care professional as well. These might include home care nurses, first responders, and others who interact with patients within the home environment. The full-service simulation center will consider the professional competencies of its constituent learners and develop such learning opportunities as appropriate.

Each of these elements can increase the realism and the effectiveness of the cases. Programs are encouraged to revisit the intended learning outcomes frequently to protect the alignment of each of the scenarios with the learner's actual experiences as he/she progresses through the continuum.

Sustained Improvement

The established center with competent to expert faculty, educators, and staff will be able to effectively implement these complex scenarios within the continuum of care case. Three possible areas of continued improvement are (1) scenario monitoring, (2) faculty development around emerging professional competencies and educational best practices, and (3) contribution back to the field by studying the learning outcomes and supporting pedagogical research.

Simulation centers that are already implementing continuum of care cases are encouraged to carefully monitor the cases, constituent scenarios, and debriefings for opportunities to more tightly align the learner responses and to detect unintended spin-off or degradation away from the stated learning outcomes. Even the best-planned scenarios require multiple iterations to stabilize within a given simulation setting, and continuum of care cases may require more cycles to achieve consistent outcomes (Figure 2.5.3).

Thriving simulation centers will invest in faculty development for all involved, including the educators, debriefers, technical staff, and other ancillary staff. A shared mental model and understanding of experiential learning within a safe environment will benefit not only the learners but also the faculty development efforts by creating a sustaining organizational culture that values lifelong learning for the educators and learners alike. Particular areas of emphasis for faculty development in this context might include interprofessional practice, communication skills, and educational best practices. Use of continuum of care cases requires an added level of flexibility and improvisational competence, which can be effective only if there is an organizational commitment to continuous self-improvement.

Finally, as mentioned in previous chapters, a commitment to innovative scenarios, thoughtful evaluation, and rigorous scholarship will set the well-established simulation center apart by contributing back to the field. Continuum of care cases offer unique opportunities for learners to experience progression of cases across settings and time frames. Studying the effectiveness of such educational interventions should become a priority as reduced duty hours and clinical experiences are increasingly limited across the health professions.

SUMMARY

Simulation-based learning is a powerful and robust educational tool that can be readily adopted to include experiences across the continuum of care that can span settings and time frames. Although there is little in the literature that defines best practices, some helpful suggestions are offered on the basis of collective experiences. New simulation centers should entertain the use of continuum of care cases cautiously, while gaining competence in the basics of simulation-based learning methodology. The established simulation centers seeking to upgrade the fidelity and realism of the learner experience will find these scenarios both challenging and rewarding, as they recreate sophisticated and coherent debriefable simulation experiences.

REFERENCES

Benner, P. A., Stuphen, M., Leonard, V., & Day, L. (for Carnegie Foundation for the Advancement of Teaching). (2010). *Educating nurses: A call for radical transformation.* San Fransisco, CA: Jossey-Bass.

Cooke, M., Irby, D. M., & O'Brien, B. C. (for Carnegie Foundation for the Advancement of Teaching). (2010). *Educating physicians: A call for reform of medical school and residency.* San Fransisco, CA: Jossey-Bass.

Dannefer, E. F., & Prayson, R. A. (2013). Supporting students in self-regulation: Use of formative feedback and portfolios in a problem-based learning setting. *Medical Teacher, 35*(8), 655–660.

Day, L. (2012). Using unfolding case studies in a subject-centered classroom. *Journal of Nursing Education, 50*(8), 447–452. doi:10.3928/01484834-20110517-03

Dieckmann, P., Gaba, D. M., & Rall, M. (2007). Deepening the theoretical foundations of patient simulation as social practice. *Simulation in Healthcare, 2*(3), 183–193.

Glendon, K. J., & Ulrich, D. L. (2000). *Unfolding case studies: Experiencing the realities of clinical nursing practice.* Upper Saddle River, NJ: Prentice Hall.

Overstreet, M. (2010). Eechat: The seven components of nurse debriefing. *Journal of Continuing Education in Nursing, 41*(12), 538–539.

Reese, C. E. (2011). Unfolding case studies. *Journal of Continuing Education in Nursing, 42*(8), 344–345.

Rudolph, J., Simon, R., & Raemer, D. (2007). Which reality matters? Questions on the path to high engagement in healthcare simulation. *Simulation in Healthcare, 2*(3), 161–163.

Svinicki, M. D., & McKeachie, W. J. (2013). *McKeachie's teaching tips: Strategies, research, and theory for college and university teachers* (14th ed.). Belmont, CA: Wadsworth Cengage.

West, C., Usher, K., & Delaney, L. J. (2012). Unfolding case studies in pre-registration nursing education: lessons learned. *Nurse Education Today, 32*(5), 576–580. doi:10.1016/j.nedt.2011.07.002

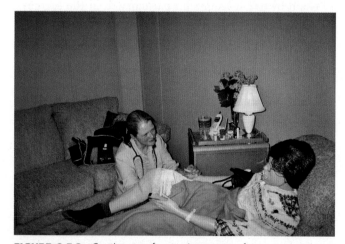

FIGURE 2.5.3 Continuum of care: Awareness of case progression is critical to appropriate wound and mobility assessment.

CHAPTER 2.6

Just-in-Time Training Programs

Anne Marie Monachino MSN, RN, CPN, and Stephanie A. Tuttle, MS, MBA

ABOUT THE AUTHORS

ANNEMARIE MONACHINO is a pediatric advanced practice nurse with 20 years' experience. She has been a nurse educator for 10 years. She joined the Center for Simulation at the Children's Hospital of Philadelphia (CHOP) in 2008 as a clinical educator but has been using simulation as a teaching methodology for many years. AnneMarie has been involved in the planning and implementation of several "just-in-time" simulation programs at CHOP.

STEPHANIE TUTTLE is the Administrative Director of the Center for Simulation, Advanced Education and Innovation at the Children's Hospital of Philadelphia (CHOP). She has a long-standing commitment to international training, and has administratively coordinated innovative projects at CHOP, including its national Simulation Education Boot Camp for first year Pediatric Critical Care Medicine Fellows, and its Operation Smile International Pediatric Advanced Life Support Courses and Boot Camp for mission members in resource-limited settings.

Acknowledgments: The authors would like to acknowledge the following people from the Children's Hospital of Philadelphia, Center for Simulation, Advanced Education and Innovation for their contributions to just-in-time training. Akira Nishisaki, MD, MSe, Dana E. Niles, MS, CCRC, Evie Lengetti, MSN, RN, Amy Scholtz, MSN, RN, WHNP-BC, CCNS-BC, and Vinay Nadkarni, MD, MS.

ABSTRACT

Just-in-time training programs provide simulation-based refresher training just before the learner needs to perform the intervention. Clinicians are tasked with learning a variety of technical psychomotor skills that may be simple or complex in nature. Often, these skills are acquired during one's initial training, and, depending on circumstances, the healthcare provider may not have the opportunity to perform the skill regularly. Allowing learners to refresh a skill or rehearse a practice guideline very near to the time it may be required is one way that simulation-based education augments clinical care. Allowing learners to practice the skill set in or near the actual location of care (just-in-place) brings additional contextual value to the just-in-time event.

This chapter describes the development and implementation of just-in-time training programs, including best methods, logistics, challenges, limitations, costs, and outcome measurements. Several examples of just-in-time simulation training programs will be cited, including the successful development and implementation of the Central Venous Catheter (CVC) Dress Rehearsal Program, Cardiopulmonary Resuscitation (CPR) Rolling Refreshers, and Pediatric Tracheal Intubation Refresher Training.

CASE EXAMPLE

It is early in the afternoon at an inpatient medical ward. The nurse reports to the physician that her patient is displaying symptoms of urinary retention. An order is placed to insert an indwelling urinary catheter (Foley). The last time this nurse placed a Foley catheter was several years ago, and although the nurse read the newly revised procedure a few months ago, she has had no hands-on exposure to the new procedure. What if immediately prior to placing the Foley in her patient (just-in-time) the nurse was able to review the procedure and deliberately practice this high-risk skill on a realistic simulator located on the inpatient unit (just-in-place), with a competent practitioner providing feedback, thereby increasing her confidence in performing this skill and decreasing the risk of harm or infection to the patient?

INTRODUCTION AND BACKGROUND

What Is Just-in-Time Training?

Simulation-based education is now recognized as an integral part of the process of training healthcare providers. This methodology is appealing to adult learners who prefer interactive, hands-on learning with immediate feedback (Decker et al., 2008). Cook and colleagues (2011) did an extensive review of the literature and found that, with rare exceptions, technology-enhanced simulation training had better learning outcomes when compared with traditional methods and is an effective method of delivering health profession education. Simulation-based training can occur in a variety of settings for several reasons: (a) introduce skill acquisition, (b) increase skill retention, (c) improve team performance, (d) promote individual or group learning, and (e) advance education. The time at which the training occurs can also vary. **Just-in-time** training programs provide simulation-based refresher training immediately before the learner needs to perform the intervention.

The term "just-in-time" has its origin in the manufacturing world and is thought to have been invented shortly after World War II by Taiichi Ohno of Toyota. After studying America's supermarkets and analyzing their production methods, Ohno created a system whereby production rates are determined by the end user rather than the producer, thereby eliminating waste and minimizing resources and time. As Toyota's gains in productivity became evident, American industrialists traveled to Japan to learn about these concepts, which have since become the industry standard (AIDT, 2001). Other fields have adapted this just-in-time concept; it has been applied to training for emerging technology needs (Kutzik, 2005), disaster preparation (Stoler et al., 2011), and simulation education.

Just-in-time training has been defined as training conducted directly prior to a potential intervention (Niles et al., 2009). In addition, this training is frequently conducted "just-in-place," at or near the location of the intervention, which provides the trainee an experiential learning opportunity that can be incorporated into clinical practice. In general, the simulation can be done in a short time using a mobile cart containing a simulator, often a partial task trainer. This educational strategy has been shown to be an effective method of training, especially for clinicians who are providing care at the bedside and may need to perform a low-volume–high-risk skill (Benedek & Ritchie, 2006; Kneebone et al., 2004; Spencer, 2003).

When Is Just-in-Time Training Appropriate?

In designing any simulation program or curriculum, the initial step is to perform a needs assessment: a systematic process to collect accurate and thorough information to determine the need and/or performance gap (see chapter 5.1 on needs assessment). This will help to establish the overall purpose of the program and determine the instructional goal. On the basis of the analysis of the information collected, educational objectives should be developed and an instructional strategy developed. If the goal involves a skill-based competency in which the learner needs to demonstrate both knowledge and performance of the psychomotor skill prior to actual clinical practice, then just-in-time training may be the answer.

SIGNIFICANCE

Benefits of Just-in-Time Training

Research suggests that simulation training can increase trainee competence (Nishisaki et al., 2007). Simulation mimics the clinical setting in that learners can demonstrate skills in the psychomotor, cognitive, and affective domains (Ross, 2012). Simulation is an effective teaching methodology, especially for task or skill training at all levels of experience (Nagle et al., 2009). Just-in-time training is not new to medical and nursing simulation; its use in clinical settings predated modern simulation technology. However, the growth of simulation technologies as a training adjunct increases the opportunities for just-in-time training. Table 2.6.1 outlines multiple advantages of just-in-time training.

Studies of long-term retention of skills (Weaver et al., 2012) have demonstrated that spaced practice, where the learner has multiple opportunities to practice a skill spaced over time, has a more positive effect on acquisition of skill than massed practice, where learning is concentrated in a short time frame. Healey et al. (1998) found that after 6 months, competence in complex tasks decreases significantly and the establishment of some method of refresher training within that time frame helps maintain proficiency. Just-in-time training, by its very nature, is a form of spaced practice refresher training. This approach supports one of the main advantages of simulation-based education. It provides the trainee or learner the chance to practice the skill on a simulator without risk to the patient.

Limitations of Just-in-Time Training

There are several limitations to just-in-time training that one should be cognizant of prior to choosing this method

TABLE 2.6.1
Advantages to Just-in-Time Training
• Provides real-time education and feedback
• Allows experiential learning
• Can be done within the clinical environment at the point of care
• May help to reinforce skill retention, which is prone to decay
• Can be done with minimal disruption to clinical obligations
• Enhances ability to provide appropriate care
• Can improve learner's confidence in performing psychomotor skill

of education. This training should be used for learners who have achieved a baseline competence level (Nishisaki et al., 2010). It is not intended as the initial training for a particular task or skill, so one must know the training level of the intended audience prior to offering the intervention. As with any simulation, just-in-time training is dependent on the availability of the faculty, the simulation equipment, and space to perform the training, all of which may be limiting factors to success. Other factors that may have an impact on the outcome of this educational method are the availability of the learners and their attitude to just-in-time training. These are obstacles one may need to overcome. Lastly, simulation education is a tool that is only as effective as the teacher, so the person conducting the training should be an expert not only in the skill, but also in the nuances of simulation as a teaching modality and associated skills, including debriefing (Weinstock et al., 2009). Educators who use the just-in-time technique should possess effective communication skills, knowledge of adult learning principles, ability to plan experiential learning activities, assessment and responsiveness to the learner's ability to perform the skill, as well as technical competence to utilize simulation resources (Galloway, 2009).

HOW TO IMPLEMENT JUST-IN-TIME TRAINING

As with other forms of simulation education, just-in-time simulation requires effort, dedicated faculty, careful planning, adequate resources, and sufficient time to accomplish the training objectives. What follows is a step-by-step plan for just-in-time training corresponding to the case example presented at the beginning of this chapter: A nurse needs to insert an indwelling urinary catheter (Foley).

1. **Needs Assessment.** The first step is to assess whether there is a need for refresher training. Learning needs may emerge in many ways, including (a) direct observation, (b) anecdotal reports, (c) potential for healthcare-associated injury to patients such as a central line–associated blood stream infection (CLABSI), surgical site infection, catheter-associated urinary tract infection, and so on, (d) noted inconsistency in practice, (e) changes to a procedure, (f) skill decay related to low-volume–high-risk technical skill, or (g) individual or group request to improve competency. In this case example, the hospital had seen an increase in the nosocomial urinary tract infection rate and several nurses on this unit reported a lack of knowledge and confidence in placing a urinary catheter related to the low frequency of performing the skill. Also, the last time this nurse placed a Foley catheter was several years ago, and although she read the newly revised procedure a few months ago, she had no hands-on exposure to the new procedure.

2. **Learning Objectives.** When the need for just-in-time training has been identified, it is essential to create learning objectives that will guide the planning of the clinical simulation program. Trainees need to know what they are expected to accomplish during the learning intervention. For task-based skill refresher training, the number of learning outcomes (1 to 2) may be less than a team-based simulation scenario. The learning objective for this case example was determined to be: To perform the correct steps of Foley insertion on a mannequin following the institutional procedure for insertion of an indwelling urinary catheter.

3. **Best Method for Training.** The best method for meeting the objectives of just-in-time training should be determined. It is important to provide the learner both the opportunity to practice the skill against a standard measurement to ensure correct application of their knowledge as well as a facilitator or simulation educator to give feedback. Since the skill in the case example had higher-level learning objectives (application level) and required a contextual application of knowledge and skill, simulation is an appropriate learning methodology.

4. **Means of Evaluation.** When designing just-in-time simulation-based training, one should incorporate an evaluation of the training to determine whether it meets the needs of the learner. A just-in-time training event that involves a technical skill requires the developer to use the most up-to-date procedure or policy when constructing the checklist or tool. The checklist or tool should be validated or assessed for accuracy and standardization by a clinical specialist in that field. If the psychomotor skill includes numerous steps, the novice and expert clinician may complete the skill differently as the more experienced clinician may have developed procedural efficiencies. Depending on the complexity of the skill, it is helpful if the content expert also highlights the key or critical steps that cannot be skipped during the performance of the clinical procedure. Even though the checklist or tool for evaluating clinical performance of a specific skill has been validated or deemed accurate by the expert, the next step is to have several people simulate the procedure using the skills checklist. This provides valuable feedback and gives a sense of how long it takes to complete the training. In the case example, the insertion of an indwelling urinary catheter skill was evaluated using a skills checklist based on the institutional procedure for insertion of a urinary catheter. An educator qualified to assess performance of this skill provided feedback to the learner.

5. **Resources Needed.** Prior to testing the measurement tool that outlines the steps of the just-in-time

training, the resources necessary to implement the specific just-in-time program must be established. Some questions to assist in planning are as follows:

- Will a partial task trainer be appropriate for the training, or does it require a full-body manne-quin? Is the simulator accessible to the point of care, or is it routinely in use elsewhere?
- Will the training occur in the simulation lab or on a patient care unit (**in situ**)?
- If in situ training is planned, is the simulator easily transportable?
- What supplies will be needed to complete the task?
- Can materials be reused, and if so, how will they be maintained?
- Where will equipment and supplies be stored?
- Who will pay for the disposable supplies?
- How many educators are needed to carry out the training?
- Who will ensure that the educators are qualified to do the training?

The training in the case example required a simulator (pelvic, full-body, or partial task trainer) that was capable of having a Foley inserted, supplies needed to complete the procedure (appropriate-sized Foley catheter for the simulator, urinary catheter insertion kit, procedure gloves, hand sanitizer, and Foley bag), a qualified educator, and an area to complete the training.

6. **Planning and Logistics.** After the audience has been identified, the objectives written, the tools to measure learning outcomes created, the simulator and necessary supplies obtained, and the appropriate educators identified, there are several additional things to consider in the planning phase prior to starting the just-in-time training.

- Has support from administration or the leaders of the group being educated been maximized? It is helpful to create a proposal that includes background information and how the need was identified, the expected time for completion, the estimated costs, the expected learner outcomes, and potential clinical outcomes.
- Within what period of time will the training take place? Is the goal to accomplish the refresher education in a day or two, over a week, a month, or even longer? This informs how much time should be allotted, especially if it is intended to be a one-time intervention.
- Will the training be mandatory for all clinicians in a specific discipline or unit, or will the just-in-time training be targeted to clinicians involved in the care of patients requiring that skill or task? This will make a difference in the approach the educators use to implement the training. For example, if training in the proper use of restraints is desired, it may be targeted to clini-cians in areas of high utilization (e.g., intensive care unit) or in areas of lower utilization (e.g., floor unit). This choice may affect the time and resources necessary to implement training.

- How will the training be tracked and by whom? Completion of the skill is sometimes easier to document on paper but may need to be in an electronic database for easy access. If the training was initiated as a result of a healthcare-associated injury or infection, it is important to ensure that the appropriate providers are educated to create a safe care environment. This seems like a simple thing, but thought must be given to the process.
- How much time will it take to complete the in-dividual training session? Learners will expect to be given a time frame that they will be away from clinical duties. An educational intervention that takes less than 15 minutes is more appealing and acceptable to direct care providers.
- Will the learner who does not complete the pro-cedure or perform the skill correctly be required to repeat the procedure/skill after receiving feed-back from the educator? Practicing a skill with meaningful feedback promotes effective learning, and repeating the skill until mastery is achieved is a desirable outcome. If this method is to be employed, the learner should be informed of the expectation prior to beginning the training.

For our Foley insertion case example, a proposal was presented to the leaders of the group monitoring catheter-associated urinary tract infections (Table 2.6.2).

CHALLENGES

While the refresher training is ideally done close to the actual time of the event, competing clinical demands may prevent the learner from taking advantage of this train-ing or contribute to an inability to concentrate due to dis-tractions. When possible, give learners sufficient advance notice so that they can integrate the training into their shift. Even with advance notice, the clinician may be unable to complete the training. If so, attempt to resched-ule the training for another time when the learner will be able to find coverage for clinical responsibilities.

Another roadblock commonly encountered is finding the appropriate space in the clinical environment to set up and perform the just-in-time training. Ideally, the learner practices the skill in a realistic setting, but you may need to improvise and use a nearby conference room or a room near the clinical area dedicated to simulation. One option is to employ a mobile cart that contains equipment/task trainers and room to perform the skill. A challenge that is not as easy to overcome is the availability of a qualified educator. It helps to have a few people who are qualified to do the just-in-time training in the event this occurs.

TABLE 2.6.2
Proposal for Foley Insertion Just-in-Time Training
Background The hospital has seen an increase in the number of catheter-associated urinary tract infections (CaUTI). In response, evidence-based revisions were made to the hospital procedure for insertion of an indwelling urinary catheter to lessen the risk of harm to the patient.
Identification of Need Nurses on the medical/surgical unit who do not routinely place indwelling urinary catheters are expressing a need for refresher training in this skill.
Proposed Education Plan Experts will develop a skills checklist for Foley insertion on the basis of the institutional procedure, and educators will be evaluated and signed off as qualified observers who can implement this education using just-in-time simulation training. Training will be offered to nurses on three medical/surgical units by six qualified educators over a 2-month period. Three simulators (one full-body and two partial task trainers) will be required as well as one urinary catheter kit and Foley catheter per person. Training will take approximately 15 minutes per person and can be completed on the ward during the nurse's assigned shift. We estimate that 120 nurses will need this training. Since this is a low-volume–high-risk skill, nurses will be required to perform the skill on the simulator correctly and will be asked to repeat the Foley insertion if mistakes in performing critical steps of the procedure are noted. The simulation center has the necessary simulators available for this training.
Approximate Cost The estimated price for supplies and educators to refresh 120 nurses on this procedure is less than the cost of one CaUTI. Keeping patients safe is our priority, and we feel that this initiative will improve clinical outcomes.

THREE EXAMPLES OF JUST-IN-TIME TRAINING PROGRAMS

This section discusses three just-in-time programs, all of which were initiated on the basis of an identified need for improvement in a psychomotor skill. Each involves the application of knowledge, all are high-risk skills with associated poor outcomes if the task is performed incorrectly, and all have the potential to be low volume so that the opportunity to perform the skill on a regular basis is decreased, thus prompting the need for refresher training.

The Joint Commission Standards defines a low-volume–high-risk duty as a rarely performed duty that carries a significant risk of hazard or harm (Summers & Woods, 2008). All three programs were designed with the intent of improving quality and enhancing the delivery of safe patient care.

Just-in-Time Simulation Training for Cardiopulmonary Resuscitation: Rolling Refreshers

Needs assessment: Researchers at a 500-bed urban children's hospital were interested in the effect of high-quality cardiopulmonary resuscitation (CPR) on patient outcomes. They were concerned because studies showed retention of CPR skills to be less than ideal with poor performance 3 to

6 months post training related to inadequate practice time on mannequins.

Learning objectives: The goal was to improve CPR psychomotor skills and provider confidence.

Best method for training: The hospital had just obtained a new defibrillator that used a force sensor and accelerometer to measure rate, depth, and quality of chest compressions while giving real-time audiovisual feedback. Using this instrument, a novel program to refresh the CPR skills of bedside providers in the Pediatric Intensive Care Unit (PICU) was developed. All bedside practitioners received baseline training on the defibrillator prior to the intervention. This just-in-time training program, which was named "Rolling Refreshers," started with the clinical staff identifying five PICU patients at risk for cardiac arrest. The multidisciplinary team (physicians, nurses, respiratory therapists) providing care for those at-risk patients (just-in-time) was given the opportunity to be refreshed.

Resources needed: A certified Basic Life Support (BLS) instructor rolled a cart equipped with a mannequin and the defibrillator to the patient's bedside.

Means of evaluation: The provider was able to practice CPR with real-time feedback until they achieved successful compressions based on American Heart Association guidelines (see Figure 2.6.1).

Planning and logistics: Training was targeted to the team of nurses, physicians, and respiratory therapists assigned to the five most critically ill patients in the unit. On a daily basis, the cart was brought to those patients' rooms and during the course of the provider's clinical shift; CPR training occurred without interruption of the provider's bedside responsibilities. Sessions lasted less than 5 minutes. In 15 weeks, 420 providers participated in just-in-time training, all of whom met CPR skill success targets. Those

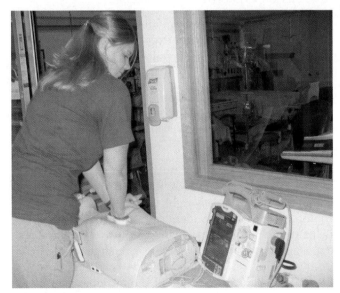

FIGURE 2.6.1 Just-in-time simulation training for CPR: Rolling Refresher cart.

SECTION 2 • Types of Simulation Programs

who refreshed two or more times per month were able to achieve CPR skill success faster on the mannequin than those refreshed less often.

Results: Evaluations of the refresher training showed the just-in-time training to be effective. When actual resuscitations were evaluated, it was found that bedside providers who were highly refreshed (more than two chest compression providers had participated in a refresher session within 90 days of event) provided significantly more chest compressions of adequate depth. Several BLS instructors in the PICU were trained to conduct Rolling Refreshers so that frontline staff can continue to refresh and be prepared to deliver high-quality chest compressions when the need arises (Niles et al., 2009). The Rolling Refresher sessions have become a mainstay in the PICU and have extended to the Emergency Department.

Just-in-Time Simulation Training on Tracheal Intubation

Needs assessment: Tracheal intubation is a life-saving procedural skill that is not performed on a routine basis, but if done incorrectly can result in tracheal intubation–associated events (TIAEs). Pediatric medical residents are expected to perform this skill during rotations in thePICU, oftentimes on a critically ill patient. However, they may have limited opportunities to achieve mastery in the skill.

Learning objectives: The learning objectives for this program were to improve pediatric medical resident participation and success in tracheal intubations and to decrease TIAEs.

Best method of training: To meet these learning objectives, a children's hospital developed just-in-time simulation-based training for residents in their PICU. In addition, they added a 10-minute airway management skill refresher training for the incoming resident at the beginning of their on-call period (Nishisaki et al., 2010).

Resources needed: An airway training station set up in the PICU training room with an experienced simulation educator with content expertise available to provide feedback and coaching.

Means of evaluation: Evaluation of this just-in-time educational intervention was achieved by measuring the first attempt and overall success rate as well as TIAEs during ICU intubations.

Planning and logistics: This simulated skill training included feedback and coaching, took the resident 10 minutes to complete, and occurred right in the PICU in a training room configured to be identical to a patient room. Participants included postgraduate years 1 to 3 Pediatric residents and postgraduate years 3 to 4 Emergency Medicine residents who were assigned to a 4-week rotation in the PICU. Four days a week, one of the two on-call residents completed the skill refresher training with coaching at the

beginning of their 24-hour on-call shift followed by a multi-disciplinary team training. The whole session lasted 30 minutes and was videotaped and reviewed by the investigators.

Results: The researchers hoped that the refresher training would contribute to positive patient clinical outcomes. They found that the overall occurrence of unwanted TIAEs did not increase during the intervention phase. However, the overall success rates and the first attempt rates were similar for the just-in-time refreshed medical residents and those concurrent nonrefreshed residents. The leaders of this program noted several limitations and challenges, and are unsure whether the negative results are related to a small sample size or whether the level of competence prior to the just-in-time training was suboptimal (Nishisaki et al., 2010). This is one example where just-in-time refresher training may be best offered to those who have a high level of proficiency in the skill.

Just-in-Time Simulation Training on Central Venous Catheters Dressing Changes: CVC Dress Rehearsals

Needs assessment: While central venous catheters (CVCs) are a necessary medical intervention for many hospitalized children, they are often associated with complications, one of which is CLABSI. Bloodstream infections are costly to treat and can have a mortality rate as high as 20% (Miller-Hoover & Small, 2009). One aspect of care in the prevention of CLABSI is CVC dressing changes, which are frequently performed by nurses. At a large urban children's hospital, patients with CVC are located throughout the hospital on inpatient wards so every nurse has the potential to perform a CVC dressing change. However, inconsistencies in practice, notably catheter maintenance and dressing change procedure, were found to be causative factors related to CLABSI.

Learning objectives: The goal was to minimize variability in the practice of CVC dressing changes and to promote a higher level of patient safety.

Best method of training: This intervention required knowledge of the procedure, technical skill, and critical thinking in the event that complications arise during the dressing change. Educators developed a just-in-time simulation-based bedside training called a "CVC Dress Rehearsal."

Resources needed: Using a mobile cart containing partial task trainers, a chest and arm equipped with a CVC, and the actual dressing change supplies, clinical educators traveled to the various hospital units and approached nurses caring for a patient with a central line and invited them to participate in a CVC Dress Rehearsal (see Figure 2.6.2).

Means of evaluation: After completing a pre-event questionnaire that assessed knowledge of the CVC policy and procedure, the nurse performed a dressing change on a simulated CVC, while the educator documented adherence

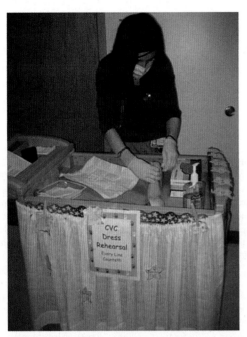

FIGURE 2.6.2 Just-in-time simulation training on CVC dressing changes: CVC Dress Rehearsals.

to the steps of the procedure and provided immediate feedback on their performance. The participants completed a postevent questionnaire that was identical to the pre-event questionnaire with the exception of a few questions pertaining to the effectiveness of the training.

Planning and logistics: The goal was to offer the training to as many nurses as possible, but the clinical educators found it challenging at times to recruit nurses to participate in the dress rehearsal owing to patient acuity and increased patient volume. While the intent was to target nurses caring for a patient with a CVC who may have to perform a dressing change at some point in their shift, other nurses on the unit were interested in the program and available to participate, so they too were offered the training.

Results: The just-in-time simulation-based CVC Dress Rehearsal program in which nurses practiced CVC dressing changes on a simulator was successful in improving nurses' knowledge and competence and increasing the consistency of practice in CVC dressing changes, thereby meeting the learning objectives (Lengetti et al., 2011).

BEEN THERE, DONE THAT: HOW CAN I CONTINUE TO IMPROVE OR SUSTAIN WHAT I HAVE ACHIEVED?

Effectiveness and Return on Investment

For programs that have already implemented just-in-time training, a well-developed process for evaluating effectiveness and return on investment should be identified. One

should assess the impact of the training and whether the time, effort, and costs of the training were worthwhile. The feedback supplied both informally and on the written evaluation can be used to improve the training. If the training is focused on a specific skill that has a potential impact on measureable clinical outcomes (e.g., CVC Dress Rehearsal or the Rolling Refreshers), explore the possibility of incorporating the just-in-time training into a research study. The following questions may assist you in the evaluation process:

- Were the learners able to demonstrate knowledge of the skill? If a cognitive examination was used, examine the results for evidence of knowledge retention.
- Were the learners able to apply that knowledge and perform the psychomotor or technical aspects of the skill? This requires a review of the data obtained from the skills checklists.
- Was the just-in-time training the best educational method to meet the learning objectives?
- Are there better types of simulation that may be used? It is helpful to query the learners immediately after the education.
- Did this simulation meet the learning objectives?
- Did the learners feel better prepared to perform this skill on a patient?

Teamwork or Communication Scenarios

While the just-in-time training detailed in this chapter focused on skill-based tasks, the more experienced educator may apply this concept to teamwork or communication-based scenarios. For instance, consider a Resuscitation Team consisting of experienced providers but with one individual newly assigned to the team. While individuals are experienced in their clinical roles (e.g., physician, nurse, respiratory therapist) and each possesses individual skills and knowledge, when one member is new to the group the level of teamwork is impacted. The ability to function optimally as a team is paramount to successfully managing a crisis. For this situation, a simulation may be planned for the Resuscitation Team prior to their first shift together or soon after, within the first week or two. This may be performed in a simulation lab designed to mimic the clinical care area or in situ in an available patient room or other clinical care area. In this case, learning objectives could center on teamwork: (a) learners will establish a team leader and assign individual roles, or communication and (b) learners will demonstrate closed-loop communication. These objectives are not as explicit as those used in the psychomotor skill activities discussed earlier, where a checklist is used to measure adherence. Attainment of these objectives is best explored through a facilitated debriefing by an experienced simulation educator immediately following the just-in-time simulation. Debriefing topics may include positive team concepts observed during the simulation as well as areas in need of improvement. One idea is to send a follow-up survey a few weeks later to the learners who participated in the simulation asking:

1. Have you responded to any code calls since the simulation?
2. If so, do you feel practicing team skills in the just-in-time simulation had any effect on your performance in the actual code? Explain.
3. Would you like another opportunity to participate in a code team simulation?

Evaluating training programs and making the necessary adjustment to meet the needs of the learners to enhance patient safety and skill retention takes time and thoughtful application of the evaluation system and are explored further in chapter 5.5. More experienced educators may need to mentor the novice or advanced beginner educator in this process. This will contribute to producing high-quality programs that play a role in enhancing patient safety and quality.

SUMMARY

Simulation as an educational method has many advantages and some challenges. Just-in-time simulation training is one type of specialized training program that helps to bridge the gap between theory and practice. With just-in-time training, healthcare providers are given the opportunity to apply baseline knowledge (theory) in a simulation of an actual event (practice) at a point in time when the information is most contextual (just-in-time). This is especially useful if the learner is familiar with the concepts and has achieved initial competence in the skill. The most effective just-in-time training provides a realistic setting that mimics the care environment, incorporates feedback on performance, and allows time for processing clinical reasoning. While incorporating just-in-time simulation-based training can be challenging, it is attainable with adequate planning and resources. Designing the training to meet the immediate needs of the individual or organization may help minimize the cost of resources and time. Ultimately, an effective just-in-time training program will demonstrate an increase in provider competence that may contribute to the delivery of safe patient care by increasing procedural success. If just-in-time training helps a practitioner who has the knowledge but is lacking confidence, all the effort of the training is indeed worthwhile.

REFERENCES

AIDT. (2006). *Just in time manufacturing*. Retrieved from http://www.aidt.edu/course_documents/Manufacturing_Skills/Just-In-Time Manufacturing

Benedek, D., & Ritchie, E. (2006). "Just-in-time" mental health training and surveillance for the Project HOPE mission. *Military Medicine, 171* (10), 63–65.

Cook, D., Hatala, R., Brydges, R., Zendejas, B., Szostek, J. H., Wang, A. T., . . . Hamstra, S. J. (2011). Technology-enhanced simulation for health professions education. *Journal of the American Medical Association, 306*(9), 978–988.

Decker, S. D., Sportsman, S., Puetz, L., & Billings, L. (2008). The evolution of simulation and its contribution to competency. *Journal of Continuing Education in Nursing, 39*(2), 74–80.

Galloway, S. (2009). Simulation techniques to bridge the gap between novice and competent healthcare professionals. *Online Journal of Issues in Nursing, 14*(2), Manuscript 3. doi: 10.3912/OJIN.Vol14No02Man03.

Healey, A., Clawson, D., MacNamara, D., Marmie, W., Schneider, V., Rickard, T., . . . Bourne, L., Jr. (1998). The long term retention of knowledge and skills. *Psychology of Learning and Motivation, 30,* 135–164.

Kneebone, R., Scott, W., Darzi, A., & Horracks, M. (2004). Simulation and clinical practice: Strengthening the relationship. *Medical Education, 38*(10), 1095–1102.

Kutzik, J. (2005). Just-in-time technology training for emergent needs. *Library Mosaics, 16,* 8–10.

Lengetti, E., Monachino, A., & Scholtz, A. (2011). A simulation based just in time and just in place central venous catheter education program. *Journal for Nurses in Staff Development, 27*(6), 290–293.

Miller-Hoover, S., & Small, L. (2009). Research evidence review and appraisal: Pediatric central venous catheter care bundling. *Pediatric Nursing, 35*(3), 191–201.

Nagle, B. M., McHale, J. M., Alexander, G. A., & French, B. M. (2009). Incorporating scenario based simulation into a hospital nursing education program. *Journal of Continuing Education in Nursing, 40*(1), 18–24.

Niles, D., Sutton, R., Donoghue, A., Kalsi, M., Roberts, K., Boyle, L., . . . Nadkarni, V. (2009). Rolling refreshers: A novel approach to maintain CPR psychomotor skill competence. *Resuscitation, 80*(8), 909–912.

Nishisaki, A., Donoghue, A., Colborn, S., Watson, C., Meyer, A., Brown, C., III, . . . Nadkarni, V. M. (2010). Effect of just-in-time simulation training on tracheal intubation procedure safety in the pediatric intensive care unit. *Anesthesiology, 113*(1), 214–223.

Nishisaki, A., Keren, R., & Nadkarni, V. (2007). Does simulation improve patient safety? Self-efficacy, competence, operational performance, and patient safety? *Anesthesiology Clinics, 25*(2), 225–236.

Ross, J. G. (2012). Simulation and psychomotor skill acquisition: A review of the literature. *Clinical Simulation in Nursing, 8*(9), e429–e435.

Spencer, J. (2003). ABC of learning and teaching in medicine: Learning and teaching in the clinical environment. *BMJ (Clinical research ed.), 326*(7389), 591–594.

Stoler, G., Johnston, J., Stevenson, J., & Suyama, J. (2013). Preparing emergency personnel in dialysis: A just in time training program for additional staffing during disasters. *Disaster Medicine and Public Health Preparedness, 7*(3), 272-277. doi: 10.1001/dmp.2011.34.

Summers, B., & Woods, W. (2008). *Competency assessment: A practical guide to the joint commission standards.* Marblehead, MA: HCPro.

Weaver, S., Newman-Toker, D., & Rosen, M. (2012). Reducing cognitive sill decay and diagnostic error: Theory-based practices for continuing education in health care. *Journal of Continuing Education in Health Professions, 32*(4), 269–278.

Weinstock, P. H., Kappus, L. S., Garden, A., & Burns, J. P. (2009). Simulation at the point of care training: reduced-cost in-situ training via a mobile cart. *Pediatric Critical Care Medicine, 10*(2), 176–181.

CHAPTER 2.7

Boot Camps

Roberta L. Hales, MHA, RRT-NPS, RN, and Stephanie A. Tuttle, MS, MBA

ABOUT THE AUTHORS

ROBERTA L. HALES is a Lead Simulation Educator for the Center for Simulation, Advanced Education and Innovation, where the focus revolves around patient quality and safety through implementation of innovative, high-quality professional education and research. She is instrumental in orchestrating in situ simulation and numerous external courses. Key external courses include pediatric critical care medicine, neonatology, trauma, and anesthesia boot camps. She serves on the International Pediatric Simulation Society as Co-chair of the Education Committee and frequently lectures on pediatric simulation-based education.

STEPHANIE TUTTLE is the Administrative Director of the Center for Simulation, Advanced Education and Innovation at the Children's Hospital of Philadelphia. She provides administrative and financial oversight for clinical training, research operations, advocacy, and fundraising. As the first staff members, Ms. Tuttle, along with Mrs. Hales, were instrumental in the creation of the Center for Simulation and collaborated on the creation of a Critical Care Boot Camp during their first year.

Acknowledgments: Akira Nishisaki, MD, MSCE, Associate Director, The Children's Hospital of Philadelphia, Center for Simulation, Advanced Education and Innovation; Vinay Nadkarni, MD, MS, Medical Director, The Children's Hospital of Philadelphia, Center for Simulation, Advanced Education and Innovation; Ellen Deutsch, MD, FACS, FAAP, Director, Perioperative Simulation, The Children's Hospital of Philadelphia, Center for Simulation, Advance Education and Innovation; Anne Ades, MD, Associate Director, The Children's Hospital of Philadelphia, Center for Simulation, Advanced Education and Innovation; Julianne S. Perretta, MSEd, RRT-NPS, Lead Simulation Educator, Johns Hopkins Medicine Simulation Center

ABSTRACT

Today's healthcare providers are rushed to get up to speed after brief training or orientation programs with very little hands-on preparation or education. With the heightened awareness of patient safety and training in an academic healthcare environment, and duty hour and other restrictions, education of the healthcare provider has become somewhat of a challenge. The development of a competent provider requires repeated participation in deliberate practice of a variety of knowledge, skills, and behaviors. Therefore, healthcare education programs must be innovative and devise strategies that maximize the learning in fundamental knowledge, skills, and attitudes, including professionalism, communication, and basic procedures, in conjunction with leadership, decision-making, teamwork, situation awareness, and management of stress to promote high-quality and safe patient outcomes. This chapter will describe an innovative educational program "Boot Camp" that utilizes the foundation of simulation-based medical education (SBME) to prepare the novice healthcare provider orienting to a new role.

CASE EXAMPLE

After several years of practicing as a pediatric anesthesiologist, I decided to broaden my knowledge and return to training to become a pediatric intensivist. One of my greatest concerns as a new pediatric critical care fellow was my uncertain knowledge base in critical care. It had been years since I had cared for a critically ill child, and now I was expected to do so with a fair degree of autonomy. My greatest fear was causing great harm to a child.

I arrived at boot camp with these preoccupations in mind, and quickly realized that the entire group had similar concerns. Some had difficulty performing procedures; others did not easily grasp physiologic or pharmacologic principles. Still others were from smaller programs than mine and were apprehensive about meeting other intensivists-in-training. I couldn't help but wonder to myself "Why are we all here?" Over the course of the weekend, the answer became clear. We were brought together to mitigate our fears through the power of experience and knowledge.

We became professionally and socially acquainted with one another and used our varied and collected experiences to benefit the group. We all left boot camp having learned and taught something. More importantly, we discovered that our concerns were shared, and the training we were going to receive over the coming years would be beneficial to our patients.

As I began my clinical service in the Pediatric Intensive Care Unit (PICU), I was astounded by how often both the concepts and the specific skills I had learned in boot camp helped me care for my patients. The team leadership and communication skills I learned, and am still trying to master, allow me to speak the PICU language—both in emergent and in everyday situations for multidisciplinary patient care.

I often remind fellows of the potential harm that exists if unchecked by knowledge, skills, and professional communication with experts and team members. And I often think fondly of those first few days at boot camp.

—Pediatric Critical Care Boot Camp Graduate Justin Lockman, MD

INTRODUCTION AND BACKGROUND

Simulation-based education is rapidly becoming an integral part of healthcare provider training. Specialized simulation training programs refer to training programs that are developed for a specific purpose or area of knowledge. This training can occur in a dedicated simulation center or in situ, which is physically integrated into the clinical environment. Variables that influence the selection of this type of training are the makeup of the intended audience, the need to authenticate the actual clinical environment, the learning objectives, and the time frame in which the learning will occur. **Boot camps** are intensive courses designed to expose learners to a cadre of cognitive, technical, and behavioral skills required to lead and manage both common and infrequent issues and crises.

BOOT CAMP

Academic healthcare institutions are complex training environments where much potential harm can come to patients. For this reason and others (e.g., work hour restrictions leading to shorter training hours, technological and medical advancements, and concerns around patient safety), training and competence-based programs are incorporating new, innovative learning methods such as healthcare simulation to promote the use of evidence-based care to improve patient and educational outcomes (Selden et al., 2010). The traditional medical model of "see one, do one, teach one" is being phased out in this age of heightened customer awareness and a focus on patient safety. Healthcare providers are expected and required to be highly functional from the start of their specialty training program. As an example, Fann et al. (2010) state, "the operating room may no longer be the ideal location for early surgical training because of the ethical concerns, time constraints, and more complex procedure performed on high-risk patients." In fact, healthcare providers' limited experience and exposure to their chosen profession and specialty, combined with their general lack of preparation to perform basic entry-level skills often leads to a wide variance in competence among trainees in fundamental knowledge, skills, and attitudes (KSAs).

In today's clinical environments, healthcare providers must quickly acquire the KSAs necessary to correctly perform in a variety of patient care situations. To meet these ongoing challenges and expectations, healthcare education would benefit from incorporating more opportunities for active learning and **deliberate practice** that promote critical thinking, analysis, and problem-solving skills to a level of mastery. SBME with deliberate practice could fit this bill.

SBME offers a safe and mistake-forgiving environment where trainees can learn from their errors without risk of harming real patients (Ziv et al., 2006). Additionally, learners have the ability to practice multiple times the psychomotor skills and clinical scenarios of their specialty in a simulated environment. For these reasons, simulation-based boot camps were created and designed to help jumpstart trainees' knowledge, psychomotor and behavioral skills, and also develop and expand their communication and teamwork adeptness. These boot camps involve learner-centric concentrated training that solely focuses on the needs of the trainees to prepare them for patient care, along with crisis resource management (CRM).

Based on the military model, boot camp is a short intense training program that focuses on preparing "recruits" with the fundamental KSAs necessary to perform their designated roles and responsibilities (Kubin & Fogg, 2010; *Merriam Webster Learner's Dictionary*, 2013). It is a concentrated, structured program for trainees to practice procedural skills and algorithms for diagnosis and management, along with the integration of behavioral skills (i.e., professionalism, communication, and leadership). The use of boot camps in various settings is well documented, including medical and nursing schools (Laack et al., 2010), surgery (Fann et al., 2010, 2013; Parent et al., 2010; Selden et al., 2010), neonatology, trauma, critical care (Nishisaki et al., 2009), anesthesiology, psychology (Foran-Tuller et al., 2012), and obstetrics (Pliego et al., 2008). Most current boot camps are offered to healthcare providers who care for highly complex patients where the risks are extremely high.

HOW TO IMPLEMENT BOOT CAMP

Boot camps are intense training events that require numerous hours and resources to develop as sound educational programs. Careful consideration must be given to the design and development of the program, starting with identifying the performance needs or gaps of the target audience. The steps in the process of developing a boot camp include the following:

1. Conducting a needs and/or practice analysis
2. Achieving consensus on instructional goals and objectives
3. Selecting the best instructional method to accomplish these goals
4. Creating course content/curriculum
5. Identifying facilitators and developing facilitator training
6. Conducting programmatic evaluation during and after completion of the program

A boot camp workgroup should be created to oversee the overall process, including development of curriculum, assessment tools, and program evaluation.

BOOT CAMP CURRICULUM DEVELOPMENT

Needs Assessment and/or Practice Analysis

The first step in curriculum development is to perform a **needs assessment** and/or **practice analysis.**

- A needs assessment is a systematic exploration to collect and analyze information, including the present state of skills, knowledge, and abilities of the current and future learners. It determines the why (needs vs. wants, feasibility), who (audience analysis), how (performance analysis), what (job/task analysis), and when (contextual analysis) for the program.
- A practice analysis is a systematic collection of data describing the knowledge, skills, and/or competencies required to competently practice a profession. The practice analysis helps to answer the questions "What are the most important aspects of practice?" and "What constitutes safe and effective care?" It also enables the development of assessments and examinations and may assist in the development of content and checklists for the boot camp that reflect the current, real-life practice of the analyzed profession. A practice analysis takes a tremendous amount of work and time. For this reason, it might be more efficient to confer with a professional society to see whether a practice analysis has been recently completed and, if so, whether the results can be shared.

No matter what type of analysis is performed, data collection tools can include observation, interviews, questionnaires/surveys, focus groups, expert opinions, evidence-based practices, and performance standards. Table 2.7.1 includes questions that may be addressed as part of the needs assessment.

In addition, a cost-benefit analysis and a contextual analysis might also be performed. No matter what method is

TABLE 2.7.1
Needs Assessment for Boot Camps

Task/Job Analysis
- What is the best and/or standard way to do this task and/or training?
- How can this topic and/or task be broken down into teachable parts?
- What steps, tasks, actions, and KSAs are required to achieve the desired state of performance?

Learner Analysis
- Who are the learners for this training?
- What entry behaviors are required of learners for this course?
- What is known about them to help design and customize this training?
- What are their current skills and knowledge?
- What other populations might benefit from this training?
- Are there any prerequisites or requirements?

used to identify the training or performance gaps, remember to thoroughly review all information in an objective manner as the analysis sets the stage for the development of overall instructional goals and learning objectives, as well as the selection of the best educational methods.

Content Development

The next step is the design and development of the program. A designated workgroup is composed of subject matter experts from the targeted specialty (e.g., critical care, obstetrics, trauma), along with simulation and technical experts. The workgroup should represent the stakeholders, including individuals who control the needed resources and services and representatives (internal and external) from all institutions involved. The scope of the group's work includes the following:

1. Development of the overarching goal and learning objectives as per the analysis.
   a. Overarching or Instructional goal
      i. What do you want the learners to know by the end of boot camp?
   b. Learning objectives at two levels:
      i. Overall objectives for the course
      ii. Specific objectives for each topic of concentration
         1. Skills station objectives, scenario objectives, didactic objectives
2. Development of the program content as per the analysis.
   a. What are the topics of concentration?
      i. No more than six to eight topic areas
      ii. Dependent on time frame
   b. Remember: Avoid overscheduling the boot camp. Including more topics does not necessarily mean a better program. Everything cannot be covered in one educational event.
3. Matching the content to the best learning method with the aim of meeting the identified learning objectives for each topic of concentration.
   a. Determine the most appropriate methodology (e.g., didactic, role-play, case-based discussion,

immersive simulation, task training, blended or hybrid learning, panel discussion, games).

b. Determine the length of time necessary to complete the identified topics keeping in mind the overall time frame for the course.

c. Develop the framework/lesson plan for didactic, skills stations, and simulation scenarios.

d. Formulate a tentative agenda/schedule for the course (see Figures 2.7.1 and 2.7.2).

e. Determine whether there will be formative and/or summative assessment.

4. Select the appropriate context (based on a contextual analysis) for each topic of concentration as

the context will have profound effects on the substance and quality of learning outcome (McGaghie et al., 2010).

a. Select the venue: simulation laboratory, classroom, in situ (if possible), combination.

b. Determine the optimum size of the group.

   i. Dependent on size of venue and number of faculty.

   ii. Keep faculty-to-trainee ratio small to provide individual attention.

c. Determine whether training will occur during the work week or during the evening or weekend.

Pediatric Critical Care Medicine
Regional Boot Camp Faculty Agenda

Friday July 26, 2013	
7:00 am to 8:00 am	**Registration: Faculty** (Colket Translational Research Building Lobby)
8:00 am to 9:00 am	**Welcome Faculty/Greet and Meet/Logistics of Boot Camp**
9:00 am to 12:00 pm	**Set-up/Dry Runs:** All Faculty (See Faculty Schedule)
12:00 pm to 12:45 pm	**Lunch**
11:30 am to 12:00 pm	**Registration: Fellows** (Colket Translational Research Building Lobby)
12:00 pm to 12:45 pm	**Welcome PCCM Fellows** **Introductions (20 min)** **Overview of Agenda (15 mins)**
12:50 pm to 2:50 pm Total = 115 mins (25 mins per procedural station)	**Airway Management Skills Stations** • 4-BVM (self and flow-inflating)/LMA stations • 4-Intubation stations (DL) • 1-Discussion (Intro to Airway Video/Airway management pearls)
2:50 pm to 3:05 pm	**Break**
3:05 pm to 3:25 pm	**Overview Simulation Based Medical Education (20 mins)**
3:25 pm to 5:25 pm Total 120 mins (25 mins per station, 5 min transition time)	**Airway Management Scenarios** (need to complete 4 stations) • 3-Simbaby Stations (Seizures) • 3-Simbaby Stations (Difficult Airway) • 3-Simman Stations (Anaphylaxis) • 1-Discussion Group (difficult airway)
5:25 pm to 6:00 pm	**Team icebreaker Exercise (30 mins): Simulation Educators**
6:00 pm to 6:15 pm	**Saturday Agenda:**
6:15 pm to 6:30 pm	**Demonstration: Glidescope and Airtraq**
7:30 pm–10:30 pm	**Facilitator Dinner (Dutch Treat)** **Fellows dinner (Restaurant suggestion)**

FIGURE 2.7.1   Pediatric critical care medicine regional boot camp faculty agenda.

(continued)

Pediatric Critical Care Medicine
Regional Boot Camp Faculty Agenda

Saturday July 27, 2013	
6:30 am to 7:00 am	**Welcome, Calisthenics, Continental Breakfast, Review Day's Agenda**
7:00 am to 7:30 am	**Airway Management Panel Discussion**
7:30 am to 8:45 am	**Team demonstration exercise /debriefing**
8:45 am to 9:15 am	**Central Venous Catherization**: Didactic: (All required to have reviewed NEJM videos on central venous catheterization PRIOR to boot camp, discussion, pearls/trouble shooting)
9:15 am to 10:35 pm	**Central Venous Catherization Skills Stations-Session 1** 10 US technique stations 3 Live US model stations 1 station for informed consent
10:35 am to 10:50 am	**Break**
10:50 am to 12:15 pm	**Central Venous Catherization Skills Stations-Session 2** US technique stations, Live US model stations, 1 station for informed consent
12:15 pm to 1:00 pm	**Lunch Delivering Bad News Panel Discussions: 8 groups**
1:00 pm to 1:30 pm	**AHA/PALS Guidelines & QCPR Update**
1:30 pm to 3:00 pm (4 rotations: 35 minutes per station, 5 minute transition)	**PALS Team Training Scenarios** (4-stations-30 mins/station) 2- BLS/QCPR (Adult half-torso) 3-Brady/asystole/PEA 3-SVT 3-VT/VF
3:00 pm to 3:15 pm	**Break**
3:15 pm 5:00 pm (4 rotations: 35 minutes per station, 5 min transition)	**PALS Team Training Scenarios** (4-stations-30 mins/station) 2-BLS/QCPR (Adult half-torso) 3-Brady/asystole/PEA 3-SVT 3-VT/VF
5:00 pm to 5:30 pm	**Debriefing of the Day**
6:30 pm to 10:30 pm	**Social Event: Cookout** (Faculty and Fellows)

Pediatric Critical Care Medicine
Regional Boot Camp Faculty Agenda

Sunday July 28, 2013	
7:00 am to 7:30 am	**Continental Breakfast & Review of Day's Agenda**
7:35 am to 7:50 am	**ACCM Approach to Shock: Review Guidelines** **Neonatal Shock Review** (All faculty required to review these guidelines)
7:55 am to 10:00 am (4 rotations: 25 mins per station with 5 min transition time.)	**Shock Scenarios** (Need to complete 4) 3 Cardiogenic Shock (Myocarditis) 3 Septic Shock (Oncology) 3 Hypovolemic/hemorrhagic Shock (Abdominal Trauma) **1 or 2 Case Discussion Stations**
10:00 am to 10:10 am	**Quick Break**
10:10 am to 10:30 am	**SCCM Trauma and Traumatic Brain Injury Guidelines**
10:30 am to 12:00 pm (No rotation: 40 mins/scenario)	**Trauma Stations** (6 stations): 8 Participants per station/2 Faculty per station) **Early TBI (ED) and Late TBI (ICU management)/Hand off** Station 1: (Early & Late TBI) Station 2: (Early & Late TBI) Station 3: (Early & Late TBI) Station 4: (Early & Late TBI) Station 5: (Early & Late TBI) Station 6: (Early & Late TBI)
12:00 pm to 12:30 pm	**Wrap Up, Evaluations**
12:30 pm	**Lunch and Departures**
1:00 pm to 2:00 pm	**Faculty Debriefing**

FIGURE 2.7.1 *(continued)*

Neonatology Boot Camp Agenda
Philadelphia, PA

Thursday July 18, 2013	
7:30 am to 8:00 am	Welcome/Continental Breakfast/Introductions
8:00 am to 8:30 am	Neonatal Resuscitation Program Basics
8:30 am to 10:15 am (30 min/station)	Skills Stations: 1. Initial Steps/BVM/Compressions 2. Intubation and LMA 3. Umbilical lines
10:15 am to 10:30 am	Break
10:30 am to 11:30 am	Introduction to Simulation and Team Training
11:30 am to 12:30 pm (45 min/scenario)	NRP Scenarios: 1. Depressed meconium- 2 mini-scenarios 2. Basic NRP (MRSOPA, Timing of Intubation and Compressions)
12:30 pm to 2:00 pm	Lunch and Delivering Bad News & Counseling at the Limits of Viability
2:00 pm to 3:10 pm 3:10 pm to 3:20 pm Break 3:20 pm to 4:30 pm	NRP+ Scenarios: 1. ELBW resuscitation 2. TGA delivery 3. Abruption/HIE 4. Case discussion
4:30 pm to 5:15 pm	What I wish had known ++++
5:15 pm to 5:45 pm	Evaluations/Debrief for Day/Tuesday Agenda
6:00 pm to ??	Dinner at Sang Kee Noodle House

FIGURE 2.7.2   Neonatology boot camp agenda.

5. Select the appropriate adjunctive materials to be used.
   a. Utilize facilitators (internal and external) to:
      i. Construct surveys (e.g., Precourse and postcourse self-reported level of confidence).
      ii. Create learning modules and pretest if preferred.
      iii. Choose relevant articles (e.g., central venous catheter placement, CRM principles).
      iv. Determine algorithms (e.g., pediatric sepsis guidelines, difficult airway algorithm).
      v. Build checklists for skills stations (e.g., airway management, central venous insertion, pericentesis, thoracentesis, chest tube insertion) (Figure 2.7.3).
      vi. Decide on the necessary videos (e.g., *New England Journal of Medicine* central venous catheterization, arterial line placement).
      vii. Construct didactic content.
      viii. Build cognitive aids, and guidelines, if wanted (e.g., handoff guidelines).
   b. Once the context and materials are determined, there should be consensus among the facilitators/faculty prior to release to trainees.
6. Design a plan for identification of the trainees who need extra help, remediation, or counseling during the boot camp.
   a. How will this take place?
   b. What time of the day will this occur?
   c. How will it be kept confidential?
   d. Who will be responsible for tracking the trainee's progress or needs?

Friday July 19, 2013	
7:00 am to 7:30 am	Welcome/Continental Breakfast/Review Day's Agenda

7:30 am to 8:45 am	**Skills Stations:**
	    1. **Chest tubes**
	    2. **Centeses**
	    3. **Teamwork and small groups**

8:45 am - 10:00 am	**Skills Stations:**
	    1. **Chest tubes**
	    2. **Centeses**
	    3. **Teamwork and small groups**

10:00 am - 10:15 am	**Break**
10:15 am to 10:45 am	**PALS Algorithms and Defibrillation Demonstration**

10:45 am to 12:00 pm	**PALS Scenarios:**
	    1. **SVT**
	    2. **Unstable Vtach**
	    3. **Bradycardia in an Intubated Neonate**
	    4. **Counseling at the Limits of Viability**

12:00 pm to 12:30 pm	**Lunch**

12:30 pm to 1:45 pm
(30 min/scenario)
	PALS Scenarios:
	    1. **SVT**
	    2. **Unstable Vtach**
	    3. **Bradycardia in an Intubated Neonate**
	    4. **Counseling at the Limits of Viability**

1:45 pm to 2:00 pm	**Break**

2:00 pm to 4:15 pm
(30 min/scenario)
	Advanced Scenarios:
	    1. **Tension pneumothorax**
	    2. **Subglottic stenosis**
	    3. **Sepsis / PPHN**
	    4. **Giving Bad News**

4:15 pm to 4:30 pm	**Wrap Up and Evaluations**

FIGURE 2.7.2 (*continued*)

Resources

As the boot camp program is developed, questions may arise in regard to the number of resources that will be needed to orchestrate the program. Table 2.7.2 includes questions that should be asked regarding resources.

Boot camps are resource-intensive programs, and some institutions may not be able undertake such a course because of cost, space, time, and resources (personnel and equipment), especially with larger numbers of trainees (Laack et al., 2010). On the other hand, high-fidelity simulators are not always necessary. The construction of inexpensive task trainers and utilization of low-fidelity mannequins and realistic environments may create the appropriate physical, conceptual, and emotional realism needed for a positive learning experience. There is no evidence that shows high fidelity is better than low fidelity. In fact, very convincing learning environments have been created with multimodal simulations where, for instance, an inanimate object is attached to a simulated patient. Regardless of the choices made, resources are an enormous part of boot camp implementation, so careful consideration of the actual needs to meet the educational goals will prevent unwarranted expenses (Figure 2.7.4).

Planning and Logistics

The main planning stage is almost complete. The learning objectives and content are developed, the time frame

Central Line Insertion Check List

Critical Steps	Completed?
Before the procedure:	
1. Obtain consent for procedure after discussing risks and benefits (signed and witnessed)	Y/N
2. Obtain supervision (if needed)	Y/N
3. Choose appropriate site and gather equipment, including appropriate line size and length	Y/N
4. Assure adequate sedation and analgesia	Y/N
5. Wear cap, mask, eye protection, wash hands, apply clean gloves	Y/N
6. Properly position the patient	Y/N
7. Enter ultrasound data, select proper probe, visualize vessel (non-sterile)	Y/N
8. Set up equipment and materials	Y/N
9. Wash hands, apply sterile gloves and gown	Y/N
10. Perform and document a time out (correct patient, correct procedure, correct equipment, correct site)	Y/N
11. Prep the procedure site and allow to air dry	Y/N
12. Sterilely drape the patient from head to toe	Y/N
During the procedure:	
13. Prepare the catheter and other equipment	Y/N
14. Prepare the US probe using a sterile cover and jelly	Y/N
15. Identify anatomic landmarks and use ultrasound guidance to perform the puncture	Y/N
16. Identify a needle tip and follow it to target vessel, avoiding adjacent structures	Y/N
17. Advance the guidewire appropriately	Y/N
18. Incise skin using a blade for dilator while keeping the guidewire safe	Y/N
19. Place the dilator to proper depth appropriately	
20. Place the catheter while maintaining contact with the guidewire	Y/N
21. Aspirate blood from each lumen and then flush	
22. Confirm correct placement (Ectopy, Pao_2, CVP tracing)	Y/N
After the procedure:	
23. Clean the site and apply appropriate dressing	Y/N
24. Document correct placement by CXR	Y/N
NOTE: We do not nick the mannequin with a blade nor suture the catheter!	

Fellow: _____   _____

Faculty: _____

FIGURE 2.7.3 Central venous catheterization checklist.

and agenda are complete, the equipment resources are selected, the venue is set, and the materials are finished. Two elements remain to be addressed: qualified facilitators and cost.

Qualified Facilitators

Facilitation has been described as a collaborative learning relationship between the learner and the facilitator within a climate of respect, mutual trust, and acceptance. It is the process of assisting the learners to critically analyze the issues, learn from the experience, and formulate conclusions. A facilitator is a catalyst who uses skillful questioning techniques to help learners draw conclusions from their personal experience and create a change (Dismukes et al., n.d.). Facilitators must encourage the learners to critique their own values and behaviors without making this scrutiny inhibiting and a personal threat to learning

TABLE 2.7.2

Resource Considerations for Boot Camps

- What type of simulators (partial, full-body simulators, animal model) will be needed?
- How many simulators will be needed?
- What consumable supplies will be needed? How will the supplies be paid for?
- How important is the high-fidelity environment?
- Where will the course be conducted? How many rooms will be needed?
- What is the layout of the room(s)? (see Figure 2.7.4)
- How many faculty and operators will be needed to provide the best educational experience?
- Who will be responsible for all the office duties (personnel database, brochure, paperwork, e-mails, ordering, welcoming letter, manuals/folders, faculty assignment grids, surveys, checklists, and other needed materials)?
- How many personnel will be needed to set up and tear down between sessions (peoplepower)?
- How will the equipment be transferred to an off-site venue?
- What kind of technical support is needed?
- Determine how employees are compensated, overtime or providing equivalent time off?

(Brookfield, 1986; Mort & Donahue, 2004). If the scrutiny is too harsh, learning is compromised, and the benefits of the session may be nullified.

Facilitators must establish the tone of the learning climate to provide a safe and conducive learning experience.

Once the ground rules and expectations are established, facilitators may assist with clarification of the learning objectives to achieve a meaningful learning session. During the debriefing session, these learning objectives are accomplished by the facilitator developing empathy or seeing through the eyes of the learner, listening and reflecting back, eliciting information with open-ended questions, and constructive feedback when needed with good judgment. However, one must be cognizant that the delivery of this feedback can be affected by the tone and transparency of the facilitator's voice, body language, and behavior. Behaviors to avoid include mocking or humiliating learners, highlighting too many key points, asking closed questions, and excessive negativism (Mort & Donahue, 2004). The facilitator's behaviors can determine the success or failure of the session because they have a deep impact on the learner's attention span, absorption of course material, enthusiasm for simulation, training in general, and the learner's willingness to participate in future training sessions (Mort & Donahue, 2004). Minimization of these detractors is imperative to maximizing the learning environment.

A key to effective boot camp facilitation is education and consensus among the facilitators regarding the type of debriefing style to be used. The facilitator discussion should occur prior to the boot camp so everyone agrees

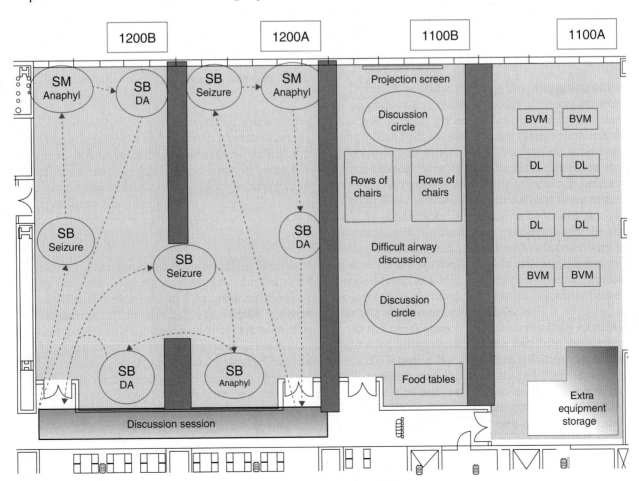

FIGURE 2.7.4 Boot camp layout: Image created by Newton Buchanan, Simulation Technician.

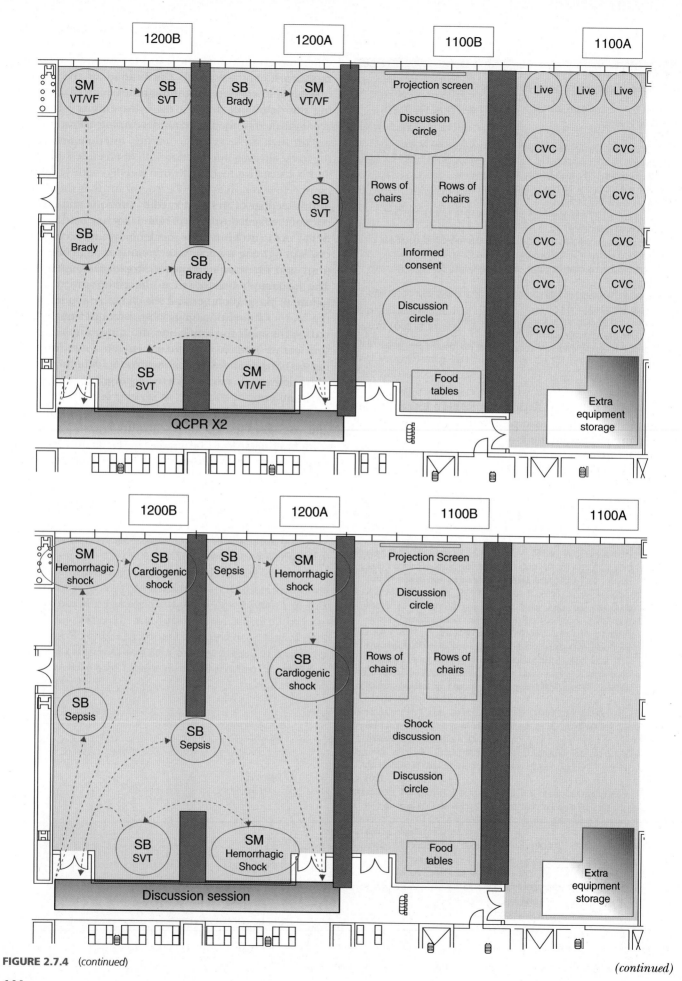

FIGURE 2.7.4 (continued)

(continued)

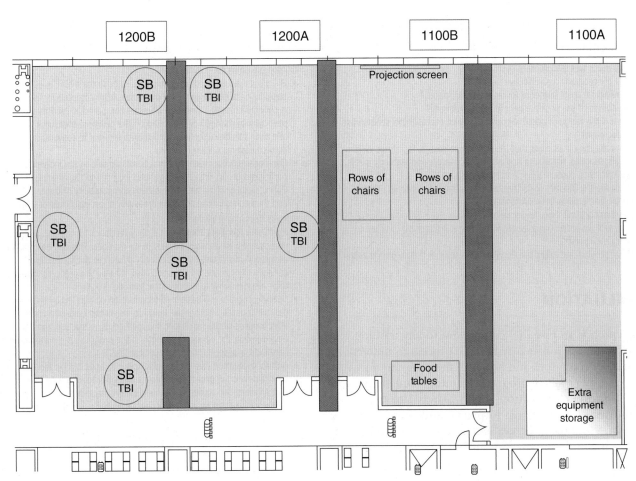

| 1200B | | 1200A | | 1100B | | 1100A |

FIGURE 2.7.4 (*continued*)

to use a similar debriefing model or at least process. Although this may be a difficult deed, it is important to exhibit a unified approach. In the end, one must be able to state that the trainees all met the same cognitive and performance objectives. To unify this approach, one could provide a facilitator guide on the content of the boot camp along with basics tips on debriefing. Table 2.7.3 includes tips on effective facilitation for boot camps.

TABLE 2.7.3

Effective Facilitation for Boot Camps

- Guide the discussion, don't direct it.
- Show respect for the learners.
- Be enthusiastic about the topic and program.
- Plan the format or structure of the debriefing.
- Ask and encourage questions and information sharing.
- Use different questioning techniques, including open-ended, overhead, direct, reflective, reverse/relay, naïve, probing, advocacy, and inquiry.
- Be clear and direct.
- Keep your own contributions/opinions/biases during the discussion brief.
- Use silence to give learners time to think about an answer or response to a question before you give them "the answers."
- Encourage the participation of quiet people.
- Don't allow one person to dominate the discussion.
- Stay neutral.
- Summarize periodically.

Effective facilitation is a complex, multifaceted process that contributes to achievement of relevant learning outcomes of the targeted learner. Facilitation requires the understanding of the adult learning principles because they have different learning approaches, depending on their level of education. It takes time and practice to master the concepts of facilitation. For this reason, it is essential to continuously monitor and provide feedback to boot camp faculty as many of them function as teachers, not facilitators, on an everyday basis. This is the only way to ensure quality and effective simulation-based education in the setting of a boot camp.

Cost

Major deterrents to implementing this type of program are resources and costs. The topic of resources has already been discussed, so this section will focus on the financial aspects of a boot camp. To determine the feasibility of instituting this program, one should perform a cost-benefit analysis. A cost-benefit analysis estimates the cost of training (including financial and human resource costs) weighed against the possible benefits that could be achieved. Questions to consider when completing the cost-benefit analysis are included in Table 2.7.4.

TABLE 2.7.4

Cost-Benefit Analysis for Boot Camps

- How much will the program cost?
- Was the program cost-effective?
- Were actual costs higher or lower than anticipated?
- How much of the possible benefit will be realized?
- What is the range of possible costs, and what makes the costs increase or decrease?
- What are the direct costs that include course design, facilitator, AV materials, supplies, travel and housing for facilitators and learners, meals, refreshments, consumables, and training space?
- What are the indirect costs that include personnel overtime, utilities, rental, and equipment maintenance?
- At what cost will it no longer be worth it?
- How will we know, once we are into it, when to back off or when to "stay the course"?
- What other things could we do with the resources that might be better?

EVALUATION

Evaluation is an essential component to any training program. Evaluation uses a systematic process to understand what a program does and how well the program does it. It is an ongoing cycle of program planning, implementation, and improvement (Patton, 1987). There are two broad categories of evaluations: formative and summative (see chapter 5.5). Formative evaluations are conducted during program development and implementation; summative evaluations are completed at the end of a program. Within these categories are several types of evaluations.

- Summative (outcome) evaluation is a systematic assessment to determine whether the program has achieved the intended goals. It helps to understand the program impact and effectiveness. The collected information determines which activities to continue and build upon and what you need to change to improve program effectiveness in the future. These measures solidify the worth of the program. The data from the summative evaluation helps achieve the buy-in needed to continue the program on the basis of the value and quality of the program. Data that may be useful for outcome evaluation is included in Table 2.7.5.
- Formative (process) evaluation assesses the design and implementation of a program to determine whether it is being executed as planned. This process can be done "on the fly" or more formally at the end of an activity. Facilitators monitor whether goals and learning objectives are being achieved for each activity. If not, what are the deficiencies or barriers impeding the learning process for the participants to master the required KSAs? Additionally, feedback can be solicited from the participants during the program, and facilitators can incorporate changes immediately, if necessary. When assessing a boot camp, some aspects to monitor include the following:

1. Educational methodology
2. Content (too much, too little)

TABLE 2.7.5

Evaluation for Boot Camps

Outcome (summative) evaluation
- Pre–post evaluation: data is collected prior to the event to establish baseline data on the outcome measures. After completion, the same data is collected. The pre- and post data are compared to identify whether participants changed or improved on the outcome measures. Additionally, data can be collected at a 6-month interval to reevaluate the outcome measures and/or retention.
- Comparison group: identify a group comparable to the individuals in the participant group, who have not been exposed to the training program. Collect demographic data to establish comparability of the two groups, and then compare the outcome measures as an individual or whole group.

Process (formative) evaluation
- Plus/Delta feedback tool: an oral daily feedback tool that can identify what went well and what needs to be changed. This can be completed at the end of the day by participants as well as the facilitators. It allows changes to be made on the spot. Also, it helps the group to think about their responsibility to improve the training program.
- Overall program evaluation: this evaluation completed by the participants evaluates whether the learning objectives have been met, the effectiveness of the facilitator, the method of instruction, the learning environment, the venue, the length of the program, the materials and handouts, and food quality (if applicable).
- Annual evaluation (the "look back" prior to boot camp): there should be a review of all program materials and prior feedback to make certain that all identified issues/problems/concerns have been addressed, and all agreed-upon changes have been implemented.

3. Length of activity (too long, too short)
4. Intensity of the activity (too hard, too easy)
5. Size of the group (too large, too small)
6. Quality of the learning activity
7. Characteristic, styles, and expertise of the facilitators

Data that may be useful for process evaluation is included in Table 2.7.5.

VALIDATION OF EVALUATION QUESTIONS

The questions on the evaluation tools define the key issues to be explored. The questions should be developed and prioritized by the program faculty and workgroup. The question development process involves determining the importance and purpose for each question. It is important to limit the questions being asked to those that will provide actionable information. There is a tendency to ask questions that are of limited value. Each question should be designed to obtain unique information. It is important to review each question to ensure that it provides useful information (Table 2.7.6). When you are reviewing potential questions, you may wish to consider the following points:

- Is each question important and/or valuable? Why?
- Is each question specific enough without needing probing for additional information?

TABLE 2.7.6

Evaluation Design Process

1. Identify and engage stakeholders.
   a. Guiding questions: Who can we identify as stakeholders? How do we engage stakeholders?
   b. Outcome of this step: List of stakeholders.
2. Identify program elements to monitor.
   a. Guiding questions: Which program elements will you monitor? What is the justification for monitoring these elements?
   b. Outcome of this step: List of program elements to monitor.
3. Select the key evaluation questions.
   a. Guiding questions: What evaluation questions will you address?
   b. Outcome of this step: List of evaluation questions.
4. Determine how the information will be gathered.
   a. Guiding questions: What information sources and data collection methods will you use for monitoring and evaluation? What evaluation research design will be used?
   b. Outcome of this step: Description of information sources, data collection methods, and research design.
5. Develop a data analysis and reporting plan.
   a. Guiding questions: How will the data for each monitoring and evaluation question be coded, summarized, and analyzed? How will conclusions be justified? How will stakeholders both inside and outside the organization be kept informed about the monitoring and evaluation activities? When will the monitoring and evaluation activities be implemented, and how will they be timed in relation to program implementation? How will the costs of monitoring and evaluation be presented? How will the monitoring and evaluation data be reported? What are your monitoring and evaluation timelines and budgets?
   b. Outcome of this step: A data analysis and reporting plan.
6. Ensure use and share lessons learned.
   a. Guiding questions: What feedback was received concerning the program? What is the evaluation implementation summary? How can we use this information to revise the program? How will this information impact internal and external communication plans? What are the lessons learned?
   b. Outcome of this step: Final summary report that is circulated among evaluation workgroup and stakeholders.

Marketing and Communication Strategy Branch in the Division of Health Communication and Marketing, C. f. (n.d.). *Gateway to health communication and social marketing practice.* Retrieved from Center for Disease Control and Prevention: http://www.cdc.gov/healthcommunication/Research/EvaluationPlanning.pdf

- Is the wording of the question sufficiently clear and explicit?
- Is the question worth asking? Does it provide useful information?

In summary, formative and summative evaluations of the boot camp provide essential information to refine the course and help prove the value and worth of the boot camp program.

ASSESSMENT

Today the sources of assessments come primarily from observational ratings. These can be subjective unless conducted under controlled conditions. Self-evaluation has been shown to be somewhat reliable but still subjective (McGaghie et al., 2010). Recent studies (Barsuk et al., 2009; Draycott et al., 2008; Seymour, 2008) demonstrate

the transfer of procedural skills to practice at the highest level (Kirkpatrick's level 4-transference). These higher levels of measurements of learning are needed to advance the effectiveness of medical education and SBME. The following assessment instruments are currently used in boot camps: self-assessment surveys, skills checklists, observation, and pre- and post-testing. Further work is needed to determine the best assessment modality for boot camps.

BOOT CAMP EXAMPLES

The three boot camps described below evolved from identified needs within the designated professional specialty. The aim of these boot camps is to expose healthcare providers to the most common psychomotor skills and crisis situations that they will encounter in their specialty. Each boot camp involves many different types of educational methodologies, including didactic, case and panel discussions, role-play, skill training, and full-scale immersive simulations.

Pediatric Critical Care Medicine Boot Camp

Owing to the acuity and complexity of their patient population, pediatric critical care medicine (PCCM) fellows are expected to have a high level of clinical competence early in their fellowship. For instance, invasive procedures are high risk, so clinical competence is necessary to prevent any unnecessary harm to the patient. In the past, demonstration of competence was performed on actual patients under the clinical supervision of the attending intensivists. However, patient safety concerns and work hour restrictions clearly limit the opportunities to perform these procedures on actual patients (Nishisaki et al., 2009). Additionally, the PCCM fellows have a higher level of responsibility and accountability for the overall management of the patients. For these reasons, a multi-institutional, PCCM first-year fellow orientation boot camp was designed. The boot camp utilizes numerous educational methods over a 2.5-day time span. The PCCM fellowship leaders from multiple institutions joined together to create the curriculum and schedule for these first-year fellows. Each participating institution provides at least one PCCM attending to participate as faculty for the boot camp. The topics of concentration in the boot camp include airway management (Figures 2.7.5 and 2.7.6), vascular access (Figures 2.7.7 to 2.7.10), resuscitation, sepsis, trauma, traumatic brain injury, and delivering bad news. A precourse and postcourse evaluation was created to evaluate the perceived effectiveness of the simulation training before, immediately after, and 6 months after the end of the boot camp. Nishisaki et al. reported that the overall training was highly rated (scores on a 5-point Likert scale >4) immediately post–boot camp.

As an example of responding to evaluative feedback from participants, the trainees (fellows) felt learning would be improved with a "train to success" strategy (e.g., repetitive training on each task or scenario) (Nishisaki et

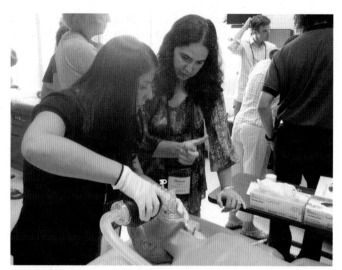

FIGURE 2.7.5   Bag mask ventilation skills training.

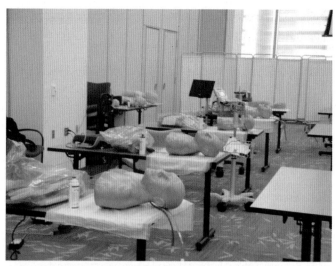

FIGURE 2.7.7   Central venous catheterization room setup.

al., 2009). After discussion, the faculty incorporated the strategy into the boot camp on day 2, and the perceived effectiveness of the training improved. This strategy is still used today in the PCCM boot camp, along with a blind-folding exercise in the team training resuscitation exercise to improve leadership, followership, and communication (Figure 2.7.11). The 6-month follow-up survey revealed that the trainees would recommend this training to others

and felt it highly improved their clinical performance and self-confidence. Today, this boot camp still performs pre- and postcourse surveys to evaluate the effectiveness and impact of the PCCM fellows training. Additionally, the curriculum is evaluated on an annual basis to integrate new practice changes or additions into the PCCM boot camp.

Neonatology Boot Camp

Neonatologists are highly trained specialists who provide comprehensive medical care to premature and high-risk infants. Neonatologists are expected to be experts in providing the state-of-the-art technologies, including mechanical ventilation, extracorporeal membrane oxygenation (ECMO), surfactant therapy, and other diagnostic and therapeutic interventions to deliver optimal care with the best possible outcomes for this tiny and fragile patient population. Just like the PCCM fellows, from the beginning of their fellowship, neonatal fellows have a high level of responsibility and accountability for the care of

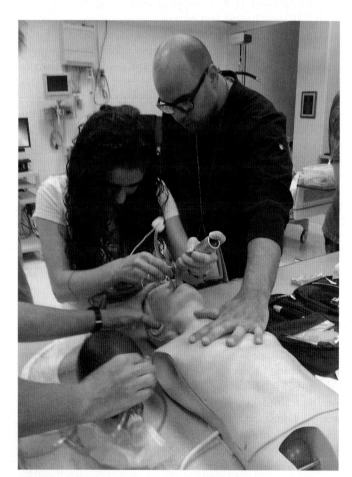

FIGURE 2.7.6   Endotracheal intubation skills training.

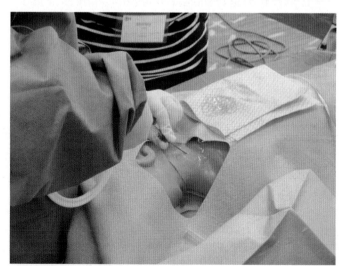

FIGURE 2.7.8   Central venous catheterization skills training.

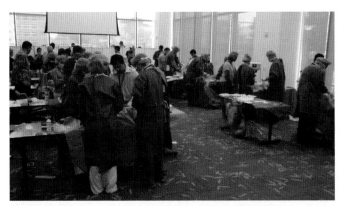

FIGURE 2.7.9 Central venous catheterization skills training.

these neonates. However, they too often arrive from their residency programs with limited experience. Therefore, a neonatology boot camp emerged from a 1-day neonatology skills training program into a full-scale 2-day boot camp, utilizing many educational methodologies. In collaboration with other neonatal fellowship programs, the curriculum was designed by assessing the perceived needs and practice of the incoming fellows. The areas of concentration

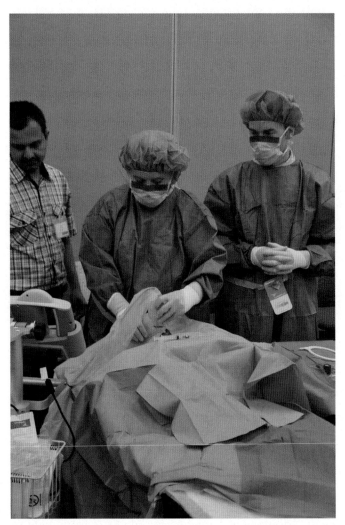

FIGURE 2.7.10 Central venous catheterization ultrasound skills training.

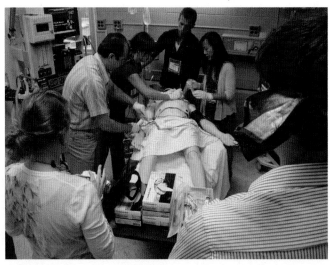

FIGURE 2.7.11 Pediatric critical care simulation team training: Blindfold simulation.

include airway management, neonatal resuscitation basics (NRP), including skill stations of the initial steps, bag mask ventilation, compressions, and intubation. Advanced skills included umbilical line placement, chest tubes, centesis, laryngeal mask airway (LMA), tracheostomy emergencies, and intraosseous placement (Figures 2.7.12 and 2.7.13). The full immersive simulations focus on basic NRP scenarios of meconium aspiration and placental abruption. Day 2 encompasses advanced scenarios (e.g., congenital diaphragmatic hernia, hydrops, Pierre Robin, and pulmonary hypertension crisis) and pediatric advanced life support scenarios on management of the most common cardiac arrhythmias of a neonate/newborn (Figure 2.7.14). Each institution sends at least one attending neonatologist to serve as faculty for the boot camp. The fellows complete a precourse, postcourse and 6-month survey of self-reported confidence on the topics in the course. Just like PCCM, there is an annual evaluation to decide whether the curriculum needs to be changed, with the purpose of keeping the boot camp aligned with current neonatal practice.

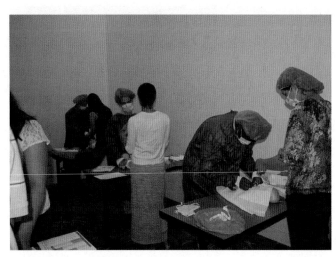

FIGURE 2.7.12 Umbilical line skills training.

SECTION 2 • Types of Simulation Programs

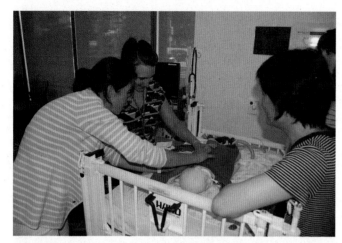

FIGURE 2.7.13 Chest tube insertion skills training.

Trauma Boot Camp

Trauma teams are a group of professionals who gather together to receive and manage trauma victims. Minimally, the core trauma team consists of 8 to 10 people: emergency department physician, trauma surgeon, general surgeon, three nurses (two at the bedside, one recording the event), a respiratory therapist, an anesthetist, and a radiographer. Additional personnel may include a neurosurgeon, orthopedic surgeon, and radiologist. Support staff includes the clerks and blood bank and laboratory personnel. It is vital that everyone knows their roles, tasks, and responsibilities, and has the psychomotor skills, equipment, and support to accomplish these. The intricacies of a trauma team and management of the complex patient necessitate frequent practice as an interprofessional team with emphasis on leadership and communication. For these reasons, a half-day trauma boot camp was developed to educate the interprofessional trauma team. Developed in collaboration with all disciplines, the boot camp agenda includes didactic lectures, hands-on skills training, and immersive simulations. Specific topics include lectures on trauma activation, team

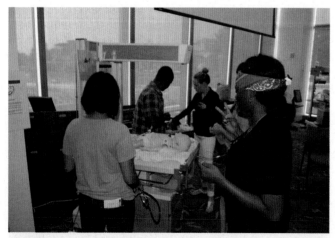

FIGURE 2.7.14 Neonatology boot camp team training: Blindfold simulation.

member roles and responsibilities, communication, blood bank protocol, and crew resource management principles; skills stations include intraosseous, hare traction splint, intubation, chest tubes, rapid infuser, and cervical collar placement; plus two immersive simulation scenarios. Each year, the trauma boot camp is evaluated by the participants for its effectiveness. The content is continuously updated by the interdisciplinary workgroup to meet the ever-changing needs of the trauma team.

CHALLENGES

A major challenge of any boot camp is the ability to measure the impact of the program on the trainees' skills transfer and resultant patient care outcomes. Assessments at these levels require more structured objective competence and performance measurement standards (Nishisaki et al., 2009). However, time is short in boot camp. It is hard to accomplish deliberate practice and **mastery learning** in time-limited sessions. In addition, while some trainees come to boot camp with a considerable amount of knowledge, simulation exposure, and skills, others do not. When it comes to education, one size does not fit all. One must adjust the content and titrate the process to accommodate both the levels of the learner. Moreover, just because the trainees are exposed to many different topics, it does not mean that all the trainees have learned all the topics equally well. As stated by an experienced simulation educator, "one must accept what boot camp is, and what boot camp is not. Boot camp can't do it all."

The second challenge of boot camp is faculty development. Faculty who do not have robust simulation curriculum embedded into their training programs often struggle with aspects of SBME. Their tendency is to teach rather than facilitate in the simulation exercises. Although there are many expert teachers, facilitating requires a different skill set. Particularly challenging is when different faculty members are teaching identical stations but using their own agenda and objectives. This can cause inconsistency in learning among the trainees. Some faculty attempt to cram as much content as possible into each learning session, while forgetting the primary goal and learning objectives for each teaching station. For this reason, it is important to have a structured guide (manual) for the faculty to use that outlines the primary learning objectives and performance standards for each of the didactic and simulation stations (skills and scenarios). The manual, in conjunction with a precourse-structured practice session, helps ensure all faculty in the boot camp teach the same content on the same level.

Boot camps are time-intensive programs that require countless hours to organize, plan, and implement. The size of the task necessitates coordination of equipment, people, and resources. Dependent on the size and location of the boot camp, it may require quite a number of people dedicated to the transfer, setup, and breakdown of equipment. Additionally, arranging for adequate equipment to meet the needs of the boot camp curriculum may take a number of phone calls to neighboring simulation centers and vendors. Similarly, it can be difficult to meet the timeline for curriculum design or redesign when trying to schedule meetings with faculty whose primary responsibility is patient care. Being aware of the necessary time commitment up front will help to ensure that the project is adequately staffed so the planning efforts are successful.

LIMITATIONS

Limitations associated with boot camps include space, equipment, faculty, time, and money. The larger the boot camp, the more resources are needed. As program directors in different specialties realize the value and benefits of the boot camp experience, more boot camps will be requested, increasing the demand on resources. This may cause increased competition for faculty, space, and equipment in the academic and healthcare community. Responding to the increased demand may result in changes in your faculty-to-trainee ratio and diminish the individuality of the boot camp program.

Limitations of time and space will have an impact on the boot camp's curriculum. If a new topic needs to be added to the curriculum, then something else might need to be removed; otherwise there is the risk of overloading the curriculum and losing the overall quality of the learning opportunities.

BEEN THERE, DONE THAT: HOW TO SUSTAIN THE PROGRAM?

A well-developed simulation boot camp provides learners with multiple opportunities to practice technical and nontechnical skills in a safe learning environment. To improve or sustain these learning outcomes, one must constantly evaluate whether the learners' benefit outweighs the expenditure of resources of personnel, equipment, time, effort, and cost to operate this intense program. For these reasons, continuous evaluation is a key factor in sustaining and improving the program. Learners should complete a precourse, postcourse, and 6-month self-evaluation to determine confidence levels in the chosen topics. Faculty should also evaluate the learners because each individual's perception of their own performance is highly subjective and can be different than reality and what objective measurements would indicate (Pliego et al., 2008). Faculty can determine whether lessons were learned by evaluating skill acquisition during performance and through extensive debriefing after each scenario to diminish misplaced confidence and correct poor technique (Pliego et al., 2008). Furthermore, program evaluation of the content and structure must occur prior to (with faculty), during, and after (faculty and learners) boot camp with the purpose of assessing what went well and what needs to be improved

or changed. This objective and subjective feedback can be obtained in many different ways: surveys, written, and oral (**Plus/Delta** method) from both learners and faculty. Also, every year the boot camp curriculum should be reevaluated to make sure it meets the ever-changing requirements of professional accrediting and regulatory bodies.

One should keep abreast of current boot camp literature and changes in educational methods to follow the evidence on what works and does not work in boot camp programs. To make learning most effective, remember to employ adult learning principles involving active learning strategies. Set realistic goals that can actually be accomplished; be careful to avoid being overly ambitious. Doing so may clutter the curriculum and decrease the efficiency and effectiveness of the program.

The second key factor to sustaining a program is faculty development. All faculty come with different levels of experience in SBME. In the beginning years of boot camps, the majority of faculty had no formal training in how to be a qualified facilitator or simulator operator. They utilized the traditional medical model to educate the trainees. Although they were all good teachers, they spent a considerable amount of time discussing and teaching the content instead of allowing the learners to learn through experience. After much discussion and feedback from the learners and experienced faculty, boot camp has become more experiential. Today, most faculty have at least some experience in SBME. Ongoing efforts to improve faculty involvement and facilitation skills, specifically with regard to boot camps, are ongoing. These include a conference call 1 to 2 months prior to the boot camp, a briefing and training/practice session (in the morning or the evening before boot camp), touchdown meetings during the boot camp, and an immediate post–boot camp debriefing to discuss any issues or concerns. These modifications mitigate many uncertainties and questions surrounding the process and structure of the boot camp program.

A third key factor related to maintaining and improving boot camps involves the participation from the institutions. Each institution should assist with the content development and provide faculty to support the program. This level of faculty involvement creates a sense of ownership, resulting in a richer trainee experience. There is usually more than one way of accomplishing a skill or handling a situation; therefore, receiving feedback and discussing different points of view will expand the trainee's knowledge base and allow them to see things from a broader perspective. On the other hand, faculty needs to avoid institution-specific protocols and concentrate on the key principles of the psychomotor skill or situation/scenario (e.g., intubation medications) to prevent institutional biases.

Networking is a significant benefit of the boot camp experience. This became apparent during the very first boot camp programs when faculty and learners joined together, creating a group-wide synergy. The simulation faculty camaraderie and sense of teamwork is strongly developed during the content development, meetings, and cofacilitating and debriefing. These strong relationships influence the substance behind the success of the boot camp program. The greatest benefit to the learners is the ability to gain knowledge from the participating faculty and other trainees, and to network with their future colleagues.

SUMMARY

The purpose of medical education is to prepare healthcare providers with the KSAs along with the professionalism needed to deliver quality patient care (McGaghie et al., 2011). Today, healthcare education is challenged to meet the needs of the trainees in this rapidly growing healthcare environment. Boot camp experiences offer an avenue to enhance the trainees' education in a structured, safe learning environment; honing in on the technical and nontechnical skills of each trainee, along with learning from the experiences of others, becomes the foundation of a boot camp program.

REFERENCES

Barsuk, J. H., McGaghie, W. C., Cohen, E. R., O'Leary, K. J., & Wayne, D. B. (2009). Simulation-based mastery learning reduces complications during central venous catheter insertion in a medical intensive care unit. *Critical Care Medicine*, 37, 2697–2701.

Brookfield, S. (1986). Adult learners: Motives for learning and implications for practice. In S. Brookfield (Ed.), *Understanding and facilitating adult learning* (pp. 1–24). San Francisco, CA: Jossey-Bass.

Dismukes, R. K., McDonnell, L. K., Jobe, K. K., & Smith, G. M. (n.d.). What is facilitation and why use it? In R. K. Dismukes & G. M. (Eds.), *Facilitation and debriefing in aviation training and operations (pp. 1–12)*. Aldershot, UK: Retrieved from Human Factors: human-factors.arc.nasa.gov/flightcognition/Publications/ChapterOne.pdf

Draycott, T. J., Crofts, J. F., Ash, J. P., Wilson, L. V., Yard, E., Sibanda, T., & Whitelaw, A. (2008). Improving neonatal outcome through practical shoulder dystocia training. *Obstetrics & Gynecology*, 12, 14–20.

Fann, J. I., Calhoon, J. H., Carpenter, A. J., Merrill, W. H., Brown, J. W., Poston, R. S., ... Feins, R. H. (2010). Simulation in coronary artery anastomosis early in cardiothoracic surgical residency training: The Boot camp experience. *The Journal of Thoracic and Cardiovascular Surgery*, 139, 1275–1281.

Fann, J. I., Sullivan, M. E., Skeff, K. M., Stratos, G. A., Walker, J. D., Grossi, E. A., . . . Feins, R. H. (2013). Teaching behaviors in the cardiac surgery simulation environment. *The Journal of Thoracic and Cardiovascular Surgery*, 145, 45–53.

Foran-Tuller, K., Robiner, W. N. Breland-Noble, A., Otey-Scott, S., Wryobeck, J., King, C., & Sanders, K. (2012). Early career boot camp: A novel mechanism for enhancing early career development for psychologists in academic healthcare. *Journal of Clinical Psychology in Medical Settings*, 19, 117–125.

Kubin, L., & Fogg, N. (2010). Back-to-basics boot camp: An innovative approach to competency assessment. *Journal of Pediatric Nursing*, 25, 28–32.

Laack, T. A., Newman, J. S. Goyal, D. G., & Torsher, L. C. (2010). A 1-week simulated internship course helps prepare medical students for transition to residency. *Simulation in Healthcare*, 5, 127–132.

McGaghie, W. C., Issenberg, S. B. Cohen, E. R. Barsuk, J. H., & Wayne, D. B. (2011). Does simulation-based medical education with deliberate practice yield better results than traditional clinical education? A meta-analytic comparative review of the evidence. *Academic Medicine*, 86, 706–711.

McGaghie, W. C., Issenberg, S. B., Petrusa, E. R., & Scalese, R. (2010). A critical review of simulation-based medical education research: 2003–2009. *Medical Education*, 44, 50–63.

Merriam Webster Learner's Dictionary. (2013, January 15). Retrieved from Merriam Webster Learner's Dictionary: http://www.learnersdictionary.com/search/boot%20camp

Mort, T. C., & Donahue, S. P. (2004). Debriefing: The basics. In W. F. Dunn (Ed.), *Simulators in critical care and beyond (pp. 76–83)*. Des Plaines, IL: Society of Critical Care Medicine.

Nishisaki, A., Hales, R., Biagas, K., Cheifetz, I., Corriveau, C., Garber, N., . . . Nadkarni, V. (2009). A multi-institutional high-fidelity simulation "boot camp" orientation and training program for first year pediatric critical care fellows. *Pediatric Critical Care Medicine*, 10, 157–162.

Parent, R. J., Plerhoples, T. A. Long, E. E., Zimmer, D. M., Teshome, M., Mohr, C. J., ... Dutta, S. (2010). Early, intermediate, and late effects of a surgical skills boot camp on an objective structured assessment of technical skills: A randomized controlled study. *Journal of the American College of Surgeons*, 210, 984–989.

Patton, M. (1987). *Qualitative research & evaluation methods*. Thousand Oaks, CA: SAGE.

Pliego, J. F., Wehbe-Janek, H., Rajab, M. H., Browning, J. L., & Fothergill, R. E. (2008). Ob/Gyn boot camp using high-fidelity human simulators: enhancing resident's perceived competency, confidence in taking a leadership role, and stress hardiness. *Simulation in Healthcare*, 3, 82–89.

Selden, N. R., Origitano, T. C. Burchiel, K. J., Getch, C. C., Anderson, V. C., McCartney, S., ... Barbaro, N. M. (2010). A national fundamentals curriculum for neurosurgery PGY1 residents: The 2010 Society of Neurological Surgeons boot camp courses. *Neurosurgery*, 70, 971–981.

Seymour, N. E. (2008). VR to OR: a review of the evidence that virtual reality simulation improves operating room performance. *World Journal of Surgery*, 32, 182–188.

Stanley, M. J., & Dougherty, J. P. (2010). A paradigm shift in nursing education: A new model. *Nursing Education Perspectives*, 31, 378–380.

Ziv, A., Erez, D., Munz, Y., Vardi, A., Barsuk, D., Levine, I., . . . Berkenstadt, H. (2006). The Israel center for medical simulation: A paradigm for cultural change in medical education. *Academic Medicine*, 81, 1091–1097.

Systems Integration

Yue Dong, MD, Juli C. Maxworthy, DNP, MSN, MBA, RN, CNL, CPHQ, CPPS, CHSE and William F. Dunn, MD

ABOUT THE AUTHORS

YUE DONG is an Assistant Professor of Medicine at the Mayo Clinic College of Medicine and a patient safety researcher and educator at the Mayo Clinic Multidisciplinary Simulation Center and the Multidisciplinary Epidemiology and Translational Research in Intensive Care group. His primary research interests include simulation-based quality improvement using systems engineering approaches to improve system performance in the ICU; using simulation as a tool to conduct usability testing; and studying the effectiveness of simulation-based medical education. He is currently the Chair of Systems Integration, Accreditation Council of SSH.

JULI C. MAXWORTHY is the former Director of the Simulation Center at Holy Names University and currently serves as the Chair of the Simulation Committee of the University of San Francisco. Juli is a registered nurse with a strong critical care clinical background and has advanced degrees in nursing administration, business, quality, and patient safety. She is currently the Vice Chair for the Accreditation Council of SSH and has been a surveyor of simulation programs since 2010. Her last clinical role was that of Vice President of Quality/Patient Safety and Risk.

WILLIAM F. DUNN is a Pulmonologist/Intensivist at Mayo Clinic (Rochester, Minnesota) and Past President of the Society for Simulation in Healthcare. He is recipient of multiple awards for clinical and educational excellence. His foundational work and leadership served to enable the Mayo Clinic to develop simulation-based learning at all Mayo sites. He continues to serve the SSH Accreditation Council, Accreditation Board of Review, Public Affairs & Government Relations Committee, and the Systems Integration Accreditation Subcommittee.

ABSTRACT

Patient safety is a sociotechnical system property, including people, technology, process, organization, and external environment. Systems integration is crucial for any healthcare organization that strives to build highly reliable delivery systems (or subsystems) that deliver safe, effective, timely, patient-centered, efficient, and equitable care—the six quality aims envisioned in The Institute of Medicine's "Crossing the Quality Chasm" report. Simulation-based education must be coupled with well-designed care process, change management strategies, and bidirectional organizational learning for successful healthcare transformation. With emphasis on improving patient and/or system outcomes by targeting multiple organizational components, this chapter strives to provide a practical framework of thinking pertaining to simulation-based systems integration initiatives that can and should occur today in high-reliability healthcare organizations.

CASE EXAMPLE

In the current era, there is an ever-increasing emphasis on improving quality and patient safety, via standardization of healthcare processes, as it has effected, in parallel fashion, improved outcomes (i.e., industrial outputs) across a wide spectrum of industry applications. Simulation applications to the *individual*, as clearly outlined elsewhere in this text, can have a great impact (because of the power of experiential learning principles, well applied) on education and standardization of performance. When applied to a healthcare *system*, the effect can be dramatically magnified. Within a given industry, product lines are commonplace. Healthcare is no different, in that many patient product lines exist, with significant opportunity (despite the intrinsic complexity) of standardization of system performance (e.g., care of sepsis, total knee replacement, myocardial infarction diagnosis and therapeutic interventions, etc.). For instance, a critical care fellowship utilizing standardized simulator-based training scenarios could guarantee that every learner treats sepsis in a standardized way with principles derived from the "Surviving Sepsis Campaign" of the Society of Critical Care Medicine, including defining performance proficiency standards in required procedures (e.g., central venous catheterization), taught within a simulation environment. By such complicated but expertly utilized iterative simulation techniques, opportunities in system improvement can, after initial identification, be attained. Thus, training programs and healthcare delivery systems may better, through the (now additional) tool of simulation as a system-level tool within the healthcare delivery organization, truly strive toward Lean Six Sigma efficiencies and excellence.

As an evolving system, a healthcare organization is constantly trying to improve its processes to adapt to the changing environment. At a medium-sized healthcare facility, senior leadership, on the basis of data it has received from a consulting company, has identified that patients are unnecessarily delayed in the emergency department, impeding optimal care. To effect the change in processes, the executive team seeks out the expertise of several departments, including simulation center, quality, risk, information technology, and emergency department leadership. The Chief Executive Officer makes a clear request: work collaboratively to determine opportunities for improvement in processes to decrease the door-to-bed time lag by 25% within the next 6 months. The team that has been assembled has their work cut out for them to meet this metric, but they know that by working together in an environment of bidirectional respect, reengineering the processes of care, they can get the job done. Five features of delays were hypothesized, measured through real-time data, and analyzed—through simulations utilizing **embedded simulated persons** with electronic identifiers, thus allowing for assessments of system response times. What was the likely outcome?

INTRODUCTION AND BACKGROUND

Simulation utilizes various engineering techniques to replace or amplify real experiences via experiential learning techniques, replicating reality toward a defined purpose. "Healthcare simulation is a range of activities that share a broad, similar purpose—to improve the safety, effectiveness, and efficiency of healthcare services" (Society for Simulation in Healthcare,). Education, assessment, research, and systems integration are major categories of applications of simulation promoted by the Society for Simulation in Healthcare (SSH), the world's largest multidisciplinary, multispecialty, international society for the healthcare simulation community.

Simulation in healthcare has been primarily used as a training and assessment tool to improve individual and team skills. This is often done utilizing various modalities (e.g., mannequins, task trainers, standardized patients, computer games, etc.) within scenarios that seek to achieve a degree of realism (see chapter 8.8, Textbox: Helping learners buy-in to simulation), thus facilitating experiential learning (Cook et al., 2011; Issenberg et al., 2005; McGaghie et al., 2011). Consistent with such uses, there are growing bodies of evidence showing learner and team improvements after training (e.g., procedure, communication, decision-making, teamwork, etc.). In contrast, patient outcome improvements and organizational changes at the *health systems* level (unit, hospital, and society) facilitated via simulation-based techniques still need further investigation and application to truly attain the incremental value potential (i.e., optimum systems impact; Schmidt et al., 2013).

Healthcare professionals are increasingly using simulation as a platform to better understand the complexity of clinical processes—for example, testing a new patient workflow process prior to clinical deployment. Such activities are primarily focused on identifying potential latent risks (due to imperfect system issues) that introduce potential for harm, and the designing of solutions to enhance system capability and improve patient outcomes. As defined by SSH, systems integration is "the integration of simulation into institutional healthcare training and delivery systems. Simulation-based processes may include quality assessment mechanisms, thereby facilitating patient safety. Simulation-based approaches can be effectively used to help evaluate organizational processes as well as individual and team performance". This chapter introduces the concept of proactively engineering various simulation applications into a system of healthcare delivery, to better serve its mission. Various simulation modalities are presented, as well as their applications to the improved integration within healthcare systems toward facilitating clearly defined and recognizable improvements in patient safety.

ENGINEERING THE HEALTHCARE DELIVERY SYSTEM

Medical Error and High Cost in the Current Healthcare Delivery System

In the 1999 landmark IOM report "To Err Is Human," it was reported that up to 98,000 preventable deaths occurred annually in the United States (Kohn et al., 1999). More recent data estimated more than 400,000 deaths associated with preventable harm to patients each year in America (James, 2013). Key quality features called for within IOM specifications are that healthcare in the United States is safe, effective, patient-centered, timely, efficient, and equitable (Committee on Quality of Health Care in America Institute of Medicine, 2001). Patient mortality due to preventable medical errors remains high. Subsequent IOM series reports have continued to point out the challenges healthcare industries (particularly in the United States) are facing in the 21st century (*Health IT and Patient Safety: Building Safer Systems for Better Care*, 2011; Olsen et al., 2007). Even after numerous efforts in quality improvement during the last 10 years, persistence of healthcare underperformance is readily demonstrable; common medical errors create 25 cases of harm per 100 hospital admissions when using Institute for Healthcare Improvement's (IHI) Global Trigger Tool for Measuring Adverse Events (Classen et al., 2011; Landrigan et al., 2010). Despite laudable transformative goals well described by Institute of Medicine (IOM) publications, costs of healthcare delivery in the United States continue to climb to record levels. Healthcare expenditures in the United States reached almost 18% of the gross domestic product (GDP) in 2011 (Keehan et al., 2011). Experts currently consider approximately one-third of total US healthcare costs to be wasted, with no added value associated (Agency for Healthcare Research and Quality, 2008). Meanwhile, large gaps remain between realities of inefficient care versus optimized potential care (Smith et al., 2012).

Complexity of the Healthcare Delivery System

Modern healthcare is conducted in a very complex environment with systems. Multiple subsystems (at the patient, provider, and process levels) are interconnected and consistently interact with other components (Shortell & Singer, 2008). The advances represented by breakthroughs, scientific discovery from clinical evidence, coupled with new diagnostics, state-of-the-art real-time patient monitors, and innovative disease management interventions, are changing the way healthcare providers are interacting with patients and each other. Information technology and devices, while offering certain efficiencies, may also paradoxically complicate the process of how to deliver care in an efficient and effective manner. Healthcare delivery complexity has also been greatly increased because of fragmented service models, specialization, and regulatory and reimbursement requirements at many levels (Plsek & Greenhalgh, 2001). Current increased penetration of mobile connectivity and social networking capability empower patients' participation. Despite offering hope for improvements in delivered care, they also increase system complexity. Family members' decision-making and personal preferences need to be considered by providers. Future healthcare delivery systems, no doubt, will be even more complex with higher prevalence

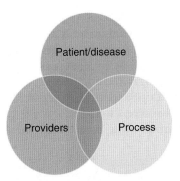

FIGURE 2.8.1 Complexity of healthcare delivery system.

of degenerative (i.e., complication-prone) diseases, aging populations, and workforce shortages. Simultaneously, large group provider practice trends will transform both patient-provider as well as provider-provider interactions. With the increasing levels of complexity, the healthcare delivery system has the potential of having increased risks of error with associated negative impacts on patient outcomes. Sir Cyril Chantler (1999) stated, "Medicine used to be simple, ineffective and relatively safe. Now it is complex, effective and potentially dangerous" (Figure 2.8.1).

The majority of healthcare research has been primarily focused on understanding disease biology and effective medications/therapeutics. However, not enough investment has been made on the actual methods of healthcare delivery *processes* that impact the degree of effectiveness and efficiency of therapies delivered to patients (Pronovost & Goeschel, 2011). Slow adoption of research identifying best practices has also limited the translation of evidence to healthcare delivery systems (Green, 2008; Westfall et al., 2007).

In the context of US healthcare reform, value-based purchasing payment requires thinking differently about how to deliver patient-centered care and to better manage patient populations more efficiently and effectively (Porter, 2009). Such systems-focused thinking will fundamentally change the way healthcare will be delivered in the future (Schyve, 2005). Strategies to improve patient safety include

> re-designing the systems of healthcare delivery to prevent errors; designing procedures to make errors visible when they do occur so that they may be intercepted; and designing procedures for mitigating the adverse effects of errors when they are not detected and intercepted. It also includes tactics to reducing errors, reducing complexity, optimizing information processing, automating wisely, using constraints and mitigating unwanted side effects of change. (Nolan, 2000)

Advances in the science of computer modeling have made simulation technology an indispensable tool in complex, high-risk industries (e.g., aeronautics, aviation, etc.) to model, predict, and examine human performance and system evaluations with consideration of the time and resource constraints. Such modeling has dramatically improved quality and safety in manufacturing and decision-making (Bertsimas & De Boer, 2005; Cates & Mollaghasemi, 2005;

Schrage, 1999). There is every reason to expect that such transformations are possible within the healthcare environment. The complex system(s) of healthcare needs to be organized in such a way that areas of identifiable patient risk are found, mitigated, and improved in an iterative process. Quality and risk departments are key members of the team as they have access to the data related to these events and can assist in ensuring that improvements are made in the system.

SYSTEMS APPROACH TO IMPROVE PATIENT SAFETY

Safety is a system property of the healthcare delivery system, with unique sociotechnical characteristics (*Health IT and Patient Safety: Building Safer Systems for Better Care*, 2011). Efficient and effective patient safety interventions need to be fully understood from the system level. Then, specific interventions within specific microsystems (people, technology/hardware/software, process, organization, external environment) can be explored, with consideration of the impact on other subsystems. Otherwise, one solution in one microsystem could create unintended consequences on other microsystems that does not necessarily improve overall system performance.

By definition, a system "… is composed of interacting parts that operate together to achieve some objective or purpose. It is intended to absorb inputs, process them in some way and produce outputs defined by goals, objectives or common purposes" (Sauter, n.d.).

Complex systems "… cannot be understood by studying parts in isolation. The very essence of the system lies in the interaction between parts and the overall behavior that emerges from the interactions. The system must be analyzed as a whole" (Northwestern Institute on Complex Systems, Northwestern University, 2011).

A complex adaptive system has been defined as having the following characteristics:

1. "Nonlinear and dynamic and do not inherently reach fixed-equilibrium points;
2. Composed of independent agents whose behavior is based on physical, psychological, or social rules rather than the demands of **system dynamics**; and
3. Agents' (individuals acting within the system) needs or desires, reflected in their rules, are not homogeneous, their goals and behaviors are likely to conflict. In response to these conflicts or competitions, agents tend to adapt to each other's behaviors. Agents are intelligent; adaptation and learning tend to result in self-organization. There is no single point of control" (Rouse, 2008).

For most of the healthcare providers, the clinical microsystems (e.g., emergency department, intensive care units, etc.) are the "sharp end" where they provide most services to most people. The clinical microsystems are the essential building blocks of the much larger healthcare delivery system (Barach & Johnson, 2006; Nelson et al., 2002, 2008). Latent risk factors are those embedded system weakness factors (staffing, resource allocation, etc.) in the working environment. Potential improvements to those systems' factors have the potential of making a great contribution to patient safety (van Beuzekom et al., 2010).

The convergence of technology from both patients and providers provides unprecedented challenges and opportunities for the healthcare industry. As we contemplate the many factors involved in a true optimal synthesis of a vast array of inputs (e.g., monitors, electronic medical record systems, provider interactions), added cognitive burdens (and potential for cognitive overload) to healthcare providers may be an additional expected component of new and evolving complexity. Regardless, the old care delivery model is on the verge of transformation, similar to what occurred in the reformation of manufacturing in the early 20th century.

Process and Workflow Redesign

In a healthcare system, the overall output has been comprised of multiple aims: safety, effectiveness, timeliness, patient-centeredness, efficiency, and equality. "The goal of the systems is to optimize—rather than maximize—the performance of each of its components in order to maximize the system's output" (Schyve, 2005). Healthcare delivery is conducted in a very diverse, distributed, and complex system of systems (patient, provider, process, hospital, payer, and regulator). Patient safety leaders emphasize the IOM's conclusion that the major cause of adverse events is poorly designed systems, not negligent individual performance (Kohn et al., 1999). The healthcare team (physicians, managers, nurses, and others) should work together to analyze and redesign flawed processes to prevent harm (Mathews & Pronovost, 2011). Such transformation will best occur top-down and bottom-up in a cohesive mission-driven way. Intervention on the provider only will not have a sustained impact on the whole system of performance without change in the delivery system. Care processes' enhancement and redesign is imperative and a more effective way to reduce patient harm than blaming individuals (Mathews & Pronovost, 2011). The systems approach focuses on working environmental conditions rather than on the errors of individuals as the likelihood of specific errors (van Beuzekom et al., 2010). Dr. Donabedian first introduced this concept of the systems approach to address complex and inefficient care delivery processes and provided a paradigm shift to address quality and patient safety (Donabedian, 1966).

The effective system interventions include designing, testing, and enhancing a system's processes so it can prevent and mitigate human errors, considering the inherent variability and vulnerabilities of human beings (e.g., distraction, fatigue, and other latent factors). Highest-value patient safety and quality care can be realized to full potential only when improvement of the underlying delivery system is accomplished (Agency for Healthcare Research and Quality, 2008).

THE SYSTEMS INTEGRATION CONCEPT IN THE ERA OF PATIENT SAFETY AND QUALITY IMPROVEMENT

Systems Integration Is Critical

Healthcare should leverage systems thinking strategies from other industries to improve the reliability of healthcare services. Patient safety is characterized by multidimensional interactions of several subsystems. Beyond solely focusing on patient- and provider-level interactions, there are unmet needs and unique opportunities that simulation-based systems integration can achieve to coordinate system-level interactions. It is critical that the various microsystems are integrated in such a way as to provide checks and balances in the system and that all levels of the organization understand and provide support to continuous improvements in the systems in which they exist.

Systems integration should incorporate the patient, providers, workflow processes, technology, and so on within a delivery system (Mathews & Pronovost, 2011). Technology is not advanced enough to make a truly comprehensive impact on healthcare delivery if the complexity of human behavior and variation is not understood and examined. In order to make the next major leap for quality improvement and patient safety, the healthcare industry must overcome the major challenges of change management and workflow redesign to achieve the potential advancements in delivery systems.

Advantage of Systems Simulation

Complexity is the new challenge for the healthcare industry. Conventional analytics and statistical modeling alone cannot handle those interconnected variables in an aggregated manner. Because of the current nature of care delivery (dynamic and time-dependent), traditional quality improvement tools (value stream mapping) are ineffective in managing random variability and interconnections and interdependencies between subsystems (patients, providers, processes). There is therefore an important opportunity for simulation modalities to provide the "glue" for these to become integrated. The transformative nature of sophisticated simulation techniques is even more relevant for the next phase of health system transformation, as it is utilized beyond domains of assessment and training. Simulation can provide a platform to analyze concepts and requirements, as well as to conduct failure analysis (constructive simulation; Schrage, 1999). Simulation has been used for electronic medical record (EMR) and device testing and implementation (simulation-based usability research) and virtual clinical trials (simulation-based disease discovery; Ahmed et al., 2011; Eddy & Schlessinger, 2003a, 2003b).

Computer simulation has been purposed as a third branch of science beyond experimentation and theory (Glotzer et al., 2008; Pool, 1992). Computer **modeling and simulation** technology is an indispensable tool in complex, high-risk industries (aeronautics, aviation, etc.) to model, predict, and examine human performance and system evaluations. Such modeling and simulation capabilities have dramatically improved quality and safety in manufacturing and decision-making. Likewise, some in the healthcare sector are now demonstrating the power of computer modeling, coupled with realistic simulation to unleash the full potential of quality improvement methods such as Lean and Six Sigma techniques (Eldabi et al, 2002; Fone et al., 2003; Kuljis et al., 2007; Young, 2005). Various computer simulation tools have been used in medicine, including **Monte Carlo** and **Markov simulation**, **discrete event simulation** (DES), systems dynamics, and **agent-based simulation** (Brailsford et al., 2009; Dong et al., 2012).

DES is among the most common **systems engineering** tools for process analysis and system optimization by many industries, including the high-reliability industries (aviation, nuclear power stations, etc.; Committee on Engineering and the Health Care System, Institute of Medicine and National Academy of Engineering, 2005; Jahangirian et al., 2010). This simulation method can reveal the mechanisms that influence complex system operation; how well the system meets overall goals and objectives; and how system performance can be improved to achieve optimization before any process improvement is introduced in the actual patient environment. It has been adopted by various healthcare settings, including patient flow management, facility planning, resource and staffing management, and so on (Baker et al., 2009; Brailsford et al., 2009; Connelly, 2004; Eldabi et al, 2007; Griffiths et al., 2010; Jun et al, 1999; Young, 2005). Most of this professional application literature emanates from engineering journals; healthcare systems seem slow to adopt modeling and simulation in medical practices (Eldabi et al., 2007; Fackler et al., 2012; Jahangirian et al., 2012). The "beer game" is a simulation game originally developed and produced by the Massachusetts Institute of Technology (MIT). It has been used in management education for decades to teach how to manage inventory in the production-distribution chain with minimal expenditure. This simulation game can help healthcare providers to better understand the concepts of complex adaptive systems, systems thinking, and process redesign (Young et al., 2004).

Medical Simulation Can Play a Greater Role in Systems Integration

Because of the complexity of the healthcare practice environment, it is often not possible, practical, and/or cost-effective to investigate all new interventions by conventional, experimental, and heuristic approaches. Adopted from other industries, simulation-based quality improvement techniques can be used as a moderately quick prototyping platform for process improvement and workflow redesign. Interventions on disease-specific, patient-specific, provider-specific, healthcare system–specific, and integrated workflow processes can be tested and improved with various custom-created scenarios. Nonlinear relationships between system components can be explored; different options of interventions can be purposed with consideration of trade-offs involving resource and time constraints. The interaction between "nature" (severity of illness, genetic predisposition) and "nurture" (hospital care delivery) can be investigated with these modalities. Interventions targeted to nature and nurture can be purposed accordingly with interaction in the simulated environment. These simulation-based quality improvements (SBQI) also greatly reduce the "time-to-market" and cost less and avoid unnecessary and potential patient harm in the conventional trial and error of the clinical environment (Young et al., 2004).

Systems simulation has several distinct advantages as learning opportunities for clinical decision support, systems analysis, and experimentation for multivariate system components that cannot be achieved by traditional quality improvement. The most commonly applied systems analysis tools enable systematic process analysis and optimization in a simulated environment. It provides novel process optimization mechanisms via engineering principles for healthcare system analysis, simulation-based drills, and workflow redesign for testing purposed interventions (virtual clinical trials or quality improvement) before clinical deployment, effectively eliminating potential patient harm.

There are two kinds of systems integrations: horizontal and vertical. Horizontal integration is defined as the integration of SBME with other patient safety endeavors in the institution. Vertical Integration includes the integration of SBQI with patient-provider processes and interactions. Simulation-based healthcare education and quality improvement are interconnected efforts to build better delivery systems.

A system of systems simulation can help to modify structures and processes to eliminate or minimize the risks of healthcare-associated injury before they have a negative impact on the outcomes of care (van Beuzekom et al., 2010; Vincent et al., 1998). Innovation and clinical integration demands that providers leverage healthcare information technology to build an integrated, accountable, and high-performance care enterprise. Simulation can serve as the catalyst for bringing healthcare delivery components together and moving agendas forward. Simulation can enable the unrealized potential of modern medicine to build an integrated, accountable, and high-performance care enterprise.

Partnership with Systems Engineering Communities

The National Academy of Engineering and Institute of Medicine of the National Academies directed attention to the issue of systems engineering and integration with their joint report in 2005, *Building a Better Delivery System:*

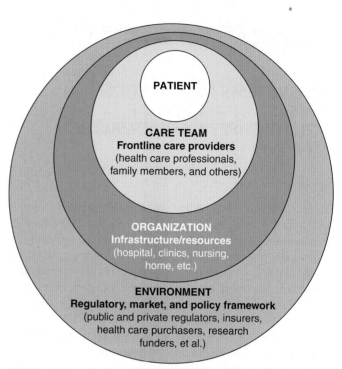

FIGURE 2.8.2 Conceptual drawing of a four-level healthcare system. (From National Academy of Engineering and Institute of Medicine. [2005]. *Building a better delivery system: A new engineering/health care partnership* [p. 20]. Washington, DC: The National Academies Press.)

A New Engineering/Health Care Partnership (Reid et al., 2005). Since then, the concept of systems integration has received much attention, yet the field requires more research. The use of simulation in systems integration provides exciting future opportunities with great potential impact (Figure 2.8.2).

The collaboration between clinicians, engineers, researchers, educators, and experts from medical informatics and management will provide a clinically relevant, systematic approach and a comprehensive solution to many of the challenging problems in clinical medicine. The systematic analysis and optimization of healthcare delivery processes coupled with simulation-based education will promote safe and high-quality patient care. The high-impact and low-cost interventions should be chosen with the consideration of a standard business value equation: Value of healthcare = (outcome + safety + service)/cost over time (Smoldt & Cortese, 2007). This capacity will offer high-impact and low-cost interventions to consider for future dissemination of scientific evidence into clinical practice. No single tool can resolve all of the problems currently faced in healthcare, but various simulation tools are important applications that, when added to the patient safety toolkits, will provide additional insight and value in quality improvement. It all needs further dissemination (Griffiths et al., 2010).

In describing the current practice and structure of healthcare delivery, the use of simulation and modeling approaches can improve healthcare delivery systems. System modeling can develop a model workflow for the medical practice that utilizes the most efficient possibilities of time of the team members, maximizing the patient encounter and delivery value. Testing system modifications via simulation modeling provides the means by which designing and testing new workflows within delivery systems can occur, without sacrificing quality. The challenge is to identify and design the specific system to assess and improve, whether it is disease or physiological processes, provider interactions, or workflow processes.

EXAMPLES OF CASE STUDIES OF VARIOUS MODALITIES FOR SYSTEM INTEGRATION

Mannequin-Based Simulators

A program utilizes in situ simulation with multidisciplinary teams of providers to introduce new processes related to intraoperative radiation therapy (Rodriguez-Paz et al., 2009). By using the mannequin simulator, the team simulates the treatment process (workflow). These simulations identify new threats and unintended consequences that could otherwise lead to patient harm. Subsequent checklists and protocols are created to prevent hazards from occurring. These activities enable the institution to prospectively identify and mitigate hazards before clinical implementation actually occurs.

Standardized Patient-Based Simulation

There are several groups employing a secret shopper (standardized patient) to go through clinics and hospital departments, similar to what a trained market researcher would do in the retail industry. The objectives vary and may include providing healthcare practice feedback to improve the efficiency and effectiveness of provider communication, noting process and procedural times, as well as understanding department-to-department flow and communication. The ultimate goal is to improve patient care, wait time, and explore other opportunities (American Medical Association, 2009).

In situ Simulation

Another team uses in situ simulation to conduct operational readiness assessment and orientation before a new emergency department moves to the new physical plant (Kobayashi et al., 2006). The simulation scenario enables participants to identify and improve several key system deficiencies (problematic placement or absence of key equipment, untested communication systems, lack of orientation, etc.). Here, simulation serves as a test bed similar to that used in auto industry crash testing to mitigate hazards before production.

Computer Simulation and Virtual Reality

A program uses a computer simulation model developed to test a new emergency department (ED) electronic patient flow "white board" that displays realistic real-time

ED operations. This activity demonstrates the unique iterative design features of computer simulation with relatively high fidelity of the ED operation, while performing such analysis at low cost toward process redesign (Pennathur et al., 2009, 2010). Engineers have also been using virtual reality (VR) systems to facilitate poststroke patient upper limb function recovery by combining VR and self-face viewing (Shiri et al., 2012). Computer simulation (DES) was also used for predicting quantitative effects of process changes in ED (Day et al., 2013). Advancements in technology are hoped to make these capabilities more affordable to stakeholders in future healthcare delivery systems.

These examples demonstrate that the system modeling approach assists in identifying and mitigating hazards (latent errors) before clinical implementation of new workflow. Here, simulation serves as rapid prototyping environment to healthcare delivery system redesign. It also educates and trains the providers to understand the concept of workflow enhancements and test the readiness of the team in a safe manner, avoiding any potential harm to the patient. Further, because of the relative low cost and no (patient) risk environment of in situ simulation, these activities should be conducted on an ongoing basis to enable quick Plan-Do-Study-Act (PDSA) cycles for quality improvement efforts in the hospital operation management (van Lent et al., 2012).

SYSTEMS INTEGRATION ACCREDITATION

How to Get Started

The key to getting started in integrating a simulation program within a system is to: (1) identify who the key stakeholders are within the simulation program, (2) identify those proponents with whom the simulation program interacts, and (3) assess the key areas of patient risk and/or liability. Organized and consistent bidirectional feedback is essential among those involved to ensure that issues are identified, resolved, and measured. This feedback structure ensures sustainability of the desired change.

Utilizing SSH's Accreditation Standards is a way to establish essential elements for a systems integration approach in your healthcare facility (Society for Simulation in Healthcare, Council for Accreditation of Healthcare Simulation Programs Accreditation Standards, n.d.). Utilizing the developed tool (see chapter 1.1) and identifying where your program is on the continuum of compliance with the standards provides a fundamental road map for the development of your program. Once it is identified where a program is on the journey, a plan can be developed to achieve full compliance with the standards.

Through multiple surveys it has been seen that one of the most challenging areas for compliance with the standards is integrating the simulation program with the organization's performance and quality improvement activities. Spending time with the performance/

quality improvement leadership can be fruitful by virtue of obtaining information about current issues and then assisting in developing a plan of correction that includes simulation. It is also critical for the simulation program to provide feedback through the performance/quality improvement committee vehicle issues that are being identified when competencies are being assessed during simulation sessions with learners. Another important step is to ensure that the sustainability of the devised plan is monitored over time to ensure that compliance is maintained.

BEEN THERE, DONE THAT: HOW CAN I CONTINUE TO IMPROVE OR SUSTAIN WHAT I HAVE ACHIEVED?

Becoming Hardwired with Integration

As mentioned earlier, there are two main types of systems integration: horizontal and vertical. If your organization has developed and implemented processes in which interprofessional teams are working together utilizing multiple simulation methods (i.e., modeling, high- and low-technology mannequins, and standardized patients) when adverse events occur and also in a proactive way to ensure that adverse events do not reach a patient in the first place (failure modes effects analysis [FMEA]), you are well on your way to being integrated. Having simulation staff routinely serve on the healthcare organization's performance improvement committees and having someone from the quality department serve on the simulation program's performance improvement committee allows the organization to feel confident that they are maximizing respective expertise as part of important patient safety conversations.

Systems integration is typically simplest in a closed system, meaning the simulation program is part of the healthcare facility or system. Systems integration can be more challenging when the simulation program is a stand-alone entity; interacting with a medical center may be difficult owing to concerns of disclosure of delicate or confidential information. One way to address this challenge is to develop a Memorandum of Understanding (MOU) articulating the quality assurance nature of the relationship between the simulation program and the medical center and have those involved sign confidentiality agreements. The possibilities of systems integration are only limited by those who have oversight of the processes.

Once You Have Obtained Accreditation in Systems Integration

After being granted accreditation in Systems Integration, it is critical that the great work that has begun is sustained over time. Sustainability can be much more difficult than initially obtaining a goal owing to "drift." Drift implies that once other initiatives get launched, other earlier initiatives

start to return to previous performance levels because of decreasing awareness of the old project and increasing awareness of the new initiative. Maintaining a high level of accountability through a system-wide approach can decrease the potential for drift.

Simulation programs can become integrated if they are intentional in their work. Some challenges with integration occur when entities merge and grow. There are great opportunities and challenges during these periods. Having a simulation program is especially important when an expansion of an area is being suggested or implemented. The ability to model workflow or mock up a potential room configuration prior to launching the build can save time and money in the long run. As these fertile relationships grow, one will be able to determine how best to shape the future potential of the organization in a safe and meaningful way.

The scope of a simulation program's patient safety influence is greatly enhanced when other entities outside of the system know of their work—for example, working with prehospital personnel as a means to decrease patient harm by integrating with these community partners. The key is whether your simulation program has bidirectional relationships with its various partners. Sounds like it would be easy, fairly simple, and straightforward, but it is anything but that.

SUMMARY

With the partnership of professionals (clinicians, educators, engineers, informaticians, etc.) from interested disciplines and specialties, various simulation tools can be adopted in the healthcare setting and provide solutions to meet the need of an integrated system. Increasingly, the adoption of health information technology will provide high-quality and real-time data for simulation and modeling of system components, thus supporting improved and informed decision-making (*Health IT and Patient Safety: Building Safer Systems for Better Care*, 2011). Education is also critical for current and future providers to adopt lifelong learning of quality improvement and patient safety science (National Patient Safety Foundation, 2010; Pronovost & Goeschel, 2010; Pronovost et al., 2009). This enables hospitals and other healthcare institutions to adapt nimbly to the environment technology, and patient healthcare stakeholders, facilitating the institution's patient-centric missions. Ultimately, shared responsibility within such a learning organization helps the system to move consistently forward toward the delivery of better care at lower cost (Smith et al., 2012).

REFERENCES

Agency for Healthcare Research and Quality. (2008, September). *Final contract report: Cost of poor quality or waste in integrated delivery system settings* (AHRQ Publication No. 08-0096-EF). Rockville, MD: Author.

Ahmed, A., Chandra, S., Herasevich, V., Gajic, O., & Pickering, B. W. (2011). The effect of two different electronic health record user interfaces on intensive care provider task load, errors of cognition, and performance. *Critical Care Medicine, 39*(7), 1626–1634.

American Medical Association. (2009). *Secret shopper patients* (Report of the Council on Ethical and Judicial Affairs). Retrieved from http://www.ama-assn.org/resources/doc/ethics/ceja-9a09.pdf

Baker, D. R., Pronovost, P. J., Morlock, L. L., Geocadin, R. G., & Holzmueller, C. G. (2009). Patient flow variability and unplanned readmissions to an intensive care unit. *Critical Care Medicine, 37*(11), 2882–2887.

Barach, P., & Johnson, J. K. (2006). Understanding the complexity of redesigning care around the clinical microsystem. *Quality and Safety in Health Care, 15*(Suppl. 1), i10–i16.

Bertsimas, D., & De Boer, S. (2005). Simulation-based booking limits for airline revenue management. *Operations Research, 53*(1), 90–106.

Brailsford, S. C., Harper, P. R., Patel, B., & Pitt, M. (2009). An analysis of the academic literature on simulation and modelling in health care. *Journal of Simulation, 3*(3), 130–140.

Cates, G. R., & Mollaghasemi, M. (2005). *Supporting the vision for space with discrete event simulation.* Paper presented at proceedings of the Winter Simulation Conference, Orlando, FL.

Chantler, C. (1999). The role and education of doctors in the delivery of health care. *The Lancet, 353*(9159), 1178–1181.

Classen, D. C., Resar, R., Griffin, F., Federico, F., Frankel, T., Kimmel, N., … James, B. C. (2011). "Global Trigger Tool" shows that adverse events in hospitals may be ten times greater than previously measured. *Health Affairs, 30*(4), 581–589.

Committee on Engineering and the Health Care System, Institute of Medicine and National Academy of Engineering. (2005). The tools of systems engineering. In P. P. Reid, W. D. Compton, J. H. Grossman, & G. Fanjiang (Eds.), *Building a better delivery system: A new engineering/health care partnership* (p. 37). Washington, DC: The National Academies Press.

Committee on Quality of Health Care in America Institute of Medicine. (2001). *Crossing the quality chasm: A new health system for the 21st century.* Washington, DC: The National Academies Press.

Connelly, L. G. (2004). Discrete event simulation of emergency department activity: A platform for system-level operations research. *Academic Emergency Medicine, 11*(11), 1177–1185.

Cook, D. A., Hatala, R., Brydges, R., Zendejas, B., Szostek, J. H., Wang, A. T., … Hamstra, S. J. (2011). Technology-enhanced simulation for health professions education: a systematic review and meta-analysis. *Journal of American Medical Association, 306*(9), 978–988.

Day, T. E., Al-Roubaie, A. R., & Goldlust, E. J. (2013). Decreased length of stay after addition of healthcare provider in emergency department triage: a comparison between computer-simulated and real-world interventions. *Emergency Medicine Journal, 30*(2), 134–138.

Donabedian, A. (1966). Evaluating the quality of medical care. *The Milbank Memorial Fund Quarterly, 44*(3), 166–203.

Dong, Y., Chbat, N. W., Gupta, A., Hadzikadic, M., & Gajic, O. (2012). Systems modeling and simulation applications for critical care medicine. *Annals of Intensive Care, 2*(1), 18.

Eddy, D. M., & Schlessinger, L. (2003a). Archimedes: A trial-validated model of diabetes. *Diabetes Care, 26*(11), 3093–3101.

Eddy, D. M., & Schlessinger, L. (2003b). Validation of the Archimedes diabetes model. *Diabetes Care, 26*(11), 3102–3110.

Eldabi, T., Irani, Z., & Paul, R. J. (2002). A proposed approach for modelling health-care systems for understanding. *Journal of Management in Medicine, 16*(2–3), 170–187.

Eldabi, T., Paul, R. J., & Young, T. (2007). Simulation modelling in healthcare: Reviewing legacies and investigating futures. *Journal of the Operational Research Society, 58*(2), 262–270.

Fackler, J., Hankin, J., & Young, T. (2012, December 9–12). *Why healthcare professionals are slow to adopt modeling and simulation.* Paper presented at proceedings of the 2012 Winter Simulation Conference (WSC), Berlin, Germany.

Fone, D., Hollinghurst, S., Temple, M., Round, A., Lester, N., Weightman, A., … Palmer, S. (2003). Systematic review of the use and value of computer simulation modelling in population health and health care delivery. *Journal of Public Health Medicine, 25*(4), 325–335.

Glotzer, S., Kim, S., Cummings, P. T., Deshmuk, A., Head-Gordon, M., Karniadakis, G., … Shinozuka, M. (2008). *International assessment of research and development in simulation-based engineering and science* (Workshop co-sponsored by National Science Foundation, Department of Energy, Department of Defense, National Institutes of Health, National Institute of Biomedical Imaging and Bioengineering, National Aeronautics and Space Administration, National Institute of Standards and Technology). Retrieved from http://www.wtec.org/sbes/#Scope.

Green, L. W. (2008). Making research relevant: If it is an evidence-based practice, where's the practice-based evidence? *Family Practice, 25*(Suppl. 1), i20–i24.

Griffiths, J. D., Jones, M., Read, M. S., & Williams, J. E. (2010). A simulation model of bed-occupancy in a critical care unit. *Journal of Simulation, 4*(1), 52–59.

Health IT and patient safety: Building safer systems for better care. (2011). Washington, DC: The National Academies Press. Retrieved from http://www.iom.edu/Reports/2011/Health-IT-and-Patient-Safety-Building-Safer-Systems-for-Better-Care.aspx

Issenberg, S. B., McGaghie, W. C., Petrusa, E. R., Gordon, D. L., & Scalese, R. J. (2005). Features and uses of high-fidelity medical simulations that lead to effective learning: A BEME systematic review. *Medical Teacher, 27*(1), 10–28.

Jahangirian, M., Eldabi, T., Naseer, A., Stergioulas, L. K., & Young, T. (2010). Simulation in manufacturing and business: A review. *European Journal of Operational Research, 203*(1), 1–13.

Jahangirian, M., Naseer, A., Stergioulas, L., Young, T., & Eldabi, T. (2012). Simulation in health-care: Lessons from other sectors. *Operational Research, 12*(1), 45–55.

James, J. T. (2013). A new, evidence-based estimate of patient harms associated with hospital care. *Journal of Patient Safety, 9*(3), 122–128.

Jun, J. B., Jacobson, S. H., & Swisher, J. R. (1999). Application of discrete-event simulation in health care clinics: A survey. *Journal of the Operational Research Society, 50*(2), 109–123.

Keehan, S. P., Sisko, A. M., Truffer, C. J., Poisal, J. A., Cuckler, G. A., Madison, A. J., … Smith, S. D. (2011). National health spending projections through 2020: Economic recovery and reform drive faster spending growth. *Health Affairs, 30*(8), 1594–1605.

Kobayashi, L., Shapiro, M. J., Sucov, A., Woolard, R., Boss, R. M., 3rd, Dunbar, J., … Jay, G. (2006). Portable advanced medical simulation for new emergency department testing and orientation. *Academic Emergency Medicine, 13*(6), 691–695.

Kohn, L. T., Corrigan, J. M., & Donaldson, M. S. (Eds.). (1999). *To error is human: Building a safer health system.* Washington, DC: National Academy Press.

Kuljis, J., Paul, R. J., & Stergioulas, L. K. (2007). *Can health care benefit from modeling and simulation methods in the same way as business and manufacturing has?* Paper presented at proceedings of the Winter Simulation Conference, Washington, DC.

Landrigan, C. P., Parry, G. J., Bones, C. B., Hackbarth, A. D., Goldmann, D. A., & Sharek, P. J. (2010). Temporal trends in rates of patient harm resulting from medical care. *New England Journal of Medicine, 363*(22), 2124–2134.

Mathews, S. C., & Pronovost, P. J. (2011). The need for systems integration in health care. *JAMA: Journal of the American Medical Association, 305*(9), 934–935.

McGaghie, W. C., Issenberg, S. B., Cohen, E. R., Barsuk, J. H., & Wayne, D. B. (2011). Does simulation-based medical education with deliberate practice yield better results than traditional clinical education? A meta-analytic comparative review of the evidence. *Academic Medicine, 86*(6), 706–711.

National Patient Safety Foundation. (2010). *Unmet needs: Teaching physicians to provide safe patient care report of the Lucian Leape Institute Roundtable on Reforming Medical Education.* Retrieved from http://www.npsf.org/LLI-Unmet-Needs-Report/

Nelson, E. C., Batalden, P. B., Huber, T. P., Mohr, J. J., Godfrey, M. M., Headrick, L. A., … Wasson, J. H. (2002). Microsystems in health care: Part 1. Learning from high-performing front-line clinical units. *Joint Commission Journal on Quality Improvement, 28*(9), 472–493.

Nelson, E. C., Godfrey, M. M., Batalden, P. B., Berry, S. A., Bothe, A. E., Jr., McKinley, K. E., … Nolan, T. W. (2008). Clinical microsystems, part 1. The building blocks of health systems. *Joint Commission Journal on Quality and Patient Safety, 34*(7), 367–378.

Nolan, T. W. (2000). System changes to improve patient safety. *British Medical Journal, 320*(7237), 771–773.

Northwestern Institute on Complex Systems, Northwestern University. (n.d.). *What are complex systems?* Retrieved from http://www.northwestern.edu/nico/about_cs.html

Olsen, L., Aisner, D., & McGinnis, J. M. (2007). *The learning healthcare system: Workshop summary (IOM Roundtable on Evidence-Based Medicine)*. Washington, DC: The National Academies Press.

Pool, R. (1992). The third branch of science debuts. *Science, 256*(5053), 44–47.

Pennathur, P. R., Cao, D., Sui, Z., Lin, L., Bisantz, A. M., Fairbanks, R. J., ... Wears, R. L. (2009). *Evaluating emergency department information technology using a simulation-based approach.* Paper presented at proceedings of the Human Factors and Ergonomics Society, San Antanio, TX.

Pennathur, P. R., Cao, D., Sui, Z., Lin, L., Bisantz, A. M., Fairbanks, R. J., ... Wears, R. L. (2010). Development of a simulation environment to study emergency department information technology. *Simulation in Healthcare, 5*(2), 103–111.

Plsek, P. E., & Greenhalgh, T. (2001). The challenge of complexity in health care. *British Medical Journal, 323*(7313), 625–628.

Porter, M. E. (2009). A strategy for health care reform—Toward a value-based system. *New England Journal of Medicine, 361*(2), 109–112.

Pronovost, P. J., & Goeschel, C. A. (2010). Viewing health care delivery as science: Challenges, benefits, and policy implications. *Health Services Research, 45*(5, Pt. 2), 1508–1522.

Pronovost, P. J., & Goeschel, C. A. (2011). Time to take health delivery research seriously. *Journal of American Medical Association, 306*(3), 310–311.

Pronovost, P. J., Goeschel, C. A., Marsteller, J. A., Sexton, J. B., Pham, J. C., & Berenholtz, S. M. (2009). Framework for patient safety research and improvement. *Circulation, 119*(2), 330–337.

Reid, P. P., Compton, W. D., Grossman, J. H., & Fanjiang, G. (2005). *Building a better delivery system: A new engineering/health care partnership* (Committee on Engineering and the Health Care System, Institute of Medicine and National Academy of Engineering). Washington, DC: Natioanl Academies Press.

Rodriguez-Paz, J. M., Mark, L. J., Herzer, K. R., Michelson, J. D., Grogan, K. L., Herman, J., ... Pronovost, P. J. (2009). A novel process for introducing a new intraoperative program: A multidisciplinary paradigm for mitigating hazards and improving patient safety. *Anesthesia & Analgesia, 108*(1), 202–210.

Rouse, W. B. (2008, Spring). Health care as a complex adaptive system: Implications for design and management. *The Bridge, 38*(1), 17–25.

Sauter, V. L. (n.d.). *Systems theory.* St. Louis: Information Systems Area, College of Business Administration, University of Missouri at St. Louis. Retrieved from http://www.umsl.edu/~sauterv/analysis/intro/system.htm

Schmidt, E., Goldhaber-Fiebert, S. N., Ho, L. A., & McDonald, K. M. (2013). Simulation exercises as a patient safety strategy: A systematic review. *Annals of Internal Medicine, 158*(5, Pt. 2), 426–432.

Schrage, M. (1999). Measure prototyping paybacks. In *Serious play: How the world's best companies simulate to innovate.* Boston, MA: Harvard Business School Press.

Schyve, P. M. (2005). Systems thinking and patient safety. In K. Henriksen, J. B. Battles, E. S. Marks, & D. I. Lewin (Eds.), *Advances in patient safety: From research to implementation (Volume 2: Concepts and methodology).* Rockville, MD: Agency for Healthcare Research and Quality.

Shiri, S., Feintuch, U., Lorber-Haddad, A., Moreh, E., Twito, D., Tuchner-Arieli, M., & Meiner, Z. (2012). Novel virtual reality system integrating online self-face viewing and mirror visual feedback for stroke rehabilitation: rationale and feasibility. *Top Stroke Rehabil, 19*(4), 277–286.

Shortell, S. M., & Singer, S. J. (2008). Improving patient safety by taking systems seriously. *JAMA: The Journal of the American Medical Association, 299*(4), 445–447.

Smith, M., Saunders, R., Stuckhardt, L., & McGinnis, M. (2012). *Best care at lower cost: The path to continuously learning health care in America.* Washington, DC: The National Academies Press.

Smoldt, R. K., & Cortese, D. A. (2007). Pay-for-performance or pay for value? *Mayo Clinic Proceedings, 82*(2), 210–213.

Society for Simuation in Healthcare. (n.d.). *What is simulation?* Retrieved from http://ssih.org/about-simulation

Society for Simulation in Healthcare, Council for Accreditation of Healthcare Simulation Programs Accreditation Standards. (n.d.). Retieved from http://ssih.org/accreditation/how-to-apply

Van Beuzekom, M., Boer, F., Akerboom, S., & Hudson, P. (2010). Patient safety: latent risk factors. *British Journal of Anaesthesia, 105*(1), 52–59.

Van Lent, W., VanBerkel, P., & van Harten, W. (2012). A review on the relation between simulation and improvement in hospitals. *BMC Medical Informatics and Decision Making, 12*(1), 18.

Vincent, C., Taylor-Adams, S., & Stanhope, N. (1998). Framework for analysing risk and safety in clinical medicine. *BMJ (Clinical research ed.), 316*(7138), 1154–1157.

Westfall, J. M., Mold, J., & Fagnan, L. (2007). Practice-based research—"Blue Highways" on the NIH roadmap. *JAMA: The Journal of the American Medical Association, 297*(4), 403–406.

Young, T. (2005). An agenda for healthcare and information simulation. *Health Care Management Science, 8*(3), 189–196.

Young, T., Brailsford, S., Connell, C., Davies, R., Harper, P., & Klein, J. H. (2004). Using industrial processes to improve patient care. *British Medical Journal, 328*(7432), 162–164.

CHAPTER 2.9

A Model for Establishing a Rural Simulation Partnership

Rebekah Damazo, RN, CPNP, CHSE-A, MSN, and Sherry D. Fox, RN, CHSE, PhD

ABOUT THE AUTHORS

REBEKAH DAMAZO is the Director and Co-founder of the Rural Northern California Clinical Simulation Center in Chico, California, and Professor of Nursing at California State University, Chico. She worked with Dr. Fox to create a rural partnership that has been in operation since 2006. The Rural SimCenter has recognition for its innovative partnership model, which includes both academic and hospital organizations. The model provides a setting for interdisciplinary practice and a sustainable business strategy.

SHERRY D. FOX is the Financial Director and cofounder of the Rural Northern California Clinical Simulation Center in Chico, California, and Professor of Nursing at California State University, Chico. She worked with Ms. Damazo to create a rural partnership of hospitals and schools of nursing, cowriting grants to establish a shared center, and helps maintain an ongoing partnership to sustain the center. This center achieved international Society for Simulation in Healthcare Accreditation in 2010.

ABSTRACT

Developing academic-service partnerships of any type is challenging. Especially in the rural setting, it is in the interest of academic institutions and community healthcare facilities to work together to maximize efforts and resources for health education and training. The advantages to creating these partnerships to provide simulation education include shared leadership, fiscal responsibility, and sustainability. This chapter describes the process of forming a collaborative partnership to support multiple users of simulation to overcome financial obstacles associated with starting a simulation center from the ground up, when individual agencies do not have the resources to implement simulation on their own. The Rural Northern California Clinical Simulation Center in Chico, California, USA will be used as a case study for an effective public-private partnership in a rural setting.

CASE EXAMPLE

The Rural Northern California Clinical Simulation Center (Rural SimCenter) formed a public-private partnership to develop a cost-effective solution for simulation education in one rural community. A school of nursing and two rural hospitals developed a state-of-the-art simulation center for a fraction of the cost of most centers. The partnership started with lofty goals, and little funding, yet has achieved an ongoing simulation collaborative that has thrived for over 8 years, offering quality simulation programs for rural health professionals and students. To promote simulation as a teaching strategy, a partnership was formed between academia (associate degree in nursing and bachelor of science in nursing) and staff development departments to train their instructors in an efficient, effective, and timely manner. The success of the partnership is exemplified by the achievement of accreditation by the Society for Simulation in Healthcare in 2010.

You work in a small community and have been charged with addressing the simulation needs of the local hospital that is seeking opportunities for interprofessional training and the health profession programs at the local college. Can California's Rural SimCenter be used as a roadmap for meeting these needs?

INTRODUCTION AND BACKGROUND

Healthcare is a rapidly changing business, and hospitals and schools are struggling to find tools to enhance their ability to keep up with the change (Campbell et al., 2001). It is widely accepted that medical simulation is an effective way for health profession students and professionals to advance their skills, as well as learn new skills in a realistic and risk-free environment. Hands-on medical simulation provides healthcare providers with valuable insight and learning. The challenge lies in the ability to translate this into an affordable and sustainable educational setting (Curtin & Dupuis, 2008).

Simulation is an expensive and time-intensive operation, yet simulation has the potential to supplement the declining resources for the education and practice of medical skills. While it is possible to use simulation methodology without elaborate mannequins or spaces, the use of simulation equipment can help create the innovative learning environment now in demand by health professionals and teams (Carney et al., 2011).

Though simulation is often considered an essential component of health professional training, this rapidly moving phenomenon has left many **rural** areas behind. The need for simulation training in rural areas is critical because healthcare institutions often lack the diverse volume of high-risk patient events that keep staff and trainees on the cutting edge of care delivery. The initial monetary outlay for suitable space, expensive mannequins, medical equipment, appropriately trained staff and the requisite audiovisual adjuncts can be daunting, even overwhelming to small hospitals and professional schools. The process of developing simulation curricula for both students and professionals using high-fidelity scenarios can be a substantial resource investment; however, these applications have the greatest potential for improving patient safety.

Many institutions are experiencing tight fiscal constraints, and simulation technologies can add hundreds of thousands of dollars in expense to already strained operating budgets. The idea that each hospital and each school should have a separate simulation program may not be practical. One possible solution is the idea that institutions could combine resources to develop a simulation program with state-of-the-art capabilities without undue financial burden on a single institution.

The initial costs of setting up a simulation program needs to be offset by high utilization, which is difficult when a single small organization tries to do this alone. Even well-planned and well-funded program are often underutilized, lacking a business plan to capitalize on a valuable resource. Cost-effective and efficient strategies must be considered by hospitals and training programs of small to modest size, to realistically embark on the simulation enterprise. One of the most feasible approaches is to form **partnerships** or alliances, to spread the cost, commitment, and utilization over more than one agency. Larger institutions can also align with smaller ones to share benefits—such as improved pricing structures.

It is in the interest of both academic institutions and communities to maximize efforts and resources for health education and training. Additional advantages of developing a partnership to provide simulation education include shared leadership, fiscal responsibility, and sustainability.

PROGRAM DEVELOPMENT

Beginning in 2005, as the national movement toward simulation program development was reaching a groundswell, faculty in a baccalaureate nursing program at a modest-sized public university realized the potential for simulation training. However, the cost of even one high-technology mannequin far exceeded the department's total annual budget for operating expenses, and space on the growing campus was at a premium, with a long queue for the state's approval of any new building. Modest state grant funding was available to assist with initial costs of implementing a program, but the issue of space could not be overcome without an external partner.

Searching out other potential simulation users, the nursing faculty invited representatives from three local hospitals, the community college, and first responder organizations to discuss the possibility of a shared simulation program. The timing was optimal. Hospitals in the region were beginning to explore the benefits of simulation for low-volume, high-risk events that the professional staff experienced rarely, but that demanded ongoing expertise to achieve optimal outcomes. Additionally, hospitals foresaw forthcoming mandates to include simulation in certification processes, such as neonatal resuscitation training. The schools of nursing were pressured to expand enrollments but lacked enough clinical sites to accommodate more students. In addition, faculty visualized exposing students to a broader range of clinical experiences than those available in small, local hospitals. They saw simulation methodology as a chance to develop the capability to achieve higher-level, standardized competencies for students. First responder organizations envisioned expanded training opportunities in a controlled setting.

As a result of early meetings, the group agreed to come together and form the Rural Northern California Simulation Partnership. Representatives from the partner organizations served as an advisory board to the project and the steering committee for simulation development. The group developed a strategy that clearly defined shared needs that might be addressed through simulation education.

This rural Northern California community serves a county with a population of 220,300 spread over 1,636 miles (2632.8 km) and serves adjacent counties that are quite rural and agrarian. The county encompasses five towns with a population ranging from 1,700 to 100,000. In the area there are four hospitals (ranging in size from 45 to 150 beds), including one regional Level 2 trauma center. There is no academic medical center or medical school in the region. A state university provides baccalaureate and master's level nursing education for about 250 students; a community college provides nursing and allied health programs. The university and the medical center are the largest employers in the region, with agriculture the other predominant industry.

Following initial discussions among seven potential partners, four committed partners emerged, consisting of the university school of nursing, the regional medical center, a rural community hospital of 100 beds, and the local community college nursing program. Representatives of the group toured two distant program to see what might be involved in setting up a simulation program, and the type of space needed. The space issue was immediately solved by the donation of space by the medical center. The simulation program (named Rural SimCenter) would be housed in a former nursing unit in a decommissioned hospital that was primarily empty with the exception of a few specialty clinics. The setting was ideal as the need to create a realistic hospital space was no longer necessary since the location was a former hospital unit. Once that start-up hurdle was solved, the Rural Northern California Simulation Center Partnership was born.

The partnership provided leverage to obtain funding from a state workforce development grant that supported modest start-up costs for 2 years. This funding allowed for a simulation project coordinator, simulation technician, and the purchase of several high-technology mannequins. The program started operations in October 2006.

There is not a single best way to implement a community partnership (Roussos & Fawcett, 2000). The first steps in Rural SimCenter's development included educator training. Initially, the partnership relied on vendor training. The Bay Area Simulation Collaborative extended a helping hand by allowing the Simulation Center Project Coordinator to attend their educator training sessions. In addition, the Coordinator attended "train the trainer" programs in other areas and attended workshops to provide a sound educational foundation.

An important step to partnership success was the development of a simulation educator training program for local educators that was based on current simulation best practices. Educators clearly require training to help them understand the pedagogy, educational theory, and effective use of high-technology mannequins. To promote simulation as a teaching strategy, the partnership worked with staff development departments to train educators in an efficient, effective, and timely manner. Professionals and educators trained side by side to develop simulation skills.

The Rural SimCenter quickly emerged as a simulation education leader in the Northern California Region. More than 40 educators were trained in simulation methods in the first year of operations. These educators came from both education and service. As a result of the growing number of simulation educators, a simulation collaborative was developed. The collaborative agreed to sponsor educational sessions twice a year, and a listserv was developed to help colleagues stay connected.

Initially, the Rural SimCenter education sessions focused on nursing students, emergency room nurses, and medical surgical nurses. The educational offerings expanded to include emergency teams, flight crews, neonatal nurses, and obstetric teams. The Rural SimCenter had 700 student visits in the first year of operation. As Rural SimCenter education developed, evaluation was a central focus.

As the initial grant funding was exhausted, the simulation program developed a partnership "buy-in" plan as well as a fee structure for non-partner users. A strategic plan was developed that looked at the overall cost of the project and set goals for the future. Throughout this process, the planning team evolved into an advisory board with representation from each partner agency. The Rural SimCenter *project* became the Rural SimCenter *program,* and the simulation program became an integral part of education in each of the partner agencies. In 2010, the program was accredited for education and teaching by the Society for Simulation and Healthcare, the only rural program receiving accreditation in the initial phase. Seven years of successful operation has resulted in useful strategies for working within a simulation partnership.

THE POWER OF PARTNERSHIP

Beal and colleagues (2011) cite common themes on which to base a healthcare partnership. These include mutual goals and a shared vision for outcomes. The government defines partnership as "the relationship existing between two or more persons who join to carry on a trade or business. Each person contributes money, property, labor or skill, and expects to share in the profits and losses of the business" (Internal Revenue Service, 2012, para. 1). This definition emphasizes the importance of mutual investment and a shared commitment to the partnership's success. In order for a partnership to thrive, it is important to establish a relationship of trust and communication. While many schools and hospitals have a shared clinical affiliation, developing a business relationship requires a greater emphasis on collaboration. Academic-practice partnerships are complex, and there is little information about how to develop and support these vital associations (Beal et al., 2011). The alliance becomes complicated because many groups are both colleagues and competitors. Balanced leadership was an important part of the Rural SimCenter development.

Granger and colleagues (2012) speak of the difficulty aligning "leadership processes and work processes" in the academic-service partnership. The success of the Rural SimCenter partnership was due in part to the history of well-established relationships among partners. The agency leaders serve on each other's advisory boards; faculty and hospital education staff meet regularly for planning nursing student clinical placements; the agencies share faculty and staff, with nursing faculty working as staff nurses, and staff nurses working as preceptors or clinical faculty for the nursing schools. Leadership and work processes were already in place and functioned quite collegially. These relationships—characteristic in rural communities—helped to address and overcome some of the typical partnership barriers.

SECTION 2 • Types of Simulation Programs

STRATEGIES FOR PARTNERSHIP DEVELOPMENT

Establish a Need

As organizations partner together, they will increase the likelihood of achieving their respective missions. While exploring potential partnerships, it is important to identify partners who will add value to the program rather than form partnerships of convenience. The premise is that a collection of people with complementary skills will produce better results, getting the project done more efficiently, more effectively, and with a shared cost burden.

The need for partnership was evident from the earliest thoughts of establishing a rural simulation program. The school of nursing could not overcome the financial challenges of building a program on its own and had no hopes of additional campus space. Additionally, the modest size (approximately 250 students) would not allow for optimal use of such a program given the enormous start-up costs. There would be many days when the program would be idle, such as the 10-week summer and 5-week winter breaks. Likewise, even as both hospitals were becoming aware of the usefulness of simulation for staff training, each hospital was focused on a major building campaign; a simulation program was not on their radar. However, by working together, something that seemed impossible for an individual organization began to seem feasible (Table 2.9.1).

Develop Shared Goals

With a shared vision, it is more likely that common objectives can be identified. Here, as in other areas of simulation, reverse engineering can be helpful, that is, "begin with the end in mind." The partners met frequently to discuss what each envisioned achieving from a simulation program. The nursing faculty desired a realistic, well-equipped setting for educating students as an adjunct to their regular clinical practica—a setting where mistakes could be made, discussed, and rectified with no harm to patients, and where students could experience a more complete range of practice and exercise their own clinical judgments; a space where all students could be guaranteed exposure to and even mastery of certain critical experiences that might never occur during the course of their scheduled clinical experiences. Hospital partners envisioned team practice that could enhance staff efficiency and effectiveness, particularly with low-volume, high-risk scenarios. Both visions converged in one single vision: "increase patient safety through improved clinical proficiency and teamwork."

Common core training needs were identified by both hospitals. For example, both hospitals offered ongoing Neonatal Resuscitation Programs (NRP) to their staff. These programs expanded from lecture-based courses to full simulation courses, both in the simulation program, and through on-site simulation in hospital settings. Partnership advantages became evident as scenarios, equipment, and resources were shared. The educators from both institutions were able to contribute to scenario design, and a stronger educational program developed.

As the Society for Simulation in Healthcare (SSH) established a process for accreditation of healthcare simulation programs, a new common goal was established. Setting a goal to achieve national accreditation for the simulation program increased the expectations and requirements for the partner educators. The partners all supported the quest for accreditation, and readily agreed to the higher standards.

Commitment to Success

Each partner was committed to the success of the Center. Frequent advisory board meetings kept everyone involved and informed. The goal to improve patient outcomes was central, and each partner was committed to this goal. According to Erickson and Raines (2011), partnership principles are grounded in "mutual respect, trust and honesty about individual interests." The partners should be able to look at the larger picture, beyond individual interests. At times each partner had to compromise. For example, the scheduling priorities set aside 2 days per week for hospital partners and 3 days per week for student training.

One rule that should be established early is the need to have some "skin in the game." Each partner should have a stake in the outcome of the simulation program and an interest in the program's success. As grant funding diminished, the program was challenged to cover the technician and simulation coordinator positions. The partners were asked to contribute an annual cash or in-kind match in the form of a **partnership fee**.

At this point, with 2 years of implementation completed, the partners were very satisfied with the outcomes attained from simulation. They readily agreed to the increased commitment. The community college, however, could not match this requirement and withdrew from the partnership. The university met its commitment by imposing course fees on students for use of the program. The partnership fee allowed the program to be able to establish an annual budget with predictable resources. In turn, the partners were encouraged to use the program more because they paid in advance for a specified number of training days. Partnerships can become "win-win" through

TABLE 2.9.1	
Education Needs Identified	
University	**Hospital**
Simulation space	Efficient use of existing space
Protect patient safety	Improve patient safety
Expand enrollment	Recruit and retain skilled personnel
Training equipment	Training equipment
Clinical sites	Certification requirements
Interdisciplinary training	Team training
Expanded training options	High-risk low-volume event training
Quality and risk management	Quality and risk management

using creative methods to strengthen their financial infrastructure and in some cases expand programs.

Establish a Stable but Flexible Environment

Both academic health professional schools and hospitals have some common elements. Both typically provide education and strive to prepare practitioners to provide excellent care to patients. However, their approaches to problem solving can lead to differences in priorities. Both education and service need to optimize opportunities through flexible processes.

Stability for the Center was achieved by agreeing to an organized schedule of usage for each partner and clear policies for how the program was to be used. However, as needed, policies were reframed or evolved. For example, the original plan was to train staff of each partnership to be able to program and run the mannequins, so each partner would provide its own technician. It quickly became obvious this policy was unworkable, and would not provide the greatest expertise or optimal conditions for maintaining the mannequins. The technician component was centralized, adding an additional cost to running the program.

Another key element in establishing a stable program was the implementation of educator training courses. Initially, the hospital educators and academic educators created separate courses to provide the necessary training in simulation methods. Having two courses was expensive and wasteful. It became evident that training needs for the two groups were similar, and in fact, the courses would be richer if the two groups were combined. The academic educators were experts in development of objectives and course design; the hospital educators provided clinical experts and current standards of practice. The courses stress collaboration between partners to maximize each contribution. Coleman et al. (2011) reports similar findings as a common bond that was created through the development of a network of capable faculty. Educators who participate and collaborate will support standardized simulation methodologies and shared teaching effectiveness. The educators embraced simulation methods that provided a stable foundation and common language for the partnership.

BEEN THERE, DONE THAT: HOW CAN I CONTINUE TO IMPROVE OR SUSTAIN WHAT I HAVE ACHIEVED?

Develop Policies

Early in the partnership, policies were developed to guide the Rural SimCenter development. Policies on priority use, educator training, supplies and equipment were necessary to make sure each partner had equal standing. Priority scheduling schemes were devised to ensure that each partner had priority access to specific days of the week. The goal was to give each partner a dependable schedule. The agreement

was that the priority days had to be booked at least 6 weeks in advance. Any open days on the schedule after the 6-week window were open to "first come, first serve" booking. This required the development of an online scheduling system that could be viewed remotely by all partners.

Other guidelines included educational policies that would determine who could hold classes at the Rural SimCenter, continued simulation training requirements for educators, policies for evaluating all the courses conducted, and advisory board attendance policies.

Develop Communication Abilities

Communication is an essential, yet difficult part of partnership development. Open communication is the basis for a strong partnership (Zahorsky, n.d.). One way communication is facilitated is through an informative website (http://www.csuchico.edu/nurs/SimCenter/index.html). The Rural SimCenter website was developed to communicate the answers to frequently asked questions as well as provide links for scheduling and course resources. The website answered common questions such as: How do I schedule a simulation session? What days are open on the calendar? What forms do I need to have my students complete?

Misunderstandings and communication errors may upset the fragile partnership balance. Advisory board meetings were an essential part of communicating Simulation Center plans, problems, and procedures. In addition to formal communications, reporting on simulation education outcomes for each partner has been a tool to support partnership involvement and document the return on investment. Each partner receives semiannual reports on the number of student/staff visits, and evaluation outcomes. Lujan reports the importance of developing and implementing procedures and tracking documentation (Lujan et al., 2011).

Assure Partner Status Is Fair and Equal

In an effective partnership, the value of each partner should be recognized. Partnerships can be comprised of partners with different assets and capabilities with the proper coordination. Each partner's contribution is valued, and each partner is treated equally. A winning business enterprise capitalizes on the strengths and skills of each partner. Clearly established procedures, developed and agreed to by the advisory board, assure that each partner has equal access to the program to meet its needs.

As the Center expanded, we have been able to invite an additional hospital partner, without limiting access to the former partners. The Rural SimCenter has different types of partner investments, but each plays an important role in simulation program sustainability. One hospital provides the space, the school of nursing provides budgetary management, a part-time faculty coordinator, and modest operating expenses provided by student course fees; two hospitals contribute an annual partnership fee. Without a balanced approach, development of an effective partnership is threatened. "When information flows freely, people trust each other and are loyal to each other," it is possible to achieve amazing results (Dent, 2006).

Essential to establishing partnership equality was the development of a business plan that clearly outlined the role of each partner, expectations, policies, and the simulation program mission and values. Dent (2006) comments that collaboration and interdependence doesn't come naturally to most organizations. The goal is to leverage connectedness (p. 1).

Competition between partners was a concern. In the case of the Rural SimCenter, the hospital partners were collaborators for improved healthcare in the region, but also competitors for their individual business interests. Located 20 miles (32.2 km) apart, the hospitals share potential consumers of medical, surgical, and obstetric care, as well as emergency services. The hospitals all had a developed working relationship as a foundation, and all hospitals provided clinical experiences for the School of Nursing. By working through the SimCenter Partnership, it was possible to set aside the fear of losing resources and shift to the strong commitment each partner had to increasing patient safety.

The advisory board structure ensured that each partner has equal representation. An important component of commitment was to include not only the leadership representatives for each partner, but also the predominant users of each partner—the end-users of the program. Nursing administration was represented on the board as well as the nursing educators. It was crucial for the educators who used the program to be able to give input to the vision as well as the operating principles. Initially, the advisory board met monthly while policies and procedures were being developed and implemented. Currently, the advisory board meets quarterly. Specialized committees were established to improve the ability to work on problems. Each subcommittee reports to the advisory board.

Sherwood (2006) states, "partnerships are founded on sharing to create an alliance for mutual cooperation and responsibility to achieve goals that are mutually beneficial" (p. 552). The quality and safety agenda is advanced through improved patient care outcomes that can result from simulation partnerships. Team building can result through collaboration to develop meaningful scenarios and learning environments through a sharing of resources. In addition, regional discussions have occurred as a result of this partnership, supporting the notion that regional simulation program can be the catalyst for discussion of competency issues in nursing, which may result in changes to the standards of care (Sportsman et al., 2009).

Develop a Strategic Plan

Early development of a business plan provided timely direction and a foundation to the partnership model. The development of a strategic plan provided the roadmap to the partnership agreement and provided the basis for business planning. The plan provides a detailed account of how the organizations will cooperate and collaborate to provide a sustainable simulation program with enhanced capabilities and diverse educational expertise. By developing a strategic plan, a strategic framework is established that will lead to a culture of partnership (Dent, 2006; Table 2.9.2).

While a partnership agreement is recommended for transparency, the agreement will not sustain the partnership relationship if the outcomes are not satisfactory for each partner (Dent, 2006). The partnership must provide recognizable benefits for all involved, with the idea that each partner's critical strengths and contributions can make the whole greater than the sum of its parts. The partnership continues, with each agency believing that the benefits are greater than if it tried to function on its own. Hospitals donate equipment and outdated supplies; hospitals bring current practice standards and clinical expertise to review and validate scenarios. The school of nursing provides updates on current research, educational expertise, and master's students and graduates who contribute to scenario validation, and to the pool of expert simulation educators for the region. The graduates of the nursing program supply the hospitals with better-prepared staff nurses, and with nurses who are familiar with and enthusiastic about simulation as part of their ongoing development of expertise. Regional workshops on simulation with national speakers on debriefing, evaluation, and research have been offered to enhance the expertise of all who are using simulation. The hospitals provide the region with more efficient, high-functioning teams, with better communication, team leadership, and safety functions, improving the healthcare for all, and providing more effective role modeling for the students they mentor.

Plan for Sustainability from the Beginning

Many established simulation program experience ongoing struggles with sustainability. Overcoming the initial start-up hurdles is not the end of the challenges for a new program. Simulators quickly become outdated, having limited lifespans, and fall prey to new technologies. Ongoing capital expenses will need to be met. A successful business plan will take these contingencies into account, with an ongoing schedule for planned replacement of equipment.

TABLE 2.9.2
Partnership Agreement Goals
1. To provide clear statement of duties and obligations related to the partnership to avoid misunderstandings.
2. To provide guidance regarding the appropriate direction if there is a disagreement among the partners.
3. To provide clarity for grants, accrediting bodies, and potential investors.

Adapted from Dent, S. (2006). *Partnership relationship management: Implementing a plan for success* (Partnering Intelligence White Paper). Partnership Continuum, Inc. Retrieved from http://www.partneringintelligence.com/documents/5.03_Partnership_Relationship_Management_WP.pdf.

If the budget does not accommodate this renewal, the plan will need to include sources of new revenue streams or community fundraising efforts.

The Rural SimCenter developed a sustainability plan through the use of partnership fees, student fees, and outside user fees to provide a consistent revenue stream for budgeting. Additionally, donations are obtained from community and service organizations committed to quality healthcare in the region.

Ongoing staffing needs demanded that the program be fully utilized, so it was essential to provide an online calendar and reservation system. A rational balance should be maintained between the ongoing investment and the hours of actual utilization, the numbers of trainees, and ultimately, the beneficial outcomes of using simulation. Dent comments, "The ability to partner successfully results in a workplace where people want to stay and contribute their best talents" (p. 9).

For programs that are underused, the power of partnerships should not be overlooked as one way of capitalizing on regional strengths and resources, to achieve maximal benefit from the investment in simulation equipment, and to maintain efficiency and expertise in simulation education. Many healthcare professionals who are not part of simulation partnerships would benefit from the team training and practice opportunities afforded by simulation. Marketing to these professionals for annual practice sessions can provide a revenue stream, and allow full utilization of a valued resource. Likewise, public health and community safety agencies are potentially eager consumers of a simulation program's expertise, for example, planning how to respond to mass casualty or pandemic events. Expertise in moulage, scenario planning, and implementation are great assets to market, to maintain revenue streams, increase the visibility of simulation, and expand potential partnerships.

SUMMARY

As evidence for the benefits of simulation for training healthcare personnel continues to amass, more healthcare agencies and educational institutions are realizing they must embrace simulation training, as part of quality and safety initiatives, and even as a recruitment and retention strategy, to achieve or maintain excellence and remain competitive. The Rural SimCenter has achieved sustainability through partnership commitment, strategic planning, and community participation.

The academic-practice partnership model has been around for more than half a century (Campbell, 2001). The idea of collaboration between academic institutions and service is a model that has had tremendous support and longevity; however, specific information about how effective partnerships are developed and the cost-effectiveness of establishing a model to support simulation program development is missing.

At the Rural SimCenter, programs have expanded and evolved into state-of-the-art simulation courses. The partnership serves as a rural model for ways in which a university and community organizations can interrelate and interact. Central lessons include the significance of sharing values and goals and the benefit of drawing on the different strengths of each partner.

This chapter summarizes strategies to achieve a highly successful partnership and includes examples of the many benefits of a simulation partnership. The emphasis is on long-term viability and full utilization of simulation program as a valuable regional resource to improve professional education and practice.

REFERENCES

Beal, J., Breslin, E., Austin, T., Brower, L., Bullard, K., Light, K., . . . Ray, N. (2011). Hallmarks of best practice in academic-service partnerships in nursing: Lessons learned from San Antonio. *Journal of Professional Nursing, 27*(6), e90–e95. doi:10.1016/j.profnurs.2011.07.006

Beal, J. A., Green, A., & Bakewell-Sachs, S. (2011). The time is right—the time is now . . . Academic-service partnerships need to be revisited. *Journal of Professional Nursing, 27*(6), 330–331. doi:10.1016/j.profnurs.2011.10.005

Campbell, S. L., Prater, M., Schwartz, C., & Ridenour, N. (2001). Building an empowering academic and practice partnership model. *Nursing Administration Quarterly, 26*(1), 35–44.

Carney, J., Maltby, H., Mackin, K., & Maksym, M. (2011). Community-academic partnerships: How can communities benefit? *American Journal of Preventive Medicine, 41*(4 Suppl. 3), S206–S213.

Coleman, P., Dufrene, C., Bonner, R., Martinez, J., Dawkins, V., Koch, M., . . . Norman, G. (2011). A regional partnership to promote nursing instructor competence and confidence in simulation. *Journal of Professional Nursing, 27*(6), e28–e32. doi:10.1016/j.profnurs.2011.09.003

Curtin, M., & Dupuis, M. (2008). Development of human patient simulation programs: Achieving big results with a small budget. *Journal of Nursing Education, 47*(11), 522–523. doi:10.3928/01484834-20081101-02

Dent, S. (2006). *Partnership relationship management: Implementing a plan for success* (Partnering Intelligence White Paper). Partnership Continuum, Inc. Retrieved from http://www.partneringintelligence.com/documents/5.03_Partnership_Relationship_Management_WP.pdf

Erickson, J., & Raines, D. (2011). Expanding an academic-practice partnership. *Journal of Professional Nursing, 27*(6), e71–e75. doi:10.1016/j.profnurs.2011.08.003

Granger, B. B., Prvu-Bettger, J., Aucoin, J., Fuchs, M., Mitchell, P. H., Holditch-Davis, D., . . . Gilliss, C. L. (2012). An academic-health service partnership in nursing: Lessons from the field. *Journal of Nursing Scholarship, 44*(1), 71–79. doi:10.1111/j.1547-5069.2011.01432.x

Internal Revenue Service. (2012). *Partnerships.* Retrieved from http://www.irs.gov/businesses/small/article/0,id=98214,00.html

Lujan, J., Stout, R., Meager, G., Ballesteros, P., Cruz, M., & Estrada, I. (2011). Partnering to maximize simulation-based learning: Nursing regional interdisciplinary simulation centers. *Journal of Professional Nursing, 27*(6), e41–e45. doi:10.1016/j.profnurs.2011.07.001

Roussos, S.T[1].,& Fawcett, S.B. (2000). A review of collaborative partnerships as a strategy for improving community health. *Annu Rev Public Health,* 21, 369–402.

Sherwood, G. (2006). Appreciative leadership: Building customer-driven partnerships. *Journal of Nursing Administration, 36*(1), 551–557.

Sportsman, S., Bolton, C., Bradshaw, P., Close, D., Lee, M., Townley, N., & Watson, M. (2009). A regional simulation center partnership: collaboration to improve staff and student competency. *Journal of Continuing Education In Nursing, 40*(2), 67–73. doi:10.3928/00220124-20090201-09

Zahorsky, D. (n.d.). *Creating a winning business partnership.* About.com. Retrieved from http://sbinformation.about.com/cs/bestpractices/a/aa030203a.htm

SECTION 3

Simulators

CHAPTER 3.1

A History of Modern-Day Mannequins

Frederick L. Slone, MD, and Samsun Lampotang, PhD

ABOUT THE AUTHORS

FREDERICK L. SLONE is the Medical Director of the Center for Advanced Clinical Learning at the University of South Florida (USF) Morsani College of Medicine and concurrently an Associate Professor of Medicine. Retired from a successful career in gastroenterology, he has been involved in simulation for medical education for the past 8 years, actively involved in obtaining accreditation for simulation at USF, and was in the first group of candidates to be recognized as a Certified Healthcare Simulation Educator (CHSE) by the Society for Simulation in Healthcare.

SAMSUN (SEM) LAMPOTANG coinvented the Human Patient Simulator (HPS) mannequin patient simulator and the Web-enabled Virtual Anesthesia Machine simulation portfolio. His contributions span the physicality-virtuality continuum of simulation, including mixed reality simulation, use of virtual humans for clinical team training, pervasive simulation on mobile devices, and race-specific pharmacodynamics modeling. His simulation accomplishments have been recognized via numerous awards, including the 2007 Society for Education in Anesthesia/Duke Award for Excellence and Innovation in Anesthesia Education.

Acknowledgments: The authors would like to personally thank the many individuals that were willing to spend their time on the phone telling their personal stories regarding the development of the mannequin patient simulators. Their stories and insight were an invaluable part of this manuscript. These individuals are cited with in-text citations.

ABSTRACT

This chapter provides a brief historical overview of the development of the modern mannequins used to simulate a full-bodied human that are computer controlled and programmable with multiple features that mimic a human patient, including, at a minimum, chest wall movement and palpable pulses. A review of the development of mannequin patient simulators gives a perspective on the varying types of motivation that led to the present-day simulators, including a short history of the various companies that produce simulators.

CASE EXAMPLE

For many, working in simulation represents part of a second career. Previously working as full-time physicians, nurses, paramedics, and other healthcare professionals, working and teaching with simulation represented a natural extension of their former full-time careers. Here is a story that may sound familiar to some of the readers of this textbook.

After having been a gastroenterologist in private practice for over 26 years and then retiring from that career, Dr. Slone began teaching at the College of Nursing and Medicine at the University of South Florida. After about a year of his new career, his wife one day asked him what he was doing in his new job. He answered that he was doing a lot of work on mannequins and programming them to simulate complicated clinical scenarios to better train students to respond appropriately in critical care situations. To this she replied, "You mean you are playing with dolls????" His ego was completely deflated. Going from Chief of Endoscopy to playing with dolls? He did not know exactly how to respond. Perturbed, he blurted out, "Yes, I am playing with dolls!" The question haunted him until one day he realized that his wife had given him a remarkable insight into why the simulation seemed such a powerful tool for teaching. All children grow up playing with "dolls" and "toy trucks and cars." A significant part of their natural learning process is basically a simulation of the reality they will eventually experience. Simulation is, in fact, a natural part of everyone's learning process.

INTRODUCTION AND BACKGROUND

Mannequins have been used for centuries to facilitate the education of health professions. However, with the explosion in technology over the last six decades, the growth in the industry has been exponential. Many of those who are working today in the field of healthcare simulation have asked about the development of the modern mannequin patient simulator. Knowing the history of these devices will provide simulation educators with a better understanding of and appreciation for these technological wonders.

HISTORY OF THE MANNEQUIN PATIENT SIMULATOR

The history of the present-day mannequin patient simulators is comprised of several different, independent paths arising from differing motivations. An interest in recreating human physiology for the purpose of training anesthesia residents was the motivation behind the earliest mannequin patient simulator.

The idea of the simulator was conceived by Dr. Stephen Abrahamson, a medical educator (Dr. Abrahamson's profession was incorrectly stated in the noted reference Cooper & Taqueti, 2004 [J. Cooper, personal communication]), and Dr. Judson Denson, an anesthesiologist at the University of Southern California in the mid-1960s. It was built in collaboration with Sierra Engineering and Aerojet General Corporation (Cooper & Taqueti, 2004), and called "Sim One." Sim One was funded by a $272,000 grant from the US Office of Education to build a prototype. With this funding, a sophisticated, full-body, remarkably lifelike, mannequin patient simulator was created. "It was controlled by a hybrid digital and analogue computer and had 4,096 words of memory. The chest was anatomically shaped and moved with breathing, the eyes blinked, the pupils could dilate and constrict, and the jaw opened and closed" (Cooper & Taqueti, 2004). The simulator was used to train anesthesia residents. Unfortunately, only one Sim One was constructed, and apparently nothing remains of it now. It was far too expensive for commercialization, and at the time the market for this type of simulation was not there (Cooper & Taqueti, 2004). It was also bulky and not easily transported because the computer controlling the simulator occupied an entire wall of a room (N. Gravenstein as told to him by J.S. Gravenstein, personal communication, July 18, 2012; Figure 3.1.1).

In the late 1980s, two independent groups, one from Stanford Medical School and the other from the University of Florida, created simulators for anesthesia training. The Stanford group was led by Dr. David Gaba, an anesthesiologist working at the VA Palo Alto Medical Center. The goals were, first, to study human performance in the operating room and, later, to train anesthesia residents. To achieve this goal, his group believed that a computer-controlled simulator would be necessary to create scenarios that would only rarely be encountered on real patients. They

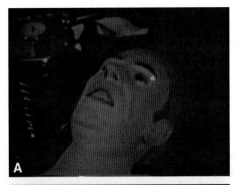
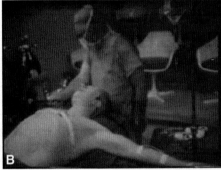

FIGURE 3.1.1   The Sim One simulator. **A.** Face. **B.** SimOne ventilating.

built the first simulator in 1987 and 1988 with an off-the-shelf mannequin with a head, neck, thorax, and two elastic lung bags. They added the appropriate tubing to carry CO_2 to the lungs. They used a wave-form generator to create EKG rhythms and wrote software to manipulate the blood pressure, pulse rate, and oxygen saturations. They then created a realistic anesthesia environment around the simulator; hence the name Comprehensive Anesthesia Simulation Environment (CASE). To guide instruction with the simulator, they developed a curriculum for Anesthesia Crisis Resource Management (ACRM) based on the aviation model of Crew Resource Management (CRM). In 1992, the Stanford group collaborated with CAE-Link to develop a sophisticated mannequin patient simulator. (CAE-Link was a descendant of the original Link Aeronautical Corporation that produced the Link trainer, the first significant simulator used in aviation.) CAE-Link later became CAE Medical Electronics, which later sold the business to Eagle of Binghamton, New York. In 1994, in collaboration with Dr. Howard Schwid and Dr. David Gaba, physiologic modeling was incorporated into the mannequin. Dr. Schwid was an anesthesiologist at the University of Washington with extensive experience in physiologic modeling. The first model of this mannequin patient simulator was introduced in 1995 (D.M. Gaba, personal communication, June 15, 2012). The mannequin was able to be intubated "and could be altered to mimic degrees of difficulty with intubation. It had palpable carotid and radial pulses, lungs that simulated behavior during spontaneous and controlled ventilation, heart and breath sounds and eyes that opened and closed" (Cooper & Taqueti, 2004). The system "allowed for automatic responses to drug interventions entered by the operator and for manual manipulation of physiologic variables" (Cooper & Taqueti, 2004). Eagle simulation eventually merged (D.M. Gaba, personal communication, June 15, 2012) with an Israeli company, Med-Sim, and the mannequin patient simulator was known as the MedSim Eagle Patient Simulator and sold throughout the world (Figure 3.1.2).

Interestingly, a few years later, the METI "Human Patient Simulator," developed by the team at the University of Florida (please see the next paragraph for details), also came on the market. Both simulators sold for about $200,000, and the sales of each were comparable over the subsequent 5 years (D.M. Gaba, personal communication, June 15, 2012). In 2000, MedSim felt that the profits in this were not nearly as much as profits in other Internet ventures, and they stopped manufacturing the MedSim Eagle simulator, and abandoned the project completely. In addition, there was no attempt by the company to sell the technology to anyone else (D.M. Gaba, personal communication, June 15, 2012). However, as a testament to the durability and utility of the product, there are some of these models that are still in use today (R.R. Kyle, personal communication, June 8, 2012). Even longer lasting than the mannequin was Dr. Gaba's contribution to the use of simulation in healthcare. The Anesthesia Crisis Resource Management program was introduced by Dr. Gaba to Harvard University in 1992 and was used to train a number of Harvard anesthesiologists (Cooper & Taqueti, 2004). Success with this method led to the establishment of a collaborative educational center dedicated to simulation-based training, and was named the "Boston Anesthesia Simulation Center," later renamed the "Center for Medical Simulation" (Cooper & Taqueti, 2004).

Another chapter in the history of the mannequin patient simulator occurred in parallel to the chapter described above. In the late 1980s, a multidisciplinary team from the University of Florida, in Gainesville, Florida, developed the Gainesville Anesthesia Simulator (GAS). The original team consisted of Dr. Michael Good, an anesthesiologist, Dr. Samsun (Sem) Lampotang (then a doctoral candidate in mechanical engineering) and Dr. J.S. Gravenstein, another anesthesiologist. This team was later joined by Ronald Carovano, Jr., MBA, and Dr. Willem Van Meurs.

The basic driving force behind the development of this simulator was to train anesthesia residents in basic clinical skills. One of the first aims of the project was to train anesthesia residents in recognizing faults in anesthesia machines. They embedded computer-controllable mechanical failures into an actual anesthesia machine. The next step was adding clinical signs and a lung simulator to their rigged anesthesia machine. This eventually led to the creation of a full-body mannequin. A sophisticated lung model was developed that mimicked the uptake and distribution of anesthetic gases. Further physiologic modeling was created to mimic human respiratory, circulatory, and cardiac physiology. The first full-bodied simulator incorporating all of these physiologic models was built in 1997. This product was originally licenced to Loral Data Systems Inc. Lou Oberndorf spun off the mannequin simulator to form a new company, Medical Education Technologies Inc. (METI), located in Sarasota, Florida, which was acquired by CAE Healthcare in 2011. The METI product was named the Human Patient Simulator (HPS), and this product competed with the MedSim Eagle simulator until the year 2000 when the MedSim Eagle simulator went out of production (S. Lampotang, personal communication, July 18, 2012; Figure 3.1.3).

The next chapter in mannequin patient simulators starts from a very different impetus. The driving force behind the next set of mannequin patient simulators was that of teaching cardiopulmonary resuscitation (CPR) to healthcare providers using computer-controlled mannequins. Three companies that were involved in this development were Laerdal, Simulaids, and Gaumard.

Laerdal Medical started as a small publishing house in the 1940s. It specialized in greeting cards and children's books. The company expanded into manufacturing wooden toys. Pioneering in soft plastics in the early 1950s, Laerdal made millions of realistic play dolls and "furniture friendly" toy cars. With the knowhow gained from producing toys, Laerdal began to make realistic wound models (Laerdal, 2012). In the late 1950s, Dr. Peter Safar and others, working at Baltimore City Hospital, developed the techniques of modern CPR. Dr. Safar was an anesthesiologist, and this prompted a Norwegian anesthesiologist,

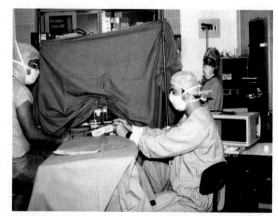

FIGURE 3.1.2 Photo of Dr. Gaba with CASE prototype.

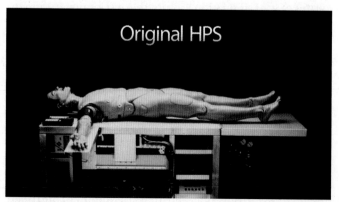

FIGURE 3.1.3 Original METI HPS mannequin. (Photo courtesy of Kim Cartlidge of CAE Healthcare.)

A MEMOIR—EARLY DAYS OF SIMULATION
Samsun Lampotang, PhD
Coinventor of the Human Patient Simulator, and Director, Center for Safety, Simulation & Advanced Learning Technologies, University of Florida

I attend the International Meeting on Simulation in Healthcare every year. Every time, I have to pinch myself when I see how well attended the meeting is, with an ever increasing number of new and creative applications of simulation, exhibitors, and products in the industry exhibit area and international attendees. Having been privileged to be at a ground zero (the University of Florida in Gainesville; the other one David Gaba's lab at Stanford University) of the rebirth of mannequin patient simulation, simulation has grown beyond even my wildest dreams when one bears in mind that when we started developing mannequin patient simulators in the late 1980s, there were only two mannequin patient simulators, the prototypes at Stanford and the University of Florida. In those early days, educators newly introduced to simulation would often ask us how many scenarios could be run on our mannequin patient simulator to understand and quantify its capabilities; our practiced (but true) answer was that the number of scenarios was only limited by the instructor's imagination. While I am not sure whether our answer was helpful, it is certainly gratifying to note that the simulation community has indeed not lacked for imagination, using simulation in ways that, ironically, I never imagined back then, such as *in situ* simulation (see chapter 2.2) and Just In Time (JIT) simulation (see chapter 2.6)!

The existential question in the nascent years was whether simulation would reach adulthood or would meet a premature demise like Sim One in the 1960s. While this may seem like paranoia now to the current generation that takes simulation in healthcare for granted, simulation was disruptive, as Jeff Cooper aptly described it. Like any disruptive technology, even if it was disruptive in a good sense as Jeff clarified, it challenged established ways of doing things and placed some outside their comfort zone. Funding for simulation in healthcare research and development was scarce. Reviewers for traditional journals were unfamiliar with the technology, making it harder to publish simulation-related papers; it was a godsend when the Society for Simulation in Healthcare launched its new journal, *Simulation in Healthcare*, providing a sorely needed outlet for simulation-related papers. In those early days when simulation was still a novelty that we exhibited in the United States and around the world, I noticed that those who embraced simulation were generally younger, while senior clinicians were a bit more reserved and literally kept their distance from the simulator. We were fortunate to have had wise influential elders in J.S. Gravenstein, MD, Ellison (Jeep) Pierce, MD, and others in the Anesthesia Patient Safety Foundation who could glimpse simulation's

potential and helped protect and nurture the flickering flame of simulation. Later, enthusiastic participants inquired about when simulation would be used for healthcare certification as it was in aviation. At the time, we considered certification the third rail of simulation, and my coinventor Mike Good and I had an agreement that we would never mention "simulation" and "certification" in the same sentence when giving demonstrations of what would eventually become the Human Patient Simulator (HPS). One can imagine the profound sense of elation in witnessing the sea change in attitudes where simulation is now a part of the required Maintenance of Certification in Anesthesiology (MOCA)!

By number of years alone and using the late 1980s as the birth of simulation in healthcare, we could declare that it has reached adulthood. I, for one, believe that simulation in healthcare is still in its adolescence partly because it still has a "crush" on mannequin patient simulators, its first love. Simulation in healthcare has so much more to offer than just mannequin patient simulation. I have been fortunate that our plans to form a company to build and disseminate our mannequin patient simulators did not materialize and that this task was instead entrusted into the capable hands of Lou Oberndorf and his team from Loral. Not being involved in the commercialization of the HPS provided me the opportunity to obtain funding to conduct hands-on research across the entire physicality-virtuality spectrum of simulation such as Web-enabled screen-based simulation, mixed reality simulations, and virtual humans for team training. Having worked with all these different simulation modalities has only reinforced my belief that simulation is not an end in itself but a means to an end, namely improved patient outcomes through simulation-based acquisition or enhancement of skills (affective, cognitive, and psychomotor). Improvement in patient outcomes directly attributable to simulation training was considered in the early days as the Holy Grail that has, in our lifetime, been shown to be attainable through the landmark papers by Draycott and Barsuk. The future of simulation is indeed bright. The best is yet to come.

REFERENCES
Barsuk, J.H., Cohen, E.R., Feinglass, J., McGaghie, W.C., Wayne, D.B. (2009). Use of simulation-based education to reduce catheter-related bloodstream infections. *Archives of Internal Medicine, 169*(15), 1420–1423.

Draycott, T., Sibanda, T., Owen, L., Akande, V., Winter, C., Reading, S., & Whitelaw, A. (2006). Does training in obstetric emergencies improve neonatal outcome? *BJOG: An International Journal of Obstetrics & Gynaecology, 113*(2), 177–182.

Dr. Bjorn Lind, to have Asmund Laerdal, the founder of the Laerdal company, create a mannequin named Resusci Anne that could be used in mouth-to-mouth ventilation. It was constructed so that the neck had to be extended and chin lifted to open the airway to allow chest movement with breathing. Safar later advised Laerdal to include an internal spring attached to the chest wall, to simulate cardiac compression (Cooper & Taqueti, 2004). Resusci Anne subsequently became the most widely used mannequin for CPR training in the 1960s and 1970s.

Of interest is the face of Resusci Anne, which anyone who did CPR training on this mannequin can vividly remember. At the turn of the 19th century, the body of a young girl was pulled from the River Seine in Paris. There was no evidence of violence, and it was assumed she had taken her own life. Because her identity could not be established, a death mask was made, which was customary in such cases. The young girl's delicate beauty and ethereal smile added to the enigma of her death. Romantic stories that speculated on this mystery were published.

According to one, her death was the result of an unrequited romance. The story became popular throughout Europe, as did reproductions of her death mask. Moved by the story of the girl so tragically taken by early death, Armand Laerdal adopted her mask for the face of his new resuscitation training mannequin, which was Resusci Anne. Asmund Laerdal was convinced that if such a mannequin was life-size and lifelike, students would be better motivated to learn this lifesaving procedure. With the introduction of Resusci Anne the company dedicated itself to advancing the cause of resuscitation and emergency care. Toy production was deemphasized, and Laerdal Medical became dedicated to resuscitation and emergency care (Laerdal, 2012; Figure 3.1.4).

In the mid-1990s, the Laerdal company was encouraged by a number of people to develop a high-technology mannequin. One of those people was Dr. Ake Grenvik, who was a colleague of Dr. Peter Safar at the University of Pittsburgh. Subsequently, Drs. Rene Gonzales and John Schaefer, also at the University of Pittsburgh at that time, developed a more anatomically correct airway and mannequin, which were manufactured by the Medical Plastics Corporation (MPL) of Texas. Laerdal acquired MPL and developed the final product, SimMan (Cooper & Taqueti, 2004; J.J. Schaefer, personal communication, June 14, 2012). SimMan was first marketed in 2001. SimMan was highly successful, and Laerdal has since greatly expanded its line of mannequins, which are used extensively throughout the world. The tetherless SimMan 3G, Laerdal's most sophisticated mannequin, became available in 2010 (Figure 3.1.5).

Simulaids began to make moulage products for healthcare in the 1960s, and Simulaids is the original name of the company. Based on a demand for products to teach advanced CPR techniques to emergency medical technicians

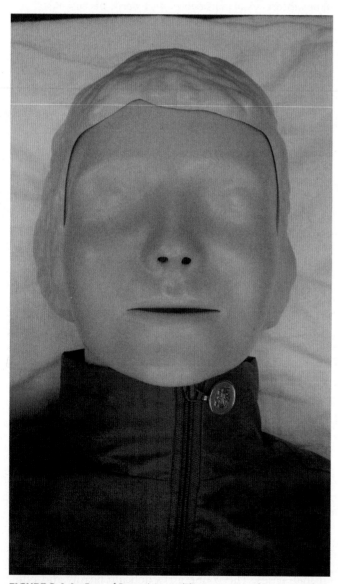

FIGURE 3.1.4   Face of Resusci Anne. (Photo courtesy of Dr. Slone of the University of South Florida.)

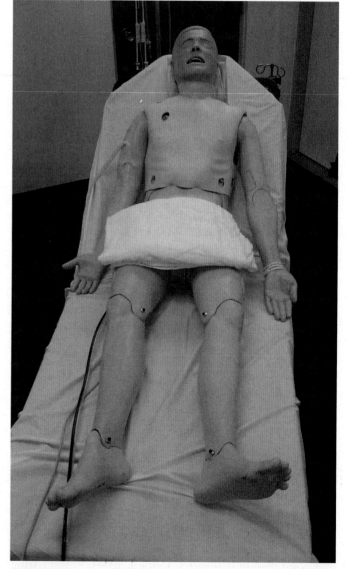

FIGURE 3.1.5   Laerdal SimMan mannequin. (Photo courtesy of Dr. Slone of the University of South Florida.)

and paramedics, they developed the 300 STAT Simulator that arrived on the scene in July 2001. This was a full-sized mannequin, 6′1″ and 200 lb, that was manually operated and included an ECG rhythm generator. This was specifically designed for Emergency Medical Services (EMS) training. Then, in January 2004, they released the PDA STAT, an electronic patient simulator operated with a Personal Digital Assistant (PDA) device. The mannequin patient simulator had to be plugged in, but had a compressor in its leg to create hydraulic pulses and lung movements. It was intubatable, had a menu of various cardiac rhythms, and pulses were present in 14 places. The mannequin was also programmable. It had a sales price of under $10,000. The product was well received and has had a steady audience of users, especially in the Emergency Medical Services world, over the years (W. Johnson, personal communication, August 7, 2012; Simulaids, 2012; Figure 3.1.6).

Another company that independently developed mannequin patient simulators is the Gaumard Scientific Company, Inc. Gaumard traces its development back to 1946, when its founder, a World War II trauma physician, recognized how polymers used in reconstructive and battlefield surgery could be used to create simulators for healthcare education. The first product was a synthetic human skeleton. In 1949, Gaumard introduced a childbirth simulator, designed at the request of the international health community, to improve the clinical competence of village midwives to reduce maternal and infant mortality and morbidity. Since that time, Gaumard has dedicated its resources to continue the development of innovative teaching simulators in nursing care, emergency care, and obstetrics and gynecology (Gaumard, 2012). In 1995, a product called Code Blue III simulators was produced that used computer controls to interact with the simulator. In 2000, Gaumard produced Noelle, a maternal and neonatal childbirth simulator. In 2004, Gaumard produced the tetherless HAL adult mannequin patient simulator (Gaumard, 2012; Figure 3.1.7).

The highly sophisticated MedSim Eagle and METI HPS mannequins were also very costly, with a price tag of approximately $200,000. This limited their use and availability to institutions that could afford this high price. In contrast, the Laerdal, Simulaids, and Gaumard mannequins ranged in price from $10,000 to $40,000. Although they lacked the sophistication of the MedSim Eagle and METI HPS mannequins, they were easy to use and had

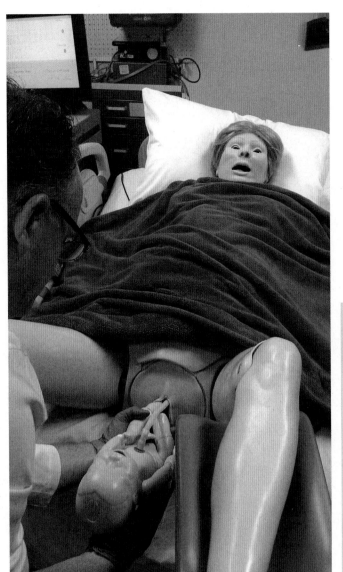

FIGURE 3.1.7 Gaumard Noelle delivering a baby at the University of South Florida College of Nursing. (Photo courtesy of Dr. Slone of the University of South Florida.)

adequate functionality to be used in a multitude of scenarios. Their affordability and ease of use created a much broader market for the mannequin patient simulators, and the popularity of the mannequin patient simulators began to grow quickly. METI, which initially had only produced the HPS simulator with a price tag of about $200,000, responded to this new market and developed the ECS (Emergency Care Simulator). This mannequin patient simulator still incorporated the underlying physiologic modeling of the more expensive HPS model and could do many of the functions of the HPS model but was priced at approximately $60,000 to compete in this growing market (Figure 3.1.8).

The development of the tetherless (can function for a period of time without cables connected) mannequins also had parallel developments. The Gaumard tetherless HAL mannequin became available in 2004 (Gaumard, 2012).

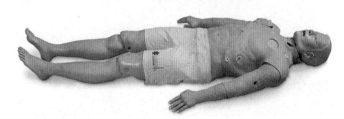

FIGURE 3.1.6 Simulaids Smart Stat Adult mannequin. (Photo courtesy of Warren Johnson of Simulaids.)

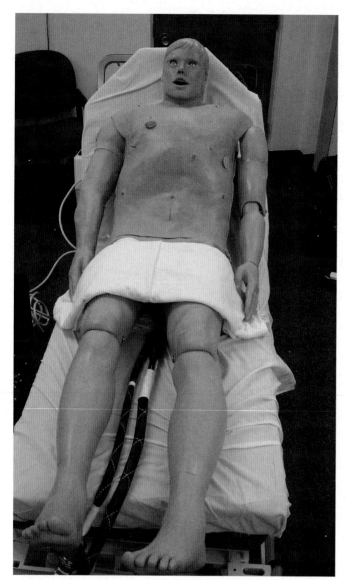

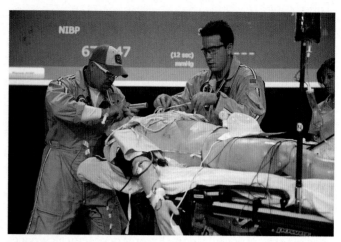

FIGURE 3.1.9   Tetherless CAE (METI) iStan being transported. (Photo courtesy of Kim Cartlidge of CAE Healthcare.)

FIGURE 3.1.8   METI ECS mannequin. (Photo courtesy of Dr. Slone of the University of South Florida.)

METI developed a tetherless mannequin that preserved the functionality of the METI ECS simulator and could be used in field training. Named iStan and introduced in 2007, the self-contained power and the compressor in its leg made it completely tetherless (R. Blumberg, personal communication, August 1, 2012). Laerdal also responded to the need for a tetherless mannequin and developed the Laerdal SimMan 3G, which became commercially available in 2010 (C. Baker, personal communication, July 31, 2012; Figures 3.1.9 and 3.1.10).

The more recent history of the development of mannequins specifically designed for combat medic training is again an interesting story of parallel development from a variety of companies and agencies.

Techline Trauma, which started in 1993 as a polymer lab that specialized in engineering services, produces the TOMManikin for military combat medic training.

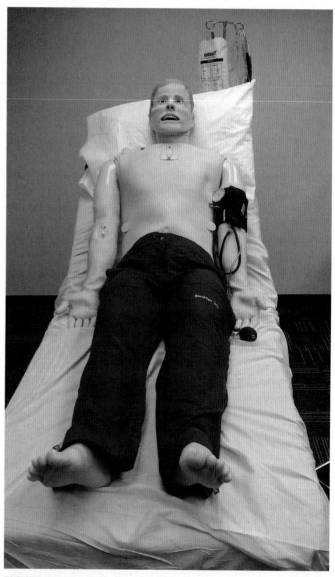

FIGURE 3.1.10   Tetherless Laerdal SimMan 3G. (Photo courtesy of Dr. Slone of the University of South Florida.)

Because of its expertise in polymers, it competed for and was awarded a grant from the US Army to develop realistic wound simulation models. A 3-year development program led to the creation of simulated wounds that could be worn by a human: without additional moulage, it could accurately simulate the most typical wounds seen in combat. In 2007, Techline demonstrated their wound models at the SOMA (Special Operations Medical Association) conference, and these models were well received. In 2010, a combat veteran by the name of Tech. Sgt. Keary J. Miller, an Air Force combat search and rescue team leader, became interested in Techline products and in creating a mannequin specific for combat medic training. Using his extensive experience as a pararescueman (United States Air Force Special Operations Command and Air Combat Command operatives tasked with recovery and medical treatment of personnel in humanitarian and combat environments [Wikipedia, n.d.-a]), Sgt. Miller designed the TOMManikin to be used in the most extreme physical conditions and to simulate the combat casualties that the military medics would most likely experience (D. Parry, personal communication, August 7, 2012; Techline, n.d.; Figure 3.1.11).

The CAE Caesar mannequin for combat medic training evolved from a physician-led engineering team in the Center for Integration of Medicine and Innovative Technology (CIMIT), a nonprofit consortium of Boston's teaching hospitals and leading universities (CIMIT, 2012). Early in the 21st century, Dr. Steven Dawson, an Interventional Radiologist at Massachusetts General Hospital, became involved in discussions with instructors training Army medics at Fort Sam Houston in Texas. At the time, the available simulators were not sufficiently rugged for use in austere conditions that the medics would be facing. The CIMIT group focused on the development of a mannequin that would be specific for combat medic training, easy to use, and rugged enough to be durable in austere conditions. The mannequin and system of training was named Combat Medic Training System

(COMETS). The initial funding for the project was from the US Army's Telemedicine and Advanced Technology Research Center (TATRC). TATRC could not provide sufficient funding to complete a working prototype. CIMIT licenced the technology to CAE Healthcare, which developed COMETS into Caesar Trauma Patient Simulator. Using expertise from civilian and military subject matter experts, Cesar was introduced at the 2011 International Meeting of Simulation in Healthcare (IMSH) in New Orleans (A. Rita, personal communication, August 15, 2012; Figure 3.1.12).

Another company involved in the production of mannequins for military combat medics is Kforce Government Solutions, Inc. (KGS), which produces the TraumaF/X line of training mannequins. These mannequins are ruggedized, untethered mannequins developed with RDECOM-ARL-STTC under the Severe Trauma Simulation Army Technology Objective. RDECOM is the U.S. Army Research, Development and Engineering Command. ARL is the Army Research Lab, and STTC is the Simulation and Training Technology Center, which conducts research and development of future training and simulation technologies to enhance the effectiveness of soldiers. The center is located in Orlando, FL, and houses engineers and scientists from the STTC, the ARL, the Army Research Institute (ARI), and the University of Central Florida Institute for Simulation and Training. The mannequins are the Multiple Amputation Trauma Trainer (MATT), a lower extremity unit that can be worn by a person to give the realistic appearance of multiple lower limb amputations. There is full motion animatronics built into the simulator so that the amputated limbs

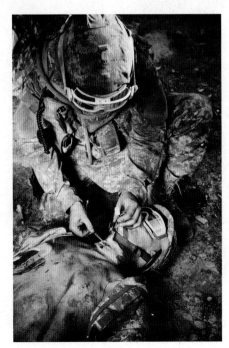

FIGURE 3.1.12   CAE Caesar undergoing a cricothyrotomy. (Photo courtesy of Kim Cartlidge of CAE Healthcare.)

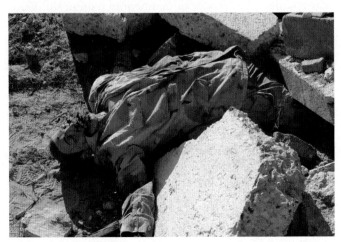

FIGURE 3.1.11   TOMManikin trapped under a collapsed building. (Picture supplied by Dave Parry, Sr. of Techline.)

move in a realistic fashion. The unit is tetherless and can be controlled remotely. In addition, an upper torso trainer with an airway is also made by this company (AirwayPlus Lifecast Upper Torso Trainer) for combat medic training. The TraumaF/X products have been awarded 2009, 2010, 2011 top merits for Army Modeling and Simulation as well as Innovation, and have also received the highest honors and awards in 2011 for National Defense Industry Association, Training and Simulation (KGS, n.d.; C. Hollander, personal communication, August 30, 2012; Figure 3.1.13).

In 2013, Gaumard introduced Combat HAL that is also designed for combat medic training in austere environments and was independently tested by the Aeromedical Research Laboratory to certify its use for in-flight training.

The software that controls the mannequin simulators has a history of its own. As mentioned, the METI products were initially based on a relatively complex underlying physiologic modeling: other products were operated primarily by manual adjustment of vital signs and key physiologic variables (see the section on the history of modeling below). Each type of operational control mode has

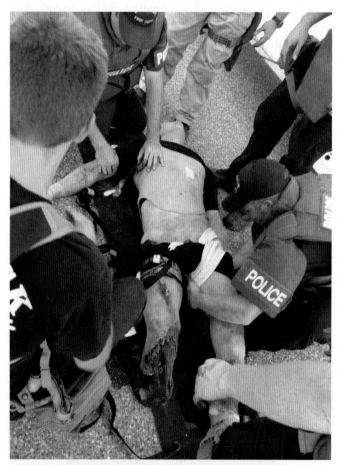

FIGURE 3.1.13   MATT trainer with APL Upper Torso Trainer by TraumaFX; Author: Ryan Lewis, Publisher: Special Tactics and Rescue Consulting, Copyright date: June 2013. (Picture supplied by Christina Witwer of KGS.)

its advantages and disadvantages. To provide the ease of the "plug in the number" model to operate, METI came out with the Müse software, which enabled the operator to plug and play but preserved most of the underlying physiologic modeling. Also, other models, such as Laerdal and Gaumard, built in some physiologic modeling that would automatically change some parameters so that the operator would not have to manually change all of the parameters to mimic a particular situation. More recently, Gaumard has produced its own underlying physiologic modeling that may be purchased as an option for many of its newer models.

In addition, it was recognized that sequences of changes in vital signs and physiology could be scripted to create realistic scenarios of different medical situations. Dr. John Schaefer, working with Laerdal, made adjustments to the software of the Laerdal simulators so that programming could be written to produce realistic trends of physiologic parameters following an action taken by a student. This helped the development of prewritten scripts that would respond to a student's actions in a realistic manner without the need for an underlying physiologic model being built into the mannequin. The prewritten script would provide the realistic modeling (J.J. Schafer, personal communication, June 25, 2012). Therefore, as concerns realism and utility of the simulators, the prewritten scripts that are available for the simulators are and will be an important part of the present and future of these simulators. Prewritten scripts that are developed with great care can mimic real-life situations accurately.

HISTORY BEHIND THE TYPE OF MODELING PRESENT IN THE MODERN MANNEQUINS

The majority of simulators that are presently available represent a mix of manual input, physiologic modeling, and state-based modeling. Which type of modeling predominates in any given model of mannequin patient simulator is dependent on the history behind that simulator.

Some of the first simulators that were built were made to train anesthesia residents. These models were made to represent human physiology (relevant to anesthesia) as accurately as possible. Multiple mathematical models of physiology and pharmacology were built into the computer software to calculate how a real patient would respond physiologically to some event. For example, if the patient was to lose a couple of liters of blood, the model would have the pulse rate and blood pressure respond appropriately. The pulse would go up and the blood pressure would decrease. Different types of physiologic models were created by Stanford University, University of California San Diego, and the University of Florida (Cooper & Taqueti, 2004; S. Lampotang, personal communication, July 18, 2012). These models were created independently of each other. Eventually, the University of Florida model became the basis of the METI HPS simulator, which considered multiple physiologic parameters in its modeling, such as systemic vascular resistance, venous capacitance, fluid volume, lung compliance, and so forth, to construct the overall physiologic modeling (S. Lampotang, personal communication, July 18, 2012). Therefore, in this model, if the simulator was made to stop breathing, it would react in a manner similar to a real patient and would eventually go into a cardiac arrest. If one parameter was changed, the simulator would automatically respond by changing the other variables on the basis of the underlying physiologic model that was programmed into the computer software (Figure 3.1.14).

On the other extreme was the development of simulators that were built on manual input. For these simulators, the operator changed all of the parameters manually on the basis of whatever the operator felt was appropriate. The Laerdal, Gaumard, and Simulaids mannequins produced in the mid-1990s and early 2000s, had a menu of different EKG rhythms and the ability to change the pulse rate,

breathing rate, and other parameters to any value without affecting the other parameters/variables (Figure 3.1.15).

SUMMARY

The history of the mannequin patient simulators reveals multiple universities and corporations working independently of each other in the creation of similar products. This parallel development is repeated throughout the history of the mannequin patient simulators and even the more recent development of the mannequins meant for combat training have had a similar parallel development. Today, multiple corporations and universities appear to be working independently of each other in developing the mannequin patient simulator of the future. Perhaps this competition among different entities is the best driving force to improve and create the products of the future, or perhaps more collaboration among these entities would improve the products more quickly. Will the future be one of development through competition or development through collaboration? Only time will tell.

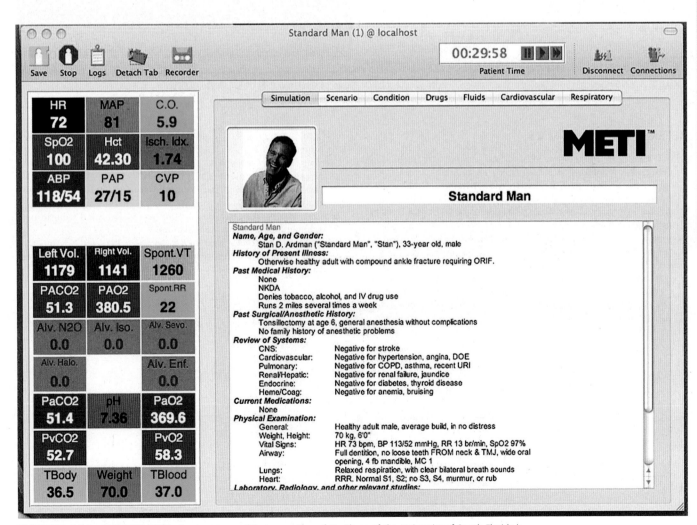

FIGURE 3.1.14 CAE METI HPS instructor screen. (Photo courtesy of Dr. Slone of the University of South Florida.)

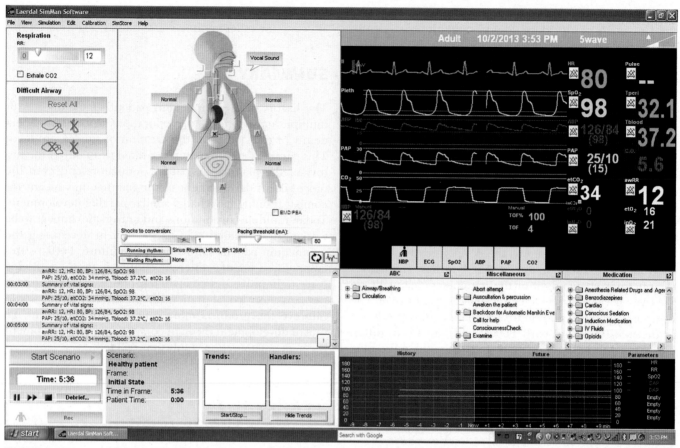

FIGURE 3.1.15 Laerdal SimMan instructor screen. (Photo courtesy of Dr. Slone of the University of South Florida.)

REFERENCES

CIMIT: Center for Integration of Medicine & Innovative Technology. (2012). Retrieved from http://cimit.org/about.html

Cooper, J. B., & Taqueti, V. R. (2004). A brief history of the development of mannequin simulators for clinical education and training. *Quality and Safety in Healthcare, 13*(Suppl. 1), i11–i18. doi:10.1136/qshc.2004.009886

Gaumard. (2012). *Gaumard history website: Our history of innovation.* Retrieved from http://www.gaumard.com/our-history/

Gaumard. (2013). *Combat HAL S3040.* Retrieved from http://www.gaumard.com/combat-hal-s3040/?utm_source=Gaumard+Scientific+Global+List&utm_campaign=63b108c140-Introducing_Combat_HAL5_9_2013&utm_medium=email&utm_term=0_9e05c233d8-63b108c140-301821342

KGS. (n.d.). *Trauma F/X.* Retrieved from http://www.kforcegov.com/TraumaFX/

Laerdal. (2012). *Laerdal history website: History.* Retrieved from http://www.laerdal.com/us/doc/367/History

Simulaids. (2012). *Smart Stat.* Retrieved from http://simulaids.com/smartstatinfo.htm

Techline. (n.d.). *TOMManikin: Techline trauma.* Retrieved from http://techlinetrauma.com/tommanikin.html

Wikipedia. (n.d.-a). *United States Air Force pararescue.* Retrieved November 24, 2012, from http://en.wikipedia.org/wiki/United_States_Air_Force_Pararescue

CHAPTER 3.2

Mannequins: Terminology, Selection, and Usage

Frederick L. Slone, MD, and Samsun Lampotang, PhD

ABOUT THE AUTHORS

FREDERICK L. SLONE is the Medical Director for the Center for Advanced Clinical Learning at the University of South Florida (USF) Morsani College of Medicine and concurrently an Associate Professor of Medicine. Retired from a successful career in gastroenterology, he has been involved in simulation for medical education for the past 8 years, actively involved in obtaining accreditation for simulation at USF, and was in the first cohort to be recognized as a Certified Healthcare Simulation Educator (CHSE) by the Society for Simulation in Healthcare.

SAMSUN (SEM) LAMPOTANG coinvented the Human Patient Simulator (HPS) mannequin patient simulator and the Web-enabled Virtual Anesthesia Machine simulation portfolio. His contributions span the physicality-virtuality continuum of simulation, including mixed reality simulation, use of virtual humans for clinical team training, pervasive simulation on mobile devices, and race-specific pharmacodynamics modeling. His simulation accomplishments have been recognized via numerous awards, including the 2007 Society for Education in Anesthesia/Duke Award for Excellence and Innovation in Anesthesia Education.

ABSTRACT

In this chapter, terminology that describes the mannequins used to simulate a full-bodied human that are computer controlled and programmable are defined and discussed. The terms high and low fidelity, high and low technology, physiologic modeling, state-based modeling, "running on the fly," manual input, scripting and finite state algorithm, are discussed in relation to their use with present-day simulators. A guide to mannequin selection to meet the user's needs and avoid misinterpretation of the mannequin's functionality, including questions to ask manufacturers when purchasing a mannequin, is provided. The chapter concludes with a review of some of the present-day research on various aspects of simulation with a peek at the potential future of mannequin patient simulators.

CASE EXAMPLE

Susan's primary interest is in the area of high-quality, evidence-based trauma care. As a faculty member interested in mannequin-based simulation, she has participated in several immersive team-based simulations. While the simulation technicians and staff at the simulation center are knowledgeable and willing to assist, she knows that it is important to her credibility with these individuals to learn the terminology and appropriate use of the many different types of equipment in use in the simulation program. How does one become familiar with the language of mannequin-based simulation? What information does one need to know about selection and use of various mannequins? With so many choices to make in regard to the use of expensive, resource-intensive equipment, how does one get started?

INTRODUCTION AND BACKGROUND

Mannequins that are computer controlled and feature chest wall movement and palpable pulses are becoming standard equipment in both academic and healthcare settings. Despite their ubiquitous nature, there are still many who are challenged by the terminology associated with these devices. Given the expense associated with these devices, there is also a need to assure that those involved with their selection and use are well versed in these matters so they make sound clinical, educational, and business decisions. In this chapter, the focus will be on mannequin patient simulators, not task trainers or other types of simulation. The topics to be covered include:

1. Terminology used in reference to the mannequin patient simulators, including low and high fidelity and modeling as it is used in reference to the mannequin patient simulators
2. A guide to selecting a mannequin
3. Present research that may help to shape the future
4. The potential future of the mannequin patient simulators

Terminology

Low-Fidelity versus High-Fidelity Mannequins

In the Merriam-Webster dictionary, one definition of **fidelity** is the degree to which an electronic device (as a record player, radio, or television) accurately reproduces its effect (as sound or picture). The term has been defined by some in the simulation literature (Phrampus, 2011) as how close something represents reality. In the simulation literature, the terms high-fidelity and low-fidelity mannequins are often used, but there is no precise definition of these terms. Fidelity (how close something represents reality) is a continuum. A few examples will illustrate this continuum. A blow-up plastic "doll" would represent a low level of "fidelity," whereas the most advanced mannequin patient simulator products available (examples: Laerdal SimMan 3G, CAE Healthcare HPS, GaumardNoelle) would be considered "high-fidelity." In between these two extremes are multiple mannequin products with variable functionality. There is no precise line that separates "high" versus "low" fidelity. Therefore, describing the functionality of a product is preferable to using the nonspecific terms of high or low fidelity.

Fidelity may also be seen as conceptual or experiential and, in this view, is often separated from technology. "Low" or "high" technology as opposed to "low" or "high" fidelity is often used. In this terminology, the technology refers to the task trainers, simulators, or other technology that is used, whereas the fidelity refers to the realism of the entire scenario as viewed by the learners (see chapter 8.8, Textbox: Helping Learners Buy-in to Simulation). The following examples illustrate this concept.

If a scenario is conducted using only a monitoring screen to portray vital signs with the remainder of the scenario being verbalized by a narrator, this would be described as low technology. However, for the learner, the narrative and portrayal of vital signs may make the scenario very realistic to the learner and therefore be a high-fidelity scenario for the learner. On the opposite end of the spectrum, a scenario may incorporate the highest-end technology mannequin patient simulator but create a scenario that is completely unrealistic for the learner. This would be "high" technology but "low" fidelity for the learner. Whether the terms of fidelity or technology are used, these terms are only relative terms. There is a continuum between the lowest technology/fidelity and the highest technology/fidelity available. There is no definitive line that separates low versus high as technology/fidelity is subjective and varies according to the user or the learning objective.

Modeling in Mannequin Patient Simulators

A term that is often misunderstood or misinterpreted as relates to the **mannequin patient simulators** is that of "physiologic modeling." The following are examples of terminology used in reference to the mannequin patient simulators:

1. **Manual modeling** (Lampotang, 2008; which some term **manual input** and which the authors believe is a more useful and accurate term; S. Lampotang, personal communication, July 18, 2012)
2. **Physiologic modeling** (Lampotang, 2008; Smith, 2008; or "mathematical modeling" based on physiology principles; S. Lampotang, personal communication, July 18, 2012)
3. **State-based modeling** (Smith, 2008; also known as finite state algorithm or scripting; J.J. Schaefer, personal communication, June 14, 2012; S. Lampotang, personal communication, July 18, 2012)
4. **"Running on the fly."**

In manual input (which is the term the authors prefer over manual modeling), the operator may "plug in" any value to a given parameter regardless of how this would affect any other parameter. As an example, if the operator sets the respiratory rate to 0, in a real person this rate will eventually affect the pulse, blood pressure, and heart rhythm of that person. However, in manual input, the pulse, blood pressure, and rhythm will remain the same until changed by the operator. Another example would be having a patient with a BP of 180/100 and in a sinus rhythm, and then changing the rhythm to a bradycardia of 30 but keeping the BP at 180/100. This can be done using manual input but would not mimic the real-life situation.

"Running on the fly" is a commonly used term. For most users, this means changing the parameters of the mannequin by manual input as the scenario unfolds, on the basis of the operator's perception of what the new parameters should be, depending on the actions of the learners. Whether or not the parameters are changed in a realistic manner or not depends solely on the operator's knowledge and observation skills. Problems with this approach include operating a scenario in an inconsistent manner across educators, distracting educators from focusing solely on teaching and possibly inputting incorrect information.

Physiologic modeling (some authorities would prefer the term mathematical modeling to simulate physiologic principles; Lampotang, 2008; Smith, 2008; S. Lampotang, personal communication, July 18, 2012), in contrast to manual input, automatically adjusts other variables in a physiologic manner when one parameter is changed. An example of physiologic modeling is as follows. If the respiratory rate is set to 0, the pulse would begin to rise initially, and eventually, when the patient becomes severely hypoxic, the pulse would slow down dramatically, and at some point the patient will have a cardiac arrest. The mannequin would react in a physiologically realistic manner to any change of a parameter.

In state-based modeling (J.J. Schaefer, personal communication, June 14, 2012), also known as finite state algorithm or scripting (S. Lampotang, personal communication, July 18, 2012), the scenario developer programs the simulator to be in one state and then to respond to an input and transition to another state. Most of the simulators presently on the market have the ability to have scenarios written and edited by the operator, prior to using the scenario in training. In scripting the scenario, the author of the scenario will assign initial values to the parameters that need to be simulated at the start of the scenario. Then, based on an action by the student, or based on time or events such as drug concentrations reaching a preset threshold, the scenario transitions to the next "state" of parameters that have been preprogrammed by the author of the scenario. By carefully scripting the scenario, the author of the scenario can reproduce an accurate physiologic representation of the scenario.

Advantages and Problems with Manual Input

The manual input simulators are easy to run "on the fly" because the operator can quickly plug in any rhythm, heart rate, blood pressure, and so forth that they wish at any time with a couple of mouse clicks. However, a disadvantage is that it can create unrealistic situations such as a simulator that quit breathing 10 minutes ago but still has a normal pulse and blood pressure. This ease of use is accompanied by the risk of **negative teaching** because the response of the mannequin is dependent on the knowledge and observation skills of the operator. If the operator manually inputs an incorrect mannequin response, the student may learn the wrong action to perform on a real patient (Lampotang, 2008; Smith, 2008; S. Lampotang, personal communication, July 18, 2012). Another disadvantage with manual input is changing all of the parameters affected in a short period of time. For example, if the respiratory rate is changed, this may affect pulse, blood pressure, end-tidal CO_2, heart rhythms, and pulmonary artery pressures. To change all of these accurately and quickly with manual input is difficult and challenging. This may produce an unrealistic simulation. A very common situation that requires changing multiple parameters at once is placing the mannequin patient simulator into asystole or ventricular fibrillation. In pure manual input, the operator would have to change other parameters, such as blood pressure, oxygen saturation, and pulmonary artery pressures to zero to be realistic. As a solution to this

problem, many of the mannequin patient simulators have some underlying physiologic states built into the software, as a convenience. For example, in the Laerdal SimMan, if the simulator is placed into asystole, the blood pressure, pulse, oxygen saturation, and so forth will all go to zero so that a cardiac arrest can be mimicked without the operator having to manually change the required parameters. This is an example of some physiologic states built into a simulator that mostly runs on manual input. Another feature to help create a more realistic manual input is creating a change that occurs over a period of time. For example, if the operator wanted the pulse to change from 180 to 80 gradually over 2 minutes, that manual input option is available on many of the mannequins.

Advantages and Problems with Physiologic Modeling

Simulators that were built on underlying physiologic modeling also have their own set of advantages and problems. The CAE Healthcare simulators, HPS, ECS and iStan, were all built on a platform of an underlying physiologic model (S. Lampotang, personal communication, July 18, 2012). An example of an advantage is the following. In physiologic modeling, a simulator would automatically respond to an action performed by a student in a physiologic way, without the operator having to program in this response or create any additional modeling. Multiple variables will change automatically, requiring no manual adjustment. This allows a consistent response to a student's action. It also allows an instructor to focus on teaching and not be distracted by having to manually change the parameters on the simulator. However, physiologic models have their own set of problems. For example, the calculation of the blood pressure for these models is based on multiple factors such as fluid volume, systemic vascular resistance, venous capacitance, and so forth and is a by-product of these other parameters. Therefore, as an operator, one cannot just "plug in" any blood pressure that one would want to portray but would have to manipulate fluid volume, systemic vascular resistance, and so forth to get the desired blood pressure. This can sometimes be difficult and time consuming. Also, there is presently no physiologic model that is completely accurate. Because of the immense complexity of real people, the present physiologic models have "gaps" where in a given situation the simulator will *not* do what a real patient would do.

In an effort to combine manual input with an underlying physiologic model, METI (later CAE Healthcare) created the Müse platform that allowed the system to override the physiology and allow the operator to "plug in" whatever parameter they would like. This allowed the simulator to have both physiologic modeling and/or manual input. Gaumard has recently produced an underlying physiologic modeling that can be used in addition to the manual input for their mannequins. Many of the other mannequins have some degree of physiologic modeling built into them. For example, if the EKG is changed to asystole and the blood pressure and pulse change automatically to zero, this represents some degree of physiologic modeling. A potential disadvantage of mixing manual input and physiologic modeling is creating unrealistic situations. For example, if the respiratory rate is at 2 breaths per minute and the pulse is set at 80, this would not be a realistic situation, and either the respiratory rate or pulse would have to change to be realistic. Therefore, mixing manual input and physiologic modeling has limitations.

The Use of State-Based Modeling

Most of the mannequin patient simulators available today have the ability to create a script to run a scenario, called state-based modeling, as described above. The simulator can be scripted to change from state to state on the basis of a student's action or passage of time, and all of the required parameters can be scripted to change simultaneously, creating a realistic physiological response. Trend handlers and event handlers are also used in state-based modeling.

Dr. John Schaefer helped to create trend/event handlers for the Laerdal mannequins to give the ability to program trends in the BP, pulse, and other responses that would mimic known physiologic responses to a given input (J.J. Schaefer, personal communication, June 14, 2012). By adding multiple trends/event handlers, realistic physiologic responses can be obtained. The following illustration will help to explain this concept. If a trend handler is created to change the heart rate by 30 beats per minute over 2 minutes if the SpO_2 drops from 99% to 94% and another trend handler is created to increase the heart rate by 15 beats per minute over 2 minutes if there is a 1 L loss of blood, then the computer would add these effects together if both events occurred, creating an automatic change in the heart rate parameter that would account for both events without having to specifically write in these parameters in the programming. In this manner, one can create a physiologic response that can change parameters automatically on the basis of the events that occur. The accuracy of state-based modeling is dependent on the expertise and knowledge of the author that created the state-based programming (Figures 3.2.1 to 3.2.5).

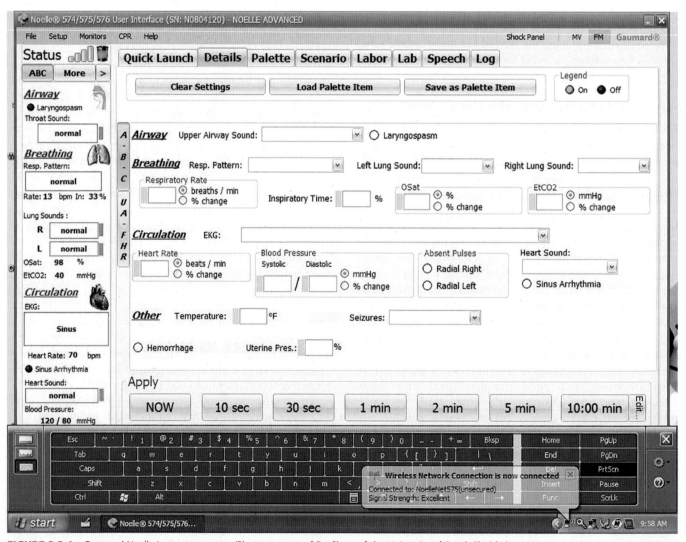

FIGURE 3.2.1 Gaumard Noelle instructor screen. (Photo courtesy of Dr. Slone of the University of South Florida.)

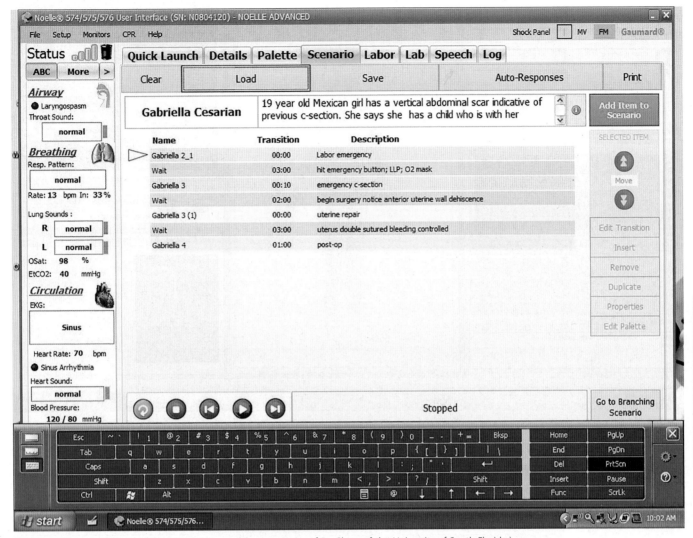

FIGURE 3.2.2 Gaumard Noelle scenario screen. (Photo courtesy of Dr. Slone of the University of South Florida.)

Determining the Type of Modeling Available in a Given Mannequin Patient Simulator

At the present time, the majority of the simulators have the ability to have manual input, state-based modeling, and some degree of underlying physiologic modeling. As concerns the degree of the underlying physiologic modeling, this varies significantly from product to product. CAE Healthcare mannequins were originally built on the basis of a significant degree of physiologic modeling (S. Lampotang, personal communication, July 18, 2012), so they tend to have more of this underlying physiologic response than the other products, but the others do have some degree of underlying physiologic response built into them. More recently, Gaumard has created an optional package for many of their products that have an underlying physiologic model to supplement the manual input model of their mannequins.

Consumers trying to select a simulator need to understand which type of modeling will best meet their educational objectives. For many of those who use simulators, manual input is sufficient to meet their educational objectives, and more sophisticated physiologic modeling is not needed.

The more extensive underlying physiologic modeling can be useful since the simulator can respond automatically to a variety of actions, saving time and effort in trying to manually input these changes or programming in these changes. In addition, these models can often correctly change parameters, such as pulmonary artery pressures, that the operator may not have the knowledge to change manually, creating a more realistic flow into the scenario. The drawback, as mentioned previously, is an unexpected response because of the complexity of real physiology that may not be accurately represented by the underlying physiologic modeling. However, at times the response may be unexpected but realistic! For example, the second author notes an occasion in Vail, Colorado, when a METI HPS simulator unexpectedly hyperventilated. This turned out to be an appropriate physiologic response to the lower oxygen partial pressure secondary to the reduced atmospheric pressure at the high elevation of Vail (S. Lampotang, personal communication, July 18, 2012).

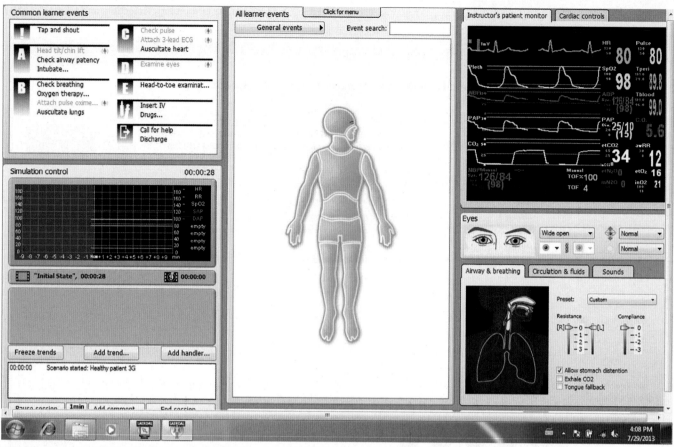

FIGURE 3.2.3 Laerdal SimMan 3G instructor application screen. (Photo courtesy of Dr. Slone of the University of South Florida.)

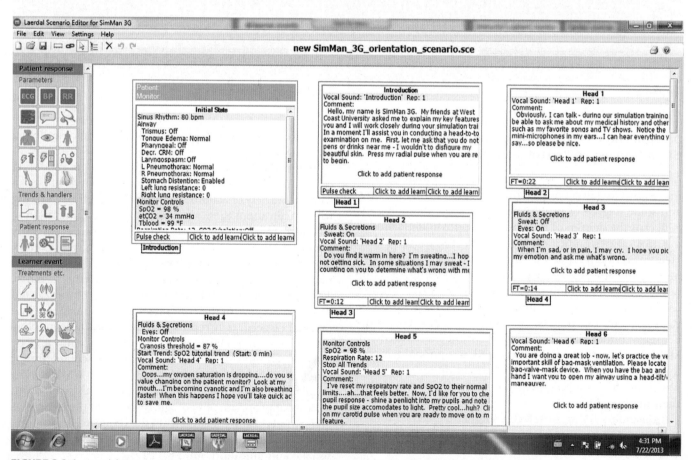

FIGURE 3.2.4 Laerdal SimMan 3G scenario editor screen. (Photo courtesy of Dr. Slone of the University of South Florida.)

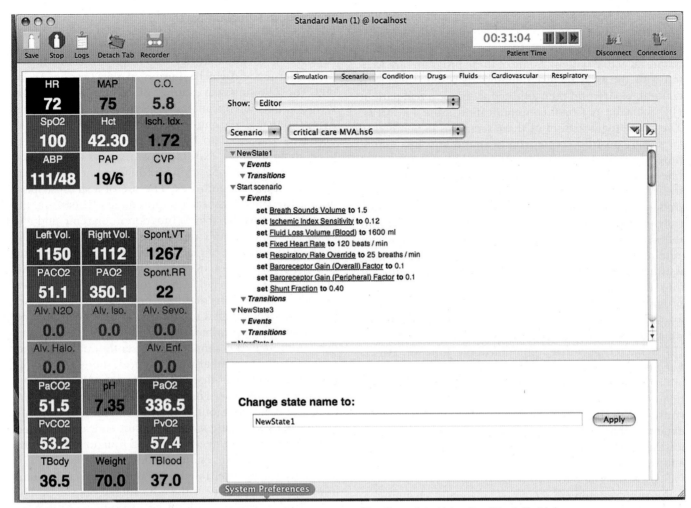

FIGURE 3.2.5   CAE Healthcare HPS scenario editor screen. (Photo courtesy of Dr. Slone of the University of South Florida.)

Determining Whether a Simulator Has Underlying Physiologic Modeling

Underlying physiologic modeling in the simulators can be tested. One can change a parameter manually and then observe whether the other variables change in a realistic manner or not. As an example of this, if the respiratory rate is set at zero, the other variables such as pulse and blood pressure should begin to change. Eventually, the simulator should go into complete cardiac arrest. If this does not occur, then most likely there is not an underlying physiologic modeling. By changing a variety of parameters, the user can evaluate what type of underlying physiology is built into the simulator software and which parameters will trigger other variables to change automatically.

Dangers of Manual Input

A danger of manual input was discussed briefly but is worth reemphasizing. It is the danger of exposing the students to negative teaching (Smith, 2008; S. Lampotang, personal communication, July 18, 2012). Different educators have different levels of understanding of what a typical physiologic response might be to any given input, and

an instructor may inadvertently be inputting a response that will teach the student an incorrect response. In addition, having to manually run the simulator and teach at the same time can be a challenge to any instructor. Simulators that are based on extensive mathematical physiologic modeling can circumvent these problems to some degree by responding to a student's input automatically and eliminating the need for the instructor to manually input a response, therefore eliminating instructor variability. Unfortunately, the mathematical modeling of physiology presently available cannot always mimic real physiology, so unrealistic responses may occur. The ideal model has yet to be created.

Prepackaged Scenarios (State-Based Modeling)

State-based modeling can be used to create a very uniform response of the simulator to a student's actions and even eliminate the need for the instructor in some circumstances (J.J. Schaefer, personal communication, June 14, 2012).

Each of the major companies has available prepackaged scenarios and educational materials for the simulators. The scenarios that have been programmed into this software represent state-based modeling, and depending upon the sophistication and completeness of the scenario written, these programs can have the ability to realistically mimic an actual patient. Some of these programs are written with the help of programmers in conjunction with content experts and then adjusted to mimic a real patient (J.J. Schaefer, personal communication, June 14, 2012). The physiologic realism of these scenarios depends to a large part on who created the scenario and how much time and effort was put into creating, validating, and fine-tuning the scenario. Another aspect of prewritten scenarios is the ability to use them for training or testing students without the need for an instructor to be physically present. A technician can load these scenarios into the simulator, and the scenario/program will then run automatically, responding to the student's input, which is either detected by the simulator's sensors or is entered into the computer by the technician. Some of these programs can then compute a score for the student in a testing situation or create a debrief log that informs which actions were correct and which actions were not (J.J. Schaefer, personal communication, June 14, 2012). Each of the companies can direct the reader to the availability of programs that they have available for their mannequins. Unfortunately, it can be very difficult for the consumer to figure out the degree of sophistication and expertise that was used to create the simulation scenarios that are available. In the future, it is the hope of the authors that users will be able to rate various available scenarios as a guide for future users.

In preprogrammed scenarios, manually changing a parameter or variable may negate the physiologic accuracy of the scenario. Many of these types of scripted scenarios are meant to be run without any operator input, and in fact while running they will lock out operator input. Therefore, it is important for the consumer of these preprogrammed scenarios to sample them before purchasing to verify that they operate in a manner that achieves the objectives that are expected.

Selecting a Mannequin

The following general questions are a guide to help in selecting a mannequin.

1. Will the mannequin help achieve the educational objectives of the program?
2. Are the human resources available that are needed to run and support the mannequin?
3. What is the cost of maintenance for the mannequin?
4. Are additional accessories needed to operate the mannequins that are not included in the purchase price?
5. What types of software products are available for the mannequin?
6. What is the overall cost of the mannequin to the purchaser?

Mannequin Selection Factors

Choosing a Mannequin to Meet Educational Objectives

In selecting a mannequin, it is important to decide who will be the learners and which educational objectives need to be met. The following is an example of selecting a mannequin to meet specific educational objectives. In a 68 Whiskey Army Combat Medic course, there are specific educational objectives that need to be met. The training must take place in austere and extreme environments and includes tourniquet placement to stop bleeding and needle decompression of a pneumothorax. The use of a stethoscope is not part of the educational requirements. Therefore, the mannequin must be able to function in extreme and austere environments and reproduce bleeding that can be stopped with the use of real tourniquets. Lung sounds and heart sounds are not necessary. There are very specific mannequins constructed to meet these objectives. Purchasing other mannequins that have many additional features but are not constructed to endure extreme environments would not be appropriate for the stated educational objectives. Although the simulators presently on the market may have an extensive array of features, there may be one feature in particular that is very important to a needed educational objective. For example, if a twitching thumb for learning how to monitor neuromuscular blockade during anesthesia training is an important educational objective, the mannequin needs to have a functional twitching thumb that is realistic enough to meet this objective. It is important for the user to evaluate the realism of the function to ensure it will meet the educational objectives. The following is a real example of an institution not evaluating the realism of a mannequin function that was essential to their educational needs before purchasing. A local EMS program purchased a very expensive mannequin for EMT and paramedic training for cardiopulmonary arrest. Unfortunately, the compression of the chest was not realistic and created a **negative teaching** situation, causing poor chest compression technique in the students. This made the mannequin useless to the program. Spending just 10 minutes to evaluate the chest compressions before purchasing would have saved tens of thousands of dollars.

To match the needs of various educational objectives, an array of mannequin types have been developed. Available mannequins include neonate mannequins, infant mannequins, child mannequins, adult mannequins, obstetric mannequins, mannequins specifically designed for anesthesia training that use real anesthetic gases and vapors, and mannequins designed to train combat medics (Figures 3.2.6 to 3.2.14). Some mannequins are tethered and others are tetherless. To best decide the mannequin needed, additional technical information can be found in the online supplement for this textbook at http://www.ssih.org/News/Defining-Excellence.

Human Resources

Personnel are needed to set up, operate, and maintain the mannequins. As the complexity of the mannequin

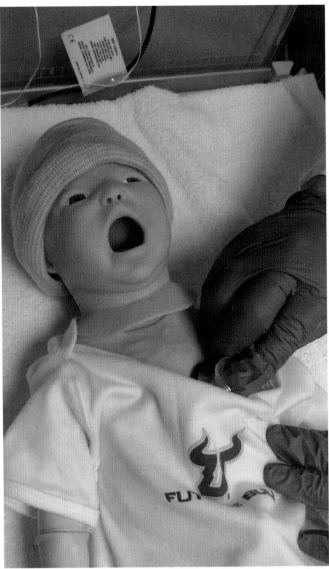

FIGURE 3.2.6 Gaumard newborn HAL being examined at the University of South Florida College of Nursing. (Photo courtesy of Dr. Slone of the University of South Florida.)

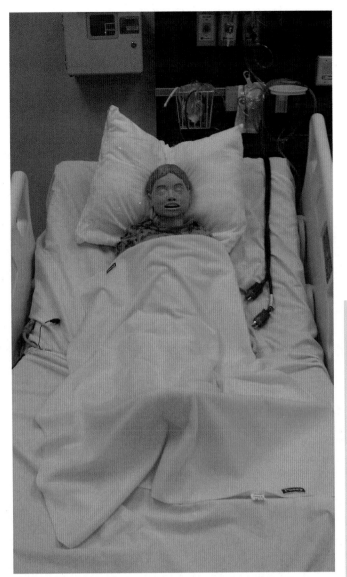

FIGURE 3.2.8 Laerdal Sim Junior in a hospital bed. (Photo courtesy of Dr. Slone of the University of South Florida.)

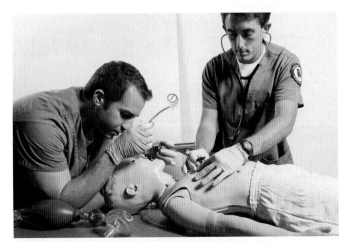

FIGURE 3.2.7 CAE healthcare PediaSIM undergoing endotrachael intubation. (Photo courtesy of Kim Cartlidge of CAE Healthcare.)

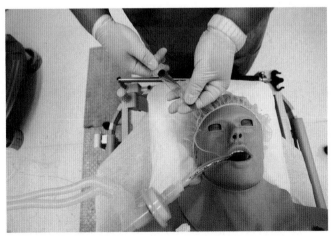

FIGURE 3.2.9 CAE healthcare HPS as part of an anesthesia scenario. (Photo courtesy of Kim Cartlidge of CAE Healthcare.)

SECTION 3 • Simulators

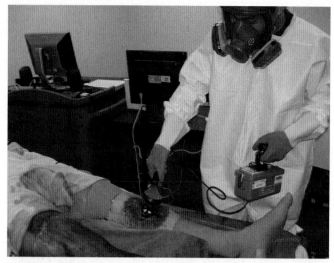

FIGURE 3.2.10 CAE healthcare iStan being used in disaster training. (Photo courtesy of Dr. Slone of the University of South Florida.)

increases, the time needed for training of personnel also increases. Features such as bleeding and secretions take more time and expertise to set up and maintain. Personnel need both appropriate training and time set aside for proper setup, operation, and maintenance of the mannequin. The cost and availability of personnel must be considered with the purchase of any mannequin. Many institutions have learned by experience that spending money on a high-technology mannequin without providing the personnel to go along with it becomes an investment with minimal return (Figure 3.2.15).

As concerns the training of the personnel to operate the mannequin, the following questions should be asked of the manufacturer.

- Is training provided as part of the purchase price of the mannequin?
- Is training provided at the purchasing institution, or is the institution required to send its personnel to workshops in other cities?
- Who pays for the travel?

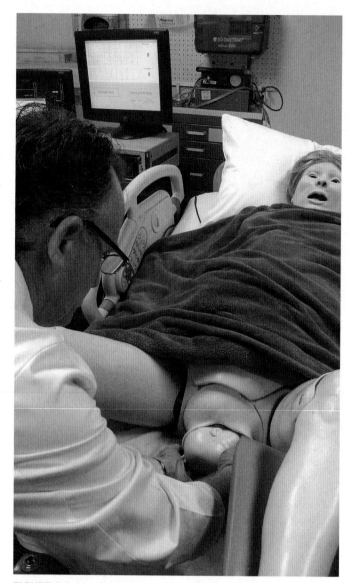

FIGURE 3.2.12 Gaumard Noelle delivering a baby at the University of South Florida College of Nursing. (Photo courtesy of Dr. Slone of the University of South Florida.)

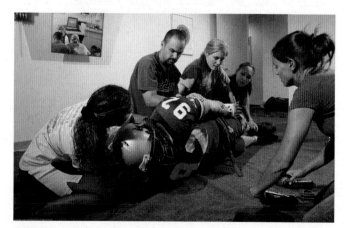

FIGURE 3.2.11 CAE healthcare iStan being used to train University of South Florida Athletic Training Students. (Photo courtesy of the University of South Florida Athletic Training Department.)

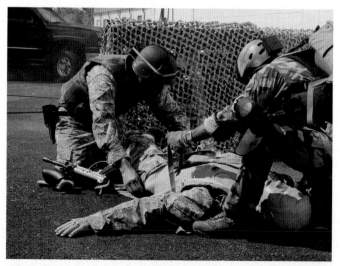

FIGURE 3.2.13 Simulaids Smart Stat Adult mannequin being used for tactical combat training. (Photo courtesy of Warren Johnson of Simulaids.)

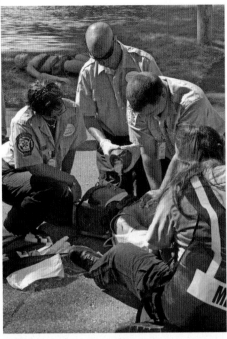

FIGURE 3.2.14 Simulaids Smart Stat Adult mannequin as part of a trauma scenario. (Photo courtesy of Warren Johnson of Simulaids.)

- Is online instruction available, and is there a cost for it?
- Is ongoing training provided for mannequin updates and upgrades?

Maintenance Costs

Maintenance contracts or repairs can be very costly and must be considered in the purchase of a mannequin. In addition to the costs of the maintenance contracts, other factors must be considered. Some critical questions to ask are as follows:

- Does the purchase price of the mannequin include any warranty period that will cover repair costs?
- What is the cost of the maintenance contract per year, and does this contract cover preventive maintenance or only repairs?
- If a mannequin breaks down, does the manufacturer send the technicians to the purchasing institution, or must the mannequin be sent to the manufacturer?
- How long will it take for the repairs to occur?
- Does the manufacturer supply a mannequin to replace the one being repaired, and if so, is there a cost for this?
- Is technical support available by phone to help solve a problem immediately?
- Sending a mannequin back to the manufacturer can mean the loss of the mannequin for many weeks and a disruption of the simulation training schedule. Having backup mannequins, replacement mannequins, or expeditious repairs is critical to any program and adds to the overall costs of the mannequins (Figure 3.2.16).

Mannequin Accessories

Whenever a mannequin is purchased, it is essential to know whether other accessories are needed to operate the mannequins that are not included with the purchase.

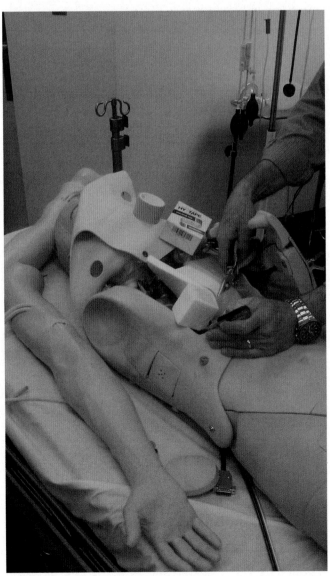

FIGURE 3.2.16 Laerdal SimMan undergoing repairs. (Photo courtesy of Dr. Slone of the University of South Florida.)

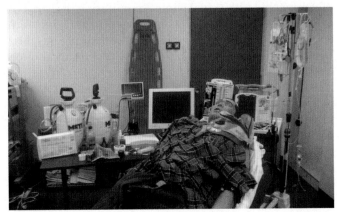

FIGURE 3.2.15 CAE healthcare iStan shown with part of the equipment needed to produce one trauma scenario. (Photo courtesy of Dr. Slone of the University of South Florida.)

SECTION 3 • Simulators

Some critical questions to ask are as follows:

- Is the patient monitor included with the purchase price?
- Does the mannequin need a compressor for its operation, and is this included in the purchase price?
- Are accessory cables, Ethernet cords, or other connecting devices needed to operate the mannequin or needed to interface with clinical monitors that may be used in simulations included with the purchase?

Some of the mannequins are made to function with real gases for anesthesia training. As an example, the HPS (CAE Healthcare) is made to use oxygen, nitrogen, carbon dioxide, and nitrous oxide. Before purchasing this type of mannequin, it is imperative that the simulation lab be equipped with the appropriate holders for the gas tanks, all appropriate gas tubing and connections, and a properly vented room and scavenging vacuum available. These accessories may add a significant cost to the mannequin (Figure 3.2.17).

Software Products for the Mannequin

Presently, there is an array of available software for the mannequins that may be included with the mannequin or can be purchased. This software may simply be prewritten scenarios for the mannequin, or may represent an entire educational program or curriculum that is made to go along with the mannequin. Some of the more sophisticated software that is becoming available represents multimedia presentations with established educational objectives that are constructed to be a self-learning module for the student that can be run with an instructor or by a technician without the presence of an instructor. These modules are designed to run large numbers of students through simulation activities with specific educational goals using a minimum number of educators (J.J. Schaefer, personal communication, June 14, 2012). Presently, there is a wide range of sophistication in the available software products, and it is prudent for the user to evaluate

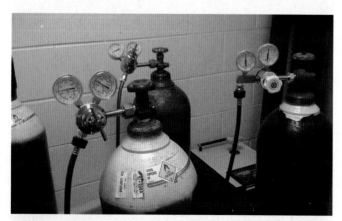

FIGURE 3.2.17 Air compressor, oxygen, nitrogen, and carbon dioxide tanks needed to supply the CAE healthcare HPS mannequin. (Photo courtesy of Dr. Slone of the University of South Florida.)

this software on the mannequin before purchasing. Good software programs can add significant value to the mannequin purchase. It is the author's hope that in the future, there will be a website dedicated to the different software programs available, with user comments to help guide other users to the programs that would best add value to their mannequins.

Overall Cost

In determining the true overall cost of the mannequins, it is imperative to add in the costs of personnel, maintenance and repairs, additional accessories, and software products to the initial purchase price. A good rule of thumb is to go with the lowest cost technology that will meet the learning objectives for a good return of investment (ROI).

Other Considerations When Purchasing a Mannequin

Mannequin Durability

The durability of a particular model of mannequin can be information that is difficult to obtain. The best practice is to contact several other institutions with the same model and question them regarding the product's durability. Some models are quite durable and easy to repair on site without the help of a technician; other models break down frequently and will be out of service for lengthy periods. It is the author's hope to have a consumer report–type website in the future to help guide purchasers regarding durability issues.

Initial Setup of a New Mannequin

Important Tip: When the vendor comes to set up the mannequin, it is best to have someone present who will be responsible for the operation of the mannequin. This person can then ask appropriate questions during the setup, help set up codes and passwords, and label/store accessory parts so they may be easily located later.

Ability to Hook up Monitoring Devices to the Mannequin

Different mannequin products have different capabilities of connecting with actual clinical monitoring devices. For example, some mannequins are made to function with actual clinical pulse oximeters and will display a pulse oximeter plethysmogram on the actual clinical monitor. Most of the mannequins presently available cannot use a real pulse oximeter and must use a "model of a pulse oximeter" that will display only on an LED screen made to mimic a clinical monitor. In a similar manner, some models may be connected to an actual 12-lead EKG machine and produce a 12-lead EKG on the actual machine, whereas most of the models will display a simulated EKG on an LED screen made to mimic the clinical monitor. If the use of actual clinical monitors are an important educational objective of the training, it is important ask about this functionality before purchasing a specific product (Figure 3.2.18).

Stated Functionality versus Functional Realism

The manufacturer and manufacturer representatives will have a list of functions that the mannequin is able to perform. However, the realism of that function may vary greatly on different mannequin products. At times the realism of the function can be so poor that it may create a negative learning situation. For example, if the chest compression function of the mannequin is either too easy or too difficult, this may translate to students performing chest compressions poorly on an actual patient. Describing the realism of any particular function is very subjective, and only the user can adequately judge whether the realism of a particular function is good enough to meet their educational objectives. Therefore, experienced users strongly suggest taking the time to go to an institution that has the particular mannequin model of interest and see firsthand how realistic the needed functions are on the mannequin. Some individuals have found that the device they are interested in evaluating is already in use in another department within the same institution. Taking the time to investigate fully before purchasing a device will save time, money, and frustration in the long run.

When the Purchaser Is Not the Same as the User

When purchasing a mannequin, problems may be created when the purchaser is not the user of the mannequin. In many large institutions, the purchaser of the mannequin may be in a financial office and have no knowledge regarding any specifics of the mannequin. Therefore, communication between the user and the purchaser must be very clear. The following are suggestions by experienced users to avoid problems.

- The user must clearly communicate to the purchaser if there are any accessories needed to operate the mannequin that are not included with the mannequin purchase. Likewise, the purchaser must clearly communicate what products are being included with the purchase price of the mannequin.
- The user and purchaser must communicate regarding the details of the service/warranty contract, and each needs to be notified prior to the end of the contract.
- The user needs to discuss with the purchaser how the account with the manufacturer is titled and clearly delineate which department is purchasing the mannequin and who the contact person will be for that particular mannequin. When multiple similar mannequins are purchased from the same company by different departments within the same institution, the company may not differentiate between mannequins that belong to different departments, each with a separate contact person. When this happens, confusion can ensue. For example, a replacement arm for one department was sent to another department with the same type of mannequin that did not need the replacement arm. It took 3 months to find and reroute the replacement arm to the department that needed it.

One Last Tip for the Users of the Mannequins Given by Experienced Users

Try out the product before buying it. If necessary, go to another institution to try it out. Be cautious about asking the vendor for a reference since they will give their best relationship that may be biased toward a particular product. Most users of the mannequins would welcome another user to try out a mannequin at their institution. The SSH list-serve can be a great place to find out who is nearby that is using a particular model. These products cost as much as an expensive automobile, and if one is going to buy an $80,000 car, it is prudent to look at a variety of makes of cars and "test drive" the cars before making the purchase.

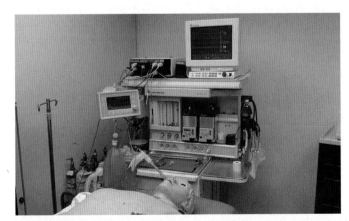

FIGURE 3.2.18 CAE healthcare HPS mannequin connected to clinical monitors and an anesthesia machine used in the operating room. (Photo courtesy of Dr. Slone of the University of South Florida.)

BEEN THERE, DONE THAT. HOW CAN I CONTINUE TO IMPROVE OR SUSTAIN WHAT I HAVE ACHIEVED?

Present and Emerging Trends and Topics in Simulation and Its Applicability to Mannequin Patient Simulators

Interpatient Variability

Simulation modeling is currently based on the concept of a theoretical average plausible human, the "standard man." For example, the Human Patient Simulator (CAE Healthcare, Sarasota, FL) is nicknamed "Stan" based on the fictitious person Stan D. Ardman, whose full name including middle initial spells out "standard man." As far as we can tell, there is currently no interpatient variability for those mannequin patient simulators that are model-driven. What this means is that if a scenario is run on a simulator with a model without patient variability, the vital signs and other symptoms in the scenario will unfold in exactly the same way (magnitude and sequence of changes) each time the scenario is run if the trainee interventions or lack of interventions occur identically in each run of the scenario.

Some of the reasons why patient variability may be desirable include:

a. Actual patients do exhibit interpatient variability, for example, interethnic variability to drugs such as propofol (Ortalani et al., 2004) and also intraethnic variability such as the need of redheads for more anesthetics (Liem et al., 2004),

b. A novice learning on a standard model (whether on a mannequin patient simulator or screen-based simulator) and running a scenario repeatedly may mistakenly conclude that patients are very consistent in their response and unconsciously "imprint" to the default parameters programmed in the standard model, and

c. An experienced clinician practicing a scenario repeatedly may not be challenged in subsequent runs if the response of the simulator can be exactly anticipated.

There have been past and ongoing efforts at diversity through the use of mannequin patient simulators of non-Caucasian ethnicity. For example, Laerdal offers some of its mannequins in light, tan, and brown skin tones and CAE Healthcare will soon provide the option of different skin colors across its product line. However, as far as we can tell from information obtained from the manufacturer, the diversity of these model-based simulators is literally only skin deep because the models underpinning the simulators are still based on patient data acquired mainly from Caucasians and do not truly reflect interethnic or intraethnic variability, at the very least in terms of pharmacokinetics and pharmacodynamics (PK/PD).

Models that display interpatient variability in pharmacokinetics and pharmacodynamics have been developed (Yavas et al., 2008) and are available without charge online at the Virtual Anesthesia Machine website http://vam.anest.ufl.edu/wip.html such as a simulation of propofol PK/PD (Lampotang et al., 2006), while others are in the process of being developed. We anticipate that eventually mannequin patient simulators will be enhanced with interpatient variability programmed into their PK/PD models as a default or optional feature.

Anatomic Fidelity

Other needs beyond anatomic fidelity may dictate the shape of mannequins used in current mannequin patient simulators. For example, electromechanical and electropneumatic equipment may need to be housed/crammed inside the torso of a mannequin, and the form factor of the equipment may require the torso to be larger than usual or disproportionate. If the learning objectives that are intended to be acquired with the simulator do not depend on anatomic fidelity, then artistic, or more accurately engineering, license may be justified. But as the lines get blurred between mannequin patient simulators and part task trainers, for example, procedural simulators that use mannequins such as HeartWorks and Vimedix, the need for anatomical accuracy in mannequins may become more pronounced. In some procedural simulators that require user intervention such as central venous line access simulators and ventriculostomy simulators, anatomic fidelity is important because trainees rely on anatomical landmarks such as the clavicle and the sternal notch and the midpupillary line to determine where to puncture the skin or drill the skull respectively.

Advances in medical imaging, 3D technology, tracking and rapid prototyping (3D printing) have made it possible to build a mannequin that is actually an identical replica of the human who was used as the model. Mannequins with high anatomic fidelity have recently become available and have been shown to improve procedural skills in subclavian central venous access (Robinson et al., 2014). These mannequins employ mixed reality technology and are called mixed simulators since they seamlessly integrate physical components with virtual components (Lampotang et al., 2012, 2013). For example, they include anatomically authentic physical components such as scalp and skulls and skin and ribs, respectively. The soft tissues of interest such as the veins, arteries and lungs and the brain ventricles and other inner brain components are virtual and do not occupy any physical space at all. On the basis of what has been shown to be possible with mixed simulators, it would be a logical development for future mannequin patient simulators to include anatomically correct outer shells (potentially produced via 3D printing) with anatomically authentic virtual components precisely underlaid below the mannequin shell, while not requiring any additional space inside the mannequin torso (Figure 3.2.19; Wikipedia, n.d.).

Affective Skills

While some current mannequin patient simulators have speakers embedded in them that allow a simulator operator to moan in pain or speak for the mannequin, these verbal interactions are not consistent and depend to a large extent on the availability and quality of a script and/or the ability of the operator to follow the script or react/improvise in response to unanticipated questions from the trainee(s). The ability to converse in a natural language such as English with a mannequin patient simulator would extend their use from acquisition of psychomotor and cognitive skills

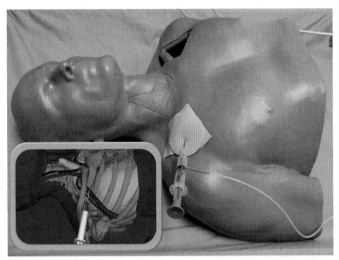

FIGURE 3.2.19 Central line trainer using mixed reality technology. (Photo courtesy of Dr. Samsun Lampotang of the University of Florida.)

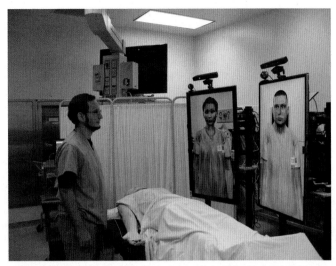

FIGURE 3.2.20 Mixed reality humans used for affective skills and team training. (Photo courtesy of Dr. Samsun Lampotang of the University of Florida.)

to include the third leg of the skills triangle (Lampotang et al., 2013): affective skills. An example of pioneering work in verbal interaction and interpersonal simulation is the Virtual Patient Factory (Filichia et al., 2011). It is an online application that can be used to generate via text entry and crowd sourcing a database of verbal exchanges that anticipates as an example all the different ways in which a patient might be asked when he or she last ate as well as all the various possible responses from the patient. As speech recognition becomes more accurate and pervasive, applications such as the VPF will most likely find their way into mannequin patient simulators (Hwang et al., 2009) and possibly extend their use to training in affective skills.

Team Training

Mixed reality humans (MRHs) can simulate not only a patient but any human. An example of an instantiation of a MRH is a TV monitor in portrait mode mounted on a sturdy frame and with physical legs (e.g., stuffed trousers, jeans, or scrubs pants) hanging below the monitor to represent the legs of the MRH (Chuah et al., 2012). MRHs build upon the interpersonal simulation work already performed using, for example, VPF. Team training and team dynamics are considered important elements of patient safety. Clinicians who are expected to work as a team should train as a team. MRHs may have a role to play in healthcare and patient safety by facilitating team training. As anyone who has attempted to schedule a team-training exercise with clinicians has experienced, there is a high likelihood of a no-show that results in cancellation of the entire exercise and wasted time for those team members who did show up for the team-training exercise. MRHs offer the promise of facilitating team training by acting as pinch hitters to simulate any last-minute no-shows or any person who is unavailable when scheduling a team exercise so that team-training exercises can occur more frequently.

The above predictions are only a quick peek at the crystal ball for simulation. Clearly, researchers in simulation will continue to exploit and adapt new technologies as they become available or more affordable to respond to training needs and advance simulation and patient safety (Figure 3.2.20).

SUMMARY: THE POTENTIAL FUTURE OF THE MANNEQUIN PATIENT SIMULATORS

The combination of new technologies being applied to the present mannequin patient simulators is likely to create the mannequin of the future.

Presently, the mannequins have a relatively realistic outer shell to give the look and feel of a real person. However, newer technologies may be able to improve this outer shell dramatically. Newer technologies have been created to more accurately reproduce the feel and look of real human tissue, to the point that the artificial tissues are able to undergo actual ultrasound or X-ray scanning and reproduce images similar to a real person.

Also, today, the inside of the mannequins is nothing but wires, tubes, and so forth, and therefore the internal organs of a human cannot be reproduced to accept interventions such as sonography or other radiologic imaging, or invasive procedures such as central line placement, lumbar puncture, thoracentesis, paracentesis, nerve blocks or other procedures. However, technology is presently available to create a virtual reality "inside" to go along with the physical outer shell of the mannequin. Through this virtual reality, the future mannequins may allow realistic physical interventions and automatically respond to these interventions. In addition, virtual reality can be used to produce realistic ultrasound pictures while using a simulated physical ultrasound probe on the surface of the mannequin.

There are several different ultrasound simulators that are presently available that could be integrated into the mannequin patient simulator.

To create better accuracy and realism in the present mannequin models, a technology called 3D printers can create an exact replica of any part of a human by acquiring a 3D image by CT or MRI scanning, and this image can be physically reconstructed into an accurate 3D physical model by the 3D printer. (Also, see the section on emerging trends and topics in simulation.) The printer lays down one thin layer of material at a time based on the 3D image, similar to how a regular printer prints out a 2D page of print, one line at a time. The layer of material hardens, and then the next layer is added to this. The process may take many hours to days depending on the complexity of the image, but will eventually produce an anatomically accurate 3D model (Wikipedia n.d., 2012). By using these models, a more exact replica of actual human anatomy can be reproduced, making the mannequin models more accurate, where needed, for training purposes. In addition, models can be accurately reproduced for many different disease states from actual humans so that accurate disease models can be produced.

Another technology that is available and is being perfected is the virtual patient. Using voice recognition technology, such as is used in the iPhone's Siri, the virtual patient can be programmed to respond to a variety of verbal inputs. There are a number of institutions that are working on and expanding the abilities of these virtual patients.

Virtual reality technology to mimic the internal workings of the patient, accurate 3D modeling of both the outer shell and virtual reality interior of the mannequin, and advances in voice recognition technology are possibilities that can realistically be added to the mannequin patient simulator in the near future. Cost restraints and technical limitations will determine how many of these functions will be able to be contained within one product versus a variety of products each targeting specific educational objectives. What is certain is that the field of mannequin patient simulation will make major advances in the near future.

REFERENCES

Chuah, J. H., Robb, A., White, C. W., Wendling, A., Lampotang, S., Kopper, R., & Lok, B. (2012). Increasing agent physicality to raise social presence and elicit realistic behavior. *Proceedings of the IEEE Virtual Reality Conference*, Orange County, CA, 19–22.

Filichia, L., Halan, S., Blackwelder, E., Rossen, B., Lok, B., Korndorffer, J., & Cendan, J. (2011). Description of web-enhanced virtual character simulation system to standardize patient hand-offs. *Journal of Surgical Research*, 166(2), 176–181.

Gaumard. (n.d.). *Combat HAL S3040*. Retrieved from http://www.gaumard.com/combat-hal-s3040/?utm_source=Gaumard+Scientific+Global+List&utm_campaign=63b108c140-Introducing_Combat_HAL5_9_2013&utm_medium=email&utm_term=0_9e05c233d8-63b108c140-301821342

Hwang, Y., Lampotang, S., Gravenstein, N., Luria, I., & Lok, B. (2009). Integrating conversational virtual humans and mannequin patient simulators to present mixed reality clinical training experiences. *Proceedings of the 8th IEEE International Symposium in Mixed and Augmented Reality*, 197–198. Retrieved from http://ieeexplore.ieee.org/xpls/abs_all.jsp?arnumber=5336466&tag=1

Lampotang, S. (2008). Medium and high integration mannequin patient simulators. In R. Riley (Ed.), *Manual of simulation in healthcare* (chap. 5, pp. 51–64). New York, NY: Oxford University Press.

Lampotang, S., Bova, F. J., Lizdas, D. E., Rajon, D. A., Friedman, W. A., Robinson, A. R., III, . . . Gravenstein, N. (2012). A subset of mixed simulations: Augmented physical simulations with virtual underlays. *Proceedings of the Interservice/Industry Training, Simulation & Education Conference (I/ITSEC)*, Orlando, FL.

Lampotang, S., Lizdas, D., Gravenstein, N., & Yavas, S. (2006). *Web Simulation of Propofol Pharmacokinetics*. Retrieved August 14, 2012, from the University of Florida Department of Anesthesiology Virtual Anesthesia Machine Web site: http://vam.anest.ufl.edu/membbers/propofol.html

Lampotang, S., Lizdas, D., Rajon, D., Luria, I., Gravenstein, N., Bisht, Y., . . . Robinson, A. (2013). Mixed simulators: Augmented physical simulators with virtual underlays. *Proceedings of the IEEE Virtual Reality meeting*, 7–10. doi:978-1-4673-4796-9/13

Liem, E. B., Lin, C. M., Suleman, M. I., Doufas, A. G., Gregg, R. G., Veauthier, J. M., . . . Sessler, D. I. (2004). Anesthetic requirement is increased in Redheads. *Anesthesiology*, 101(2), 279–283.

Ortolani, O., Conti, A., Chan, Y. K., Sie, M. Y., & Ong, G. S. Y. (2004). Comparison of propofol consumption and recovery time in Caucasians from Italy, with Chinese, Malays and Indians from Malaysia. *Anaesthesia and Intensive Care*, 32(2), 250–255.

Phrampus, P. (2011). Training. In J. Sokolowski (Ed.), *Modeling and simulation in the medical and health sciences* (chap. 8, p. 140). Hoboken, NJ: John Wiley & Sons.

Robinson, A. R., Gravenstein, N., Cooper, L. A., Lizdas, D., Luria, I., & Lampotang, S. (2014). A Mixed-Reality Part-Task Trainer for Subclavian Venous Access. *Simulation in Healthcare*, 9(1), 56-64.

Smith, N. (2008). Physiologic modeling for simulators: Get real. In R. Kyle & B. Murray (Eds.), *Clinical simulation operations, engineering and management* (chap. 49, pp. 459–467). Oxford, UK: Academic Press.

Wikipedia. (n.d.). *3D printing*. Retrieved September 23, 2012 from http://en.wikipedia.org/w/index.php?title=3D_printing&oldid=513929285

Yavas, S., Lizdas, D., Gravenstein, N., & Lampotang, S. (2008). Interactive web simulation for propofol and fospropofol, a new propofol prodrug. *Anesth Analg.*, 106(3), 880-883.

CHAPTER 3.3

Standardized Patients

Tamara L. Owens, MEd, and Gayle Gliva-McConvey, BA

ABOUT THE AUTHORS

TAMARA L.OWENS is the Director of the Clinical Skills and Simulation Centers at Howard University. She serves on key curriculum committees for the university as well as on the Simulation Task Force for the Association of American Medical Colleges. She is a Past President for the Association of Standardized Patients Educators. Ms. Owens has more than 17 years as an administrator and educator in the standardized methodology field.

GAYLE GLIVA-McCONVEY is the Director of Professional Skills Teaching and Assessment at Eastern Virginia Medical School. Since 1973, she has developed and integrated the Standardized Patient (SP) methodology in healthcare and various professions. She has numerous publications, presents at national and international conferences, was a founding board member of ASPE, served on the BOD for 8 years and was President from 2012 to 2014. She represented ASPE on the SSH certification executive committee and the Terminology & Concepts committee.

The authors would like to acknowledge Kathryn A. Schaivone for her input in this chapter.

ABSTRACT

Throughout the healthcare industry, confidence is growing in the validity and uses of a spectrum of simulation modalities for teaching and assessment. One modality in this spectrum is Standardized Patients (SPs), and consistent with other simulation modalities, learners are immersed into a safe and controlled environment in which they can engage in activities crucial for their individual development as well as activities that increase team building skills. SPs, when used in conjunction with other educational strategies, can substantially improve the quality of the learning environment and lead to healthcare professionals who are better equipped to safely practice in a variety of clinical settings.

Integrating SPs into health professions education provides valuable hands-on learning experiences in live patient–based encounters. Educators introduce sessions with SPs to bridge the gap between the textbook learning and real-patient clinical experiences, encompassing several perspectives and incorporating both cognitive and affective domains. Education and clinical assessment can be enriched by incorporating SPs as evidenced by increased learner satisfaction and outcomes (Dearmon et al., 2013). Medical, nursing, hospital-based clinical training, and allied health professions recognize the value of SPs in learning experiences, noting the results to be more objective, more systematic, and more consistent from learner to learner.

Trained SPs realistically portray patients, and can reliably and accurately record data on learner performances in history taking, physical exam techniques, and patient education. Because SPs are not healthcare providers, SPs are able to remain unbiased and follow criteria to objectively document learner performance. The unique nature of the SP encounter also allows the learner the opportunity to get immediate feedback on communication techniques and hear the patient's perspective. Knowledge of and experience with the efficacy of SPs and how to effectively incorporate them into training can enhance educational programs. However, the challenges some educators face in designing a robust and effective curriculum using SPs is understanding the breadth and depth of this methodology. The theoretical concepts and practical implementation outlined in this chapter can benefit educators ranging from novices to experienced persons.

CASE EXAMPLE

A quality improvement (QI) study at a rural hospital validated a concern of the administration, noting deficiencies in the ability of the midwives to effectively prioritize during obstetrical emergencies. Previous in-service lectures did not yield the desired results in improvement in patient outcomes. Faced with a challenge of how to bridge the gap between theory and practice, the QI education team began considering alternative strategies. After reviewing materials on educational modalities, the group decided to implement teaching with Standardized Patients (SPs). The hospital retained the services of an SP educator to conduct staff development sessions on the use of SPs in labor and delivery. Training sessions were conducted with midwifery and nursing staff to increase their confidence and comfort in handling emergencies. Focusing on refining history taking, communication and time management skills with the use of SPs demonstrated an improvement in the ability of the midwives to effectively prioritize the data collected. Over time the QI team will continue to evaluate the competency of the midwives by looking at patient outcomes.

INTRODUCTION AND BACKGROUND

The use of **Standardized Patients** (**SPs**) in healthcare education began in the 1960s in Los Angeles, California, with Dr. Howard Barrows. Barrows, a neurologist at the University of Southern California, was interested in standardizing the assessment of the clinical competence of medical students and residents. He trained an artist's model to portray a patient with multiple sclerosis. She was examined by learners and asked to provide her feelings from a patient's perspective. He described this early effort in an article in the *Journal of Medical Education* titled "The Programmed Patient: A Technique for Appraising Student Performance in Clinical Neurology" (Barrows & Abrahamson, 1964). In the late 1960s, at the University of Southern California School of Medicine it was decided that the term "simulated patient" was more accurate as the person portraying the role was not giving a fixed performance, as suggested by the term "programmed" but responded to context as a real patient would during the interview and examination by different learners. Howard advocated that properly trained SPs provided structure and objectivity to the encounter and that SPs could be coached to provide constructive feedback on the professional manner or interpersonal skills as experienced from the patient's point of view to the learner. Howard originally defined the simulated patient as:

> a person who has been carefully coached to simulate an actual patient so accurately that the simulation cannot be detected by a skilled clinician. In performing the simulation, the simulated patient presents the "gestalt" of the patient being simulated; not just the history, but the body language, the physical findings and the emotional and personality characteristics as well.

The acceptance of the SP as an educational instrument was evident as medical schools started to integrate them in undergraduate curricula. In the early 1970s, SP programs began to emerge throughout the United States and Canada.

On a parallel path, in 1972 in Arizona, Dr. Paula Stillman, a pediatrician, was inspired by the work of Ray Helfer, who, motivated by Howard's work, trained "programmed mothers" to work with his medical students.

However, his process of providing **feedback** was complicated and too subjective for Paula, so she developed her own instrument, by teaching her mothers to give consistent and authentic histories, while thinking of structured checklists that were to be completed after the interaction. Paula referred to them as "**patient simulators**" and "**paraprofessionals**." She successfully demonstrated that well-trained paraprofessionals/patient simulators could effectively teach interviewing skills, verify that a skill was acquired to a level of competency, reliably evaluate the students and provide uniform learning experiences without clinical faculty. Paula also introduced **Patient Instructors** (**PIs**) who were not simulating a patient case, but using their own normal bodies to teach learners how to perform a comprehensive and accurate physical exam using a checklist generated by clinical faculty (Wallace, 2006).

Paula's approach to using patient simulators/PIs to complete content, communication, and physical examination checklists immediately following the encounter and Howard's approach to using simulated patients who portrayed a patient with interpersonal feedback gradually merged into the SP modality we now commonly utilize.

While the evolution of the terms simulated patient (patient simulator) and standardized patient overlapped in the 1980s, these terms continue to be used interchangeably. In the United States, the term "standardized patient" is prevalent, and internationally "simulated patient" continues to be the accepted term. For the purposes of this chapter, we will use the term SP to mean standardized patient and will use this definition:

> individuals who are trained to portray a patient with a specific condition in a realistic, standardized and repeatable way (where portrayal/presentation varies based only on learner performances). SPs can be used for teaching and assessment of learners including but not limited to history/consultation, physical examination and other clinical skills in simulated clinical environments. SPs can also be used to give feedback and evaluate student performance. (Association of Standardized Patient Educators [ASPE], n.d.)

During the early 1990s and into the 2000s, a significant milestone for the modality/methodology was the research and implementation of SPs in high stakes national exams in North America. In 1992, the Medical Council of Canada developed a licensing examination using SPs in the Medical Council of Canada Qualifying Examination (MCCQE) to assess knowledge, skills and attitudes essential for medical licensure in Canada prior to entry into independent clinical practice. In 2004, The United States Medical Licensing Examination (USMLE), sponsored by the Federation of State Medical Boards (FSMB) and the National Board of Medical Examiners (NBME), began Clinical Skills testing of graduating medical students. The Step 2 Clinical Knowledge (Step 2ck) portion of the USMLE assesses medical knowledge, skills, and understanding of clinical science essential for the provision of patient care under supervision. Step 2 Clinical Skills (Step 2cs) uses SPs to test medical students and foreign medical graduates on their ability to gather information from patients, perform physical examinations, and communicate their findings to patients and colleagues. It represents the basic patient-centered skills that provide the foundation for the safe and effective practice of medicine. Examinees must pass the Step 2cs to be licensed to provide medical care in the United States.

Internationally, SPs are more commonly trained as *simulated* patients to incorporate more of their own personal backgrounds in their roles, and used in teaching where the impact of performance may differ from learner to learner. When using a SP in these types of sessions, authenticity tends to be more important than consistency (Bokken, 2009) with an emphasis on facilitative instruction from the eyes of the patient. SPs for evaluation and assessment of learner skills are less prevalent outside North America.

EDUCATIONAL ADVANTAGES OF THE SP METHODOLOGY

SP encounters are incorporated in the healthcare curriculum to allow for repeated deliberate experiences. When SP educators working with faculty integrate the theory of deliberate practice, they design SP encounters with the outcome of the learner attaining and improving skills. Deliberate practice (Ericsson et al., 1993) is a process by which experiences are specifically designed to improve performance. The learner is an active participant in the educational process. The settings for these activities are safe and nonthreatening, allowing the anxiety of the learner to be reduced so confidence can grow. Learners have an opportunity to apply knowledge and skills attained in an appropriate and realistic context. From these experiences, faculty and educators are able to teach and evaluate universal competencies that are the foundation of skills needed for effective growth and development of the learner. Learners are able to improve performance in response to feedback they have received by SPs, faculty/educators, and self and peer evaluation.

The SP modality offers the following advantages to the learner, the faculty, and the curriculum:

Advantages to Learners

- Reduces learner anxiety and eliminates risks
- Focus is on individual performance
- Immediate feedback that is standardized, clinically unbiased, and trained
- Hears patient's perspective that is integrated into specific feedback
- Authentic and real world—SP reacts to learner skills and performances as would a real patient
- Deliberate and repeatable experiences
- Active and engaging learning
- Offers practice with difficult patients and sensitive topics and examinations
- Allows opportunities to perfect skills
- Provides a transition to real patients

Advantages for Educational Program/Curriculum

- Availability in curricular schedule
- Assesses and reinforces curricular goals
- Provides feedback about teaching effectiveness
- Supports predefined course objectives
- Supports preset performance criteria
- Allows programmatic assessment of overall curriculum
- Flexibility—used at all levels of healthcare training
- Provides a reproducible, fair, and reliable experience for all students, allowing teaching and assessment of core skills to complex skills
- Provides opportunities for learners to work in emergency conditions
- Ability to monitor the continuum of learners' development
- Eliminates the risk of mistreatment of real patients

Advantages for Faculty

- Faculty control of content and complexity
- Relieves and reduces faculty of time-consuming instruction and assessment of basic skills
- Provides quantitative and objective feedback about student performance and applied skills not available through other methods
- Ease of scheduling similar clinical experiences
- SPs reliably and accurately document learner performance, reducing faculty time in real-time and multiple observation

Integrating SPs into the curriculum allows the learners to master skills and increase confidence. As a result, the curriculum is strengthened and reinforced to enhance learning.

Standardized Patient Roles and Activities

The flexibility and controllability of the SP methodology allows for the ability to integrate SPs into all healthcare curricula. The integration can be for teaching and instructional purposes or for assessments, either formative or summative. Furthermore, the role of an SP in the curriculum has been refined over the years. SPs are used not only in simulating and assessing learners but are becoming more accepted in the role of teacher and facilitator. This expansion is a result of several external forces such as an increase in class size and accreditation requirements, decrease in clinical experiences and faculty and restricted resident hours. The decision as to what role the SP will have and his/her scope of responsibilities will depend on the goals and objective of the course and the simulation activity embedded within the course.

The scope of SP duties may include, but is not limited to, the following:

- Teaching and Instruction Activities
  - Case portrayal—the SP's primary responsibility is to realistically perform a case or scenario in the role of a patient, and observe learner skills to provide feedback.
  - Facilitator—experienced SPs may be trained as facilitators in the process of a learner moving through a case or learning a skill. SPs can be used in problem-based learning, team-based learning, small groups, and so forth.
  - Teaching Associate—known as Patient Instructors (PI) or **Physical Examination Teaching Associates** (**PETA, PTA**), **GYN Teaching Associates** (**GTAs**), and **Male Urogenital Teaching Associates** (**MUTAs**), these SPs are extensively trained to teach comprehensive physical examination techniques, communication skills, professionalism, GYN and genitourinary clinical skills.
- Assessment Activities
  - **Formative**—SPs are trained to provide immediate qualitative feedback to learners focusing on details of content and performance. Scores are generally not the focus of the formative assessment, but the SP may complete a checklist as a stimulus for feedback. Scores may be discussed in feedback and used in low stakes activities.
  - **Summative**—SPs are trained to complete a checklist used to collect qualitative data and scores. Data is used to determine a learner's proficiency and is generally not provided immediately after completion of the assessment. Scores are provided at a later date. SPs used for summative assessment are trained and monitored to recall information with significant accuracy.
  - Remediation—advanced SPs are trained to meet the needs of the learner exhibiting deficiencies.
  - **Unannounced or "mystery" patients**—"the use of unannounced standardized patients as an approach to the research and practice of clinical performance assessment *in vivo* provides both the direct observation and control of standardized patient assessments and the naturalistic and nonreactive properties of assessment in practice" (Swartz & Colliver, 1996).

As programs have grown and SPs have become more experienced, a rich resource of lay educators has emerged. SPs portray various characters, teach, debrief, and assess. Utilizing these skills, many programs are training the SPs in roles other than "patients." They are now simulated health professionals (doctors, nurses, technicians, etc.), family members, clinical faculty, healthcare administrators, and more (discussed at the end of this chapter). In using the same methods of training, these advanced roles can be successfully integrated into a range of experiential situations.

HOW TO INCORPORATE SPs INTO THE CURRICULUM

A well-constructed curriculum achieves the goals, objectives, and the learning outcomes of the institution. The same is true for integrating SP experiences in courses. At the course level when educators and faculty are considering incorporating SP experiences into the curriculum, the objectives must be ever present in discussion and design.

Designing a course with an SP experience occurs in much the same way as designing a course without an SP experience. Noel Meyers and Ducan Nulty eloquently stated the essence of what educators want to design for learners in an article in 2008 for *Assessment & Evaluation in Higher Education*. They stated: "To maximize the quality of student learning outcomes we, as academics, need to develop courses in ways that provide students with teaching and learning materials, tasks and experiences which:

1. are authentic, real-world, and relevant;
2. are constructive, sequential, and interlinked;
3. require students to use and engage with progressively higher-order cognitive processes;
4. are all aligned with each other and the desired learning outcomes; and
5. provide challenge, interest and motivation to learn."

Integrating deliberate SP experiences into the curriculum will achieve this goal. There are many models for curriculum development, but essentially most have the same elements for the process. The process for curriculum development is a dynamic, iterative, and continuous process.

As faculty begin to think about integrating SPs, a careful review of the appropriateness of the SP experiences, where these experiences are placed in the curriculum, and the outcome expected is needed. This includes a clear alignment, coherence, sequence, continuity, and integration from top to bottom. Figure 3.3.1 details this process (Curriculum Resources, 2012).

Rationale/Curriculum Need

The process begins with a statement as to an identified need in the curriculum. It should speak to a learning

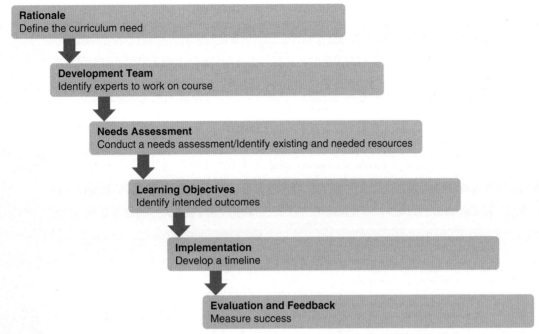

FIGURE 3.3.1 Details the process whereby faculty begin to think about integrating SPs. A careful review of the appropriateness of the SP experiences, where these experiences are placed in the curriculum, and the outcome expected is needed. This includes a clear alignment, coherence, sequence, continuity, and integration from top to bottom.

problem or issue that the curriculum will address, including any observational data to support the need. The statement should be as clear as possible, including any factors that perhaps contributed to the need. For example, learners may demonstrate a lack of skill in decision making and communicating. The need is for the learners to acquire knowledge, practice, receive feedback, and be assessed. *Will integrating an SP experience be the solution for the need?*

Integrating SP encounters into health professions education curricula should be the appropriate solution for the need described. SPs allow for careful identification of cognitive, psychomotor, and affective knowledge and skills. The answer will drive the development process and ultimately achieve the learning objective. The answer to the question above is yes. Integrating an SP experience into the curriculum will address the need of student's ability/inability to demonstrate the skill of communicating with patients. The SP experience will allow students the opportunity for deliberate practice on communication skills in a simulated environment and receive immediate feedback from a patient's perspective.

Development Team/Experts

A critical part of the planning is the identification of a curriculum development team or an expert in curriculum design. In some institutions, it will be the **Standardized Patient Educator**. At institutions who do not have an SP educator, it is incumbent upon whoever is training SPs to fill the role of the SP educator and implement the SP methodology. These individuals bring their expertise and knowledge to give input and manage the integration

within the curriculum. Who are the key individuals at your institution that need to be part of this process? When looking at improving learning and assessment across the healthcare continuum, it has been, currently is, and will be an educational journey, which can also be described as curriculum theorizing. It is during the journey that the development team/expert must look at the big picture and be visionaries of the curriculum. Their mindset can focus on the endless possibilities of the SP integration and work toward a consensus as they examine the complexities and multidimensional aspects of specific curriculum and course situations. At the end of the process, the development team/expert will have a curriculum matrix that shows the integration and alignment of SPs into individual courses and overall curriculum (Figure 3.3.2).

Needs Assessment

"A targeted needs assessment is a process by which curriculum developers apply the knowledge learned from the general needs assessment to their particular learners and learning environment" (Kern et al., 2009). The targeted needs assessment provides information to determine educational objectives based on facts and foundation and establishes baseline data. This part of the process will help the development team/expert document what they already know about the curriculum and build on that. In building the course, identify what resources are essential for integration specifically for SP experiences as they are unique and very different than a lecture. The following six areas should be considered during this process. A more detailed explanation of each area is covered in chapter 5.5.

SP CURRICULUM INTEGRATION

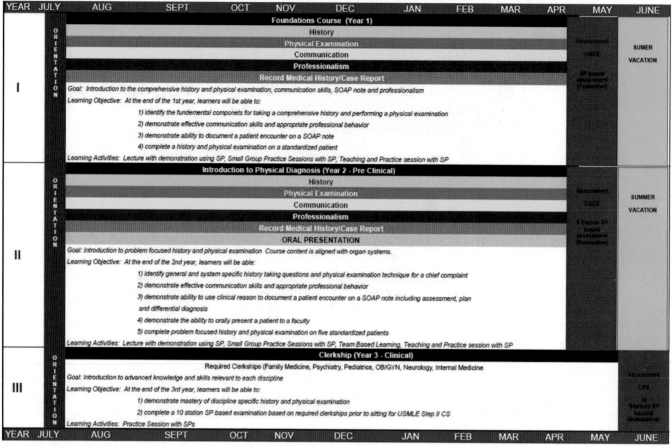

FIGURE 3.3.2 SP curriculum integration.

1. Expertise Availability—The expertise needed to integrate SPs into the curriculum includes an individual(s) who is knowledgeable and educated in the SP methodology. Is there an existing SP program or department within the institution with an SP educator? If an SP program does not exist, a decision is needed on who will take on this role and how personnel and SPs will be secured for the curriculum.

2. Funding—SPs are the highest-fidelity simulator; therefore, integrating SPs will impact the annual operating budget. The development team/expert should determine how much funding is available as it will help to set priorities for the integration and the funding source. Consistently, SP compensation will depend on the region and the task expected of the SP.

3. Staff—identification of how much human capital will be required for the SP experience. The purpose is to make sure the appropriate staff is in place for sustainability for the required SP activities. The most reoccurring pitfall is starting with minimal staff support, and as the SP activities grow, the staff support does not reflect the SP activities.

4. Facility—identification of where the SP experience will take place. Is there dedicated space available, or will the experiences take place in existing classrooms throughout the campus?

5. Technology—the type of technology required to conduct SP experiences. Effective technology integration is achieved when the use of technology is routine and transparent, allowing for total immersion into the experience, and when technology supports curricular goals.

6. Curriculum Scheduling—One of the most challenging factors in integrating SPs in the overall curriculum is where the SP experience will be put in an already busy course schedule. Depending on the objectives and format for the SP experience, the length of time for the experience will be established. Is there time in the course curriculum scheduling to accommodate this teaching session as well as all other components of the course?

The needs assessment is a critical step that requires time, strategy, and thoroughness. The results of this process will help to shape the intended educational objectives strategically.

Learning Objectives

The learning objectives for an SP integrated curriculum describe what the learners will be able to do that they were not able to do before. The learning objective establishes measurable behavioral outcomes. The objectives may be either general or specific, with the general objectives being appropriate at the course or program level. More specific objectives are used at the session level and are considered performance objectives. The performance objectives are categorized as knowledge, attitude, behaviors or skill. Figure 3.3.3 shows an example of how the educational objective at the institutional level is achieved on the basis of the performance objectives at the course level.

The learning objectives clearly state what the learners should be able to do (perform) after leaving the course. At the end of the curriculum, the institutional educational learning objective will be achieved.

Implementation/Timeline

The implementation phase is layered with several key issues that should be considered for a smooth launch. Although the use of SPs has been in place for numerous years, there are still pockets of hesitancy and resistance. "Effective implementation of innovations requires time, personal interaction and contacts, in-service training and other forms of people-based support" (Fullan & Pomfret, 1977). Recognition that the integration may produce a certain amount of anxiety may be minimized by organizing the implementation into manageable events (milestones) and by setting achievable goals.

In integrating SP experiences, many logistical issues that are inherent have to be considered. To begin with, the decision of "when" the SP experience would be integrated into the curriculum and individual courses must be made. Will it launch at the beginning of the next academic year or

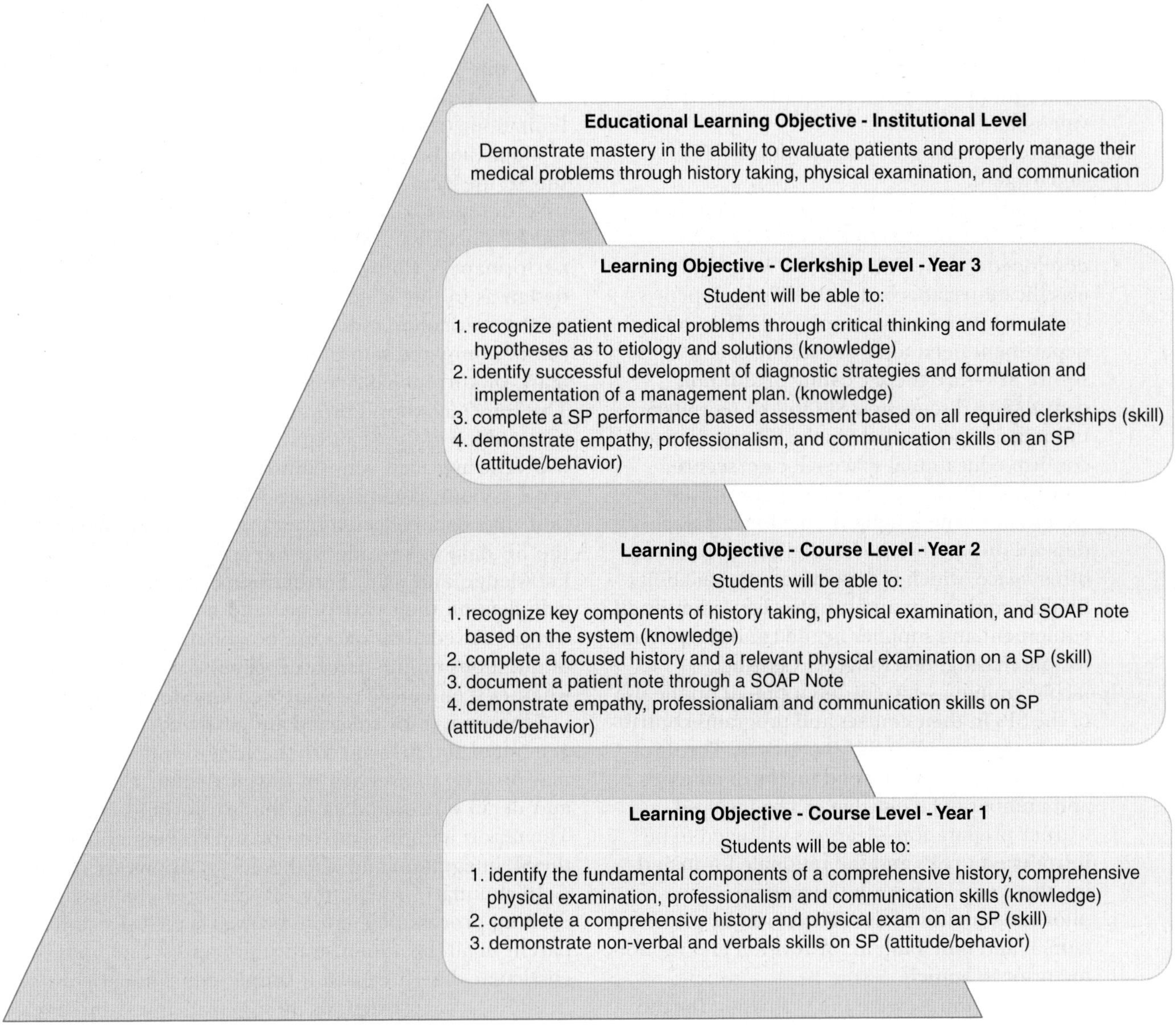

Educational Learning Objective - Institutional Level
Demonstrate mastery in the ability to evaluate patients and properly manage their medical problems through history taking, physical examination, and communication

Learning Objective - Clerkship Level - Year 3
Student will be able to:
1. recognize patient medical problems through critical thinking and formulate hypotheses as to etiology and solutions (knowledge)
2. identify successful development of diagnostic strategies and formulation and implementation of a management plan. (knowledge)
3. complete a SP performance based assessment based on all required clerkships (skill)
4. demonstrate empathy, professionalism, and communication skills on an SP (attitude/behavior)

Learning Objective - Course Level - Year 2
Students will be able to:
1. recognize key components of history taking, physical examination, and SOAP note based on the system (knowledge)
2. complete a focused history and a relevant physical examination on a SP (skill)
3. document a patient note through a SOAP Note
4. demonstrate empathy, professionaliam and communication skills on SP (attitude/behavior)

Learning Objective - Course Level - Year 1
Students will be able to:
1. identify the fundamental components of a comprehensive history, comprehensive physical examination, professionalism and communication skills (knowledge)
2. complete a comprehensive history and physical exam on an SP (skill)
3. demonstrate non-verbal and verbals skills on SP (attitude/behavior)

FIGURE 3.3.3 An example of how the educational objective at the institutional level is achieved on the basis of the performance objectives at the course level.

immediately? The date can be changed; however, deciding on an appropriate date will allow for a draft timeline to be rolled out. The items that need to be included in the timeline are listed below. The items should also include identification of an individual who will be responsible for each task.

1. Launch Date: Determine the date for the SP experience to start.
2. SP Integration Approval: Will a presentation of the SP experience to the department or curriculum committee be required for approval? If so, identify the steps from presentation to approval.
3. Secure Resources: The identification of existing resources and which of those resources that need development. Each item will be dependent upon other departments within the institution, requiring an idea of their specific timelines.
   a. final operational budget
   b. finalize course materials—identify what course materials are needed for faculty, SPs, and learners. The materials may include, but are not limited to, SP training materials, faculty instructional guides, learner prerequisite materials, videos, and so forth.
   c. finalize technology—consult with the IT department.
   d. hire staff—consult with HR process and timeline. Do new job descriptions need to be developed for the SPE and SPs? What will the classification status be for the SPs (independent consultant versus employee)? Does a legal department need to be consulted?
   e. secure SPs—are there existing SPs? If not, consult and discuss how SPs will be recruited, trained, and scheduled for the SP experience.
   f. confirm educational space—locate, secure, and schedule the educational space for the SP experience. The length of time for this step will depend on whether it is in dedicated space or other space, which is dependent on availability.
   g. finalize equipment and supplies list—identify all equipment and supplies needed and the process for purchasing, receiving, and storing.
   h. faculty training—faculty development on the use of the SPs in their courses and programs contributes to the success of the experience. The duration of training will depend on the experience and number of faculty that will be involved.
   i. learner preparation—learners will need to be introduced to SPs and the rationale for including these experiences in the course.
   j. pilot test—a pilot of the SP experience prior to launch and time built in for revision and repiloting prior to launch.
   k. final evaluation—create the evaluation for the SP experience, and determine the time needed for analysis, reporting, and revision before the next launch.

The best-laid plans are met with unexpected challenges. Developing a flexible implementation plan that is reviewed and modified along the way is the most practical and effective approach for success.

Evaluation Plans/Measuring Success

"Evaluation and feedback, closes the loop in the curriculum development cycle. The evaluation step helps curriculum developers ask and answer the critical question, Were the goals and objectives of the curriculum met?" (Kern et al., 2009). The team must close the loop on the SP integration by building in the evaluation process at the beginning. The steps to close the loop are to first develop the evaluation, collect the data, and report back. Ideally, the individual who will design the evaluation, collect the data, perform the analysis, and generate the report will be on the development team. This individual will guide the development team in making sure the goal and objectives for the SP integration are connected to the outcomes. Also, this individual will assist in defining the purpose, scope, and tools for the evaluation as well as in identifying limitations (time, resources, technology, funds).

Data can be collected from various sources, including the SP, the faculty, and the learner. The information can be used to report back to the educational stakeholders. From the SP checklist, the data provides feedback on learner performances (individual and group) and overall course design as to the achievement of the objective and impact on the curriculum. Additionally, data from the SP checklist can be compared with preexisting data or used as a benchmark of current skills and for comparison in the future. This information will provide a pre- and postview as to the value added of the SP integration into the course. However if preexisting data is not available, the collected data will serve as both baseline and evidence of validity for integration. The data collected from the faculty will complement the SP data to provide further insight into the learner's knowledge and skill. Furthermore, the learner can provide data on their experience and beliefs if the objectives were achieved. This data can be obtained through a series of questions on the perceived value of the integration and whether it enhanced or improved knowledge and skills.

Moreover, once collected and analyzed, a report can be generated and presented to the administration. The report may provide an overview of the curriculum design process and detail outcome data at the learner and course level. The report identifies next steps and recommendations for the SP integration and whether any revisions are required.

In summary, integrating SPs can be a challenging and exciting process. The entire process is inclusive and transparent of all the administrative processes. The basis of the curricular design can be a simple educational construct. In addition to instructional design principles, the development of an SP experience includes adult education theory and experiential learning principles in the design. Success depends on a plan, a map, and an outcome.

STANDARDIZED PATIENT MODALITY DEVELOPMENT—THE SPECIFICS

As outlined previously, many medical schools and institutions employ a Standardized Patient Educator (SPE) to work with faculty to design SP activities, develop cases and accompanying materials, train SPs, and implement the SP-based encounters. At institutions who do not have an SP educator, it is the responsibility of whoever is training SPs to implement the SP methodology, thereby filling the role of SPE.

Case Construction and Writing

Depending on the objectives of the course and SP session, case construction may include several components: the SP training case (summary or protocol), the SP checklist and accompanying materials. SP educators often develop a case writing template, which provides a prescribed format for constructing each component and aspect of the case. The Association of Standardized Patient Educators (ASPE, n.d.), the National Board of Medical Examiners, and others have case writing templates available as a guideline when constructing a comprehensive and trainable case.

Similar to other simulation modalities, the selection of the case to be developed for training the SP is based on curricular goals and objectives, and the learner tasks are clearly defined to meet these objectives. Other components to be clearly identified as the case is being developed are the following: the type of documentation and reporting of learner performance by the SP; learner orientation, behaviors or skills the learner is to practice or demonstrate; accompanying materials (i.e., lab results, X-rays, charts, etc.) and the components of SP feedback (content and communication checklists). The role of the SP to meet the activity objectives is also defined in the case and reinforced in training sessions

A simple way to think about the construction of a SP training case is to dissect a patient chart from the patients' perspective. The SP training case includes:

- patient demographics (age, gender, body type, race, socioeconomic/educational level, etc.)
- a standardized opening statement that the SP must memorize verbatim and say to all learners at the start of the encounter
- history of presenting illness, PHM, FM, SH, ROS, signs and symptoms to be exhibited (if applicable)
- relationships (personally and professionally)
- patient affect, demeanor, mannerisms, and personality
- standardized questions/challenges to be asked if the learner does not address an issue (assessing knowledge base)
- Interaction guidelines for the SP are also specified in the case:
  - pacing of information,
  - reactions to learner questions,
  - how to respond to various learner approaches and how to answer unexpected questions,
  - cases that include the portrayal of a family/team member define the emotional/professional response to each member with specific verbal and nonverbal behaviors appropriate for the role and relationships.

Once the training case has been completed, the case author (SPE, faculty SME) "pilot-tests" the case, and revises as needed before training the SP.

In many cases, SPs may be trained to collect the data used to evaluate the learner. On the SP checklist are all the concrete tasks the learner should be able to perform at the end of the course. Each task has predefined criteria that the SP uses to rate each item. This checklist is memorized by the SPs, and after the encounter they complete it on behalf of the faculty, documenting the questions that were asked, if the student performed certain skills, and the techniques they demonstrated. SPs are extensively trained to obtain a high inter-rater reliability and accuracy when completing the checklists for high stakes examination.

Cases may include scenarios that are designed to improve the current knowledge and skill; for example, a second-year Nurse Practitioner student working with an SP may be asked to demonstrate competency by integrating history taking and appropriate physical exam in a focused encounter. A case of this type might be integrated into a diagnosis and management course. The NP student will gain insight on his/her performance in the diagnosis and management of, for example, acute back pain. These types of cases are designed to evaluate the current level of performance toward improvement. Encounters in which the learner needs to perform at a more advanced level to determine whether they are ready to progress to clinical placement or advancement are best with cases designed for use in a Clinical Performance Exam (CPE). Skill-based assessment alone often evaluates procedures and techniques but cannot address or include higher-level problem-solving processes that are necessary; consequently, the SP case is typically multifaceted to include data collection, assessment, and clinical reasoning.

Training of Standardized Patients

Standardized patient training is a multistep process to ensure reliable, consistent, and accurate portrayal of a case or character. While details such as length of time and number of sessions needed to train an SP for a case, or whether or not to have the SP memorize the case prior to arriving at the initial training session, vary among educators, certain principles never change.

1. The training is done over several sessions to provide time for the SP to practice and assimilate the case details.
2. During the first session, SPs are coached: on the key learning objectives, the expectations of the SP, the details of the case history; to simulate the physical symptoms, discuss the gestalt of the character,

the standardized questions, interaction guidelines, and the parameters of feedback. If the SP is completing a checklist, the checklist and checklist parameters/guide are reviewed. An enhancement for training may be a video/recording of the role. Reviewing the recording is efficient and effective for standardization of patient portrayal—with a cautionary note. Selection of the recording to be used is done with care. The recording must demonstrate the specific details the SPs are to portray in the case. SPs will replicate incorrect information or incorrect portrayal actions because they will now have the "picture of the patient" on the recording in their mindset. It is sometimes difficult to "undo" what the SPs observe on a recording.

3. A second session addresses SP questions, case and checklist grey areas, fine-tuning and refinements, and practice—including simulating physical findings (if present). Feedback is again reviewed to meet the objectives of the encounter.

4. Whether in a third session or during the second session, a "dry run" or "dress rehearsal" is conducted in which each SP has an opportunity to portray the patient while observed by the case author/trainer, complete a checklist, and provide feedback. The focus is on standardization of performance, inter-/intrareliability, and accuracy while completing the checklist and constructive/specific feedback. It is preferable that a person who is blind to the case to assess the realism conducts the dry run and determines whether the simulation is authentic and plays out the way it was intended. Experienced SPs are an excellent barometer to see the efficacy of the case and portrayal.

5. Exposure to "different leaner styles" will assist in the SPs' ability to portray the case, provide specific feedback, and discriminate checklist items.

6. The number of sessions and the amount of training depends on the activity and objectives. Higher stakes exams require more extensive and intensive training, practice, and standardization. There may be four to six sessions of training, video role-plays, review of checklists and rating scales, and a higher level of standardization for case portrayal. A more tempered approach to training is common for formative evaluations and formative teaching sessions.

7. If more than one SP will perform the case, ideally they should be trained together. Group training allows each SP to see the performance of their peers and enables performance direction that all SPs will follow. Keeping the encounter standardized allows every learner an equal opportunity to demonstrate his or her skills in key clinical and interpersonal areas.

8. When training an SP to portray a family/team member they will be trained in how to respond to various cues of learner performance and to each member of the team. In all encounters, attention is given to specific verbal and nonverbal behaviors appropriate for the role and directives regarding how to answer learner questions.

9. The faculty is responsible for development of assessment tools and any written materials or notes the learner will be expected to complete as part of the SP encounter.

In summary, through rigorous training, SPs come to understand that they must work from the same information and facts and deliver the responses in the same way to each learner. Refinement training allows for practice to ensure believable and consistent portrayal of someone with a particular condition/problem and reactive to learner approaches. The goal of training is to: (1) achieve consistent and accurate portrayal, (2) instill the SP with the characteristics, behaviors, and history of a real interaction, (3) produce sufficient realism to elicit the desired clinical performance, (4) review techniques for constructive feedback, and (5) maintain reliability and accuracy of checklist completion.

EXAMPLE

In a SP case of an 18-year-old female with abdominal pain, the portrayal needed from the SPs may be that of a shy, college student, embarrassed by having a sexual encounter with a friend and is now worried about pregnancy or illness. One SP portraying that case might be older than 18 years old who has never been to college and is married with one child. The real-life perspective of that individual SP is not the same as that of the patient in the case. How the SP views the world is different from her case patient. Consequently, the well-written case and training help the SP understand the gestalt of that patient. This allows her to accurately portray and to evaluate the interpersonal communication skills of the learner in a manner that is true to that 18-year-old patient in a standardized way.

Feedback and Debriefing from Standardized Patients

It is difficult for real patients to provide constructive and objective feedback to people who are involved in their healthcare. Since SPs are not actually suffering from the disease/condition and not reliant on the provider, it allows them to take a step back and assess the interpersonal skill of the learners. However, this is not a natural skill, so SPs need to be trained to give learners skillful, constructive, and individualized feedback on their performance. While feedback may be included in case training, many SPs are trained in a separate session(s) specifically focused on feedback techniques and principles. SPs incorporate various debriefing techniques such as the use of learner self-reflection, providing specific behavior-based examples, reinforcing strengths, and defining areas for improvement.

When training SPs to provide feedback, various instruments and guidelines are available to ensure they are objectively evaluating interpersonal communication skills and techniques. The various approaches to SP feedback range from structured and standardized Likert scale instruments to unstructured open formats. However it is standard procedure that SP feedback includes the viewpoint of the patient the SPs are portraying and patient perspective, and assesses the learners' ability to demonstrate empathy, negotiate care and active listening. Specific and consistent training of SPs ensures they understand the criteria and benchmarks they should follow when determining the effectiveness of learner communication and interaction.

Feedback from the SP should be provided only at the end of the encounter. If the objective is for the learner to treat the SP as a real patient and demonstrate development of the patient-provider relationship, it is confusing and distracting to have the SP go in and out of role during the encounter. The switching from patient to debriefer (providing feedback) back to patient can have a negative impact on the learner, and the simulation is no longer perceived as real or representative of learner performance when with a real patient. At the end of an encounter, the SP can communicate directly with the learner by giving verbal or written feedback by completing a communication checklist that will provide a document of learner performance and a source for discussion.

Ensuring Reliability and Validity of SP Encounters

While computerized patient simulators can be programmed through their software with such accuracy that any concerns about reliability are removed from the educational experience, the same is not true for SPs. Because SP encounters include portrayal of the same case by different SPs, faculty may have concerns about reliability and human error. It is during the development process of the case and, most importantly, the training and quality assurance check of the SP that reliability measures can be implemented to ensure a fair and equitable experience for all learners.

Attention to validity and reliability are crucial when developing SP sessions. Case validity indicates that the case is representative of the domain and the factors are congruent with learning objectives. It is during the training of the SPs that the faculty can assess the validity of the case and experience. By actually performing the case in training and completing postencounter notes in much the same way as a learner would do in an actual session, faculty are better able to judge the validity of that particular case.

Preparation of Learners

The use of SPs like any other educational strategy may be built in a stepwise manner. It is more effective for learners to be adequately prepared to work with SPs and in the appropriate context. It is less productive to have learners encounter an SP for the first time in testing situations. An effective way to begin using SPs is in the classroom in the first year of training. Faculty can model a provider-patient interaction immediately following didactic sessions. Learners can also work with the SP in a small group setting, thereby reinforcing to the entire class interactions that are positive and those that need improvement. Moving along a continuum of different formats of SP encounters throughout their education allows learners to progress through various stages of development in a nonthreatening manner. Also, in moving along the spectrum of encounters, learners gain experience with the modality and are better equipped when they reach the stage of one-on-one encounters and high stakes assessment.

Prior to an SP encounter, laying the groundwork with learners begins by sharing the objectives for session, expectations, and housekeeping items. Learners are reminded that, although SPs are portraying a patient with a condition, disease, or problem that is not their own, they are people and are to be treated as a real patient. From the moment the learner meets the SP until the end of the debriefing and feedback, they are with a patient with needs, concerns, and opinions.

Assessment of Learner and Curriculum Performance

The University of North Carolina Teaching and Learning Center defines assessment as the systematic collection, review, and use of information about learner performance to improve their overall knowledge, skills, and attitude. SPs are a reliable source of data collection on the tasks performed by the learner during the patient encounter (Vu et al., 1992). This information, communicated back to the learner can then be used to improve current and future performance. The data can be scored by the faculty responsible for grading and used to provide scores and statistical performance feedback to learners.

While SP encounters can be used as a method of teaching, and for formative or summative evaluation, the results from an SP-based assessment provide additional information that can be used to:

- determine whether or not intended session objectives set by faculty have been achieved,
- unveil relevant issues that can impact the course and educational experience,
- determine whether competency-based objectives are being met, and
- assess the overall curriculum ability to meet expected outcomes.

Types of Standardized Patient Assessments and Testing

In reviewing the literature, there are several terms referring to comprehensive exams using SPs to assess the competency of learners. The terms **Clinical Skills Assessments** (**CSA**), Clinical Performance Exam (CPE), and Objective Structured Clinical Exam (OSCE) are sometimes used interchangeably but are in fact different assessment strategies. While all of these testing approaches incorporate the assessment of clinical skills using SPs, some are broader in scope than others.

CPEs and CSAs (including the high-stakes Step 2cs) can be either formative or summative assessments of overall competency. Examinees must demonstrate the ability to apply clinical knowledge, skills, and attitude in a patient encounter. In a CSA or CPE, the learner will be challenged, for example, to care for a patient with abdominal pain. The examinee would be required to demonstrate all aspects for the care of the patient to include history taking, physical exam, diagnosis, treatment, and effective communication with the patients. The stations tend to be longer than 10 minutes, depending on the tasks required of the examinee. SPs are painstakingly trained to portray cases in a realistic manner with accuracy and reliability. If multiple SPs are portraying a case, their affect, presentation of symptoms, and responses to student questions must be standardized across all SPs. Additionally, they must portray the case the same way with every student they see during the testing day.

An OSCE, first described by Harden et al. (1975), can also be used for formative or summative testing and typically focused on specific competencies and skill mastery. As an assessment method, it is based on objective testing and direct observation of student performance during short (historically less than 10 minutes) task-based encounters. While originally OSCEs did not include SP-based stations, over the years SPs have become an active part of the multistation assessment. The primary differences between an OSCE station and a Clinical Skills Assessment (CSA) are timing and the specificity of the aims/tasks for the learner. OSCE tasks tend to be more clearly defined for the learners in order to undertake one specified aspect of the clinical encounter. Using the abdominal pain case as an example, the learners in an OSCE might be asked to demonstrate competencies limited to the abdominal exam in order to assess their physical exam techniques. Another short station may provide pregnancy test results, should the faculty want to assess the counseling and communication skills of the examinee. If SPs are used to complete a checklist in these short stations, they require the same diligence in training, as would the longer CSA and CPE.

Sustaining the SP Experience

Sustaining quality SP experiences for learners requires implementing Continuous Quality Improvement (CQI) initiatives, program evaluations, and keeping abreast of latest innovations. CQI initiatives ensure that standard operating procedures are in place.

Principles utilized by business and industry are likewise applicable to education and the SP modality/methodology.

- Ensuring linkage of SP encounters to institutional and educational objectives
- Prioritizing the demonstrated need for SP encounters relative to other initiatives, programs and priorities
- Using facts and data to address student and institutional performance to support actions at all levels of decision making
- Creating accountabilities, expectations, roles and responsibilities for the institution
- Conducting regular reviews of performance and implementing evaluations after session
- Ensuring visible, active feedback mechanisms to learners, educators, and stakeholders
- Monitoring and including innovative immersive SP activities
- Continuing education of SPE and faculty

After systematic and strategic review, the SP experiences may need to be periodically adjusted for learner differences, class size, and funding.

Implications for Educators

This chapter focused on high-fidelity simulations in the form of the SP modality. With the goal of developing a more competent and confident healthcare provider, providing current and future learners with SP experiences can optimize learning and practice. There are pros and cons to the utilization of any form of simulation. Roger Kneebone (2005) is cited as saying that as the climate of clinical education places more emphasis on simulation as a safe substitute for practicing on real patients, the range of available simulations will increase, and it is now that we must examine what the characteristics of a successful simulation are in terms of learning and clinical outcomes. Resourceful educators will utilize multiple teaching and assessment strategies and select those that allow learners to demonstrate a range of competencies.

An emerging combination of SP and other simulation modalities such as Hybrid Simulations is discussed in another chapter. Implementing the SP methodology with other simulation modalities requires the same strategic planning, thoughtful development, and methodical training of the SP/family member/team member and faculty.

BEEN THERE, DONE THAT: HOW CAN I CONTINUE TO IMPROVE OR SUSTAIN WHAT I HAVE ACHIEVED?

Although SPs' origin is in healthcare, they have also been used in other professions. Such expansion stimulates creative thinking on the part of the medical institutions to solicit additional work for their center and SPs. The investment in time and energy into exploring new endeavors

	History taking interviewing	Physical exam	Communication	SOAP note/ patient note	Systems	Professionalism ethics	Reasoning problem solving	Disease recognition and detection	Patient education counseling	Team building	Cultural considerations	Research
Dentistry	X	X	X	X	X	X	X	X	X	X	X	X
Medicine	X	X	X	X	X	X	X	X	X	X	X	X
Nursing	X	X	X	X	X	X	X	X	X	X	X	X
Pharmacy	X	X	X	X	X	X	X	X	X	X	X	X
Allied health	X	X	X	X	X	X	X	X	X	X	X	X
Psychology	X	X	X	X	X	X	X	-	X	X	X	X
Residents	X	X	X	X	X	X	X	X	X	X	X	X
Social work	X	-	X	X	X	X	X	-	X	X	X	X
Humanities	X	-	X	-	X	X	X	-	X	X	X	X
Business	X	-	X	-	X	X	X	-	X	X	X	X
Law	X	-	X	-	X	X	X	-	X	X	X	X
Divinity	X	-	X	-	X	X	X	-	X	X	X	X
Education	X	X	X	-	X	X	X	-	X	X	X	X
Military science	X	X	X	X	X	X	X	X	X	X	X	X
Basic science	X	-	X	-	X	X	X	X	X	X	X	X

FIGURE 3.3.4 Professions and domains into which SPs have been effectively integrated.

and adapting the SP methodology to conduct experiential sessions benefits the institution in multiple ways:

- Advancing beyond healthcare challenges and improves the performance of the individuals who work as standardized patients,
- It keeps experienced SPs by providing additional work,
- It further develops SP skills, and
- It generates revenue for the institution.

Many programs are expanding to include work with nonmedical professions such as social services, k-12 education, law, and customer service training. Unique opportunities are available for SPs to work with market research companies, healthcare training, electronic healthcare companies, and pharmaceutical research.

Performing a market analysis and needs assessment of the community can provide information about the range of possible opportunities. As one example, law firms often run training and mock trials for their legal staff prior to the start of a case. SPs can memorize significant amounts of information and can portray a defendant, subject matter expert, or plaintiff in a mock trial. Undergraduate college students may want to practice interviews for medical or law school, where SPs can portray faculty interviewers and provide feedback to the candidate on their professional interview.

Figure 3.3.4 identifies professions and domains into which SPs have been effectively integrated.

SUMMARY

The integration of valid methodologies will facilitate the preparation of professional, caring, and creative healthcare providers and professionals. Integration of SPs into the curriculum and other types of simulation is not a substitute for learning experiences in the real world or clinical setting. It is this broad range of experiences—didactic, computer simulation, human patient simulators, and SPs—that prepare healthcare providers for the safe care of patients in the clinical setting. SP can also prepare professionals for more effective communication in their daily lives and with collegial interactions encountered in any work situation. The SP methodology is unique as it can be adapted for use with both medical and nonmedical training in multiple settings with all levels of learners and can provide the learners with individual experiential opportunities.

REFERENCES

Association of Standardized Patient Educators. (n.d.). *Standardized patient definition.* Retrieved from http://aspeducators.org/terminology-standards

Barrows, H., & Abrahamson, S. (1964). The programmed patient: A technique for appraising student performance in clinical neurology. *Journal of Medical Education, 39*(8), 802–805.

Bokken, L. (2009). *Innnovative use of simulated patient for educational purposes* (Doctoral dissertation). Datawyse, Maastricht University, Maastricht, Netherlands.

Curriculum Resources, (2012). Aligning and Building Curriculum. Retrieved December 10, 2012 from http://gototheexchange.ca/index.php/curriculum-at-a-program-level/overview-of-program-development

Dearmon, V., Graves, R. J., & Al, E. (2013). Effectiveness of simulation-based orientation of baccalaureate nursing students preparing for their first clinical experience. *Journal of Nursing Education, 52*(1), 29–38.

Ericsson, K. A., Krampe, R. T., & Tesch-Römer, C. (1993). The role of deliberate practice in the acquisition of expert performance. *Psychological Review, 100*(3), 363–406. doi:10.1037//0033-295X.100.3.363

Fullan, M., & Pomfret, A. (1977). Research on curriculum and instruction implementation. *Review of Educational Research, 47*(2), 335–397. Retrieved from http://eric.ed.gov/?id=EJ166914

Harden, R. M., Stevenson, M., Downie, W. W., & Wilson, G. M. (1975). Assessment of clinical competence using objective structured examination. *British Medical Journal, 1*(5955), 447–451. Retrieved from http://www.bmj.com/cgi/content/abstract/1/5955/447

SECTION 3 • Simulators

Kern, D. E., Thomas, P. A., & Hughes, M. T. (1998). Curriculum maintenance and enhancement. In *Curriculum development for medical education* (p. 272). Baltimore, MD: Johns Hopkins University Press.

Kneebone, R. (2005). Evaluating clinical simulations for learning procedural skills: A theory-based approach. *AAMC Academic Medicine Journal of the Association of American Medical Colleges, 80*(6), 549–553. Retrieved from http://www.ncbi.nlm.nih.gov/pubmed/15917357

Swartz, M. H., & Colliver, J. A. (1996). Using standardized patients for assessing clinical performance: An overview. *The Mount Sinai Journal of Medicine New York, 63*(3–4), 241–249. Retrieved from http://ovidsp .ovid.com/ovidweb.cgi?T=JS&CSC=Y&NEWS=N&PAGE=fulltext&D= med4&AN=8692171

Vu, N. V., Marcy, M. M., Colliver, J. A., Verhulst, S. J., Travis, T. A., & Barrows, H. S. (1992). Standardized (simulated) patients' accuracy in recording clinical performance check-list items. *Medical Education, 26*(2), 99–104. Retrieved from http://ovidsp.ovid.com/ ovidweb.cgi?T=JS&CSC=Y&NEWS=N&PAGE=fulltext&D=emed2 &AN=1992130436

Wallace, P. (2006). Following the threads of innovation: The history of standardized patients in medical education. *Caduceus, 13*(2), 5–28.

CHAPTER 3.4

Using Embedded Simulated Persons (aka "Confederates")

Jill S. Sanko, MS, ARNP, CHSE-A, PhD(c), Ilya Shekhter, MS, MBA, CHSE, Richard R. Kyle Jr., MS, and David J. Birnbach, MD, MPH

ABOUT THE AUTHORS

JILL S. SANKO is pursuing a PhD in nursing. For the last decade, Jill has been dedicated to simulation-based education and research. Most recently, she worked as a research and simulation education specialist at the UM-JMH Center for Patient Safety. Prior to that, Jill spent 8 years at the National Institute of Health, where she was Associate Director of the NIH Simulation Service and conducted clinical research for NHLBI.

ILYA SHEKHTER is educated in biomedical engineering and business administration. He has been the Simulation Manager at the UM-JMH Center for Patient Safety since 2004. He contributes expert knowledge and experience in the design, implementation, maintenance, and evaluation of simulation-based learning systems. Before coming to Miami, he was the senior simulation engineer at the University of Rochester Medical Center, where he was instrumental in designing, opening, and operating the Rochester Center for Medical Simulation.

RICHARD R. KYLE holds degrees in biomedical engineering and physical chemistry. He helped to develop the first patient simulation facility and teaching program at the Uniformed Services University. Along with Bosseau Murray, he cocreated the textbook *Clinical Simulation –Operations, Engineering and Management*. His fundamental educational principle is "there is no learning without mistakes, so use simulations to make mistakes safely and on time."

DAVID J. BIRNBACH is the Vice Provost and Professor of Anesthesiology, Obstetrics and Gynecology, and Public Health and Epidemiology at the University of Miami (UM); Associate Dean, Patient Safety, and Quality at the UM Miller School of Medicine; Chief Patient Safety Officer at the UM Hospital; and Director of the UM-Jackson Memorial Hospital Center for Patient Safety. He has published in the area of simulation and patient safety and earned recognition from the Society for Simulation in Healthcare.

Acknowledgments: The authors would like to thank the experts who agreed to participate and who supported them during this project. They also thank their initial panel of experts for their input, and patience. They extend a special word of thanks to: Dr. David Birnbach, Maureen Fitzpatrick, Dr. Paul Heinrich, Nancy Muldoon, and Dr. Daniel Raemer.

ABSTRACT

From the perspective of a simulation program the effectiveness of a training program may be seen as the product of three components: the training platform, the skills of the educators, and the curricular integration (Issenberg, 2006). If any of these components is missing or deficient, the overall result will be diminished, and effective training may not occur. For example, it is not uncommon for an institution to purchase an expensive simulator only to see it sit unused because the faculty and staff are not adequately trained in the use of the equipment or the proper methods to integrate simulation into healthcare education.

One group of simulation staff for which proper training is vital is that of embedded simulated persons (ESPs), also known as simulation confederates. Simulation programs that lack training and assessment of ESPs do their learners and their programs an injustice, robbing them of the full spectrum of engagement and learning that can take place in a well-rehearsed, well-rounded, and well-acted simulation experience. This chapter provides 10 recommendations aimed at improving the performance of all levels of ESPs from novice to experts, as well as enhancing the effectiveness of scenario coordinators who guide ESPs scenario production personnel who interact with ESPs and simulation center directors who employ ESPs. Using these recommendations will help to develop and improve clinical training programs.

SECTION 3 • Simulators

CASE EXAMPLE

A cohort of 2nd-year medical students was participating in a simulation exercise as part of their comprehensive assessment. In one 20-minute exercise, teams of students were asked to assess and start treating an acutely ill patient with evidence of poor perfusion and shock. An embedded simulated healthcare provider was available to help them accomplish various clinical tasks. To differentiate the various types of shock, the students were expected to connect a Swan-Ganz catheter to the monitor, measure systemic vascular resistance (SVR), and proceed with generating a differential diagnosis. One team of students seemed puzzled by the catheter. Instead of giving the students the SVR value and encouraging them to proceed with the assessment, the embedded simulated provider decided to demonstrate how the catheter worked. The demonstration took most of the allotted time, preventing the students from completing their training assignment.

INTRODUCTION AND BACKGROUND

Attention comes first, learning after attention is focused. And learning is primarily action.

Dewey et al. in Bricken (1991)

Before discussing the best practices of acting while facilitating learning in healthcare simulation, it is necessary to define the terms used for individuals assigned to directly interact with learners within the simulation scenario. Although these roles exist to help guide the presentation of the training objectives, the underlying training purposes of these roles are frequently not revealed to the learners. The intentional influence of a role on the learners may be positive, negative, or neutral, depending on the learning objectives of the scenario. There is variability in the nomenclature as well as strong opinions about the correct terms that should be used for these participants in the simulation who directly interact with the learners. The following terms are frequently used: **actor, confederate, embedded actor,** scenario guide, scenario role player, simulation actor, **simulated person, and standardized participant.** These terms as well as their relative virtues and drawbacks are listed in Table 3.4.1.

Many prefer the simple term *confederate* to refer to everyone (other than professional standardized patients) that interacts with the learners on the simulation stage. This term has long been used in both psychology and simulation, however, as a result of changing terminology that is a more precise description of the role, the term "embedded simulated person" or "ESP" will be used for this chapter.

For simulation to be most effective as a teaching technique, learners must focus their attention upon the

TABLE 3.4.1

Various terms used for individuals who interact with learners

Term	Pros	Cons
Actor	• Denotes a skill set needed to be effective • The term is clear to a lay audience	• Takes away from the serious nature of simulation • Downplays technical skills required of certain clinical and educator roles
Confederate	• Long history of use both in simulation and psychology literature	• Is viewed as an emotionally charged term that has a negative connection with the American Civil War • Denotes an accomplice in tricking the participants • Suggests experimenting with the participants
Embedded actor	• Denotes a skill set needed to be effective as well as the concealed nature of the role	• Takes away from the serious nature of simulation • Downplays technical skills required of certain clinical roles • Awkward term, unfamiliar to people
Embedded simulated person	• Embraces different types of simulated persons: healthcare provider, patient, or family member • Denotes active simulation role	• Awkward term, unfamiliar to many people • Umbrella term, not specific
Scenario guide	• Describes one aspect of the role, which is to assist the learners to interact with the simulation environment	• Evokes the idea of a passive learner experience in simulation
Scenario role player	• More closely defines the role of the person in the learning experience	• Awkward construct because the learner might also be playing a role
Simulation actor	• Denotes a skill set needed to be effective and specifies simulation as the acting domain	• Ignores technical skills required to play the role
Simulated person	• Includes a reference to simulation	• Vague • Not widely used
Standardized participant	• Emphasizes the consistency required for presenting scenarios to multiple groups of learners	• Is often used for nonstandardized participants • May be confused with standardized patient • The word "participant" usually refers to a learner or a research subject, thus adding another possible source of confusion

learning objectives of the clinical scenario and perform critical actions. It is in this way that they demonstrate their current level of competency. A study of learners' perceptions of real and fictional cues in simulation reported that learner engagement was strongly influenced by the role-playing competency of simulation ESPs (Dieckmann et al., 2007). Unlike standardized patients (SPs) who are trained extensively in advance of their performances and often engage in learner assessment (Walker & Weidner, 2010), the roles of ESPs are often filled by any available personnel who are quickly briefed on their role and scripted lines only moments before entering the "stage" to act an untried role within a larger, unfamiliar ensemble. The ESPs' interactions are meant to inform and guide the learners' understanding and choices along the arc of the scenario's training objective. While instructors spend significant time on crafting a compelling clinical scenario and fine-tuning the technical aspects of the simulation, they are often unaware of the detrimental effect of poorly prepared ESPs on the **realism** of a scenario, the ability for learners to suspend disbelief and ultimately learning. In their study, Dieckmann et al. (2007) suggest training simulation personnel in the basic theatrical concepts of role-playing may help improve the learners' level of engagement and learning through simulation.

Given their essential mission in making simulation a success, individuals who serve as ESPs should learn and strive to implement universal team-member competencies and adopt individual best practices. As team members, all ESPs should have:

1. An intimate understanding of the learning objectives of the scenario, including assessment tool items,
2. A respect for the learners' current level of training, and
3. A complete knowledge of scripts for all the roles, not just their own. As an individual, the confederate should be aware of his or her assigned impact on the learning experience and ultimately the educational outcome.

TEN BEST PRACTICES FOR ACTING IN SIMULATION

It takes many individuals to create and deliver an effective simulation experience. Regardless of their assignment, individuals who author, direct, produce, and evaluate simulation scenarios should be aware of best practices in the field. When educators develop scenarios, they establish the purpose for ESPs and define words and actions that the ESPs should and should not say and do. When simulation coordinators guide the live performance, they emphasize moment by moment what is and is not important for the learners to

---

CONSIDER THIS

USING VOLUNTEERS

Laura K. Rock, MD
Pulmonologist and Critical Care Physician, Beth Israel Deaconess Medical Center (BIDMC) Instructor, Harvard Medical School and the Center for Medical Simulation Director of Simulation Programs, BIDMC Department of Medicine. Dr. Rock has designed and taught numerous courses, including procedural training, "rapid response" management of clinical emergencies, and an ICU communication course for promoting effective and empathic communication between doctors, nurses, and family members.

Margaret Hinrichs, MEd
Coordinator and Trainer, Beth Israel Deaconess Medical Center Family Meeting Project Volunteers

Trained volunteers are a feasible alternative to employing paid actors. Effective communication and empathy are among the most important skills for health professionals. It is imperative to practice these skills in simulated environments with people who are prepared to create realistic situations, react and offer feedback. Communication training programs may incorporate former patients or family members of former patients to play these roles in simulated conversations and provide feedback to learners. The real-life emotional experiences of the volunteers bring an authenticity to the role play, offering much more compelling feedback to the learners. In addition, the cost savings are considerable.

VOLUNTEER SELECTION

Volunteers can be recruited from a variety of sources. The Hospital Volunteer Office may refer potential volunteers, clinicians may recommend patients or family members they have treated, or hospital employees who have experienced being a patient or family member may be interested in the project. Hospitals often have a Patient and Family Advisory Board consisting of former patients who may be interested in enhancing the communication skills of hospital clinicians.

AN EXAMPLE OF A VOLUNTEER TRAINING PROCESS

A professional trainer with experience training SPs or actors screens potential candidates and provides initial and ongoing training to ensure high quality role-play and effective feedback.

A new volunteer is screened through e-mail and phone contact with the trainer. The trainer and the volunteer review the course learning materials and cases to become familiar with the process and characters before the volunteer observes sessions with the trainer. The new volunteer debriefs the observed simulated meetings and feedback sessions with the trainer and the volunteers who participated, sharing observations and reactions to the role-play and feedback. The new volunteer is offered an opportunity to observe and debrief course sessions until they feel ready to participate for a role. The trainer attends course sessions to provide ongoing support and feedback to volunteers.

LOGISTICS

Each simulated conversation includes one to three volunteers. At least 10 volunteers are needed to reliably run a weekly course. The volunteer schedule should be established

(continued)

USING VOLUNTEERS *(continued)*

approximately every 3 months. Reminders should be sent to volunteers each week by e-mail.

TIPS FOR A SUCCESSFUL VOLUNTEER PROGRAM

Volunteers must feel comfortable in the role-play and offering feedback. The debriefing with the volunteer following role-plays should be conducted in an informal, supportive atmosphere. The trainer must be accessible for volunteers to contact as needed to discuss the cases, feedback, or any thoughts or concerns. The training should reinforce volunteers' positive efforts, as they are not professional actors. They are donating their time for a cause they believe in, and it takes time to develop the skills to play their roles well.

STRATEGIES FOR EFFECTIVE VOLUNTEER ROLE-PLAYING AND FEEDBACK

1. Feedback should be very specific.
2. Limit comments to behaviors that are remediable.
3. Limit feedback to the most important one or two skills.
4. Use descriptive nonevaluative language (avoid "good," "bad," or "better").
5. Describe how the behavior made you feel rather than what the learner did or said (use "I" statements).
6. Discuss the behavior, not the individual.
7. Connect a specific behavior to a specific emotion, for example:
   - "When you (turned away, nodded, laughed, interrupted me, stood up . . . [a specific behavior]) then I felt (ignored, listened to, upset, rushed, intimidated . . . [specific emotion])."

- "When you asked me how I was coping and then interrupted me I felt like you didn't really want to know how I felt."
- "When you noticed I was sad and said you could see how hard this was for me, it made me feel like you were really trying to understand how I feel."

8. Family member (volunteer) feedback may be more learner-centered and facilitated by focusing their feedback on what the learner identified as challenging or chose to practice.
9. When giving feedback, be emotionally neutral.
10. Volunteer family members or patients should stay in character throughout the course and avoid casual interactions with faculty or learners.

CHALLENGES AND LESSONS LEARNED

- Volunteers bring a wonderful authenticity and have real emotion drawing from their own experiences, but they are usually not skilled actors and may not be able to evoke a specific response or replay a challenging moment for deliberate skill-building practice.
- Volunteers may be unreliable as schedules and levels of interest change.
- It takes several months for volunteers to feel confident and relaxed and play their roles naturally.
- It takes time to learn how to give constructive feedback.
- Volunteer quality will benefit by limiting recruitment to those volunteers who anticipate being able to commit to at least 1 to 2 years of participation.

focus their attention on. When simulation production personnel produce live simulation events, they make real the learning objectives of the authors and coordinators. When ESPs interact with learners on the simulation stage, they are the living embodiment of the scenario's training objectives. After the simulation scenario is complete, when evaluators discuss with the learners their observed actions, the evaluators emphasize what is and is not important for the learners to focus on during future learning efforts.

Using best practices can assist these individuals in a number of ways. Educators can use best practices to inform their creative efforts when authoring simulation scenarios. Simulation coordinators can use them to inform their leadership efforts when selecting and directing ESPs. Production personnel can use best practices to inform their efforts when producing simulation scenarios. ESPs can use them to inform their teaching efforts. Evaluators can use them to inform their selection of the more important lessons for the learner to practice. In addition, after a simulation is complete and the team comes together for the after-action review, best practices can be used to inform their constructive criticism.

The following are 10 practices to consider when acting in simulation.

1. *Do allow learners to make mistakes: There is no better setting for mistakes than simulation.*

Mistakes indicate an individual's current boundary of competence. The goal of *training* simulations is for learners to safely expand their zone of competence on a rational schedule. This is in contrast to the goal of *testing* simulations where learners are expected to present their best possible patient treatment behaviors. Learners that do not make mistakes during training simulations are demonstrating what they have learned before, not what they are learning now. Preventing learners from making mistakes in training simulations or criticizing them for those actions does not decrease the likelihood of occurence during actual patient care.

Healthcare providers tend to have well-developed reflexes for protecting actual patients from novice learners. These same reflexes, when applied in simulation-based learning environments, actually interfere with the learning process. An example of this patient-protective reflex at work in a simulation environment is the clinician acting in the role of a confederate, who focuses on the patient's condition (as they would in real life) and neglects to observe the learner's behaviors while reflexively providing the learner with too much information (or by completing a task the learner is expected to complete). Such added help negates the powerful learning that comes to a learner from directly experiencing negative consequences of an incorrect action or inaction. ESPs who are also healthcare providers must recognize that they have this patient-protective reflex and thus must explicitly script and diligently rehearse realistic negative consequences for the purpose of having the learners experience the "something is wrong here, what should I do?" situation.

Rehearsals uncover patient-protective reflex errors in the ESPs' scripts and in their acting. Before each simulation event, the scenario coordinator should confirm that all the ESPs are prepared for their performances as individuals and as team members. Practice runs should focus on the information they should and should not reveal as well as how to respond to expected questions and requests from the learners.

2. *Do not Ad-lib for drama's sake: There's a time and a place, for but it's not usually in simulation.*

Ad-libbing (any dialogue or action that had not been previously agreed upon or rehearsed) for drama's sake can present learners with conflicting or incorrect information. Simulation ESPs should be careful to avoid unintentionally misdirecting the learners' attention away from the preestablished learning objectives through episodes of unscripted information or action. Should unintended lulls in the scenario need to be filled, ESPs should focus on educating rather than entertaining through ad-libbing. Prepare ESPs with clinically nonrelevant yet easily recalled background facts for each role (e.g., marital status, profession, recent travels) that they can inject into conversations when needed to further the training objectives. Having authentic facts available gives the ESPs a familiar scaffold to assist in keeping their role-play nondistracting and the action flowing toward the intended learning objectives. In addition, adopting the approach commonly used in improvisational theatre to accept rather than deny what is going on in the experience can assist in creating realistic scenarios.

The following is an example of how ad-libbing can lead learners off track. In a scenario where the objectives were to have an anesthesiology resident consent, perform preoperative assessment, and experience an antibiotic reaction in an elective presurgical patient, a confederate nurse—upon noticing a cup filled with water that was used in a prior simulation and was inadvertently left on the bedside table—stated, "Oh I guess Mr. Green didn't like his ginger ale this morning." This ad-libbed information about what the patient *might* have drunk that morning caused the learner to write orders to cancel the surgery and talk to the nurse about the importance of preoperative Nothing by Mouth (NPO) orders, rather than consenting the

patient and administering the preoperative antibiotics. A better approach for the confederate to use upon finding the cup filled with water that would have aligned with the objectives could have been, "I guess Mrs. Green left her cup of water here when she visited earlier." This comment aligns with the objectives by keeping the learners focused on completing the task of a preop consent and assessment, is plausible, and accepts the finding of the cup of water that was left out inadvertently.

3. *Do adapt to learner behaviors: The scenario should be scripted, but learners' responses are unpredictable.*

While the scenario script is the primary guide for the ESPs' actions and words, it is often necessary for ESPs to creatively adapt their actions and words in order to realign the ongoing scenario with the learners' actions and words. Whenever unplanned occurrences happen, creative adaptability, which differs from ad-libbing, should be employed to guide the learner back on track.

For example, a trainee once asked a confederate respiratory therapist if the patient had dentures. Per the script, the patient was a 24-year-old male who had just eaten lunch, was found in respiratory distress, and had no significant medical history. Not having anticipated this question, but thinking on the fly, the nurse confederate answered, "No, he is 24." As soon as she got the statement out of her mouth, the trainee removed the teeth out of the mannequin and proceeded to intubate him. Trying to integrate this unexpected action by the trainee into the scenario and to keep the learner on track to discovering the "real" issue (a foreign body obstruction), the confederate smiled and said, "Oh, I guess I missed that on the admission history. I assumed that a 24-year-old wouldn't have dentures."

4. *Do use communication devices: They help keep ESPs and scenario coordinators on track, but beware of their pitfalls.*

Communication devices (wireless one-way or two-way voice or text devices, mobile or wired telephones) allow in-the-moment passing of information and instructions between off-stage faculty in the control or observation rooms and on-stage ESPs. This is especially helpful in situations when unexpected questions crop up or changes to the script are necessary. However, the unexpected intrusion of unfamiliar communication devices into the learners' perceptions can produce unintended consequences. Wireless headsets can disorient ESPs engaged in two different conversations simultaneously. Likewise, learners easily disengage when the confederate to whom they are speaking suddenly diverts attention toward the hidden voices in the headset. Also, the persistent visual presence of a wireless headset on a confederate can suggest to

MAINTAINING PSYCHOLOGICAL SAFETY FOR EMBEDDED SIMULATED PERSONS

Janice C. Palaganas, PhD, RN, NP

In healthcare simulation, embedded simulated persons (ESPs) may be placed at risk if you assign them to portray a role without knowing whether or not the ESPs are able to emotionally manage the role or exit it once the simulation is over.

To explore how to keep ESPs psychologically safe, while maintaining the quality of the simulation, acting instructors, formally trained actors, SPs, ESPs, and SP trainers were interviewed. On the basis of these interviews, the following five suggestions to support psychological safety were developed.

SUGGESTIONS TO SUPPORT ESP PSYCHOLOGICAL SAFETY

Suggestion 1. Seek experienced resources. Where possible, have someone with ESP-facilitated simulation experience available during the recruitment, selection, training, and debriefing of the ESP.
Eliciting information from someone that could indicate their fit for a role takes some knowledge of the challenges of ESP-facilitated simulations. It often takes experience to gain the sensitivity and skills necessary to elicit and understand an individual's psychological state. New programs often do not have individuals with this level of experience. If you do not have experienced individuals on staff, we suggest you consult with others who do. Expand your network to seek other experienced resources who can guide you through your processes.

Suggestion 2. When interviewing or auditioning individuals for a given role, get to know the person to determine if they have any real-life experiences that relate to the scenario in which they will participate.

Case Example 1: Exiting the ESP from the Role
A husband and wife played the roles of a male, obese, diabetic, nonadherent simulated patient and his simulated wife who is frustrated with having to care for him. After the simulation, the real-life couple informed the simulation staff that the performance felt so real since he was obese, diabetic, and nonadherent to his medications and his wife was frustrated with having to care for him. This is often a source of daily arguments for the two of them.

Screening someone for a given role is crucial to the simulation. The goal of this process is to determine whether their experiences will enhance their portrayal or interfere with it. Prior to an audition, you should provide the details of the scenario. Some questions you might want to ask as you choose the right person for the role are:

1. Have you ever been in a situation similar to the scenario in this simulation? Or do you know anyone who has?

   If the person has, ask them to tell you about the experience. Pause and let them tell you their story. What you're looking for is any emotional response the person has when telling their story. When interviewing a potential ESP, you are attempting to see that they have the emotion that you are looking to produce in a given case. If any emotion arises when they are talking about a similar situation they may have been in, find out how the person feels about portraying a case that is so close to them emotionally. You will have to make a determination at this point about whether or not you want to bring them in for an audition before deciding whether or not to hire them for the role. It is important to make these determinations up front, before you start training so you avoid putting someone in a situation where they might

lose their emotional control. In the event this occurs, they won't be able to carry out the requirements of the role. If the role is intense, it is critical to choose somebody who has acting skills to pull off a naturalistic performance.

2. How do you think you'll "drop" into this role?

   Actors and SPs are trained to "drop in" to a role using conjured images, thoughts, music, or other techniques. When exiting a role, it will be important to reverse this by revisiting the technique they initially used and exit out of that technique. For example, an actress thinks about the death of her mother to elicit tearing and sadness; when exiting the role, she will usually call her mother to confirm that she is okay.

3. How do you typically exit your role?

   Actors and SPs are trained to "exhale it out," after performing an intense role. Techniques include exhaling, shaking, stretching, or cognitive re-centering methods.

   With this information, you can gauge the risk of using this person for the role. As much as possible, the ESP should not realistically live the situation you are simulating. A solution to case example 1 is assessment and prevention (e.g., assess the similarities in the simulation to the similarities at home and choose another standardized patient and standardized wife).

   When selecting an ESP, you must audition the individual. An interview or conversation is not an audition. You should have the potential ESP run through the actual case. Auditioning can answer the question: Can this person portray the case?

Suggestion 3. Remind the person.
Remind the person before the simulation starts that immediately following the exit of the learners, you or a staff member will invite them to exit the role.

Suggestion 4. Engage in role exiting with the person. Debrief the person after the simulation. Debrief the scenario with ESP(s).
Prior to the simulation, it is important to work with the person to see if they can come up with something that may work for them. After the learners have exited the simulation, encourage the person to perform the method they use to exit the role to make sure that they have reversed the conditions of that technique. If the planned methods do not work, you may need to continue working with the person to determine ways to help them exit their role.

For the debriefing, find a quiet place and just talk with them. Let them say what is on their minds. You can ask, "How are you doing emotionally?" "Say more about that," or "What was your personal experience in this?" For collective feedback and idea sharing on a scenario, you can also debrief with all ESPs who played the role simultaneously. Some questions you can ask include: "How did that feel?" "Did it bring anything up for you?" "Do you have any concerns?" "How did you drop into your role?"

Case Example 2: An Unexpected Breach in Psychological Safety
A young woman portraying abdominal pain was great during the interview and audition, and was selected for training and underwent the simulation. She was crying throughout the simulation, unable to fulfill the role. The simulation was stopped, and she informed the simulation staff that her father had died in that hospital for abdominal aortic aneurysm. When asked

why she did not share this during the interview, she stated, "Well, it was two years ago. I thought I was over it."

If you are concerned with any kind of threat to the psychological safety of the ESP, some questions and language you could use include:

- "Have you felt like this before? What did you do to help yourself?"
- "Are you present?"
- "What were the highlights for you?"

If you are still concerned after engaging with the ESP, you can refer the individual to a professional resource. This may be the same psychological support resource you have for your learners/students, staff, center, or institution. Many programs have on-call resources to assist on-site and off-site when needed. Talking often helps a person to exit a role. When someone is not a trained actor, you may need to engage more; actors are often trained to deal with exiting a role. ESPs often appear to resolve their high emotional state. You will need to use your judgment and ask the ESP to judge themselves. If you feel it is appropriate for the ESP to leave the simulation and your program, you should clearly ask if they are in a good emotional state to leave: "Are you okay to get on the road and drive home?" If you have concerns about the psychological impact on an ESP during a simulation event and you feel unsettled after they have left despite using some of the techniques above, you might consider following up with the ESP if you feel it is appropriate.

Suggestion 5. Bring closure to the role.

Case Example 3: Bringing Closure to the Character
A simulation was created from an actual case where a nurse initially performed a medication administration error. After the course, the embedded simulated nurse told the simulation staff that she often sees members of the staff who were learners in the simulation and, during clinical shifts, she wonders if they confuse the simulated event with a real event by thinking, "There's that nurse who made that real drug error!"

Similar to case example 2, if an actor is worried about confusion between the role and the quality of their acting, they are trained to use methods that bring closure to the role (e.g., laughing loud after the scene is closed; Yakim & Broadman, 2000). In healthcare simulation, to maintain the realism of the case, we often ask our ESPs to stay in the role until learners have left the simulation, giving no opportunity for this type of role closure immediately after the simulation. There are other ways to allow a person to formally exit the role. In simulation, it should occur after the learning event (usually after the learner debriefing) and in a very apparent way. As much as possible, formally close the role with the learners by making it conscious. Some ways to do this include inviting him/her at the end of the debriefing and publicly thanking them for their role or having him/her stand at the doorway with the debriefers or faculty to say goodbye to learners.

The psychological safety of ESPs is often overlooked. The implementation of these five suggestions may help guide the development of processes that offer a psychologically safe environment for ESPs.

REFERENCES

Yakim, M., & Broadman, M. (2000). *Creating a character: A physical approach to acting.* New York, NY: Applause Theatre Book.

learners that the confederate might not be competent, that the simulation team leader might not have prepared for their lesson.

As part of their review after the scenario, faculty should discuss the degree to which the learners were distracted by any unfamiliar communication devices used in the scenario. If such communication devices are to be used, ESPs and instructors should practice before the learners' lessons and gain proficiency in using them covertly. Mobile phones or online bedside computers with the option to silently text can be unobtrusive communication devices. The former are easily concealed, and the latter can be scripted to blend well within scenarios at institutions that use them in real clinical areas. Remember, technology, no matter how costly or clever, is a poor substitute for the ESPs, the scenario coordinator, and the rest of the simulation team knowing the training goals and learning objectives of the scenario, as well as how their own and others' roles contribute to the stated training goals and learning objectives.

5. *Do know your learners: Their level of training should guide the ESPs' words and actions.*

Knowledge of the learners' demographics (current or intended clinical profession, current year in training, as well as gaps in knowledge, skill, and attitude) should guide the ESPs role-playing. Within the scenario, "helping" cues should be adapted to match the learning objectives and the learners' level. Problems arise when the simulation challenges and cues are not matched to the learners' current competencies. For example, when training medical students who may not know how to use a defibrillator, their decision to use the device to defibrillate the patient may be sufficient and the confederate may offer to help them to use the device. On the other hand, post-graduate physicians would be expected to recognize the need to defibrillate and should already know how to use the defibrillator appropriately. Learners can become frustrated instead of enlightened when the clinical challenges and ESPs' responses are directed far above or below their current level of competency.

Every simulation should include a debriefing, with the learners describing their experiences and the lessons they extracted from the simulation. Every debriefing with learners should conclude with questions for the learners about the level of clinical challenges, ESPs' role portrayals, and their overall engagement with the simulation. After the learners are excused from their debriefing, the simulation should conclude with a debriefing with the trainers. In the trainer's debriefing, everyone who contributed to the scenario production should gather to review what went well, what did not, what to keep, and what to change.

6. *Do use realistic props and costumes: They always tell a story and provide valuable clues.*

Learners assume that everything they perceive within a simulation is intentional and valid. Thus, setting the stage for simulation includes making sure the ESPs' appearances as well as the **props,** equipment, and room environment present information to the learners appropriate for the scenario's intended purpose. Before each simulation, the scenario coordinator should meet with the ESPs to review the intended purpose for their character's clothes and tools. The great value added to every simulation presentation by these small details is all too easily overlooked or minimized, especially by ESPs who do not participate in simulations routinely and by scenario coordinators new to simulation. The simpler the details the better, but be sure the details are not so simple that the informing message is not presented clearly and correctly. Save confounding communications for scenarios specifically devoted for teaching the problems of unnecessarily complex communications.

It is easier for ESPs to immerse themselves into a believable character and easier for learners to engage their attention when ESPs are dressed in role-specific attire. Attire may include the character's name and position on an ID badge and appropriate "tools of the trade" (i.e., stethoscope, surgical mask, sterile gown). Examples of useful props are clipboards, tablet computers, and phones with texting capabilities. They are both esthetically acceptable (i.e., found in real clinical arenas) and functionally useful to hide information (such as lab values, medical history, or medication lists), which may be difficult for the confederate to remember.

7. *Do commit to the character: ESPs are playing roles to send messages to the learners, not playing themselves.*

To be accepted by learners as legitimate and to engage them in learning through simulation, it is important for ESPs to commit to "being the character." It is a skill that takes deliberate practice to master, and can be made more challenging (especially for the novice confederate) when it conflicts with what they do in both their professional and personal lives. ESPs should remember that their reason for role-playing is to play a character in a scenario in order to support the learning objectives, and to answer questions and respond to the learners in the manner of the assigned character. Just before the start of the scenario, help the ESPs commit to their character by having all ESPs, simulated patients, and SPs introduce themselves to each other in character. Other strategies can be implemented to ensure a quality performance. The first is to purposefully, thoughtfully, and whenever possible cast for the role. Just like in the professional world of acting, not every actor is equally suited for every role. The Wizard of Oz was originally written for Shirley Temple, not Judy Garland, but the movie just does not work the same when one imagines Shirley Temple in the role, does it?

Second, just prior to sending a confederate on to "stage," take a minute to engage the confederate in an in-character conversation about something that might actually be happening to the character just prior to the scene they are about to play. For example, the rushed nurse who needs to urgently leave to pick up her sick child may have just had a conversation with the school who has called about the sick child. Actually calling the confederate who will play the rushed nurse and role-playing a conversation between a mother and a school nurse can go a long way in helping the confederate get into character.

Third, within every scenario, whenever ESPs meet learners for the first time, an orientation to the scene should take place. To accomplish this, the confederate should complete five statements as one continuous phrase of engagement:

1. State the character's name,
2. State the role being portrayed,
3. State the role the learners are to portray,
4. State where they are, and
5. State what is happening.

For example: "Hello. I am *Fred*, the *CT Technician*. I understand you are the *Rapid Response Team*. Thanks for coming so quickly to *radiology* after I called you. This lady started having *difficulty breathing after her scan*." This language may seem contrived, but every encounter in real life begins with individuals automatically seeking answers to these fundamental "Who, What, Where, and Why" questions, so expect learners to seek the same answers in simulation encounters. The sooner the learners find answers to these questions, the sooner they can start focusing their attention on the educational purpose of the simulation scenario. As a counterexample, imagine a learner in a Rapid Response Team scenario. When the learner enters the simulation, the confederate, playing the CT Technician, just stares at the learner, speechless. Has the need for interprofessional communication during a crisis supported or negated the instructor's training objectives that were focused on individual resuscitation skills? Alternatively, if the training objectives are related to effective communication during a crisis, imagine the impact on the learners' development by doing this scenario twice, first with a "mute" CT Technician, then with a fully informing one.

Learning objectives such as where to find information or how, when, and whom to call for help often use a "non-initiating yet competent follower" character to engage the learner's leadership skills. Highly competent clinicians can make the best and the worst teaching ESPs in these simulations. Their wealth of knowledge about real treatment mistakes, both drawn from their own experience and observed in others, can prepare them to present invaluable learning "mistakes" as well as creatively adapt to a wide range of unexpected events during simulation. However, the highly competent clinician's hard-won reflexes to detect dangers and promptly respond to protect real patients from learners' mistakes can reduce time and opportunities for the learners to extend themselves within the simulation. See no. 1.

As it goes against the self-identity of most ESPs, the "noncompetent" or the "not forthcoming" character is one of the harder characters to portray. Yet scenarios often use these difficult roles to elicit independent thoughts and actions from learners. Because of this, it is important to develop a robust set of "if–thens" (e.g., If a learner does X, then Y occurs) for the scenario so that the experience progresses in a smooth and standardized manner.

Learning how to work with difficult personalities is no less important than is learning how to diagnose and treat difficult illnesses and injuries. Simulating difficult personality types and the management challenges they create are done best with ESPs. The scenario coordinator can help ESPs who struggle with playing these "difficult" characters by reminding them that they are not that difficult person in reality, but are only playing that difficult person for the sake of improving the trainees' learning. The coordinator and confederate might both know an actual difficult person for the confederate to use as a seed or reference for building their own difficult role portrayal.

The scenario coordinator can be very helpful when the confederate must shed the difficult character persona at the end of that scenario and prepare for adopting a new persona. Unlike SPs who usually portray one character and should never interact with learners when out of character, ESPs often portray several different roles and often have real interactions with learners outside of the simulation. To help ESPs change into their next role and to help the learners accept the ESPs in that new role, the difficult characters have to be "flushed out" of both the ESPs and the learners. Thus, at the end of the learners' debriefing, the coordinator should introduce the learners to the real person that just portrayed that difficult character, and remind everyone that the difficult character was intentionally placed in the scenario for the purpose of improving the trainees' competence, was not punishment for anyone, and is not the real person standing before the learners.

8. *Do pay attention to nonverbal cues: Emotional responses contribute to learning.*

Learners respond not only to ESPs' speech and actions, but also to their subtle nonverbal cues. These cues often project an emotional message. It is important, therefore, that all ESPs deliberately project nonverbal cues that are appropriate for their character's behaviors.

Professional actors do not generate anger, for instance, but instead imagine a trigger that would produce angry emotions from their character (Soto-Morettini, 2010). Professional ESPs are taught to commit themselves 100% to the situation rather than focus on emotion itself. For novice ESPs (as many simulationists are), it may help to have them ask themselves, "*How have I behaved in situations like this?*" or "*How have I seen others behave in situations like this?*"

Inadequate or inappropriate emotion makes it difficult for the learners to take the simulation seriously enough to commit themselves to their own expected role. ESPs who are unsure of their acting skills for a given role often do not show enough emotion. As an example, imagine a tense resuscitation situation, the patient is dying and the person unsure how to portray a competent code leader says in a deadpan tone, "call-for-help." Would this command be taken seriously? If so, what assumptions might the learners make about the condition of the patient, about their own responsibilities toward caring for this patient, as well as understanding this code leader? ESPs must study and exhibit emotional cues that reinforce the messages of their words and actions. Laughing and silly comments that are *out of character*, as well as acting as if the exercise is entertainment instead of education, will most likely keep learners from achieving the desired learning objectives. Humor is best saved for the debriefing, when everyone can share in the release of tension.

Committing to the role, setting the stage, taking the simulation event seriously, and presenting message-reinforcing emotional cues are all important assignments. The confederate must also maintain the character throughout the scenario. Sometimes, nonprofessional ESPs feel drawn out of character when learners are unsure what they can and cannot do with the various devices, props, and people, or when they are confused about where the boundaries of the simulation lie. A thorough orientation to the simulation center, simulator, props, and boundaries can minimize common mistakes made by ESPs that cause unintended learner uncertainty or negative learning.

In addition, there are techniques that ESPs can utilize to help guide confounded learners through their uncertainty. For example, if learners are unsure whether they are responsible for administering drugs or operating the defibrillator and these are not explicit teaching objectives of the scenario, then the confederate can offer to assist in this task. If the learner's behaviors clearly indicate uncertainty, then a confederate's statement such as *"I can administer the medication"* or *"I can operate the defibrillator for you, just let me know what settings you would like."* works well to prevent the learner from becoming distracted and disengaged by items and issues outside the scenario's primary learning objectives. Also, scriptwriters can make use of affirmation techniques that the ESPs can use to keep the learner on the right track. For example, *after* the trainee verbalizes what they have perceived and interpreted, the confederate can reaffirm: *"Yes, the patient does have a pulse"* or *"Yes, I am hearing crackles"* or *"Yes, the rash has gotten worse in the last few minutes."*

Simulation can reveal learners' observable behaviors, but not their thoughts and feelings that triggered those behaviors. Thus, during every debriefing, instructors should explicitly ask learners about what they did or did not perceive and what interpretations they made. The learners' comments will speak volumes for how well the simulation team produced the teaching cues that were intended. Most learner distraction caused by confederate confusion can be eliminated, or at least greatly reduced, by designing, rehearsing, and refining the teaching objectives of simulation scenarios.

9. *Do not be the star of the show: Simulation is all about the learners' improving.*

Never be the star of the show—*the learner is the only star.* All ESPs, no matter what their job title is in real life, perform for the learners' benefit and are there to support the teaching objectives. Everyone in simulation must operate under one common directive: orient and deliver all their energies and abilities toward guiding the learners toward aligning with the teaching objectives.

One example of a confederate stealing a learning opportunity is highlighted in the following scenario. A simulation called for two ESPs a nurse and a physician, each acting in the roles of their respective professions. The learner arrived and began asking questions. To everyone's complete surprise, the physician started speaking with an Italian accent. This change caught the entire team off guard, as he is usually very serious, and did not have an Italian accent. Everyone was so distracted by the confederate's actions that the resulting consequence was a reduction in clinical learning. Further, the learner left feeling the simulation-based learning experience was a wasted educational opportunity. In this case, one show stealer distracted everyone else from the scenario's teaching objectives, turning an educational event into entertainment.

10. *Do find ways to improve: Rehearse before, debrief and evaluate after simulation.*

Video reviews can be excellent tools for performance analysis and assessment for both clinical learners and simulation ESPs. Novice as well as expert ESPs should expect to see themselves making mistakes. Additionally, they should be aware that viewing oneself on video can be anxiety provoking. Invariably what is seen is something unfamiliar if not also unwelcome, which can become a fixation point. This can produce mechanistic changes to external appearance in acting rather than the more important internal corrections to motivation and role objectives that produce believable behaviors. Reviewing one's self on video is a skill that has its own associated learning curve, and takes deliberate practice to learn what is important to focus on and what is not.

BEEN THERE, DONE THAT: HOW CAN I CONTINUE TO IMPROVE OR SUSTAIN WHAT I HAVE ACHIEVED?

The video review tool "Actions, Communication, and Teaching in Simulation—the **ACTS Tool**"* (see Appendix A) is designed to help ESPs improve their performances. The tool provides a multistep approach to performance improvement. Using the ACTS tool, ESPs should first watch themselves in a video seeking to identify ways to improve their contribution to the learners' attainment of the scenario's teaching objectives, not to improve their acting for their ego's sake. Second, ESPs should solicit feedback from learners and peers following each performance. At the end of every session, the learners' grading faculty can be excused from the room and a nonacting simulation production member can ask the learners what improvements should be made to the ESPs' performances. Specific areas to be explored include:

1. How can we make the presentation more effective?
2. How can we make the scenario more acceptable, that is, a better fit with the learners' current level of competence?
3. Ask peers to "score" acting performances using an objective evaluation tool (*like the ACTS tool*).
4. Critical feedback can be gathered from learners during the debriefing session, but anonymous surveys are recommended to gather constructive criticism rather than gracious praise (*see Appendix B for recommended survey questions*).

---

*The ACTS tool is a tool developed by our team that can be used in self-assessment or in peer assessment to evaluate acting performance. This tool is not yet validated, but work is being done to validate this tool.

Everyone in the simulation production team should always know what the ESPs in the scenario are going to do next. There are no exceptions. Note that the simulator operator is another confederate on the stage, the one "wearing" the outward appearance of the simulator device. This is why prescenario script discussions and rehearsals are vitally important. If changes must be made during the simulation, as will happen to the best prepared simulation teams, make every attempt to surreptitiously catch the attention and warn the others in the simulation presentation that you are about to redirect the event. A phone call from the off-stage scenario coordinator to an on-stage confederate is a good way to privately share such notices while the confederate stays in character in plain view of the learners. Like many things in life, practice makes permanent, so practice the best behaviors. Practicing to perfect simulation performances is no exception. Developing good presentation skills for one character will transfer well into other roles.

Practicing takes many forms—especially when developing new scenarios. Once the scenario script-writing phase is completed, new scenarios should undergo at least three rehearsals before the first production with the intended learners. The first rehearsal is a technical rehearsal for the people responsible for props and equipment. This rehearsal is needed to find and refine all material requirements (e.g., all batteries that should be fully charged or discharged and in place are in fact so; all intentionally broken, missing, incomplete devices are in fact so). The second rehearsal involves just the simulator operators to execute the simulator behaviors within the environment created in the first rehearsal. The third rehearsal is with the full complement of personnel, each in full costume, using stand-ins for the learners. Ideally, a faculty member blinded to the scenario design should be a stand-in learner to help uncover problems in the scenario progression or the acting presentations before the real learners do.

This sequence of three distinct rehearsals will help reveal mistakes as well as opportunities for improvement. They will also assist the ESPs to focus upon their learners' behaviors and not upon their own anxieties. All simulation scenarios have errors that become evident only during performances. Most of these errors will surface during formal rehearsals designed to exorcise errors. Foregoing formal rehearsals will result in these errors being inflicted upon the intended learners. In this case, the learners suffer all the negative learning that results from the defective training experience. As the training team will expend most of its time and attention correcting the learners'

confusion, there will be little opportunity for them to learn the intended lessons and improve their performances before the next unprepared simulation-enhanced training event. In contrast, well-rehearsed simulation presentations are powerful teachers of what it means to be a prepared professional.

SUMMARY

Producing efficient, well-designed simulation experiences that result in substantive learning takes time, effort, and know-how. Through discussions and surveys in the simulation community, it has become evident that a list of best practices would be beneficial for both novice and experts in the field of simulation-based education. Further work is in progress on gathering more evidence for these best practices, including the use of the ACTS tool as a reliable and valid instrument for the assessment of acting in simulation-based education.

REFERENCES

Bricken, W. (1991, June). Training in VR. In T. Feldman (Ed.), *Virtual reality '91: impacts and applications.* Proceedings of the First Annual Conference on Virtual Reality. London, UK: Meckler.

Dieckmann, P., Manser, T., Wehner, T., & Rall, M. (2007). Reality and fiction cues in medical patient simulation: An interview study with anesthesiologists. *Journal of Cognitive Engineering and Decision Making,* 1(2), 148–168.

Issenberg, S. B. (2006). The scope of simulation-based healthcare education. *Simulation in Healthcare,* 1(4), 203–208.

Soto-Morettini, D. (2010). *The philosophical confederate: A practical meditation for practicing theatre artists* (pp. 113–153). Chicago, IL: The University of Chicago Press.

Walker, S. E., & Weidner, T. G. (2010). The use of standardized patients in athletic training education. *Athletic Training Education Journal,* 5(2), 87–89.

ACTS TOOL REFERENCES

Creating a character rubric. Assessment Dr26B.I

Tomalin, J. E. (2006, June). *A video self-assessment tool: Improving acting skills and monologue performance.* An unpublished dissertation, Capella University, Minneapolis, MN.

ONLINE RESOURCES

http://www.ehow.com/how_4406429_be-good-actor.html

http://www.articlesbase.com/art-and-entertainment-articles/how-do-you-become-a-good-actor-or-actress-8886.html

http://www.associatedcontent.com/article/128564/what_makes_a_good_actor_physical_actions.html

http://findarticles.com/p/articles/mi_m4467/is_8_54/ai_64705682

http://www.isbe.net/ils/fine_arts/drama/stage_I/Dr26BI.pdf

SECTION 3 • Simulators

The ACTS Tool*
(Actions, Communication, and Teaching in Simulation)

Learner Discription: _____

Confederate Role Discription: _____

Brief Scenario Stem: _____

Objectives for the scenario:

1.
2.
3.
4.
5.

Directions for use: All values awarded should be based on how well the confederates (actors) remained aligned or deviated from the learning objectives established for the scenario.

Notes-Comments:

Helpful Definitions:

Ad-libbing: any dialogue or action which had not been previously agreed upon or rehearsed.

Flexibility (adaptability): Adjusting acting (responses and actions) to align with learners' behaviors, actions or questions while remaining aligned with the objectives of the scenario/learning experience.

Topics	Outstanding 6	Good 5	Adequate 4	Fair 3	Marginal 2	Poor 1	Inadequate 0
Verbal Characterization	The confederate's verbal communication (speech inflection, rate, intensity, clarity, and word choice) was clear, supported learning objectives and enhanced realism.		The confederate's verbal communication was mostly clear and largely consistent with reality; however, any inaccuracies did not impact learning.		The confederate's verbal communication was often unclear, often conflicted with the objectives and may have negatively impacted learning.		Appeared wholly unprepared to play the role and unaware of the learning objectives.
Non-verbal Characterization-Emotions	The confederate's non-verbal and emotional portrayal of the character added to the realism of the scenario. The confederate not only played the action but used set/ support realism.		The Confederate relied on a limited number of choices for physical behaviors and emotion. While problems with non-verbal communication were present there was no impact to learning.		The confederate's non-verbal communication and emotional portrayal interfered with the learning. Inappropriate non-verbal detracted from the realism.		Appeared wholly unprepared to play the role and appeared unaware of the objectives of the case.
Flexibility/adaptability	Used appropriate flexibility, steered clear of ad-libbing and all deviations, remained consistent with the objectives of the case.		Sometimes used appropriate flexibility and may have used some ad-libbing. Conveyed some inconsistent information but did not negatively impact the learning.		Never used flexibility and relied mostly on ad-libbing, which conveyed information which conflicted with the objectives. Learning was negatively impacted but not entirely lost.		Appeared wholly unprepared to play the role and unaware of the learning objectives.
Use of attire, props and set pieces	Used the attire, props and set pieces as an extension of the character which added to the realism of the scenario.		Used props intermittently to support learning objectives. Contribution of attire to character portrayal was limited. Utilized props in a limited capacity.		Use of props conflicted with learning objectives. Attire conflicted with role. Props were used as crutches detracting from realism of scenario.		Appeared wholly unprepared to play the role and unaware of the learning objectives.
Interactions with participants and other confederates/ patient (simulator)	Interactions were completely in line with the objectives. Interactions added to the learning and realism of the scenario.		Interactions were mostly in-line with the objectives. The learning opportunity was not interrupted by the interactions.		Interactions were out of line with the learning objectives. Interactions affected the learning opportunity negatively.		Appeared wholly unprepared to play the role and unaware of the learning objectives.

Over all (based on your gestalt): _____

RESOURCES

1. Establishing a convention for acting in healthcare simulation: merging art and science, Simulation in Healthcare. August 2013, Vol8, Issue 4. P 215–220
2. Making the Most of your confederates Chapter _____ in Excellence in Healthcare Simulation......

APPENDIX B

Postscenario Survey—Acting, Staging, and Production of Simulation-Based Education

1. The scenario was realistic.
   a. Completely disagree
   b. Mostly disagree
   c. Somewhat disagree
   d. Neither agree nor disagree
   e. Somewhat agree
   f. Mostly agree
   g. Completely agree
2. The actor(s) in the scenario presented were realistic.
   a. Completely disagree
   b. Mostly disagree
   c. Somewhat disagree
   d. Neither agree nor disagree
   e. Somewhat agree
   f. Mostly agree
   g. Completely agree
3. The environment/setting was realistic.
   a. Completely disagree
   b. Mostly disagree
   c. Somewhat disagree
   d. Neither agree nor disagree
   e. Somewhat agree
   f. Mostly agree
   g. Completely agree
4. It was easy for me to suspend disbelief—it was easy for me to behave as if I were caring for an actual patient in a real clinical environment.
   a. Completely disagree
   b. Mostly disagree
   c. Somewhat disagree
   d. Neither agree nor disagree
   e. Somewhat agree
   f. Mostly agree
   g. Completely agree

Procedural Training

Daniel A. Hashimoto, MD, MS, and Roy Phitayakorn, MD, MHPE (MEd), FACS

ABOUT THE AUTHORS

DANIEL A. HASHIMOTO is a general surgery resident at the Massachusetts General Hospital who has been engaged in surgical education research since 2006 and completed a master's degree in translational research with a focus in surgical simulation at the University of Pennsylvania in conjunction with the Imperial College of London. His research interests include identifying objective measures of technical skill and investigating the translation of training methods from outside fields to surgery.

ROY PHITAYAKORN is General/Endocrine Attending Surgeon at the Massachusetts General Hospital, and Director of Surgical Education Research. He is a faculty member of the National Surgeons as Educators course from the American College of Surgeons, and a consultant for Harvard Macy International and the American Board of Surgery. Dr. Phitayakorn has focused on surgical education research since 2004; his research interests include procedural simulation, the assessment of nontechnical skills, and stress monitoring/management in surgery.

Acknowledgments: The authors of this chapter would like to thank Dr. Ernest Gomez for his input regarding custom procedural simulation and collaborating with nonclinical departments. They also thank the Center for Medical Simulation for all their valuable help and collaborations.

ABSTRACT

Procedural simulation is designed to teach the technical skills and knowledge required for the safe execution of a clinical procedure. It spans a range of techniques from individual skill training to group and multidisciplinary training. A curriculum should be utilized to guide the educational sessions and ensure standardized learning across trainees. Within a curriculum, education should be structured to first ensure acquisition of cognitive knowledge before advancing to structured technical skills training that emphasizes educator feedback and trainee rehearsal of skills. A five-step process of teaching technical skills allows trainees to build skill and confidence through modeling, tight coaching, loose coaching, debriefing, and following a practice plan for continued improvement. This model can be expanded to include more complex procedural simulations that can include patient-specific simulations and interprofessional collaborative projects. As trainees improve their performance beyond basic competence, theoretical models of expert performance acquisition such as deliberate practice can be utilized to enhance skills toward mastery.

CASE EXAMPLE

You are the program director of a community hospital residency program. You have been approached and asked to set up a procedural training program for internal medicine residents to learn the skill of paracentesis. The department chair for medicine would like to have this program developed and in place by the start of the new academic year. That is only 3 months from now. When asked about being provided with additional resources to accomplish this project in the desired time frame, your chairman tells you that he is unable to substantially increase your training budget. How will you proceed? (See Box 3.5.1 on the next page for resolution.)

SECTION 3 • Simulators

INTRODUCTION AND BACKGROUND: DEFINING PROCEDURAL SIMULATION

Procedural simulation is a training method that incorporates cognitive knowledge and technical skill into a precise sequence of actions that are both safe and efficient. Procedural simulation can target any level of learner, ranging from beginners to advanced practitioners. Indeed, with the ever-increasing complexity of technology and its rate of implementation, procedural simulation provides a standardized venue in which individuals and teams alike can learn and rehearse technical skills in a safe environment that poses no risk to patients.

Procedural simulation has long been utilized in fields outside of medicine, particularly in high-stakes industries that emphasize safety and reliability. The airline industry is perhaps the most recognized and celebrated in its championing of procedural simulation for pilots and flight crews. Pilots can prepare step by step for various procedures such as takeoff, landing, or even crisis management. The Federal Aviation Administration now requires flight simulation as part of the credentialing process for pilots, and simulation time is a prerequisite before accumulating flight hours in an actual aircraft (Page, 2008).

Not surprisingly, the military and many police departments have also begun to utilize procedural simulation to prepare for everyday occurrences and rare disaster events alike. For example, the Defense Advanced Research Projects Agency (DARPA) has developed virtual simulations to train soldiers in decision-making skills for combat situations (Chatham, 2007); and disaster relief training now emphasizes procedural simulation (Slattery et al., 2009). Simulation exercises in these fields help soldiers and first responders to better understand execution of situation-specific incidences such as planning entry into a danger

zone and/or extricating personnel and victims from a dangerous environment.

With other high-stakes industries adopting and mandating procedural simulation, it is no surprise that medicine and its specialties have also turned to simulation to improve training with the goal of reducing patient morbidity and mortality related to errors. Procedural training can be integrated into other forms of simulation to enhance its educational potential, including boot camps (chapter 2.7), in situ simulation (chapter 2.2), and mobile simulation (chapter 2.3) among others. This chapter will provide readers with an understanding of the key concepts in procedural simulation, a framework for beginners to implement procedural simulation, and recommendations on expanding preexisting procedural simulation programs to include more complex clinical scenario simulations.

THE HOW-TO: GETTING STARTED WITH PROCEDURAL SIMULATION

By conducting a needs assessment first, a program director can focus a program's resources (including faculty time) to determine what knowledge and skills are most needed by the target learners. Chapter 7.1 details the process of conducting a needs assessment to identify themes, skills, and procedures that may need to be addressed.

For programs looking to start procedural simulation programs, many medical specialty societies have resources for getting started in simulation (see Table 3.5.1). Resources vary from listings of journal articles, textbook chapters, and other publications to full curricula that are ready to be implemented "off the shelf."

A highly regarded example of a standardized curriculum for simulation is the one provided by the American

TABLE 3.5.1

Professional Societies with Procedural Simulation Resources

Society for Simulation in Healthcare	http://ssih.org/
American College of Surgeons/ Association of Program Directors in Surgery	https://www.facs.org/ education/program/ apds-resident
International Nursing Association for Clinical Simulation and Learning	https://inacsl.org/
American Society of Anesthesiology Simulation Education Network	http://education.asahq.org/ Simulation-Education
Society for Academic Emergency Medicine Simulation Interest Group	http://www.emedu.org/sim/

College of Surgeons (ACS) and the Association of Program Directors in Surgery (APDS). The ACS and APDS collaborated to release a simulation-based curriculum meant to facilitate the incorporation of simulation into surgical training programs. This curriculum is standardized into three phases that combine Web-based tutorials with low-cost, low-technology simulators to address the teaching of basic skills, advanced procedures, and team-based competencies (Korndorffer et al., 2013). Phase I addresses basic surgical skills and techniques ranging from suturing and knot tying to chest tube placement and bowel anastomosis. Phase II of the curriculum is designed to teach procedures such as hernia repair, cholecystectomy, and colon resection. Finally, Phase III focuses on team-based work (Scott & Dunnington, 2008).

Over half of all surgery programs in the United States currently use portions of the ACS/APDS curriculum (Korndorffer et al., 2013). In consideration of individual programmatic needs, programs may find that modifying components of available "off-the-shelf" curricula, such as the one provided freely by the ACS/APDS, or developing in-house curricula may be the best option for integrating procedural training with program goals (Mittal et al., 2012).

THE PHASES OF PROCEDURAL SIMULATION

Phase 1: Building Cognitive Knowledge

To generate a systematic method of learning and gaining proficiency in a skill(s), one should first develop a base of knowledge about the skill(s). Preliminary cognitive knowledge allows the learner to become familiar with the context in which a procedure occurs. Furthermore, providing a cognitive framework to learners creates a set of expectations and goals for performance. Cognitive knowledge that learners should acquire prior to participating in procedural simulation includes, but is not limited to:

1. Assessing the appropriateness of a procedure
   a. What are the indications for performing this procedure?
   b. What clinical, laboratory, or radiologic data supports the decision to perform this procedure?
   c. Can this procedure be performed safely in the selected patient?
2. Understanding relevant anatomy to safely and efficiently perform the procedure
   a. What landmarks should be identified prior to beginning the procedure?
   b. What positioning will help execute this procedure in a safe and expeditious manner?
   c. Are there danger zones in the anatomical area of this procedure that could harm the patient if the procedure is not executed correctly?
3. Knowing the instrumentation used to perform the procedure
4. Understanding the key steps and decision nodes of the procedure
   a. What may occur during the course of the procedure that would change the usual execution of the remaining steps?
   b. What signs/symptoms would lead one to abort the procedure?
5. Understanding management of the patient after the procedure
   a. What is the expected course of recovery from the procedure?
   b. What are potential complications that may occur or be detected after the procedure?

Preprocedural training knowledge content can be delivered in a variety of ways. A popular method of delivering cognitive knowledge is through a lecture or didactic format. Alternatives to this method include assigned reading of textbooks, primary journal articles, or in-house syllabi. However, with modern technological tools, the concept of the "**flipped classroom**" can be applied to teaching procedural skills knowledge.

The flipped classroom is a concept that emphasizes individual study in a learner's free time (i.e., homework) followed by protected, directed instruction by a preceptor (Tucker, 2012). The flipped classroom can utilize a wide range of content delivery systems ranging from low technology online videos to complex computer-based simulation software such as that utilized by the American Heart Association to deliver Part 1 of HeartCode Advanced Cardiac Life Support (ACLS) training. The education literature suggests that online learning can lead to a 25% to 60% increase in retention rate compared with traditional in-classroom methods (Means et al., 2010). Within the medical literature, Web-based training has also been demonstrated to be effective (Lee et al., 2012), and many professional societies now offer Web-based coursework (Scott & Dunnington, 2008).

A formal knowledge curriculum, delivered in whatever manner an educator chooses, is an essential component in procedural training to introduce important concepts to the learner. The best media to deliver content will be dependent on each program's needs and resources. Of greater importance than the medium of content delivery is the content itself.

The introductory knowledge curriculum should provide clear learning goals and objectives, deconstruct the procedure to be learned, and thoroughly explain the equipment that will be utilized. Although this portion of the curriculum does not need to be exhaustive, it should provide the learner with a cognitive framework that will facilitate learning the indication for the procedure(s) as well as a basic understanding of the steps of the procedure onto which technical skills can be built.

Phase 2: Practice and Types of Rehearsal

Once learners have obtained the knowledge base necessary to understand the procedure, technical skills training can commence. The Center for Medical Simulation (CMS) uses a five-step approach to technical skills training in procedural simulation:

1. Modeling/Demonstrating
2. Tight Coaching
3. Loose Coaching and Practice
4. Debriefing
5. Prescribing for the Future

Step 1

The first step in technical skills education involves educator(s) modeling or demonstrating the procedural skill. Demonstration should occur in a stepwise manner to allow the learner to reflect on his/her cognitive knowledge pretraining. While the literature suggests that experts may have difficulty verbalizing their thought process during a procedure owing to internalization of knowledge (Arora et al., 2011), it is important for the educator to think aloud during any demonstrations to convey the timing of key steps and decision nodes. This will assist the learner in understanding cues throughout the procedure that reflect correct performance.

If the learners are complete novices, it is important to model only the most essential steps so as not to overwhelm the learner. However, if the learners already have some proficiency in the procedure, after modeling we will typically offer extra tips on how to position one's body when doing the procedure to maximize efficiency of movement. We also often demonstrate and discuss common mistakes and pitfalls that may occur throughout a procedure. This allows learners to understand not only the right way to perform a procedure, but also how to avoid moves that are incorrect and potentially dangerous for the healthcare provider or the patient.

Step 2

Tight coaching following demonstration is defined by close educator contact and feedback. At this stage, the coach should emphasize individualized practice techniques to develop the fundamental skills necessary to execute the key steps of a procedure. We expect that the learners will rehearse the procedure many times during this step with many opportunities for directed feedback that may include more modeling by the coach. This cycle of modeling with feedback builds on work conducted in the athlete training literature that demonstrates greater skill acquisition and retention using tight coaching than a prepractice demonstration model that emphasizes multiple attempts at rehearsal with little feedback between repetitions (Weeks & Anderson, 2000).

Step 3

Loose coaching follows the initial learning that occurred under tight coaching. Unlike tight coaching, where more immediate guidance was required to ensure correct execution of procedural steps, loose coaching places greater emphasis on allowing an individual to practice the steps on his or her own. This freedom allows the learner to develop and hone techniques over multiple repetitions. Most importantly, learners have the opportunity to make mistakes in a safe, low-risk setting and gain recognition about how to avoid these mistakes in the future. Coaches should restrain their feedback to allow learners to internalize technical skills and develop a personalized understanding of the procedure.

Coaches are typically faculty and subject matter experts, and their time can be very expensive for a simulation program to secure. As an alternative, resident physician or medical student peer teaching has been shown to be an effective mechanism of instruction for some types of procedural training (Duran-Nelson et al., 2011). The effectiveness of peer teaching may be related to Noel Burch's four stages (Table 3.5.2) of competency learning, wherein peer tutors may be at the "consciously competent" stage of skill acquisition and thus be best equipped to relate to learners (Evans & Cuffe, 2009).

For programs that cannot supply close supervision and feedback as described in the tight coaching step, rehearsal of skills through independent practice is another

TABLE 3.5.2	
Burch's Four Stages of Competency Acquisition	
Stage	**Learner Status**
Unconsciously incompetent	Unaware of what is lacking in knowledge/skills to address incompetency
Consciously incompetent	Beginning to understand why he/she has not gained competence in a skill
Consciously competent	Understands and can verbalize his/her skill set while executing these skills
Unconsciously competent	Has internalized knowledge and skill and can perform a procedure well but has difficulty explaining or teaching the procedure as the knowledge has become "second nature"

Adapted from Peyton, J. W. R. (1998). *Teaching and learning in medical practice.* Rickmansworth, UK: Manticore.

alternative. Feedback through tight and loose coaching is preferred as it provides an opportunity for learners to correct mistakes and/or optimize the execution of the procedure under guidance. Nonetheless, any practice is better than none at all, and independent practice at least allows for learners to rehearse the technical skills (Giglioli et al., 2012). However, in general, the lack of feedback precludes continued improvement in performance of a procedure, especially for learners who have difficulty gauging their own performance and adjusting the execution of the procedure to meet external benchmarks.

For simulation programs that have limited space or resources or for learners with limited time for procedural practice, mental imagery may be employed to decrease the cognitive load of performing a procedure. Mental imagery has been demonstrated in the sports and surgical education literature to be an effective adjunct to physical practice. This technique involves the mental rehearsal of each step of a procedure using vivid visual and tactile cues from a practice script developed by an experienced clinician (see Figure 3.5.1). Research has demonstrated that mental imagery can be superior to didactic training alone (Arora et al., 2011; Blair et al., 1993). Thus, mental imagery can serve as a potential alternative, and certainly an adjunct, to deliberate or independent practice after didactic training.

Phase 3: Assessment and Evaluation

The final essential component in the delivery of procedural skills training is assessment and evaluation, and these are addressed in Steps 4 and 5 of the approach to teaching procedural skills.

Step 4

Debriefing is a structured period of posttraining feedback and discussion between the educator and the learner(s).

Clipping and cutting the cystic duct and artery
You ask the nurse for the 10 mm clipper which you gently introduce into the epigastric port. You place it behind the cleared area of the duct, making sure you can see its back jaws. Ensuring it's as flush to the cystic duct as possible: you carefully position it close to the gallbladder. Slowly and deliberately you close the clipper and hold it there for a few seconds. You open it and are satisfied to see your clips safely in place. You place two further clips on the stay side, each time making sure you can see the back jaws of the clipper.

You see the artery now, darker, pinkish red and thinner than the duct You take the clipper back and clip the artery. This feels a lot easier to clip than the duct. You put one clip towards the gallbladder and two on the stay side.
You remove the clipper. You then introduce some scissors into the port, and still retracting with your left hand, you slowly cut between the clips on the duct then the artery

FIGURE 3.5.1 Excerpt from a mental practice script. (Image reproduced with permission from Arora, S., Aggarwal, R., Sevdalis, N., Moran, A., Sirimanna, P., Kneebone, R., & Darzi, A. (2010). Development and validation of mental practice as a training strategy for laparoscopic surgery. *Surgical Endoscopy, 24*[1], 179–187.) Red text represents visual cues, green are kinesthetic cues, and amber are cognitive cues

Debriefing provides the learner with constructive criticism on which to reflect on his/her performance. As discussed previously, a short form of debriefing occurs throughout the tight and loose coaching phases of learning. However, postprocedural training debriefing assumes a more formal mechanism through which final words of advice and criticism are provided to the learner.

The goal of the debriefing session is to provide a supportive, blame-free environment conducive to educating the learner. Keeping this in mind, procedural training educators should approach debriefing with the aim of identifying and reinforcing proper execution of procedure steps, while also explicitly stating areas that need continuing improvement. Genuine curiosity may help skills trainers determine why certain parts of the procedure are more difficult for some types of learners. The debriefing period is also an ideal time for the educator to receive feedback about what parts of the training sessions worked well and/or need improvement. Please refer to chapter 8.2 on Debriefing for more detailed information.

Step 5

Following the debriefing period, the educator should explain to the learners what is expected of them for the immediate future. It is often helpful at this point to explain to the learners when their formative and summative assessments will occur (if applicable) and how often/in what manner the learners are expected to practice/rehearse before their assessments.

OTHER CONSIDERATIONS IN PROCEDURAL TRAINING

Complex procedural training is very similar to basic procedural training, but requires development of greater cognitive and technical skills. These procedures go beyond typical bedside procedures such as central venous catheters, skin biopsies, and urinary catheter placement to more involved procedures such as entire surgical operations. While the complexities of the procedures are certainly increased, the tenets of the CMS training model still hold. Cognitive knowledge should be acquired first, followed by modeling of the procedure.

While complex procedures have traditionally been taught through an apprenticeship model of graduated responsibility, a more structured stepwise approach allows for standardization of learning. Stepwise training by difficulty allows a learner to conquer the simpler steps of a procedure and build knowledge, technical skill, and confidence before attempting maneuvers that require greater dexterity (Hashimoto et al., 2012). By increasing the level of difficulty at each step, learners can continue to be challenged in the learning process and avoid becoming discouraged by failure early in the training process.

The three phases of procedural simulation outlined above emphasize the role of an educator or coach, particularly for phases 2 and 3. Understandably, some institutions may not have the freedom in their budget to hire a dedicated procedural simulation educator (please see chapters 4.2 and 4.3). This is especially true for institutions that host procedural simulations for different specialties—a situation where one educator may not have the appropriate experience to teach a wide array of skills. Furthermore, faculty may be unable or unwilling to commit time to teach procedural simulations (please see chapter 4.5 on How to Create Buy-In for tips on securing institutional buy-in).

With procedural simulation, educational goals can vary from teaching introductory knowledge to advancing skill beyond competency and toward mastery. Identification of mastery is difficult in the clinical arena. Unlike fields such as athletics where organized, standardized contests crown superior athletes, medicine does not have standardized competitions. Halm et al. (2002) found that the volume of cases may correlate with outcome in procedures. However, overall data does not support the use of reputation, title, and years in training to determine expertise as experts identified in this manner have been found to perform on par or actually worse than amateurs (Ericsson et al., 2006, 2009; Schaverien, 2010). Morbidity and mortality statistics or measures of blood loss and operative time have also been considered to be performance measures (Ericsson, 2004; Norcini et al., 2002). However, these metrics are often not publicly available and thus must be collected from individual studies of departments and individuals. Thus, at this point in time, achievement of mastery is a theoretical concept in procedural simulation without strict performance criteria to guide training. As trainees gain competency in procedures, educators are encouraged to have learners further minimize errors and maximize efficiency (see below on integrating theory into practice) as a surrogate measure of mastery.

BEEN THERE, DONE THAT: ADVANCING PROCEDURAL SIMULATION

Custom Procedural Simulation and Interprofessional Collaboration

Recent advancements in virtual reality technology (described at greater length in chapter 3.7) and materials engineering make it possible for learners to engage in custom and patient-specific procedural training. Such technological advancements push the boundaries of procedural training and allow educators to deliver increasingly complex procedural simulation that is more directly applicable to individual patients.

One way to expand a department's procedural simulation program is to collaborate with departments outside of

medicine. For example, collaborations with business schools can lead to improvements in leadership, team skills, and communications training. Similarly, from an equipment and technology perspective, engineering departments can be of tremendous value in assessing the potential technological enhancements to a simulation program.

At the University of Pennsylvania (Penn), collaboration between the Department of Surgery and the School of Engineering and Applied Sciences has led to multiprofessional surgical simulation that addresses research questions in both surgical education and haptic engineering for robotic platforms. Engineers at Penn have developed a haptic feedback device for the Intuitive Da Vinci Surgical System (DVSS) that allows users to feel the vibrations being experienced by the robot's instruments and have also designed an abdominal simulator for use with the DVSS (Figure 3.5.2). Particularly relevant is an ongoing study that involves complex procedural training in robotic bariatric surgery using custom organ models of the abdomen to simulate bariatric procedures such as sleeve gastrectomy and gastric banding. These models are utilized to provide surgical residents with procedural training in robotic bariatric surgery prior to rotating on the bariatric surgical service as Clinical Year 3 and 5 residents (Gomez et al., 2013). Such collaboration empowers educators to tailor simulations to a specific need while contributing to advances in education technology.

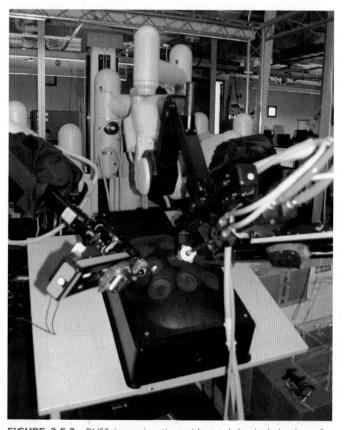

FIGURE 3.5.2 DVSS in conjunction with an abdominal simulator for procedural training in robotic bariatric surgery. (Image reproduced with permission from Dr. Katherine J. Kuchenbecker and Dr. Ernest Gomez of the University of Pennsylvania.)

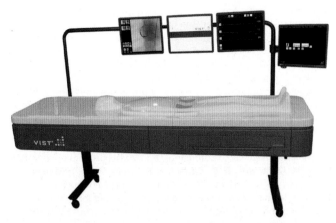

FIGURE 3.5.3 Mentice VIST Simulator System. (Image reproduced with permission from Mentice AB.)

As technology has improved, some simulators have evolved to allow for simulation of specific, individual patients. Virtual reality (VR) trainers, particularly those that involve image guidance, have advanced to the point that patient-specific CT scans, X-rays, and MRI images can be uploaded onto these trainers. Certain VR trainers can then render these patient images into a functional simulation that allows the learner to rehearse a scheduled procedure repeatedly (Figure 3.5.3). These simulations provide the learner with the ability to experiment with different approaches and techniques in a safe environment before attempting a novel or potentially difficult procedure in an actual patient (Padua et al., 2013).

Integrating Theory into Practice

For institutions looking to push learners beyond initial skill acquisition and toward "mastery," deliberate practice has been shown to be one of the more effective combinations of coaching and practice. Deliberate practice has gained popularity both in the lay press (Gladwell, 2008) and in the academic literature (Crochet et al., 2011). First described by K. Anders Ericsson in musicians, deliberate practice is described as effortful practice that is guided by an educator or coach who can provide specific feedback on weaknesses in performance and prescribe practice activities to address those weaknesses (Ericsson & Charness, 1994). As learners improve on the identified areas of performance, new feedback and practice activities are provided to address other weaknesses. Thus, as different weaknesses in performance are addressed, overall performance of a procedure increases.

Deliberate practice has been shown to improve skills beyond basic proficiency as specific feedback on performance and directed practice allows for continuing improvements in performance. Literature in fields as wide ranging as music, sports, surgery, and medical student education has demonstrated the effectiveness of deliberate practice in improving both technical and cognitive skills (Ericsson, 2007; Moulaert et al., 2004). Given the evidence suggesting the effectiveness of deliberate practice, it should be considered as a form of practice to be utilized in procedural training if possible.

While deliberate practice has been demonstrated to be an effective means of improving performance, there are drawbacks that must be taken into consideration. Particularly relevant to medical training are the time commitment required of faculty, the synchronization of availability between educators and learners, and the cost (whether calculated directly as faculty cost or loss of clinical revenue from faculty participation) of organizing multiple faculty-supervised practice sessions (Crochet et al., 2011). While larger institutions may absorb such costs, some training programs may find the resources required by deliberate practice to be too restrictive. In such cases, the frequency of feedback and coaching may be reduced to accommodate constraints. Prescriptive feedback with skill-specific practice assignments and engaged learners who are motivated to rehearse are key to the successful implementation of deliberate practice in procedural training and progression of skill toward expertise.

SUMMARY

Procedural training, as it relates to simulation, involves imparting the knowledge and technical skills needed to successfully perform a clinical procedure. The complexity of the procedure can range from simple intravenous blood sampling to difficult surgical operations.

Procedural training is best executed in a methodical manner that focuses first on delivering the cognitive skills necessary to understand the procedure and then focusing on teaching the technical skills required to perform each step. Tight and loose coaching should be utilized to build skill and confidence in the learner before transitioning the trainee to rehearsal sessions. Constructive feedback is encouraged throughout the learning process, and debriefing at the end of procedural training is useful for both the learner and the educator. Following the debriefing period, the educator should prescribe suggestions for continued learning in perfecting a procedural skill.

As educators become more adept at organizing procedural simulations, more complex procedures and patient-specific simulations can be utilized to enhance procedural education. Procedural simulation is a powerful tool through which learners can learn and hone technical skills in a safe, supportive environment that prioritizes patient safety by focusing on prevention of technical-error-related morbidity and mortality.

REFERENCES

Arora, S., Aggarwal, R., Sirimanna, P., Moran, A., Grantcharov, T., Kneebone, R., & Darzi, A. (2011). Mental practice enhances surgical technical skills. *Annals of Surgery, 253*(2), 265–270.

Blair, A., Hall, C., & Leyshon, G. (1993). Imagery effects on the performance of skilled and novice soccer players. *Journal of Sports Science, 11*(2), 95–101.

Chatham, R. E. (2007). Games for training. *Communications of the ACM, 50*(7), 36–43.

Crochet, P., Aggarwal, R., Dubb, S. S., Ziprin, P., Rajaretnam, N., Grantcharov, T., . . . Darzi, A. (2011). Deliberate practice on a virtual reality laparoscopic simulator enhances the quality of surgical technical skills. *Annals of Surgery, 253*(6), 1216–1222.

Duran-Nelson, A., Baum, K. D., Weber-Main, A. M., & Menk, J. (2011). Efficacy of peer-assisted learning across residencies for procedural training in dermatology. *Journal of Graduate Medical Education, 3*(3), 391–394.

Ericsson, K. A. (2004). Deliberate practice and the acquisition and maintenance of expert performance in medicine and related domains. *Academic Medicine, 79*(Suppl. 10), S70–S81.

Ericsson, K. A. (2007). An expert-performance perspective of research on medical expertise: The study of clinical performance. *Medical Education, 41*(12), 1124–1130.

Ericsson, K. A., & Charness, N. (1994). Expert performance: Its structure and acquisition. *American Psychologist, 49*(8), 725–747.

Ericsson, K. A., Charness, N., Feltovich, P. J., & Hoffmann, R. R. (2006). *The Cambridge handbook of expertise and expert performance.* Cambridge, UK: Cambridge University Press.

Ericsson, K. A., Nandagopal, K., & Roring, R.W. (2009). Toward a science of exceptional achievement: Attaining superior performance through deliberate practice. *Annals of the New York Academy of Sciences, 1172,* 199–217.

Evans, D. J. R., & Cuffe, T. (2009). Near-peer teaching in anatomy: An approach for deeper learning. *Anatomical Sciences Education, 2*(5), 227–233.

Giglioli, S., Boet, S., De Gaudio, A. R., Linden, M., Schaeffer, R., Bould, M. D., & Diemunsch, P. (2012). Self-directed deliberate practice with virtual fiberoptic intubation improves initial skills for anesthesia residents. *Minerva Anestesiol, 78*(4), 456–461.

Gladwell, M. (2008). *Outliers: The story of success.* New York, NY: ePenguin.

Gomez, E. D., McMahan, W., Hashimoto, D. A., Brzezinski, A., Bark, K., Dumon, K. R., . . . Kuchenbecker, K. J. (2013). *Vibrotactile haptic feedback improves performance during robotic surgical simulation: A randomized controlled trial.* Paper presented at the Clinical Congress of the American College of Surgeons, Washington, DC.

Halm, E. A., Lee, C., & Chassin, M. R. (2002). Is volume related to outcome in health care? A systematic review and methodologic critique of the literature. *Annals of Internal Medicine, 137*(6), 511–520.

Hashimoto, D. A., Gomez, E. D., Danzer, E., Edelson, P. K., Morris, J. B., Williams, N. N., & Dumon, K. R. (2012). Intraoperative resident education for robotic laparoscopic gastric banding surgery: A pilot study on the safety of stepwise education. *Journal of the American College of Surgeons, 214*(6), 990–996.

Korndorffer, J. R., Jr., Arora, S., Sevdalis, N., Paige, J., McClusky, D. A., 3rd, & Stefanidis, D. (2013). The American College of Surgeons/Association of Program Directors in Surgery National Skills Curriculum: Adoption rate, challenges and strategies for effective implementation into surgical residency programs. *Surgery, 154*(1), 13–20.

Lee, J. M., Fernandez, F., Staff, I., & Mah, J. W. (2012). Web-based teaching module improves success rates of postpyloric positioning of nasoenteric feeding tubes. *JPEN Journal of Parenteral and Enteral Nutrition, 36*(3), 323–329.

Means, B., Toyama, Y., Murphy, R., Bakia, M., & Jones, K. (2010). *Evaluation of evidence-based practices in online learning: A meta-analysis and review of online learning studies.* Washington, DC: U.S. Department of Education.

Mittal, M. K., Dumon, K. R., Edelson, P. K., Acero, N. M., Hashimoto, D., Danzer, E., . . . Williams, N. N. (2012). Successful implementation of the American College of Surgeons/Association of Program Directors in Surgery Surgical Skills Curriculum via a 4-week consecutive simulation rotation. *Simulation in Healthcare, 7*(3), 147–154.

Moulaert, V., Verwijnen, M. G., Rikers, R., & Scherpbier, A. J. (2004). The effects of deliberate practice in undergraduate medical education. *Medical Education, 38*(10), 1044–1052.

Norcini, J. J., Lipner, R. S., & Kimball, H. R. (2002). Certifying examination performance and patient outcomes following acute myocardial infarction. *Medical Education, 36*(9), 853–859.

Padua, M. R., Yeom, J. S., Lee, S. Y., Lee, S. M., Kim, H. J., Chang, B. S., . . . Riew, K. D. (2013). Fluoroscopically guided anterior atlantoaxial transarticular screws: A feasibility and trajectory study using CT-based simulation software. *Spine Journal, 13*(11), 1455–1463.

Page, R. (2008). Lessons from aviation simulation. In R. Riley (Ed.), *Manual of simulation in healthcare* (pp. 37–49). New York, NY: Oxford University Press.

Schaverien, M. V. (2010). Development of expertise in surgical training. *Journal of Surgical Education, 67*(1), 37–43.

Scott, D. J., & Dunnington, G. L. (2008). The new ACS/APDS skills curriculum: Moving the learning curve out of the operating room. *Journal of Gastrointestinal Surgery, 12*(2), 213–221.

Slattery, C., Syvertson, R., & Krill, S. (2009). The eight step training model: Improving disaster management leadership. *Journal of Homeland Security and Emergency Management, 6*(1), 1547–7355. doi:10.2202/1547-7355.1403

Tucker, B. (2012). The flipped classroom: Online instruction at home frees class time for learning. *Education Next, 12*(1), 82–83.

Weeks, D. L., & Anderson, L. P. (2000). The interaction of observational learning with overt practice: Effects on motor skill learning. *Acta Psychologica, 104*(2), 259–271.

CHAPTER 3.6

Hybrid Simulations

Dawn M. Schocken, MPH, PhD(c), CHSE-A, and Wendy L. Gammon, MA, MEd

ABOUT THE AUTHORS

DAWN M.SCHOCKEN is the Director of the Center for Advanced Clinical Learning (CACL) at the University of South Florida (USF) Morsani College of Medicine in Tampa, Florida, and a Certified Healthcare Simulation Educator. Under her guidance, CACL, a founding member of the USF Health Simulation Consortium, has achieved national recognition as a fully accredited simulation center. Ms. Schocken serves on several national committees and specializes in hybrid simulation with an interprofessional team.

WENDY L. GAMMON is an Assistant Professor of Medicine at the University of Massachusetts (UMASS) Medical School and Director of the UMASS Standardized Patient Program. Under her leadership, the program provides standardized patients for teaching, assessment, and curriculum, and faculty development to the UMASS clinical and academic communities. Ms. Gammon also provides standardized patient services and academic consulting to several New England healthcare training programs and serves as a peer reviewer for MedEdPORTAL.

ABSTRACT

This chapter explores the utilization of hybrid simulation in teaching and assessment in the healthcare education and training setting. The opportunity to re-create complex clinical situations in which healthcare professionals can safely practice management of these situations makes hybrid simulation a valuable educational asset. Running sophisticated scenarios that highlight serious patient challenges allows the healthcare professional or trainee to become immersed in skill development, enhancement, proficiency, and mastery without untoward effects on patient care.

Hybrid simulation is a process of selection and implementation. Scenarios are developed on the basis of what is known, what has been experienced, what is anticipated to happen, and any known knowledge or performance gaps among healthcare students or professionals. Resources are selected on the basis of the scenario. This chapter provides an overview of the methodology along with an outline of questions that will help determine when a hybrid simulation is appropriate.

CASE EXAMPLE

When preparing to run simulations for practicing teams in the labor and delivery suite, it becomes apparent that having only the high-technology simulator in the room will not be adequate to simulate a complex obstetric clinical scenario. More realism is necessary to meet the learning objectives that include early recognition of fetal distress, preparing for an emergency Cesarean section, dealing with a disruptive family member, and delivering bad news. Blending the high-technology simulator with standardized patients to provide a real face and voice for the birthing mannequin and play the role of the family members along with embedded simulated persons to play other needed healthcare team members, and the addition of a task trainer to perform a fetal maneuver will both enhance learning and heighten the learners' retention of skills.

INTRODUCTION AND BACKGROUND

When more than one type of simulator is used in a simulation, it is called a hybrid simulation (Issenberg et al., 2004). The most common hybrid simulation combines a mannequin (in the role of a patient) with one or more standardized patients (SPs). The combination of methodologies typically enhances the realism of the scenario while providing additional challenges that allow the learner to become immersed in the learning experience. In a hybrid simulation, the SPs may portray the patient at different times in the scenario, a family member, or anyone else associated with the patient. Depending on the educational objectives, SPs can portray a vast array of emotions, testing the learner's ability to handle not only the medical needs but also the emotional and psychosocial needs of the patient and others. Hybrid simulations can also include various combinations of immersive or virtual simulations with task trainers or low-technology simulators.

Hybrid simulation was developed almost as soon as the high-technology simulator arrived on the scene. Having a full body mannequin in crisis was made much more real with the addition of a crying family member, a screaming infant, or the noises of a critical care unit. The addition of humans (SPs) to the human patient simulator allowed the learner to develop a sense of urgency that was not always present with a simulator alone. As simulators have become more sophisticated, the educators, too, have become more sophisticated in scenario building. (See the example on the next page for a rich demonstration of using hybrid simulation to reinforce a common hospital task: managing a patient code).

When learners read about how to do something, they can envision how they might respond. When those same learners are immersed in a hybrid scenario with voice, emotion, and action included, the learner, or team of learners, can work to resolve the medical crisis and manage the entire scene in a safe environment. Simulations that integrate various modalities permit adult learners to practice skill sets in realistic scenarios to a level of perfection, allowing in-depth learning to occur.

As an example, disaster simulations typically use a hybrid approach. Communities want to be sure that their disaster teams are in a state of preparedness. Using multiple simulators and SPs in various stages of triage allows a team of emergency workers to practice timely and efficient care and management of the multiple wounded (Kneebone, 2003). The simulation can then be studied independently to improve the team's ability to manage the disaster. This allows the team to build confidence in its ability to handle a disaster, should one occur.

Hybrid scenarios can be set up in either the simulation lab or in situ, allowing the learner or team of learners to practice their skill set, demonstrate proficiency, or demonstrate deficiencies that may need to be remediated. Hybrid simulations can be used from the initial phase of learning a rudimentary skill through proficiency demonstration of the most sophisticated task (Noeller et al., 2008). They can be used in both the teaching and the assessment phases of learning, and are frequently coupled with debriefing and learner reflection.

METHODS

Not every educational objective requires a hybrid simulation to be addressed effectively. As with all educational efforts, it is important to start with a clear articulation of

the goal of the effort. With the educational goal in mind, learning objectives can be developed. From these, the specifics of the simulation experience can be determined and an appropriate simulation methodology selected. Asking the following series of questions will help determine whether a hybrid simulation is appropriate:

1. What are the goals for this simulation?
2. What are the learning objectives?
3. What level of learners will be involved in this simulation?
4. What clinical or professional competencies are being addressed?
5. Where will this simulation take place?
6. Will this simulation be used for teaching, demonstration, assessment, or high-stakes testing?
7. What level of fidelity is needed in the scenario to achieve the learning objectives?
8. What functions and roles are necessary to achieve the desired end-points?
9. What simulators, ESPs, and SPs are available for use?
10. How will you evaluate whether the educational goals have been met?
11. Who will conduct the debriefing session?

Once these questions are answered, a determination can be made as to which simulation methodology— physiologically responsive mannequin, task trainer, virtual simulation, static mannequin, SPs, or hybrid—would be most effective and efficient. As with other simulation methodologies, hybrid simulations require the development of a complete simulation scenario with supporting documents for SPs and ESPs. Additionally, the scenario needs to provide complete directions related to the interface between the various simulation technologies.

When a decision is made to use a hybrid simulation, the level of preparation and rehearsals is heightened to ensure the simulation team is well prepared for the event. (See chapter 3.2, 3.3, 3.4, and 8.2 on preparing to use mannequins, SPs, ESPs, and debriefing.) Taking the time to review each detail of the simulation in rehearsals will allow for fine-tuning the acting, timing, and transitions. A well-rehearsed scenario can run like clockwork, affording the opportunity to observe learner behaviors and performance when the scenario is run live.

Hybrid simulations can be done in situ (actual clinical setting) or in the simulation lab (attempting to make the scene as real as possible). Unlike scenarios that use a single simulation methodology, hybrid simulations require more coordination and more experienced members of the simulation team to be effective. Preparation is even more critical than in single modality simulations as the interfaces and transitions between methods must be practiced. To prepare for the simulation, early access to the simulators to be used is essential. The facilitator may need a high-technology mannequin that can run a demonstration of a disease state. The recruitment of ESPs to enhance realism (e.g., nurses in the emergency room, a phlebotomist to draw blood, a nurse anesthetist to assist in the labor and delivery suite) may be required. Standardized patients to act the role of the patient or family member may need to be recruited. And all of these pieces must learn to work well together.

Evaluations of the hybrid simulation scenario can be done on multiple levels. As in simulations that use a single methodology, the educator can evaluate whether the learners reached the objectives. The learners can evaluate whether they felt the hybrid simulation was useful or too complex. The SP can evaluate whether there was effective communication between themselves and the learners as well as with ESPs and the simulation coordinator. A preceptor can watch the hybrid simulation while it is ongoing to complete an evaluation to determine the effectiveness of the simulation on the learner's performance. An independent observer can be brought in to determine the efficiency and overall effectiveness of the simulation in meeting the scenario objectives (Issenberg & Scalese, 2008).

THEMES FOUND IN THE FIELD

Simulation-based education complements traditional medical education in patient care settings, enhances postgraduate education, and assesses the licensed practitioner's competency. Introducing hybrid simulations at all levels of healthcare practice allows the healthcare professional to develop and refine individual and team-based clinical and professional competencies. While research in the field needs improvement in terms of rigor and quality, high-technology hybrid medical simulations have been shown to be educationally effective (Noeller et al., 2008).

Hybrid simulation is primed to provide the learner with a rich, dynamic experience, with a real-time feel and real-time patient flow that can then be reviewed, debriefed, and repeated until proficiency and mastery is reached. As our healthcare system continues to become more complex, offering hybrid simulation to mimic complex patient experiences allows healthcare to practice integrating the knowledge, skills, and attitudes necessary for high-quality, patient-centered care.

EXPERT'S CORNER

DOCUMENTATION FOR SIMULATION (EMR/EHR)
Pamela B. Andreatta, EdD, MFA, MA
President, Society for Simulation in Healthcare (2015)

There are three important connections to be made between electronic medical/health records (EMR/EHR) and simulation. The first is that simulation can be useful in orienting clinicians to the uses of an EMR/EHR system in clinical practice. This is not a trivial issue, especially as systems are integrated, updated, and modified within the healthcare environment. The complexity and (ironically) proprietary configurations of EMR/EHR platforms, coupled with the necessity to accurately enter and access patient information during the provision of care, render this task essential for patient safety and quality of care. As such, instruction in the uses of EMR/EHR systems fits well within a simulation-based context because it facilitates that engagement during the provision of care, without the potential to adversely affect patient data during training. As with all other areas where patient safety is a high priority, the greater the extent to which personnel can master their abilities in a simulated context, the more likely errors due to unfamiliar practices will be averted.

The second connection to simulation is the potential for EMR/EHR data to be used to create or re-create training scenarios that serve to mitigate or remedy risk in applied practice. Many simulation programs facilitate this process in the aftermath of near miss or adverse and sentinel events, with the intention of reviewing what led to the outcomes and remedying any deficit areas through targeted training. Although this practice has significant value for healthcare providers, it tends to be a reactive process rather than a proactive one. Assembling de-identified libraries of cases informed by clinical variables from EMR/EHRs would begin to establish the types of proactive instruction that serve to develop the critical thinking skills that are essential for both common and unusual situations. The more variable and detailed case libraries are, even for a single clinical

presentation (e.g., myocardial infarction), the more learners will have the opportunity to develop complex diagnostic reasoning and clinical management skills. Case libraries built upon real patient data will provide more impactful training scenarios *because* they are based on real data, and therefore best replicate the applied clinical environment.

The third potential connection between EMR/EHR information and simulation is the ability to transfer data describing patient-specific anatomy, physiology, pathology, or injury to a simulated rehearsal context prior to performing an actual clinical procedure or implementing a therapeutic course of action. For example, MRI data could be used to model a patient's difficult airway before surgery to help anesthesiologists determine the safest approach to intubating. Likewise, imaging data could be used by surgeons to try alternate approaches to difficult dissections using virtual reality modeling before performing the procedure in an operative context. Physiological modeling could be useful for simulating potential responses to drugs and other therapies, the intent of which is to improve efficacy while reducing adverse interaction effects. In this way, EMR/EHR information can be used to simulate the actual patient and allow clinicians to customize care in a way that best meets the patient's needs, while minimizing risk.

As with any disruptive technology, EMR/EHR systems and their integration into applied clinical practice will continue to change over time. We will likely see numerous other opportunities to utilize the benefits of both EMR/EHR and healthcare simulation in a synergistic manner as each construct continues to mature in its application. To the extent each development can benefit patient safety, clinician safety, and quality of care, better healthcare will result for all.

BEEN THERE, DONE THAT: HOW CAN I CONTINUE TO IMPROVE OR SUSTAIN WHAT I HAVE ACHIEVED?

Hybrid simulations take practice to implement correctly. Each time a hybrid simulation is run, there may be a new set of learners. Making the simulation effective and exciting for them requires the simulation faculty to demonstrate a sense of passion for student learning even if this is the fiftieth time the scenario has been run. With an eye to moving the learner from skill learning to skill development, to skill proficiency, and ultimately to skill mastery, hybrid simulations need to be carefully constructed. Fine-tuning the scenarios, enhancing the embedded simulated persons' (ESPs) range of emotions, adding additional ESPs to play professional roles, placing moulage on the mannequin to enhance the realism, and sharing more advanced scenarios with colleagues will all improve on the momentum developed with the first simulation. Staying abreast of the newest technology, learning how to make the simulations look more real, embracing new skill sets,

and reading the simulation literature will identify new concepts that can be incorporated into the scenarios.

Many sustainable simulation programs today are marketing hybrid simulation opportunities to academic, clinical, and affiliated healthcare training programs, both within their own institutions and in the geographical region. A strategy to incorporate hybrid simulation into the portfolio of simulation offerings is to encourage, nurture, and facilitate collaboration between course directors, program faculty, and administration. Individuals who are familiar with the value of hybrid simulation readily become early adopters and champions. However, even where there is support for the concept, it is important to be aware that there can be challenges to using hybrid simulation beyond the obvious financial and space considerations. For example, faculty support might be lacking because of the increased time and effort this form of simulation requires.

Working closely with key core educators in the development of the hybrid simulation scenarios assures the success and continued relevance of this teaching modality. Success can be achieved through a collaborative approach.

EXAMPLE: ACUTE MYOCARDIAL INFARCTION WITH CARDIAC ARREST

Location: Emergency Department
Chief complaint: "Bad chest pressure for the last hour, now I feel like I am going to die!"

Scenario Phase 1
Patient Information: Volunteered
You are a 67-year-old male who began to have chest pressure about 1 hour ago. It got progressively worse, and you felt weak and somewhat short of breath, so you told your wife, who brought you straight in to the ED. Now the pressure is quite severe, and you feel horrible, almost like you are ready to die. You are very frightened.

Other Patient Information: All Other Historical Information Below Is Given Only When Asked
   Chest pain: Pressure feels as if someone is sitting on your chest. It is in the middle of your chest, and there is no radiation of the pain to your arm or jaw; it is all in your chest. You have never had pain like this before. On the pain scale it is 10 out of 10. It has gotten progressively worse since it started, and nothing relieves it. You were walking up the stairs in your house when it started. You immediately went back downstairs and sat down in a chair, but the pressure kept getting worse.
   Shortness of breath: Along with the pain you have had increasing shortness of breath, and now you feel short of breath just lying there.
   Sweaty: You broke out into a sweat, as the pain got worse.
   Past history as relates to heart disease: Never had a heart problem that you knew of.
   Physical exercise: You normally walk about 20 minutes a day; no other significant exercise beyond that.

Past medical history:
1. History of hypertension for 10 years and have been on Diovan 80 mg daily and HCTZ 12.5 mg daily.
2. History of Type 2 Diabetes Mellitus diagnosed 5 years ago. You are on Metformin 500 mg twice a day. Your glucose (finger stick) runs at about 120 mg per dl fasting and about 140 mg per dl 2 hours after eating. You cannot remember your HgbA1C.
   Surgical history: Appendectomy at age 18.
   Review of systems: Negative for all other than what is stated above.
   Social history of pertinence: You are married and live with your wife; you have two grown children.
   Smoking history: You finally quit smoking about 2 years ago but smoked one-half pack per day for 45 years prior to that.
   Alcohol history: You drink about three glasses of wine per week with dinner.
   Sexual history: Noncontributory.
   Family history of pertinence: Father died of a heart attack at age 62. He was diabetic, hypertensive, and a smoker. Mother died at age 88 after she fell and broke her hip.
   Medications: Diovan 80 mg daily for 5 years. Hydrochlorothiazide (HCTZ) 12.5 mg daily for 10 years. Metformin 500 mg twice a day for 5 years.
   Allergies to medications: No known allergies.
   Physical exam: Initial vital signs: Pulse = 130 beats per minute; Respiratory Rate = 30 breaths per minute; Blood Pressure = 85/40 mm Hg; Temperature: 98.2°F (36.8°C).

EXAMPLE: ACUTE MYOCARDIAL INFARCTION WITH CARDIAC ARREST (continued)

Mannequin Presentation
- Vital Signs are as reported above.
- The monitor will show a wide-complex tachycardia at a rate of 130.
- Chest: Clear
- Heart: S4 gallop sound
- Abdomen: Within Normal Limits
- Extremities: Within Normal Limits except unable to feel dorsalis pedis, posterior tibial, or radial pulses
- Diaphoretic

Scenario Phase 2
The student should recognize that the patient is in a wide-complex unstable tachycardia with hypotension, and initiate synchronized cardioversion at this time. If the student does this, the patient will go into a sinus rhythm and be stable and able to talk for 1 minute but will then go into pulseless ventricular tachycardia (V-tach) and require immediate defibrillation. If the student does not initially cardiovert, the mannequin will go directly into pulseless V-tach in 1 minute.

Once in pulseless V-tach, Cardiopulmonary resuscitation (CPR) should be initiated, and the student will have to perform CPR and direct the nurses to help in a team effort.

The student will run the code. The code will run as follows: CPR for 2 minutes, then a rhythm check. The mannequin will be in ventricular fibrillation (V-fib) at that time and require a shock followed by epinephrine or vasopressin. This should be followed by 2 minutes of CPR, after which the patient will be in V-fib and require a shock followed by amiodarone 300 mg given intravenously. After 2 minutes of CPR, the rhythm will convert to V-fib again and require a shock. After this shock, the cardiac monitor will show rhythm of pulseless electrical activity (PEA) at a rate of 50 beats per minute, but the student should perform CPR for 2 minutes before rechecking the rhythm. When the rhythm is checked, it will be PEA at a rate of 50 beats per minute. At this point, the student should not deliver a shock but should administer epinephrine 1 mg and do two more minutes CPR, followed by another rhythm check, which will be PEA. Atropine 1 mg should be administered as CPR is resumed.

At this point, if the student has not already considered the causes, the student will be prompted by the nurse to look for causes for the PEA by asking, "Why is this patient in PEA?" The student should list the causes of PEA (first, the immediately reversible causes, and then those that are not immediately reversible).

In response to inquiries, there will be no hypoglycemia, no hypothermia, no hyper- or hypokalemia, no hypoxia, no hypovolemia, and no significant acidosis other than the acidosis expected at this point in the code. There will be no trauma, no tamponade, no tension pneumothorax, no toxins, and no pulmonary thrombosis.

When the cause of the PEA is noted to be a massive coronary thrombus, the scenario will end.

Final diagnosis: Acute Myocardial Infarction with ventricular tachycardia (VT) followed by ventricular fibrillation (V-fib) and finally pulseless electrical activity (PEA).

Evaluation Tools
For the purposes of this case, two tools will be used:
1. Precode: critical action list
2. Postcode: The American Heart Association Megacode Testing Checklist 3 for Tachycardia to VT/Pulseless VT to PEA

PreCode Critical Action List
____Asked about location of chest pain
____Asked about severity of pain and quantified on a 1 to 10 scale
____Asked about pain radiation
____Asked how long pain present
____Asked about past history of heart disease
____Asked about medications at home
____Asked if any allergies to medications
____Asked what you were doing when the pain started
____Asked if you had or have shortness of breath with the pain
____Examined the heart in four areas
____Examined the chest bilaterally
____Feels for a pulse
____Checks a BP
____Taps and shouts the patient before initiating CPR

Postcode AHA Megacode Testing Checklist 3 for Tachycardia to VF/Pulseless VT to PEA (Field et al., 2010)
____Ensures high-quality CPR at all times
____Assigns team-member roles
____Ensures that team members perform well
____Starts oxygen if needed, places monitor, starts IV
____Places monitor leads in proper position
____Recognizes unstable tachycardia
____Recognizes symptoms due to tachycardia
____Performs immediate synchronized cardioversion
____Recognizes VF
____Clears before ANALYZE and SHOCK
____Immediately resumes CPR after shocks
____Appropriate airway management
____Appropriate cycles of drug–rhythm check/shock–CPR
____Administers appropriate drug(s) and doses
____Recognizes PEA
____Verbalizes potential reversible causes of PEA/asystole (H's and T's)
____Administers appropriate drug(s) and doses
____Immediately resumes CPR after rhythm and pulse checks
____Identifies ROSC
____Ensures BP and 12-lead ECG are performed, O_2 saturation is monitored, verbalizes need for endotracheal intubation and waveform capnography, and orders laboratory tests
____Considers therapeutic hypothermia

Engage the stakeholders. Meet with faculty to listen and learn not only what they teach but how they teach it, and what their overall and specific goals and objectives are for a particular course or group of trainees. Learn about the clinical "pearls" they want learners to absorb and take away by the end of the session.

Start small. Work with faculty to identify a single concept or skill exercise already in the syllabus, and determine where a hybrid simulation could enhance and supplement that existing learner experience. Starting with an overly ambitious hybrid simulation will increase the risk for confusion, expense, or even failure. An example of an ambitious initial effort would be to start with a multistation, high-stakes examination where all stations blend simulation modalities of SPs, sophisticated mannequins, and task trainers. With so many moving parts combined with the learner's heightened sense of stress during this graded activity, it would be more advisable to begin with a single multimodality teaching simulation. This would allow both faculty and learners to gain proficiency and comfort with the modality before moving to more expansive hybrid scenarios.

As an example, an existing course has a session introducing or reviewing a procedural skill such as inserting an intravenous (IV) catheter. Currently, the content is presented as a lecture in a large group format with PowerPoint illustrations shown on a large screen. This is followed by a short video showing a clinician starting an IV on an actual patient. The learners are then assigned to the lab for self-directed practice on skin trainer blocks. Embracing the benefits of hybrid simulation, the faculty could provide the content using an SP with a part task skin trainer attached to the arm and draped to look like an actual IV insertion site. This hybrid simulation would also provide an opportunity for faculty to role model clinical skills beyond the technical challenges of starting an IV. Communication in its many forms is now recognized as a major component of clinical competence. Using this methodology, the faculty can demonstrate how to address the communication challenges of preparing the patient for the procedure, providing patient education and demonstrating facilitative behavior through reassurance and empathy.

SUMMARY

Hybrid simulation can be as sophisticated or as simple as you wish to make it. You can create a rich learner experience with thoughtful consideration of what you wish to have the learners achieve. Making the scenario exciting, interesting, and challenging draws the learners into the event, and allows individuals and teams to practice, demonstrate proficiency, and walk away with a sense of confidence in having acquired or perfected the targeted competency. Hybrid simulations allow individuals and teams to work just as they work in actual clinical settings. When done well, hybrid simulations contribute to the number of "teaching moments." When combined with deliberate practice, this method can ultimately result in enhanced patient safety and increases the overall quality of patient care.

REFERENCES

Field, J. M., Hazinski, M. F., Sayre, M. R., Chameides, L., Schexnayder, S. M., Hemphill, R., Samson, R. A., … Vanden Hoek, T. L. (2010). Executive summary: 2010 American Heart Association guidelines for cardiopulmonary resuscitation and emergency cardiovascular care. *Circulation AHA, 122* (18 suppl. 3), S639.

Issenberg, S. B., McGaghie, W. C., Petrusa, E. R., Gordon, D. L., & Scalese, R. J. (2004). *Features and uses of high-fidelity medical simulations that lead to effective learning: A BEME systematic review* (BEME Guide No. 4). Dundee, Scotland: Association for Medical Education in Europe.

Issenberg, S. B., & Scalese, R. J. (2008). Simulation in health care education. *Perspectives in Biology and Medicine, 51*(1), 31–46.

Kneebone, R. (2003). Simulation in surgical training: Educational issues and practical implications. *Medical Education, 37*, 267–277.

Noeller, T. P., Smith, M. D., Holmes, L., Cappaert, M., Gross, A. J., Cole-Kelly, K., & Rosen, K. R. (2008). A theme-based hybrid simulation model to train and evaluate emergency medicine residents. *Academic Emergency Medicine, 15*(11), 1199–1206.

CHAPTER 3.7

Virtual Simulation

Eric B. Bauman, PhD, RN, and Penny Ralston-Berg, MS

ABOUT THE AUTHORS

ERIC B. BAUMAN has held numerous academic, public safety and industry positions specific to game-based learning and simulation. Dr. Bauman is a Registered Nurse, Fire Service Division Chief, and founder of Clinical Playground, LLC. He is also a Fellow at the University of Wisconsin–Madison School of Education, Department of Curriculum and Instruction and Games Learning Society. Bauman's research interests focus on hybrid learning that moves between the physical and virtual worlds.

PENNY RALSTON-BERG has been designing online courses since 1997. She has also served as a technology trainer and design consultant for K-12, community college, higher education, and nonprofit groups. Penny is currently a telecommuting instructional designer for the Penn State World Campus. Her primary research interests are games and simulations for education and how learner perspectives of quality impact online course design.

ABSTRACT

This chapter introduces the reader to the concept of simulations taking place in a virtual or digital environment and the importance of game-based learning mechanics and activities as an integral part of multimedia digital environments. We begin with a discussion of contemporary terms and definitions common to the genre of game-based learning. This discussion also introduces readers to contemporary pedagogy specific to learning within digital environments. The relationship between game-based learning and learner motivation is discussed, as is the concept of fit from the perspective of the integration of digital games and digital learning environments and related technology into clinical curricula. Finally, evaluation of virtual simulation and game-based learning is addressed from multiple perspectives, including learner success, educator performance, and curriculum evaluation.

CASE EXAMPLE: FORENSIC NURSING

As part of a forensic nursing course, students have an option to view an autopsy, which may or may not include a sexual assault examination. The autopsy is a key experience where all the roles of forensic nursing are tied into the collection of evidence to assist in closing a case. An autopsy is a limited opportunity for face-to-face students when the occurrence does not match student availability or there is not enough room in the morgue to invite more than four students to view the procedure. Students at a distance have no opportunity to view the autopsy unless they happen to be close enough to travel to the location where the observation has been arranged. Educators of the forensic nursing course would like to:

• Provide an opportunity for more students to experience an autopsy and sexual assault examination.
• Illustrate an accurate virtual representation of the coroner/forensic pathologist, forensic photographer, and nurse roles in the autopsy process.
• Provide a detailed view of how evidence is identified, collected, and preserved during the autopsy process, which is crucial for the justice system.
• Demonstrate the value of discovering the cause of death, as well as preventing death.

They believe some type of game or simulation may fill these gaps. Their questions include:

• Are game elements or simulations more appropriate?
• What are the elements of an effective game or simulation?
• How will we ensure good curricular fit?
• What types of evaluation should we consider?

(Case example courtesy Alicia Swaggerty, Penn State World Campus)

INTRODUCTION

The aim of this chapter is to introduce the reader to the concept of virtual simulation and game-based learning or learning opportunities provided in digital virtual environments. We argue that learning necessarily takes place during play (Botturi & Loh, 2008). We also argue that the term "serious games" is misplaced even in the context of clinical education and prefer the term game-based learning. Educators new to game-based learning or serious games will find many of the elements that promote good simulation experiences discussed elsewhere in this text are congruent with the facets of good games or good game play (Bauman, 2007).

> As researchers and educators began to delve more into video-games and complex learning dynamics that take place during game play, it is important for the educational community to clarify what game means in order to facilitate clear dialog with other learning domains and the videogame industry.
> *Botturi and Loh (2008, p. 2)*

Promoting engaging learning opportunities found in created spaces (Bauman, 2007), including digital environments and video games, can be fun. Nothing is lost in terms of educational merit by creating learning experiences that are enjoyable. The terms "serious games" should not be misunderstood to mean devoid of fun. We argue that leveraging technology, including games, to create active learning experiences increases learner engagement (Gee, 2003).

This chapter will begin by introducing the reader to contemporary terms and theory supporting game-based learning. Throughout this section of the chapter we will provide examples that help to situate these terms and theories to clinical education. The next section of this chapter will discuss the concept of learner motivation for game-based learning.

The later section of this chapter will go on to discuss the notion of "fit" in terms of the curriculum in general and with other forms of technology, specifically eLearning platforms. We will also discuss the use of digital environments and game-based learning as a function of hybrid or mixed method learning strategies.

Finally we will discuss learner, faculty, and curriculum evaluation as it relates to game-based learning occurring within digital environments. While this chapter does not provide an in-depth discussion of academic evaluation, it will introduce readers to games as a mechanism for data collection.

TERMS AND DEFINITIONS FOR GAME-BASED LEARNING AND DIGITAL ENVIRONMENTS

Digital Natives and Digital Immigrants

Prensky (2001) originally developed and discussed the terms *digital native* and *digital immigrant*. These terms, now well over 10 years old, seem more important today than they did 10 years ago and illustrate an important challenge. All traditionally aged learners are **digital natives**. Digital natives are those people that grew up immersed in digital technology. They have likely spent more time playing video games than reading by the time they begin college (Prensky, 2003). The digital native leverages digital technology intuitively. "*Digital natives* are fluent in the language of the digital environment. They possess an innate sense of media literacy" (Bauman, 2012, pp. 79–80).

Digital immigrants generally represent those who were born prior to the digital media explosion. Digital immigrants wrote term papers on a typewriter. They took college exams in person and penned them in "blue books" provided by teaching assistants to large classes. For many digital immigrants, the Scantron fill in the bubble multiple-choice exam was still a novelty when they were in school or entered the academic workforce. Digital immigrants remember the invention of cordless phones. The first cell phone they purchased certainly was not a smartphone. Digital immigrants are being forced to adapt to the increasingly prevalent digital environments. Ten years ago, it was still possible to resist the inclusive nature of digital environments. This is no longer the case in mainstream academia or healthcare. It is simply no longer possible to thrive as a clinician or academician without some degree of digital and informatics literacy.

It is possible for digital immigrants to adapt to the digital world, but they face the same challenges that many nonnative speakers encounter when they arrive in a new country. The challenge moves beyond a simple language barrier. It includes the challenges associated with immersion into a new sociocultural environment. Immigrants are biased by their previous lived experiences. They carry the artifacts of the old world with them and use those to form opinions about their success and failures negotiating the modern and rapidly advancing digital world. For many digital immigrants, achieving native levels of digital literacy is beyond their reach (Bauman, 2012; Prensky, 2001).

The challenge for leadership and faculty is particularly acute because they are outnumbered. Even if leadership does not fully understand the importance of technology at the native level, leadership must appreciate the important role that digital technology has come to play in educational and clinical processes. Failure to meet learner, expectations in terms of how curricula will be delivered and how learning will be supported will drive the best and brightest students to those institutions able to negotiate, integrate, and leverage digital technology effectively (Bauman, 2010, 2012).

Ludology

The word "ludic" originates from the Latin word *ludis*, meaning game. **Ludology**, a relatively new term, refers to the study of games in general. However, the term is more often used informally in the context of video games. Frasca (2001) argues that the goal of ludology is to understand games and video games, both from a formal perspective and as part of the larger media ecology. Defining game study as a mechanism of ecology encourages teachers to examine how game technology, specifically digital game or application technology, plays a role in the human and, more narrowly, learner experience.

Broussard (2011) defines ludic pedagogy as the manner in which games teach players to play. From this perspective, we can reframe Broussard's definition of ludic pedagogy to examine the manner in which games teach learners to learn. This is an important question because learners cannot learn to become clinicians without being acculturated to the professions they hope to join. This is to say one cannot become a baseball player without learning how to play baseball. Further, one cannot learn to play baseball by reading baseball rulebooks—you must play baseball.

Gamification

Deterding et al. (2011) define **gamification** as ". . . the use of game elements in non-game contexts." Deterding et al. go on to discuss the difference between play and games. Games are in general constrained by rules and a system of rewards or consequences for mission success or failure, whereas the term play tends to be more free form and represents a broader, less rule-bound activity. Gamified applications or curricula aim to encourage targeted behaviors and provide incentives for completion of tasks that might be undesirable or boring.

Attempting to define gamification, let alone apply it to academic healthcare, remains challenging. Many faculty and staff may initially resent the need to coax essential behaviors relevant to healthcare out of their learners. Clinicians routinely engage in boring, mundane, uncomfortable, and even undesirable tasks and behaviors. Some of these tasks and behaviors are essential to patient safety and best practices. Our students must learn these skills and behaviors in order to move from prenovice, to novice, to expert. By embracing gamification to engage challenging topics we may be able to emphasize important content that might otherwise be ignored. The key to engaging learners through gamified homework is to promote the *intrinsic* value of mastery, rather than the *extrinsic* nature of most course work. Learners are extrinsically motivated to complete assigned tasks found in the curriculum because they are receiving a grade. They are intrinsically motivated when successfully completing an assignment represents deeper meaning and validates and reinforces something that the student is already committed to.

For example, rewarding a nursing student who has quickly and efficiently mastered introductory clinical skills during early clinical experiences with more of the same by increasing their patient load is really just another take on the skill and drill, where the reward for finishing a math worksheet is to be assigned another similar math worksheet. The reward for mastery of introductory material should be to level up, to move forward to more challenging material and related tasks. In the case of our nursing students, it should be to assign them to more challenging patients, not simply more patients.

Virtual Environment versus Game-Based Environment

Of themselves, virtual environments or worlds do not have any inherent purpose other than to provide an environment in which to be. They are often very aesthetically pleasing and accurately represent existing spaces. However, without the inclusion or embedding of activities, games, or simulations to give virtual worlds purpose, learners are left needing a reason to be there (Ralston-Berg & Lara, 2012). In terms of instruction, games provide opportunity for learning to take place within a **virtual environment**.

Game-based environments must provide facets of game design, including narrative and a system of rewards for accomplishing specific tasks and objectives. Game-based learning uses virtual environments to stage the game just as a theater is used to stage a play (Bauman, 2010, p. 186). In other words, the created digital environment represents a virtual theatrical set where a game can take place. From a clinical perspective, the operating room, also known as an operating theater, only represents the place where the surgery takes place. While it provides support for the surgery in very precise ways, the operating room is not the surgery and cannot complete the surgery on its own.

Created Environment or Space

Created spaces are environments that have been engineered, built, or programmed to accurately replicate an actual real-world existing space, producing sufficient authenticity and fidelity to allow for the suspension of disbelief. This term is not unique to digital or game-based spaces. Mannequin-based simulation laboratories and standardized patient clinics are created spaces. These spaces are either fixed, in the case of mannequin-based simulation laboratories resembling elaborate theatrical sets, or exist only within a virtual reality or **game-based environment** as a **created environment or space** (Bauman, 2007, 2010, 2012; Bauman & Games, 2011; Games & Bauman, 2011).

Metagaming

Metagaming is the use of out-of-game resources and strategy to promote in-game success (Carter et al., 2012). In many traditional teaching and evaluation contexts, we might consider this cheating. In the context of game-based learning, metagaming is often rewarded. In the game world, players move through multiple levels of a game based on their game-play achievement. As players demonstrate competency by meeting benchmarks, they are allowed to advance through the game narrative. The game does not know or care how players meet in-game benchmarks. This is to say, the player must demonstrate achievement through competency, and how the player obtains the knowledge to do this is irrelevant. In-game success requires a combination of both acquired knowledge and the ability to deploy related skills in order to solve the challenges occurring in the game.

Clinical practice is distributive. We understand that healthcare has become very specialized. What we want and expect students to learn is how to make informed decisions that will drive desired outcomes. We do not want students or clinicians to guess what to do when they encounter new or unfamiliar clinical challenges. We want them to access information and resources to effectuate patient care in a safe and effective manner. In actual clinical practice, clinicians are in fact metagaming all of the time. Consults, labs, literature reviews, and diagnostics associated with actual care are consistent with the concept of metagaming and can be exploited and reinforced in game-based learning environments.

Minigames

Minigames are games within games. They exist within video games or virtual environments. Minigames can serve to inform players of important information, support in-game processes, or drive engagement with the game experience. In general, they provide players with just-in-time information, orient them to an environment, or teach players specific skills required to negotiate the environment. For example, in the game Grand Theft Auto, the early missions focus on teaching the player how to play the game. The first mission focuses on spatial in-world orientation and begins with walking to a location in the virtual world, while later missions may present players with a bicycle to ride, a car to drive, and even a plane to fly. These skills are needed in order to interact with the game environment and engage the player in more meaningful game play.

Imagine a game based on a hospital environment. Playing the game might initially involve transporting patients among departments throughout the hospital. This mission is not really about clinical education; rather it serves to orient the player to the virtual environment to support more meaningful future in-game encounters. Later, players might be asked to use various types of equipment found in the hospital. For example, a player might be asked to get the crash cart and use the defibrillator. This mission encourages the player to interact with the environment, to figure out how to use the defibrillator and to explore the contents of the crash cart. In this type of game, the real mission assignments map back to curriculum objectives and might ask the players to respond on different types of clinical emergencies with varying levels of complexity based on past successful game play. Without using the embedded minigames as tutorial and orientation tools, players will not be adequately prepared for more meaningful lessons.

Designed Experience

From an educational perspective, **designed experiences** encourage learners to learn through performance. Teachers and instructional designers create designed experiences with structured activities for targeted audiences that facilitate predictable interactions to promote anticipated actions and consequences. Activities included in designed experiences should support authentic narratives that represent the clinical professions, which learners hope to join. Theme parks like Disney are so successful because guests do not simply stand in line for rides; rather, guests have an embodied experience. You do not simply ride the Pirates of the Caribbean; you experience it as a pirate. At the Disney princess breakfast, children do not simply eat mouse-shaped pancakes with Disney characters; they embody the character and role of the princess through performance (Bauman, 2010, p. 185, 2012).

In actual clinical experiences, students are evaluated through their performance. However, students in actual clinical settings are not nurses or physicians; they are clearly identified as students. Thus, they never really get to perform as licensed clinicians during supervised clinical experiences. In game-based environments, students become the clinician. Not only do students play the role of their future profession, they can play the role of other disciplines. In this way, the nursing student can play the role of the medical resident, the medical resident can play the role of the charge nurse, and the paramedics can play the role of the triage nurse. Virtual and game-based environments allow learners to better understand their future role, as well as the roles of the many other types of professionals they will work with. Further, framing clinical learning activities through designed experiences supports interprofessional education. Providing future clinicians with the opportunity to learn together in authentic situated environments will promote valuable skills that will prepare nurses, physicians, and others with the needed experience to work together. Interprofessional educational opportunities are essential to redesigning flawed clinical processes that represent very real threats to patient safety and job satisfaction (Leape, 2009; Leape et al., 2012).

Ecology of Culturally Competent Design

Bauman and Games (2011) developed the **ecology of culturally competent design** with video games in mind. The ecology of culturally competent design provides a framework to design new video games and virtual environments for educational purposes and evaluate existing ones in the context of practice professions. Bauman and Games provide unique perspectives on multi- or interprofessional practice environments and their cultural contexts. They move beyond the traditional perspectives of cultural competence to acknowledge the importance of interprofessional education in accounting for not only the distinctive cultural contexts of these professions, but also the lived experiences of those who come to occupy these professions. The ecology of culturally competent design is comprised of four elements: **activities**, **context**, **narrative**, and **character**.

Activities

Activity is essential to learner engagement. Without anything to do in virtual environments, students find little utility associated with them. Virtual environments that lack activity may be aesthetically interesting, but have a limited ability to engage participants. Activities provide the game or engagement facet of digital environments. The most powerful and meaningful activities are situated to promote environmental and psychological fidelity. They account for and promote authentic social and behavioral facets of practice, culture, and diversity. Higher levels of authenticity are achieved when activities are derived from expert knowledge of the communities and individuals represented within game-based environments (Bauman, 2010; Bauman & Games, 2011; Games & Bauman, 2011).

Context

Context refers to the way learners are able to interact with digital environments. Well-designed experiences taking place in game-based environments provide context that is fluid and malleable. Context is defined and redefined by player interaction occurring among others coinhabiting the environment as well as the environment itself (Bauman, 2010; Bauman & Games, 2011; Games & Bauman, 2011). For example, if a student fails to attend to the "rights of medication administration," a situated consequence may occur later during game play. The consequence in this example might be a function of programming. However, another student coinhabiting the same environment might be in the position to prevent this practice error, thereby avoiding a potential sentinel event and consequence.

Narrative

Narratives should situate player or learner identity within the game environment. Narratives must be intentional and integrated so that they support lessons that map back to the curriculum objectives. Ultimately, the role of narratives in game-based environments is to engage learners so that experiences provided by a game provide important cues for pattern recognition that can be recalled during actual clinical performance. Narratives should be used to illustrate important patterns that can later be recognized and recalled to make sense of real-world experiences during future learning opportunities and actual clinical practice (Bauman, 2010; Bruner, 1991; Games & Bauman, 2011; Gee, 2003). The authors argue that narratives should be used in the same way during traditional mannequin-based simulation. In fact, it is possible for a narrative to begin in a virtual world and extend into a mannequin or standardized patient laboratory.

Character

Character is the role that a learner is playing during sophisticated levels of game play. It represents a unique in-game identity. Gee (2003) refers to this in-game identity as the projective identity. The projective identity is the negotiation of a player's in-game existence with the player's actual real-world identity. In created environments, designed to support professional or clinical education, character moves one step further. Learners must negotiate who they are as a person—perhaps a medical student or respiratory therapist—with the character they are playing in the game, which represents the affinity group they hope to join when they begin practicing professionally (Games & Bauman, 2011; Figures 3.7.1 and 3.7.2).

MOTIVATION FOR GAME-BASED LEARNING

Much of the discussion in the serious games or game-based learning movement focuses around learner engagement. In other words, can games be used to engage learners, and how well does a game engage learners? Deterding (2011) argues "playing games is the prototypical example for an autotelic, intrinsically motivating activity . . . ." By autotelic we mean that playing the game provides a purpose in and not apart from itself. While players may be learning a variety of content specific to a given curriculum during game play, mastering the game becomes synonymous with mastering the content.

Denis and Jouvelot (2005) argue that intrinsic motivation pushes participants or learners to "act freely" pursuing a given activity for the sake of the pursuit. Intrinsic motivation requires learners to be innately satisfied. Extrinsic motivation takes place because of outside factors like reward or consequence. Games that are engaging offer players something more than a badge. Educational content that is engaging offers the learner something more than a grade. Engaging content or experience is innately satisfying.

Intrinsic motivation provides learners with a sense of autonomy and includes facets of effective game design and best educational practices such as activity and creativity. Knowledge transfer becomes extrinsically motivating when it is done to meet benchmarks that lead to hierarchical task-based learning. In a curriculum that leverages extrinsic motivators, students complete one task not to master the said task, but to gain access to more of the curriculum. Access to more information and eventually access to the profession is based on compliance rather than deep meaning that demonstrates content and context mastery. Figure 3.7.3 juxtaposes the differences between intrinsic motivation and extrinsic motivations.

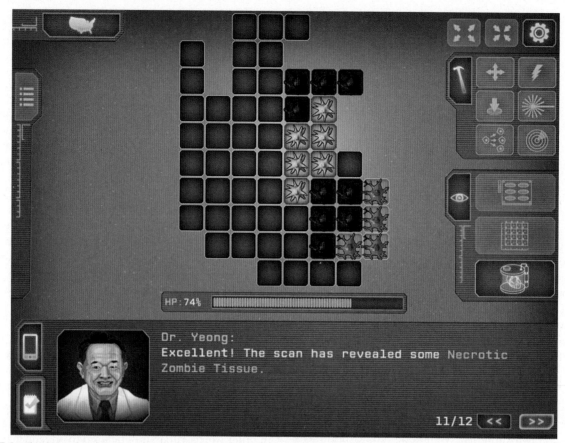

FIGURE 3.7.1 This screenshot from ProgenitorX, courtesy of the Wisconsin Institutes for Discovery, Learning Games Network, and Games+Learning+ Society, illustrates the four elements in the ecology of culturally competent design. The player's *character* is a scientist and member of The Progenitor X Defense Force working to save infected humans. Other scientists within the game, such as Dr. Yeong, provide the *narrative* and story elements. The game is played within the *context* of a world overrun with zombies where laboratory work is crucial to saving lives. The player completes *activities* within this environment to save the infected humans.

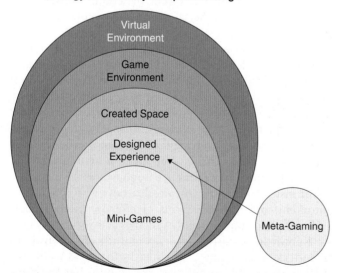

FIGURE 3.7.2 Illustrates how various definitions are related to one another in the context of the Ecology of Culturally Competent Design. (Modified from Bauman, E. B., & Games, I. A. [2011]. Contemporary theory for immersive worlds: Addressing engagement, culture, and diversity. In A. Cheney & R. Sanders (Eds.), *Teaching and learning in 3D immersive worlds: Pedagogical models and constructivist approaches.* Hershey, PA: IGI Global and Games, I., & Bauman, E. [2011]. Virtual worlds: An environment for cultural sensitivity education in the health sciences. *International Journal of Web Based Communities, 7*(2), 189–205. doi:10.1504/IJWBC.2011.039510.) Copyright Eric B. Bauman & Penny Ralsont-Berg All Rights Reserved.

In creating or integrating games and simulations into the curriculum, it is important to consider intrinsic motivation. Key questions include:

- Does the activity represent practices the learner currently uses or will use in the future?
- Does the activity include opportunities for the learner to make decisions based on relevant situations?
- Do those decisions have varied and appropriate consequences?
- Does the learner receive immediate feedback from the game or simulation?

By addressing these questions, learners will experience more intrinsic motivation in the game or simulation.

Selecting Games and Simulations for Curricular Fit

Curricular fit bridges motivation and objectives. By "fit" we mean the degree to which a game enhances or supports the course and curricular objectives. Instructional designers often refer to this as alignment. Games should not be incorporated solely to add perceived excitement or elements of fun. Games can be fun and engaging, but their first priority should be to provide an integrated,

Intrinsic	Extrinsic
Reward comes from mastery	Tangible reward
Goals are clear, meaningful and situated	Goals assigned
Progress is intuitive, apparent and immediate [real-time or just-in-time]	Progress is determined or assigned outside of the current activity
Endorses or reinforces behavior you are already committed to or hope to engage in the future – <u>Represents player agency</u>	If you complete this task you will be given access to another task – <u>Hierarchical direction</u>
Autonomous	**Directed**

Active learning	Creative		Shallow	Compliance
Deep meaning			Outcome driven	

FIGURE 3.7.3 Juxtaposes the differences between intrinsic motivation and extrinsic motivations. Copyright Eric B. Bauman All Rights Reserved.

meaningful, instructionally valuable activity that promotes intrinsic motivation in learners to meet learning objectives. Specific tasks or objectives within the game must fill gaps or challenges in the curriculum in order to motivate learners to participate. Without this bridge, learners may see the game as "busy work" or a distraction from the measured learning taking place in other parts of the course.

We previously discussed a mini-game in which players are asked to respond to different types of clinical emergencies. This type of game addresses the challenge of allowing learners to practice making decisions in a safe environment prior to actual clinical practice. In this case, the teacher would not select just any role-play or decision-making game, but rather one that directly relates to the intent and context of the lesson so that objectives, content, activities, and assessments within the lesson are aligned or have a good fit. The game that is relevant, contextual to the lesson, and perceived as valuable by the learner is engaging. Learners are actively thinking, deciding, and practicing behavior they will engage in the future, as opposed to simply playing and going through the steps to finish the activity. When a learning activity is relevant, contextual, and valuable, it exemplifies intrinsic motivation (Figures 3.7.4 and 3.7.5).

The company Johnson & Johnson produced and released the Happy Nurse game as part of their campaign for the Future of Nursing. Happy Nurse debuted around National Nurses Week and was billed as a stress relief tool for nurses. The game, originally Web-based, is now available as a mobile application. Happy Nurse is a traditional roller-style game. The player can customize their avatar and begin playing the game. The game is a race against the clock that has your avatar jumping over beds, hampers, crash carts, and IV poles. While Happy Nurse provides some level of entertainment and does have a facet of game play that supports good hand hygiene, it lacks a narrative and is not situated to best practices found in nursing. The game provides a distraction from practice but does not reinforce good practice. Completing level one simply gives you access to level two, but the game does not become more situated. For this reason, even though it supports one facet of nursing practice, hand hygiene, it is seen as a poor fit in meeting global objectives related to best practices of nursing. Assigning a game like this to students might be seen as an unsituated filler, and as an assigned task is only extrinsically motivating. Students would complete it because it is assigned, but it would not actively engage them in making decisions about nursing practice.

The first step to ensure good curricular fit is to define clear, meaningful goals and objectives. Then analyze existing materials, activities, and assessments for any gaps for challenges in the instruction. Is a defined objective not adequately addressed by existing curricula? Do parts of the curricula present challenges to learners? Do students have particular difficulty with certain parts of the curricula? These gaps and challenges are opportunities to supplement the existing curricula with game-based learning. Another aspect to consider is enhancing or adding more interest to existing materials. We previously mentioned gamification as an option for mundane, uncomfortable, or undesirable materials and tasks. Use of games in this situation can make such materials more engaging and in turn provide more motivation for students to learn.

Considerations of Fit:

- Clear meaningful goals and objectives
- Fill gaps in instruction
- Support challenging material
- Enhance or add interest to existing materials
- Raise engagement for less desirable materials or tasks

Fit: Integration with eLearning

When integrating game-based learning into curricula delivered via eLearning as opposed to face-to-face, the same considerations of fit and alignment with learning objectives still apply. The main difference is that in eLearning the teacher is not present to judge understanding or coach participation. To accommodate learners with varying time zones or availability, the game-based learning should be "standalone" with no need for supervision or synchronous participation with other players. The game should be integrated into the existing learning management system (LMS) as seamlessly as possible. In other words, if it

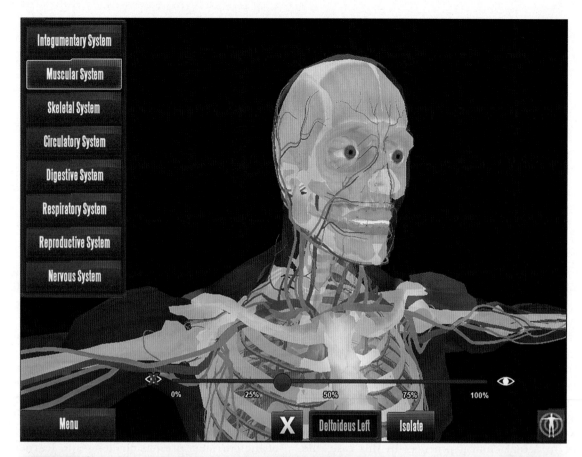

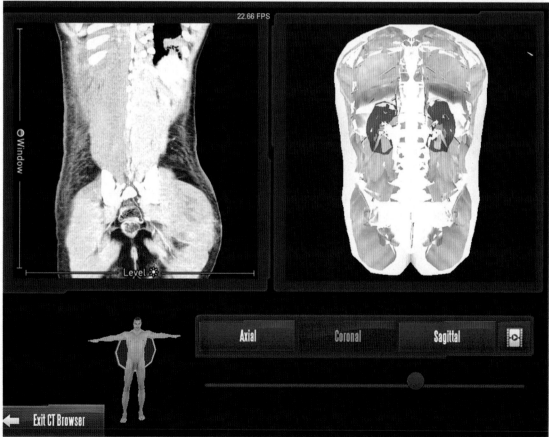

FIGURE 3.7.4 and 3.7.5   These screenshots from Anatomy Browser, courtesy of the Wisconsin Institutes for Discovery, Learning Games Network, and Games+Learning+Society, engage the learner in activities that support curriculum objectives specific to anatomy. These activities also connect the student via a learning activity that is relevant and contextual for clinical practice. In this way, the player might also see the activity as intrinsically motivating.

is possible to embed the game or link to the game from the existing LMS, students will have a smoother transition between the curricula to the game and back again. When using third party software or applications, this is not always possible, but should be investigated to ensure ease of navigation between systems. Any costs, extra time for installation, or other requirements of third party applications must also be provided to the learner in advance, preferably before the course starts. Appropriate instructions and orientation must be provided to acclimate learners to the system, as well as practice rounds that teach players how to play are especially important for distance students. Players should also be made aware of any help systems or staff available if they have difficulty during game play. Teachers may also consider a debrief discussion of some kind after game play. This is consistent with best practices in simulation-based education in which players reflect on what they learned from the game experience.

Fit: Game-Based Learning as Hybrid or Mixed Methods Learning

The same considerations for fit and eLearning also apply to hybrid or mixed methods learning. With hybrid delivery, teachers have more flexibility in the coordination of existing curricula, game play, and debrief sessions. For example, the teacher may choose to use face-to-face or synchronous meeting time for game play and then use some sort of asynchronous technology such as a discussion board or blog to allow learners to debrief and reflect on their experiences. The reverse is also possible. The educator may choose an asynchronous game experience in which students play at any time from any location. Then face-to-face or synchronous time could be used for a group reflection, debrief, and sharing of lessons learned.

In a hybrid learning scenario, students might begin a lesson in a game-based or virtual reality environment and transition to a live, in-person educational environment like a traditional fixed, bricks and mortar simulation laboratory. Students could begin triaging patients at the scene of a multicasualty emergency incident existing in a game-based environment and then begin accepting these same patients (now represented by mannequin or standardized patients) into the simulation laboratory. In this way, the lesson begins in a digital environment and transitions to a live face-to-face environment.

Resources and Fit

Another aspect of fit is the need for resources. The constraints of time, budget, available staff, and available technology can impact the games or simulations selected for integration. For example, using a face-to-face simulation requires mannequins, space, and technical staff. Creation of online games and simulations for eLearning requires a diverse team of experts, including instructional designers, game designers, graphic artists, media specialists, programmers, and content experts. Learning objectives are most important in determining curricular fit, but availability of resources must also be factored into the decision.

EVALUATION

Games integrated into curricula must map back to lesson objectives and meet students' learning needs. Evaluation provides the means to ensure objectives were met and learner needs were effectively addressed. Healthcare strives to follow best practices when providing patient care and should also strive to follow best educational practices. This means that a sound course of evaluation should be followed when it comes to curriculum changes, including the introduction of new technology like virtual simulation and game-based learning. Evaluation of technology supporting course objectives such as games and simulations can validate design decisions or provide feedback for revision of future iterations of course content and related technology.

Digital games and environments are very good at collecting data. Evaluation has always been a function of game play. The nature and design of digital games allows for sophisticated data collection based on learner performance. Game engines are data driven. Digital worlds exist as a consequence of computer code. Environmental change and how players interact with the environment occur on the basis of manipulation and processing of data. Variables like time-in-state and if/then commands supported by branching narratives drive player experience. By tracking this experience, evaluators can study decision-making points, learner experience path through variables, and in the case of repeated experience, changes in the number of steps or time to successful resolution of the presented problem.

Commercial video games provide an ongoing evaluation of player proficiency and mastery. This evaluation drives players experience and supports the game narrative. Players cannot advance through the game without mastering in-game skills that help them meet predetermined benchmarks. Even in Massively Multiplayer Online Games (MMOGs), where players enjoy a large degree of autonomy, the game-world rewards players for exploration and discovery and often provides some sort of consequence for inaction or unproductive in-world play. This process occurs as a function of continuous player evaluation (Gaydos & Bauman, 2012).

Learning necessarily takes place during play. Lessons might be anecdotal and informal, or they may be highly structured designed experiences taking place in sophisticated created spaces (Bauman, 2007). You cannot be a good hockey player without learning the rules and skills of the game. You can be a very strong weightlifter, but without understanding the rules of the contest, you cannot be a successful weightlifter. In any type of game or contest, players are evaluated on the basis of performance. Evaluation of performance is based on rules and expectations of mastery. This type of evaluation is consistent with clinical practice. Performance in clinical practice is based on expectations defined by communities of practice. Intuitions codify expectations into rules or standardized operating practices resulting from evidence-based practice.

Learner Success

Learner achievement is perhaps the hallmark of an academic success. Learner success in any given course or clinical environment represents only one variable in the complex matrix of learner achievement. Achievement can be measured in different contexts. Graduate education often focuses on professional advancement and the development of successful research programs. Undergraduate clinical education is fundamentally about preparing learners for clinical practice. Evaluation of learner success in the context of preparation for practice moves beyond grade point average (GPA) and class rank. Success is also measured by variables such as licensing, certification, residency, and job placement.

It is important to understand how variables of evaluation map back to curriculum. Learners who achieve high GPAs but struggle to pass licensing exams or secure appropriate career employment have not met the litmus test for success. To this end, games should not be introduced to learners as part of an educational social trend. Rather, they should be used to address curriculum gaps or challenges related to other variables that define achievement and learner success. For example, games being used as a mechanism for professional acculturation may prepare learners for the transition of learner to clinician and job placement. If a game can better prepare learners for licensure exams and increase first time pass rates by even a few percent, its utility would be considered significant. At the very least, games should provide measurable, situated supplemental opportunities that hold intrinsic value for learners.

Educator Performance

Games allow participants to cocreate knowledge by interacting with digital environments and other players coinhabiting the game or instructional space. In some cases, educators will take active player-character roles during academic game play. The educator should understand that learners will evaluate them on the basis of the game experience and the technology that supports the integration of games into their courses. Video games should not be integrated into curricula to replace teachers. Teachers are responsible for facilitating learning experiences in traditional learning spaces and in digital spaces. Teachers must understand the games and supportive technology that they choose for their courses to ensure that they are relevant, hold instructional value, and promote learning

objectives. Teachers must also be sure games are thoroughly tested for functionality and stability prior to implementation with learners; provide necessary instructions, orientation, and background information for learners' success; and make learners aware of any support or help available to players.

Courses and Curriculum Evaluation in the Context of Game-Based Learning

Educators who are comfortable using mannequin-based technology understand the importance of developing new simulation scenarios and that implementing existing scenarios is an iterative process requiring continuous refinement. This is also true when integrating virtual simulation and video games into curricula. Course and curriculum objectives should come first. Everything else, including how and where to integrate virtual simulation and video games, should follow. As discussed previously, the notion of "fit" is extremely important. We argue and believe that virtual simulation and game-based learning can be an effective part of clinical education, but should be subject to continuous evaluation to ensure that it provides a synergistic effect on course and curriculum objectives.

BEEN THERE, DONE THAT

When educators first begin to delve into games and simulations, they often do so with limited resources, budget, and time constraints. In such circumstances, efforts focus on design and implementation, while evaluation drops to a lower priority. Minimal evaluation often results in a more superficial, summative evaluation at the completion of a project. Those experienced with games and simulations in education see the value of formative evaluation throughout the design and development process as well as summative evaluation at the end of the learning experience. Planned formative evaluation throughout the process gathers valuable feedback and data, which shapes future iterations of the game or simulation. It is also important to evaluate all aspects of the game or simulation, including fit, alignment to objectives, and educator performance, and not limit evaluation only to learner performance. These are all parts of the formal evaluation plan.

SUMMARY

In conclusion, we support and advocate the integration of games and simulation into clinical and continuing education curricula throughout the health sciences. This chapter introduced and discussed a variety of terms and definitions that frame virtual and game-based learning in the context of clinical education. We discussed strategy for the integration of virtual and game-based learning by emphasizing the importance of "good fit." Further, we emphasized the need to evaluate all aspects of virtual simulation and game-based learning when it is integrated into clinical curricula from multiple perspectives.

It is our hope that this chapter contributes to existing education processes. Leveraging technology like mannequin-based simulation and game-based learning requires a mixed approach that uses game technology to address gaps and challenges in curriculum content and delivery. Successful integration of new technology requires organized forethought and team approach to promote successful learning experiences. At a minimum, collaboration with content experts, instructional designers, and the faculty responsible for teaching courses will help to ensure that the integration of games and simulations into the curriculum promotes learner success.

REFERENCES

Bauman, E. (2007). High fidelity simulation in healthcare (Doctoral dissertation). *University of Wisconsin–Madison. Retrieved from Dissertations & Theses @ CIC Institutions database.* (Publication No. AAT 3294196 ISBN: 9780549383109 ProQuest document ID: 1453230861.)

Bauman, E. (2010). Virtual reality and game-based clinical education. In K. B. Gaberson & M. H. Oermann (Eds.), *Clinical teaching strategies in nursing education (3rd ed.).* New York, NY: Springer.

Bauman, E. B. (2012). *Game-based teaching and simulation in nursing & healthcare.* New York, NY: Springer.

Bauman, E. B., & Games, I. A. (2011). Contemporary theory for immersive worlds: Addressing engagement, culture, and diversity. In A. Cheney & R. Sanders (Eds.), *Teaching and learning in 3D immersive worlds: Pedagogical models and constructivist approaches.* Hershey, PA: IGI Global.

Botturi, L., & Loh, C. S. (2008). Once upon a game: Rediscovering the roots of games in education. In C. T. Miller (Ed.), *Games: Purpose and Potential in Education* (pp. 1–22). New York, NY: Springer.

Broussard, J. E. (2011). *Playing class: A case study of ludic pedagogy (Doctoral dissertation).* Louisiana State University, Baton Rouge, LA.

Bruner, J. (1991, Autumn). The narrative construction of reality. *Critical Inquiry, 18,* 1–20.

Carter, M., Gibbs, M., & Harrop, M. (2012, May 29–June 1). Metagames, paragames and orthogames: A new vocabulary. *FDG'12,* Raleigh, NC.

Denis, G., & Jouvelot, P. (2005, June). Motivation-driven educational game design: Applying best practices to music education. In *Proceedings of the 2005 ACM SIGCHI international conference on advances in computer entertainment technology* (pp. 462-465). New York, NY: ACM.

Deterding, S. (2011, May). Situated motivational affordances of game elements: A conceptual model. In *Gamification: Using game design elements in non-game contexts.* CHI 2011 Workshop, Vancouver, BC.

Deterding, S., Dixon, D., Khalid, R., & Lennart, N. (2011, September 28–30). From game design elements to gamefulness: defining "gamification". In *Proceedings of the 15th International Academic MindTrek Conference: Envisioning Future Media Environments* (MindTrek '11) (pp. 9-15). New York, NY:ACM. DOI=10.1145/2181037.2181040 http://doi.acm.org/10.1145/2181037.2181040

Frasca, G. (2001). What is ludology? A provisory definition. Retrieved from http://www.ludology.org/2001/07/what-is-ludolog.html

Games, I., & Bauman, E. (2011). Virtual worlds: An environment for cultural sensitivity education in the health sciences. *International Journal of Web Based Communities, 7*(2), 189–205. doi:10.1504/IJWBC.2011.039510

Gaydos, M., & Bauman, E. B. (2012). Assessing and evaluating learning effectiveness: Games, sims and Starcraft 2. In E. Bauman (Ed.), *Games and simulation for nursing education.* New York, NY: Springer.

Gee, J. P. (2003). *What videogames have to teach us about learning and literacy.* New York, NY: Palgrave-McMillan.

Leape, L. L. (2009). Errors in medicine. *Clinica Chimica Acta, 404*(1), 2–5.

Leape, L. L., Shore, M. F., Deinstag, J. L., Mayer, R. J., Edgman-Levitan, S., Meyer, G. S., & Healy, G. B. (2012). Perspective: A culture of respect, Part 1: The nature and causes of disrespectful behavior by physicians. *Academic Medicine, 87,* 845–852.

Prensky, M. (2001). Digital natives, digital immigrants. *On the Horizon, 9*(5), 1–6.

Prensky, M. (2003). *Digital game based learning. Exploring the digital generation.* Washington, DC: Educational Technology, US Department of Education.

Ralston-Berg, P., & Lara, M. (2012). Fitting virtual reality and game-based learning into an existing curriculum. In E. Bauman (Ed.), *Games and simulation for nursing education.* New York, NY: Springer.

CHAPTER 3.8

Repurposing of Equipment

Shad Deering, MD, and Taylor Sawyer, DO, MEd

ABOUT THE AUTHORS

SHAD DEERING is a board-certified perinatologist who is currently stationed at the Uniformed Services University in Bethesda, MD. He is the Assistant Dean for Simulation Education and the Deputy Medical Director for the USU Simulation Center, and serves as the Chairman for the Army Central Simulation Committee, which is responsible for oversight of simulation for Graduate Medical Education in the Army and trains over 35,000 providers a year at their 10 training hospitals.

TAYLOR SAWYER is a board-certified neonatologist at the University of Washington/Seattle Children's Hospital. He received his Master's in Education from the University of Cincinnati, where his thesis research was on the use of video review during simulation debriefing. His research interests include defining optimal debriefing methodologies in medical simulation and the use of simulation for procedural and team training in neonatal resuscitation.

Acknowledgments: The views expressed here are those of the author(s) and do not reflect the official policy or position of the Department of the Army, Department of Defense, or the US Government. Dr. Deering created the Mobile Obstetric Emergencies Simulator, which the US Army has patented and licensed to Gaumard Scientific, FL.

ABSTRACT

Have you ever had trouble finding a commercially produced simulator or task trainer to meet your needs? Have you ever felt you could create a piece of simulation equipment yourself for a fraction of the cost that a manufacturer charges? Have you ever repurposed or modified a mannequin or task trainer? Many in the simulation community have answered "yes" to these questions.

Repurposing and modification of simulation equipment is a common practice within simulation programs worldwide. This can be done by modifying simulators to fit a new use, or by using the item as it is in a new way. In this chapter, practical tips and a "how to" on simulation equipment repurposing are provided. Examples of several published simulation equipment modification and repurposing are also provided, as well as things to consider before modifying the simulation equipment in your program. The chapter concludes with a discussion regarding the sharing of repurposing experiences with the simulation community and/or partnering with industry to make your repurposed equipment available to others. The following case example illustrates just one of the various ways in which healthcare educators and researchers have repurposed, or modified, simulation equipment to meet their needs.

CASE EXAMPLE

The NOELLE mannequin (Gaumard Scientific) is a birthing simulator that comes equipped with a birthing motor that automatically expels a simulated fetus to provide a lifelike delivery simulation. In 2006, obstetric educators at the Anderson Simulation Center at Madigan Army Medical Center, investigating the use of simulation to improve technical and teamwork skills, repurposed the NOELLE and used the simulator as part of an integrated mobile obstetric emergency simulator (MOES) system. The repurposing of the mannequin was conducted to provide an integrated obstetric simulation and debriefing package that could be distributed to all military medical programs with delivery service.

The team started by adding a video system to record simulation exercises and integrating an audience response system to allow for a standardized debriefing. Additionally, the NOELLE mannequin itself was modified by removing the original birthing motor and installing a reciprocating motor that allowed the mannequin to visibly shake to simulate an eclamptic seizure; a feature not included on any birthing mannequin on the market at the time. Development of the MOES system was funded through the military and external grants, and a total of 54 systems were built. The MOES device was widely distributed throughout the military for obstetrical team training and is currently in use at every hospital with a delivery service in the US Army, Navy, and Air Force (Deering et al., 2009). Based on the success of the system within the military, the MOES training system has recently been patented and licensed from the Army Medical Command by Gaumard Scientific and is now commercially available.

INTRODUCTION, BACKGROUND, AND SIGNIFICANCE

Throughout the long history of healthcare simulation, equipment has been hand produced on a small-scale basis by medical educators or artisans (Cooper & Taqueti, 2004; Owen, 2012). It is only in recent decades that medical educators have relied on industry to mass produce and supply medical simulation mannequins and task trainers. Prior to the commercialization of healthcare simulation, educators interested in conducting simulation training were required to independently develop and create the simulation equipment they needed. This was often accomplished by developing task trainers from scratch, or repurposing existing medical equipment or devices in a new way. The inventor spirit and the "mad scientist" tinkerer present in these early healthcare simulation users remain ingrained in simulation educators today.

In the modern era, the reasons for repurposing simulation equipment are many, but commonly include the need for a simulator that is not otherwise available, a perceived lack of fidelity or efficacy in what exists on the market, or a desire to develop an equivalent simulator for less cost than purchasing the device from industry. For these reasons, and many more, people involved in healthcare simulation continually seek to **repurpose** and/or **modify** equipment to meet their specific needs.

Within the Technical Reports section of the journal *Simulation in Healthcare*, one can find numerous reports of innovative and imaginative examples of repurposing and modification of simulation equipment. Some of these include: (1) the report by Hellaby (2011) on the modification of the Laerdal SimMan, which allowed the mannequin to demonstrate hives as part of an anaphylaxis simulation, (2) a report by Heiner (2010) who described a model for skin abscess identification and management wherein a simulated abscess was filled with simulated pus allowing the user to incise, drain, and pack the wound, (3) the report by Perosky et al. (2011), who described their efforts to create a low-cost simulator for learning to manage postpartum hemorrhage in rural Africa, (4) several reports from the Evanston Northwestern Healthcare, Center for Simulation Technology and Academic Research (CSTAR) in Evanston, Illinois, including an innovative design for an epistaxis simulator, a low-cost cricothyrotomy simulator using a sheep trachea, and an inconspicuous portable audio/visual recording system attached to an IV pole (Pettineo, Vozenilek, Kharasch, Morris, et al., 2008; Pettineo, Vozenilek, Kharasch, Wang, 2008; Pettineo et al., 2009). These are just a few examples of the numerous published reports of simulation equipment repurposing. Certainly, countless numbers of unpublished modifications and/or repurposing have been conducted over the past decades.

Despite the growing number of available mannequins and task trainers on the market, there will always be gaps between what is commercially available and what educators need to create realistic and effective training. Additionally, there will always be a lag in time between the development of a new medical procedure, device, or technology and the commercial production of simulation equipment to augment training. Thus, there will always be a need for the modification or repurposing of simulation equipment. All too often, healthcare simulation educators depend upon commercial vendors to produce the simulators and task trainers they need to provide realistic training, while sometimes forgetting that the simulators they desire could be created independently at much less cost and perhaps with more fidelity.

THE "HOW TO . . ."

Repurposing simulation equipment most commonly involves modifying it in some way to fit a new use, or by using the item as it is in a new or innovative way. The variety of ways to repurpose and/or modify simulation equipment is limited only by one's imagination. In general terms, there are four basic ways in which to repurpose simulation equipment. These include the creation of a simulator or task trainer de novo (*creation*), addition of new pieces or functionality to existing equipment (*addition*), the removal of parts or functions from a simulator (*subtraction*), or the combining of two or more simulators together to improve functionality (*integration*). In this section, we examine each of these methods, and explore examples of what other investigators have done with regard to each of these types of repurposing.

Creation

Creation is the most novel method of repurposing equipment and involves the development of a new and unique piece of simulation equipment from the ground up. The components used to create the new simulator can be pieced together from existing simulation equipment, or, if needed, taken from common medical, hardware, or household items. If novel and useful enough, these new simulation devices can be patented and marketed to the simulation community. More information on partnering with industry is included in the next section of this chapter.

An excellent example of creation is the independent development of the Ventriloscope by Dr. Paul Lecat. In 2008, after realizing the limited amount of physical findings available to learners during a standardized patient exam, Dr. Lecat developed a simulator, the Ventriloscope, to simulate cardiac murmurs on live patients. To do this, he used a stethoscope and equipped it with a digital receiver and transmitter. Using the device on a live patient, the Ventriloscope transmitter can send a sound file wirelessly to the receiver in the stethoscope and provide a realistic murmur while the learner auscultates a live patient or mannequin. Based on successful use in both standardized patients and on simulators, the Ventriloscope is now marketed commercially (Lecat's SimplySim, n.d.).

Addition

Addition is the most common method of repurposing equipment. It is typically done in an attempt to add increased functionality or fidelity to an existing simulator or task trainer. The addition can be made with parts or pieces from another simulator, pieces of repurposed medical equipment, or off-the-shelf materials from a hardware or craft store, depending on the needs and budget of the developer. Addition, like other types of modification, often requires developers to partially or fully dismantle their simulation equipment in order to expose the inner workings and provide an area for the upgrade. In some cases, one must remove some of the existing equipment to make room within the simulator for the additional functionality.

Multiple examples of simulation repurposing by addition can be found in the literature. One example is the work by Sawyer et al. (2009) involving the addition of an umbilical catheter task trainer to the standard Laerdal SimBaby. This modification was done to repurpose the infant simulator for use as a newborn simulator, which would allow the placement of an emergency umbilical catheter during neonatal resuscitation training. To accomplish this, an umbilical catheter task trainer was scavenged from a low-technology mannequin, equipped with a drainage port, and integrated into the abdomen of the SimBaby (see Figure 3.8.1A, B). This modification was felt to

provide a realistic umbilical catheter task trainer, as judged by a panel of neonatologists. Another example of repurposing by addition is the work of Pettineo et al. in creating an epistaxis simulator (Pettineo, Vozenilek, Kharasch, Morris, et al., 2008). To create the model, the Center for Simulation Technology and Academic Research (CSTAR) team repurposed an older CPR Trainer by adding IV tubing, and a bag of normal saline with simulated blood. The model provided realistic epistaxis simulation that was able to simulate hemostasis in response to proper positioning of nasal packing.

Subtraction

Subtraction is another common type of simulation equipment repurposing. It is simply the removal of some parts or pieces from a simulator. Subtraction is typically completed in order to simplify an existing simulator by removing functionality that is deemed either poorly functional or nonessential by simulation users. Subtraction sometimes precedes addition. In these cases, the removal of existing equipment is completed to make room for the addition of another piece of equipment. An example of subtraction is the work by Deering et al. (2009) described in the case example at the beginning of this chapter. In this case, the developers removed the existing birthing simulator motor from an early model Gaumard NOELLE simulator because they perceived that the mechanism took too long to deliver the infant simulator and the ability of the simulator to have an eclamptic seizure mechanism was felt to be more important for training. In place of the motorized birthing simulator, the investigators simply used a manual method of holding the infant simulator within the mannequin by hand, or using a nylon strap wrapped around the infant's body. This was felt to provide an important improvement in the birth experience fidelity for trainees, in terms of realistic resistance felt during the baby's delivery and the increased control that the staff had in timing the delivery during the simulation.

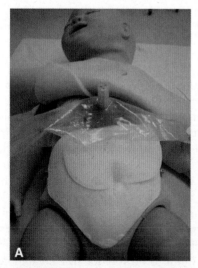 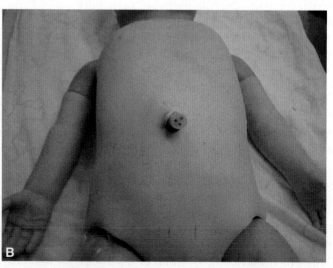

FIGURE 3.8.1   A. Internal view of modified SimBaby (Laerdal Medical) with umbilical cannulation task trainer in position. **B.** Mannequin with skin replaced and umbilicus exposed.

Integration

Combining the components and/or functions of two or more simulators together is a method used by simulation innovators that we term *integration* and often referred to as "hybrid simulations" (see Terms of Reference). Integration is used at times when two different simulators are available that can each do a key task but an educator desires one complete simulator that integrates both, or when specific parts of two simulators perform well and an educator combines the best of both simulators into one. By combining the best functionality of different simulators, educators can often overcome perceived difficulties with functionality and fidelity. An example of integration completed by one of the authors (S. Deering, unpublished work, 2012) involved the combination of a laparoscopic body form together with simulated pelvic organs in order to create a hybrid laparoscopic hysterectomy simulator.

For laparoscopic simulation, there are several available basic task training boxes for the Fundamentals of Laparoscopic Surgery (FLS) tasks. There are also virtual reality simulators that simulate certain procedures, mostly specific to general surgery, with cholecystectomy being the most common. For gynecology, and other specialties, there are many relatively common surgical techniques for which basic or virtual reality simulators either do not exist or do not have the necessary degree of fidelity and haptics. Additionally, most virtual reality simulators do not include tasks that are done outside of the abdomen, such as the cervical cuff being closed from below through the vagina as is sometimes done with laparoscopic hysterectomy. Because of the lack of commercially available devices, some simulation innovators have started to work on hybrid models combining physical task trainers with basic box trainers. These have the advantage of providing real-life haptics, providing surgeons with the opportunity to use their actual instruments (though most of the internal organ models currently available do not allow for the use of all energy sources), and are limited only by the cost of the consumables and the availability of the physical models. At our institution, we have initiated a project to combine a laparoscopic abdomen

---

EXPERT CORNER

SIMULATION IN UNDERRESOURCED COUNTRIES
Mary D. Patterson, MD, MEd
President, Society for Simulation in Healthcare (2010)

The Helping Babies Breathe project, focusing on resuscitation of depressed newborns, has demonstrated that simulation in low-resource settings can be effective in improving mortality of infants in the perinatal period (Goudar et al., 2013; Msemo et al., 2013). Focusing on training traditional birth attendants in the recognition and treatment of the depressed infant, the Helping Babies Breathe project develops expertise in the people most likely to be able to intervene when an infant is born: the traditional birth attendant.

There are many horrific candidate conditions to consider for the next big push for simulation in low-resource settings. Let me suggest that we think about traumatic injuries. Trauma is the leading cause of death for young people worldwide, accounting for 5.8 million deaths annually (more than from malaria, tuberculosis, or HIV/AIDS combined). Like neonatal asphyxia and postpartum hemorrhage, it disproportionately affects those in low- and middle-income countries, with 90% of the deaths occurring in low- and middle-income countries (de Ramirez et al., 2012). As devastating as the mortality is, the morbidity that results from trauma: 63 million Disability Adjusted Life Years (DALYs) annually (Sakran et al., 2012).

The absence of infrastructure in low-resource settings requires that we develop creative alternatives to existing models for trauma care in high-income countries. For example, in Madagascar, taxi drivers have been successfully trained as first responders in the absence of a prehospital emergency medical services system (Geduld & Wallis, 2011).

Similar to the Helping Babies Breathe Project, it is likely that nonhealthcare responders will offer the best chance of success in much of the world (Sakran et al., 2012). Given the shortage of trained paramedics, physicians, and nurses in low-resource settings, simulation training needs to focus on those who are in close proximity when injuries occur.

Employing simulation to improve the care of trauma patients in low-resource settings is likely to be a more difficult challenge than that of resuscitating the depressed infant. Trauma may be blunt or penetrating, involve burns, shrapnel and blast injuries. It often occurs in settings of natural and civil chaos. Nonetheless, implementation of the Advanced Trauma Life Support (ATLS) course in Trinidad resulted in the mortality for severely injured patients decreasing from 67% to 34% (Ali et al., 1993, 1994).

The management of trauma in low-resource settings is a "wicked" problem; there is not likely to be a single solution. Improvement in trauma outcomes is likely to result from the aggregation of marginal gains and local solutions. The simulation community has the ability to develop the multiple ingenious solutions that will be required to address this devastating epidemic.

REFERENCES

Ali, J., Adam, R., Butler, A. K., Chanq, H., Howard, M., Gonsalves, D., . . . Williams, J. I. (1993). Trauma outcome improves following the advanced trauma life support program in a developing country. *Journal of Trauma, Injury, Infection, and Critical Care, 34*, 890–898.

Ali, J., Adam, R., Stedman, M., Howard, M., & Williams, J. I. (1994). Advanced trauma life support program increases emergency room application of trauma resuscitative procedures. *Journal of Trauma, Injury, Infection, and Critical Care, 36*, 391–394.

Geduld, H., & Wallis, L. (2011). Taxi driver training in Madagascar: The first step in developing a functioning prehospital emergency care system. *Emergency Medicine Journal, 28*(9), 794–796.

Goudar, S. S., Somannavar, M. S., Clark, R., Lockyer, J. M., Revankar, A. P., Fidler, H. M., . . . Singhal, N. (2013). Stillbirth and newborn mortality in India after helping babies breathe training. *Pediatrics, 131*(2), e344–e352.

Msemo, G., Massawe, A., Mmbando, D., Rusibamayila, N., Manji, K., Kidanto, H. L., . . . Perlman, J. (2013). Newborn mortality and fresh stillbirth rates in Tanzania after helping babies breathe training. *Pediatrics, 131*(2), e353–e360.

de Ramirez, S. S., Hyder, A. A., Herbert, H. K., & Stevens, K. (2012). Unintentional injuries: magnitude, prevention, and control. *Annual Review of Public Health, 33*, 175–191.

Sakran, J. V., Greer, S. E., Werlin, E., & McCunn, M. (2012). Care of the injured worldwide: trauma still the neglected disease of modern society. *Scandinavian Journal of Trauma, Resuscitation and Emergency Medicine, 20*, 64.

SECTION 3 • Simulators

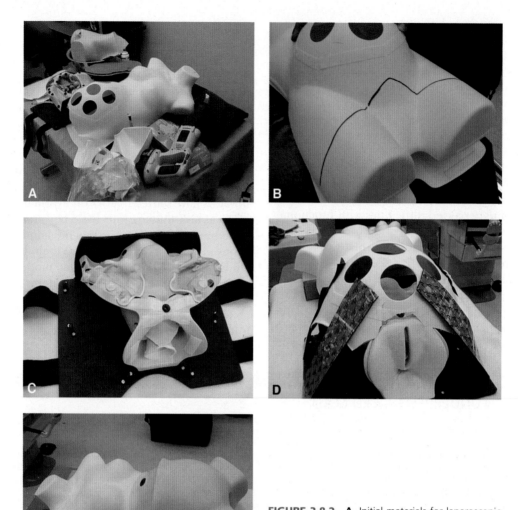

FIGURE 3.8.2 **A.** Initial materials for laparoscopic hysterectomy simulator. **B.** Laparoscopic shell modification (Delletech.com). **C.** Internal anatomy—limbs and things advanced surgical uterus. **D.** Laparoscopic simulator model for laparoscopic hysterectomy, assembled. **E.** Final prototype laparoscopic hysterectomy simulator.

"shell" with realistic internal organs to train residents in the performance of a laparoscopic hysterectomy. Photos of the design and build sequence can be seen in the images below (Figure 3.8.2A–E). The final prototype was used in training and allows the learner to use actual instruments and perform a wide range of gynecologic laparoscopic procedures.

BEEN THERE DONE THAT: HOW CAN I CONTINUE TO IMPROVE OR SUSTAIN WHAT I HAVE ACHIEVED?

Those who have repurposed or modified a piece of simulation equipment and have found that it met their educational need, or functioned as well as (or better than) a commercially available item, should consider sharing their experience with others in the simulation community. There are multiple venues in which this can be done, and the options to share are expanding all the time. Some options include posting a description of your modification online (see list of websites at the end of this chapter), presenting your work as an abstract at a national or international simulation meeting, conducting a workshop using your simulator at a medical meeting, and/or publishing a description of the materials and methods.

Given the significant growth and interest in medical simulation, and the recognition that innovation by subject matter experts that are actual end users may create the next best simulator, there are now many national meetings at which simulation technology abstracts are being presented. The annual International Meeting on Simulation in Healthcare (IMSH) is the largest and most well known of these, and has a specific track for technology innovation abstracts. However, because simulator modifications may have narrow applicability within a single medical specialty, when considering places to present your modifications as an abstract, it is also advisable to look within your specialty meetings, both on a local and on a national level. This is especially relevant when the modification relates to residency training and/or assessment as this is a key area of focus at this time. Novel, inexpensive, modifications to simulators are very valuable to program directors trying to meet Accreditation Council for Graduate Medical Education (ACGME) requirements regarding assessment and competency evaluations, especially in light of the new milestones requirements.

Many specialties are now also integrating simulation training demonstrations and courses into their local and national meetings. If you have a simulator modification that addresses a specialty-specific need, these meetings may be a good opportunity to both use the simulator and also get feedback from peers that can help make it even better. There are also simulation committees for many specialties, and working with your specialty's national organization is another way to bring helpful modifications to other's attention.

Publication is perhaps the most effective way to share your experiences and success with a repurposing or modification. The Technical Reports section of the Journal *Simulation in Healthcare* is a prime venue for such reports. Additionally, individual specialty journals are now beginning to publish reports on the development of novel simulators, especially if they relate to residency education and/or patient safety initiatives. Publishing in a journal related to your specialty will likely get the information out to more providers that can and will actually benefit from the work. To strengthen reports of simulator modifications, it is advisable to include not only a description of the modification, but also a report on your experience in using it, feedback from its use, and the evaluation forms you used. This will make it much easier for others to utilize your work rather than having to re-create evaluation forms on their own, and increase the likelihood of the work being published.

Collaborating with industry is a powerful way to make your simulation repurposing/modifications available on a wider scale. However, several things should be considered when collaborating with industry regarding a simulator repurpose/modification. First, it is important to check with your institution on their rules and regulations regarding intellectual property. If you are developing a new technology with your hospital or simulation program during normal "duty" hours, this may apply to you. While the rules regarding inventions may seem restrictive at first, there can be advantages as many institutions, especially academic centers, may be willing to lend support to the project. This support may range from purchasing more equipment to improve your initial design, grant support for validation and implementation, to assistance with patent applications and/or licensing agreements. Knowing the rules from the beginning is the key to making the process go smoothly.

While medical simulation has many examples of repurposed simulators, most of these are not adopted and produced by companies and distributed. This may be a result of many factors. First, if the simulator addresses a very specific need and the potential market for resale is small, then companies may not be interested in or able to invest a significant amount to develop and market it. Second, if the simulator you have created is inexpensive and easy to create, industry may not be able to make it better without it costing significantly more, and it would therefore not be profitable for the manufacturer.

Despite these barriers, there is significant potential for new simulators or modifications to be picked up and produced by industry. Remember that medical simulation companies are continually reaching out to providers to try to determine what is really needed in the marketplace, and innovative solutions like the modifications discussed in this chapter may be things that industry is interested in pursuing. Your input and clinical knowledge is worth a lot, especially in lending credibility to the simulator's use and fidelity.

Considerations

Several things must be considered prior to repurposing simulation equipment. Of primary consideration is the technical skill of the individual performing the repurposing. As already discussed, modification and repurposing may require a great deal of disassembly, modification, and reassembly of simulation equipment in some circumstances. Without a certain amount of baseline technical and mechanical skill, a well-intentioned repurposing can easily result in a broken and nonfunctional simulator. Unfortunately, no user manual exists on how to perform specific modifications and/or repurposing. However, most reports published in the Technical Reports section of the journal *Simulation in Healthcare* provide detailed descriptions of the authors' work that are intended to provide a user's guide to conducting the repurposing. Additionally, several online resources and blogs have arisen over the past decade devoted to assisting simulation educators, technicians, and administrators. Many of these contain useful information on simulation equipment repurposing. A list of online equipment repurposing resources is provided at the end of this chapter. Other considerations when repurposing equipment include the cost of the repurposing, the time commitment to perform the repurposing, and warranty issues.

The cost of modifying or repurposing a simulator depends on several factors. These include the cost of the simulator itself, the cost of any additional materials, and the upkeep and maintenance costs associated with the modification. Prior to repurposing or modifying a piece of simulation equipment, each of these should be considered.

Time is a precious resource within a simulation program. A considerable amount of time can be spent repurposing or modifying a simulator to meet a specific educational goal. When devoting a simulation program's personnel time to a simulator modification, the payback for that time must be considered. An important consideration in this calculation is, how much use will the repurposed piece of equipment get? If the answer is more time than it takes to perform the repurposing, then there may be an advantage to the repurposing. However, if there will need to be several hours devoted to performing a modification to a simulator that will be useful only to a select group of learners a few times a year, then one must consider the return on investment in performing the repurposing.

Simulation equipment warranties must also be considered prior to performing a repurposing or modification as this voids service warranty contracts. Since some simulation equipment is expensive and costly to repair, service warranty contracts are often provided with equipment purchases. A common statement included within a simulator's user manual is something like: "Caution: Changes or modifications not expressly approved by the manufacturer could void the user's warranty." Prior to repurposing or modifying an item with an existing service contract, one should considering reviewing the service contract or contacting the manufacturer to determine whether the planned modification will affect the warranty. This is an especially important consideration for full-body high-technology simulators that may cost several thousand dollars. As a place to begin, consider working on older simulators that are out of warranty, have been damaged, or are getting ready to be replaced.

SUMMARY

In this chapter, we have reviewed the repurposing of simulation equipment and attempted to provide concrete examples and a relatively simple "how to" guide for anyone interested in pursuing this. With the continued rapid changes in medical simulation training needs and technology, we are confident that the types of innovation discussed in this chapter will continue to improve training and drive the specialty forward.

REFERENCES

Cooper, J., & Taqueti, V. (2004). A brief history of the development of mannequin simulators for clinical education and training. *Quality & Safety in Health Care, 13*(Suppl. 1), i11–i18.

Deering, S., Rosen, M., Salas, E., & King, H. (2009). Building team and technical competency for obstetric emergencies: The mobile obstetric emergency simulator (MOES) system. *Simulation in Healthcare, 4,* 166–173.

Heiner, J. (2010). A new simulation model for skin abscess identification and management. *Simulation in Healthcare, 5*(4), 238–241.

Hellaby, M. (2011). Anaphylaxis simulation session: Seeing is believing. *Simulation in Healthcare, 6*(3), 180–183.

Lecat's SimplySim. (n.d.). Retrieved from http://www.simply-sim.com/faqs.php

Owen, H. (2012). Early use of simulation in medical education. *Simulation in Healthcare, 7,* 102–116.

Perosky, J., Richter, R., Rybak, O., Gans-Larty, F., Mensah, M., Danquah, A., . . . Andreatta, P. (2011). A low-cost simulator for learning to manage postpartum hemorrhage in rural Africa. *Simulation in Healthcare, 6*(1), 42–47.

Pettineo, C., Vozenilek, J., Kharasch, M., Morris, W., & Aitchison, P. (2008). Epistaxis simulator: An innovative design. *Simulation in Healthcare, 3*(4), 239–241.

Pettineo, C., Vozenilek, J., Kharasch, M., Wang, E., Aitchison, P., & Arreguin, A. (2008) Inconspicuous portable audio/visual recording: Transforming an IV pole into a mobile video capture stand. *Simulation in Healthcare, 3*(3), 180–182.

Pettineo, C., Vozenilek, J., Wang, E., Flaherty, J., Kharasch, M., & Aitchison, P. (2009). Simulated emergency department procedures with minimal monetary investment: Cricothyrotomy simulator. *Simulation in Healthcare, 4*(1), 60–64.

Sawyer, T., Hara, K., Thompson, M., Chan, D., & Berg, B. (2009). Modification of the Laerdal SimBaby to include an integrated umbilical cannulation task trainer. *Simulation in Healthcare, 4,* 174–178.

ONLINE RESOURCES FOR SIMULATION EQUIPMENT REPURPOSING

SSH: http://ssih.org
Behind the Sim Curtain: http://www.behindthesimcurtain.com
Healthy Simulation: http://www.healthysimulation.com
SimGHOSTS: http://www.simghosts.org
HealthySimAdmin: http://www.healthysimadmin.com
Simulation Innovation Resource Center: http://sirc.nln.org
California Simulation Alliance: https://californiasimulationalliance.org
Games & Simulation for Healthcare: http://healthcaregames.wisc.edu
Clinical Playground Blog: http://clinicalplayground.com
UNE Sim Log: http://blog.une.edu/simlab
One Stop Simulation: http://www.onestopsimulation.com

CHAPTER 3.9

Warranties or Fix-It-Yourself?

Marcus Watson, BSc (Hon), Grad Dip CS, MS, PhD, and Dylan Campher, Cert AT, Adv Dip Perf., Dip PM, Dip Buss. Management, Grad. Cert. Healthcare Simulation

ABOUT THE AUTHORS

MARCUS WATSON leads the Queensland Health Clinical Skills Development Service, Australia's largest healthcare educational and research simulation program. His 20 years' experience include: working with computer-based simulation, high-end immersive simulation, serious games, and distributed learning; leading research on applying Human Factors; consulting on the development of simulation programs internationally. Additional titles include: founding member and past Chair of the Australian Society for Simulations in Healthcare; contributor to the HWA NHET-Sim program; Director on the Board of Simulation Australia.

DYLAN CAMPHER graduated as an Anesthetic Technician and Auto-Transfusionist. He has experience in program management, program design, instructing, and simulator development and has developed and implemented 40 new simulation facilities, including the Graduate Certificate in Healthcare Simulation, and contributed to the HWA NHET-Sim. Coauthor of the book *Medical Crisis Management: Improving Performance Under Pressure*, he is an Executive Member of the Australian Society for Simulation in Healthcare (ASSH) and Simulation Australia Professional Development Committee member.

ABSTRACT

The technical skills required to service and operate education technologies, including simulators and audiovisual, have the potential to enhance the educational outcomes and influence the cost of simulation programs dramatically. This chapter focuses on the technical considerations for the delivery of simulation-based programs by examining different models of supporting the technical requirements. The work examines industry warranties, outsourcing technical support and in-house technical programs as delivered by simulation services. Examples of in situ simulation, simulation programs, and skills development services are used to illustrate the skills, technologies, and contractual and logistical considerations required to deliver simulation in healthcare. The potential savings through in-house maintenance and repairs can be significant; however, understanding the skills, scale, and redundancy requirement is crucial to sustaining simulation capabilities.

CASE EXAMPLE

It is 9 minutes into the first scenario of the program, and you can cut the tension in the air with a scalpel. The pitch of the pulse oximeter drops against the background din of anesthetic alarms; then suddenly the patient's chest fails to rise.
The chief educator looks at the mannequin operator and asks:
"Dan what happened?"
Dan replies:
"I am not sure; potentially, one of the pneumatic valve blocks has failed."

In the room the anesthesiologist gives a confused glance to the surgeon as the monitor continues to indicate respiration and expired CO_2 but the chest lies dormant.
The chief educator states:
"Dan, I'll get them into the debrief room, you've got 20 minutes to fix it."

Minutes later, Dan has the mannequin's skin off, and inside it doesn't look good.

- Could this happen in your program?
- If this happens in your program what are your options?
- Can your team fix anything that goes wrong?
- Do you have a backup or redundancy mannequin?
- Do your warranties ensure external support that can step in at short notice?
- Have you planned your program to be resilient to technology failure?
- Do you have a spare valve block or repair part in stock readily available?

INTRODUCTION

As simulation programs increase in complexity, greater attention must be paid to the support process required to ensure sustained high quality outcomes. To guarantee the right outcomes, a simulation **program** should manage preventive maintenance and the repair of the technologies through internal and external providers. Simulation programs should expect technology to fail, with planned redundancies in the facilities equipment or alternative solutions to ensure sustainability of the program. In addition, knowing the strengths and weaknesses of the technologies will ensure simulation procurement meets the programs' training requirements. Such analysis should extend to understanding the usage and technical training required to operate and maintain the programs' equipment efficiently.

WARRANTIES AND SERVICE LEVEL AGREEMENTS

Before buying any product it is important to understand how to maintain and repair the equipment across its life cycle. Many simulation programs start by buying their simulation equipment with warranties and service support. Few simulation programs fully analyze the impacts of these agreements on their delivery capacity prior to their first call for assistance to the manufacturer or service provider. It is at this point that they get the first hint of the return on investment in the warranties and service support. If the educators and **program directors** do not understand the impact of maintenance and repairs, leaving warranties and service level agreement management to your legal service puts simulation delivery at risk.

Manufacturers of simulation equipment provide warranties and encourage service agreements because they have a vested interest in their products being useful (Hogreve & Gremler, 2009); however, they must still maintain a profitable business. Many manufacturers do not have effective models of equipment failure rates and expected maintenance costs over the life cycle of their products. This is not surprising in a new, rapidly growing industry where the technical skills of the end user impact on product sustainability. Warranties and service level agreements may not cover all replacement parts, may not guarantee the time to repair and return the simulator. Taking the time to model the cost of maintaining your equipment and identifying how warranties and service level agreements will impact delivery is crucial to effective simulation programs. Also, for many simulation products any modification of equipment voids the warranty, which limits the ability to tailor devices for training needs.

SERVICES, CENTERS, AND IN SITU SIMULATION PROGRAMS

The strategies used to manage educational technologies will vary depending upon the size of the program and the opportunities for collaboration. Many simulation programs are a small-scale operation with a limited number of staff. In situ programs are often based around a single simulator, while many simulation centers have only a few items of simulation equipment. With the right person it is possible to acquire the technical skills to do most, if not all, of the maintenance and repairs of the simulators. There are still many risks involved with this approach as the right person may be hard to find and hire or replace if they leave. The lack of equipment redundancy can also impact a program's processes and training as not every problem can be fixed immediately.

Finding the balance between external and internal maintenance and repair is difficult and likely to change as simulation programs evolve. The Queensland Health Clinical Skills Development Service (CSDS) model is presented in this chapter as an example of a programmatic approach to support the educational and technical aspects of simulation (http://www.sdc.qld.edu.au/). This chapter focuses on the technological aspects; however, in actuality, the educational and technical elements are codependent in the CSDS model.

CSDS started its life in 2004 as the Queensland Health Skills Development Centre, a large, well-equipped facility that in 2007 was still struggling to deliver the volume of training expected. Among the issues, the center suffered from a burden of warranties that covered the many items of equipment procured since the center was built. In some cases, expensive warranties covered equipment that had never been used for training over the first 3 years of the service. Further, simulators were distributed at affiliated sites with varied levels of use and with only limited technical support. Even with the highest level of warranties, equipment failures continued to impact on training as contract providers would require some notice to do site visits or to take the equipment away for up to 4 weeks for repair.

There were many contributing factors, including: capital funding models that drove procurement on an opportunistic rather than programmatic approach, there was no modeling of simulation technologies against training requirements, and a lack of information on equipment failure rates and maintenance requirements. As with many simulation centers of the time, the approach had been: buy the simulators and try and find a use for them. However, the sheer scale meant that the cost of the warranties and repairs to support the equipment grew significantly. To support the diversity of training required of CSDS and to increase access to simulation, the service needed to move away from external support of its simulation equipment and invest in a more robust and flexible operational model.

CSDS conducts hundreds of programs annually at the Skills Development Centre in Brisbane, supports a growing number of **Skills Centers** and **Pocket Simulations Centers** (in situ and hospital-based programs) across the state (41 in June 2013), and provides an equipment loan library of simulators. The experience at the CSDS in developing many centers and in situ programs combined with the management of fleets of simulators has allowed CSDS to develop a service model to increase access to simulation while reducing the cost per use. The technical component of the service model is based on four key themes.

1. Maintenance and repair
2. Redundancy and distribution
3. Usage and training
4. Procurement and evaluation of products

Maintenance and Repair

Many types of technology add to the ability to create great simulation programs, but they also add potential risks to the effective delivery of a program. CSDS manages more than 1,800 items of simulation equipment, including part-task trainer, fixed and mobile audiovisual, virtual trainers, and more than 300 mannequins. The size of the **fleet** is further complicated by distance between sites; the furthest Thursday Island is 2,185 km (1,358 miles). The equipment is managed using a database capturing location and usage and maintenance schedules. Core to all equipment management is the **Inspection, Preventive, Maintenance (IPM)** program. The maintenance schedule devolves into the three levels: (1) Functional checks, (2) Replacement of parts, and (3) Complete Replacement of all parts (Table 3.9.1).

IPM1 is conducted four times a year and includes a thorough inspection procedure, which identifies potential repair issues that may need to be conducted earlier to prevent potentially expensive repair components. This cycle

TABLE 3.9.1		
IPM Requirements		
IPM	**Details**	**Frequency**
1	Functionality check	Four times per annum
2	Replacement of parts	Twice per annum
3	Complete replacement of all parts	Once per annum

also focuses on replacement and repair of some minor components and cosmetic deformities such as chest and arm skin replacement. This first level of IPM is conducted at all sites by all trained **simulation coordinators** and educators as first-line operators. An example of an IPM1 can be seen in Figure 3.9.1.

IPM2 is conducted twice a year and includes all the elements of IPM1, plus the replacement of commonly worn parts of the simulator, and includes a full replacement of pneumatic bladders and any software upgrades required for the simulator. The second-level schedule requires a more advanced maintenance practitioner and is conducted at the main Brisbane site by a team of Simulation Coordinators led by a highly experienced **Simulation Educator**. IPM2 is the pivotal component of the schedule and results in the most preventive means for ongoing repair issues with all simulators.

IPM3 is conducted once a year at the Brisbane site and is overseen by the Simulation Educator with the Maintenance and Repair **portfolio**. The level 3 IPM results in a complete breakdown of the simulator down to a mere shell and replacement of all components. The ability to completely deconstruct a simulator requires a highly advanced knowledge base of not just the technical components, but how they relate to being used in the clinical simulation setting. The requirement to have a skilled practitioner in simulation education delivery combined with technical knowledge and ability has been instrumental in conducting this level of IPM.

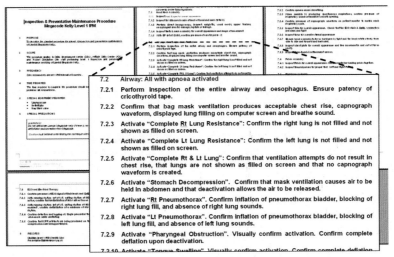

FIGURE 3.9.1 Example Inspection and Preventive Maintenance Procedure Level 1 IPM.

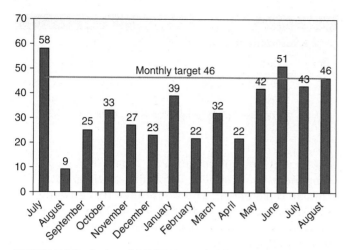

FIGURE 3.9.2 Review of CSDS IPM completed.Data used to adjust Simulation Educators' portfolios of work to ensure preventive maintenance schedules as met and reduce equipment overheads.

The frequency of preventive maintenance and repair is based upon data collected from the usage of each type of simulator, which changes with the age of the simulators. Preventive maintenance is critical because, first, it improves the quality of the training by detecting equipment failures before they occur, thereby reducing interruptions, and, second, it reduces minor issues becoming major repairs. In CSDS's first full year of data collection it became clear through both the IPM reporting and cost analysis that increased technical support recourses were required (Figure 3.9.2). Changes were made to the Simulation Educators' portfolios to ensure adequate time was allocated to preventive maintenance.

Repairs are conducted in a similar manner to maintenance, with minor fixes conducted at local sites but major repairs, such as the replacement of a motherboard, performed at CSDS. On the basis of fleets of simulators CSDS has modeled failure rates and repair costs for each item. These costs are used to inform future procurement, loan library costs, and life cycle management. Approximately 20% of the CSDS simulation fleet is salvaged equipment seen to have reached the end of the product's life or were considered unserviceable by service providers. Many of these simulators predate CSDS and have been recovered from hospitals where they lay broken and unused for many years. Data on the costs of repairs is also used to inform decisions on the procurement of spare components, for example, to buy in bulk or to maintain the minimum number or purchase replacements as needed when equipment fails.

Redundancy and Distribution

Vital to the effectiveness of the CSDS maintenance and repair program is the redundancy and distribution model. Equipment is owned and managed in fleets by CSDS but distributed across the Skills Centers and Pocket Simulation Centers. Every simulator has a redundancy; in most cases it

is the same type of product. In the case of virtual trainers, the redundancy can be an equivalent task on another type of virtual trainer with complementary functionality. By managing equipment in fleets and moving them around the different sites, Skills Centers and Pocket Simulation Centers (managed and owned by the local health service) have access to not just a few different simulators but hundreds of different simulators. Using the redundancy model maintenance cycles does not impede training time as a simulator of like type is shipped to the site for use that day without any training or opportunity for training lost.

TIPS FOR SHIPPING EQUIPMENT

Logistics is a highly competitive industry; if you do regular business with a particular carrier you can get substantial discounts on shipping.
Be prepared to use multiple companies, as some will provide better service to different destinations.

So a skills program may have permanent access to "mannequin type A" on the basis of their volume of training delivery. Instead of a single "mannequin type A" based at their site, they may have several different "mannequin type A's" move through the program over the course of a year as they are exchanged through the maintenance program. The same skills program may loan for short periods of time many other simulators during the year to deliver a wider scope of training.

The advantages of central management and distributed delivery include:

- When equipment breaks beyond local skills to repair, it is replaced quickly
- Access to a broad range of simulators is larger than any stand-alone center could provide
- Regular major services do not interfere with training, as a replacement simulator is provided when the simulator is brought in for service
- Costs are reduced as the replaced simulator does not have to go back to the same site
- The technical skills required for preventive maintenance can be maintained at the Skills Centers and Pocket Simulation Centers through communication with the technical experts, the CSDS simulation provider training package, and online support
- Innovations in maintenance, repair, and modifications are easily shared
- The cost of maintenance is significantly reduced compared with external warranties which, depending upon the equipment, maintenance and repair costs, can be reduced between 70–95% in CSDS's experiences. These savings are calculated based on a 2013 analysis of 50 random CSDS simulation item covering part-task trainer, mannequins, and virtual reality.
- Can maintain equipment external providers are either unwilling or unable to support

The disadvantages of central management and distributed delivery include:

- Requires investment in equipment management databases and administrative processes
- Requires educators to relinquish personal ownership of their simulators
- Requires contractual agreements between the Skills Centers, Pocket Simulation Centers, and CSDS
- Requires significant scale to be efficient and sustainable

The CSDS model of redundancy applies not only to equipment, but also to the skills in maintaining the equipment. This requires a balance between ensuring redundancy in the number of people trained to maintain each item of equipment and the opportunity to practice repairs. In determining the number of people whom CSDS has trained to conduct repairs, the service has taken into account staff rosters, leave entitlements, and provisions for turnover of staff.

Usage and Training

Internationally, the extent that individuals working in simulation engage with equipment maintenance varies considerably, with some educators leaving all technical support to service providers and others knowing their simulator intimately. Methods for acquiring the skills to maintain simulation equipment can vary between supplier delivered training programs, apprenticeship at another skills program, and even self-taught. The CSDS has a programmatic approach to ensure the Skills Centers and Pocket Simulation Centers have enough local skills to support the equipment. This is achieved through three elements: first, a requirement for a minimum of two local staff to undertake a short course covering technical simulation; second, online support through e-learning and data sharing; and third, regular contact with expert technical staff at CSDS (Table 3.9.2). Over time, some Simulation Educators at the Skills Centers and Pocket Simulation Centers have developed skills that go beyond preventive maintenance and minor repairs to do innovative work on modifying simulators. In one example, a Simulation Educator in a Cairns Pocket site developed a modification to a full body mannequin venous arm, allowing for a dialysis machine to be connected to the mannequin while in operation and performing team-based scenarios to train dialysis nursing and medical staff (Hudson et al., 2012). In another example, staff at the CSDS Brisbane site modified both tibial (leg) and humeral (arm) bones to allow for intraosseous insertion techniques on full body mannequins. Many of the more experienced users have interfaced the pneumatic system of the simulators to control bladders to move arms and legs of once static mannequins, and even to create arterial blood flow using nothing more than the mannequin's software-driven valve blocks to perform this complex and highly desired feature. Developing this advanced skill normally takes many years of training with simulators and knowing intimately how they operate and function.

Simulation Program Operation

The Simulation Educators and Coordinators working at CSDS receive more training from internal programs (including a Graduate Certificate of Healthcare Simulation) as well as significantly more training from simulation manufacturers (Figures 3.9.3). Achieving a detailed understanding of each type of simulator's strength and weakness for these staff has proven effective in supporting both curricula design and maintenance planning. The use of the right simulator for the task can improve training outcomes and at the same time reduce equipment repair and maintenance cost. For example, the use of an expensive high-end mannequin simulator designed for anesthesia training for Advance Life Support training will increase maintenance costs and may be less effective in chest compression training than a basic mannequin designed for the task (see chapter 3.2 on Mannequins). It would be difficult for many simulation programs to justify the range of simulators required to optimize maintenance efficiency, as each device is unlikely to get enough use. However, even if the simulation program does not have enough scale to optimize equipment usage, models of equipment use are valuable to inform purchasing and maintenance training requirements.

The Skills Centers and Pocket Simulation Centers provide CSDS with monthly equipment usage reports. Data on

TABLE 3.9.2	
Minimum Simulation Coordinator Training Requirements Involve the Completion of the Following Short Courses	
Introduction to Simulation Training	**Simulation Coordinator Training**
General overview of simulation-based education (1 day)	Technical aspect of simulation delivery (4 days)
Targets faculty, simulation coordinators and educators	Targets simulation coordinators and educators
• Overview of simulation-based education • Simulation environments and equipment • Facilitators' role in simulation • Education principles and theories • Facilitation skills and techniques • Introduction to debriefing	• Set up, quick check, IPM, use, pack up, trouble-shooting of part-task trainers, full body mannequins, and AV systems • Hazard ID and risk management • Moulage • Using course documents to set up and run simulations

SECTION 3 • Simulators

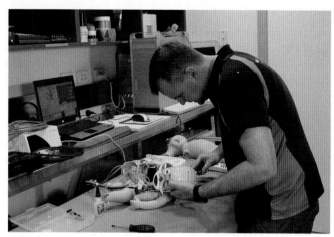 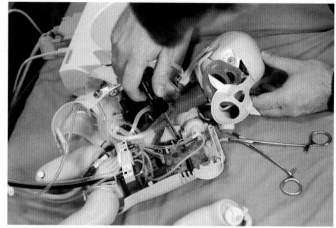

FIGURE 3.9.3 Simulation Educators at CSDS are trained to conduct all IPM 1, 2, and 3, covering the full range of simulators managed by the Service.

equipment use is employed by CSDS to model equipment breakage rates from which both redundancy requirements and maintenance costs are calculated. On the basis of several years of data collection, CSDS has reliable data on breakages and costs. For example, average maintenance and repair costs of one common birthing trainer are AU$188 a day of use (the skins tear and are expensive to replace), while a common low-end mannequin costs only AU$5 a day of use. In some cases, it has been cheaper for CSDS to replace an entire fleet of simulators with another product. In at least one case, the annual cost of consumables for the original product was greater than the combined costs of the fleet replacement annual consumables of the new product.

Procurement and Evaluation of Products

Simulators are often expensive acquisitions, and there is a tendency for educators to want the latest product with all the new bells and whistles. Most simulation programs' ability to evaluate a product is very limited. Common methods of evaluation are demonstrations by the manufacturer, hiring consultants who claim expertise in simulation, asking people who have already purchased the product or, more rarely, trial the product for a short period. Such approaches are very limited and have led to many simulators gathering dust in storage around the world. A needs and utilization assessment prior to purchase may help programs achieve cost-effective procurement. Questions that can guide programs in this assessment include:

- Who will use the product and how?
- How does the product compare with other simulators?
- How often will the product be used?
- Can the product be misused?
- Are there safety issues to consider?
- Can the simulation program afford the consumables?
- Does the simulation program have the skills to maintain this product?
- Who will do the repairs on the product?

- Can the simulation program afford the repairs?
- How often does the product break, and how will this impact on training?
- Do we know and can we contact a program that has used this product?

The service level approach at CSDS is a programmatic evaluation of equipment to identify training limitation, safety issues, and information to inform the cost modeling for consumables, maintenance, and repairs. All new products are reviewed by a team of Simulation Educators, Coordinators, Lead Faculty, and clinical subject matter experts. Typically over a 2-week period, the product is reviewed by 10 or more staff examining the fidelity, flexibility, and sustainability of each device. Although there is a significant cost in salaries to conduct such a detailed analysis, the cost saving in procuring the right products can outweigh the initial investment. This is especially true when buying simulators and audiovisual systems in fleets. Organizations may perform a "head-to-head" testing, where multiple vendors are invited to bring their product for staff and faculty to trial and provide input into which equipment can help service their learners' needs. An alternate approach is a "loan library service," where clients can borrow equipment at a cost and under certain conditions to trial and use.

The process usually involves stripping and rebuilding the product to identify safety issues, areas of fidelity to investigate, and likely maintenance issues and costs. For each product, a list of critical areas of fidelity (e.g., depth of chest compression, force required for chest compression, feel of compression, etc., for CPR) are identified by an interprofessional team and assessed against performance requirements. The number of critical areas of fidelity can be significant, depending on the complexity of the mannequins. As part of the evaluation process, the products are also used in simulations to identify technical issues, potential changes to delivery, and to seek staff feedback on simulators' impact on realism. CSDS has also worked with a range of research to do more in-depth product evaluations as part of curricula design.

The results of the CSDS evaluation process have been significant for procurement, safety, and curriculum design. Queensland Health is a large employer with around 45,000 frontline staff, most of whom annually require either Basic Life Support training or Advance Life Support training. Evaluations demonstrate low-cost part-task trainers and mannequins can do the task better than expensive mannequins and decrease maintenance cost significantly. In another evaluation, it was identified that there was a potential safety issue that led the manufacturer to do worldwide recall of the product to correct the issue. Given the product was in use by many centers for a year prior to the CSDS evaluation, it raises concerns about technical knowledge and safety requirements as simulators become more complex. A third evaluation found three of the latest wireless mannequin products were not suitable replacements for an older tethered mannequin for physiotherapy training. This was in part because of the inbuilt compressors producing unbalanced and incorrect leg weights. As the manufacturer has ceased support for the older model, CSDS has purchased a stockpile of parts and expects to extend the life cycle of the product out to 12 to 15 years.

The findings from the evaluation are also feedback to the manufacturers. CSDS has identified issues in the majority of products evaluated so far, and in many cases there are design flaws that have to be rectified by the manufacturer before CSDS would purchase the product. In most cases, the manufacturers are prepared to update their products in view of both the scale of purchasing conducted by CSDS and the beneficial flow on effect to other customers. The evaluations create a win-win scenario, with the manufacturers improving the quality of their products and CSDS acquiring the right products.

BEEN THERE, DONE THAT: EXTERNAL SERVICE PROVIDER VS. FIX-IT-YOURSELF

Striking the balance between external service providers and fix-it-yourself will be different across most simulation programs. There are many advantages to having a high level of technical skills to conduct the work in-house, including quality, reliability, and improvements associated with large cost saving. However, acquiring and retaining the high level of technical skills provides a risk that needs to be managed. The CSDS model of simulation support is more efficient and effective than managing so many simulators through warranties and external service agreements. The CSDS model requires a high volume of training and a large fleet of simulators to justify enough staff to ensure redundancy of skills. Investments in equipment databases, negotiations with other skills centers and in situ programs all come with a cost and take time to achieve.

There may be other avenues to achieve the efficiency; potentially, industry could loan or lease products to simulation and in situ programs allowing them to move from site to site. Another model would be collaborative, where through contractual arrangements the equipment, maintenance, and product management is distributed across multiple simulation centers. An alternative would be the establishment of a consortium where simulation centers and in situ simulation programs agree to pool their service support funding into a central entity that manages all equipment.

SUMMARY

Whether your simulation program uses a service provider and warranties or in-house support, it is important to understand the costs and risks associated with sustaining the technical side of simulation programs. Given the variability of simulation programs and the services provided, these costs and risks differ from program to program, and an analysis should be performed within each program. Around the world, too many simulators are collecting dust in cupboards and storerooms as a result of insufficient planning for equipment procurement and maintenance. The future of simulation in healthcare should include programmatic approaches to increasing access, reliability, and sustainability of simulation technologies.

REFERENCES

Hogreve, J., & Gremler, D. D. (2009). Twenty years of service guarantee research: A synthesis. *Journal of Service Research, 11,* 322–343.
Hudson, D., Dunbar-Reid, K., & Sinclair, P. M. (2012, March–April). The incorporation of high fidelity simulation training into hemodialysis nursing education: Part 2—A pictorial guide to modifying a high fidelity simulator for use in simulating hemodialysis. *Nephrology Nursing Journal, 39*(2), 119–123.

SECTION 4

Funding

CHAPTER 4.1

Where's the Money, Sources of Revenue

Jennifer A. Calzada, MA

ABOUT THE AUTHOR

JENNIFER A. CALZADA directs the Tulane Center for Advanced Medical Simulation and Team Training. Ms. Calzada has her bachelors degree in Communications, and her masters degree in Media Studies prepared her for working in advertising and marketing for 20 years. In 2008, she joined the Tulane School of Medicine. Using her experience in sales, marketing, communications, training, and business development, Ms. Calzada has launched a new simulation center and has built a new client base.

ABSTRACT

Healthcare simulation programs can be expensive operations to fund at start-up and require substantial ongoing financial support for personnel and equipment maintenance as well as capital expenses (e.g., equipment and structural upgrades). More and more institutions are expecting their simulation programs to help fund their own operation. This chapter will review several different sources of revenue that are available for both new and established simulation programs.

CASE EXAMPLE

As the manager of the simulation center, you are responsible for a medium-size simulation program with multiple types of learners using multiple simulation modalities. The simulation program is now 8 years old, and you have begun to notice that **grant funding**, which in the past had accounted for approximately 40% of the operating budget is now becoming harder to obtain. You know that **institutional support** will sustain the center, if needed, but that source of funding would be minimal and would not increase over time. As such, you are looking for additional **revenue** opportunities to replace decreasing levels of grant funding as well as help support expansion and equipment upgrades.

INTRODUCTION AND BACKGROUND

There are two different business models for medical simulation centers—the first is built and sustained solely for the purpose of training the institution's own constituents, and the second seeks to wholly or partially raise funds from external sources. This chapter will primarily address the latter situation, but first a few points on simulation centers that serve internal learners.

If the simulation program serves only internal learners, then its funding sources will come from within the institution. Some simulation centers are wholly funded by the institution's administration, but be aware that this funding source is subject to cuts and changes and may not remain a consistently reliable source of funding. Another approach to internal funding is to assign the expense based on usage volume across specialties and departments. For example, if the surgical residency program accounts for 20% of the activities in the simulation center, the surgical residency program would be assessed an amount equal to 20% of the simulation budget. If the institution allows it, this method of funding the center places **expenses** within the departments that are receiving the value of the education and training. This method can provide greater immunity to budget cuts, as the departments utilizing the center may be more likely to fight to maintain funding.

Even if the program starts with internal funding, keep in mind the start-up and **annual maintenance costs** for simulation centers increase every year, forcing more and more centers to seek a portion of their funding from external sources. As the number of large-scale simulation centers grow in numbers, the difficulty of securing external funding increases. Therefore, identifying as many revenue opportunities as possible becomes critical.

BIRTH OF A SIMULATION IDEA

Healthcare simulation is currently experiencing a dramatic rise in usage, and careful and thoughtful preplanning is not always undertaken. Sometimes, simulation centers come into being simply to demonstrate an organization's commitment to appear on technology's leading edge; for competitive reasons to attract students, residents, and staff; or to appease large donors.

Even centers that were born out of one of these purposes can take advantage of many of the opportunities presented in this chapter. A review of existing resources may yield many possible opportunities. Programs in their planning phase have the benefit of being able to tailor their plans and resources to take advantage of as many opportunities as desired.

It cannot be stressed enough that determining opportunities that are available to a simulation program should follow the established and accepted mission and vision. By doing so, the program is setting a guiding plan that should be accepted not only by program management, but also by those with the responsibility for institutional oversight. With an accepted vision and mission, center management is able to determine how the desired requirements for facility space, equipment, staffing, faculty and educator support, and ongoing budgetary support will be accommodated.

REQUIRED FUNDING

How much is needed to start and maintain a simulation center? The easiest and best answer is: whatever it takes to achieve the desired vision and mission goals. The harder answer is: it all depends. There are very few published examples of simulation center financials, likely due to the proprietary and competitive nature of the industry. However, several published examples are given here.

The first example provided in this chapter comes from a published look at the cost of construction and operation for the Canadian Simulation Centre, Sunnybrook Health Science Centre at the University of Toronto. The start-up cost was $665,000 CAD ($619,300 USD) from 1994 to 1995, and the sample maintenance costs totaled $167,250 CAD ($155,764 USD) for 1995 to 1996 (Kurrek & Devit, 1997). For a comparison with 2013 dollars, based on inflation indexes, see Table 4.1.1. The second, and more

TABLE 4.1.1
University of Toronto Centre Costs
Centre Start-up Costs
1996 $665,000 CAD (approximately $619,300 USD)
2013 $916,642 CAD ($892,196 USD)
Centre Annual Operation Costs
1996 $167,250 CAD (approximately $155,764 USD)
2013 $167,250 CAD ($224,391 USD)

recent, example presented here is from the Kanbar Simulation Center at UCSF School of Medicine, a 1,800 square feet (167.2 m^2) facility meant to serve the UCSF School of Medicine community. The proposed **start-up capital** in 2007 to 2008 was $497,526 USD, and annual expenses started at $211,727 USD and are projected to increase to $424,408 USD by FY 2012 to 2013 (University of California, San Francisco School of Medicine, 2008). A third is from a larger-scale simulation center, which is the Tulane Center for Advanced Medical Simulation and Team Training, which is 14,000 square feet (1,300.6 m^2). Opened in January 2009, with a nearly $3-million USD initial build budget, it currently has an annual operating budget of more than $700,000 USD.

Additional insight into funding can be found in the 2011 Association of American Medical Colleges (AAMC) Survey on Medical Simulation in Medical Education. While the survey did not query start-up costs, as it was surveying existing simulation centers, it does give a more recent glimpse into annual operating costs of simulation centers and even distinguishes between those based on medical schools versus teaching hospitals. The survey found that for fiscal year 2009, hospital-based teaching centers had operating budgets under $250,000 for 57% of the respondents, and under $500,000 for 75%. Medical school-based centers were more spread out, with budgets from under $250,000 up to $1,000,000+ (Figure 4.1.1) (Passiment et al., 2011). It should be noted that these results are limited by the fact that annual budgets are not necessarily correlated with facility size, staff levels, or program size and scope. Once the vision and mission are developed for a center and requirements to meet these goals are determined, including facilities, equipment, staffing and budgeting, only then can educational opportunities be appropriately considered (Figure 4.1.1).

OPPORTUNITIES GO BOTH WAYS: REVENUE UP OR EXPENSES DOWN

Institutional leadership for almost any simulation program will have ideas for opportunities to expand, and this will most often involve revenue generation from a variety of sources. Unless there are specific institutional reasons why this is not the case, saving on expenses equally affects

SECTION 4 • Funding

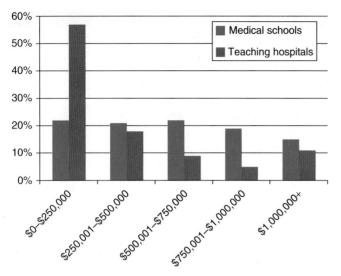

FIGURE 4.1.1 Annual operating budget.

the center's availability of financial resources. Increasing revenue is generally the preferred method to improve a center's bottom line. Not only does revenue generation provide for the opportunity to break even or, better yet, produce a profit, there is also the not so subtle positive public relations effect of having significant revenue. Even in the business world, everyone loves a winner and wants to be associated with a center that is financially successful.

However, for the purpose of internal budgeting and providing justifications to leadership, driving down expenses can be just as valuable, as it can have the same effect on the bottom line. Especially for programs that are suffering from degree of bloat or waste, cost cutting and clearly linking expenses to mission is a necessity. A note of caution: driving down expenses is most valuable when it is done by saving the expense on items (or personnel time) that would otherwise be an actual expense. The expense should ideally be one that is critical to the center's operations, not an optional extra that was perhaps donated. Having a da Vinci robot donated provides a tremendous saving when it was a planned and budgeted item. Having one donated when there was no plan or budget to purchase one is still a fantastic donation, but not necessarily helping to improve the budgeted bottom line, because there is no associated expense that is being eliminated. In fact, having an item donated that was not planned, can increase expenses if the item carries any annual maintenance, service, or usage costs.

There is a third category of opportunities that should be considered, those that will not result in any revenue and will not save expenses (they may even incur expenses) but will generate **public relations capital**. While considerably harder to quantify, opportunities for adding high PR value should be considered, and they may lead to future options owing to good press. For example, the Tulane Center for Advanced Medical Simulation and Team Training created a rural emergency department training program and ran it several times for no cost as a means to test the

curriculum. Press coverage of this course in New Orleans and a rural newspaper has led to contracts to run this same course (for a fee) for other facilities.

BEFORE REVENUE GENERATING OPPORTUNITIES ARE CONSIDERED

By now, the center has developed and approved a vision and mission, and a plan for budgeting, staffing, facilities, and equipment. In addition to this, there are several other considerations for each opportunity that are listed here.

Simulation Modalities

Depending on the **simulation modalities** available at the center, certain opportunities may exist. The most commonly used modalities for healthcare simulation are: standardized patients, full-scale mannequins (low, medium, and high technology), partial task trainers, computer-based or virtual reality-based simulations, embedded simulated persons, team training, and game-based simulation (see other chapters throughout this textbook).

The center should have an up-to-date list of modalities it can provide and their associated costs and availability. For example, partial task trainers will have an up-front cost and little ongoing or per usage costs, compared with standardized patients, where the cost is per usage and must be part of every training plan. When center educators are well versed in both the appropriate use of various forms of simulation as well as the cost of using each methodology, they can make scenario design decisions that are educationally sound as well as fiscally conservative.

Staffing Levels

The largest portion of a program's annual budget is often staffing costs, including full-time and part-time staff, and educators. This is often two-thirds to three-quarters of a program's ongoing operating budget. An accurate picture of staffing levels, availability, and capabilities is necessary to plan many revenue opportunities.

Equipment

Certain opportunities will require specific equipment and supplies. If a center does not have this equipment already available, then a specific opportunity budget should be planned to determine whether purchasing the necessary equipment will be offset by the projected revenue stream.

Accreditations, Certifications, and Credentials

Some revenue opportunities require specific **accreditations**, certifications, or credentials. Just as with equipment, if these do not already exist, creating a business plan can help determine whether seeking the necessary approvals will be offset by projected revenue.

FUNDING OPPORTUNITIES (YOUNG CENTERS)

What type of opportunities (both revenue and expense saving) should a newly opened center consider?

Institutional Funding

Many centers will derive all or a significant portion of their funding from their own institutional sources. How much and what percentage of total funding required will likely be a decision made by institutional leadership above a center's management; however, center leadership should play an active role in shaping and influencing these decisions.

Example

The percentage of funding from institutional ownership varies from 0% (in the case of the Center for Medical Simulation, which became a separate entity from Harvard in 1999; The Center for Medical Simulation, 2013) to 100% for many centers and every level in between. Institutional funding at the lowest levels puts a center into a significant revenue generating business model, which has not proven to be easy and increases the risk that a center will financially fail. A recent example is the Humboldt Bay Regional Simulation Center, which closed operations in 2012 after 3½ years when the single grant funding source concluded the initial nurse training project.

How much institutional funding does a center need? At the very minimum, funding to cover annual staffing, supply needs, and minimal equipment maintenance. This level may allow a center to remain open, but will not provide an opportunity for additional growth of the program unless specific changes are made to the program.

How to Get Funding

Before a simulation center opens their doors, a decision will have been made by institutional leadership on how much and to what percentage they will support the on-going funding needs. If not fully supported, the best way to increase this source of funding is to survey similar institutions (be sure leadership considers them similar) for their level of internal funding. Consistently providing this information to leadership can sometimes help the case for maintaining or increasing funding.

Pro

A secure internal source of funding can relieve a program director from having to perform any type of sales role in seeking external revenue. It will relieve day-to-day financial pressures and allow the center to focus on training and education to fulfill their mission.

Con

It is hard to say there is a downside to having internal funding; however, attention does need to be given on a regular basis to keeping the program a top priority to the institution and top of the list when the time comes for budgeting. No funding source, internal or external, should be assumed to continue year after year. Taking the time to regularly do internal public relations on program accomplishments can help maintain internal funding. The focus of the program also should be limited to the needs of the institution. This is difficult in simulation since many external partnerships and opportunities may present themselves to leadership.

Departments/Practice Plan/ Risk Management

Another form of institutional support comes from the departments of internal users of a simulation center. In the 2009 AAMC survey, 13% of medical school-based centers and 16% of hospital-based centers reported this type of support (Passiment et al., 2011). While this is another form of internal funding, it sometimes comes with different challenges than funding directly from administration.

The first challenge will be determining whether the program can charge other internal departments for usage. Generally, this will be an institutional policy. The ideal answer is yes, because charging for a service helps build perceived value. Most often, this decision will be provided to the simulation program director by institutional leadership.

How to Get Funding

If a center is required to allow internal usage at no charge, keep track of "fair market" charges by department and any actual expenses that may be incurred on their behalf. This report should go to institutional leadership at least annually and may help with a policy change. Often, leadership is not aware of the expenses incurred.

Pro

If the institutional decision is made to allow charging internal departments, and simulation activities are a priority, the program director's job will be made that much easier. However, keep in mind that if the program is allowed to charge other departments for usage but simulation is not an institutional priority, the program's leadership will essentially be trying to sell their services to internal departments. Be careful not to price the program beyond reach, or departments may simply choose not to participate in simulation.

Con

While not a con to the simulation program to the overall institution this is not technically revenue, but really transferring funds between departments. Depending on an institution's accounting system and whether they are a for-profit business, this may not be allowed by generally accepted accounting rules.

Practice Plan

Institutions with a **Physician Practice Plan** may have an opportunity for support by providing certain credentialing and remediation services.

Example

The simulation program can provide credentialing for all physicians for central venous catheter placement to help prevent central line associated bloodstream infections (CLABSI). A simulation program can also provide **physician remediation** after certain sentinel events. These are two examples where an agreement can be forged with the Physician Practice Plan to provide support on a per person basis for certain procedural trainings.

How to Get Funding

Meet with the Practice Plan manager, and understand their concerns and goals regarding credentialing and remediation situations. Do the same for local hospital leadership and the credentialing committee. Understanding local hospital and group practice goals can help a program determine which needs they can help meet.

Pro

Procedural training and credentialing can become a nearly automated process that is planned in detail and can be executed whenever needed with relative ease.

Con

Process approval should be given by the institution's general counsel to ensure credentialing is set up correctly. While the process can be a management and regulatory minefield, once set up correctly, changes should not be necessary unless regulations change. Extra care must be taken to ensure that every training encounter follows procedures exactly.

Can a program receive support from a hospital's **risk management** department? In a word, yes! While this varies by institution, there are more and more examples of fee reductions given by risk management for providing certain types of training. A meeting with risk management leadership is well worth the time to determine specific opportunities.

Example

Hospital Corporation of America (HCA) provides reductions in premiums for hospitals that participate in Team-STEPPS training with staff and physicians and improve patient safety performance (The Agency for Healthcare Research and Quality, 2013).

How to Get Funding

Just as with Practice Plans, program leadership should meet with Risk Management to determine what issues they have, where they might be able to share savings from programs offered, and then determine whether a business plan can be developed around these opportunities.

Pro

Many of these savings are very new, and institutions may not even be aware of them. Providing proof of expense reductions after training at a simulation center may help gain a hospital as a client if the savings outweigh the training cost.

Con

Finding savings opportunities can require extensive legwork on the part of the simulation center. Owing to the way many hospitals plan departmental budgets (departments are budgeted in isolation), there may not be enough savings in a single department to convince them to spend dollars on training. In this situation, finding a way to look at aggregate savings may be an option.

Local Institutions

Local, related institutions are another source for both revenue generation and expense saving. Other medical schools, nursing schools, hospitals, allied health schools, paramedic training and providers, home health providers, long-term care facilities, and all other healthcare professionals need some level of ongoing learning, training, or certifications.

Understanding who is in the market, what their needs are, and what their own resources are should be the first step in a business plan. The plan should also include a look at any other simulation programs in the market that can provide these same services. Know the potential and the competitive landscape before approaching anyone with a business opportunity.

These healthcare institutions may provide a source of revenue by selling training courses that meet their needs. They may also provide expense saving by establishing a partnership where they provide the simulation program educators or donate expired supplies or used equipment that can eliminate planned expenses.

Local Government

Just as there are federal and state grants, there are sometimes grants funneled through local governments. In addition to grants, consider partnering with local governments for disaster training or surge capacity planning.

Example

A simulation program can partner with the local health department to run an annual disaster drill for healthcare professionals.

How to Get Funding

Meet with local health department and first responders to find out their plans for **disaster and emergency drills** to determine how the simulation center can become a partner.

Pro

While this example is likely a low revenue opportunity, it can be very high PR value to both the center and the institution.

Con

This can require tremendous planning and has the potential of allowing government officials to take control.

State Government

The AAMC survey found that 11% of medical school-based centers and 3% of hospital-based centers received state government funding (Passiment et al., 2011).

Example

State government departments can be a prime source for grant funding. Many state hospital associations or departments of health and hospitals individually fund state initiatives for nurse training, patient safety, emergency training, disaster planning, and other healthcare-related training opportunities.

How to Get Funding

Determine what mechanism state **funding announcements** utilize, and subscribe to those lists. Many state grants are actually federally funded, and announcements can be found on grants.gov.

Pro

Government grants can often be used to partially cover staff, equipment, training courses, and many other expenses, directly associated with the project.

Con

Announcements are not frequent, the lead time to complete the application is short, and the competition can be significant. Without a grant writer on staff or under contract, government grants can be difficult to win.

Federal Government

AAMC survey results showed that 3% of medical school centers and 6% of hospital-based centers receive funding from federal grants (Passiment et al., 2011).

Example

Just as with local and state governments, federal departments can be a prime source for grant funding.

How to Get Funding

A program within an institution likely has a department that could help inform program leadership of how to get government funding. Grants.gov is the primary funding announcement for federal government grants in the United States. Primary funding sources for simulation centers are DHHS (Department of Health and Human Services), DOD (Department of Defense), and AHRQ (Agency for Health Research and Quality). However, other agencies should not be ignored. Keywords can help refine searches, and common keywords include simulation, medical procedures, healthcare training, patient safety, and medical practice.

Pro

Just as with state grants, federal grants can cover directly associated expenses to a project.

Con

Again, even more so than state grants, federal grants are highly competitive, and application times require a rapid turnaround. This source of funding can be one of the most resource intensive, both during application and during grants management.

Corporate Grants/Foundations

After institutional sources, corporate grants and foundations are the most significant funding sources in the AAMC survey, with 40% for medical school-based centers and 25% for hospital-based centers (Passiment et al., 2011).

Separate from government grants are funding sources from corporations and private foundations. These sources often give specific funds on an annual basis, but funding tends to be highly focused on an area of interest to the corporation or foundation. Private corporations with business

FUNDING FOR HEALTHCARE SIMULATION RESEARCH

Debra Nestel, BA, PhD, FAcadMEd CHSE-A
Board of Directors, Simulation Australia

The vibrancy of the healthcare simulation research community does not reflect the highly competitive and seemingly scarce funding for our field. Given that much of our work "saves" rather than generates income for institutions (i.e., promotes patient safety and limits the financial costs associated with healthcare errors), it can be especially difficult to "sell" our mission in cash-strapped economies. Further, many of our research endeavors have an indirect impact on patient safety. In this brief commentary, I review approaches to obtaining funding for healthcare simulation research. I assume you already have your research idea, so I will move straight to the proposal and then sourcing funds. However, I need to acknowledge the breadth of healthcare simulation activities and research—it includes, for example, simulations that model healthcare systems, task trainers that support the acquisition of psychomotor skills, large-scale first responder *disaster* simulations, team-based crisis resource management immersive simulations, and simulated (or standardized) patient-based communication scenarios, and so much more. Therefore, each simulation activity has its own particular funding context. I simply offer general considerations in obtaining research funding to explore this expansive field.

With any written grant or funding proposal, there are some common themes—be clear about your goals and your research questions/hypotheses, articulate your methods, outline the potential impact or strategic gain, and show your competitive edge. Ensure you demonstrate how your research meets a need. Justify your budget, be realistic about milestones against time frames, and include a dissemination strategy. Know your audience, so contact the funder ahead of submission to express your interest and air your ideas. This can lead to a better understanding of the funder's intent. Just as scholarly writing is different to preparing educational materials, so too is grant writing—work with others who have had success and established a track record. It is probably worthwhile intermittently attending workshops on grant writing to refresh your approach. Keep your CV as a dynamic document, and review it each time you submit for funding. It will very likely need shaping for the funder. Make yourself invaluable to the project. Try to obtain feedback from your colleagues or institutional research support (if you have any) before submitting. Writing grants is time-consuming and if you are unsuccessful, be prepared to carefully rewrite for a new funder. Although disheartening, even a 10% success rate is to be celebrated!

As for funding sources, look to all the traditional research bodies associated with universities and institutes. Funding for healthcare simulation is likely to be in response to specific calls. The Australian healthcare simulation community has had significant investment from a government body concerned with health workforce planning and reform. There may be occasions when a government agency has funds that need to be spent quickly and you are asked to make a bid—having some loosely drafted ideas filed away can be just the thing to roll out at short notice. Make sure you are in the communication loop to be made aware of these calls. Sign up to electronic lists of funding opportunities.

Consider your professional association(s) and your local institution for seed and other small pots of money. If you generate income from courses, think about allocating a portion of your income stream to research. These funds might be enough to support piloting a really good research idea—enough to test feasibility in order to work up a full proposal for external funding. You might also look to healthcare and professional indemnity insurers, simulator manufacturers, and education-oriented technology companies to fund your research. If you have a particular patient population in mind that may benefit from your research, then seek out opportunities with organizations targeting that population group (e.g., diabetes, heart disease, mental health support/research foundations, etc.). Think about linking up with engineers, educationalists, information technology specialists, artists, industrial designers, and others involved in simulation—this can help to widen the scope for sourcing funds and can lead to really exciting partnerships.

It is also important to connect with your healthcare simulation community by participating as a member, attending conferences and other events, reading news releases on professional websites, and scanning a wide range of journals. Chances are that the people you meet at conferences, read about in the news, and contribute to journals will be those reviewing your applications and the papers you write postresearch. They are also likely to be your future collaborators. Find ways to showcase your ideas and work locally, nationally, and internationally.

When you are successful with funding, make sure you deliver. In my experience, projects are rarely implemented exactly as planned (document and justify any changes) and often end up with unanticipated results. This is also acceptable and often more exciting than what was planned. Although it is ideal to have a program of research, sometimes you have to *follow the money*. Having established a track record in delivering on your research, you are in a stronger position to have people buy your ideas. It is so satisfying to work through the whole process from idea generation through dissemination and to see your ideas translated into clinical education and practice. And, sometimes, into directly improving patient outcomes.

---

that overlaps with medical education or training equipment may provide **equipment grants** (see chapter 4.7 on obtaining grants).

How to Get Funding

Listings of foundations can be found on foundationcenter.org, and universities have development departments that are familiar with the larger ones. Become familiar with foundations that have interests that cross over with the program's capabilities. Just like foundations, make yourself familiar with corporations in the medical and simulation field, especially any located near the program.

Pro

Like government grants, these funds can be used for a variety of reasons and can be quite significant per year.

Corporation equipment grants can provide equipment and supplies that would otherwise have been included in a program's expense budget.

Con

Like government grants, foundation awards can be highly competitive. Foundations also tend to have specific areas of interest and a narrow focus. As more simulation programs open, corporation grants are also becoming increasingly difficult to secure.

Philanthropy

Private donations also are a large funding source, with 26% of medical school-based programs receiving funds and 16% of hospital-based programs (Passiment et al., 2011). Whether restricted (can be used only for a designated purpose) or unrestricted, private donations can be quite a boon for a simulation program at both the start-up phase, for any expansion or annual expenses (see chapter 4.6 on Fundraising).

Example

There are many reasons a private donor may wish to make a donation; among them could be a graduate from a medical school interested in providing support for a simulation program in that medical school, or a former patient interested in contributing toward a hospital-based program.

How to Get Funding

Securing philanthropic donations can involve a tremendous amount of time and effort and is usually facilitated by the Development department. Meeting with the institution's Development management and ensuring they understand the benefits and needs of the simulation program is the best approach.

Pro

Unrestricted money is strictly a gift, and restricted money is a gift for a specific purpose. Either way, it is additional funding and, depending on the amount, can be structured to provide an ongoing endowment.

Con

Securing philanthropic donations is difficult and time-consuming, and the institution may have greater needs beyond the simulation program.

For-Profit Entities

Six percent of medical school-based programs and 1% of hospital-based programs report receiving funding from for-profit entities (Passiment et al., 2011), which are most often vendor sources.

During a simulation program's start-up, this source of funding will be especially important. While having simulators themselves donated is not common, donations of related equipment are possible. Advanced planning definitely makes a difference in this situation.

Example

Planning donation requests at the time of significant affiliated hospital purchases are ideal. For example, if the affiliated hospital is purchasing 10 new high-definition laparoscopic towers, advanced planning allows the simulation program leadership to request that a number of towers for educational use be added to the negotiation.

How to Get Funding

A close relationship with both the purchasing department and members of each specialty who are making equipment decisions is key. It is certainly possible for simulation programs to approach vendors for donations on their own, but it is more likely when it is tied to a large hospital purchase.

Pro

Donated vendor equipment is typically positive for the simulation program although the program does need to consider whether additional personnel may be needed to run the equipment as well as the budget implications for any needed maintenance or supplies.

Con

While not exactly a negative, one difficulty is with the rapid increase in the number of simulation programs there is also an increase in these types of "asks." More vendors are moving to agreements for annually renewing "loaners," and not outright donations. While the end result can be even better, as the program will always have the newest model, it does mean the program must assume liability and maintenance costs for a piece of equipment that the institution does not own.

Retired Equipment Donations

Most simulation programs are either based in or affiliated with a hospital, or even serving a consortium of hospitals. This gives the program the potential access to retired equipment, which may not be the latest model, but is generally more than functional and will allow the program to expand capacity. Care should be given to ensure the acceptance and use of retired (old) equipment does not result in less than acceptable learning experiences for the participants in the program's simulations.

SECTION 4 • Funding

Example

Nearly every piece of equipment at a hospital is retired at some point, and often before it is truly unusable. Examples can include operating room tables, stretchers, patient beds, defibrillators, suction pumps, and thousands more items. Many of these items will be in working order for simulation purposes. This is not an expense saving that can generally be planned for, but over time it can save simulation program money by receiving items that would eventually need to be purchased.

How to Get Funding

Meet with the hospital inventory management to determine how retired equipment is currently disposed and whether it can be donated to the simulation program especially if the program is part of a non-profit, this is generally an easy process. Meeting with administrators in hospital departments can also make the program's "wish list" known. Before taking an item, be sure to ascertain the working condition and whether it will work for simulation, as some of the equipment can be large and difficult to move.

Pro

Retired equipment is often in acceptable working order for simulation.

Con

There is not much of a negative to free equipment, unless the equipment uses outmoded technology that would confuse learners, is not in good working condition, or if the center is lacking storage space. Then hard decisions will need to be made as to how important a donated item might be or how cost effective it would be to fix the item.

Expired Supply Donations

Just as with retired equipment, hospitals supplies expire on an even more frequent basis. Simulation programs utilize many of the same supplies, and training with identical brands to an affiliated hospital is beneficial to a program. While programs can reuse some types of supplies, with a large volume of training, certain supplies need to be constantly replenished.

Example

Nearly every item in a hospital, from gloves to saline bags, and medications to complete procedure kits, carries an expiration date. Removing soon-to-expire items is vital for hospital inspections, and regulations do not allow expired items to be used on patients even by charities desperate for supplies. Making the right contacts can result in these supplies being donated to a simulation program.

How to Get Funding

Meeting with hospital inventory managers and, in this case, nurses from every unit (or any with needed supplies) is key. Nurses in the unit are most often the ones removing soon-to-expire items from the floor. Tulane's example to facilitate this process is to supply large plastic tubs with lids and the program's phone number on the outside. One was delivered to each hospital unit with instructions to call when it is full. Currently, the flow of expired supplies has removed a need to purchase supplies in 90% of the trainings.

Pro

Just as with equipment, free supplies can have a positive impact on the program.

Con

Be prepared, once units are used to this process, for a flow of supplies that can be overwhelming. A space and a process need to be established to sort through bins immediately and dispose of supplies that cannot be used and incorporate the rest into existing inventory. There should be extra caution taken regarding expired medications. There are regulations (state and institution) that must be reviewed and considered. Medications also have trace amounts that may effect simulation equipment or pose danger from simulation (e.g. if a learner places a medication vial in his or her pocket and takes it to the clinical setting). Contents should be emptied before being accepted, as real medications are a risk and a violation of pharmaceutical hazardous waste regulations. Bottles should be marked for simulation only.

Film Industry/Commercial Work

If the center is in a locale that has regular feature filming or commercial filming, there will be location scouts and film commissions who cover the area. Sometimes, a hospital or doctor's office environment is needed, and if the center has re-created this "look" (remember it doesn't have to be functional), scheduling filming will certainly be easier than in an actual patient care facility.

Example

Examples can range from an advertising agency shooting a 30-second commercial about a hospital to a feature film with scenes in a healthcare environment.

How to Get Funding

Consult a local film society, film commission, or advertising federation to get the center (with sample photos) listed. Sit back and wait.

Pros

Filming activities often require little staff time, planning, or development. Often, filming can be done at odd hours when the center is normally not busy. Fees charged can be significant.

Cons

Large shoots can overrun time, can change a shooting schedule, and can be destructive with heavy film equipment, camera tracks, and lights. Damage provisions should be clearly stated in the contract. Crews will want a tightly controlled environment. "Quiet on the set" will mean other trainings may not be able to run in adjacent rooms. Depending on institutional policy, this type of filming may not be allowed at the center or may be controlled by institutional leadership.

FUNDING OPPORTUNITIES (EXPERIENCED CENTERS)

Individual/Group Courses

Revenue generated by holding courses at a simulation program was reported by 33% of AAMC medical school-based programs and 17% of hospital-based programs (Passiment et al., 2011). While a large percentage of programs reported receiving funding from courses, this does not mean the funding accounts for a large percentage of their annual budget.

Group or individual courses are often one of the first revenue opportunities that program management considers undertaking. It seems obvious to simply run what was created for internal learners for an external, paying, audience. What is not always obvious is that this revenue opportunity can be resource intensive and can result in low (or worse, negative) margins.

Example

A program has created and tested a half-day advanced airway management course for their anesthesiology residents. The program is considering offering this course to outside healthcare professionals for a registration fee. What needs to be considered are the time and expense to market the course, the time to answer questions and discuss details with institutions, details such as how registration will work, how payments will be accepted, cancellation policies, confidentiality agreements, customer disputes, and, most importantly, whether the market will bear a registration fee that will cover supplies, equipment wear and tear, faculty costs *and* allow a profit for the program.

How to Get Funding

Start with courses already run at the program for residents or senior-level learners. Considering which of these courses can be adapted for external learners is the shortest route to having a viable product. Consider first approaching similar users in the region, for example, residency programs without a simulation program.

Pro

Can be an easy win to provide training already created for external clients at a cost. Providing the same course can have a shorter lead time and less paperwork and resource requirements than those offering continuing medical education (CME) and continuing education units (CEUs). Profit with smaller attendance is still viable.

Con

Simulation still does not have a well-proven efficacy for many practicing healthcare professionals, and convincing them to pay for trainings can be difficult and time-consuming. Additionally, charges required to cover costs and faculty time can be too steep for individuals or small groups. Lack of CME/CEU certification can hurt attendance.

CME/CEU Courses

Continuing Medical Education (CME) or Continuing Education Units (CEU) are common certification units for courses that satisfy annual ongoing learning requirements for physicians, nurses, and other healthcare professionals. Providing these credits can greatly enhance interest in a course, as physicians and nurses are required to achieve a certain number each year. However, meeting the guidelines to offer credits can be paperwork intensive and expensive for an institution without a department to handle such processes.

CME and CEU courses involving simulation can be a profitable way to generate revenue, as courses with credits can charge a higher fee per learner. However, this either requires an internal department that is accredited to issue CME and CEU certificates or will necessitate the cost of contracting externally. Not having a credential department does not preclude this option, as many medical associations will issue certification for courses aimed at their specialty. This latter option should be considered before third-party CME/CEU providers, as this final route can be quite expensive.

For example, an advanced course specifically for surgeons might qualify for a CME Joint Sponsorship Program with the American College of Surgeons (ACS), who are accredited to provide CME credits. Their cost is $375 USD and $200 USD per credit with no per certificate (or per learner) fees. This could make a single-day course issuing 7.0 CME credits a cost of $1,775 USD (American College of Surgeons, Division of Education, 2013).

Third-party CME management companies often have application fees in thousands, not hundreds, of dollars, as the application process is quite extensive. Many also charge a per learner fee of $10 to $100 USD per learner and additional administrative fees. Total costs from a third-party company can easily run $3,000 to $5,000 USD for a single course.

Whichever method of issuing CME/CEU certificates is used, it should be noted that planning for these courses requires both significant paperwork and lead time. A meeting with the issuing authority can provide details on all requirements, but plan for a 6-month lead time.

Example

Almost any course run by a simulation program can be turned into a CME/CEU course, with enough lead time and content planning. For example, a laparoscopic course planned for residents can become a CME laparoscopic course for surgeons.

How to Get It

The path to having a viable CME/CEU product is similar to planning individual or group courses, with the added layer of the credentials process, which will add significant lead time for application approval.

Pro

CME/CEU courses are able to charge higher per learner fees, and when marketed correctly can achieve high attendance. Popular and profitable courses can easily become annually attended seminars.

Con

These courses require a long lead time, significant paperwork, and issuing authority expenses must be considered in budget planning.

Vendor Courses

Medical supply and equipment vendors of all types want a realistic space to demonstrate new products and train healthcare professionals on the correct usage of their existing line. Demonstrations are also done for their own internal employees, especially sales and marketing, to expose them to the correct demonstration and usage of the companies' products in the healthcare environment. Some of these training sessions are held directly in hospitals and practice settings, but increased regulation and privacy concerns can make this difficult and scheduling impossible. A second option is to hold these sessions in a hotel meeting room, but this option lacks any sense of realism.

A simulation center that has gone to any lengths to recreate a patient care environment can provide a demonstration and training venue that is free from any patient privacy concerns and likely has less scheduling conflicts than a typical hospital.

Example

An ultrasound vendor is releasing a new model of bedside, portable ultrasound machine, and wants to demonstrate the model for local physicians considering the purchase. A patient bed and an ultrasound task trainer could be all that are required.

How to Get It

Consider vendors the center already works with. Next consider any vendor whose products can be adequately demonstrated at the center. Nearly any healthcare vendor is going to have demonstration, sales, or training needs on either a regular or at least product launch basis. Start with the sales representative for vendors you currently work with. A second starting point is any vendors who have regional headquarters or offices located in your market.

Pro

Vendors are aware of the increasing difficulty in trainings within patient care areas and the downside of a plain hotel meeting room space. Priced right, this type of client can become a regular source of revenue. Additionally, if the vendor has a product line that the simulation program is considering purchasing, training space can be provided in lieu of equipment or supply donations.

Con

While not specifically a con, as more simulation programs open in a region, more competition will exist for this business.

Product Demonstrations/Testing/Patents/Licensing Development

While on its surface this opportunity seems similar to vendor product demonstrations and trainings, there are some specific differences that must be considered.

Example

A vendor (or even an inventor) still in development wants to test a potential new product at a simulation center owing to lack of access in a hospital.

How to Get It

A university-based center will likely have a Technology Transfer or Development department that will have contacts in this area. Otherwise, look for any regional business incubator non-profits, entrepreneur groups, biomedical engineering departments, or local business schools.

Pros

This is very likely to require little or no staff time. Remember to require they bring or pay for any supplies consumed. If inventors are internal to the institution, the center will likely not derive any revenue, but may have some PR benefit from being the development and testing location if the device is ever produced.

This is an avenue that is not likely to generate significant revenue; however, more importantly, it is an opportunity to make connections with potential inventors. This is important, as they can become partners when someone at the center identifies an opportunity to develop a new product such as a novel task trainer.

Cons

Each instance is likely a one-time deal, so chasing the business is often not worth the time. The major consideration is that product testing, by its nature, can potentially cause significant damage to simulation equipment. Contracts with damage fees or replacement costs should be developed and signed and considered in package pricing.

Simulation Training for Medical Conferences

Simulation centers located in urban areas with frequent medical conferences may benefit from renting out space around the dates of the conference for demonstrations and hands-on training. Either vendors or the conference association itself wishes to create add-on mini-courses as pre- or postconference.

Example

During an infection control conference, a vendor may wish to hold hands-on training for a new product line. Typically, these are done in a meeting room at a conference center, but a nearby simulation center can provide a more realistic environment and more productive training, and generate more interest in the training itself.

How to Get It

Meet with the local convention and visitor's bureau and convention center staff. They have sales people who are working with conferences, often years in advance, and a tour of a simulation center for them can be another valuable tool to help sell a particular market to conference organizers. A second route, but more time-consuming, is to watch for local conference announcements and contact planners directly. This is generally too late to secure pre- or postconference options, but this approach can lead to a list of vendors to whom you can offer the option of realistic demonstrations or trainings.

Pro

These types of trainings will generally be fully supported by the conference organizers or vendors, and the simulation center is simply providing the space and equipment. Vendors may even bring in extra equipment to supplement what already exists.

Con

Conferences have long planning timelines, often years, and convincing organizers to have a group leave the conference facility is sometimes difficult. Scheduling should also be carefully handled, as conference attendees are notorious for signing up for sessions and not attending. Equipment and space may also incur damages that need to be accounted for with an agreed process for how to deal with such an event.

Long-Term Partner Contracts

In addition to revenue generation from local institutions, these same institutions can also become partners, and long-term agreements can be valuable to both institutions. Experienced programs should explore these types of agreements as they can provide long-term revenue, expense saving, and potential research partners.

Example

A simulation program can contract with residency programs in the region to run intern boot-camp trainings every year, consisting of procedural station rotations before they begin significant patient interaction. Residency programs can use this training to both demonstrate their preferred procedural method and to assess intern proficiency.

Long-term agreements with local partners can also become expense saving opportunities. For example, a simulation program can contract with faculty at other institutions to help teach courses (after adequate educator training), in exchange for simulation time for their students. This traded time can be limited to days or times when the program is not normally busy, thereby saving educator expenses and utilizing unused time.

One caution to this latter expense saving opportunity: Providing "free" training time to an institution can devalue simulation training and preclude the institution from ever being willing to pay for the services. Be sure this expense saving does not cannibalize a potential revenue client.

How to Get It

Any local institution that is considered a potential client should also be considered a potential long-term partner.

Pros

If revenue is charged, it is external to the institution and true revenue. Long-term agreements can cut down on the time needed to sell course-by-course.

Cons

Once the concept of trade deals and partnerships is introduced, it can often be poached by institutional leadership for mission goals beyond the simulation program. These institution-wide missions may take away specific simulation revenue opportunities, but add value to the parent institutions.

ACGME Resident Training

The Accreditation Council for Graduate Medical Education (ACGME) rules allow some procedure trainings done in simulation to count toward competency requirements. Depending on an institution's patient mix, there may be certain procedures that are more difficult for residents to experience.

How to Get It

For any institutions with residents, a meeting with GME leadership can determine which procedures are less frequently seen in the current patient mix. If these procedures can be appropriately simulated at the program an ongoing resident training program can be created.

Pro

Even if there is no revenue charged, this type of advanced procedural training is the type that can easily be turned into training programs for external learners.

Con

If the residency program is part of the simulation program's own institution, there will not likely be a revenue gain.

New Team or Facility Testing

Newly formed healthcare teams, group practices, clinics, and even hospitals benefit from testing of their staff and procedures before providing patient care. Simulation program teams are in a unique position to help provide this team testing.

Example

In anticipation of opening a clinic, the team can be brought to a simulation program and scenarios similar to what will be seen in the clinic can be run through on medium and high-fidelity mannequins.

How to Get It

Knowledge of the local healthcare market and planned openings is necessary.

Pro

This type of service can and should carry a significant price tag, as the curriculum planning could be time-consuming.

While the opportunities are not likely to come along often, depending on the size of the facility, a large number of teams can be tested.

Con

The flip side is that a large facility can require a large volume of teams to be tested in a very short time frame. Additionally, be prepared for the question of in situ testing to come up. If the center is not prepared or not willing to conduct in situ simulation, this needs to be discussed up front.

RELATED BUSINESS LINES

AHA Certification Courses

Hospital staff, nurses, and physicians all require some type of American Heart Association (AHA) certification renewals on a biannual basis. More and more healthcare settings are requiring additional certifications for staff, and not all provide the training in-house.

Example

There are three levels of involvement with AHA certifications for a simulation program. At the lowest level of resources, credentialing and costs, a staff member is certified as an educator in one or more AHA disciplines, and courses are offered through the program. The next level of commitment is when a center becomes a Training Site and has many educators affiliated with them as a site (these are not necessarily employees) and derives some revenue from courses these educators conduct, either at the center or elsewhere. The largest commitment in resources, costs, and credentials is for a center to become an AHA Regional Training Center. This means that not only are educators affiliated, but also the center must take on oversight of other Training Sites in the region.

There are specific credentialing requirements for all three examples, and both the Training Site and Training Center levels have specific liability insurance requirements. However, all are likely already met by a simulation center's staff and institution.

Pro

AHA certification is required for healthcare professionals in hospitals, and that requirement is expanding to more and more roles. Renewals are every 2 years, and many hospitals do not provide certifications internally. The AHA allows instructors, Training Sites, and Training Center to set their own prices, and this line of business can be both high volume and profitable. The recent addition of computerized testing allows centers to have even greater flexibility in scheduling certifications and is less dependent on having educators.

Con

AHA certification courses and Training Site or Center management can be labor intensive and will require at least one FTE staff position, depending on the size of the program. Management of this training is highly detailed, and oversight is paperwork intensive. However, this is not unusual for other areas of healthcare, and staff with experience is likely used to this.

Other Certification Courses

While AHA and International Liaison Committee on Resuscitation (ILCOR) certifications are the most widespread in healthcare, there are several other certifications that can take place in a simulation program, if the program meets the requirements.

The American College of Surgeons requires several different certifications for various subspecialties—Advanced Trauma Life Support (ATLS), Pre-Hospital Trauma Life Support (PHTLS), Fundamentals of Laparoscopic Surgery (FLS), and the forthcoming Fundamentals of Robotic Surgery (FRS) and Fundamentals of Endoscopic Surgery (FES). The American Society of Anesthesiologists requires Maintenance of Certification in Anesthesiology (MOCA) courses.

In addition, there are many other certifications across specialties and disciplines, and the trend will grow in the future with more opportunities to provide advanced training courses. These courses, like AHA certifications, have specific requirements in locations, instructors, and Course Directors.

Example

ATLS and PHTLS courses are offered throughout the country on a monthly basis and are required for paramedics, surgeons, and emergency physicians. Partnering with the department of Surgery can likely provide qualified instructors, and most simulation programs would likely meet facility and staffing requirements.

How to Get It

Just as with the AHA, there are specific requirements for each accrediting body for applying to run courses, resources and Instructors available, and facilities and equipment.

Pro

ATLS courses often charge rates of $1,000 USD per learner and higher, and nearly all of the equipment and supply needs would be found in a larger simulation center. ASA MOCA courses range from $1,500 to 2,000 USD per learner, and if you have a robust anesthesiology simulation program, your courses are likely well on their way to meeting requirements.

Con

These courses are resource and labor intensive, and some are 2-day courses. While total revenue per course can be high, so can expenses if not managed carefully. They are also specifically regulated by their accrediting bodies, and application process can carry an expense of a few thousand dollars and can require months of up-front work.

For the Novice

By now, hopefully you have generated a list of ideas for sources of funding to help support your simulation program, but where do you start? Start with a meeting of the program's leadership. There should be agreement on which revenue opportunities will be pursued and how they are prioritized. It is also an opportunity to keep the program's primary mission in mind. It is likely not revenue generation, and the pursuit of partial funding should keep this mission top of mind so opportunities can be considered that will complement current activities and not interfere.

An important next step is to meet with the parent institution's leadership to ensure everyone is fully aware of any specific policies that would impact on a decision to pursue certain revenue streams. Lastly, keep in mind the power of a pilot test. Before getting to the point of marketing a course, make sure it is the strongest course possible. Offering it free to an initial small group can provide valuable, external feedback and gain supporters and positive feedback to help sell the course to others.

Finally, remember, this is not about selling courses, certifications, credits, or credentials—it is about offering the opportunity to increase patient safety and enhance patient outcomes.

BEEN THERE, DONE THAT: ADVICE FOR AN EXPERIENCED SIMULATION PROGRAM OPERATION

What if you're an established simulation program that has been training medical students, residents, nursing students, or hospital staff for years? In this case, you have an even greater advantage when you begin to offer training to outside individuals or institutions. Years of experience can hopefully be translated into meaningful and measurable data, which can be turned into a rational business case for using your program.

Start with what the program does best. What is the best course or program offered? Now look at why it is the best course. Is there data supporting improved performance after course completion? Increased patient safety? Reduced harm or error? Improved student new skill acquisition or procedural retention? This data makes the case for why others would want to come to your program to take this training.

SUMMARY

Simulation programs have proliferated over the last decade, but programs that are staffed and equipped right, driven by data, and managed with a vision for growth still have an advantage. The best of these programs can require significant funding to maintain their status at the forefront of a growing industry. That requires revenue, and just like a personal portfolio, the more diversified the sources of revenue, the better the chance the program has to maintain a steady pace of growth into the future.

REFERENCES

The Agency for Healthcare Research and Quality. (2013). *National Implementation of TeamSTEPPS Program Webinar 16: The impact of TeamSTEPPS implementation on medical liability.* Retrieved from http://teamstepps.ahrq.gov/webinars/webinar16.htm

American College of Surgeons, Division of Education. (2013). *American College of Surgeons CME Joint Sponsorship Program.* Retrieved from http://www.facs.org/education/jsp/index.html

The Center for Medical Simulation. (2013). *History of CMS.* Retrieved from http://www.harvardmedsim.org/about-history.php

Kurrek, M. M., & Devit, J. H. (1997). The cost for construction and operation of a simulation centre. *Canadian Journal of Anesthesia,* 44(11), 1191–1195.

Passiment, M., Sacks, H., & Huang, G. (2011, September). *Medical simulation in medical education: Results of an AAMC survey.* Washington, DC: Association of American Medical Colleges.

University of California, San Francisco School of Medicine. (2008, November). *Kanbar Simulation Center Mt. Zion Facility.* Retrieved from http://medschool.ucsf.edu/medicaleducation/KanbarReport2007.pdf

SUGGESTED READINGS

Bank of Canada. (n.d.). *Inflation calculator* and *currency converter.* Retrieved from http://www.bankofcanada.ca

Rosen, K. R. (2008). The history of medical simulation. *Journal of Critical Care, 23,* 157–166. doi:10.1016/j.jcrc.2007.12.004

Society for Simulation in Healthcare. (n.d.). *Find a member.* Retrieved from http://www.ssih.org

Society in Europe for Simulation applied to Medicine. (n.d.). Retrieved from http://www.sesam.ws

CHAPTER 4.2

Establishing a Simulation Program Budget

Stephanie A. Tuttle, MS, MBA

ABOUT THE AUTHOR

STEPHANIE A. TUTTLE is the Administrative Director of the Center for Simulation, Advanced Education and Innovation, at the Children's Hospital of Philadelphia, since 2005 to establish the program. The Board of Trustees had approved a business plan, but while launching the program, she identified gaps in the initial budget and embarked on the challenge of generating a workable budget for the first and ensuing years.

ABSTRACT

A budget is an estimate of income and expenditures for a set time period. Developing a budget establishes not only a financial plan for the organization but an operational one as well. This chapter will provide general guidelines for the development of an initial simulation program budget and ongoing planning for later years. Since policies and practices of each institution vary, only general concepts will be considered. It has been assumed that a needs assessment for the institution has been completed, and a survey of the landscape has been performed to understand what the projected staffing and equipment needs will be for the program. Key aspects of operating and capital budgets will be discussed. Basic definitions for accounting terms will be provided as well as items that may be included in each category. It is recognized that objectives and settings for programs vary significantly, and budget considerations for various institutional situations will be covered, that is, hospital-based vs. university-based. A sample budget spreadsheet with common categories will be provided. While this chapter will not address more complicated accounting statements and transactions, suggested references for the basics of these budgeting facets are provided at the end of the chapter.

CASE EXAMPLE

A hospital leader shares with you that the institution has created a steering committee to explore the possibility of establishing a simulation laboratory to enhance the training programs for clinical staff as a means to improve patient safety. A needs assessment has been done, and he would like to enlist your help with generating the initial and projected 5-year budget to include in the business plan they are drafting. Additionally, he would like to recruit you to administer the program, implement the budget, and assist with ongoing budget planning and projections. Although you have several years of experience as a clinical nursing education specialist, you are not familiar with the budgeting process. You wonder, where can you find a layman's guide to establishing a simulation program's budget?

INTRODUCTION

A majority of simulation programs are located within larger institutions (hospital, university, military, etc.), where a finance or accounting office oversees the institutional budget and provides guidance for budget development and management to the departments. As a result, budgeting for a simulation program is generally not a complicated process once basic concepts are understood.

A budget conventionally covers a specific period of time, typically a **fiscal** year. The defined fiscal year will vary from institution to institution and often will not match, for example, the calendar or academic year. Fiscal planning will include two types of budgets: operating and capital. Operating budgets capture the day-to-day operating revenue and expenses. Capital budgets include higher cost items that have a sustained use and value over time, such as simulation equipment. They also include facilities construction

283

or renovations. In the following sections, both budget types and their components will be discussed as well as considerations for future planning. Regardless of how an institution manages the overall budgeting process, either by spreadsheets or by more sophisticated financial planning software, the basic components of budgeting are the same.

OPERATING BUDGET

Figure 4.2.1 provides an example of an operating budget where various line items are captured. There are literally hundreds of potential categories to track revenue and expenses. However, for departmental budgets, most

SIMULATION CENTER	FY 2013 BUDGET
GROSS REVENUE	
TOTAL OTHER OPERATING REVENUE	
TOTAL REVENUE	
EXPENSES:	
Salary & Wages	
700100000 S&W PHYSICIAN	*238,000*
700300000 S&W NURSE	*38,308*
700400000 S&W ALLIED PROFESSIONAL	*54,080*
700500000 S&W CLERICAL & SECRETARIAL	*44,782*
700600000 S&W OTHER	*511,076*
701000000 S&W OVERTIME	
Salary & Wages	**886,246**
Other/Outside Labor Expenses	
702250000 S&W UNIV P/R	*62,178*
Total Salary Other/Outside Labor Expenses	**62,178**
TOTAL S&W LABOR EXPENSE	**948,424**
Supplies Expense	
750000000 Drugs	*400*
755000000 Iv Component Supplies	*200*
756000000 Medical & Laboratory Supplies	*65,000*
771000000 Minor Equipment	*30,000*
820000000 General Supplies	*500*
822000000 Office Supplies	*6,000*
823000000 Forms	
TOTAL SUPPLIES EXPENSE	**102,100**
Purchased Services and Other Expenses	
809000000 Repairs & Maintenance	*6,000*
809100000 Service Maintenance Contracts	*100,000*
828000000 Duplicating & Printing	*700*
833000000 Travel & Conference	*6,000*
851000000 Purchased Services	*12,000*
851004500 Purchased Serv-Courier Servcs	
863000000 Special Functions	
873000000 Misc Expense	
TOTAL PURCHASED SERVICES AND OTHER	**124,700**
Fringe Benefits	
716500000 Fringes University Payroll	14,052
TOTAL FRINGE BENEFITS	**14,052**
TOTAL DEPRECIATION	
GRAND TOTAL - EXPENSES	**1,189,276**

FIGURE 4.2.1 An example of an operating budget where line items are captured.

institutions limit the categories to approximately 15 to 20. Programs may be funded by various sources; research budgets and sometimes donated funds are managed separately from operating budgets and adhere to the restrictions of the funding sources.

REVENUE/INCOME

Many programs are wholly funded by their institutions, in which case, actual revenue or income would be a rare occurrence, if happening at all. For other programs there is an expectation that the center generate revenue or income to offset expenses or even to bring in a profit to the institution (see Chapter 4.1). **Revenue and income** refer to the positive flow of money into a business. Revenue includes money that has been earned through the provision of services or sale of goods manufactured by the business. Income is generally the increase in assets or decrease in liabilities. Assets, for example, are items of value for the business, such as a building or property. Liabilities are a responsibility or debt that results in an outflow of cash.

If the program is fully funded by the institution, a projection of estimated revenue or income will not be included in the operating budget, and it will consist solely of expense categories and, potentially, recovery of expense. In this case, following negotiation of the annual budget with the parent institution, the program will be expected to manage to budget rather than to manage the anticipated revenue. If the program is expected to raise revenue through courses or special activities, or is partially funded by undesignated donations or grants, these projections will appear at the top of the operating budget as revenue.

Designated research awards, special purpose funds and donations will be tracked separately from the center's operating budget and will have their own individual budgets to allow individual accounting for funds from each source. If the program is supported by various departments, divisions or colleges, the anticipated support from those sources should be listed at the top of the operating budget to assure the creation of a balanced budget.

EXPENSES

Salary and Wages

Salary and wages capture all staff funded by the operating budget and often represents the largest component of a budget. Salary and wages are compensation paid to employees for services provided. Generally, "wages" is a term used to designate payment on the basis of a rate per hour, day, or week worked, for example, "Mr. Smith is being paid $12.00 per hour worked." Salary is quoted on a yearly basis, for example, "Mrs. Jones is being paid $24,960 a year."

Wages may be paid weekly, bi-weekly, and so forth. It is also possible that one or more staff members may be supported by funds from another source, such as a research grant or home department, as with a part-time medical director. In this case, only the salary supported by the simulation program should appear in Salary and Wages. This expense category will contain various staffing categories as designated by the institution, such as physician, nurse, allied professional, clerical, and so forth. Programs that are affiliated with a university may separate out university payroll physicians from hospital salaried physicians. The operating budget generally includes the salary sum for each category and not the individual staff as line items.

Benefits

If the institution includes the cost of fringe benefits as part of each department's operating budget, a line item will be included for this. Often, benefits are not included in departmental budgets, but in some other administrative budget such as Human Resources. If the institution is affiliated with a university, however, although hospital staff benefits may not be listed, there may be a separate line item for university benefits.

Fringe benefits are often calculated as a percentage of total salary for an employee category. Be cognizant that there may be different fringe benefit rates across the institution, depending on the staff members' department and relationship to the institution. Again, only the amount of fringe benefits relative to the staff salary supported will appear in the operating budget.

Supplies

Budgeting for supplies for a simulation program is similar to personal budgeting. When someone purchases a new or used automobile, they also need to consider what other financial impact it will have on their personal expenses. Does this purchase increase or decrease their personal operating expenses, and if so, in what areas. Possibly, they have bought a more fuel-efficient car, which will result in a decrease in gas expense. Or maybe their previous vehicle was 5 years old, and this one is new, so they now need to anticipate paying more for car insurance. As a program plans their budget for the coming year or a period of years, they need to consider the impact that operating changes, such as additional equipment purchases, possible additional space or staff, or an increase in training courses, will have on the operating budget, and adjust accordingly. For example, the purchase of a new mannequin may require the addition of an annual maintenance fee or a budgeted amount for unanticipated repairs or even repair of normal wear and tear. The new equipment might have a replaceable component such as skin, the cost of which will need to be added to the ongoing budget. The addition of a new course may increase consumables such as needles or intravenous tubing or require the purchase of specialized equipment not already owned.

In the category of supplies, expenses are often broken down into expense **subaccounts** to allow for better planning, tracking, and capturing actual expenses at a more detailed level. Allowable subcategories may vary by institutions, but generally include Medical and Laboratory Supplies, Minor Equipment, Office Supplies, and General Supplies. Medical and Laboratory Supplies commonly includes consumables. If the program is affiliated with a hospital, a central supply department may be able to provide medical supplies such as resuscitation cart drug trays, needles, intravenous components, gowns, masks, gloves, medical gases, and so forth. For other programs, they may not have access to a central supply department and will need to purchase these items for external vendors. In these situations, you may also need to budget in related categories such as drugs or intravenous components.

The Minor Equipment category captures equipment of a noncapital nature. Each institution will have a per-item cost over which an expense is considered capital. It may be $5,000 higher or lower. Equipment that falls under this level will be budgeted under minor equipment. This may include task trainers, specialized carts, stretchers, and so forth. The Office and General Supplies category includes the estimated expense for items such as copy paper, mock medication labels, batteries, and so forth.

Purchased Services

Common categories under Purchased Services include Repairs and Maintenance, Service Maintenance Contracts, Duplicating and Printing, Travel and Conferences, and Other Purchased Services. If a center decides to purchase Service Maintenance Agreements, it can represent the second largest expense in a program's budget after salary and wages. For equipment not covered by agreements or warranties, a budget estimate should be made annually for ongoing repair and maintenance. Duplicating and printing would include expenses related to photocopying in the center or utilizing the services of a copy center for course material, brochures, and so forth. When projecting budgets for travel and conferences, refer to the institutional policies regarding what can be reimbursed and international travel. Other purchased services may include consultants, standardized patient actors, and so forth.

Miscellaneous Expense Subaccounts

Other expense subaccounts that may not be used on an ongoing basis, but should be regularly considered, are marketing, presentation/audiovisual services, computer hardware or software, shipping and freight, catering, or rent and utilities. These are by no means the only categories that should be considered, and it is quite possible a center, depending on their objectives, learners and setting, may have a number of additional categories to include. Other considerations for operating budgets will be discussed in the Budget Planning section.

CAPITAL BUDGET

Capital budgeting includes consideration of higher cost items that have a sustained use and value over the time that they will be used, or space planning, facilities renovation or construction, including construction materials. Each institution will have guidelines regarding what qualifies as a capital expense. It may be an item that is over $5,000 or a set dollar amount that is higher or lower with a useful life of a certain number of years. Examples would be medical equipment such as anesthesia machines, high-fidelity mannequins, defibrillators.

If the capital budget is being prepared to create a physical simulation laboratory, in addition to all of the equipment the program will need to launch the course, the budget should also include the architect design expense for the new space and costs related to renovation, construction, and building materials.

Each institution will have a capital budgeting cycle. It may coincide with the operating budget planning cycle, or it could begin several months earlier. Depreciation of capital expenditures will be discussed later in the chapter.

BUDGET PLANNING

Operating Budget

In advance of opening a simulation program, as part of developing the business plan for the new program, a needs assessment should have been completed. Through a review of the needs assessment and business plan, staffing levels, equipment, space and related facilities costs will be identified. These projections will assist with generating the operating budget for the initial year. Business plans typically include a 5-year plan. This will provide information on the foundation for years 2 through 5 in accordance with the expansion outlined in the plan.

An example of a projected 5-year budget is shown in Figure 4.2.2. Limited staff may be budgeted for year 1 as the program begins operations. In subsequent years, as the program becomes more established, the institution comes to recognize the value of simulation and requests incorporation of simulation into training activities increase. The budget in the Business Plan would outline the estimated increase in personnel, equipment, consumables, and so forth on the basis of the projected growth of the program.

During the initial year or during subsequent years, review and planning will be necessary to project adjustments that need to be made to the operating budget and planned capital expenditures. When any type of budget is developed, institutional practice may to be "straight line" expenses (spread evenly) across 12 months or to project a variable flow of expenditures or capital purchases over months or quarters that adjusts to seasonal changes. For example, reflecting increased expense (potentially revenue) associated with the increased training provided new residents and fellows who start in early summer. The

	Year 1	Year 2	Year 3	Year 4	Year 5	Total
STATISTICS						
FTEs	1.5	3	3	3	3.5	3.5
Courses taught	65	100	140	200	260	765
Estimated enrollees	800	1,200	1,600	2,000	2,500	8,100
REVENUES						
Fundraising	$75,000	$25,000	$25,000	$50,000	$75,000	$250,000
Course enrollment	$0	$0	$0	$0	$25,000	$25,000
Total Revenue	$75,000	$25,000	$25,000	$50,000	$100,000	$275,000
EXPENSES						
Labor						
Salaries	$200,000	$279,200	$290,368	$301,983	$336,562	$1,408,113
Benefits	$56,000	$78,176	$81,303	$84,555	$94,237	$394,272
Non-Labor						
Purchased services	$20,000	$0	$0	$0	$15,000	$35,000
Supplies	$33,000	$24,000	$32,000	$40,000	$50,000	$179,000
Service maintenance	$0	$15,000	$15,000	$20,000	$25,000	$75,000
Other	$20,000	$5,000	$5,000	$5,000	$10,000	$45,000
Total Operating Expense	$329,000	$401,376	$423,671	$451,538	$530,799	$2,136,384
Total Operating Support Needed	($254,000)	($376,376)	($398,671)	($401,538)	($430,799)	($1,861,384)
Capital	$108,000	$40,000	$25,000	$0	$0	$173,000
Total Resources Required	($362,000)	($416,376)	($423,671)	($401,538)	($430,799)	($2,034,384)

FIGURE 4.2.2   An example of a projected 5-year budget.

additional expense in these months would be justified as relating to allowing the new staff to improve their medical skills and gain confidence.

Once the budget is developed, it will be important to monitor monthly or quarterly expenses, not only to ensure the accuracy of charges, but also to make adjustments to the flow of the remaining expenses for the year to ensure the budget is not exceeded. A common report provided by Finance and Accounting departments will be the Monthly Financial Report. This is frequently a spreadsheet that displays the approved budget as projected across the 12 fiscal months and the actual posted expenses for each month. There will be columns for the year-to-date budget and expenses as well. Actual expenses will include **accrued expenses** (those expenses that have been incurred, but have not yet posted to the account). The latter is important since it provides a more accurate representation of the budget status.

The calendar for fiscal planning for each institution will vary, but there are several common processes, historically based budget planning and zero-based budgeting.

Historically Based Budget Planning

In this budget planning process, the institution will identify a time to "close the books." This is a process where an accounting period is closed by accruing expenses not yet paid and removing any deferred items. For operating budget planning, the accounting period may be at the end of the second quarter or possibly at the end of the 7th month. This 6- to 7-month period is used to estimate the projected budget for the coming fiscal year. Often, the institution will provide the program with a draft budget for the coming fiscal year based on actual expenses from the chosen accounting period plus planned expenses for the remainder of the current fiscal year. Adjustments will need to be made for planned expenses that did not occur but will during the balance of the current fiscal year. This will also be the time for revisiting the strategic plan for the coming year and adjusting staffing and operating expense projections based on consultation with center staff regarding anticipated replacement of equipment, planned increases in training that will result in an increased need for supplies, new minor equipment that needs to be planned, expected conference travel, and so forth. The assembly of this information will help establish the draft budget to submit through the institution approval process.

Zero-Based Budget Planning

A different approach to the budget planning process is zero-based budgeting. In this budget process, the department is provided a target budget total by the institution. This number may be initially generated by the process described above, but in this situation, it may be adjusted up or down, depending on financial climate and constraints, as well as institutional expectations for departmental or overall institutional revenue and expenses. With this technique, the manager starts with zero dollars in each line item and must build the budget, providing explanations and justification for each amount added. This method provides for close scrutiny of all previous and anticipated expenses and the opportunity to trim costs in certain areas rather than a blanket increase across all categories. A balanced budget would hit the target provided by the institution.

Identification of the causes behind variances will be discussed below along with providing rationale to senior leadership.

Capital Expenses

Capital expenses are items or equipment that have a purchase cost above a certain amount and a life expectancy of several years, usually 3 to 5. This type of expense also includes design costs related to renovations or new building construction, construction costs, and building materials. For ongoing capital expenditures, an institution may provide a lump sum annually that can be used at the discretion of the center director, or they may require the submission of requests for prioritized individual items. In the latter, the requests may be submitted to the Purchasing Department for vendor bidding, or the program may request quotes from vendors and submit an estimated budget amount for that item. In this case, the vendor and actual piece of equipment have been identified. When submitting individual item requests, it is important to remember to include any training, shipping, and installation costs that might be required. Often, the program will be asked to project the quarter the purchase will be made for capital planning purposes. Policies will vary by institution, but if there is a vendor or equipment change in a capital request, senior management approval will often be required. Additionally, if not all capital funds are expended in a fiscal year, there may be an opportunity to request carryover to the coming fiscal year.

BEEN THERE, DONE THAT: HOW CAN I CONTINUE TO IMPROVE OR SUSTAIN WHAT I HAVE ACHIEVED?

The basic development and understanding of the budgeting process is relatively easy. Where skill and experience come into play is as the program grows and expands and planning is needed, as well as possibly justification for additional resources to senior leadership. In the following sections, pitfalls will be discussed along with considerations to be taken to assist with more accurate budget planning.

Avoid Fiscal Year Confusion

Experienced managers become adept at keeping multiple calendars straight, for example, fiscal, academic, and annual. However, it might be difficult for other staff to think in these terms. For example, when discussing a potential purchase for the next fiscal year with a medical director, a recommendation may be made to purchase a piece of equipment in

2015. It will be important to clarify whether calendar or fiscal year is being suggested. This may become especially confusing in preparing a 5-year plan. It may help to talk months and annual calendar and convert to fiscal year later. It is very difficult for people not used to thinking in fiscal periods to make the conversions during conversation.

Be Mindful of Accruing Expenses

In most cases, an expense is not entered into the accounting books until the item or service has been paid. Accrued expenses are those that are entered into the accounting books before payment. This process is utilized where documenting these unpaid expenses allows for more accurate representation of the current status of the budget. For example, for whatever budget planning approach you use, it is important to have as accurate as possible a picture of the status of the budget. Normally, a finance department will not include accrued expenses; however, when a historical snapshot is to be taken to assist with budget planning, they will frequently ask you to provide them with expenses that payment is anticipated on but do not yet appear on your monthly expense statement.

Monitor Various Revenue Sources

There are various types of funding available for creation and ongoing support of a simulation program. If a program is fully funded by its institution, there is generally not a revenue line for this. If the program is part of an academic institution, it may be funded by various departments who contribute a determined amount annually to cover program operations. In this scenario, it would be helpful to list these entities at the top of the budget so receipt of the funds can be tracked and the balance of funding and expenses monitored over time. This can also be achieved by using the combined funds as a target for budget development.

Another arrangement may be that partial funding is being provided from external sources such as foundation support, private donors, corporate grants, and research awards. If these funds are unrestricted, meaning that the source has not put limitations on how they may be spent, they may be grouped with the institutional funds for budget planning. If there are sources that have set limitations on how their funds may be used, a separate account and budget will need to be set up for each source, and the budgets will need to be tracked separately. Remember that the institutional indirect cost rate, costs related to administration and personnel, will need to be applied to the total funds provided, and only the remaining funds are available for the budget.

Ongoing Expenses and Fees

Whether planning next year's budget or adjusting the 5-year budget projection, it is important to remember the impact that purchases or changes this year will make in coming fiscal years. If a mannequin is purchased with capital funds this year, it will likely come with a 1-year maintenance warranty. An often forgotten expense is to budget for the renewal of that equipment's warranty at the appropriate time in the coming years. The same concern applies to certain software licenses where a one-time purchase is made, but a monthly or yearly license fee is required. As equipment is purchased, the expense for the warranties will grow significantly. Although many vendors will offer discounts as the number of purchases increase, warranties frequently become the second biggest expense in a program's budget after personnel.

Recovery of Expense

Recovery of expense occurs when part of a purchase price or expenses related to an occurrence are recovered and added as a line item in the budget expenses. This may occur if a piece of equipment is leased to another institution and that institution makes monthly payments that recoup the cost of equipment for you. Another example might be where you host a course for other institutions. Rather than charging tuition, you might invoice each institution for their fair share of the course expenses. This payment would also be added to the recovery of expense line item.

Budget Variance Justification to Senior Management

The importance of tracking variances and determining their cause was discussed earlier in this chapter. Depending on the size of the variance, justification may be necessary to senior management. A careful monitoring of monthly budget reports is recommended. Regardless of how careful your finance department may be, errors do occur. It is far easier to identify these errors, such as mischarged expenses or duplicate charges, as they happen and have them quickly resolved. Delay may decrease the opportunity to identify the true target for the expense or revenue.

Once the possibility of errors has been ruled out, variance in a subaccount should be analyzed, and the root of the cause identified. Maybe a safety event has resulted in the creation of a new course with a large target audience and requires additional staff or consumable supplies. Possibly there has been a shift in the training schedules within a supported unit or an increase in cancellations due to high patient acuity and census that has not allowed learners to be free for educational activities. If you are not already aware of the circumstances, monthly training records and discussions with the educators will help identify the reason for the variance. Many institutions report training activity as contact hours (The course duration times the number of learners taught; see chapter 5.2 on Metrics). Review of the statistics may demonstrate an increase or decrease in expenses and hourly staff expense as the training numbers fluctuate. This data, supplemented by explanations from staff, is often useful in explaining variances to management.

Workforce Productivity Metrics

Many institutions are now measuring workforce productivity as an opportunity to look for ways to improve work processes and provide leaders with ways to make informed business decisions. Workforce productivity is calculated as the ratio of productive hours over the appropriate unit of service. Productive hours are calculated using the actual paid hours for salaried and hourly staff in the center for a period of time, often a month. In hospitals or academic centers, the unit of service designated for the simulation program may be Patient Visit Days or Inpatient Days, something that is used across the institution. This is a unit that is not directly under the control of the program, and the impact of adjustments to staffing levels or process changes may not be measurable. In this situation, it would be beneficial for the program to develop its own metrics.

One opportunity may be to track educator time spent on various large categories such as Setup and Breakdown of Equipment, Course Development, Teaching, Paid-Time-Off, Administrative Tasks, and Personal Education. If the educators are salaried employees, it may also be helpful to record the actual hours worked. Comparison from month to month of the overall percentage of educator time in each category can be helpful to identify the need to hire another technician to assist with course setup or possibly offloading administrative activities to office administrators to free up time for development and teaching. An unexpected increase in development may require a look at processes to identify potential efficiencies. Tracking actual hours versus budgeted hours helps identify trends in course load and possibly the need to add additional educator staff.

A refinement of this data collection may include projecting what personnel resources will be required for specific courses and then comparing them with the actual time spent on those courses. This is often complicated by the significant variation for one course development to another and the inability to plan for courses that are added during the year and not anticipated during earlier planning.

Once data is collected, it can be analyzed in various ways to demonstrate where educator time is being spent and whether they are working over capacity. It is also possible to link time spent to monthly contact hours; however, if the center does distributed training, it is possible that they may not be physically present at many training courses even though they participated significantly in the course development and early course conduct.

Depreciation

Capital expenditures are generally depreciated over time, and this devaluation expense may be captured in the institutional budget or in the individual department's operating budget as an expense line item. Calculation of depreciation varies among institutions and may be calculated over 3 to 5 years. The Finance or Accounting Office will be able to provide the rate used at a specific institution for inclusion in a department budget.

SECTION 4 • Funding

SUMMARY

Because many simulation programs exist within a larger in-stitution, budget management and planning need be a dif-ficult task. The institution's finance or accounting office will be there to answer questions and provide support during the planning and development process of the initial budget and will assist with annual budget planning and creation. Despite how careful an institution's finance department may be, it is important to review the monthly expense reports they provide to confirm that erroneous expenses have not been applied and expenses have been documented correctly. As experience grows, managers will become increasingly comfortable with identification of factors behind monthly variations and, if necessary, explaining and justifying them with senior management. Gaining experience with tools such as workforce productivity will also provide data to jus-tify addition of staff as the simulation program expands. Budget administration does not need to be complex, but it does require time for careful review and management.

SELECTED READINGS

Lesser, A., & Lesser, G. (2011). *Basic accounting simplified: A primer for begin-ning and struggling accounting students.* Indianapolis, IN: GSL Galactic.

Piper, M. (2013). *Accounting made simple: Accounting explained in 100 pages or less.* Lexington, KY: Simple Subjects.

CHAPTER 4.3

Creating a Fee Structure

Aisha Jamal, CPA, Kelly D. Wallin, MS, RN, and Jennifer L. Arnold, MD, MSc, FAAP

ABOUT THE AUTHORS

AISHA JAMAL is a Senior Project Manager in the Strategic Planning and Business Development department at Texas Children's Hospital. A Certified Public Accountant, with a background in accounting and over 6 years of experience in healthcare finance, she performs and conducts complex financial and statistical analysis for executive leadership and builds financial models for many of the organization's top strategic initiatives. She has leveraged this experience to create and enhance a robust fee structure for the Simulation Center at Texas Children's Hospital.

KELLY D. WALLIN serves as the operational director for the Simulation Center at Texas Children's Hospital. In that role, she is responsible for financial management of the program as well as daily operations, simulation program development, and strategic planning for the center. Since opening the center in 2009, increasing requests for Simulation Center services by external entities led her to partner with the hospital's financial experts to develop a robust and flexible pricing model.

JENNIFER L. ARNOLD is the medical director of simulation program at Texas Children's Hospital. She is an assistant professor in pediatrics, division of neonatology, at Baylor College of Medicine and Texas Children's Hospital. At Texas Children's Hospital, in addition to direction of the simulation program, she is the course director for the simulation-based Neonatal Resuscitation Program, the Integrated Fellows Simulation Training Program and has led the development of simulation-based clinical systems testing initiatives to utilize simulation to identify potential latent threats to patient safety in hospital environments.

ABSTRACT

Using a five-phase process, simulation programs can build a financially sound fee structure consistent with the program's mission and financial needs. Programs should follow the pathways presented for evaluating key elements in the program such as operational activity, organizational goals, and financial philosophies, and for making key decisions that will drive the pricing model. Financial metrics and ratios such as "cost per operating hour" can be built into worksheets, spreadsheets, and other tools for calculating cost and adding markups or discounts to reach a final price. This chapter will present an overview of necessary "ingredients" to consider when building a fee structure for simulation services, and a "recipe" for building a pricing model that meets the needs of the program.

CASE EXAMPLE

SimCenter ABC is a hospital-based simulation program that opened in 2009 with an 8,600 square feet (798.9 m²) main facility, dedicated staff and equipment, and an operating budget completely funded by the hospital. Hospital leaders believed that investing in a high-technology simulation program was an operational expense important to their mission of supporting excellence in patient care, education, research, and safety. Therefore, the operating budget was built as an expense center rather than a revenue center without expectation that the program support itself through fees-for-services. Although a goal for the simulation program was to develop a fee structure to offer programs for external learners in the future, the initial strategic plan focused on supporting the simulation needs of the hospital and its internal staff and physician providers.

Immediately after opening, SimCenter ABC leaders began receiving requests from external entities (e.g., individuals, hospitals, schools, community groups) willing to pay to use or send staff to participate in simulation program activities. With a long list of internal priorities to address in the first few years after opening, a budget that fully supported operations, and no fee structure yet developed, the program's leaders determined that they would hold off pursuing any of these opportunities unless persuaded by a change in circumstances or a particularly compelling request. Within 1 year of opening, both of those persuasive factors presented themselves: (1) The local and national economy went into recession resulting in hospital budget cutbacks, and (2) The hospital was asked to provide simulation training to the city's 5,000 emergency medical service providers.

Given the new circumstances, SimCenter ABC leaders decided that, to sustain as well as continue to grow their new program they would need to place a higher priority on developing ways to offset at least some of the operational cost of running their simulation program. Although they had already made some progress toward that goal by pursuing grant opportunities, there was still no real pricing model or structure for processing financial transactions on a fee-for-service basis. In addition, the professional backgrounds of the program's staff and leaders were in clinical and technical fields rather than finance, thereby limiting their internal resources for building an effective fee structure—where would they even start?

Their journey forward led them to engage experts from the organization's financial, legal, and compliance departments to assist in building a pricing model, financial transaction workflow, and legal agreements. There were many questions to be answered and decision points along the way, including:

- What capacity does the program have to add external learners?
- How are costs calculated for simulation activities in a way that captures direct as well as indirect expenses?
- Once costs are calculated, how are decisions made about market value, markups and discounts, and final pricing?
- How is the income processed when the simulation program is not set up to be a revenue center?
- Should internal users be charged to recoup expenses to support budget?

It turned out that there were many financial, legal, ethical, and philosophical aspects to consider in developing a financially sound simulation program fee structure. SimCenter ABC's journey has progressed in phases as the program developed pricing for its first project, then refined the process and model to use space more efficiently and robustly as additional opportunities arose. Today, the SimCenter ABC team knows they will need to continue to monitor and refine their model as circumstances inevitably change, but they look forward to continuing the journey.

INTRODUCTION, BACKGROUND, AND SIGNIFICANCE

Even the most financially well-positioned simulation programs can encounter financial concerns, and may need to generate revenue to stay operationally viable. In order to generate revenue, a simulation program will need to have a fee structure in place to quickly and easily identify what resources can be leveraged and what potential revenue streams are available. Concerns surrounding funding or fiscal viability don't need to be the primary motivation around the generation of a fee structure. A simulation program that serves as an academic center of excellence will want to maintain a level of standing within the academic community, and there are always motivating factors to be recompensed for the outstanding level of services being provided. Thought should be given as to what competing organizations are doing to ensure that an institution is not underselling its services, especially if your program offers superior services or training.

Very little is found in the current literature to provide specific direction for building a simulation program fee structure. Kyle and Murray (2007) and Levine et al. (2013) discuss the conceptual foundations for overall business models, but stop short of offering practical guidelines, procedures, and tools to price services. Simulationists are, however, nothing if not resourceful, and a review of

networking via e-mail and listservs reveals frequent queries related to how programs price their services and how they determine their fees. Even if one could amass a spreadsheet of pricing points from various simulation programs through survey and networking, there are still many considerations related to individual organizations, regions, and markets that influence final decisions on pricing.

This chapter provides an overview of how to formulate a fee structure for a simulation program. A step-by-step process is offered that includes individualized options for strategizing an approach based on technical financial components (e.g., computing operating cost ratios, facility utilization rates). Several strategic options are presented, and the corresponding benefits and challenges to each approach are highlighted.

PLAN OVERVIEW

A fee structure for a simulation program is a pricing schedule that shows the dollar amounts charged for various courses, workshops, and other activities. It is an essential tool to help potential clients examine services and courses offered. There are five key phases necessary to develop a simulation program fee structure (Figure 4.3.1). Each phase and the steps within are critical to the process and ultimately lay a

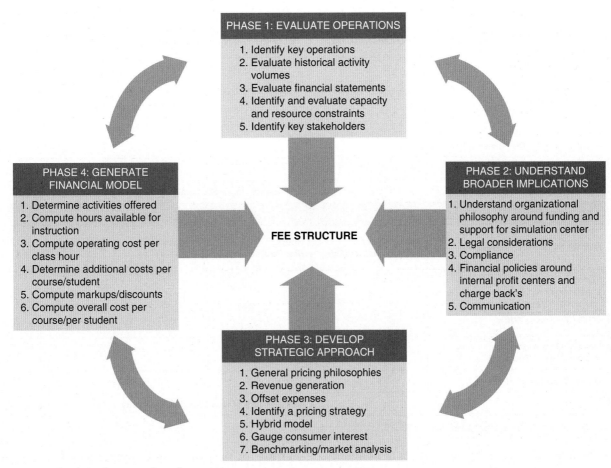

FIGURE 4.3.1 Five phases for generating a fee structure.

framework for a fee structure template that can be customized for pricing out all types of activities and courses. The five key phases for fee structure generation are:

1. Evaluation of simulation program operations
2. Understand broader implications
3. Develop a strategic approach
4. Generate the financial model and fee structure
5. Final analysis and decision-making

PHASE 1: EVALUATION OF SIMULATION PROGRAM OPERATIONS

Evaluating the operations of a simulation program is the first step to creating a fee structure. There must be a good understanding of both the operational and financial data in order to establish an accurate and comprehensive baseline assessment critical to building a fee structure. Programs should consider adopting a consistent methodology, if not already available, to appropriately track the necessary data. The five key tasks in evaluating the operations of a simulation center include identifying key operations, evaluating historical activity volumes, evaluating financial statements, evaluating capacity and resource constraints, and identifying key stakeholders. These will become the building blocks for a successful fee structure template.

Task 1: Identify Key Operations

Begin by determining courses and services (e.g., activities) to be offered. Consider whether the program is interested in renting out space, whether simulation staff and equipment will be included as part of that rental, and whether simulation staff will provide trainings or consultative services. Ensure that a comprehensive list is generated that shows all simulation activities, existing and planned, available for internal and external clients. In our case example, it was useful for SimCenter ABC to separate the "chargeable" activities from those that are "noncharge-able." Chargeable activities are provided to external (and possibly select internal) clients for a fee. A fee is not collected for noncharge-able activities; these may be internal activities funded by the hospital's annual allocation to the simulation program, or they may be activities offered as a community benefit. As discussed later in this chapter, it is helpful to identify community benefit activities for the purposes of governmental reporting. A sample list of activities for SimCenter ABC is included in Figure 4.3.2.

Task 2: Evaluate Historical Activity Volumes

Historical activity volumes will vary from one program to another, depending on how recently the simulation

Activity Name (Chargeable)	# of Learners (Per Course/Activity)	Hours (Per Course/Activity)	Frequency (Per Year)	Annual Hours
Fire Department Course (External Users)	12	8	12	96
High-Fidelity Neonatal Resuscitation Program	24	16	12	192
Proposed Course on Pediatric Advanced Life Support (External Users)	8	4	2	8
Site Tour	24	1	1	1
			Annual Hours of Chargeable Activity	297

Activity Name (Non-Chargeable)	# of Learners (Per Course/Activity)	Hours (Per Course/Activity)	Frequency (Per Year)	Annual Hours
Pediatric Advance Life Support (Internal Users)	8	4	12	48
Acute Care Mock Code	24	8	24	192
Intensive Care Advanced Procedural Skills Training	16	2	48	96
Onsite Workshop	24	1	6	6
			Annual Hours of Non-Chargeable Activity	342

FIGURE 4.3.2   A sample list of activities for SimCenter ABC.

program became operational. If a program is in its infancy, there may be little historical activity to review, and projections will need to be developed to determine what the program is capable of offering based on capacity, equipment, and staff. A new simulation program will want to ensure that key metrics are captured from the inception of the program so operations and activity growth can be tracked over time.

The case example highlights a simulation center that has been operational for several years. Evaluating the historical activity volumes for SimCenter ABC will also determine the facility utilization rate, which shows the extent to which the facility's potential for offering services are being used. An existing program may already have a methodology for tracking the time spent on activities and courses. Refer to columns two, three, four, and five of Figure 4.3.2, which includes fields to capture the number of learners per activity, instruction time per activity, and annual frequency of activity. Based on networking with other simulation programs, a national benchmark for course and instruction time for a simulation program is 70%, with the remaining 30% of time spent on program development and documentation. By having a well-documented list of time spent on all the activities being conducted at a simulation center, a program can evaluate how well they align with national standards.

Task 3: Evaluate Financial Statements

Evaluating the financial statements, specifically the statement of operations, will help administrators understand the general nature of a program's financial structure. The

purpose of the statement of operations is to show how a program uses resources to provide various programs and services. This analysis will determine whether the simulation program is an expense only department or whether there is real or potential revenue to offset operational expenses; the proportion of revenue to expense can then be calculated. If a program is margin neutral, enough revenue is being made to offset expenses without generating any profit or margin. Review as much historical financial data as is available to evaluate trends and growth patterns from both a revenue and an expense perspective. A new program can review monthly financials rather than annual financials as a starting point. A sample Statement of Operations for SimCenter ABC is provided (Figure 4.3.3).

Programs may also utilize the financial statements to begin computing preliminary financial metrics and ratios. For example, benefits as a percentage of salaries can be determined and, if multiple annual financial statements are available, a percent growth can be determined:

- Percent growth from prior year = (Current expense line item amount − Prior year expense line item amount) ÷ Prior year expense line item amount
- Benefits as a percent of salaries = Benefits expense line item ÷ Salary expense line item

Task 4: Identify and Evaluate Capacity and Resource Constraints

Identifying capacity and resource constraints will help determine the pace and tempo at which operations can

SimCenter ABC

DATA IS FOR ILLUSTRATIVE PURPOSES ONLY

Operating Revenue

Operating Revenue	0
Total Stimulation Center Revenue	**$0**

Operating Expenses

Salaries	$450,000
Benefits	$148,000
Professional fees	$50,000
Supplies	$35,000
Purchased services	$25,000
Utilities & maintenance	$35,000
General & administrative	$25,000
Depreciation & amortization	$150,000
Total Stimulation Center Operating Expense	**$918,500**

**Operating Margin/(Loss) = Operating Revenue - Operating Expenses	**($918,500)**

FIGURE 4.3.3   Sample statement of operations.

be conducted. Simulation programs may have different primary constraints, or limiting factors, depending on resources (e.g., rooms, equipment, educators, technicians) available. The most common constraints are rooms and educators. SimCenter ABC has eight simulation rooms but only three educators, so the primary constraint is educators; the number of educators available limits the number of courses that can be offered. This primary constraint will be important for computing hours available for courses (see Phase 4, Exercise 1).

Task 5: Identify Key Stakeholders

It is critical to identify key stakeholders in the simulation program and to continually reassess as the fee structure is being determined. Stakeholders that influence the programming and operations of the simulation program are important to consider. For a hospital-based simulation program, key stakeholder(s) may include:

1. Clinical departments—Clinical departments provide the core learner groups for a hospital-based program and, depending on program structure, may also be the primary source for simulation educators.
2. Treasury—Programs should consider the forms of payment that will be accepted. If credit card or wire transfer payments are considered, engaging the treasury team will ensure the appropriate equipment and processes are in place for implementation.

3. Information services—Programs should engage information services for developing a strategy for online marketing, advertisements, and payment portals if desired.
4. Finance/Accounting—Programs should consider how payments will be accepted and how receipts will be processed. Either the simulation program staff or an institutional finance/accounting team commonly performs these functions. Engaging the finance/accounting team early will ensure the payment process is set up appropriately and will assist in determining classification of revenue and revenue flow. Revenue must be classified and assigned to an account. In many instances, simulation revenue falls into an "Other Operating Revenue" category. If simulation revenue is placed in an operational cost center that is swept from year to year, budget appropriately to ensure funds are adequately spent within the fiscal year. Working closely with the finance and accounting teams will help answer questions surrounding grants, philanthropic revenue, fund flow, and internal payments if necessary.

By identifying key stakeholders and liaising with these groups early in the process, the simulation program will be well situated for the next phase, understanding the broader implications. Stepping back to look at the bigger picture will prompt more questions and will also help identify additional key stakeholders, such as legal, compliance, and government relations.

PHASE 2: UNDERSTANDING BROADER IMPLICATIONS

Partnering with stakeholders will raise many questions that may not have been addressed. To move ahead, there will be a need to understand the organizational philosophy around funding and support for the simulation program. It is important to determine whether the larger organization views the simulation program as a mission-supporting cost center or whether there are expectations for the simulation program to generate revenue. Understanding the organization's view of internal profit centers and charge backs will also inform policy on providing services for internal clients (e.g., clinical departments).

In the case example, SimCenter ABC was a hospital-based simulation program that was viewed as a cost center and completely funded by the organization. Any external client revenue generated, however, was intended to offset operational expenses and allow for operational expansions, including additional staff and equipment. The financial policies for this organization were very clear: there were no internal profit centers or processing charge backs within the organization because they have no real impact on the broader operating margin. All departments within the organization were focused on one mission, and internal profit centers just added complexity in terms of administrative processes and paperwork. A decision was made to charge external clients only to offset costs while being mindful of what the market can bear. This became a key element in choosing a pricing strategy.

For most simulation programs situated within a larger organization, financial and administrative leadership will make these decisions. Through this process, additional organizational offices may be identified as potential stakeholders. SimCenter ABC identified the legal and compliance departments as additional key stakeholders. It was critical to work with the legal and compliance teams because there were viable concerns around disseminating pricing information. For example, there were questions around price fixing, particularly with organizations viewed as having contractual or political partnerships with SimCenter ABC's parent organization. The Stark Law imposes limitations on certain physician referrals by prohibiting referrals of designated health services ("DHS") for Medicare and Medicaid patients if the physician (or an immediate family member) has a financial relationship with that entity. SimCenter ABC's parent organization was a tertiary care center, so any discount offered to an organization that referred patients to the parent organization could be seen as an incentive for referrals and not being in compliance with the Stark Law (see http://starklaw.org/).

Understanding the broader implications for fee structure creation was a significant phase for SimCenter ABC. Only by working with key financial and administrative leadership was SimCenter ABC able to answer key questions and gain a true understanding of what their organization would permit from a pricing standpoint.

PHASE 3: DEVELOPING A STRATEGIC APPROACH

At this stage, an approach and philosophy around pricing will have been identified. These should guide a pricing strategy to meet the outlined objectives. There are numerous pricing strategies available, and a few are listed below for reference.

- "Loss leader pricing" is when a product or service is sold at a low price (at or below cost) in order to stimulate other potential business. This can help gain visibility, community credibility, or it may help expand or potentially capture additional market share.
- "Market-oriented pricing" is when a price is set after conducting analysis and research based on the target market. For instance, evaluating what other simulation programs charge per hour or per course, and then setting a price either above or below that amount to meet the desired objective.
- "Penetration pricing" includes an initial plan of low price setting in order to gain customers and then raising prices once market share is gained.

Once a pricing strategy is chosen, there are numerous options for computing a course or activity price. An approach can be as simple as charging a flat fee for any activity regardless of resource utilization. Alternatively, a very detailed and labor-intensive process of identifying individual elements of a course or service may be computed to determine the overall charge. For our case example, SimCenter ABC decided to compute an overall cost of operations on an hourly basis and then layer in additional costs unique to the course in addition to a scalable markup depending on the client. This approach was a hybrid between a flat operating cost per hour and a more detailed itemization of specific course costs. It utilizes the simplicity of a flat fee structure while maintaining consideration for key elements that may alter the delivery price.

Gauging client interest is important for setting prices, as initially it may be better to start with key courses that are in high demand and then add to the pricing menu as demand for additional courses grows. Networking with peers may help gain a better understanding of which courses are most likely to fill up and how many courses should be included in the pricing menu. At some point, a simulation program will face capacity or resource constraints, and it is important to generate a pricing structure where the conceivable demand will not outpace the supply.

Benchmarking and market analysis will be helpful in determining whether prices being considered are reasonable. One of the struggles faced by SimCenter ABC was the availability of pricing data. Most simulation programs do not make fee structures and pricing information publicly available. SimCenter ABC engaged other centers through networking and listserves to determine comparable pricing. It became apparent, however, that this practice could be viewed as colluding to fix prices which raised another legal and compliance issue. A safer alternative may be to research data that is publicly available and leverage that information to the best possible degree while being mindful that it may be incomplete or imperfect.

PHASE 4: CREATING A FEE STRUCTURE

All the tools and data necessary for creating a fee structure are now in place. The key tasks for this phase include computing the hours available for work, computing an operating cost per hour, computing a cost per course and per student, and determining whether there will be markups or discounts applied to the pricing structure. An Excel file template for creating fee structure can be found online at http://www.ssih.org/News/Defining-Excellence.

Exercise 1: Compute Hours Available for Work

Total working hours per year can be calculated by considering the number of business days available for delivering courses each year. The sample calculation for SimCenter ABC is provided in Figure 4.3.4.

A widely accepted benchmark among simulation programs is to reserve 70% of available time for delivering simulation courses and 30% of available time for planning, pre- and postcourse activity, professional development, and performance improvement activities. For SimCenter ABC, this means that 1,428 course hours are available for delivering courses (70% of 2,040) per year. The total hours for delivering courses should be multiplied by the primary resource constraint, or limiting factor, determined in Phase 1, Task 4. For SimCenter ABC, the primary

constraint is educators. Because SimCenter ABC has three educators, two of whom only spend half their time teaching courses, 1,428 hours is multiplied by 2, resulting in 2,856 available hours for course delivery (Figure 4.3.5).

Exercise 2: Compute Operating Cost per Hour and per Course Hour

Start by leveraging the financial statements evaluated in the third task of Phase 1. Each line item of the financial statement (including total operating expenses) should be divided by the total center hours (from Figure 4.3.5) to determine operating cost per center hour (Figure 4.3.6). Likewise, each line of the financial statement (including total operating expenses) should be divided by the total course hours (from Figure 4.3.5) to determine operating cost per course hour.

This exercise will provide an upper and lower threshold for pricing. For SimCenter ABC, it is best not to charge any client less than $225 USD per center hour because that is the minimal cost to run the simulation center on an hourly basis; charging less than $225 USD per hour would generate a loss. This is not the price per student or per activity; this is the price per hour. This amount can be used if the flat fee pricing strategy was chosen so that at minimum, $225 USD per hour will be charged for any activity provided by the simulation program. However, if SimCenter ABC utilized the higher threshold of $321 USD per center hour, the total cost for development and delivery is being recouped. Any amount charged beyond $321 USD per hour ensures that not only are all costs being recouped but a profit is being made. Once upper and lower thresholds have been set, select the price per hour that reflects a baseline that most adequately meets the objective of your simulation fee structure. To cover costs, use the lower threshold; to start generating profits, use the upper threshold. This can be the platform from which to build prices for each course.

	Oct	Nov	Dec	Jan	Feb	Mar	Apr	May	Jun	Jul	Aug	Sep	Yearly totals
# of business days per month[1]	23	21	22	23	20	21	22	22	21	23	21	22	261
# of holidays[2]	0	1	1	1	0	0	0	1	0	1	0	1	6
Total working days per month[3]	23	20	21	22	20	21	22	21	21	22	21	21	255
Total working hours per month[4]	184	160	168	176	160	168	176	168	168	176	168	168	2,040

Key:

[1] Count of Monday – Friday working days per month

[2] number of holidays per month for your organization

[3] number of business days per month less number of holidays

[4] Total working days × 8 hours per day

FIGURE 4.3.4 Calculation of working hours. *Excel template can be found online at http://www.ssih.org/News/Defining-Excellence*

SECTION 4 • Funding

	A	B	C	D	E	F
1	Resource[1]	% Effort[2]	Annual Center Hours[3]	Total Center Hours[4]	Delivery Benchmark[5]	Total Course Hours[6]
2	Educator 1	1	2040	2040	70%	1428
3	Educator 2	0.5	2040	1020	70%	714
4	Educator 3	0.5	2040	1020	70%	714
5						
6				4080 [7]		2856 [7]

Key:

1 Constraining resource, identified in Phase 1, Task 4

2 Percentage of constraining resource dedicated to delivering course. For educators, this would be percent effort dedicated to instructing. This may not be applicable for other constraining resources (e.g., rooms)

3 Annual number of center hours available to center (from Figure 4.3.4)

4 Total center hours (Percent Effort × Annual Center Hours)

5 Delivery benchmark indicates amount of time program spends on delivering courses. Benchmark used is 70%.

6 Total hours available to deliver courses by SimCenter ABC.

7 Though not shown in this example, number of hours for vacation, personal time, or other time away should be deducted from the total center and total course hours.

FIGURE 4.3.5 Determining total course hours per educator. *Excel template can be found online at http://www.ssih.org/News/Defining-Excellence*

Data is for illustrative purposes only			
	Annual expenses	Operating cost per center hour[1]	Operating cost per course hour
Salaries	$450,000	$110	$157
Benefits	$148,500	$36	$52
Professional fees	$50,000	$12	$18
Supplies	$35,000	$9	$12
Purchased services	$25,000	$6	$9
Utilities & Maintenance	$35,000	$9	$12
General & Administrative	$25,000	$6	$9
Depreciation & Amortization	$150,000	$37	$52
Total Operating Expenses	**$918,500**	**$225**	**$321**

Key:

1 For case example, center hours are 4,080 (see Figure 4.3.5, cell D6).

2 For case example, course hours are 2,856 (see Figure 4.3.5, cell F6)

FIGURE 4.3.6 Example of calculating cost per center hour and cost per course hour. *Excel template can be found online at http://www.ssih.org/News/Defining-Excellence*

CONSIDER THIS

A QUICK WAY TO ESTIMATE COST/HOUR
Christine S. Park, MD, and Paul J. Pribaz, MS

For an established simulation program, a quick and easy way to determine an approximate baseline cost of providing service (a break-even price) is to take the prior year's operating budget and divide by the total hours of operation, divided again by the number of discrete simulation spaces. For example, a two bay simulation program may have a $600,000 annual budget, which, divided by 2,000 hours of annual operation and two rooms, equals $150/room/hour. Note that this figure should be used only for internal consideration, as it does not include several allowable components of cost that should be included in calculating the price charged, most significantly depreciation expense.

A program may be tempted to consider charging a "membership" price, perhaps based on headcount or potential users, to utilize service on an ad hoc basis. However, this model is problematic for several reasons. First and foremost, it does not comply with the federal costing guidelines, as the prices paid are not allocable to the activity. Second, without a careful administrative strategy, some users will receive more benefit than others, whether because of being proactive in reserving space or a better communication strategy.

Exercise 3: Compute a Cost per Course and per Student

Use the data generated in Phase 1, Task 1 (Figure 4.3.1), to compute a cost per course. The example that follows will compute a cost per course and per student for SimCenter ABC's High-Fidelity Neonatal Resuscitation Course. To ensure total costs are considered, any additional supplies needed for this course are included.

Example calculations for Neonatal Resuscitation Course are outlined below.

Step 1: Determine an overall cost per hour for operating the simulation center
$321 USD per hour (using upper threshold for hourly pricing)

Step 2: Multiply the cost per hour times the number of hours in the course
$321 USD per hour × 16 hours = $5,136 USD per 16-hour course

Step 3: Determine any unique course-specific elements that need to be included, such as meals, parking, consultants, embedded simulated persons licensing fees and supplies, to name a few.
$500 USD per 16-hour course

Step 4: Take the sum of the overall cost per hour and the unique course-specific elements
$5,136 + $500 = $5,636 USD per 16-hour course

Step 5: Divide the result obtained in Step 3 by the number of students in the given course
$5,636 USD per 16-hour course ÷ 24 students = $234 USD per student per course

Exercise 4: Compute Markups or Discounts

Once an overall cost price per course and per student is generated, evaluate each rate for potential markups so that all course revenue can be maximized. In addition to markups, also evaluate the course for potential discounts. Discounts for partner organizations may be beneficial but should be evaluated with the Stark Laws in mind and in conjunction with senior leadership in regard to an overall pricing philosophy.

SimCenter ABC determined the best way to avoid potential Stark Law violations or compromising situations was to offer only marginal discounts (10% or less) to organizations with which there were established relationships. Since the goal of SimCenter ABC was to generate the maximum potential revenue, a markup was applied to most courses. However, the markup had to be within reason, so the markup percentages varied according to the number of learners per course, and the frequency with which the course was being offered. We evaluated comparable simulation programs to ensure our prices would not be above the market or industry standards.

PHASE 5: FINAL ANALYSIS AND DECISION-MAKING

After baseline course rates, discounts, and markups have been determined, the following points should be considered before finalizing the fee structure:

- Degree of profitability for the venture
- Degree of interest from external clients based on price
- Overall cost-benefit analysis
- Value of "community benefit" versus "fee-for-service"
- Impact of grant funding

Once pricing for each course is in place, programs should determine whether this will be a profitable venture for your program. If there is no consumer demand, no interest in the courses offered, or an inability to bring in external learners, the likelihood of generating revenue may be low. If the amount of revenue generated is immaterial but the corresponding level of effort either for the simulation program or other teams within the organization is too high, it may no longer be financially viable for the organization to pursue this effort. Conducting a cost-benefit analysis may be beneficial in determining overall strategy for the simulation program. Programs may decide that generating some profit is better than no profit at all or that generating a loss is worth the exposure. This is not an exact science, and the final decisions should be made by simulation program and organizational leadership on the basis of work from the prior phases.

SECTION 4 • Funding

PROS AND CONS OF APPROACH

There are positives and negatives of the "hybrid" approach taken by the case study example, SimCenter ABC. This method is a simple way to compute prices as it utilizes a flat per hour fee (upper threshold for hourly pricing) and adding in additional pricing components. A potential negative is that there is a level of "double dipping" since the overall operating cost per hour is inclusive of all financial statement line items, yet course-specific elements were added. Since the philosophy for SimCenter ABC was to maximize potential course revenue, this was not necessarily problematic. The course price inflation was justified by the need for expansion and items that may not have appeared in the historical financial statements. However, the overall decision to utilize this approach came from a need to maximize potential course revenue, yet have a flexible and easy way to compute course prices by only changing very few variables. As SimCenter ABC moves forward and develops new courses, they can easily compute new prices based on more current data.

BEEN THERE, DONE THAT: HOW CAN I CONTINUE TO IMPROVE OR SUSTAIN WHAT I HAVE ACHIEVED?

There will be an adjustment period after the development of a fee structure, because developing prices that seem reasonable may not necessarily attract clients as expected. Prices may need to be adjusted depending on client reaction. Programs should be mindful of other alternatives and consider investigating opportunity costs, especially as activity nears capacity, to ensure the simulation program is taking advantage of the best available options. Opportunity cost is defined as the value of the best alternative forgone. This isn't always a monetary value. For example, if a simulation program is capacity constrained and has to choose between two courses to be provided, there may be potential cost, revenue, or even relationship implications from those choices.

If a course only generates minimal profits, and the complexity of billing and administrative paperwork becomes intolerable, programs should evaluate other options. For instance, grant funding may generate more revenue or exposure than external client activity. Another option for generating simulation program exposure and value may be reporting activity as a community benefit. Programs may partner with the organization's Community Benefits team to determine whether simulation program activity meets the appropriate criteria for being reported as a community benefit. Community benefit operations include costs associated with assigned staff and community health needs and/or assessment, as well as other costs associated with community benefit strategy and operations. There is a three-step process and list of questions that an organization must follow to determine whether a program or activity should be reported as a community benefit. Additional information can be found at http://www.chausa.org/communitybenefit/what-counts

SUMMARY

Developing a simulation program fee structure may seem like an overwhelming task! There is no one right way to develop a fee structure, and it may vary depending on organizational mission and objectives. Care should be taken in identifying the organizational philosophy around funding and partnership with key stakeholders. The process of evaluating operating costs and determining a pricing strategy provides an opportunity to understand programmatic capacity, resource constraints, and opportunities for growth. Once established, the fee structure should be reevaluated as needed to remain competitive while continuing to work toward programmatic goals.

REFERENCES

Geissel, T. S. (1990). *Oh, the places you'll go!* New York, NY: Random House.

Kyle, R. R., & Murray, W. B. (Eds.). (2007). *Clinical simulation: Operations, engineering, and management.* San Diego, CA: Academic Press.

Levine, A. I., DeMaria, S., Schwartz, A. D., & Sim, A. J. (Eds.). (2013). *The comprehensive textbook of healthcare simulation.* New York, NY: Springer.

CHAPTER 4.4

How to Write a Thorough Business Plan

M. Scott Williams, PhD, MBA, and Danyel L. Helgeson, MS, RN

ABOUT THE AUTHORS

M. SCOTT WILLIAMS is the Associate Superintendent of Instruction and Student Services at Tulsa Technology Center in Tulsa, Oklahoma. He holds a PhD in Occupational Studies from Oklahoma State University, an MBA in Business Administration from Northeastern State University, and a BBA in Management from Northeastern State University. Scott's previous experience includes work as a business consultant, management instructor, campus administrator, Chief Workforce Officer, Director of Workforce Development, and Dean of Academic Affairs.

DANYEL L. HELGESON recently completed her tenure as Interim Associate Dean of Allied Health and Chief Nursing Officer at Riverland Community College, where she provided local and statewide leadership in simulation, allied health, and nursing education. She received her MS and BSN from Winona State University in Winona, Minnesota. Danyel currently attends Yale University, where she is enrolled in the Doctorate of Nursing Practice Program in Leadership, Management, and Policy.

ABSTRACT

Simulation programs around the world often operate as small businesses anywhere from one employee and a mannequin, to moderate/large businesses with multiple sites, multiple mannequins, and employees. Unfortunately, many simulation programs have not applied a crucial business best practice—the development, implementation, and evaluation of a business plan. This chapter will provide an overview of the two common forms of business plans: the start-up plan and the operational plan. The significance of business planning, how to write a plan, and what considerations should be evaluated are presented. A template of a business plan will be provided. Additionally, plan improvement, sustainability, best practices, and challenges will be identified.

CASE EXAMPLE

SimCENTER has been operational for 6 years. They are experiencing multiple issues affecting the functionality of their high-technology simulators, audiovisual equipment malfunctions, and computer crashes owing to outdated systems. Downtime related to nonfunctional equipment recently cost the simulation program one major training contract and reduced service to the School of Medicine by 20%. A general financial assessment indicates that additional funding to update the technology and equipment in the center must be sought. Without a new funding source, it is likely that major stakeholders will be unable to utilize the core products—the high-technology simulators and task trainers at SimCENTER. Lenders have indicated that the simulation program must present a business plan to be considered for funding. SimCENTER was built with grant funds, and a business plan was not developed at the time of inception.

Leaders at SimCENTER determined that the creation of a business plan was imperative to ensure the future of the institution. You are the manager for SimCENTER and have never written a business plan. Where does one start?

INTRODUCTION AND BACKGROUND

The healthcare simulation literature is abundant with architectural drawings of simulation centers, audiovisual layout diagrams, and lists of simulators necessary to outfit a center, but what seems to be needed operationally is information regarding business planning for a simulation program (Kyle & Murray, 2007). With the quick rise of simulation programs (and the centers that house them) and fairly abundant funding during the 2000s, managers and educators were able to build centers without a business plan to secure start-up funding. Since the economic downturn, funding for these programs has decreased in many areas, grant availability and accessibility has decreased,

301

competition for money has increased, and yet simulation programs still require funding to sustain and grow. A realistic business plan has never been more valuable or more necessary.

Additionally, the opportunity for Healthcare Simulation Programs to become accredited by the **Society for Simulation in Healthcare** has reinforced the need for a mindful approach to program organization and management. Core Standard Two, *Organization and Management*, of the Accreditation Standards of the Council for Accreditation of Healthcare Simulation Programs, lists the specific need for simulation programs to have "an organizing framework that provides adequate resources (fiscal, human, and material) to support the mission of the Program" and that "there is a plan designed to accomplish the mission of the Program" in which "the goals for the future of your program and how they will be achieved (e.g., business plan/strategic plan/operational plan)" are identified (Society for Simulation in Healthcare, 2013).

This chapter will provide an overview of the two common forms of business plans, the significance of planning, how to write a plan, and what considerations are included in the process. A template of a business plan will be provided. Additionally, plan improvement, sustainability, best practices, and challenges will be identified.

PLAN OVERVIEW

A business plan is a written document that provides an in-depth overview of the business, in this case, a Healthcare Simulation Program. Business plans are typically found in two common forms, each serving a specific purpose for which the business or organization was completed. These include a start-up business plan, which is commonly used as a selling document, and an operational business plan, generally developed and maintained as a management tool. It is important to note that the two types of plans are not mutually exclusive. A start-up plan can develop into and be retained as an operational business plan, for example.

While there are differences in a business plan as it relates to specific content, there is a general theme that can be observed with regard to the specific sections that are addressed in the plan. These include a product and service plan, a marketing plan, a management plan, an operating plan, and a financial plan. The product and service plan identifies and describes the product and/or service. The marketing plan outlines the target market, describes the unique characteristics of the target market, and the strategy behind how the product or service will be presented to that market. A management plan summarizes how the business itself will be managed and led as it pursues the marketing plan in delivering the product or service described in the product and service plan. The operating plan entails what strategies management will pursue in operationalizing said practices. The financial plan is the core underpinning of the other sections of the business plan. It contains **pro-forma** accounting statements under varied scenarios. This is typically seen as an Income Statement, a Cash Flow Statement, and a Balance Sheet. If the plan is a start-up plan, then the pro forma statements make projections for the first 3 years, with the first year having monthly totals and the remaining 2 years illustrated in quarterly segments. The scenario typically includes the best case, the worst case, and the most likely. If the plan is an operational business plan, then a single set of accounting statements for the most likely scenario is often used.

SIGNIFICANCE

Regardless of the type of plan, a well-written, detailed business plan for your simulation program will provide great benefit at the start of the program and as part of the day-to-day operations and management. A quality start-up plan will increase the likelihood of securing appropriate funding for the site, equipment, and human capital. An operational plan provides a clear picture of where and how money moves through the program, the strengths and weaknesses of the program, and the current and future opportunities and threats to the program.

THEMES

In the business world, it is a fundamental expectation that a business will create, maintain, evaluate, and revise a business plan if it is to succeed. When proceeding with business planning, be aware that much of the planning texts available tend to focus on business planning for individual, small businesses and not large institutions or simulation programs.

While these texts provide an accurate overview of business planning and are excellent resources, writing a plan is a time-consuming process. Program managers may want to consider hiring a consultant to assist with the planning process. Networking with other program managers (especially accredited programs) may also be beneficial. A business plan is usually considered an internal, confidential document, so be aware that others may not be able to share their plan (Covello & Hazelgren, 2006a, 2006b; McKeever, 2005).

PLAN COMPONENTS AND CONSIDERATIONS

This section will address the components of a business plan and provide questions for your consideration. Please note that these components and considerations are not specific to any one type of plan. Further additional information should be added to a plan over time, especially as the start-up plan evolves to an operational plan or changes occur.

The following section should serve as a guide, and all elements may not necessarily be relevant to your type of simulation program. The development of a plan should be approached with a strategy to customize the plan to the unique and specific needs of your simulation program. All areas discussed in the following sections are demonstrated in the appendix of this chapter.

Executive Summary

The Executive Summary of a Business Plan is a one- or two-page distillation of your entire plan, and is usually the last section to be written. A first-time reader should be able to read the Summary by itself and know what your plan is all about. The Summary should stand alone and should not refer to other parts of your plan. Remember, most readers will never get any further than your Executive Summary, so make it count! The Summary includes an introductory paragraph introducing the Executive Summary. Include a brief summary of your Company Overview. Then provide brief summaries of your Product Description, Marketing and Sales, Operations and Management, and Financial Plan sections.

EXPERT'S CORNER

INTERACTING WITH BOARDS

Bonnie Driggers, MS, MPA, RN
Board of Directors, Society for Simulation in Healthcare

Developing and implementing a business plan for your simulation program may require approval by your organization's Board of Directors or Board of Trustees. It is important to understand how best to interact with the board and understand their role.

First, get to know the board members—who they are, what their passions are, what specific competencies they bring to the board, and how they, through other groups, might support or block your agenda. Who is the finance wizard? Who has clinical competency? Who knows the safety literature? Who knows what simulation in healthcare is? This is good information on the off chance you get an expected or unexpected opportunity to interact with a board member or the board as a whole.

But one caution: know your organization's rules and culture related to contacting individual board members. Board members are volunteers who often have limited time, so make the most of the time that you have them. Be respectful of their time by being concise in your message, utilizing key points (15-second elevator speech or the use of executive summaries), while offering greater detail as desired. Find a champion on the board to keep informed about your program.

When interacting with the board, remember that the role of the board is mission-driven, with responsibility far broader than your specific program. Linking your program to larger organizational initiatives (e.g., safety, lean, or quality) may demonstrate interdependence and be seen favorably by the board. Also, find out the committee structure of the board and how you might link to a committee. One strategy is to volunteer a member of your staff or simulation advisory team to serve on the committee(s) that you think will provide greatest visibility for your program to decision makers.

When seeking financial approval for your program, ongoing funding, or funding for expansion, be prepared with data to support your request. Creating legitimacy for your program requires that you understand the value of the program for various stakeholders. The value can be defined through data that you collect and share. Data may take many forms, from utilization, to testimonials, to research reporting potential returns on investment, or literature reporting best-known practices, mandates from regulators, legal, and ethical groups, to annual reports of activity- and program-specific outcomes (Barsuk et al., 2009; Cohen et al., 2010; Draycott et al., 2006; Patterson et al., 2013; Siassakos et al., 2009; Wheeler et al., 2013; Young-Xu et al., 2013).

Boards have a fiduciary responsibility, which includes being good stewards of the organization's finances so they will look for a return on investment (*ROI*). With funding comes responsibility and accountability. The board will ask what impact the funds provided have had, and you will need to be prepared with data to answer the questions. They will also want to know what the consequences of not funding a program will be, so be prepared to answer the question in your business plan or when presenting your proposal.

Be sure to have a strategy for keeping the board informed. You may consider inviting the board to see the simulation facility. Inviting the board to attend simulation center tours, especially when there is community or political exposure, can be beneficial. If your organization has a "take your child to work day" or some other family-oriented activity, invite the board of directors to visit and participate.

Most importantly, boards don't like surprises, so anticipate their need for information. They also like options, as they are regularly presented with competing priorities and requests. Phased proposals are usually appealing, so should be considered when possible.

In conclusion, have a solid, anticipatory business plan, and keep the board informed of any variances. Business plans are a vehicle to obtain funding, keep boards current over time, and support sustainability. They also serve as a guide for short- and long-term planning and for holding programs accountable. Creating and maintaining relationships with board members and the board as a whole is important to obtaining funding for programs and for program sustainability over time.

REFERENCES

Barsuk, J. H., Cohen, E. R., Feinglass, J., McGaghie, W. C., & Wayne, D. B. (2009). Use of simulation-based education to reduce catheter-related bloodstream infections. *Archives of Internal Medicine, 169*(15), 1420–1423.

Cohen, E. R., Feinglass, J., Barsuk, J. H., Barnard, C., O'Donnell, A., McGaghie, W. C., & Wayne, D. B. (2010). Cost savings from reduced catheter-related bloodstream infection after simulation-based education for residents in a medical intensive care unit. *Simulation in Healthcare, 5*(2), 98–102. doi:110.1097/SIH.1090b1013e3181bc8304

Draycott, T., Sibanda, T., Owen, L., Akande, V., Winter, C., Reading, S., & Whitelaw, A. (2006). Does training in obstetric emergencies improve neonatal outcome? *British Journal of Obstetrics and Gynaecology, 113*(2), 177–182.

Patterson, M. D., Geis, G. L., Falcone, R. A., LeMaster, T., & Wears, R. L. (2013). In situ simulation: Detection of safety threats and teamwork training in a high risk emergency department. *BMJ Quality & Safety, 22*(6), 468–477.

Siassakos, D., Crofts, J. F., Winter, C., Weiner, C. P., & Draycott, T. J. (2009). The active components of effective training in obstetric emergencies. *British Journal of Obstetrics and Gynaecology, 116*(8), 1028–1032.

Wheeler, D. S., Geis, G., Mack, E. H., LeMaster, T., & Patterson, M. D. (2013). High-reliability emergency response teams in the hospital: improving quality and safety using in situ simulation training. *BMJ Quality & Safety, 22*(6), 507–514.

Young-Xu, Y., Fore, A. M., Metcalf, A., Payne, K., Neily, J., & Sculli, G. L. (2013). Using crew resource management and a "read-and-do checklist" to reduce failure-to-rescue events on a step-down unit. *The American Journal of Nursing, 113*(9), 51–57.

Company Overview (Healthcare Simulation Program Overview)

The Company Overview is a brief (one or two pages) description of the company (or program) you have founded or want to establish. How is it (or will it be) organized? Is it (or will it be) a sole proprietorship, partnership, or corporation? If a program, will it be a free-standing program or situated within a larger division or organization? What are your ambitions for the company or program? Will it always be a small one, or do you want to grow it into an international giant? Upon reading this section, the reader should have a good idea of where you are and where you are going with your company. Please note that the Company (or Program) Overview is the reader's introduction to your plan.

The Overview section includes an Introduction, Mission Statement, History and Current Status, Markets and Products, and Objectives. The Introduction should include an introductory paragraph introducing the company or program, current name, and location. The Mission Statement is a short (one paragraph) inspirational statement of the vision and goals you have for your company or program. Be sure that your mission statement is succinct and content-rich, and excites your readers. In the History and Current Status subsection, outline the history and current status of your company or program. If this is a start-up plan, you probably do not need to include this subsection. For Markets and Products, in one or two paragraphs, answer the following questions: What market(s) needs will we address? Who are our target customers? What products and services will we sell? What are our current sales and current products (if any)? What are the boundaries of our business? In the Objectives subsection, spell out the objectives of your company or program in a single paragraph: Where are we going? What are our goals for the organization (keep it small, grow it big, etc.)?

Industry and Market Analysis

Similar to the other sections in the plan, you will first need an Introduction to the overall Industry and Market Analysis section. Following the general Introduction, you will have the Industry Analysis. In this subsection, summarize the industry in which you will compete. Most of the research you do for this subsection will probably be in a library or on the Internet, and will come from the healthcare simulation literature, educational and government statistics, and healthcare and simulation organizations. Other great sources of information about an industry are suppliers who sell to the industry, equipment manufacturers, and accrediting bodies. Upon completion, your analysis will provide a "big picture" overview of the size and scope of your industry. How do we define our industry? How is the industry segmented? How are the segments defined? What are current trends and important developments? Who are the largest and most important players? What problems is the industry experiencing? What national and international events are influencing our industry? What are the growth forecasts?

The Industry and Market Analysis section of your plan will make or break the prospects for your venture. A great idea is meaningless if you cannot find customers. Carefully drafted and logical financial projections are irrelevant if nobody buys your product. In the Industry and Marketing Analysis section, you must convince first yourself, and then the reader, that there is indeed an eager market for your product. This section will probably be in four subsections: an Industry Analysis, a Market Analysis, a Customer Analysis, and a Competitor Analysis in that order.

The next subsection is Market Analysis, which includes an Introduction, the Market, and Market Trends. In your Market Analysis subsection, you explain the market in which you will be competing. This is not the place to go into detail about your ideas and concepts, but to carefully and analytically describe the larger environment in which you will be participating. Be sure to identify voids in the market that are currently not served, and that you presumably will be filling. Identify your place in emerging healthcare simulation markets.

Include an introductory paragraph to the Market Analysis subsection. When addressing the market, what is the market and how large is it? What industries, companies, or educational institutions currently service this market both regionally and nationally? Market trends should address where the market is headed. Is it growing? Stagnant? Declining?

Following the Market Analysis is the Customer Analysis subsection. Who are the customers in this market? How is the market segmented? What motivates the customer to decide that your simulation program is the right one for them? The research you do for this subsection will be with customers and potential customers. It is imperative that you do sufficient customer research to convince potential investors (and yourself) that customers will indeed come flocking to your simulation program. Customer research can include simply talking with potential customers to get reactions to your product idea, conducting focus groups, undertaking walk-up or mailed surveys, putting up a mock demonstration of your concept and soliciting customer feedback, and so on. Be creative in finding ways to get honest customer input about your product or service.

Included in this subsection is an Introduction. Following that, the Direct and Indirect customers need to be identified. Who are your *direct customers* (the customers that pay you for your product or service)? Carefully define the attributes and characteristics of these customers. For individual consumers, identify age, gender, socioeconomic status, interests, jobs, needs, and/or other attributes as appropriate. For business customers, identify industry, type, size, location, and/or other attributes as appropriate.

Who are your *indirect customers*, if any (the ultimate consumer of your product or service)? Carefully define the attributes and characteristics of these customers. For individual consumers, identify age, gender, socioeconomic status, interests, jobs, needs, and/or other attributes as appropriate. For business customers, identify industry, type, size, location, and/or other attributes as appropriate.

Lastly, the Competitor Analysis subsection addresses competition. In this section, identify your direct and indirect competitors. Compare and contrast your business to these competitors. How will you differentiate your customers from your competitors? Why will customers switch to or select you? How quickly and how effectively can your competitors respond to your business?

Again, an introduction is necessary, followed by Direct Competitors. Identify your *direct competitors* (competitors that sell similar products or services to your potential customers). Carefully define the attributes and characteristics of these competitors and their products/services. For direct competitors, identify size, location, target market, and other important characteristics. For their products or services, identify price, quality, features, distribution, and other important attributes.

Identify your *indirect competitors*, if any (competitors that sell related products or services that may substitute for your product or service). Carefully define the attributes and characteristics of these competitors and their products/services. For these indirect competitors, identify their size, location, target market, and other important characteristics. For their products and services, identify price, quality, features, distribution, and other important attributes.

Marketing Strategy

The Marketing Strategy subsection is where you show how you are going to fit into the market structure you just finished describing. What are the unmet needs in the simulation marketplace, and how are you going to fill them? How will you differentiate your product or service from your competitors? What unique features, benefits, or capabilities will you bring to the marketplace? What is your target market? Who will want to use your simulation program? Who are your customers? Why will they buy your product or service? What are the unique selling points of your product? How will you set prices? What distribution channels will you use? How will you communicate with your internal and external customers (promotion and advertising)? What "sales" strategy will you employ (your own sales personnel, manufacturing reps, telephone solicitation, etc.)? In short, given the previous market, customer, and competitor analyses, what are your strategies for connecting with your target market?

For the Introduction to the Marketing Strategy section, lay out the presentation of your marketing strategy, and then move on to explain your strategy for defining your target market. Describe the unmet needs of your target customers that your product/service fulfills or the problems that it solves. What segment of the market are you targeting? What characteristics define your target customers? How big is your target market? What share of the market will you capture? Who are your customers? End users? Distributors? Retailers? (Interesting notions for a simulation program to consider.) What needs does your product fulfill with your target market? What problems are you solving for these customers? What evidence do you have that potential customers want your product? How will you position your product or service with these customers? What evidence do you have that your target market wants or needs your product or service?

Describe how your product or service has been designed and tailored to meet the needs of your target customer, and how it will compete in your target market. What specific product/service design characteristics meet the needs of your customers? What differentiates your product in your target market? How does it differ from that of your competitors? What are the strengths of your product/service? Weaknesses? Why will customers in your target market buy (use) your product rather than the competition's? How will you differentiate yourselves from your competitors? Why will customers switch to or select you? How quickly and how effectively can your competitors respond to your business?

Explain your pricing strategy and why it will be effective with your target customer in your marketplace. What is your pricing strategy? Why? How does your pricing strategy compare with your competition? What evidence do you have that your target market will accept your price?

Describe your distribution strategy, and explain why it is the best for your marketplace. How will you distribute your product or service? What distribution channels will you use? Why? How will you gain access to these channels? Explain your advertising and promotion strategy. It is critical that you inform your target market about the availability of your product or service, and that you continue to communicate your benefits to that market. How will you advertise and promote your product or service? How will you communicate with your customers? Advertising? Public relations? Personal selling? Printed materials? Other means of promotion? Why will this strategy be effective in reaching your target customer?

Depending on your business, sales may be a critical component of your success. Even a simulation program that is funded by the academic unit needs to "sell" itself—to its learners, program directors, department chairs, and administrators. Remember, "nothing happens until the sale is made." An effective sales strategy is critically important for most manufacturers, publishers, software firms, and many service providers. And, ultimately, simulation programs are service providers. Do not overlook the importance of formulating an effective sales strategy! How will your product or service be sold? Personal selling? TV or Internet advertising? Trade show booths? Direct mail? Who will do the selling? An internal sales force? Manufacturer's representatives? Telephone solicitors? How will you recruit, train, and compensate your sales force? How will you support your sales effort (e.g., internal staff, service operations, etc.)?

Operations and Management

The Operations section outlines how you will run your business and deliver value to your customers. Operations is defined as the processes used to deliver your products and services to the marketplace (learners!) and can include manufacturing, transportation, logistics, travel, printing, consulting, after-sales service, and so on. In all likelihood, about 80% of your expenses will be for operations, 80% of your employees will be working in operations, and 80% of your time will be spent worrying about operating problems and opportunities. Be sure that you carefully link the design of your operations to your marketing plan. For example, if high quality will be one of your comparative advantages in the marketplace, then design your operations to deliver high quality, not low costs. Remember that you will probably have to make trade-offs with your operations. It is impossible to have the lowest cost, highest quality, best on-time performance, and most flexibility in your industry all at the same time. Often, higher quality means higher costs, lower costs mean less variety and less flexibility. Be careful how you make these trade-offs so that you can deliver products to the market in accordance with your marketing plan.

As in the other sections, an introductory paragraph to the Operations section is necessary. This can be a good place to paint a brief and attractive picture of how a hypothetical customer will interact with your business. This is especially effective for service businesses, that is, Healthcare Simulation Programs.

In this subsection, describe how you will fulfill your marketing strategy using operations and how you will use operations to add value for customers in your target market. How will you win in the marketplace on the dimensions of cost, quality, timeliness, and flexibility? Which dimensions will you stress, and which will you de-emphasize?

Describe how your company will be organized. How will you be organized? What does your organizational chart look like? What is the ownership structure of your company? Will you have a board of directors? Who will be on it? What will be their role?

Describe the founders and principal managers who will run your program. Who are the key managers (Include resumes in the Appendix)? What will be their duties and responsibilities? What unique skills do they bring to the venture? How will they be compensated? What additions to the management team do you plan? When? Who are the content experts, curriculum developers, simulation technicians?

Financial Management

The Summary of Financials section should be the frosting on a cake. You have outlined a great business concept, demonstrated a real need in the marketplace, shown how you will execute your ideas, proven that your team is just right to manage the venture, and now you will show how much money everyone is going to make. Note, however, that if your business concept is weak, or there is not a market, or if your execution is poor, or if your management team is incompetent, then your financial plans are doomed to fail. If you have not convinced your readers by now in the strength of your concept, then they will not be convinced with your financials.

Having said this, it is important that you have strong, well-constructed financials. If you cannot show that your great concept is going to make money (or at least break-even) and have outcomes vital to improving healthcare, your readers will quickly lose interest. To construct your financials, we highly recommend that you start with your development and operations plan to create a schedule or timetable of development and operational activities. From these development activities, you can then create cash flow projections, income statements, and pro forma balance sheets for at least 3 years into the future. As a rule of thumb, your financial projections should extend far enough into the future to the point where your business has achieved stable operations. The first year of your financial statement projections should be month-by-month because cash flows are critical in the early stages of any start-up. Second- and third-year financial statements should be quarterly. If possible, it is useful to include best-case, expected-case, and worst-case scenarios with your financials. This allows you and your readers to explore the upside potential and downside risks of your venture. Be sure that your financial projections are congruent with the other sections of your plan.

The Financial Management section should be a discussion and description of your financial projections—put the actual financial spreadsheets in the appendices. Describe the timing and amount of investment that you will require to achieve your plans. Then demonstrate that this investment is a good one by showing that profits, assets, and **return on investment (ROI)** are all favorable as the business progresses. When readers are finished with this section, they should be anxious to fund or sustain your simulation program.

As always, a brief introduction to the Summary of Financials section is necessary. When addressing the Initial Equity and Capital, address what significant start-up costs are required and what level of equity will be contributed to the business. For the Financial Forecast subsections, summarize your financial forecasts. Include detailed statements in appendices, including income statements, cash flow statements, and balance sheets. Generally, include statements for 3 years into the future. The first year should include forecasts by month, and the second and third year should include quarterly forecasts. You may also wish to include other financial documents such as valuation calculations as well as best-case, expected-case, and worst-case scenarios.

The break-even point (BEP) is simply where sales are equal to variable costs plus fixed costs. If a company had no fixed costs, then a BEP would not be necessary because sales would automatically cover the variable costs, assuming you priced the product/service at cost or above. However, by having fixed and variable costs, the company has to experience financial loss up to a specific volume. Thus, the point of sales volume that covers all costs is the BEP, where Sales = Variable Costs + Fixed Costs. This tool also shows your company's responsiveness to price—for example, if you lowered your price, then the margins would shrink, causing the BEP to dramatically shift upward. The Break-Even Point subsection should provide the critical information in both dollar figures as well as quantity. Provide an overview of your given assumptions and outlined figures as well as include graphical illustrations in the appendix. Figure 4.4.1 shows a graphical illustration of the BEP.

If applicable, what is the current condition of your governing body or head organization's finances? Have grant dollars or an endowment been leveraged? This can provide stability to the plan. Include a balance sheet (in the appendix) and address any negative factors, for example, high levels of debt, lack of assets, and so on.

What financial risks are inherent to your plan? How do you intend to minimize these risks? How will you avoid financial pitfalls? What is the worst-case scenario, and how will you respond?

References

Include sources of information used in your business plan for this section. References should be as up-to-date as possible.

Appendices

The appendices are where you should collect all of the documentation that supports the body of your business plan. As with the plan as a whole, it should be complete, but succinct. Include those documents that are required (e.g., financial projections), those that are helpful (e.g., results of marketing studies), and those that assist in selling your idea (e.g., letters of interest from potential "customers" who will use your simulation program). Do not include lots of tangential information such as newspaper clippings or tables of data unless they really serve to bolster your plan. One way to deal with information that is voluminous and/or lengthy (such as a large market research study) is to summarize it and note in the plan that the complete document is available upon request.

Template

See Appendix for Complete Business Plan Template.

BEEN THERE, DONE THAT: HOW CAN I CONTINUE TO IMPROVE OR SUSTAIN WHAT I HAVE ACHIEVED?

Improvement and Sustainability

The business plan, if implemented as a management tool, can provide an insightful perspective into the product or service an organization is offering. This applies to the overall strategy as well as operational administration. Continued development and review of the plan can prove effective in terms of improving and sustaining the simulation program.

It is imperative that management of the simulation program recognizes the need for the business plan to be a "living" active document that is continually revised and utilized. Responsibility for the plan depends upon the organizational structure of the simulation program. It is important that responsibility is identified in a formal manner (in a job description, for instance) and outcomes are identified to ensure that the plan is continually developed, reviewed, and utilized. Identification of operational policy and procedure is warranted so that all stakeholders are familiar with how the plan is used, how feedback is solicited, and how changes occur.

Best Practices and Challenges

There are many elements that exist in business planning. While these can vary significantly, depending upon industry, commonality among standards can be easily identified. First, the author should be concise and effective in the construction and verbiage of the plan. Knowing the audience (e.g., a grant committee, external funding source, or internal staff and administration) is essential to ensuring that the intended message and analysis is received as it is intended. Second, it is important that significant attention is given to how each part of the plan fits together to complete the overall model. If one element

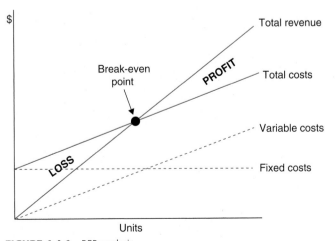

FIGURE 4.4.1 BEP analysis.

SECTION 4 • Funding

is weak in the overall plan, it may be a cause to render the venture unfeasible. For example, if the author is confident that the BEP can be easily achieved given market forces and financial projections but there are errors in operational delivery, it can then be determined to address the deficiencies or decide not to pursue the said initiative.

SUMMARY

Business planning within the simulation discipline is a critical component of laying the foundation for success. The business plan is not necessarily a tool used only for seeking venture capital. Rather, it is a management mechanism that allows for effective analysis of the strategy for start-up, growth, and sustainability. From a holistic perspective, it is imperative that the organizational leader be privy to the characteristics of the industry and market, develop a marketing strategy that will enable the organization to capitalize upon the said characteristics, understand how to align operations and management in doing so, all while maintaining a firm grasp of the financial implications of such contingencies.

ONLINE REFERENCES

Covello, J., & Hazelgren, B. (2006a). BEP analysis. Retrieved from http://technewsrprt.com/2012/11/27/break-even-point-an-in-depth-analysis-in-business-studies/

Covello, J., & Hazelgren, B. (2006b). *The complete book of business plans: Simple steps to writing powerful business plans* (2nd ed.). Naperville, IL: Sourcebooks.

Society for Simulation in Healthcare. (2013). *Accreditation standards of the council for accreditation of healthcare simulation programs.* Wheaton, IL: Author

Kyle, R., & Murray, W. B. (Eds.). (2007). *Clinical simulation: Operations, engineering and management.* Burlington, MA: Elsevier.

McKeever, M. (2005). *How to write a business plan* (7th ed.). Berkeley, CA: Delta Printing Solutions.

ONLINE RESOURCES

Babson College: http://define.babson.edu/

Kauffman Foundation: http://www.kauffman.org/Section.aspx?id=Entrepreneurship

The U.S. Small Business Administration: http://www.sba.gov/category/navigation-structure/starting-managing-business/starting-business/how-write-business-plan

SUGGESTED READING

Bygrave, W., & Zacharakis, A. (Eds.). (2009). *The portable MBA in entrepreneurship* (4th ed.). Hoboken, NJ: Wiley.

APPENDIX

Business Plan

COMPANY NAME

Logo

This business plan is intended solely for informational purposes to assist with providing a due diligence investigation of the project. The information contained herein is believed to be reliable, but the management team makes no representations or warranties with respect to this information. The financial projections that are part of this plan represent estimates based on extensive research and on assumptions considered reasonable, but they are of course not guaranteed. The contents of this plan are confidential and are not to be reproduced without express written consent.

Table of Contents

EXECUTIVE SUMMARY

(Introduction)

Product Description

Marketing and Sales

Operations and Management

Financial Summary

COMPANY OVERVIEW

(Introduction)

Mission Statement

History and Current Status

Markets and Products

Objectives

INDUSTRY AND MARKET ANALYSIS

(Introduction)

Industry Analysis

Market Analysis

(Introduction)

The Market

Market Trends

Customer Analysis

  (Introduction)

  Direct Customers

  Indirect Customers

Competitor Analysis

  (Introduction)

  Direct Competitors

  Indirect Competitors

MARKETING STRATEGY

(Introduction)

Target Market Strategy

Product/Service Strategy

Pricing Strategy

Distribution Strategy

Advertising and Promotion Strategy

Sales Strategy

OPERATIONS AND MANAGEMENT

(Introduction)

Operational Strategy

Company Organization

Management Team

FINANCIAL MANAGEMENT

(Introduction)

Initial Equity and Capital

Financial Forecasts

Break-Even Point Analysis

Balance Sheet

Risks and Assumptions

SECTION 4 • Funding

REFERENCES

APPENDICES

Table of Appendices

Support for Product/Service Description (e.g., diagrams, pictures, etc.)

Support for Marketing and Sales Plan

Support for Operations and Management Plan

Resumes of Management Team

Financial Statements

- Income Statement (3 years)
- Balance Sheets (3 years)
- Cash Flow Statements (3 years)
- Ratio Analysis (3 years)
- Other Supporting Financial Statements
- Break-Even Point Analysis Graphs

CHAPTER 4.5

How to Create Leadership and Organizational Buy-In

Katie Walker, RN, MBA, and Ian Curran, BSc, AKC, MBBS, FRCA, PgDig MedEd (distinction)

SECTION 4 • Funding

ABOUT THE AUTHORS

KATIE WALKER is the Director of the New York Health and Hospital Corporation's Simulation Program. Prior to this appointment in December 2011, she was the Program Manager of a national simulation program being established in Australia through the peak government agency, Health Workforce Australia. She coconvened the 2010 International Meeting on Simulation in Healthcare in Phoenix, Arizona, and the first Asia-Pacific meeting on Simulation in Healthcare in Hong Kong in May 2011.

IAN CURRAN is the Senior Clinical Advisor at the National Health Service's (NHS) Health Education England. His role covers national policy and strategy development, particularly in relation to educational excellence, human factors, innovation, and reform. As London's Dean of Educational Excellence, he led the multiaward-winning Simulation and Technology-enhanced Learning Initiative (STeLI). This flagship workforce development initiative won the prestigious Health Service Journal's (HSJ) Award for Patient Safety in 2009 and the BMJ Award for Excellence in Healthcare Education in 2011.

ABSTRACT

Concepts drawn from health management, general management, and business literature are useful for those interested in creating "buy-in" for simulation projects. Theories and tools such as the NHS Leadership framework, PESTLE analysis (Tshabalala & Rankhumise, 2011), force field analysis (Paquin & Koplyay, 2007), Porter's Five Forces and value-based healthcare (Ormanidhi & Stringa, 2008), Moore's Strategic Triangle (O'Hare, 2006), disruptive innovation (Christensen et al., 2009), and contagious commitment (Shapiro, 2003) provide valuable information that leaders can use to develop strong messages as well as understand the market and the factors that impact on program opportunity, development, and delivery.

Drawing from the literature and binational experience, this chapter will explore the challenges of leading sustainable large-scale change through effective institutional and systemic leadership. Using selected case studies, a wide range of strategic and operational leadership issues will be explored. By offering personal insights and by referencing tools and concepts the authors have found useful, this monograph will offer a practical framework for current and future leadership development. Leadership and buy-in will be approached from two perspectives. The first examines factors that influence institutional leadership. The second is about creating champions in organizations.

CASE EXAMPLE

The basic business plan has been written. It includes the potential courses that might be delivered from a proposed new learning center called The Clinical Simulation Center. The funding has been dedicated from the state government for the development of the center with a goal to provide simulation education to 60,000 clinicians throughout the state. The vision for the center came from a keen and well-respected physician writing a compelling case saying that patient safety will be improved if this new training technique called healthcare simulation was adopted. The reason that the State Health Minister wanted to embrace the vision was that patient safety was a key political issue for him. There had been many high-profile clinical errors reported in the media, and the simulation program was seen as a potential panacea to solve the problem, ease his pain, and report that his government was going to make a difference to patient care.

INTRODUCTION AND BACKGROUND

Human behavior is infinite in its variety and effectiveness. Many leaders are particularly challenged by their organizational responsibility to optimize human behavior and so ensure operational success. A critical insight for leaders is to understand their role in creating the appropriate climate and productive conditions that enable their team or organization to succeed. This is not a simple or straightforward recipe, but one that must be cultivated and nurtured, built upon with experience, pragmatism, and adaptability. Every **leadership** situation or context is unique, and so the relative merits or demerits of individual leadership concepts must be assessed for worth or value. Indeed, flexibility and adaptability are key attributes of successful leaders. As there are many forces and factors at work in most operational contexts, it is imperative that leaders develop as clear an overview as possible of the "ballpark" or, perhaps, the "battlefield."

In the pursuit of operational excellence in simulation programs, it is helpful to consider the challenges in two principal domains: the internal or organizational domain and the external or wider sociopolitical domain. Successful institutional leadership requires that leaders adopt an outward-facing gaze, or consideration for the external leadership challenges that they face. This will typically include, but not be limited to, consideration of influencing and negotiating at a high level, strategic and political planning, and insights. The key to success in this outward-facing domain is a deep understanding of the needs of those with whom you are seeking to influence, exploring what their needs are, and how your program will solve their challenges or problems. Good institutional leaders see their organization or program in a wider operational and strategic context; understanding what can be achieved or delivered and how it is seen through the eyes of others are key skills for effective leaders.

Leaders cannot work in isolation. They need the support of advocates and champions to advance the collective agenda or mission. Nurturing champions in healthcare simulation is an art and a science. It takes patience, determination, and endurance to identify and nurture effective advocates and champions. **Champions** can be directly or indirectly involved in the core business and may be representative of a healthcare profession, specialty, or perspective. You will need different champions for different tasks, so you will need to recruit widely.

Once potential champions are identified, it is essential to ensure that they understand the vision of the program, are able to support the time schedule to work in the program, and remain dedicated to the program. These commitments are imperative to the success and sustainability of programs. To be effective, Peshawaria (2012) references the importance of seeking and harnessing the energy within organizations. Part of the key to developing internal leadership is articulating the vision and mission

of the organization and the development and establishment of effective teams.

CREATING BUY-IN AMONG YOUR INSTITUTIONAL LEADERSHIP OR HOW TO BEHAVE IN WAYS THAT INFLUENCE YOUR INSTITUTIONAL LEADERSHIP

The English National Health System Leadership framework (NHS, UK, n.d.) describes the seven elements required for effective leadership: demonstrating personal qualities, working with others, managing services, improving services, setting direction, creating the vision, and delivering the strategy. In the case study described earlier, the vision and strategy had been developed; however, it was only by working with others (i.e., stakeholders) that the program was able to grasp a solution that would meet the needs of those in the hospitals served. It was expected that a state-of-the-art simulation program would be developed and all courses would be delivered from that center. Stakeholders were hamstrung by staffing shortages, so the only way that staff could attend simulation programs was if the simulation programs were delivered to them, which led to an "on the road" simulation program (see chapter 2.3). That program has grown to service hospitals throughout the state. This was not a direction that had been initially planned, and if it were not for working directly with stakeholders, a great opportunity would have been missed. Being adaptable and able to consider the needs or challenges of others will mean that solutions are more client-facing and valued (Figure 4.5.1).

Useful leadership capabilities include openness, curiosity, listening, questioning, critical thinking, understanding, pragmatism, adapting, wise judgment, linking the program to clear deliverables, setting targets, achieving set targets, researching and reporting, and using meaningful metrics to demonstrate value. **Force field analysis**

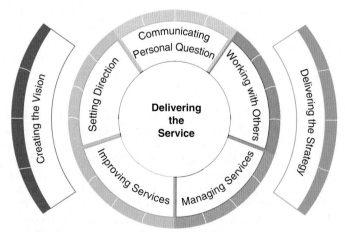

FIGURE 4.5.1 NHS leadership framework.

is a principle developed by Kurt Lewin in 1951 that provides a framework for looking at the factors (forces) that influence a situation, originally social situations (Paquin & Koplyay, 2007). It looks at forces that are either driving movement toward a goal (helping forces) or blocking movement toward a goal (hindering forces). It is interesting when spearheading a new project to identify what the driving and restraining forces are and what the present and desired states are and whether there is a discrepancy between them. Force field analysis is a useful tool to examine the variables in planning and implementing a change program, and will undoubtedly be of use in project planning and team building, particularly when attempting to overcome resistance to change.

Lewin assumes that in any situation there are both driving and restraining forces that influence any change that may occur. In the development of the national program, the driving forces for change were the need to increase clinical placement capacity, provide access to interprofessional education, and create learning environments for students in rural and remote environments. The restraining forces were the health professional schools that had been teaching the same courses for many years using lecture and didactic methods and did not see the need to change. The difficulty in developing and providing interprofessional learning experiences is due to accredited curricula and scheduling challenges and the acceptance that in lieu of sufficient data that simulation was an efficient and effective method of training health professional students. Analyzing these forces and monitoring was key to rolling out a successful program(Figure 4.5.2).

FORCE FIELD ANALYSIS – KURT LEWIN

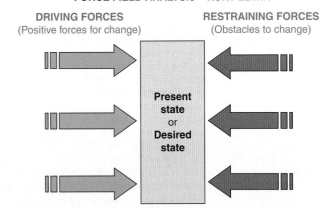

FIGURE 4.5.2 Force field analysis.

Understand and Examine Driving and Restraining Forces

Healthcare leaders must be cognizant of the internal and external forces that are present in their environment to position new innovations in healthcare for sustainability. In 1979, Michael Porter developed a framework for industry analysis and business strategy development. It is called **Porter's Five Forces**, and it determines the intensity of competitors and therefore how attractive a market is in terms of overall industry profitability. Porter has subsequently turned his attention to the healthcare system. He has developed a model for value-based healthcare delivery. He says that reforms in the healthcare system must be about value—improving patient health outcomes and delivering them more efficiently. He proposes that currently

SECTION 4 • Funding

EXPERT'S CORNER

HOW TO CREATE CHAMPIONS
Paul E. Phrampus, MD, FACEP
Past President, Society for Simulation in Healthcare (2013)

There are several different types of program champions—those who advocate for a program, those who fund a program, and those who lead the work and encourage others to do the same. In simulation, champions are an important part of any successful simulation program. These individuals often shoulder the responsibility of developing and delivering educational programs. In addition, they employ creativity, grit, and hard work to help simulation programs obtain buy-in and credibility while they grow in importance and relevance in the context of the stakeholders they serve.

An important part of the leadership function within simulation programs is to find ways to identify, attract, and nurture the growth of these types of champions. The structural nature of simulation programs varies tremendously, but some common principles of champion growth can nonetheless be recognized. Consider the following areas of leadership that are critical in creating champions: intrinsic and extrinsic motivation and lowering systematic barriers.

INTRINSIC MOTIVATION

Intrinsic motivation resides within the potential champion and is expressed as a desire to support the simulation program. For some, this includes the desire to engage in teaching, research, or other activities germane to healthcare simulation. Simulation leaders can exploit this intrinsic motivation by maintaining the simulation program at a high level of visibility so that potential champions are aware of the simulation program's capabilities and successes. Leaders in the simulation program should remain actively vigilant in identifying potential champions and, after identification, inviting these potential champions to participate in a simulation event. This will often inspire thoughts and ideas that encourage potential champions to become more engaged in the simulation program. Another way to fuel intrinsic motivation is to facilitate an active mentoring program in which potential champions can be mentored by an experienced simulationist and, ultimately, serve as a mentor to those following behind.

EXTRINSIC MOTIVATION

Management of extrinsic motivating factors is an important job for the simulation program leadership. Effective management of these extrinsic factors ensures sustainment and longitudinal participation of the simulation champions. Extrinsic motivators are those factors external to the champion that encourage them to grow. These may include promotion or salary increases but do not necessarily need to be associated with a direct financial motivation. A title alone may serve as a motivational factor; however, the position must be one of relevance and managed by the leader with expectations of performance whether or not there is direct financial compensation. Public recognition in the form of news stories or other directed communication should not be underestimated as it can increase the visibility of the champion's efforts. Busy programs should be cautioned that this recognition can be inadvertently overlooked by assuming that everyone is aware of the champion's participation and investment in the program.

Simulation program leaders should also ensure that they are informing the stakeholders to whom the champions report. For example, if a champion from a clinical department has created or is in the process of creating substantial contributions, it is important to inform the relevant department chairperson on the true efforts being put forth by the champion. Often, such leaders are aware that their faculty member is participating in simulation, but are largely unaware of the amount, complexity, and dedication of effort being put forth by the individual. This awareness may lead to downstream increases in compensation, protected time, and other forms of recognition that help the champion continue to grow within the simulation efforts in which they are involved.

LOWERING SYSTEMIC BARRIERS

Lowering the barriers for participation in a simulation program is the third broad focus of leadership associated with creating simulation champions. Attention should be paid to the administrative burden, standard processes, and other items that can be identified to allow the simulation champion to be productive in a way that aligns with the intrinsic and extrinsic motivating factors described previously.

First, the staff of the simulation program should be cognizant of those efforts that can contribute to the successes of the simulation champions. Many simulation programs regard the ultimate customer or client as the learners who participate in the simulations. Over time, we have identified the ultimate consumer of our simulation program to be the course directors and facilitators who carry the "heavy lifting"

of the creation and execution of new simulation programs. They are our simulation champions. When resources are aligned to assist the simulation champion in these efforts, the participants experience programs that yield the best possible outcomes.

Carefully analyzing the actual work that comprises the creation of a successful simulation program from the brainstorming of an idea, to the execution of the course or program over time is important. Recognizing common areas of administrative tasks, operational tasks that can be automated or guided by carefully developed templates can greatly assist the simulation champion. Normally, simulation champions are intrinsically motivated by conducting the education and the successes that it accrues to the participants in the program, but less so by the administrative tasks necessary to create success.

While every successful simulation effort counts on robust involvement of instructors and faculty members, many of the behind-the-scenes tasks such as scheduling, collection of data, reminder systems, evaluation processes, and quality improvement initiatives are repetitive tasks from an administrative perspective but are critically important. Finding ways to assist the simulation champion to minimize their efforts in the conduct of these administrative tasks can help lower the barrier to the simulation champion's ability to put significant efforts and investments into the program. Examples of such may include sending reminder e-mails to participants in programs, the ability to print reports germane to their faculty evaluation process, and the ability to print reports aggregating student data, evaluations, and effectiveness of the simulation program. When leadership helps to lower the champion's administrative burden by minimizing the amount of time spent on such tasks, the simulation champion will have more time to focus on new and innovative ways to teach and/or assess participants in the simulation programs.

In summary, it is important that leaders of simulation programs engage in the active identification and development of simulation champions. This will maximize the possibilities for high-quality simulation activities as well as help to create potential for growth of the program. Three fundamental focus areas include (1) appealing to that which intrinsically motivates the potential champion, (2) nurturing and helping to create visibility and a mission-critical nature of simulation to other leaders of the organization in which the simulation program exists, and finally (3) being mindful and creative with regard to providing solutions that help to lower the administrative barriers to the simulation champions' ability to achieve their goals.

healthcare delivery is not aligned with patient value, suggesting that healthcare organizations need to better organize delivery around the patient's personal needs and medical condition. This implies that healthcare organizations should deliver care through effective multidisciplinary teams that take responsibility for the entire care cycle, and vigorously measure patient outcomes and the costs of providing effective care.

Simulation can be used as a powerful method for examining clinical processes and operational implementation. With

simulation there is the ability to rehearse best practice and so achieve efficient and value-based healthcare delivery. A key strategic insight for simulation-based leaders is that they must always understand the value of the program or intervention they are offering. Successful leaders first seek to understand the value proposition of their activities. Once these objectives are clear, the operational process can be developed to provide efficient provision of the program. Understanding the difference between cost, value, and efficiency is an attribute that sets good leaders apart.

I HAVE THE BUY-IN: NOW HOW DO I SUSTAIN IT?

First, Think about the Value Your Program Is Delivering

Both private organizations and government are now clearly seeing the need to ensure that the programs being funded and delivered are providing value for their customers. A method of doing this is by having the political legitimacy of leadership at the highest level, and also from the "on the ground" staff that will be actively involved in delivering the program, by constantly nurturing the operations of the program and by creating a clear value proposition. This method is a theoretical model called "Moore's Triangle" (Moore, 1995). Michael Moore, an academic from the Harvard Business School, developed this model in the early 1990s (Figure 4.5.3).

The national simulation program that used this model to underpin its strategic direction and operations is now in its third year, and it has grown and flourished. Each principle or point of the triangle was considered and nurtured. In a practical sense, this is what happened. The top vertex of the triangle underlines the importance of establishing political support and legitimacy. Most funded programs will endure the challenge of establishing support in an authorizing or governing environment. Achieving and securing political legitimacy can unlock enormous support and resources. The funding for the national program was committed, as the Health Minister, at the highest level who, once convinced, saw the vision and then applied a practical approach (dedicating millions of dollars to simulation) to support the effort. Having this legitimacy and accountability caused stakeholders to really think about how simulation could be used most effectively in their context.

The right vertex refers to value and performance management. There was a particularly challenging problem: a shortage of clinical placements that was causing direct pain to the system and to government. There was a dire need to increase clinical placement capacity within the hospitals

for health professional students, the hospitals were overrun with students, and there was no surplus capacity for clinical placement–based training. Simulation was seen as a practical, achievable, and desirable solution to this "wicked" problem. The idea was to build new or build on current simulation programs to create simulated clinical environments so that the students would use simulation as another clinical setting to practice their knowledge and skills in order to be work-ready when they completed their degrees.

The left vertex of the triangle is about nurturing resources and building organizational capacity and capability. It is essential to develop a process that ensures good governance and accountability by each program for its funding. This involves clear contracting, performance management frameworks, and clear performance indicators. This requires that where possible, clearly demonstrated outcomes for the program were identified to reflect the goals of the project. There were ongoing reporting mechanisms so that it was clear how the funded projects were progressing against milestones and that they were meeting the required outcomes.

To sustain support, you need to think about **Moore's strategic triangle**. Does your program have political legitimacy from your funders, your peers, and all stakeholders? Are you creating value through the program by monitoring its performance? Are you sustaining the program by continually nurturing its operations?

NURTURING CHAMPIONS: HOW TO CREATE ADVOCATES AND ALLIES THROUGHOUT YOUR INSTITUTION

> Entrepreneurs [Champions] are simply those who understand that there is little difference between obstacle and opportunity and are able to turn both to their advantage.
> —*Niccolo Machiavelli*

Creating **buy-in** requires that leaders articulate their points in a memorable and effective way. Building champions in organizations relies on leaders having the communication skills to impart their ideas in a way that "sticks." To be successful, one's ideas need to be memorable. Specifically, it is also essential to understand what you are offering and how it might or will be seen by others. Successful communicators are often able to see matters from the perspective of other key stakeholders including, most importantly, commissioners. ("Commissioners" is meant to signify someone who has an official charge or authority to do something. In this case, it might be the potential funder or others associated with the project that operate at a high political level.)

Heath and Heath (2007) suggest that there are the same themes or attributes shared by successful or memorable ideas. They have developed the "SUCCESs" acronym, which includes the following concepts for getting buy-in or making points "stick."

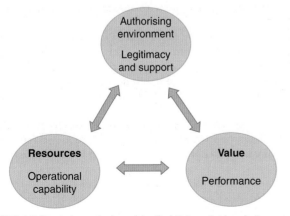

FIGURE 4.5.3   A theoretical model called "Moore's triangle."

Simple—keep any messaging simple.

Unexpected—use surprise or impact for maximal effect and engagement.

Concrete—use specifics, including key data, detail, and descriptions, to engage the recipients of the message, but be selective; many a powerful message is lost in the swamp of too much data.

Credible—examples must be plausible and believable also.

Emotional—themes and messages are more memorable if people can invest "emotional effort and capital" in the story.

Stories—the power of the narrative should not be overlooked; well-crafted coherent stories, especially if emotionally engaging, are efficient routes into people's memories. Successful stories are easy to deploy and easy to remember.

What is your SUCCESs story for your program? (See EXAMPLE)

In addition to the SUCCESs tool, another useful method for scanning the environment is the PESTLE analysis (Tshabalala & Rankhumise, 2011). This approach includes six key areas of understanding that effective leaders can use to create buy-in.

Political—understand the static and dynamic political forces in play.

Economic—understand the current economic setting. Is it a time of growth and investment, or are austerity measures in force?

EXAMPLE

In London, a large-scale simulation program was developed and implemented called STeLI. The acronym STeLI stands for the London Simulation & Technology-enhanced Learning Initiative. STeLI started as a small-scale initiative of a few hundred thousand pounds; it started small, delivered on time and to budget, building organizational capacity and a reputation for being able to deliver. At its core, STeLI's leadership set out a compelling vision for patient safety and human factors team training in healthcare. Using stories from healthcare and other industries and by focusing upon safety and quality of care, STeLI was able to garner increased political support and legitimacy. It offered a vision of a systemwide solution for patient safety training. The educational method happened to be simulation-based, but this was not the main focus of the message to commissioners. It was, however, useful as it offered a contemporary, innovative, visual solution to safety issues, and this was useful in attracting engagement at a local hospital and political level. This program developed into a pan-London workforce development program, and had an impact in every acute hospital and mental health hospital in London. It ran successfully for 6 years, delivered over 500,000 training episodes, 600 projects, and over 3,000 academic outputs, and secured funding in excess of £35 million. The STeLI program was entered in a number of national and international awards, winning the BMJ Award for Excellence in Healthcare Education and the national HSJ Award for Patient Safety. This multiaward-winning regional program had several workstreams, including an educational capacity and capability arm that included programs such as curriculum integration, faculty development, facility development, and specific course and training program development. In addition, key themes to the success of the program were around creating effective buy-in from individuals, teams, departments, and organizations.

The way that the project leader and team were able to steer this initiative was primarily through stakeholder engagement, and this played out by annual conferences, showcase and staging events, and Master classes. Policy development sessions, conferences, and workshops were also delivered.

One of the key success factors for STeLI that became clearer over the years was the importance of building communities of practice and networks of learning. This amounted to a strategic communications and engagement workstream that involved formal goals around relationship management. This was about understanding that it was valuable to invest time in building relationships, to invest in people, and really understanding that forming key relationships is essential for establishing sustainable support and buy-in.

Another key aspect of STeLI was the importance of formal education commissioning and structured contracting of education providers locally. Performance management of all providers was required, and this involved having clearly communicated and contracted expectations, which were formalized through specific goals, objectives, and contracts, to ensure that everyone clearly understood the mission, vision, and values of the program.

A strong governance framework was developed. This created credibility, accountability, and responsibility for everyone who was part of the program team. Contractors were engaged to deliver leadership development courses. This gave support to leaders through mentorship, coaching, and availability of advice and guidance. When spearheading a new program such as STeLI, there can never be too much communication. The communication strategy included a dedicated website, blogospheres, learning environments, and social networks. These clearly aided the dispersing of information and gave stakeholders multiple forums for communication and access of shared resources.

All of these elements added to create a distributed community of practice, working in local organizations, with local responsiveness, to common principles and goals. By supporting local ownership and employing more facilitative approaches, STeLI was highly successful in achieving buy-in rather than a more directive or command-and-control approach, which was minimized. It offers a highly successful distributed leadership model.

Use the SUCCESs acronym to project an idea that will stick! Keep it SIMPLE, use an UNEXPECTED approach (a simulation is great for this), CONCRETE—use specifics including data, ensure CREDIBILITY by using plausible examples, use EMOTION through anecdotal feedback from happy participants, and tell STORIES—don't overlook the power of the narrative.

Social—understand public expectations, lobby groups, what are the positives and negatives of the initiative (i.e., safety requirements, demand, unmet need, outrage, media pressure, etc.).

Technical—understand opportunities, restrictions, and limitations, especially the cost, implementation, and any ongoing maintenance costs.

Legal—understand any mandatory or statutory elements in your jurisdiction. These elements can be both blockers and enablers.

Environmental—understand ecological or sustainable aspects of the initiative.

BEEN THERE, DONE THAT

Successful simulation leaders must keep looking forward; it is essential to understand your purpose or your value to the healthcare system you serve. What are the current challenges in the healthcare sector? What are the emerging technologies? What are the new ways of doing things? What are the educational solutions or opportunities you might offer to meet these challenges?

Successful simulation leaders understand disruptive innovation. Simulation and immersive training were disruptive innovations to the traditional educational methods of lecturing and small-group teaching. The value of simulation over these more established educational methods is its experiential nature and impact, the behavioral focus, and the ability to tailor learning opportunities to the needs of individual learners or teams. Immersive simulation training is safer than exposing real patients to real novice students, particularly in relation to procedural skills. Simulation offers a unique and valuable opportunity to move the steep and dangerous part of the professional learning curve away from patients and the service.

A **disruptive innovation** is an innovation that creates a new paradigm, opportunity, or market (Christensen et al., 2009). By definition, a disruptive innovation must offer or add value to the established way of doing things. Disruptive innovations eventually go on to disrupt an existing market (over a few years or decades), often displacing earlier techniques or technology. The term is used in business and technology literature to describe innovations that improve a product or service in ways that the market does not expect, typically first by designing for a different set of consumers in the new market and later by lowering prices in the existing market.

A sustaining innovation differs from a disruptive innovation as it does not create new markets or value networks but rather only evolves existing ones through efficiency, offering better value. This means that the firms within the sector will compete against each other's sustaining improvements. Sustaining innovations may continue to evolve, or they may be transformational.

One of the key reasons effective change initiatives sometimes fall short of expected gains is that leaders fail to involve and engage with members of the community of practice or employees and so fail to embrace and understand their perspectives. This phenomenon leads to the people who are expected to implement the initiative feeling discounted and disconnected, and ensures that leaders will not get the input that would be very valuable for their mission. Often associated with this suboptimal outcome is authoritarian or pace-setting leadership behavior that demands, directs, or orders teams but does not explain why. There is emerging evidence from sociology and business literature that building shared purpose, shared ownership, and shared vision can be very powerful in building **contagious commitment** (Shapiro, 2003). This term is used to describe how through meaningful engagement it is possible to motivate participants, employees, or stakeholders to become impassioned advocates of change, instead of resistant blockers. This more facilitative and enabling leadership style is being advocated as the leadership style for the 21st century.

SUMMARY

Leadership, understanding buy-in, creating champions, and nurturing advocates are all key to the successful establishment and sustainability of new simulation centers and programs. The importance of building contagious commitment is particularly true when introducing an innovative development or tool such as simulation particularly to perhaps skeptical funders or commissioners where the perceived evidence for cost-effectiveness and efficiency has not been clearly demonstrated.

There are many leadership frameworks, principles, and models that can assist those who are starting out on these challenging leadership journeys. Seasoned simulation proponents can achieve greater success, deliver more value, and achieve sustainability if they address many of the issues discussed in this chapter. It is vital for all leaders to understand and recognize the unique challenges and many different contexts and ever-present opportunities they face.

This chapter has identified several models useful in guiding leadership development, has shared leadership experiences, and encourages readers to be brave and inquisitive in exploring their own leadership challenges and capabilities. The journey, though at times daunting, will be worth it.

REFERENCES

Christensen, C., Grossman, J. H., & Hwang, J. (2009). *The innovator's prescription: A disruptive solution for health care.* New York, NY: Mc-Graw Hill.

Heath, C., & Heath, D. (2007). *Made to stick.* New York, NY: Random House.

SECTION 4 • Funding

Moore, M. (1995) Creating Public Value: Strategic management in government, Cambridge, MA, Harvard.

NHS, UK. (n.d.). *Leadership framework.* Retrieved from http://www.leadershipacademy.nhs.uk/discover/leadership-framework

O'Hare, M. (2006). Environmental agencies' funding sources should follow their diverse business models. *The Policy Studies Journal, 34*(4), 511–532.

Ormanidhi, O., & Stringa, O. (2008). Porter's model of generic competitive strategies. *Business Economics, 43*(3), 55.

Paquin, J.-P., & Koplyay, T. (2007). Force field analysis and strategic management: A dynamic approach. *Engineering Management Journal, 19*(1), 28.

Peshawaria, R. (2012). Energizing the organization: From Hesselbein and Company. *Leader to Leader, 2012*(63), 19–25.

Shapiro, A. (2003). *Creating contagious commitment: Applying the tipping point to organizational change.* Hillsborough, NC: Strategy Perspective.

Tshabalala, D. B., & Rankhumise, E. M. (2011). What impact do economic issues have on the sustainability of small, medium and micro entrepreneurs? *Journal of Management Policy and Practice, 12*(1), 108–114.

CHAPTER 4.6

Fundraising: A Potential Additional Source of Income for the Research and Educational Activities of a Healthcare Simulation Program

Guillaume Alinier, PhD, MPhys, PgCert, SFHEA, CPhys, MInstP, MIPEM
and Jean Claude Granry, MD

ABOUT THE AUTHORS

GUILLAUME ALINIER's career in healthcare simulation started in 2000 at the University of Hertfordshire (UK), where he holds a full Professorship since 2011 and was leading all aspects of simulation developments. He was instrumental in designing, fundraising, and running the University's large multiprofessional simulation center accessed annually by 10,000 students, professionals, and visitors. Guillaume is active internationally, supporting center developments, and recently joined Hamad Medical Corporation Ambulance Service, Qatar, which is rapidly developing into a world-class prehospital care service provider.

JEAN-CLAUDE GRANRY, Professor at the University Hospital of Angers (France), is the founder of the French simulation society ("Société Francophone de Simulation en Santé - SoFraSimS"). Prof. Granry serves as a simulation expert for the French Higher Health Authority (HAS), where he published two national reports about the state of the art of simulation in healthcare and good practice recommendations in simulation education. In 2009, he received two prestigious distinctions: "Chevalier de l'Ordre National du Mérite" and "Chevalier de l'Ordre des Palmes Académiques".

ABSTRACT

The fact that "simulation" can be used to promote safer patient care delivery is seen as a noble cause worthy of being the recipient of generous donations and sponsorships; however, substantial gifts rarely just happen. Fundraising is a specialized activity that requires a range of skills from a dedicated team, substantial time investment, an established and reliable list of influential contacts, networking skills, and perseverance. This chapter covers the fundamentals of fundraising and explores aspects from both sides of such initiatives (from the donor and the benefactor's perspective) in the context of the delivery of simulation-based education. Information as to how to put together a fundraising campaign with full documentation will be shared as well as considerations about what may convince potential donors to support a simulation initiative. Finally, a series of questions will be shared to provide additional information and tips for people new to fundraising as well as for simulation programs that have already been the recipient of generous private or corporate donations, whether it was financial or in the form of equipment or expertise.

CASE EXAMPLE

You are excited about your recent appointment as the director of your hospital's new simulation center. While you are aware that multiple sources of funding are necessary to build a **sustainable** simulation program, your background as a healthcare professional did not prepare you with the knowledge and skills to obtain the funds needed to not only get the project launched but also to ensure that it is fiscally sound. You contact the chief financial officer and work with her/him to get the budget started, but you also look at other simulation centers and note that many are raising funds from outside donors and benefactors. Through research you find that successful programs have intentionally developed the expertise and infrastructure to recruit and retain donors committed to the goals of healthcare simulation. Knowing that the viability of your center depends upon a diversified revenue stream, you commit yourself to becoming a proficient fundraiser.

INTRODUCTION AND BACKGROUND

Simulation is often perceived as being an expensive educational methodology because of its time-consuming and human resource–intensive nature, yet by not providing this type of experience for learners, there is the risk of allowing for an inadequately skilled workforce to treat patients, and this can be significantly more costly. This is increasingly recognized at government level and has resulted in several countries rolling out national simulation training initiatives or publishing guidelines about simulation-based training for health care professionals (Alinier and Platt, 2014). The establishment of even a basic simulation program and its ongoing support requires a significant financial investment (Fritz et al., 2008). Simulation does not always require the use of very advanced and specialized technology, which can be costly, but the staff employed to facilitate the training is a significant and ongoing expense that cannot be ignored or compromised. Beyond these direct costs, additional funds may be required for the purchase of equipment, technological solutions, and course development. Provided a program is run by adequately qualified, simulation-trained, and resourceful staff, a great deal can be achieved with modest resources before moving on to the more high-end products. Regardless of the ambition, even a basic simulation program making use of mostly standardized patients, moulage, and task trainers requires a setup and operational budget. These extrinsic limitations (Meguerdichian et al., 2012) are often the most significant financial burden of a simulation program and still limit the broad adoption of simulation-based education in healthcare.

Fundraising is usually a means by which to collect a large amount of money to start a new project or program, expand an existing one, or revitalize a current one. This chapter will be particularly relevant to anyone about to venture into fundraising for any of the examples mentioned above and seeks a positive outcome. Fundraising can be defined as the purposeful effort of gathering financial donations/contributions toward a particular cause or project (The Free Dictionary, 2013). It is an activity commonly conducted by official charities and other entities, often to benefit the community, a particular cause, a group in need and for which monetary and other forms of donations would be highly beneficial. Fundraising is an exercise that has been done on many occasions to support the development of clinical simulation facilities and the purchase of expensive pieces of equipment for training purposes (Alinier, 2007, 2008; Henderson & Hassmiller, 2007; Meek, 2008). Many

simulation programs report relying significantly on institutional subsidies and income obtained from philanthropic donations, foundations, grants, private malpractice insurers, and commercial sources (Huang et al., 2007; Pratt et al., 2005). This chapter will only cover the core aspect of fundraising, which by virtue of raising people's awareness of a need for support for a particular project may also attract other forms of support such as industry sponsorship and philanthropic donations, whether corporate or private. Although grants can be applied for with the same aim as a fundraising campaign, the process varies greatly from country to country and hence will not be addressed in this chapter. Grant writing is covered in chapter 4.7.

SIGNIFICANCE

Government funding of academic institutions has decreased over time worldwide, and to maintain their level of operation, they are forced to rely on other additional sources of income. In addition to increasing student fees, academic institutions are very often relying on endowments, donations, land development, real estate investments, research contracts, business initiatives, copyrights, and patents (Orkodashvili, 2007). Their strength in these various areas largely depends on their existing resources, portfolio of activities, and established reputation in certain areas upon which they can levy new and profitable contracts.

Beyond the initial costs of setting up a simulation program, simulation-based education requires a high level of commitment on the part of any institution owing to the associated costs of running sessions with a relatively high staff-to-participants ratio. To that effect, some simulation-based initiatives or programs could be or are even totally reliant on some form of fundraising or external financial support on an ongoing basis (Huang et al., 2007). However, it is common for the initiation of a simulation program to be significantly reliant on private or corporate donations, and hence the need to be able to prepare a robust case in the form of a fundraising campaign.

THEMES

Various Forms of Fundraising

Various avenues exist to attract external support. This support can take different forms such as sponsorships and

philanthropy and may be accessible from different sources. Sponsorship can be in the form of material support (loan or donation) for a work, an event, or a person to exercise the activity of general interest and potentially derive a direct benefit from it. This may be in the form of free provision of otherwise expensive technological or scientific expertise or technology belonging to the sponsor or their financial support directed toward skills sponsorship to pay for the required personnel, resources, and links to a network. Sponsorship can also be presented as financial support toward covering all or part of the costs associated with a specific project or specific staff salaries. It is also possible to negotiate for the donation or long-term loan of equipment or other forms of physical resources. The forms of sponsorship are usually done either in exchange for recognition of the corporate or industrial sponsor for marketing purposes or because the supported activity directly or indirectly benefits the sponsoring organization (i.e., research and development work). Sponsorship may also be provided without the intent of attracting public attention. This would be a form of philanthropic sponsorship or corporate philanthropic giving, sometimes interpreted as altruism (Zhang et al., 2010). While not being enforced in the majority of countries like economic and legal responsibilities, such types of donation are relatively common, often strategic, and viewed as a sign of good corporate citizenship (Zhang et al., 2010).

Philanthropy may result from a fundraising campaign and is a form of donation toward an idea, event, action, or realization of an important project that is done to better humanity, and usually involves some sacrifice as opposed to being done for a profit motive. This is what differentiates this act from sponsorship. Acts of philanthropy include donating money or valuables to a charity or a nonprofit organization, volunteering time to a humanitarian activity, or raising money through various activities to donate to research. Enhancing the training experience and clinical competencies of healthcare students and professionals clearly qualifies as being for the betterment of humanity and is hence a worthy philanthropic cause. It is worth considering that both healthcare and education figure among the reported domains that receive the most funding from foundations (Srivastava & Oh, 2010). Other forms of fundraising can also be adopted such as special events (educational or entertaining). For academic or healthcare institutions, organizing and hosting conferences can help generate income (Pratt et al., 2005) as well as raise the profile of an institution.

Why Do Individuals Partake in Sponsoring and Philanthropy?

Donors and sponsors become involved in sponsoring or philanthropy for multiple reasons. For example, they may become involved for purposes of social responsibility, visibility, advertising, image enhancement, marketing strategy, employee retention, building corporate relationships, facilitating teamwork, indirect support in return, or individual or collective recognition (internal and external objectives), or for tax rebate or deduction. Several of these potential reasons fall under the category of profit maximization (Brammer & Millington, 2005) and are part of a strategy (Zhang et al., 2010). In the case of a purely philanthropic act, the donor may inform the receiving institution that they do not want to receive any visible form of acknowledgment for their contribution to the fundraising campaign. This is usually seen on donors' boards marked as "Anonymous donor."

For the beneficiary benefits can be used to: build a new simulation facility or update an existing one, conduct a project, gain the ability to offer a new service, acquire additional resources to better meet the needs of existing programs, receive assistance in support of a current or future project, benefit from external expertise, and enhance collaboration opportunities.

Exploring Strategies and Benefits Behind Successful Fundraising

Companies and individuals usually do not easily part with their hard-earned money unless they really value the cause for which support is sought, have great faith that the group will manage the donations and project well, and believe it will be successful in achieving its ultimate goal. Alternatively or in addition, it may benefit them in another way or they may feel the need to fulfill a duty of corporate social responsibility (in the case of a company) or charity (mainly in the case of an individual).

Programs with a track record of an already successful program or simulation training initiative embarking onto a capacity building project are likely to be favorably looked upon by potential donors (Pattillo et al., 2010). An external mark of recognition such as that received when awarded accreditation by a professional body or respected society (such as being recognized by the Society for Simulation in Healthcare [SSH] as an accredited simulation program) provides a declaration that a program has met the highest standards in the industry (SSH, 2012).

Having a clear understanding of the local financial and tax system can be extremely helpful as some special situations may prove beneficial to either or both the donor and the benefactor in the form of tax rebate or matched government funding (Kaye, 2008; Pharoah, 2011; Zhang et al., 2010). These can be powerful arguments that can sway the decision of a potential donor, as it could be seen as an additional gain to them for supporting the fundraising campaign.

Being able to make a case that resonates with donors such that they respond to a fundraising campaign is crucial. Examples that may "speak" to the community are the ethical and proven benefits of simulation in the delivery of patient care through demonstrated improved patient outcomes (Barsuk et al., 2009; Draycott et al., 2008) and the opportunities offered of addressing the real shortage of teaching sites (Cleary et al., 2010).

SECTION 4 • Funding

Another key factor behind successful fundraising is knowing whom to contact and which companies are likely to respond to the fundraising campaign. It is reported that larger companies in consumer-focused industries are more likely givers than other companies (Brammer & Millington, 2005). Institutions that rely on nongovernmental external support usually have an individual or an entire department specialized in raising external funds (Daly, 2013). Other than wealthy potential donors and figureheads, the alumni population constitutes a constantly growing target population (Gallo, 2012). Fostering the alumni's loyalty to a university seems to be a determining factor in how much support a university is going to receive (Orkodashvili, 2007). Developing and maintaining an intimate relation with alumni or other potential donors through events, news brochures, and other communicative means has become a key strategy of educational institutions to diversify their income streams (Gallo, 2012). The sophistication of this type of activity has become a profession in the sector with actual fundraising targets (Daly, 2013; Proper, 2009). The responsibility of such activities is often absorbed by what may be called Alumni, External Relations, or Communications departments. Such a department may have among their core responsibilities to drive or at least support fundraising activities. The efficiency of the solicitation and established relationship may be determinant factors of the generosity expressed by alumni and donors (Belfield & Beney, 2000; Gallo, 2012; Weerts & Ronca, 2009), although there is a real effect of accumulative advantage whereby rich and prestigious institutions usually attract more donors than other institutions (Orkodashvili, 2007). Fundraisers develop relationships over time and through this learn when it might be most appropriate to contact companies or individuals, depending on their circumstances and annual budget allocations.

One should also consider what can be expected from whom (foundations, individuals, companies) when it comes to fundraising. As a fundraiser, it is important to know exactly what is needed (money, expertise, equipment, or a mixture of some of these) and be able to identify appropriate potential donors that match with the identified needs. Then comes the important question as to how best to formally approach the targeted sponsor or donor, how to write the sponsorship request or fundraising brochure, and what incentives can be put forward. Potential donors will be flattered to receive an invitation from a senior member of staff of the institution conducting a fundraising campaign, and hence are more likely to be responsive to it.

It is sometimes preferable to negotiate long-term loans of equipment from entities over donations (financial or equipment) or have a combination of both. The latter approach has already been successfully implemented (Alinier, 2007), providing mutual benefits to both parties while ensuring that some assets (preferably those with a long-term currency and low maintenance costs such as beds) actually belong to the program. Such donated items count toward institutional assets, whereas items on loan may never be accounted for from a financial or institutional income point of view. In addition to becoming obsolete over time, the maintenance of purchased equipment can be very expensive. In the case of a long-term loan, it remains the responsibility of the manufacturer to maintain their equipment. By providing this equipment, the manufacturer provides the learners with a piece of equipment that they may ultimately purchase once they complete their course and are in a position of purchasing authority in a health care institution. Another beneficial arrangement is the negotiation of a sponsorship or donation contract over a period of time such as 2 or 3 years. From a budgeting perspective, this ensures recurrent financial support over a period of time as opposed to receiving a large lump sum payment given by a donor.

Projects of Interest to Potential Donors

A potential donor is always interested to know how their financial support will be used. When equipment is provided by a sponsor or donor, it is easy to show how it was utilized and by whom. Money, on the other hand, could potentially be used for anything, and the donor usually needs some form of reassurance and recognition to feel comfortable about providing. When they are told their financial donation contributed to the purchase of a specific piece of equipment, they may appreciate seeing it actually visibly recorded somewhere in the form of a small recognition plaque. It is essential that these funds that have been provided for a specific purpose are used and that this use is documented in a formal way to ensure there was no potentially perceived inappropriate use of the funds.

Major donors, whether private, corporate, or foundation, might be interested in providing support in setting up a new facility or expanding a current program, and offer to provide an **endowment** worth having the program named after them. Specific research projects may also prove attractive to potential donors, but if a corporate sponsor comes forward, one must consider whether there are any possible conflicts of interest.

Benefits to Donors and Sponsorship Opportunities

Different types of sponsorship opportunities can be offered to potential donors and partners:

1. Major partner
   Support at this level would be substantial and may result in the establishment of an exclusive relationship. Partners are often offered association in activities and possibly an invitation to participate in decisions (e.g., member of board of directors, participation in working meetings). There may be a naming opportunity for major sponsors in relation to a facility, activity, or staff position.
2. Project partner or sponsor
   Support provided depends on the nature of the project. Benefits are related to the identified project only.

3. Service partner or in-kind supporter
   An example of this would include insurance, necessary materials, accommodation, and various supplies. Benefits are typically based on the value of the partnership.

Benefits that can be offered to donors include the following:

1. Visibility
   - Logo included or sponsorship noted on promotional materials: posters, flyers, invitations, tickets, website, catalog, program, newspaper, or other publication.
   - Logo included in advertising (Web, TV, or radio).
   - Association with the media campaign, invitation to speak at the press conference, listed in the press release and press kit.
   - Presence on site (e.g., signs, banners), naming, access, and even exclusivity. This may attract future customers as learners become accustomed to their products or equipment (marketing opportunity).
   - Attendance at the inauguration event: speaking, signage, gifts.
   - Recognition toward an individual.
2. Public relations
   - Guided tours, provision of reception rooms for guests of the sponsor.
   - Invitations to the opening or other formal events.
   - Collaboration on current or future projects.
   - Team spirit strengthened between the sponsored team and donor organization.
3. Internal communication
   - Articles and pictures in company newsletter.
   - Gaining access to the sponsored facilities and resources, free entrance for staff.
   - Involvement of some staff in the implementation of the project.
4. External communication
   - Authorization for the sponsor to use the logo of the sponsored program in its communications and brochures.

Role of Simulation in Fundraising

Apart from being used in education of healthcare providers, simulation can also be used in other business or administrative activities such as for selection, recruitment, and training purposes. Simulation can therefore be used to help in fundraising. For example, scenarios can be created to simulate potential communication experiences between potential donors and staff, thus providing the individuals who will be meeting with potential donors the opportunity for deliberate practice (Alinier & Platt, 2014).

Another potentially important role for simulation to obtain the support of donors is to conduct demonstrations of the type of learning experiences additional funding will help support. Even with limited resources, through the use of standardized patients for example, realistic simulated encounters will help laypersons understand what the ultimate goal of the overall project is.

THE "HOW TO . . ."

Start a Fundraising Campaign

The first step in the process is to ensure that all immediate stakeholders are consulted to determine the exact scope of the fundraising campaign. This includes determining specific details related to the goal and scope of the project that is seeking funds. This applies whether funds are being solicited for general support or for the development of a new program, research project, or facility. The itemized list may include capital elements (nonrecurrent items) or operational elements over a set period of time (i.e., to the completion date of the project). Capital elements could include the purchase of expensive pieces of equipment or buildings required for a new facility or the renovation of an existing one. On the other hand, operational costs can be used for replacement of disposable items, project staff salaries, maintenance contracts, running costs, and, if applicable, funds for the dissemination of the project outcomes to cite only a few. Past that stage, it is time to start discussions with the institution's fundraisers to actually develop the formal fundraising campaign that will appeal to potential donors.

Attract Donors or Sponsors

One approach is to organize events to which you can invite potential donors or sponsors and show them what you would like to achieve and what has already been achieved thanks to donations already received. This may include achievements supported by external donations in a totally different domain to the one for which you are trying to raise funds. Bringing to their attention how their donation may be benefited by other donors, directly or indirectly, can also be a powerful method to demonstrate that extending support to your project would be a positive action. It could include showing them how a project, room, facility, or building has been named after the major donor as a sign of recognition, showing a prominently positioned donor's board listing all their names, or pointing out pieces of equipment with a recognition plaque mentioning thanks to the individual or company who donated it.

Public events also provide great opportunities for potential donors to meet with the institution's leadership and begin to develop relationships. If donors see that a project receives direct support from the executives of the institution, they often realize that the project is perceived to be of high importance, and they are more likely to help in whatever way they can.

Write a Fundraising Document

Writing a fundraising document or brochure should provide sufficient information so individuals can understand what the project is about, what the current context is, and why its realization is so important. It should be just the appropriate length and use terms that can be understood by everyone. The team developing the fundraising documentation should be mindful that some large companies may receive as many as 100 such sponsorship invitations per month and one wants to make sure that theirs stands out in a positive manner. A clear, concise, and well-organized document is more likely to be read in its totality, and hence it increases the chances of the project being supported. A cover letter usually accompanies the brochure and should be customized to the recipient, be as clear and concise as possible, and inspire confidence. Having received and reviewed the information provided, the potential donor should feel compelled to meet the project leader to explore how they could support the project.

Structure the Fundraising Document

The front cover of the brochure should include the title of the project, with possibly an explanatory subtitle. The benefiting institution or organization should be clearly identifiable by its full name and logo. It is also an appropriate place to provide the contact details of the project leader or institutional fundraiser. If a fundraising event is being organized, it can also be prominently advertised with the date and exact location.

The document itself can be divided into several parts:

1. Presentation of the project leader from the fundraising organization; introduction of the currently secured sponsors (with their authorization) if appropriate and applicable; other information that brings credibility to the quality and the reliability of project and its team (e.g., experience, previous achievements).
2. Presentation of the project: background and objectives, description, practical information (e.g., location, date, duration). Include any identified future prospects.
3. Public campaign activities.
4. Budget presented in outline format.
   - Income: grants, in-kind support already obtained, own revenue, sponsorship sought.
   - Expenses: wages, fixed costs, and other miscellaneous expenses related to the event.
5. Partnership opportunities and fundraising target: This is the most interesting part for corporate or business partners. It must be very clear, innovative, and as attractive as possible.

Goals, interests, wishes, benefits, financial resources, methods, and function of official sponsorships vary from one company to another. It is therefore suitable to make proposals to the greatest possible number of companies and leave the door open for discussion. Proposed benefits put forward to potential industry partners can be listed as bullet points but state explicitly whether these are negotiable. The ideal outcome may be a long-term agreement with a single partner, although it may not always prove practical owing to conditions that the company may impose. For example, it would be important to consider whether it is a good idea to use only a specific brand of medical equipment if that brand is totally absent from the local market—learners might not be familiar with the devices, and it would potentially distract them from the core learning objectives of their simulation session. This is why it is valuable to consider cosponsorships, occasional or temporary sponsors, as well as in-kind services. These may allow the program to affiliate with the various companies that equip the surrounding hospitals and healthcare settings.

The intended fundraising target is highly dependent on the sponsors that are eventually attracted to support the project. The specified fundraising amount can be offset by the support received through equipment donations or loan, for example. Amounts of fundraising can be linked to offered benefits. For example, a financial donation of $1,000,000 can be linked to the naming of a facility.

In addition to the document described above, once a dialogue has started, additional materials can be provided. These might include product brochures, press releases, curriculum vitae, programs, promotional materials, photos, and floor plans.

Ensure the Sustainability of a Simulation Program

Strategies have been developed to ensure sustainability, support new programs, or build capacity of simulation programs (Alinier, 2008; Pattillo et al., 2010). As such, it is not unusual for simulation program to diversify their income streams by becoming involved in funded research or developing some form of commercial activity portfolio whereby they offer continuing professional development to staff from other institutions, or they may even rent out the environment for short periods as a film set. Well beyond the realm of fundraising, this significantly calls upon other skills such as finance, management, program development, marketing, evaluation, and leadership.

BEEN THERE, DONE THAT: MAINTAINING A RELATIONSHIP WITH EXISTING KEY DONORS?

Institutional fundraisers are usually very good at developing a relationship with donors, but they need to be supported by the teams who benefit from the funds raised. This involves keeping fundraisers, and through them donors, informed of the success stories that emerge from funded projects. This may include external marks of esteem received by a program (i.e., accreditation by SSH), key publications directly emerging from a sponsored research project, or receipt of positive media attention. It may also be beneficial to organize a public event showcasing what a program has achieved after a period of time following completion of the fundraising campaign.

Depending on the type of donor (foundation, private, or corporate), various avenues exist to maintain and build upon existing relationships. An industry partner may be interested in being offered access to your training facility for a short period of time as a training venue for their staff or customers or to shoot a short video clip about a new piece of equipment, whereas a private donor may welcome a personal tour of your facility to see the piece of equipment purchased with their financial contribution to the fundraising project.

In time, other initiatives will be identified that will be the object of a future fundraising campaign. Knowing your donors and their personal interests will position you to present these opportunities to them.

SUMMARY

To be successful at fundraising requires specific knowledge and skills. Building a successful fundraising campaign requires significant planning so that there is a compelling case for giving with a clear message, set expectations, and goals. Fundraising needs to target the right audience of potential donors, which may include companies or individuals to whom the message will be of interest and the potential return appealing.

Established institutions may have staff specialized in managing fundraising campaigns and maintaining a relationship with key donors. This can be a very time-consuming activity, and success partially depends on the relationships that have been established with the potential donors and the trust they place in the people leading the project. Philanthropic donations and funds obtained through fundraising typically do not represent a stable form of income that will guarantee the sustainability of a simulation program unless the funds are in the form of a substantial endowment. Totally relying on this form of income in the long-term places the staff directly linked to the program under great pressure and uncertainty of continuous employment. To develop more secure income streams, seeking sponsorship contracts with key partners for periods of at least 2 to 3 years at a time is optimal.

REFERENCES

Alinier, G. (2007). Enhancing trainees' learning experience through the opening of an advanced multiprofessional simulation training facility at the University of Hertfordshire. *British Journal of Anaesthetic and Recovery Nursing, 8*(2), 22–27.

Alinier, G. (2008). Prosperous simulation under an institution's threadbare financial blanket. In R. R. Kyle & W. B. Murray (Eds.), *Clinical simulation: Operations, engineering, and management* (1st ed., pp. 491–493). San Diego, CA: Academic Press.

Alinier, G., & Platt, A. (2014). International overview of high-level simulation education initiatives in relation to critical care. *Nursing in Critical Care, 19*(1):42–49.

Barsuk, J. H., Cohen, E. R., Feinglass, J., McGaghie, W. C., & Wayne, D. B. (2009). Use of simulation-based education to reduce catheter-related bloodstream infections. *Archives of Internal Medicine, 169*(15), 1420–1424.

Belfield, C. R., & Beney, A. P. (2000). What determines alumni generosity? Evidence for the UK. *Education Economics, 8*(1), 65–80.

Brammer, S., & Millington, A. (2005). Profit maximisation vs. agency: An analysis of charitable giving by UK firms. *Cambridge Journal of Economics, 29*(4), 517–534.

Cleary, B. L., Hassmiller, S. B., Reinhard, S. C., Richardson, E. M., Veenema, T. G., & Werner, S. (2010). Uniting states, sharing strategies: Forging partnerships to expand nursing education capacity. *The American Journal of Nursing, 110*(1), 43–50.

Daly, S. (2013). Philanthropy, the new professionals and higher education: The advent of directors of development and alumni relations. *Journal of Higher Education Policy and Management, 35*, 23–33.

Draycott, T. J., Crofts, J. F., Ash, J. P., Wilson, L. V., Yard, E., Sibanda, T., & Whitelaw, A. (2008). Improving neonatal outcome through practical shoulder dystocia training. *Obstetrics and Gynecology, 112*(1), 14–20.

Fritz, P. Z., Gray, T., & Flanagan, B. (2008). Review of mannequin-based high-fidelity simulation in emergency medicine. *Emergency Medicine Australasia, 20*(1), 1–9.

Gallo, M. (2012). Beyond philanthropy: Recognising the value of alumni to benefit higher education institutions. *Tertiary Education and Management, 18*(1), 41–55.

Henderson, T. M., & Hassmiller, S. B. (2007). Hospitals and philanthropy as partners in funding nursing education. *Nursing Economic$, 25*(2), 95–100, 109, 155.

Huang, G. C., Gordon, J. A., & Schwartzstein, R. M. (2007). Millennium conference 2005 on medical simulation: A summary report. *Simulation in Healthcare, 2*(2), 88–95. doi:10.1097/SIH.1090b1013e318053e318066.

Kaye, T. (2008). The gentle art of corporate seduction: Tax incentives in the United States and the European Union. *Kansas Law Review, 57*, 93–156.

Meek, T. (2008). Anaesthetic simulators: Making the most of your purchase. *Current Anaesthesia & Critical Care, 19*, 354–360.

Meguerdichian, D. A., Heiner, J. D., & Younggren, B. N. (2012). Emergency medicine simulation: A resident's perspective. *Annals of Emergency Medicine, 60*(1), 121.

Orkodashvili, M. (2007). Higher education funding issues: US/UK comparison (Munich Personal RePEc Archive, Paper 16417). Retrieved from http://mpra.ub.uni-muenchen.de/id/eprint/16417

Pattillo, R. E., Hewett, B., McCarthy, M. D., & Molinari, D. (2010). Capacity building for simulation sustainability. *Clinical Simulation in Nursing, 6*(5), e185–e191.

Pharoah, C. (2011). Private giving and philanthropy—their place in the Big Society. *People, Place and Policy Online, 5*(2), 65–75.

Pratt, N., Vo, K., Ganiats, T. G., & Weinger, M. B (2005). The San Diego Center for Patient Safety: Creating a research, education, and community consortium. In K. Henriksen, J. B. Battles, E. S. Marks, & D. I. Lewin (Eds.), *Advances in patient safety: From research to implementation* (Vol. 4: Programs, tools, and products). Rockville, MD: Agency for Healthcare Research and Quality.

Proper, E. (2009). Bringing educational fundraising back to Great Britain: A comparison with the United States. *Journal of Higher Education Policy and Management, 31*(2), 149–159.

Society for Simulation in Healthcare. (2012). *SSH Accreditation of Healthcare Simulation Programs.* Retrieved from Society for Simulation in Healthcare website: http://ssih.org/accreditation-of-healthcare-simulation-programs

Srivastava, P., & Oh, S.-A. (2010). Private foundations, philanthropy, and partnership in education and development: Mapping the terrain. *International Journal of Educational Development, 30*(5), 460–471.

The Free Dictionary. (2013). Definition of fund raising. Retrieved from http://www.thefreedictionary.com/Fund+raising

Weerts, D. J., & Ronca, J. M. (2009). Using classification trees to predict alumni giving for higher education. *Education Economics, 17*(1), 95–122.

Zhang, R., Zhu, J., Yue, H., & Zhu, C. (2010). Corporate philanthropic giving, advertising intensity, and industry competition level. *Journal of Business Ethics, 94*(1), 39–52.

CHAPTER 4.7

Grant Writing

Sandrijn M. van Schaik, MD, PhD

ABOUT THE AUTHORS

SANDRIJN M. VAN SCHAIK designs and tests simulation programs and runs an active research program focusing on interprofessional teamwork and communication. She has extensive grant writing experience and has successfully competed for a variety of different grants for her various projects. These include small institutional awards at her home institution, as well as substantial external grants, including the Josiah Macy Jr. Foundation Faculty Scholarship Award and Stemmler funding from the National Board for Medical Examiners.

Acknowledgments: With appreciation for the UCSF Kanbar Center Simulation and Scholarship group for their thoughtful comments.

ABSTRACT

Funding in healthcare is under stress from many sources. Finding alternative funding sources is key to survival for simulation programs globally. This chapter provides information about how grant funding can support simulation, where to look for grant funding, and how to write a competitive application. A compelling grant should address an important problem that is in line with the funding agency's priorities and be clearly written with a concise problem statement, sound methodology, and a reasonable budget. Common pitfalls are discussed.

CASE EXAMPLE

You are an experienced simulation educator known for your creative ideas for innovative approaches to simulation-based education. The administrator of your simulation program at the academic medical center approached you this morning to inform you that she would like for you to take the lead role in writing a grant to support your simulation work. You are pleased to be asked and excited by the opportunity, but are not sure what grant to apply for nor how to write a compelling grant application. Complicating the matter, you are not exactly sure for what to ask. Who can help you get started? Where can you find further information?

INTRODUCTION AND BACKGROUND

Grant funding can be an effective way to augment the support of simulation programs. Most organizations that provide grant funding are interested in innovative approaches or research aimed at improving either educational or health outcomes. Applying for a grant can therefore be a great way to fund new program development as well as research efforts that study the impact of such programs. Grant funding is typically short term (<3 years) and often not renewable; thus, if grant funding is used for development of new programs, a strategy to ensure sustainability of the program after the funding ceases needs to be developed. Regardless of the source of grant funding, the granting organization will want to see that the proposal addresses an existing need or gap, and it is of the utmost importance that a proposal has a clear problem statement. The key to successful **grant writing** is to ensure that the problem statement matches the funding priorities of the organization providing the grant, and that the proposed project offers a sound and feasible way to approach this problem. Sections in this chapter will discuss sources of revenue, fundraising, and other ways to obtain funding besides grants.

SOURCES OF GRANT FUNDING

There are a wide variety of organizations to consider when applying for funding. Some grant sources explicitly mention simulation in the **request for applications** (**RFA**). An example of an RFA specifically targeted at simulation is the RFA issued by the United States National Institute of Health (**NIH**) in conjunction with the Agency for Healthcare Research and Quality (**AHRQ**), entitled "Advances in Patient Safety through Simulation Research" (AHRQ, 2013). More often, simulation will be mentioned as one of several possible acceptable strategies to achieve certain desired outcomes. For example, the MedEvac Foundation International awards grants to support the development of education projects, such as those involving human simulators, to benefit the critical care transport community (MedEvac Foundation International, 2013), and the American Academy of Pediatrics supports research that furthers knowledge in the area of neonatal resuscitation, including research that studies whether simulation is an appropriate method of teaching and evaluating the necessary skills of resuscitation (http://www2.aap.org/nrp/science_RGP-YIA.html.). Even if simulation is not mentioned in the RFA, but the proposed project addresses the problem or need identified by the **funding agency**, the application may still receive favorable review. In this regard, it is important to remember that simulation is a relatively new strategy, and the granting organization may not have considered simulation as a possible approach when issuing the RFA. It can be helpful to look at proposals from previous grantees (often a brief synopsis or at least a title is available on the granting organization's website) or to contact the organization before putting a proposal together.

To find potential sources of grant funding, it is wise to think broadly about the problem the project is addressing. Consideration of stakeholders who could benefit from the project can help identify potential funding agencies. For example, nursing societies may have funding mechanisms to support projects that enhance nursing education, those focused on pediatric research may award proposals that improve child health, and community-based organizations may have funds to promote education of the public or enhance access to healthcare. A variety of organizations have scholarship awards for faculty development, which can provide (sometimes substantial) salary support. Several search engines exist to help with identification of funding opportunities, including the global engines Cos Pivot (http://pivot.cos.com/.), The Foundation Center (http://foundationcenter.org/.), SPIN Funding Opportunities Database (http://infoedglobal.com/solutions/grants-contracts/spin-funding-opportunities/), and ResearchResearch (http://www.researchresearch.com/.). Some of these search engines and databases require an institutional subscription. A good place to start your search for possible grants is the development office at one's own institution. This office often has a wealth of information on local, national, and international funding opportunities.

How to Get Started

Writing a grant starts with identifying the problem the grant application will address, and doing so in terms that will resonate with the funding agency's priorities. While it does not make sense to write a grant that targets a different problem than the one the agency is interested in,

experienced grant writers can often help you view a problem from different angles that makes it suitable for a variety of funding opportunities.

The first step is therefore to brainstorm with one or more people who have successfully competed for grants before. This does not necessarily have to be someone with experience in writing simulation grants; in general, people who have written grants for education or quality improvement projects will have sufficient expertise to provide valuable advice. At university-affiliated institutions, dean's offices often have information about who at the institution has received grants. If there is a medical education or grants office, individuals in these offices can be a source of information and support. Alternatively, successful grant writers can be located through professional networks, through websites maintained by funding agencies, and by paying attention to listed funding sources in peer-reviewed publications (Figure 4.7.1).

Writing a Compelling and Cohesive Story

Grant applications undergo competitive review; the ratio between submitted proposals and funded awards varies but can be as low as 1 in 10. It is therefore critical that a grant application tell a compelling and cohesive story that will convince reviewers of the importance of the proposed project. A clear problem statement that matches the priorities of the funding agency is essential, but this may get lost if the proposal is poorly written. Most organizations set forth clear guidelines that describe the required components of an application, and such guidelines should be followed closely. Typically, a proposal has at least the following components, which will be discussed in detail below: (1) introduction and background section with rationale, (2) **specific aims** or objectives, (3) methods, (4) anticipated outcomes and impact, and (5) budget and **budget justification**.

Introduction and Background or Rationale

This section should describe the problem statement or research question and clearly outline why this problem or

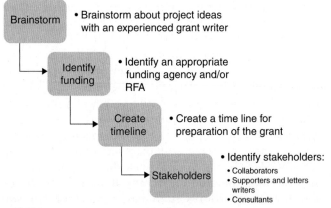

Writing a grant: first steps in the process

- Brainstorm → • Brainstorm about project ideas with an experienced grant writer
- Identify funding → • Identify an appropriate funding agency and/or RFA
- Create timeline → • Create a time line for preparation of the grant
- Stakeholders → • Identify stakeholders:
  - Collaborators
  - Supporters and letters writers
  - Consultants

FIGURE 4.7.1 Writing a grant: first steps in the process.

question is important in light of the funding agency's priorities or RFA. It should include a recent, relevant, and concise review of the literature and highlight the gaps that exist that the proposed project will fill. Depending on the scope of the project and the priorities of the funding organization, this can be a gap that is universally true (e.g., "it is not known how often simulation-based team training needs to be repeated to achieve optimal retention of teamwork skills"), or a gap that exists locally or in one area (e.g., "despite evidence in the literature that teaching novices central line insertion with the use of simulation reduces central line infections, at our institution such training is currently not available"). While a large, international funding organization might be interested in supporting research that addresses the former gap, the latter may get support from a local or regional agency.

A proposal for an educational research project should mention the **conceptual framework** for the study, which is the theoretical context for the study question (Beckman & Cook, 2007). The last sentence of the Background/Rationale section should clearly summarize the gap and the overall goal of the proposed project: "The project proposed in this application aims to address gap X by doing (or studying) Y."

Specific Aims or Objectives

The overall goal of the project should be broken into specific aims, or objectives; these are the measurable outcomes of the project. If the proposal is to develop a new simulation program, what outcomes will be measured to assess the impact of the program? These should be outcomes that are relevant and directly related to the innovation; outcomes lower on Kirkpatrick's evaluation model (e.g., learner's satisfaction) are often less compelling than those at the top of Kirkpatrick's hierarchy (e.g., changes in patient health; Beckman & Cook, 2007). As an example, assessing the impact of simulation-based neonatal resuscitation training could involve evaluation data from participants, skills assessment during subsequent simulated resuscitations, skills assessment during real-life resuscitations, or changes in outcomes after neonatal resuscitations.

Similarly, the specific aims for a research study break the study question into the specific, measurable ways in which the study hypothesis will be tested. For example, the study question "do high stress levels during simulation training interfere with learning?" can be broken up into specific aims that describe in detail who will be studied, how stress will be measured and modulated, and what instruments will be used to assess learning.

Methods

An RFA may have specific instructions on what to include in the Methods section. Typically, this section includes information about subjects and settings, procedures, and statistical analysis. If the project includes an innovation and/or intervention, this should be described in detail. If preexisting instruments are used, a brief description of available validity information with references should be included; if new instruments are developed for the purpose of the project, there should be a plan for validity testing (Downing, 2003).

The Methods section of a research study should start with the study design: is the study observational or interventional, quantitative or qualitative in nature? Consultation with educational research specialists is recommended to confirm that the methodology is appropriate, will provide answers to the research question, and is clearly described. For quantitative research, justification of sample size, if possible based on power calculation, as well as a description of the sampling strategy should be included. Consult with a statistician to get help with identification of appropriate statistical tests and to ensure that potential confounders are accounted for.

Anticipated Outcomes and Impact

This section should describe the possible outcomes of the project, including potential problems and how these will be addressed. It should be explained how the project outcomes will be disseminated; will study results be presented at conferences and/or submitted for publication? If the project involves development of new curriculum or assessment tools, how will these be distributed to other potential users? The section should also discuss the expected impact of the project. Going back to the original problem statement or research question, what will happen once this project has addressed the problem or question? Depending on the scope of the project and the priorities of the funding agency, this should be described in terms of impact on a local, national, or global level, or in terms of impact on the field. Lastly, there should be a plan for sustainability after completion of grant funding, which should link to the budget and explain how different budget items will be funded (unless no longer needed) after the end of the grant cycle.

Budget and Budget Justification

Check carefully what is allowed as part of the grant; this can vary greatly between different funding agencies and even between different grants offered by the same organization. Make sure that the budget is realistic and accurate; all budget items should be required to perform the proposed project, and quotes should be included when appropriate and possible. Personnel costs, if allowed, should be reasonable in light of the scope of the work. Some funding agencies only allow so-called direct costs to be included in the budget, whereas others allow **indirect costs** (administrative and other overhead costs incurred by the institution of the grant recipient); these are often capped at 10%. While there is no point in creating

SECTION 4 • Funding

a budget that is too low, overbudgeting will reduce the credibility of the proposal. Many institutions require grant applications to be reviewed by their contracts and grants department days to weeks before the submission deadline, so make sure to check institutional guidelines in this regard (Figure 4.7.2).

Guidelines, Fine Print, and Other Details

Perhaps the second most important aspect of writing a successful grant application, after a compelling problem statement, is close attention to guidelines set forth by the funding agency. Read and follow guidelines carefully, and if anything is unclear, contact the funding agency for clarification. Remember that writing a high-quality grant takes time; create a timeline for the application process, and build in ample time to collect elements of the application that are dependent on others, such as quotes and letters of support, if required. Make sure letter writers have clear information about the project and why their support is requested; sometimes it may be advisable to draft a letter to ensure that it has the essential elements. For projects with an element of research involving human subjects, institutional rules regarding human subject research should be followed, and many granting agencies want to see documentation that this has been done.

Common Pitfalls

The most common, serious pitfalls in grant writing have been discussed above: a problem statement that is not relevant to the funding organization, and a proposal

that is poorly written. When discussing the problem statement, it is important to have a good idea about the scope of the project, which should be neither too broad nor too narrow, and realistic in light of the time allotted and the funding provided. It is helpful to create a timeline for the project and include that with the proposal. If resources are required that the grant will not provide, it should be clear how these resources will be obtained, and letters of support from relevant people should be sought. For example, if the proposal requires new equipment currently not available in the simulation program but the grant does not allow equipment purchases, it should be clear how this piece of equipment will be acquired. If the project involves a new program that requires significant time in the curriculum of a school, a letter of support from the school's dean is in order. In short, reviewers want to see evidence that a project is truly feasible, and that the specific aims or objectives will indeed be met. Along the same lines, reviewers want to see evidence that the group responsible for the project, the principal investigator (**PI**) and other project personnel, have the qualifications and experience to complete the project as planned. That does not mean that junior, inexperienced grant writers cannot get funding, but it does mean that proof of adequate mentorship by experienced people is in order.

As mentioned earlier, even with a sound problem statement and a compelling, feasible idea, a grant application can fail if it is poorly written. Grant reviewers, in general, appreciate proposals that are written in concise, clear language, without jargon and complex abbreviations. Consider, if the information is publicly available, who the reviewers are: what is their background, their area of expertise? Avoid making bold statements such as "we are the first to introduce this new approach" or "there are no published studies looking at this problem," because you risk that if you have overlooked something, you offend a reviewer. Better language to use is, for example, "to our knowledge, ours is a novel approach" or "there is a paucity of data about this problem." For similar reasons, what is presented in the application should be accurate and up to date, again an argument to consult with experienced researchers, statisticians, and the like when preparing a proposal. If there is anything unclear in the RFA, contact the program officer at the funding agency. It is always better to verify than to assume, and potentially irritate the reviewers with an application that is incorrect or incomplete.

BEEN THERE, DONE THAT. HOW CAN I CONTINUE TO IMPROVE OR SUSTAIN WHAT I HAVE ACHIEVED?

The most experienced grant writers will admit that grant writing is a skill, which needs practice to become proficient. As with any skills, the principles of deliberate

Components of a Grant*

- Problem statement
- Background and rationale with literature review
- Specific aims or project objectives
- Methods, including analysis
- Time line
- Anticipated outcomes and barriers
- Impact and plan for dissemination
- Budget with justification
- Supporting documents: letters, CV, etc

*This list is not all-inclusive and grant writers should follow the guidelines in the RFA closely, using the terminology and organization of sections as outlined by the funding agency.

FIGURE 4.7.2 Components of a grant.

practice apply: reflection and feedback are essential to get better (Ericsson et al., 1993). Rejection is never pleasant, but reviewers typically provide comments, and reading those comments carefully can be tremendously helpful, so if a proposal gets rejected, be sure to see whether comments are available. It can also be helpful to get in touch with previous grantees, ask to see their proposal and whether they have any specific tips. Have other people read the proposal, including people who are relative outsiders, who can confirm that the language is clear and the proposal easy to follow. Many organizations offer grant writing workshops at annual conferences, and a workshop on writing effective medical education research grant proposals can be found on MedEdPORTAL (2012). Additional useful references are the article by Bordage and Dawson (2003) on educational research design and grant writing and the 12 tips on grant writing published in *Medical Teacher* (Blanco & Lee, 2012).

Because grant writing is an acquired skill, it is often wise to start small. Many institutions have internal grant mechanisms, and while they may not have large sums of money to offer, the experience with grant writing can be worthwhile. In addition, having previous funding mentioned on your resume helps with credibility to obtain future awards. While not unheard of, it is unlikely for a first-time, junior grant writer to receive a large, competitive grant such as a National Institute of Health R-series grant, unless supported by senior investigators with extensive experience. The higher the sum of money involved, the more likely it is that the funding agency will want to see preliminary data, prior publications, and other evidence that the money will be well spent. It is therefore wise to consult with previous grantees and pay attention not only to the project, but also to the evidence of support and feasibility that was submitted as part of the proposal. To be eligible for large grants,

projects typically have to have considerable impact; hence, proposals with a broad scope or clear generalizability, including multi-institutional applications, are often desirable.

SUMMARY

Grant funding can provide resources to support work in simulation, in particular, new program development and research. Considering the competitive nature of the grant application process and the effort that goes into writing an application, it is advisable to plan ahead and take the time to prepare a compelling proposal. Identifying appropriate resources including a solid network of (experienced) people to support both the application and the actual project will greatly increase the chances that the project will be awarded funding, and subsequently successfully executed.

REFERENCES

Agency for Healthcare Research and Quality. (2013). *Funding announcements*. Retrieved from http://www.ahrq.gov/funding/research/announcements/index.html

Beckman, T. J., & Cook, D. A. (2007). Developing scholarly projects in education: A primer for medical teachers. *Medical Teacher, 29*, 210–218.

Blanco, M. A., & Lee, M. Y. (2012). Twelve tips for writing educational research grant proposals. *Medical Teacher, 34*, 450–453.

Bordage, G., & Dawson, B. (2003). Experimental study design and grant writing in eight steps and 28 questions. *Medical Education, 37*, 376–385.

Downing, S. M. (2003). Validity: On the meaningful interpretation of assessment data. *Medical Education, 37*, 830–837.

Ericsson, K. A., Krampe, R. T., & Tesch-Römer, C. (1993). The role of deliberate practice in the acquisition of expert performance. *Psychological Review, 100*, 363.

MedEdPORTAL. (2012). *RIME grantsmanship: How to write promising grant proposals*. Retrieved from https://www.mededportal.org/publication/9069

MedEvac Foundation International. (2013). *Education grants*. Retrieved from http://www.medevacfoundation.org/

SECTION 4 • Funding

CHAPTER 4.8

Working with Vendors

David M. LaCombe, BSM, CPLP, and Graham Whiteside, BSc (Hons) Nur Sci, DipHE MHN, RMN, RGN

ABOUT THE AUTHORS

DAVID M.LACOMBE joined Laerdal in 2006, following a 20-year career in Emergency Medical Services. His passion for patient safety and healthcare simulation began while working at the University of Miami School of Medicine. David's experiences as a Laerdal customer strongly motivated him to join the company. In his current role, he plays a strategic role in shaping the Emergency Care Portfolio to meet customer needs. David has a B.S. in Business Management.

GRAHAM WHITESIDE worked as a General & Psychiatric Nurse in England for 14 years and has spent the past 13 years working in the medical device & simulation industries in the UK & North America. Graham is fascinated by the power of positive and negative learning experiences, team work training, immersive training environments, the use of IT and emergent technologies in healthcare and simulation-based education. He is motivated by the potential for simulation to enhance clinical communication, teamwork and improved patient care outcomes.

Declaration of Interest: David LaCombe is the Emergency Care Portfolio Director for Laerdal's Americas Region. Graham Whiteside is the COO of Limbs & Things, Inc., a Task Trainer and Simulator design, manufacturing, and distribution company located in Savannah, GA, USA.

Acknowledgments: DL: I gratefully acknowledge my wife Kathryn and son William—you are the center of my universe. Through your love and daily teachings, I am a better person. I am also grateful to the many mentors, both intentional and accidental, who have taught me along the journey. Finally, I wish to thank Dr. Michael S. Gordon for his profound impact on my understanding of teaching and learning—Michael, I am forever in your debt. GW: I am proud to acknowledge my wife Helen, and my children, Ellie and Charlie, for their love, support, and tolerance of my work schedule. You make all the hours of sacrifice worthwhile! Plus, my grateful thanks to Margot, Nic, Tim, Nick, Debbie, Christer, the Limbs and Things Worldwide Team, and my colleagues and friends in the Simulation Industry for their support and encouragement in my career. I would also like to thank the clinicians, educators, and simulationists who have shared their expertise with me throughout my clinical and commercial career, which has fed my interest in simulation and my desire to positively influence patient care in an indirect way.

ABSTRACT

Working with vendors is an important component of all Simulation Center operations. The broad, and growing, simulation industry and plethora of product options and services can be overwhelming for novices and experienced managers alike.

This chapter seeks to help the reader to appreciate the value of the tacit knowledge held by vendors so that they may incorporate vendor expertise into Center operations. It also aims to aid the experienced Center Manager to understand how to share their simulation expertise with vendors to improve the art and science of simulation options.

CASE EXAMPLE

Andrea Browne is the newly appointed Manager of Immersive Learning at a university-based center for allied health education. Her vast experience as a nurse, manager, and educator helped her stand out from other applicants. Andrea is well versed in adult learning theories and teaching strategies. She taught nursing and medical students at a previous job and has some experience in facilitating simulations. Unfortunately, Andrea is about to experience a challenge she is not prepared for—she must lead the Center's acquisition and implementation of healthcare simulation technology. The Dean for Health Programs directed Andrea to chair a cross-functional technology committee charged with selecting vendors and equipment. Her authority is limited—she does not supervise the committee members, and the Dean will make the final decision on equipment.

Drawing upon her experience as an educator, Andrea knew the committee should first determine user needs. The committee members, however, believed they already understood the user's requirements and wanted to tour other simulation centers to view "best practices." This was the first sign of friction. Andrea accompanied the committee on tours and continued to advocate for speaking with potential users to determine their unmet needs. To no avail, Andrea observed the committee discussing educational tools and practices without really understanding what problem they were trying to solve.

Immediately following one of the tours, the committee experienced an upset when one of the members scheduled a meeting with vendors to review simulator technology. The meeting invitation was the first indication to the team that their organization was speaking to the industry. Andrea was deeply worried that the committee was not prepared to speak to vendors. She believed that the committee members were acting in silos and that things were moving too fast. Despite expressing her concern to the committee, several members suggested that there was no harm in speaking to vendors—the meeting would occur next week.

Andrea's concerns became apparent to the committee when two things happened: first, the vendors asked a lot of questions that the committee could not answer. In some cases, the committee members gave conflicting information to the vendors. Secondly, the Chair of the Foundation partnering on the project expressed concern to the University President that the foundation would not fund any project without first reviewing a detailed plan. The President and Dean were embarrassed and assured the foundation that the project plan would be reviewed and increased leadership would be provided to the technology committee.

INTRODUCTION, BACKGROUND, AND SIGNIFICANCE

Opening and expanding a healthcare simulation program may feel overwhelming even to the experienced manager. Without a well-developed plan, the experience may be likened to being dropped into a foreign country—the language is different, the culture is confusing, and people are impatiently waiting for you as you struggle to open a borrowed map.

This chapter contains principles and practices that, if applied, will simplify your technology adoption journey. The authors provide a unique perspective on the use of technology to support learning needs. Because they both work for technology companies, they are able to describe the industry's perspective on working with vendors.

Much like traveling, it is advisable to prepare before wandering into the unknown. Navigating the technology landscape without a plan increases the risk of getting lost. The advice contained in this chapter is organized into two themes: *Technology Planning* and *How to Select Vendors, Services, Products, and Solutions.*

The heart of the first theme includes principles that call for developing an understanding of user needs and creating value propositions for stakeholders. Once these core principles are addressed, the manager may define use models, develop technology plans, and begin a budgetary process.

The second theme is about engaging vendors. It begins with a description of vendor types, including capabilities, then moves into how and when to contact them. Next, a framework for selecting the right solution for your organization is presented.

Many excellent texts describe the ideal way to research, plan, and implement a simulation program at a local level (Doyle et al., 2008; Jeffries, 2007; Lewandowski, 2008) or a consortium level (Jeffries & Battin, 2012). This chapter adds to this knowledge base by helping the reader understand the structure and capabilities of vendors in the broadest sense so that you may get the very best out of your vendor relationships.

Vendors produce a wide range of educational products, including didactic materials, task trainers, augmented and virtual reality trainers, computer-based simulations, full-body mannequins, courseware, debriefing and learning management systems. Vendors also bring a unique perspective to the simulation program that is based upon years of experience and exposure to multiple simulation-based programs. For instance, vendors who supply audio-visual tools for debriefing are often involved with a greater volume of program planning than even architects or consultants and at a much deeper level (Doyle, Carovano, & Anton, 2008).

A vendor's ability to draw upon their existing customer's practices, coupled with business acumen and diverse product portfolios, has created an industry-wide tacit knowledge around simulation that is extensive.

The mutual codependence between buyers and those that produce solutions for them is recognized. Just like symbiotic relationships found in nature, balance must be sought to ensure both parties benefit from the interaction. The authors trust that this chapter helps buyers create the optimal environment when dealing with vendors. For the continued prosperity of both species, we call for each party to listen carefully, seek to understand needs, and collaborate on solutions that help to enrich the lives of others.

THEMES: THE HOW TO . . .

Theme 1: Technology Planning

On planning, American Army General Dwight Eisenhower (1957) said, "plans are worthless; planning is everything." Eisenhower's wisdom is highly relevant to simulation program managers. A strategic plan or technology plan is never really complete. Revisions occur because the landscape frequently changes. However, the process of ongoing planning is priceless. Planning forces one to assess where they are and compare that to where they want to be. The gaps, or distance between current state and future state, are the tasks that need to be managed.

Respected leader and author Steven Covey (2004) described a habit known as "Begin with the end in mind." This habit is about imagination—the ability to envision in your mind what you cannot yet see with your eyes. Recall the case study where Andrea Browne was tasked with opening a new immersive learning program. Don't you agree that Andrea had to demonstrate imagination as she initially described the vision for the program? When planning is properly conducted, imagination is replaced in iterations with plans, timelines, and budgets.

A word about efficiency and effectiveness for planners: Neither dream too long nor hasten the planning process. Visionaries with clear plans who cannot direct the actions of others are valueless, so too are those who squander time creating the perfect plan. The effective planner understands the value of planning and acts with a sense of urgency to get plans in action.

Imagine what would happen if Andrea could not explain the vision to vendors. How likely would the technology providers understand the required solution? Knowing this risk underscores the critical need to begin planning before engaging vendors. The plan need not be complete, but the canvas should have some detail, specifically mission and desired outcomes, both of which are based on user needs.

Experienced instructional designers, entrepreneurs, and leaders share a common understanding. They know that successful solutions are born from unmet user needs. Begin with the user in mind when planning your simulation solution. Know what pains them and what keeps them awake at night.

A Framework for Selecting the Right Solution for Your Organization

Selecting a solution to a problem often requires striking a balance between many complementary factors illustrated in Figure 4.8.1. A solution delivers value when it helps to make organizational impact. The Framework supports value-based design and purchasing decisions.

Take care not to conclude on user needs too quickly. The needs statement, or user requirements statement, must be based on fact. The planner should focus first on the "Why" before "How" and "What." People (executives and other decision makers) do not buy what you do; they buy why you do it (Sinek, 2009).

The Framework's foundation is about the "Why." Using a traditional gap analysis process, the problem is studied and measured. Sample questions may include "why are patients getting infection during central line insertions?" and "why are new graduates making medication errors?" The baseline

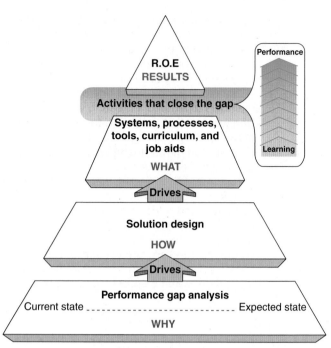

FIGURE 4.8.1 Why to results framework.

measurement establishes the current state while the desired state described the stakeholder's expectations—from these measurements, the value proposition is born.

Too frequently, a customer will approach vendors with a statement such as "we want to build a 4,000 square feet (371.6 m^2) simulation program." "OK, can you tell me why?" asks the vendor. The customer replies, "Sure, we want to teach using simulation." From this point, little good can happen without hitting the pause button. Planners and vendors alike need to understand why the institution is investing in simulation.

Tip: Resist the temptation to conclude that all performance deficiencies are due to lack of knowledge. Be wary of stakeholders that open a "why" discussion with statements like "we need a training program that . . ." Be sure to consider operational and cultural factors before assuming that all performance deficiencies are caused by a lack of knowledge. Training will not be impactful when employees possess knowledge and skills but have operational obstacles that prevent them from applying it on the job.

The "How" section of the Framework describes the processes within an organization to design, develop, and implement training. Organizations with well-defined instructional design processes usually start with "why" questions and apply the answers in a disciplined and multi-iterative approach. When discipline and processes are lacking, the organization typically struggles to create timely and impactful programs.

Tip: A perfect solution is the enemy of a good-enough solution. It is preferable to roll out a solid draft, measure the solution's impact, and adjust as needed rather than waiting for the perfect solution that may never materialize.

The discipline demonstrated in the "How" phase drives outputs in the "What" phase. Courses, job aids, and simulation scenarios are examples of services and products that help to achieve results. The goal of all training should be to effect changes in behavior. Thus, one should take great care to select the technology that supports the desired results.

Tip: Vendor representatives can make relevant suggestions about "What" when they understand your "Whys."

Use the Value Proposition to Build Allies

A stakeholder is a person, or group of people, with an interest in a project or enterprise. Starting, or growing, a simulation program requires influential stakeholders who align themselves to your endeavor. Getting allies to buy in depends on your ability to communicate a clear value proposition—a short statement that clearly communicates the benefits your "customer" gets for using your product, service, or idea (MindTools, n.d.).

Building a simulation program is not a goal. It is an activity, and it is not an activity that excites those that have to pay for it. Effective goals, the ones that do excite payers, solve unmet needs, are measurable, and bring value to the organization. Try this sample goal instead: "ABC Hospital seeks to build a simulation program to shorten the transition to practice process for graduate nurses while ensuring the competence of new team members." Better? Do you think this goal will create excitement? You bet it will. Time and competence can be measured. Knowing these goals also sets the actions of planners and vendors on a synergistic path.

Identifying stakeholders starts easily but then requires some imagination. The most obvious stakeholders are those who have a known requirement to consume your product, and trust us, you are creating a product.

Potential stakeholders

- Clinicians needing training to satisfy, earn, and maintain privileges
- Learners with limited clinical opportunities
- Teams needing practice to maintain infrequently used skills
- Healthcare providers seeking continuing education
- Community-based groups
- Patients
- Risk managers
- Patient safety advocates
- Academic programs seeking supplemental training
- Medical device companies
- Physician and insurance groups

The above stakeholders have diverse needs—clinicians, students, and the community at large may benefit from your program. Each may help support your program if you can deliver value to them. Consumers will pay when value is apparent.

An Exercise in Establishing Value

Step 1: Know your customer—In this case, let us imagine the primary customer to be a nurse manager for a hospital operating room. The manager has several new staff; she is concerned that the staff may struggle fitting into the fast-paced surgical environment. She wants to build a strong team in a short time.

Step 2: Know your product—Understanding the customer's needs, you may leverage the experience and resources of the simulation program to solve an unmet need. Your solution may consist of evidence-based, standardized surgical simulations that may be conducted in the simulation lab or the actual OR. Teams may train together to build cohesiveness.

Step 3: Know your competitors—Your competitors require off-site training consisting of lectures and some role-playing with participants from multiple organizations. **Note:** Think broadly when identifying potential competitors. Sometimes, competitors work for the same organization. They may compete for funding and other resources. Consider transforming the internal competitors into collaborators. This may be an opportunity to gain efficiencies.

Step 4: Distill your value proposition—Completing the first three steps defines the problem, formulates a solution, and analyzes the competitive landscape. Now it is time to pitch your value proposition. Here is a sample value proposition: *The simulation program may conduct team building simulations in your actual OR. Schedule a simulation like a case—you'll improve team effectiveness while minimizing cost and disruption to your department.*

Now, repeat this exercise for each of the identified stakeholders. The sum of this activity should be a clear understanding of who your customers are, what they need, and how you may help. Using this information, you may continue to develop business, marketing, and communication plans. Share the statements with stakeholders, partners, and vendors—repeat the statements often to help build a shared mental model that describes why you exist.

Tip: Refine value-based statements so that they are memorable and impactful.

CASE STUDY: Reflection

How did Andrea's Technology Committee's failure to establish a clear value proposition affect the project? What would you do differently?

After stakeholders buy in to a vision, they will soon want to understand specific details about the metrics, or measurable outcomes, for the simulation initiative. For a new project, the metrics might initially be focused heavily on opening a program. Then, after the grand opening, a new set of metrics is required.

Outcome Measures

As the popular song "Any Road" by George Harrison (Mendes, 2008) says, "If you don't know where you're going, any road'll take you there." Investors want to know the figurative "road" you are taking while attempting to meet the objective. The value proposition is a promise—it tells others, especially buyers, what they get for investing. Few buyers invest without understanding how the promise will be delivered. Establishing realistic milestones and measurable goals improves the likelihood for success.

Establishing measurable goals for learning activities makes sense, but what measures need to be communicated to technology vendors? Consider organizing goals into two broad categories: preparing to open the program and operating the program.

Technology providers can be valuable resources when they are aware of the project goals. Because they participate in technology projects on a daily basis, providers may leverage previous experiences to assist you. Sharing the short-term and long-term goals with providers helps to inform and focus them on what matters most to your program.

Preparation Goals

- **Delivery of equipment**—When does the equipment need to be delivered? Is there more than one location for delivery? Should the order be shipped complete, or may components be shipped as they are ready?
- **Installation of components**—Some technology solutions may include components from different vendors. In such cases, it is important to be clear about your expectations for installation of each part.
- **Integration of components**—Coordinating the integration of systems requires advance planning and ongoing **project management** activities. Determine whether your organization has internal expertise available to lead, or at least assist, for the planning and execution of technology integration tasks. Large projects with multiple or complex systems may require the services of a third-party system integrator. Ask the individual vendors for recommendations of integration firms that consistently meet their client's expectations.
- **Initial user training**—What are the learning and performance requirements for successfully operating the technology? Decisions about in-service training can make or break the implementation process. Give deep consideration to the types of users and their specific needs. A vendor's generic class may not be suitable for all users. A custom solution may be required. Also, ongoing training should be considered when technology is used infrequently or when turnover, or growth, is expected.
- **Rehearsal for opening**—Knowing the operational basics of a technology solution is different than demonstrating how to harness technology to achieve a learning goal. Plan to rehearse as a team before using the technology with customers. Ask a representative from the technology provider to be on-site when you rehearse. In some cases, this may require a fee to ensure that a technologist or educator is present.

Even when fully immersed in the planning to open a simulation program, the manager needs to keep an eye on long-term outcome measures. Sharing these measures with technology providers moves conversations from equipment components into a contextual framework for how the program will operate as a successful learning enterprise.

Operating Goals

- **Leading indicators of success**—The financial world uses leading indicators as a measurable factor that changes before the economy starts to follow a trend or pattern. An educational enterprise may use enrollment and satisfaction as early indications that customers value the provided services. Leading indicators must not be confused with definitive learning and performance outcome measures; however, they are helpful to indicate whether the "ship is headed in the right direction."

  Tip: Consider faculty's demonstrated ability to load and control a programmed scenario using a simulator as a leading indicator of success.

- **Learning outcome measures**—You cannot manage what you cannot measure. A widely adopted model for measuring training was developed by Donald Kirkpatrick. The Kirkpatrick Model (Kirkpatrick & Kirkpatrick, 2006) includes four levels that progressively measure training participants' reaction to a program through the sponsor's **return on expectations**. Solution providers have a vested interest in understanding how their customers envision success—the Kirkpatrick Model is one method to communicate training effectiveness.
  - **Level 1**—To what degree did the learners react favorably from the training?
  - **Level 2**—To what degree did participants acquire the intended knowledge, skills, attitudes, confidence, and commitment on the basis of their participation in the training?
  - **Level 3**—To what degree did participants apply what they learned during training when they are back on the job?
  - **Level 4**—To what degree did targeted outcomes occur as a result of the training and subsequent reinforcement?

  Tip: The simulation program may establish benchmarks for each level and measure actual programs against the benchmarks. The practice of establishing benchmarks may support discussions with solution providers about meeting curriculum tools and implementation of full solutions rather than a piecemeal approach.

Well-written outcome measures describe an end point. Their limitation is that they cannot illustrate how the work gets accomplished. Using the learning outcomes as a destination, the manager should next plan a use model that shows how many moving pieces contribute to the final product.

Create a Use Model

Describing how customers will use, and pay, for the simulation program forces the planner to take several logistical dimensions into consideration. The dimensions are learners, curriculum, facility, staff, and finance. The use model is helpful when planning a new facility as it will reveal technology needs to support the vision. The formula is also beneficial to existing facilities because it helps to illustrate key logistical parameters.

- **Learners**—How many potential learners will attend programs per day, per course, per semester, per year? What is the interval of time a cohort will use the facility?
- **Curriculum**—Determine what skills and simulations are required to support the learning needs. Technology should support the curricula. Thus, the technology plan and vendor discussions can occur only after understanding the learning and performance needs.
- **Facility**—What are the types and functions of rooms that support teaching and learning? What is the capacity of each room?
- **Staff**—Categorize staff into a few simple functions, including instructional staff, technical staff, and administrative staff. Identify the staff's aggregate hourly rate.
- **Finance**—Determine the direct costs associated with a class, a course, and a curriculum. Also, consider the revenue sources including the following:
  - **Recurring revenue**—This is the most valuable form of revenue. Using subscription-like agreements, the simulation program has reliable income to pay expenses such as salaries, curriculum costs, warranties, and supplies. The most common source of recurring revenue is an internal department that agrees to fund the program, in part or whole, for ongoing training. Try to avoid the "cost-center" moniker as it does not adequately describe the enterprise's value.
  - **Transactional revenue**—The pay-as-you-go model is well suited for individuals that seek an individual class or program. This form of revenue is more difficult to project, especially during the inception of a program with no historical data in individual transactions.
  - **Quid pro quo**—Bartering for services is an acceptable form of payment, especially when the value of both parties' resource is mutually understood. Consider providing services in exchange for space, equipment, expertise, and endorsement as needed. Be sure to communicate the value of the exchange as none of the aforementioned examples are free.
  - **Project revenue**—This class of revenue describes projects performed by the program that consume resources, have value, and require a clear deliverable. Hosting a workshop, creating a video, and designing a course for a third party are examples of project revenue.

Even the most conservative use models obviously incur cost. The simulation manager must understand the costs and create a budget to support the planned activities. Often, sales representatives will ask questions about funding. Do not be offended when a representative asks you whether your initiative is funded—they need this information to update a forecast on the probability that you will award them business. The forecast supports decision making about manufacturing, shipping, and service delivery. It is helpful to have open and honest discussion about your goals and budget with vendors. The input you provide helps them to suggest the most appropriate solutions.

Budgeting to Support the Use Model

There are two common methods for calculating costs for managing expenses. They are known as the top-down and bottom-up approaches.

- Using the *top-down model*, a fiscal or management authority provides a concrete amount of funds to pay for the simulation activities. Using this budget amount, the simulation manager prioritizes where to apply the funds. He or she then informs stakeholders about what can be accomplished using the budget resources. This model is commonly used when new programs open and their value and revenue streams are not well established.
- The *bottom-up model* is built on the assumption that the simulation program will pursue specific initiatives during a budget period. Thus, the budget reflects the total costs to pursue the initiatives. This model exists in well-established programs where recurring revenue streams are secured.
- Budgets are often described as *operating* and *capital.* The operating budget is typically set for a calendar or fiscal period. Salaries, rent, utilities, and travel expenses are common items in an operating budget. A capital budget is designed to purchase durable items that will last for several years and cost more than $1,000. New simulator and hospital beds are examples of capital funds (Table 4.8.1).

This chapter's first theme places significant value on understanding user needs. Prior to contacting a vendor, the buyer and users should make an effort to understand foundationally how technology supports learning and performance goals. The goal is not necessarily to know every nuance about technology or how simulation supports andragogical learning theory. Rather, customers having a sense of focus and prioritization can help the vendor to present relevant options.

So, When Is the Right Time to Contact a Vendor?

There is no single answer that fits all situations. However, you will know you are ready when you can, at least superficially, speak to the questions in Table 4.8.2.

TABLE 4.8.1

Ten Considerations for Purchasing Simulation Resources

1. **Needs drive technology purchases.** Procure technology that supports learning and performance needs. Make sure the technology is easy to use, and don't let individual features excite you too much.

2. **Think big picture.** A fully loaded simulator might contain an excess of features that will not substantially drive learning outcomes higher than a sufficiently equipped simulator. Use the savings to invest in complementary resources like task trainers, data management, standardized curricula, and faculty development.

3. **Know the total cost of ownership.** Warranties, courseware, installation, and consumables all contribute to the solution's total cost. Be sure to compare apples with apples when comparing solutions from multiple vendors.

4. **Consider the overall value proposition.** Purchasing a simulator is long-term investment. It is important to understand how the solution will deliver value to your customers. Ask vendors how they may provide additional value through services, courseware, and other support.

5. **Avoid the feature trap.** There is a fine line between "need to have" and "nice to have." Features add value—they also add cost and complexity. Realistic humanistic features are a topic of frequent discussion in the healthcare simulation market. Consider how a feature contributes to educational efficacy. Avoid emotional decisions about a simulator's hairstyle or color.

6. **Calculate consumables and disposables.** Moulage and the deliberate practice of skills consume supplies. Budget for replacements on the basis of the use model.

7. **Mechanical things need maintenance and repair.** Repeated handling and invasive procedures can take their toll on any patient. Be sure to budget for time to maintain your investment. Simulators need preventative and unplanned service just like cars and aircraft.

8. **Making the complex simple costs.** As solutions are procured over time, the need to integrate multiple individual components becomes increasingly apparent. At some point, the program will incur cost to harmonize apples and oranges in one shared environment.

9. **Implementation requires support.** Few solutions make a material impact without deliberate, and ongoing, activities to support adoption by users. Consider budgeting for training, time to practice, and rehearsal before the full adoption reaches a critical tipping point.

10. **Be a good steward.** Simulation programs are often built with other people's money. Foundations and taxpayers appreciate investments that create value. Simulators remaining in shipping containers or sitting on shelves don't help save lives, and this makes buyers leery of future requests. Buy what is needed, and use what you have to make a difference.

Theme 2: How to Select Vendors, Services, Solutions, and Products?

About Vendors

Simulation vendors were identified by Doyle et al. (2008) as the healthcare simulation education industry and were described as:

> . . . commercial firms who provide technology, services and educational solutions to users of healthcare simulation.

In this chapter, the authors chose the term vendor to simplify communication about a broad range of commercial firms, including solution providers, distributors, and others.

TABLE 4.8.2

Questions Vendors May Ask During the Initial Meeting

1. Tell me about your goals—what are you trying to fix...improve... reduce? Tell me about the current state, and then tell me about what things look like after we implement the solution.

2. Describe why the organization is interested in simulation—check all that apply.
   - Improve individual competence
   - Reduce risk of harm to patients
   - Improve clinical teamwork
   - Assess and improve systems and processes
   - Limited availability of clinical training sites
   - Meet a regulatory requirement—explain
   - Other—explain

3. Who are the simulation program's customers and what are their needs?

4. Who are the stakeholders and what are their expectations?

5. How does simulation fit into the organizational strategy and goals?

6. Describe the organizational culture—is it ready to adopt simulation?

7. What are the technical requirements?

8. What is the scope of the project? Timeline?

9. Is the project funded?

10. How will purchasing decisions be made and by whom? Will the organization solicit competitive bids or sole-source the solution?

11. What is the amount budgeted for the capital expenditure?

12. Are operating funds budgeted for disposable and consumable supplies?

Vendors are structured to provide products and services that reflect market needs. The needs are determined from user stories, clinical and educational literature, guidelines, and standards. Vendors may also use Instructional Systems Design and Human Factors methodology to create solutions that support learning and improved performance.

The vendor's organizational structure may range from not-for-profit status to for-profit; some are privately held, and others are publicly traded companies. While vendors may operate in highly competitive markets, it is common for competitors to work collaboratively in the interest of helping mutual clients. Vendors support the healthcare education industry through grants and workshops; some partner with other industry leaders to develop comprehensive solutions with the goal of making a significant impact on patient outcomes.

The types of companies supporting healthcare education include the following:

- **Manufacturers**—Produce and sell products directly to the market or through distributors. They manage their own product and warranty issues, and may even provide custom product development services. Manufacturers may produce a single product or portfolios of products that form solution bundles.

- **Manufacturers/distributors**—Companies as described above that also sell other manufacturers' products chosen to fill gaps in their product offering that fulfill user requirements. Will often have preferential relationships with suppliers that enable them to support all product and warranty issues and can often provide unique product combinations as a single-source supplier.

- **Distributors**—Companies that sell products manufactured by others and add value to product dispersal through their subject matter expertise and/or marketing capabilities. May have a well-informed and grounded understanding of the healthcare simulation industry, or a superficial interest in simulation but a wide footprint in the education or healthcare industry. Product and warranty issues are usually referred to the manufacturer.

- **Resellers**—Most often nonspecialist education or healthcare suppliers who provide products as a sourcing service. They can often run multiple lines of products that may or may not be in related markets. Product and warranty issues are almost always referred to the manufacturer.

- **Consultants**—Individuals or teams that have a range of relevant expertise within the healthcare, education, and simulation industries, who might be engaged to consider organizational-level issues and make recommendations on future organizational design, structure, and practice.

- **Consolidators/solution providers**—These companies offer turnkey solutions to organizational needs by drawing on the resources of varied contractors, experts, and product manufacturers. They may be considered to provide a high value proposition as they can assist with the sourcing and implementation of services.

- **Technology transfer/seed companies**—Companies that grow out of an academic institution's drive to commercialize a product that is developed in-house and bring it to the market for the greater good and commercial profit.

When to Engage Vendors

Vendors play key roles in the selection, acquisition, and implementation of technology. Knowing when to contact a vendor and how to engage them is historically learned by trial and error. This section provides tips for successful interactions at various milestones.

- **Information gathering**—The vendor's websites and printed literature may provide detailed specifications about products, accessories, services, and pricing. In some cases, user stories, testimonials, and white papers may be available—these resources provide additional details about implementation and outcomes.

  Tips:
  - Subscribe to user groups and forums—these online communities may provide tremendous value through sharing of knowledge and information. Your institution's e-mail exchange may permit you to create rules that automatically organize mails from vendors into specific folders. This helps to manage information without adding volume to your e-mail inbox.
  - Ask the vendor's representative to explain volume or multiyear pricing. These data are typically not available on websites.

- **Consultation**—Vendors may provide professional consultation about educational methodologies, technology integration, faculty development, and facility design. These services may range in their sophistication and cost. Given the volume of existing customers, even vendors without professional consultation services may share information about the institution's experiences with technology implementation.

  Tips:
  - Review the qualifications of consultants and ask for client referrals.
  - Review the consultation agreement. Determine the terms, methodologies, deliverables, cost, and value.
  - Determine whether the vendor proposes to outsource the consultation services.

- **Demonstrations**—Tradeshows, product showcases, and vendor customer centers are examples of where users may experience a hands-on review of product and solutions. Demonstrations are useful to introduce a product; specific features and capabilities may be observed in action. However, an evaluation of the product may take longer if the evaluation is to occur on-site and in the context of normal operations.

  Tips:
  - Determine objective evaluation criteria on the basis of current and potential user needs.
  - Include actual users in the evaluation of the solution.
  - Visit other users who adopted similar solutions—ask for balanced reporting on the pros and limitations of the solution.

- **Quotes**—Deny the temptation to conclude that the word quote is synonymous with price. The type of information contained in a quote may vary significantly among vendors. Simple quotes may contain price and warranty information, while others may include detailed information about integration of the solution as well as performance guarantees. Pricing is one component of an overall value proposition. As quotes are received from multiple vendors, the evaluation of value rests with the purchasing authority—this is a potentially risky time for the institution. Select a solution on price only and you may experience integration, usability, and quality problems down range.

  Tips:
  - Ask the vendor to show the **total cost of ownership** for the solution. Warranties, accessories, and consumables add to the cost.
  - Evaluate each item's value through an operational lens. Up-front costs may cause sticker shock, and it may be tempting to strike them from the **purchase order**. Be sure to evaluate the potential consequence for each decision.
  - Ask the vendor about purchasing options including leasing, volume discounts, multiyear discounts for software services, and other helpful financial services that help simplify acquisition.

- Be realistic about asking for donations and unusually large discounts. In order for such requests to be considered, the value proposition to the vendor must be clear and commensurate with the value being requested by the client.
- **Order processing**—Many manufacturers have introduced "**Just in Time**" or "**Lean Manufacturing**" processes that create inherent **lead times** for order fulfillment, which are rarely hidden and generally discussed up front by representatives. Firm curriculum and project management will enable you to consider these as you plan your procurement. For instance, ensure that the vendor lead times, net payment terms, and intended go-live dates are abundantly clear to your Procurement Department so they know that there is a sense of urgency. It is not uncommon for delayed PO processing to cause significant delays in product ordering. In turn, this will help your vendor to source raw materials, plan manufacturing, installation, and team resources to address your needs.

  Tip:
  - Identifying potential "bottlenecks" in your procurement processes will simplify your ordering processes and reduce supply chain issues greatly.
- **Order fulfillment**—Some technology-based products require formal installation and training from the manufacturer, while others may be taken out of a box and used once the "Directions for Use (DFU)" have been thoroughly read and understood. It is advisable to ensure that your procurement team understands your "product needed by dates" and the lead time of the manufacturer to reduce delivery lag.
- **Product or service issues**—When products malfunction or break, or when users have questions about functionality, the vendor may offer tiers of technical support ranging from DFU, online forums, and live representatives. Some support services may be complimentary, while others require a subscription.

  Tips:
  - Place printed DFU in an accessible location. Upload electronic copies onto a shared Web-based workspace. Obtain electronic support documents from the vendor's website.
  - Encourage users to review the DFU prior to calling the vendor's Technical Support Line.
  - Record the product's serial number and the institution's account number in a conspicuous location—the vendor's representative may ask for this information at the onset of the technical support call.
  - Document complaints with the vendor's Technical Support Representative. This input helps to drive continuous improvement activities.

Product Selection Guidelines

Be Clear about Needs and Requirements

Determine must-have, optional, and undesired features. Features drive cost up. As the cost to acquire a product increases, its value to the organization must be commensurate. Staying focused on organizational goals will help to mitigate excitement about features.

Evaluate Solutions Using Objective Criteria

The requirement-based evaluation approach should accommodate the comparison and contrast of solutions from multiple vendors. Potential measures include the following:

- **Usability**—What skills do users need to possess to operate the solution? How are users trained to operate the solution? What training and performance support aids exist (job aids, tutorial videos, checklists, etc.)?
- **Accessibility**—Are licenses required? If so, what is the cost per license?
- **Durability**—How many procedures may be performed before the solution needs preventative maintenance?
- **Portability**—Does the solution need to be movable? How long should it take to prepare the solution for movement? How many people are required to move the solution?
- **Quality**—How well is the solution constructed?
- **Serviceability**—What components may be replaced, or serviced, by the user? Is special training required to access service components? How does the vendor perform preventative maintenance, and how often should the service be performed?
- **Total cost of ownership**—What consumables are needed, and what is their cost? What is the cost and value of the warranty?
- **Interoperability with existing systems**—Does the solution output data in a format that is compatible with other systems? Are there special power requirements?

Consider the Vendor's Track Record

What experience does the vendor have with implementing the solution in similar institutions to yours?

BEEN THERE, DONE THAT: HOW CAN I CONTINUE TO IMPROVE OR SUSTAIN WHAT I HAVE ACHIEVED?

There are many educators and simulation technicians with experience that are driven to innovate and design products, or who wish to influence simulator and simulation designs with vendors. All vendors welcome such dialogue and are often inundated with "good ideas."

Product innovation and design is an **iterative** process, whereby a proposal and review process is repeated with the aim of approaching a desired goal, target, or result. Each repetition of the process is called iteration, and the results of one iteration are used as the starting point for the next iteration. This requires a firm commitment to time and resources from all parties involved and can be much longer than you might expect, even with modern, rapid prototyping processes.

The main arenas for more involved end user and vendor discussions generally revolve around three areas:

- Ideas generation
- Product proposal review or beta testing
- Formal technology transfer agreements

These are examined briefly below and are designed to be food for thought for end users. You may find that a periodic team review of your current programs and the products used within them will generate great feedback for vendors, all of whom welcome structured, objective, and factual feedback on their products and services.

Ideas Generation

Vendors understand that opinion leaders and experts of simulation practice are best positioned to understand the needs of their specialty and evolving best practice issues. At the same time, vendors are exposed to multiple sites and sources of feedback on evolving practice, and frequent review of these can also result in the identification of previously unidentified needs. In discussing your ideas with a vendor, they will wish to understand the "Why? How? What?" (Sinek, 2009) of your idea. This will then be developed to cover the commercial considerations around the material and resource needs of a project, the methodology of dispersal, and promotion of any new product.

The iterative process described above will help both parties to identify a "road map" of product evolution (or revolution) that accounts for the long-term needs of the clinical/educational environment. By providing the "Why?" of an idea, you can help the vendor to identify the "How?" and "What?" of the innovation.

Product Proposal Review or Beta Testing

Vendors will often seek feedback at two stages of a product's evolution: (1) the review of a "Functional Requirements Documents," "Project Requirements Specifications," or "Scope of Work Documents" and (2) the Beta Testing of a prototype. The commitment to this process must never be underestimated by the end user, so you should ensure that the aims of the process you are involved with are clearly understood within your own organization.

Generally, the needs of an organization and vendor collaboration on a product idea deserve the following considerations:

- Commitment—Number and type of practitioners involved and the time period of their involvement.
- Delivery dates—Product development is a long-term project management process, which will have many soft and concrete checkpoints. Ensure that your organization can work within these needs and deliver reports on time.

- Local versus global appeal—Vendors will often have an eye on the global appeal of a product, but will be very interested in how your local clinical policy, practice, and guidelines as well as your education and simulation processes impact upon the product development. It is also important to consider the global/generalizable nature of your feedback on the proposal, while recognizing that products need to appeal to the widest possible section of the market and therefore may lack some facilities that you desire.

Technology Transfer

Vendors recognize the emerging role of Technology Transfer Departments within many Education and Healthcare organizations and respect their role in developing and protecting the inventive process. As mentioned before, vendors wish to make an informed decision on the "Why? How? What?" of any idea you propose; however, in promoting a product within a Technology Transfer Framework, a vendor will also expect you to address the following data collection needs:

- Clinical data on the size of the issue your idea/product addresses.
- Identify a curriculum (if any) that supports the need to address the issue.
- Identify any literature that relates to the idea you wish to propose and the conclusions you have drawn from the papers identified.
- Drivers that address the issue, including evolving programs and funding opportunities.
- The frequency that the procedure is practiced and by whom within the multidisciplinary team.
- How many trainees locally, within specialty practice, and globally might require training in the procedure?
- What do you think is a realistic cost for the mass production of any resulting product?
- What do you think is a realistic price for the resulting product?
- What do you think is a realistic sales volume for the resulting product?

Aligning these considerations in a briefing document will allow you to communicate most effectively with the vendor you approach. Bear in mind that even with these details in hand, the time from idea to product launch may best be measured in years and not weeks.

SUMMARY

Vendors represent an undeniable source of knowledge about their products and services, including how they are used effectively across the globe. This "tribal knowledge" can be of benefit to any simulation program team and may help the reader to avoid repeating the perceived mistakes of others.

SECTION 4 • Funding

This chapter was designed to provide the reader with suggestions covering two themes: (1) Technology Planning and (2) How to Select Vendors, Services, Products, and Solutions. The processes associated with these themes can seem daunting, particularly for a new manager, but also for an experienced one. The authors recognize that it is easy for Program Managers to become overwhelmed by choice and the proactive nature of vendor sales teams.

Technology Planning is best managed if the Center Manager and their team have a clear understanding of their user's needs and can relate these needs to a positive value proposition that is supported by easily identifiable outcome measures. If the reader is able to condense their user's needs into a set of targeted and focused preparation and operational goals that support a clear Simulation Center "Use" and "Budget" model, they will be able to engage in direct and honest communications with their vendors. This can eliminate a great deal of frustration and ensure that you receive excellent customer service.

You may wish to consider Return on Expectations as a way to focus your team rather than the traditional Return on Investment process, as the latter is too tightly focused on financial benefits that may not be easily linked to simulation or training outcomes.

Selecting Vendors, Services, Products, and Solutions is a complex process. The reader should be prepared to ensure that they understand not only the aims of the training program, the product and services required, but also the nature of the vendor under consideration. Consider your internal customer and vendor as partners in your plans. Be sure that you understand their structure, capabilities, and limitations, as this will help you to manage everyone's expectations within a structured procurement/program that will breed confidence in your Center.

Engage with your vendors in a direct and honest manner periodically throughout your planning and operational processes. Whether you are standing up a new program like Andrea or managing an established program, your vendors should be considered as long-term partners, but do not expect them to underwrite local budget deficits. Cost management will be one of the user's biggest challenges throughout the Simulation Program and Budget Year. Careful consideration of the "Total Cost of Ownership" of any product or service will enable you to maximize your investments and ensure you get the most out of and for your money.

REFERENCES

Covey, S. R. (2004). The 7 habits of highly effective people. New York, NY: Simon and Schuster.

Doyle, T., Carovano, R. G., & Anton, J. (2008). Successful simulation center operations: An industry perspective. In R. R. Kyle & W. B. Murray (Eds.), *Clinical simulation: operations, engineering and management* (pp. 479–488). Boston, MA: Elsevier.

Eisenhower, D. D. (1957, November 14). *Remarks at the national defense executive reserve conference* (Online by G. Peters & J. T. Woolley, the American Presidency Project). Retrieved from http://www.presidency.ucsb.edu/ws/?pid=10951.

Jeffries, P. R. (2007). *Simulation in nursing education: From conceptualization to evaluation.* New York, NY: NLN.

Jeffries, P. R., & Battin, J. (2012). *Developing successful health care education simulation centers: The consortium model.* New York, NY: Springer.

Kirkpatrick, D. L., & Kirkpatrick, J. D. (2006). *Evaluating training programs: The four levels* (3rd ed.). San Francisco, CA: Berrett-Koehler.

Lewandowski, W. E. (2008). Success with clinical simulation = assessment + planning + implementation. In R. R. Kyle & W. B. Murray (Eds.), *Clinical simulation: operations, engineering and management* (pp. 471–478). Boston, MA: Elsevier.

Mendes, D. (2008). *George Harrison—Any road* [Video file]. Retrieved from http://www.youtube.com/watch?v=mePp1l299EE

Mind Tools. (n.d.). *Creating a value proposition* [Web log comment]. Retrieved from http://www.mindtools.com/CommSkll/ValueProposition.htm

Sinek, S. (2009). *Start with why: How great leaders inspire everyone to take action.* New York, NY: Penguin.

SECTION 5

Management

CHAPTER 5.1

Business Needs and Assets Assessment

Sandra J. Feaster, RN, MS, MBA, and Jennifer A. Calzada, MA

ABOUT THE AUTHORS

SANDRA J. FEASTER is the Assistant Dean for Immersive and Simulation-based Learning at Stanford University School of Medicine. Over the past 8 years, she has opened and managed two key simulation centers at Stanford, the 1,500 square feet (139.4 m²) Goodman Surgical Simulation Center (which is an ACS AEI level 1 accredited center) and the 28,000 square feet (2601.2 m²) Goodman Immersive Learning Center. She is active in the Society for Simulation in Healthcare and the American College of Surgery Accredited Education Institutes.

JENNIFER A. CALZADA is the Administrative Director for the Tulane Center for Advanced Medical Simulation & Team Training at the School of Medicine. She has worked in advertising and marketing for 20 years, and in 2008 made a career change by joining the Tulane School of Medicine as the Sim Center's day-to-day Director. Her unique perspective and experience in marketing, communications, training, and business development have proved useful in launching a new Sim Center.

ABSTRACT

This chapter discusses how to identify your business needs and assets using the investigative method of asking who, what, where, when, why, and how. By asking these questions early on when planning a new program, or even for an established program, this process will help you develop or reflect on your audience, educational goals, and finances, and will help drive the decision on what assets to acquire and maintain. We will discuss examples, including purchasing equipment, acquisition by collaborating with departments, and expanding a current program to a high-revenue CME program based on the needs of a specialty or a geographic opportunity. By looking at opportunities and risks from a variety of perspectives, this chapter aims to give the reader some pearls to ponder and an organized process to dive deep into your business needs.

CASE EXAMPLE

In August 2010, the Stanford School of Medicine opened its doors to the Li Ka Shing Center (LKSC) for Learning and Knowledge, the new home to the medical school, and the 28,000 square feet (2601.2 m²) Goodman Immersive Learning Center (ILC). The ILC was designed to accommodate exercises and activities primarily (but not limited to) for undergraduate medical education/medical students (**UGME**), graduate medical education/residents (**GME**), and continuing medical education (**CME**). The ILC was designed to offer multiple modes of immersive and simulation-based activities, including mannequins, embedded simulated persons (**ESPs**), and partial task trainers. During the planning phase for the program, mannequin-based simulation was used sparsely for UGME, somewhat for GME (particularly anesthesia and emergency medicine), and very little for CME (outside of instructor courses). Given that, identifying the business need for the future and the asset requirements were quite daunting to the planning team and required a vision into the future of immersive and simulation-based learning that many of us still did not know (Gaba, 2004).

Meeting with department heads, faculty, and staff in the early and mid-2000s to discuss simulation was challenging. Many of the faculty who taught medical students only had familiarity with the use of ESPs for clinical skills exercises and assessment, and only a small handful could imagine how to use mannequin-based simulation in their curriculum to either replace or repurpose their current educational activities. Faculty who primarily taught residents could not imagine how the standardized Patient (SP) program could benefit residents and how to use ESPs to assist in the education process. Today, requests are received several times a year to use standardized Patient's SPs for a variety of resident activities, such as delivering "bad news to a patient," obtaining consent, and so on, and more mannequin-based simulation is being integrated into the medical student curriculum.

It is difficult to predict the future; we do not have a crystal ball. Considering business needs and completing assets assessment provide guidance as we set our focus on educational needs of our learners. How can you obtain a similar outcome in your program? Our mantra is from a quote by Zig Ziglar, who used the phrase "what could you do if you didn't know you couldn't" (Zig Ziglar quote, n.d.).

INTRODUCTION

Do you know your institution, **customers**, learner population, **competitors**, resources, unique qualities, assets, and the simulation industry? If not, you should. The success and sustainability of your simulation program is dependent on a thorough assessment of the business needs and a deep understanding of both your tangible and intangible assets (Galati & Williams, 2013, chap. 46; Seropian et al., 2013, chap. 45).

Whether you are starting up a new simulation center as described by Horley (2008), expanding your center, or perhaps focusing on in situ simulation activities, a needs assessment and review of your assets should be performed. Often, centers are built or a space is repurposed for simulation. Then, or even before, simulators are purchased or donated without a clearly developed business plan or vision for the learning needs or activities that will or should take place in the center. Hospitals tend to be quite cautious in their planning of equipment acquisition, and perhaps mirroring some portion of that model could serve those in the simulation business well (David & Jahnke, 2005).

These are the situations where in a year or two down the road, simulators may end up stored in the back of an equipment closet or become the "forgotten" either because they do not meet the needs of the program, the staff is untrained in how to use/repair them, or that particular simulator has no champion. This is particularly true in cases where the simulator requires frequent or extensive maintenance, requiring a level of funding that was never in the strategic plan or the operating budget. Any new or expanded program must include a plan for ongoing support. It is the philosophy of "who cares and who pays" (Box 5.1.1).

DON'T MAKE PURCHASING SIMULATORS LIKE PURCHASING "THAT SPECIAL CAR"

Here is an analogy for thinking about purchasing simulators. Think in terms of someone that requires transportation to and from work. Let us assume the person has a fixed transportation budget, but spends every dollar on "that special car." They have not planned for fuel, oil changes, and maintenance, not to mention parking. This approach definitely leads to going back to riding the bus, while the car sits. Spending every dollar you have on the newest simulator (even if someone is enamored with it) with nothing planned for maintenance and ongoing support will leave you teaching from PowerPoint or having a simulator as your "objet d'art" in your program. Think carefully and strategically before making that purchase.

As in the book *Alice in Wonderland*, Alice comes to a fork in the road and asks the Cheshire Cat, "Would you tell me, please, which way I ought to go from here?" "That depends a good deal on where you want to get to," replies the Cat. "I don't much care where," she replies. "Then it doesn't matter which way you go," states the Cheshire Cat (Carroll, n.d.).

UNDERSTANDING RISK

Instead of relying on random opportunity when building a program, take a step back and develop an intentional plan to address the development and growth of simulation activities in your institution or facility. The plan may have inherent risks, either known or unknown, but at least you can begin to prepare for those risks. This helps develop a baseline planning framework, which can be adjusted as

SECTION 5 • Management

BOX 5.1.1

CASE STUDY: GROUP PURCHASING

At Stanford's Immersive Learning Center (ILC), there are two key simulators that were purchased in conjunction with other departments. The first was Harvey, the Cardiopulmonary Patient Simulator, which was copurchased by the ILC and the Department of Medicine; the other was the CAE Medical VIMEDIX TEE/TTE and FAST Ultrasound simulator. This simulator was copurchased by the ILC and the Departments of Surgery and Anesthesia. This was a strategic decision and a way to engage the various departments.

When making such decisions, you will need to decide whether other departments that did not share in the purchase can or should use the equipment. Who pays for the warranty and maintenance should also be determined in advance. This will require some thought and agreement at the time of the purchase. A service-level agreement (SLA) is an option to ensure that everyone fully understands the agreement and there is a document that can be used in the future.

the plan is developed and operationalized (Merton, 2013). No plan is risk free, but exploring the potential landmines before proceeding is prudent in any business venture. It is better to do it right the first time than do it over. Major risks to be mindful of include, but are not limited to:

1. **Financial risks**—This is hugely important when choosing the space, equipment, and personnel. Being able to sustain financial solvency on an ongoing basis is even more important. Considerations regarding space include the actual physical plant, any building costs, retrofit costs, and the ongoing facility fees (maintenance, utilities, etc.). Equipment also has similar risks to consider (how and who will use the equipment, how will it be repaired, who will pay warranties, etc.). Personnel have another broad spectrum of consideration ranging from the right people to do the right job, the cost of such personnel, and the long-term plan for personnel (such as a growth plan, clinical ladder, or other retention strategies).

2. **Opportunity risks**—You will need to determine whether to focus on serving one learner group (e.g., residents, nursing, or medical students) and giving up the opportunity to partner with industry or another more financially attractive group (i.e., outside learners, certification courses, etc.). Conversely, you may want to include all potential opportunities with a matrix of the best mix for your needs. Thinking about these opportunities well in advance may serve the program in the long term.

3. **Political risks**—Often the most difficult and possibly the least obvious risk associated with those you may have influence on, such as specific faculty members, administrators, new deans, and donors. Specific faculty members may be strong mentors and your rainmakers for others to join. Conversely, they could impact your program negatively by talking with others and being subversive with other faculty, administration, or others. It is wise to align politically with supportive and well-respected individuals. Politics change often, and knowing your allies and those who are not strong allies can be very important down the line.

CONDUCTING A NEEDS ANALYSIS

Regardless of whether it is new business or business expansion, you need to ask a number of questions to help guide thinking and provide a framework to develop alternatives. One mechanism simulation educators and administrators should know involves the six Ws of information gathering. The six Ws are often thought of in terms of journalistic inquiry, but they can also help develop a framework and hone the thinking about exploring business needs (Suzuki, 2005). The six Ws, listed here, can help provide focus and clarity as the plan is developed or refined.

1. Who
2. What
3. When
4. Where
5. Why
6. How

WHO	**Consider the following when you are asking the question "WHO are your":**
	Learners
	Customers
	Stakeholders
	Competitors

Identifying your customers, **learners**, **stakeholders**, competitors, and the like will help guide your thinking—knowing who they are today, but also keeping in mind who they could be well into the future. The "who" can be a major factor in making a decision regarding what equipment to purchase, how to configure space, and what staff expertise is necessary. Knowing the "who" relative to who is going to use the space is extremely important and can be a significant driver for revenue and expense expectations. You will need to ask yourself the following questions:

- Who determines **what equipment** you will require, and how is that matched with the learner population?
- Who determines the **level of fidelity** and sophistication needed in equipment? Are you training novice learners with their first exposure to procedures or practicing professionals who want to advance their skills and communication techniques?
- Who determines the **volume of equipment** you require, how many learners will you be teaching, over what period of time on a procedure or activity? If ultrasound training is extremely important, how many ultrasound machines and of what type? Do you need to augment that with virtual reality ultrasound or task trainers that are ultrasound compatible?

  Again, knowing who your learners are and how you will pay for your assets and supplies is key to formulating your plan.
- Who determines **the staff** you must hire? Will you need technicians to run high-technology simulators and complex audio/video (AV) systems or only to maintain and set up task trainers?

Below, we will discuss several of the "whos" and the potential impact each has on the space, program, and/or long-term sustainability.

Learners

For this purpose, learners are defined as those participating in the simulation activity or exercise in the program. They can be early learners (nursing, medical, or allied health), residents, practicing clinicians (nurses, physicians, therapists, etc.), or industry partners (sales reps or marketing teams learning what it is like to be in an operating room, acute care, and/or intensive care unit setting). Understanding and developing a matrix of learner groups will help in the long term to develop a pricing strategy, workflow, and space and asset requirements. Keep in mind a long-term strategy as well, and envision what activities may look like in 5 or 10 years. It is hard to imagine looking ahead 10 years. It is likely that the space will be intact, but the learning may be very different.

Customers

Customers are those individuals who request use of the simulation program (departments and faculty, CME/CEU, and industry). These customers may or may not pay for the use of the program. That depends on the program's financial model. In some instances, donor funding may be used to build infrastructure, and another source provides an annual operating budget. Simulation programs that partner with industry may have other financial models, and may pay for the use of the program and use it for training their staff or their customer. In still other models, specific departments may pay for resident training as part of their GME funds. Some sites also charge lab fees for students; this is often seen in nursing schools. In all of these models, those who pay and use the program will likely drive the asset requirements. If you are building and equipping your program with a particular paying customer or learner population in mind, it will drive your business one way. If you are building a program with unspecified customers or learners, your business may be driven in an entirely different direction. Again, thinking forward to who pays today and in the future will be essential to the program's sustainability. (See chapter 4.1 for a more detailed assessment of possible customers who may generate revenue.)

Another great opportunity for revenue-producing customers is CME or CEU. These activities can generate revenue and help pay for space, personnel, and equipment. These activities generally produce higher revenues than learner activities, and thus CME/CEU as a key customer may be something that you would want to cultivate and grow. However, one must be mindful of the asset requirements needed for these activities as there may be very different requirements requested on an infrequent basis.

Stakeholders

Stakeholders are those who have a specific interest in the center. This interest could be financial or pedagogical (e.g., dean, faculty, donor). A dean could be a key fundraiser, stakeholder, and supporter of the program. Also, there could be a naming donor that is supportive (both in concept and financially) and supports the program. Many centers are built and initially equipped with philanthropic funds. However, once the bricks and mortar fund-raising activities are completed, ongoing operational requirements cannot be forgotten. That is when a Program Manager often begins to hear requests for "return on investment," and the ability to become revenue producing, or at least being cost-neutral, becomes the next big hurdle.

Faculty as stakeholders can also be key. Often it is the zealot with a vision who guides the direction of the program, and faculty can be your best cheerleaders both internally and externally. The champion faculty member(s) can be helpful in raising money, developing new curriculum, and getting others excited about simulation. Often, these early adopters will springboard others to develop new activities or repurpose a "tired" curriculum. The peer-to-peer enthusiasm cannot be underestimated or overlooked.

Stakeholders can also create potential risk in three key areas: finance, opportunity, and politics. Each must be taken into consideration. There are various tools that can be used to help you identify and map your stakeholder(s); the link provided (http://www.stakeholdermap.com/) is just one of many resources that are available to help identify the impact stakeholders may have. Developing a stakeholder map can be an extremely helpful exercise and a great reference tool that can serve you and others well in years to come.

Competitors

It is important at the beginning of the journey, or actually anytime during the journey, to think of all of the possibilities that may occur internal or external to your program, and the impact, if any. This includes the potential competitive climate that may be present or could arise. For example, consider that you have a program that provides GME activities to anesthesia residents and a new hospital is being built that contains an operating room simulation suite, which is adjacent to the new surgery suites. Would this be viewed as complementary or competitive? How would that affect your program activities, equipment, and supplies? Is there a potential that you could have equipment that goes unused? These are questions that you need to think about. This type of scenario could happen with internal departments, within your hospitals or university system, and competing programs in a geographically close area. Do you have alternative plans if a particular learner population leaves?

More simulation programs are seeking opportunities to improve their revenue stream and are thus developing programs and training where learners need specialty certification such as Advanced Cardiac Life Support (ACLS), Advanced Trauma Life Support (ATLS), and Maintenance of Certification (MOC) activity. These certification programs can be added as a business unit to a simulation center to generate revenue that helps offset the expense of training internal learners. Other countries have different models as well, so again there is tremendous variability (Box 5.1.2).

SIMULATION PROGRAM COMMITMENT AND DIRECTION

While the case study of developing a MOCA course was a straightforward example of adding a new course to an already existing training activity at the Tulane Simulation

---

BOX 5.1.2

BUSINESS EXPANSION FOR PROVIDING MAINTENANCE OF CERTIFICATION COURSE

The Tulane Center for Advanced Medical Simulation & Team Training made the decision to apply for American Society of Anesthesiologists (ASA) Endorsement. The following discussion highlights Tulane's **needs analysis** and ultimate business decision based on the Six Ws Model.

The case to become an ASA-endorsed center is based on the ASA's Part 4 Maintenance of Certification in Anesthesiology (MOCA) requirement for all practicing anesthesiologists. This ongoing maintenance requirement means there will be a consistent need for simulation programs to provide advanced anesthesiology training. Because MOCA centers must be endorsed, it also means future competition is likely to be kept to a minimum.

WHO

Anesthesiologists who need to complete an MOCA course are both the learner and customer. ASA MOCA courses carry a significant registration fee, and for Tulane, the competitive landscape was an easy decision as there is a lack of endorsed centers in the Southeast region of the US. Had Tulane been located in a market with an existing endorsed center, a review and analysis of board-certified anesthesiologists in the region would help determine whether the market could bear another endorsed center.

WHAT

ASA MOCA courses follow a specific curriculum plan with well-defined assessment expectations. Tulane was already running compatible training for internal learners, so there would not be a need to create dramatically different curriculums.

WHEN

ASA MOCA courses run a full day and would necessitate some offerings running on Saturdays, a day when the Tulane Sim Center is typically not open. This consideration required planning flextime for the simulation tech role.

WHERE

ASA MOCA courses require high-technology simulation mannequins, AV recording and monitoring equipment for remote viewing, and space for debriefing a small group. The Tulane Sim Center is already set up for this level of course and resource needs, so the decision was easy to make to hold courses within the Sim Center.

WHY

There are several reasons that were considered in the decision to apply to become an ASA-endorsed center. First and foremost, the courses would be revenue-producing. Because the courses require similar resources to Tulane's existing anesthesiology residency training, these courses were looked at as a source to help generate funds to maintain that training. Second, Tulane's own anesthesiologists (and those from two other partner institutions) have MOCA requirements and becoming an endorsed center allows those to be met at home. Finally, ASA MOCA courses fit within the mission of the Tulane Sim Center to provide national-level training and certifications for healthcare professionals.

HOW

Because the Tulane Sim Center was already providing nearly compatible training to the anesthesiology residency of two institutions, there were minimal additional resources that were required. This made up-front funding requirements low, with the exception of the application costs, which would be covered after running a single paid ASA MOCA course. Ongoing financing is covered by course revenue, and the high-fidelity simulator has an existing backup should there be a temporary equipment failure.

Center; it is illustrative of the considerations for any planned program expansion. Questions that one should think about include: Will there be consistent learner/customer needs? Who are the competitors for these learners? What will the expansion consist of, and how different is it from the current workflow of our offerings at the program? Is the expansion planned to fit within current operations in terms of time and space, or is it additional? Why is this expansion being considered? And, finally, how will the expansion be funded and financed on an ongoing basis? It is necessary to have the vision for what you are committing the center to offer and a planned direction for the future. Answering a few of the questions below may help.

	WHAT does your center offer?
WHAT	Education
	Training
	Certification
	Assessment

Are you using simulation activities for education, training, certification, and/or assessment? Are you training medical students, residents, or nurses or allied health professionals? Are you part of a medical school, nursing school, hospital, or an independent program? Is there a movement for developing interprofessional education activities?

Knowing the user base or "the who" will help determine "what" you are offering. Purchasing a $100,000 virtual reality surgical simulator if you are teaching medical students may provide you with a "cool simulator" that gets you a lot of interest from students and visitors. But is it an asset that you want to purchase and maintain? Which learners will use it, and are they the learner population you want in your center? What makes a worthwhile purchase? Part of identifying and obtaining your assets should focus on what you intend to offer and to which audience. Also, the learner population will often drive the fidelity of the simulator that is required. Do 2nd-year medical students really need to learn to central line insertion using an expensive ultrasound trainer (that may require costly replacement skins) and expensive central line kits? And, if it is not a fully immersive learning experience (from gown and gloves, to ultrasound, to insertion), is there really a purpose in that activity? Is there a clear learning objective for the activity? If not, then further discussion should occur with faculty and the activity adjusted accordingly. It is often helpful to have an associated cost with each activity to help faculty determine whether they are paying for the activity, whether it is in alignment with the learning objectives, and worth the expense.

Programs often have challenges when a donor wants to purchase an expensive or complicated simulator because it is of interest to them. Consideration has to be given to the warranty, maintenance, training of staff, and how and who will use it. Often, these types of assets can be costly, both in dollars and staff time. It may also not be appropriate for your learner population. Understanding why a donor wants that particular simulator and knowing the plans for support of the simulator is key. You do not want, nor can you afford, an expensive asset just because it was the special interest of an individual (following the money). The purchase of equipment should be based on your learner population, learning objectives, operating budget, and the requisite support. Sometimes you have to "just say no," but the political risk could be high. Again, the risks must be assessed and weighed. Try to find an opportunity to change the mind of the donor or faculty that want the expensive/cool simulator and find a common ground. But think carefully before saying yes or no. There are many simulators still in their boxes collecting dust and taking up space, and you do not want to have or be one of them.

Understanding the support you can expect from your administration, deans, departments, and faculty for your mission can be key to the infrastructure capabilities of your organization. Do you have what you need and/or can you find and resource what you want? You could embrace the entrepreneurial spirit that Schlesinger et al. (2012) describe in their article "New Project? Don't Analyze—Act." This approach recommends taking small, quick steps to get your initiative off the ground. You know your environment, people, and resources—it is up to you and your team to make this a reality. Just be aware of your risks.

Vision without execution is hallucination.

Thomas Edison

WHAT ARE YOUR ASSETS (BOTH TANGIBLE AND INTANGIBLE)?

Identifying your tangible and intangible assets can be key to positioning your center activities and "what you offer, and to whom."

Tangible assets can be defined as items that have a physical form. These can be simulators, AV equipment and systems, medical equipment and supplies, and even a building or physical space. You may be known for being the only center with a particular simulator or asset. That may create a high draw of a particular learner population that you can exploit. You may be a center that focuses on a specific skill or specialty such as surgery, anesthesia, ultrasound, and so on.

Intangible assets are defined as reputation, name recognition, and intellectual property such as knowledge and know-how, patents, and so on. These should not be taken lightly. Intangible assets can be a major differentiator and provide competitive advantage to your program or activities. It can be a faculty member who has national recognition, or the institution itself. Stanford is known for its Associate Dean, David Gaba, MD. Dr. Gaba teaches several courses that are highly sought out, well received, and are revenue producing. The Stanford name and other well-known universities or centers can bring a certain cache or seal of approval. Accreditations by the Society for Simulation in Healthcare, the American College of Surgeons, the American Society of Anesthesiologists, and others provide important "seals of approval" for simulations programs. Take advantage of the opportunities that name recognition and accreditation afford, and highlight your tangible as well as intangible assets. Hint: List your accreditations on your website and all collateral material. Celebrate your success and hard work with others. Work locally, think globally.

	WHEN do you provide exercises and learning opportunities?
WHEN	24/7 access. What is your threshold for missing or broken equipment? What purpose does 24/7 access serve?
	Weekends
	Evenings

This is always an interesting conversation and elicits strong opinions. Should students have 24/7 access, and if so, for what purpose? Does a surgical resident want to hone their laparoscopic skills while they have some downtime if they are on call, does a medical student want access to the center, and to practice what? Studies have shown that practicing and hardwiring poor technique can be unhelpful and could be dangerous, because as Gladwell (2008) states and provides numerous examples throughout his book, practice is the thing you do that makes you good. It is wonderful that students wish to get their 10,000 hours of practice. But it needs to be well thought out what level and type of practice warrants 24/7 access and the consequences of offering such access.

Supplies and Equipment Can Develop Legs

You must be prepared to have instruments and materials disappear if around-the-clock access is provided. Camera surveillance may prevent some of this loss, but often with open access (even with limited badge or key access), assets do disappear or get broken and that must be a budget consideration. You will need to know your threshold for replacement assets. Has this been budgeted? What is your policy for damage?

	WHERE are you providing the learning?
WHERE	Stand-alone independent center
	Center inside a hospital or healthcare facility
	Refurbished space
	In situ

This is an important question whether you are building a new center or expanding/refurbishing a current center. If you are inside the hospital, can the learners drop in to practice (e.g., surgical warm-up), do you have the ability to run quick in situ scenarios (e.g., bedside rounds for medical or nursing students to fill in the learning gap)? It is also an important question to ask as you purchase equipment and supplies. A key consideration if your center is in the hospital facility—do you use expired supplies and equipment that could migrate to the clinical location? What are the safeguards in place against that happening? Could the space be repurposed for emergencies? These are just a few things to consider.

If your learner population is, for example, Emergency Medicine learners, what is the requirement for emergency room equipment? Can you get the same equipment that is used in the clinical environment, thus enhancing training and patient safety? Do you need real gasses for your exercises, or are you in a space that will need to be approved by any agency (e.g., OSHPD)? Do you have plans to expand to another learner group like surgery or anesthesia, and will you need new or different equipment for such activities, and will the space be adequate?

Could your space be repurposed in 5 years to accommodate new activities or direction? This is an important consideration because the more flexible the space, the better positioned you are to enable a variety of learning potentials that may not have been considered. Think of the possibilities—an open space can be an acute care room, emergency room, operating room, and so on. Purchasing equipment that will be used immediately is wise, and if the space is flexible for reconfiguration, you can repurpose it for a different audience and purchase equipment later. If the space has only one use, you are much more limited to what you can offer, so think flexibility equals sustainability.

If the design and build stage has not started, or the center is still in the early stages of design, you will want to understand the intended use, including the learner population, teaching purposes, room use (animals, cadavers), as well as any accreditation or regulatory requirements of the space (locker rooms, restrooms, air handling system, gas scavenging, etc.). You will also need to consider room and crowd control as well as ingress and egress of people, equipment, and supplies. Another financial consideration is determining who is responsible for facility maintenance (lights, cleaning, etc.). If this is the responsibility of the center, be sure this is added into the financial model and that you are fairly compensated for such. Starting up a simulation center is covered elsewhere, but these are just a few tips to keep in mind as you review your business needs and assets.

	WHY do you do the things you do?
WHY	Learner assessment
	Training and certification
	Revenue producing
	Education for hospital(s)
	Team training

A written road map will help you determine why you are doing what you do. Remember *Alice in Wonderland*. If you are to make strategic decisions and long-term plans, you need to understand where you are going and why.

If your goal is to produce revenue, that will take you down a path of certifications, larger group activities, increased marketing, and active solicitation of participants. This is when a clear assessment of your tangible assets is important in your planning. Do you need video capture and archiving for learner assessment? If you are doing assessments for medical students, do you have a policy in place for video archiving? Is there a cost for storage? Why are you archiving? Are there regulations or accreditation processes that you need to be aware of?

Consider your AV system—how does it fit into your asset funds? How will you update your AV system in the future? Do you need an expensive and intricate system, or just bare bones? What mannequins do you have, and what is the expected fidelity and life of your mannequins? Which simulators and programs add value to the activities that will take place in the center today and in the future? If your focus is surgical task training, do you really need an expensive mannequin if your objective is to just provide skills enhancement? If you are offering Team Training, what are the expectations vis-à-vis fidelity of the mannequin, equipment, and space? It should be as close as possible to the real environment so the team can focus on teamwork, not figuring out how to work a new defibrillator (that should be taught at another session).

The competitive climate of simulation activities is growing. So knowing why you are doing something is very important. Are you part of a mission-driven organization, committed to teaching students or looking for a way to make revenue, or both? Developing your road map should address these questions with honesty and clarity while keeping an eye to the horizon for what is in future, because it will change.

BEEN THERE, DONE THAT: HOW CAN I CONTINUE TO IMPROVE OR SUSTAIN WHAT I HAVE ACHIEVED?

	HOW will you maintain and sustain your assets?
HOW	Know your funding source
	Know your finances
	Celebrate your successes

Whether you are funded by course revenues, individual departments, the dean's office, the hospital, philanthropy, or other sources, you will need to think outward to sustainability. It is imperative that you understand your operations, equipment, and staff capabilities. Tracking productivity and profitability will be a key indicator of your success and ability to manage your center.

There are many different metrics you can track for that will be indicative of the center's success and sustainability.

These are only a few, but will give you an idea of ways to promote and keep your success top-of-mind with your funding sources. Simulation program productivity tracking may include the following:

- Monthly space usage based on percentage used
- Monthly space usage based on total hours in use
- Monthly and annual total number of courses run
- Monthly and annual number of unique learners
- Monthly percentage of time (or total hours) specific, major simulators are used

Simulation program profitability tracking may include the following:

- Revenue and profit per individual course
- Revenue and profit per budget line or cost center or category of courses (i.e., all Anesthesiology MOCA courses)
- Revenue and profit totaled per simulation room, simulator, or course (whichever is most appropriate for your center)

These and other metric topics will be covered in greater detail in a variety of chapters, but it is clear that you need to follow and track your metrics, and use them to your advantage to celebrate what you do!

SUMMARY

By using the investigative technique of Who, What, When, Where, Why, and How, you can start asking important questions to help you determine your business direction and asset requirements. In some simulation programs, there is an unfortunate tendency to take leftover, old, or damaged equipment, used or outdated supplies and attempt to make lemonade from the lemons you receive. Some of these items are the lifeblood of a simulation program, but knowing what to keep and what to refuse are equally important. Involving key stakeholders and developing a rich road map for your learner population and needs will guide your asset collection. Being armed with your requirements will make it easier to negotiate with industry, your hospital, or other entities to get equipment and supplies that are current and pertinent to the activities that will occur in the program.

REFERENCES

Carroll, L. (n.d.). *Which road do I take.* Retrieved from http://www.goodreads.com/author/quotes/8164.Lewis_Carroll

David, Y., & Jahnke, E. (2005). Medical technology management: From planning to application. *Conference Proceedings IEEE Engineering in Medicine and Biology Society, 1,* 186–189.

Gaba, D. M. (2004). The future vision of healthcare in simulation. *Quality and Safety in Health Care, 13*(Suppl. 1), i2–i10.

Galati, M., & Williams, R. (2013). Business planning considerations for a healthcare simulation center. In A. I. Levin, S. DeMaria, A. D. Schwartz, & A. J. Sim (Eds.), *The comprehensive textbook of healthcare simulation* (pp. 625–640). New York, NY: Springer.

Gladwell, M. (2008). *Outliers.* New York, NY: Little, Brown and Company. Chapter 2.

Horley, R. (2008). Simulation and skill centre design. In R. H. Riley (Ed.), *Manual of simulation in healthcare* (pp. 3–24). New York, NY: Oxford University Press.

Merton, R. C. (2013). Innovation risk. *Harvard Business Review, 91*(4), 48–56.

Schlesinger, L. A., Kiefer, C. F., & Brown, P. B. (2012). New project? Don't analyze—Act. *Harvard Business Review, 90*(3), 154–158.

Seropian, M., Driggers, B., & Gavilanes, J. (2013). Center development and practical considerations. In A. I. Levin, S. DeMaria, A. D. Schwartz, & A. J. Sim (Eds.), *The comprehensive textbook of healthcare simulation* (pp. 611–624). New York, NY: Springer.

Suzuki, C. (2005). A template for questioning: a learning exercise used for workplace training in listening. *Listening Professional, 4*(1), 3.

Zig Ziglar quote. (n.d.). What you could do if you didn't know you couldn't. Retrieved from Creators.com: http://www.creators.com/lifestylefeatures/inspiration/classic-zig-ziglar/what-you-could-do-if-you-didn-t-know-you-couldn-t.html

CHAPTER 5.2

Policies and Procedures

Thomas A. Dongilli, AT, Ilya Shekhter, MS, MBA, CHSE, and Jesika S. Gavilanes, MA

ABOUT THE AUTHORS

THOMAS A. DONGILLI, Director of Operations at the Peter M. Winter Institute for Simulation, Education, and Research (WISER) at the University of Pittsburgh and the University of Pittsburgh Medical Center (UPMC), and Co-Chair of the 2014 International Meeting on Simulation in Healthcare (IMSH 2014), manages all operations of WISER. He led the efforts in creating the first SSIH Policy and Procedure Manual for Simulation Centers and has authored book chapters on simulation center design and management.

ILYA SHEKHTER, Medical Simulation Manager at the University of Miami-Jackson Memorial Hospital (UM-JMH) Center for Patient Safety, trains faculty and staff on the setup and maintenance of the patient simulators and associated information and audiovisual systems, curriculum development, and applications of simulation technology. He works with physicians and nurses from different clinical departments to help them create simulation courses based on the curricular needs of their learners and has run thousands of simulation-based training sessions.

JESIKA S. GAVILANES is the Statewide Simulation Operations Manager at the Oregon Health and Science University Simulation and Clinical Learning Centers (SCLC). She develops policies and procedures in relation to simulation and clinical skills training, including scheduling, utilization data reporting, equipment maintenance, and space utilization. Jesika has been involved with simulation facilities across the country assisting with logistics, operations, and simulation implementation. She is a member of the Society for Simulation in Healthcare (SSH).

Acknowledgments: Daniel Battista, MBA, Jordan Halasz, ASEE, Juan-Manuel Fraga-Sastrias, MD, MEmergMgt, MA, DHlthSc, Jeanette Wong, RN, MPA, Valerie M. Howard, EdD, RN.

ABSTRACT

The number and complexity of simulation programs have grown exponentially over the past 10 years. The need for structured use and efficient management of these programs and facilities is becoming increasingly important. This chapter will focus on the identification and implementation of standardized policies and procedures common to most simulation programs. Simulation center environments offer challenging issues to those who have to manage and operate the facilities. It is important that simulation managers take into consideration the many variables involved in running a simulation program and address best practices used by industry leaders. Policies and procedures on topics such as administrative considerations, budgeting, educator training, off-site use, curriculum development process, video recording, and conflict of interest will be covered. Creating a policy and procedure manual can be a daunting process. This chapter will identify steps to get started and help shape the composition of an effective manual.

CASE EXAMPLE

Today, as you review the upcoming events with the staff at the Simulation Center, there is a collective groan when you mention that Instructor Jones will be working on Thursday. When you ask about their response, they tell you that she is difficult to work with and increases the stress level on everyone including the students. You recall that the evaluations for this instructor have not been good. You think about your options for dealing with this situation. You could provide this individual with more training, let the situation slide, or ban her from the Simulation Center. As a relatively new manager, you wonder how to proceed in a way that will be supportive and fair to the individual, knowing you want to act in a way that is consistent with actions taken in similar situations in the past and into the future. You decide to check the Center's Policy and Procedure Manual to see whether it provides guidance regarding the actions managers should take in a situation like this one. As you open the manual, what will you find?

INTRODUCTION AND BACKGROUND

Regardless of the industry or the domain, the advantages of having formal policies and procedures cannot be underestimated. Some simulation program managers, however, may not believe that having formal policies and procedures help their operations, and prefer to keep management flexible.

There are many considerations when developing policies and procedures for a simulation program. Whether you are running out of a closet or a 30,000 square feet (2,787 m^2) center, policies and procedures maintain standards and assure consistency. Policies and procedures provide guidelines that facilitate the smooth operations of the facility and help ensure that learners and simulation team members are literally all on the same page.

A sample policy and procedure manual from the WISER Center at the University of Pittsburgh is provided in the Appendix. To support the development of policies and procedures specific to simulation programs, the Society for Simulation in Healthcare (SSH) convened a number of administrators from simulations programs around the world to outline key components of policies and procedures from a global perspective. The result was the SSH Simulation Center Policy and Procedure Manual Template (http://ssih.org/membership1/ts-toolbox). Simulation program managers may find this a useful guide.

THE "HOW TO . . ."

Before You Get Started

Since most simulation programs exist within a parent organization, the program may need to follow some or all of the parent organization's policies. If an organization-level manual exists, make certain you have it available as you prepare to create a policies and procedures manual for the simulation program.

Consider the following steps prior to starting the creation of the manual:

1. Obtain any institution's policies on the topics you plan to include in the simulation program manual. This will help ensure your policies are aligned with your parent institution's policies.
2. Touch base with your human resource and legal departments to see whether there are any pitfalls or ideas they may have for you as you develop the manual.

3. Ensure that any policies created by your center can be enforced by your center or referred to the parent organization.

Policy and Procedure Categories

Policies articulate the rules that govern the operations of an organization. **Procedures** describe general operating processes and include how specific policies are implemented. Procedures evolve over time as new processes are created.

The following information can be utilized as a guide to assist you with the creation of your own simulation center policy and procedure manual. For each section, there is a list of topics and an explanation of each topic. The details included in each topic should help you understand its application and purpose.

General Information

- **Mission statement:** A statement specific for the simulation center yet in alignment with the parent institution, for example, university or hospital. A mission statement is brief and states the purpose of your simulation center. Mission statements often include a purpose statement, audience served, and types of activities or services.
- **Vision statement:** Can be the same vision statement as the parent institution. The vision statement reflects a larger ambition in that it defines where you want to be in 5 to 10 years.

(Please refer to chapter 5.3 Writing and Implementing a Strategic Plan for additional information on mission and vision statements.)

- **Governance—organizational chart:** Identifies the stakeholders and defines specific reporting lines within the simulation center, and delineates the level of authority for reporting, evaluations, and decision making. Please refer to chapter 5.3 Writing and Implementing a Strategic Plan for additional information.
- **Decision-making process:** Defines how decisions are made regarding equipment purchases, prioritizing projects, resolving scheduling conflicts, and other disagreements or uncertainties. This section goes hand in hand with the organizational chart.
- **Required disclaimers and pre-event statements:** This policy addresses outside presenters who may be a guest educator for a simulation-related class or event hosted or sponsored by the university or hospital. This policy ensures that the material presented is in

alignment with the program's values, and the simulation program is represented well. The primary purpose is to protect the reputation of the simulation program and respect the philosophy of using simulation-based learning.

- **Required event or course acknowledgments:** This policy addresses using the name of the simulation program when presenting projects to external audiences. The policy should clearly state when, how, and by whom these presentations must be approved, and if nonfaculty are presenting, then this must be cleared with the director of the simulation program. The intent of this policy is to ensure that the simulation program has quality representation at all times.
- **Simulation facility "Brand" use policy:** A policy stating how the simulation program is to be acknowledged in documents to establish consistency, for example, if you have a specific name and sequence you want to be included in published writings. The statement should include guidelines regarding when the simulation program needs to be acknowledged in a publication.
- **Hours of operations:** A clear statement identifying when the simulation center is open for business. Be sure to consider the setup and cleanup time needed when scheduling simulation sessions. The policy should address use times for internal and external customers and a mechanism to prioritize these when conflicts arise.
- **Simulation program terminology:** A listing of simulation terms used by the program. For example, a session may be defined as a series of scenarios followed by a debriefing or a single scenario followed by a debriefing. It is a tool to have clear, concise, and consistent taxonomy used within the facility by all. Please refer to the Glossary for the terms of reference.

Administrative Information

- **Support staff and contact tree:** The contact tree is helpful in case the program needs to shut down in an emergency, and helps with the contacting of staff, educators, and participants.
- **Personnel policy:** This is typically set by the entity that governs the program; however, because of its business needs, the program may have individual policies that are either more stringent or more lenient than the parent institution. For example, while overtime may not be allowed in general, special consideration can be made for courses where the program may charge a fee and allow for overtime. Similarly, the program should specify whether its vacation, leave of absence, workers compensation, and travel policies differ from those of the parent institution.
- **Scope of work and description for each personnel classification:** This section provides direction on roles and functions in the program. The size of the simulation team may vary depending on funding, space, and the priority stakeholders of a given program.

- **Organizational chart:** This is necessary to show the reporting structure within the program and, if applicable, how the program fits within a larger organizational structure.

Course Directors/Educators

- **Educators training:** Standards should be established for teaching within your simulation program. In particular, the development and delivery process of simulation-based educational programs should be standardized. Central to this standardization is educator training, which consists of two major components: course content and using simulation technology for teaching.
  - Course content
    It should be the responsibility of the course author to develop and validate course content and to identify instructors who will be teaching the courses. It should also be the responsibility of the course author to train these educators on the course content. An example of course creation methodology can be found at http://www.edpsycinteractive.org/topics/cognition/cogsys.html.
  - Simulation technology
    Courses can utilize various pieces of equipment within the simulation program. Most course authors are not expert on the equipment. Simulation staff should work with the course author and educators on teaching them how to utilize the equipment pertinent to their courses and/or to offer a member of the simulation staff to be part of the simulation team during the course. Refer to chapter 3.2 Mannequins: Terminology, Selection, and Usage for additional information.
- **Code of conduct:** Educators, learners, and staff are expected to act professionally and abide by rules. The course educator has the right to remove any participant from a course and the program. Simulation staff, after consultation with management, should also have the right to remove anyone (e.g., educator, learner) who is disruptive to operations. You should explain and document your process for removal as well as managing complaints. Course participants are expected to arrive for class academically prepared. Participants are expected to participate in class discussion and complete assignments as designated.
- **Course development policy:** There should be a standardized template for creation of courses. There should be no exceptions to this process as it ensures standardization and quality.
- **Evaluation policy:** All courses should have an evaluation component. Most simulation programs ask for a "General" section of the evaluation, where participants can comment on the program, its infrastructure, and staff. A course-specific component will address the course content, quality, and effectiveness of the simulation sessions and lectures. In the final

component, each educator should be evaluated. This policy should specify who should review evaluations and who should have access to them.

- **Course registration:** This section should explain how participants and educators register for courses or any other events. More specifically, the section should state what information (such as course name, course date/time, department, and professional title) needs to be collected during registration.
- **Equipment utilization:** This section should include policies on equipment utilization with specific do's and don'ts. For example: *DO NOT use pen on any mannequin within the center. Make sure you shut all projectors off when you leave for the day.*
- **Educator travel:** If educators travel on behalf of your simulation center, you should establish clear polices on such items as who is paying for the travel, shipping of equipment, and key contacts to assist that educator.

Scheduling Courses and Rooms

- **Approval process:** All initial courses or events should be approved by operational or administrative leadership of the simulation center. There are typically three main components to the approval process.
  1. Does this course meet the training missions of the program?
  2. What are the financial arrangements for this course? Or are you going to do this without financial support?
  3. Can this course be taught effectively using simulation or components of simulation?
- **Process:** Once a course has been created, the scheduling of the course can occur. Most programs now utilize some form of a reservation process. This section should explain the process for requesting a course and might include an information collection form with room, equipment, and staff requirements.
- **Notification:** Once a course has been approved, the educator should be notified. From there you should establish whose responsibility it would be to notify the participants. This should be clearly outlined in this section.
- **Priority of use:** Many simulation programs operate under a "First Come, First Serve" policy. Others give priority based on funding sources. Whatever the policy is, you should explain it here. You might also consider including a statement that courses can be cancelled at the discretion of the program.
- **Cancellation policy:** There are three issues to consider when cancelling a course.
  1. Notification of the simulation program
  2. Notification of educators
  3. Notification of participants

The details of who will contact which group should be clearly outlined. Example: A course is cancelled. Educator calls to notify the program. The program e-mails and calls all participants. This policy should also specify the time frame for cancellation and under what circumstances the user will be charged for cancelling a course.

- **Recording of scheduled events (i.e., calendar structure and information):** The simulation program should have a policy regarding maintaining an accurate account of what courses ran at the center, dates of the course, number of participants, departments, and so on.
- **Arbiter of scheduling conflicts:** This policy should explain how a scheduling conflict between two or more courses is resolved and who has the final say in the dispute. This section should also explain how the center handles complaints from educators or learners.
- **Severe weather:** Most simulation centers are affiliated with a medical center, hospital, college, or university and should follow their department's policy for severe weather and closures. In this section, you should explain the process for simulation center staff, educators, and participants.

Tours

- **Requesting tours:** Tours require time and resources. This policy should state the program's willingness to provide tours and an overview to requesting tours. This policy should include the process for scheduling and requesting tours, the contact person, and the specific areas that the person would like to visit. When placing a request for a tour, consider the audience visiting and their individual learning needs.
- **Tour requirements:** This policy should cover the specifics regarding each tour. Consider including time frames for tours, length, minimum and maximum numbers in each tour, photography, and, depending upon the needs of the visitors, charging a fee.
- **Tour cancellation:** This policy should state that the tours need to be cancelled within a certain time frame of the tour date. Consider the resources and needs of the individual center when determining this time frame.

Equipment

- **Loaning of equipment:** A policy statement describing who may borrow equipment, the type of equipment available for loan, the responsibility of the individual/department who is borrowing the equipment, the return policy, and any terms/fees that need to be included. In addition, a form should be created with a process of completion (name, contact information, pickup date, return date, any special instructions regarding the loaned item, etc.) and a tracking system to follow up on missing items.

SECTION 5 • Management

- **Standard program equipment:** A description of the basic equipment available for use at the program, how to access the equipment, how to use the equipment, and how to return the equipment. In some instances, the equipment may require an orientation prior to use. If this is the case, you may want to consider a sign-off form to document that the user has been trained and understands the use of the equipment.
- **Acquisition policy and process:** This provides a description on to request equipment. A form is likely required. This may include a statement of need and rationale, and who may benefit from the acquisition. The policy would state how requests are prioritized and the decision-making process in acquiring new equipment.
- **Maintenance and care of equipment:** There may be one overall policy identifying the individual(s) who is/are responsible for the maintenance and care of the equipment, the frequency of the maintenance, including any warranty work. Then there should be specific maintenance and care instructions for each different piece of equipment, for example, what type of chemicals can and cannot be used, and how to disassemble and reassemble. This may just be the user guide that comes with the equipment, but it must be available for the user. This section should also describe a process to document every usage and cleaning as well as rate any deterioration or damage on a scale (e.g., from 1 to 5). Once the item is rated a certain level, a purchase order would be generated to replace the worn-out item.
- **Breakage and repair (internal and external):** The policy needs to state the reporting procedure to alert the Operations Manager of the broken piece of equipment. A form may be used in this process that describes how the equipment broke and what was being done when it broke. This information may be helpful in identifying patterns if equipment is breaking on a regular basis. The repair policy identifies who may be responsible for the repair, for example, warranty, maintenance agreement, personal responsibility.
- **In situ versus in-facility use:** Depending on the program, there may be two dedicated sets of equipment—one for in situ and another for in-facility use. Either way, there needs to be an inventory of the equipment, supplies, and a regular maintenance check of the equipment.

Supplies

- **Acquisition:** This section should state who is responsible for making certain that all supplies are available for a given course/session and when their availability needs to be confirmed. One may work directly with the hospital supply warehouse for supply acquisition.

If supplies need to be purchased through an outside vendor, ordering 1 month prior to its need is ideal. International programs should consider importation and customs delays in devising their policies. Please refer to chapter 3.2 Mannequins: Terminology, Selection, and Usage and 3.8 Repurposing of Equipment for additional information on purchasing simulation equipment and supplies.

- **Organization:** Supplies will be organized by the Simulation Program Operations Team with clear labeling and understanding of where items live. Organizing with the use of colors, letters, or numbers with a map and clear descriptions is essential. Depending on courses/programs, disciplines may consider organizing supplies by course/program.
- **Inventory:** Routine inventory of supplies should be conducted and documented in a format that the facility and infrastructure support. A database or excel spreadsheets organized by skills lab training or simulation sessions is an option.
- **Budget source:** Funds that come from participant lab fees can be used to offset the supply cost. When facilities are first starting, it is important to track costs to better understand the sustainability needs and expectations. Budgeting is discussed in depth in chapter 4.2.
- **Usage and reusage:** In simulation and skills sessions, there are many items that can be reused. There should be a standardized description of which items will be reused and which items will be thrown away. For example, one could reuse an intravenous flush; however, needles would be disposed of in the sharps container.

Note: It is important to partner with your local hospitals and clinics to acquire supplies that are expired for patient use but can be used for training purposes. Sometimes, having a conversation with your surplus partners will result in a huge cost savings that will help with sustainability efforts.

Scenarios

- **Scenario development:** The program should develop a standardized scenario template that may be used by course directors to develop simulation-based cases describing case presentation and narrative, pertinent patient history, chief complaint, appropriate student responses, and so on. Once completed, the scenario template may be used by the program's simulation staff to program and prepare for the course. It is strongly suggested that the simulation staff receive the completed scenario template no later than 1 month prior to the program. The course author should review and validate the programmed scenario at least a week in advance of the course. More detailed information on scenario development is available in chapter XX, and Kyle and Murray (2008, chaps. 57–59) and Jeffries (2007).

- **Scenario structure:** The structure of the scenario template must be one that encompasses all aspects and pertinent physiology of the patient, equipment, supplies, and necessary case information and best standardizes the experience for multiple groups. Some recommendations include, but are not limited to:
  - Case title
  - Goals and objectives/debriefing points
  - Patient chief complaint
  - Patient information (name, age, gender, weight, height)
  - Case presentation (information given to the participant prior to the beginning of the case)
  - Vital signs
  - Past medical history
  - Medications
  - Allergies
  - Events (actions taken by the participant)
  - Result of event (decrease in BP, increase in HR, etc.)
  - Staff needed
  - Staff roles and Environments
  - Equipment/props needed
- **Authorship:** This policy should outline which authors of a scenario are recognized on the basis of their involvement with the development and implementation of the case.
- **Ownership:** This policy establishes whether a scenario developed by an external author may or may not be used by the simulation program as part of their portfolio of simulation cases. In general, the program should adopt the parent institution's policy on intellectual property.
- **Audiovisual storage:** This policy addresses the length of time that an audiovisual recording of the scenario is to be kept. These guidelines should take into consideration whether the recordings will be used during the course for debriefing or saved for future review and research. The policy should be standardized for all audiovisual recordings. It is recommended that the program seek advice regarding this issue from legal counsel. Additionally, the policy should reference **confidentiality** of the recording. Should there be a desire to use a recording for viewing by others not involved in the case, a written release should be obtained by the participants involved. While most video recordings are legal with or without consent, laws governing audio recordings vary by state and country. The program should be familiar with the recording laws in their jurisdiction.
- **Utilization of scenarios:** There should be a policy stating that it is the responsibility of the authors of the scenario and the Course Director to ensure the case follows current acceptable standards of care and hospital policy. It is suggested that resources used in the preparation of the scenario be listed.

- **Clinical quality assurance:** There should be a policy that scenarios continue to be updated to ensure they follow the current clinical standards of care. As these standards change, revisions to the scenario need to be made.
- **Debriefing:** Debriefing is the most critical component of the simulation exercise. It is recommended that the program develop a policy and procedure to allow participants to reflect on their performance during the scenario and receive constructive feedback about their performance. Audiovisual technology and playback should also be considered as part of the debriefing process if feasible and available. In certain circumstances, the best educators may not necessarily make the best debriefers. As such, the policy should address whether educators involved with debriefings need to take a formal course on the structure and art of debriefing.

Operations

- **Start-up and shutdown process:** The policies in this section should include step-by-step instructions for accessing the facility, disarming any security alarms, turning on and turning off every simulator model, and audio and video recording and presentation equipment. The policies should specify what categories of users are qualified to open up the center and whose responsibility it is to shut everything down. Furthermore, it should be stated who is expected to clean up after simulation activities. It is very helpful to the users to include photos of the procedures and equipment as well.
- **Security of information:** This section should address where printed and digital information related to simulation activities should be stored and who will have access to the files. Specific policies should address storage simulation scenarios, sign-in and attendance records, video records, equipment manuals, maintenance logs, and purchasing documentation.
- **Simulator maintenance:** A separate maintenance policy should be developed for each simulator. It should include daily, weekly, monthly, and yearly tasks related to keeping the simulator operational. Also, attached to each policy should be a maintenance checklist template. The policy should identify staff members who are responsible for performing each maintenance task.
- **Course supplies:** Supplies will be organized by the simulation program staff with clear labeling and understanding of where items are stored. Organizing with the use of colors, letters, or numbers with a map and clear descriptions is essential. Depending on courses/programs, disciplines may consider organizing supplies by course/program. Ideally, each course should have a bin with supplies and props needed for it. A policy should be in place to notify

the person in charge of replenishing supplies when a particular item is depleted.

- **Course preparation:** For each course, a set of precourse checklists should be developed that specify what tasks need to be accomplished and when. For example:
  - 1 month before the course
    - Schedule the course, send out invitations
  - 1 week before the course
    - Confirm attendees, educators, and staff participants
  - 1 to 2 days before the course
    - Prepare paperwork
    - Check supplies
    - Remind participants
  - The day of the course
    - Configure simulator
    - Configure AV equipment and software

The policies should state who is responsible for each task—whether simulation program staff or the client department.

- **Course turnover:** Similar to course preparation, this section should include postcourse checklists that specify what tasks need to be accomplished immediately after the course completion (e.g., shutdown equipment, cleanup, file paperwork) and what needs to be done later (e.g., follow-up surveys, CME/CE certificates).
- **After-hours access:** The policies should state under what conditions access to the simulation program is allowed outside of regular business hours. The following questions should be addressed: What activities are allowed after hours? Whose approval is needed to allow after-hours simulation? Who is allowed to conduct after-hours simulation? How are expectations for after-hours activities different from regular daylight activities? What information needs to be recorded in a log?

Video Recording and Photo Release

- **Confidentiality:** Every participant in simulation and clinical learning must sign a program-specific confidentiality, video recording, and photo release form. The policy should state the importance of confidentiality, the details of what the expectations of the facility are in terms of participation, and to fully disclose how videos and photos will be used. The following information should be acquired and maintained for a determined period of time (if it is a student course, then their name and cohort information should be collected and maintained through date of graduation). The expectations need to be clearly defined.
- **Forms:** Forms should include the policy information needed for the below topics. These should be

provided to participants before they are involved with their first simulation activity. In some cases, these forms may be compiled into one and may be administered after the fact as a reminder (an example of this could be mock codes in the hospital setting).
  - Confidentiality (see detailed information below)
  - Video recording/photo release (see detailed information below)
  - Video reviewing policy (see detailed information below)
- **Consent:** The program should have a policy in place that ensures that each participant reviews the consent form and signs it at the appropriate time.
- **Video recording policy:** The program should have a policy in place that ensures that each participant is aware of the recording policy determined for the varying simulation courses. The participant should be informed and sign it at the appropriate time.
- **Video distribution policy:** The program should have a policy in place that clearly states if and when video will be distributed. The policy should also address to whom videos will be distributed to.
- **Video retention and deletion:** The program should have a policy in place that clearly defines if and when videos will be retained, destroyed, and deleted. This may vary depending on the level of the participants. For example, videos of learners will be saved (according to School or Institution policy) until successful graduation and 1 year past the date of attendance, whereas clinician's videos will be immediately deleted unless otherwise communicated. Participants must have clear communication and understanding of this process.

Course Observation

- **Observation of simulation policy for course participants:** This policy should explain how and where course participants can observe simulation involving their peers. In particular, it is important to emphasize the confidentiality policy that protects participants from judgments and opinions of their performance. The participants should pledge not to discuss each other's performance in simulation scenarios outside of the simulation program. Another reason for confidentiality pledge is to ensure that participants do not divulge scenario information to other participants.
- **Observation policy for nonparticipants:** This section should describe what procedures need to be followed for the protection of the learners, educators, and staff. Who is allowed to approve observation by nonparticipants? Is it the Program Director or course educators, or both? How far in advance must the request for observation be made? Under

what conditions are the observers allowed to take still pictures or video? Are observers allowed into the control room? Into the debriefing room? Are observers allowed to interact with simulation staff and participants?

- **Required disclaimers and pre-event statements:** Observers need to be told of confidentiality expectations. Just as students are expected to pledge confidentiality, so too should the educators and simulation staff pledge not to divulge information on learners' performance outside of the program.
- **Required event or course acknowledgments:** This section will include any sponsorship information or an explanation that simulation is a teaching, not a testing tool (if appropriate). Also, the program might state that taking a simulation course does not necessarily translate into achieving competency in the clinical arena.

Fiscal

- **Fee structure for use (internal and external use):** It is important to set up a pricing structure for internal and external users of the program. This is an opportunity for the program to have additional income. Internal users typically are given a lower rate for the use of the program because they have supplied the initial backing for the facility or are the primary users of the program. External users can be charged at a rate that the market will bear depending on the geographical location of the simulation program.
- **Required reporting (type and frequency) and to whom:** Each simulation program is typically required to provide some sort of report to either the governing body of the simulation program or the department/hospital where the program sits. This report may be something as simple as how many days the program is used to a breakdown of how much each user group used the facility and what courses are run there. It is important to make sure that from the beginning accurate and detailed records are kept of the financial doings of the program as well as the use of the facility.
- **Annual budget reporting requirements:** The budget is one of the most fundamental infrastructure documents of a simulation program. Each program has different requirements that they must provide, and here is where that information would be placed—everything from staffing requirements to projected direct/indirect costs to confirmed or potential income for the upcoming fiscal year.
- **Required fiscal year–end documents:** In this section, a list of year-end documentation that must be reported should be provided. Examples are purchases that were made for the year, income for the year, and any other fiscal documents that are needed to report to the program's stakeholders.

- **Purchase and acquisition procedure:** The procedures for purchasing are described in more detail above in the Equipment and Supplies sections focused on acquisition.
- **Reimbursement process:** Reimbursement of expenses typically falls under the policy of the institution that hosts the simulation program.
- **Financial accounting:** This section would be guided by the program's governance structure.
- **Conflict of interest:** This section covers specific rules on dealing with **conflict of interests** that may impact the integrity of the courses.
- **Purchasing equipment:** Purchasing equipment is a major expense in operating. In this section, the proper steps for requesting the purchase of a piece of equipment and the actual process that is involved with purchasing equipment are listed. Please refer to the chapter 4.8 Working with Vendors on purchasing for additional information.
- **Purchasing approval process:** Some purchases are approved at the administrative level, whereas some are required to have much higher approval. The processes that are needed for any purchase should be included here and should have details on what the approval steps are as well as what can be done in case a purchase has been denied.
- **Payroll:** In this section, key payroll contacts should be indicated as well as the process for employees to be paid.

Courses

- **Course approval process:** Each course should be approved by the appropriate personnel and be routed through an approval process. Most courses need to meet the following criteria: funding available (who will pay for development or course running at the center), makes sense (medically), meets the mission of the simulation program, can be performed within the simulation program or in situ, and you have or can purchase supplies or equipment to manage the course.
- **Funding and course financials:** All courses cost money to develop and run. The simulation program should create a course development form for use by administrative personnel as well as sharing this information with the potential user. This form should include supplies, development time, and actual time in the program, and administrative considerations such as copies, binders, catering, and other incidental expenses.
- **Mandatory elements of a course:** In this section, you should describe the key elements of a course and what is expected for each element. The example below shows a set of core elements for a course. Once you have decided what elements are needed, you should explain them in further detail.
  - Course Description
  - Course Objectives

- Precourse Material
- Day of course Content
- Postcourse Assessment (Hertel & Millis, 2002)
- Assessment
- **Continuing medical education:** On the basis of the program's mission, you should describe what your policy would be for obtaining CME/CEs for courses. You should also establish a process for obtaining these credits and establish a relationship with the CME department.

Remediation

- **General remediation policy:** If simulation is used for remediation, then participants should be aware of that from the beginning of their involvement. The program should have a policy in place that explains the process of remediation training.
- **Policy for educators:** If simulation is used for remediation, then educators need to be aware of it and be consistent with its use. Ideally, a simulation expert should work with educators to determine whether simulation is the best route for a remediation.
- **Policy for participants:** If simulation is used for remediation, then participants should have the information and access to the policy at their first simulation encounter and at any time in the future.
- **Documentation:** A standard form should be created for documentation and keeping track of the dates and details of the events that led up to the remediation and the remediation itself.
- **Ethical guidelines:** If simulation is used for remediation in a given situation, there should be a policy in place that clearly states whether this will affect a learner's current or future employment.

Customer Relations Policies

- **Dispute resolution:** This policy should explain how a dispute is processed and resolved and who has the final say in the dispute. This section should also explain how complaints from educators or learners will be handled.
- **Marketing of program:** This section should specify the following:
  - Who is allowed to initiate customer (client) solicitation; what are the differences between approaching an internal customer (within the institution) and an external customer (outside the institution)?
  - Through what channels can the program's services be promoted?
- **Policy on use of program's name:** The policy should state the official name of the program and its acronym to be used in all communications and publications. It might also be helpful to list names and acronyms that should NOT be used. If the program has a word mark, logo, seal, or color motif, they should also be spelled out in this section.

- **Web usage:** This section should describe the following:
  - What information belongs on the program's website? Who decides?
  - Who is in charge of updating content on the website?
  - Who is responsible for replying to Web requests?
- **Information dissemination:** This section should explain how information about the program's services is disseminated (such as printed materials, Web, and e-mail), and if information is disseminated to a wide audience, whose approval is needed.
- **Official media policy:** Often, a simulation program works with the public relations department of its parent institution. Therefore, the following questions should be addressed in the policy:
  - What is the procedure for media requests?
  - Who is authorized to talk to the media?
  - What activities are members of the media allowed to observe?

Travel and Meeting Attendance

- **Travel:** See above in Course Directors and Educators category for additional information. Clearly defined processes for travel are key to the facility's overall success and continued networking. This section should also explain the approval process for travel.
- **Meetings:** This section should specify under what conditions a staff member can travel to attend a meeting, describe the approval process, and list the pre- and postmeeting expectations. It may be necessary to state how many meetings per year an employee can attend and how many people can be away from the program at the same time.
- **Reimbursement policy:** The reimbursement policy is usually the same as the university or health system in which the program resides.
- **Covered expenses:** Expenses that are typically covered are meals (usually a maximum per diem has been determined), airfare, hotel, rental car/taxi/transit, mileage, parking, and purchases that may be needed for meeting (i.e., copies, abstract poster).
- **Priority scheduling in case of conflict:** If an individual is to attend a meeting and a conflict arises, the director should determine whether the conflict is a higher priority than the meeting.

Research Policy

- **Institutional Review Board (IRB) policy:** Researchers will follow the IRB policies within their organizations. All expected paperwork and timelines will be followed per protocol. Please refer to section 9.2 Simulation Research Considerations for additional information.
- **General Guidelines if different from institutions:** Learners/participants must have informed consent for involvement in research. There are specific institutional guidelines that must be followed.

- **Security:** Researchers will follow the security guidelines outlined in the review process for both hardcopy checklists and also for other research data collected. Any videos used in research will be kept locked and confidential per institutional protocol.
- **Fiscal impact:** Principal investigators (PI) need to partner with simulation teams within their institutions to better understand the resources that are needed to conduct simulation-focused research. It is important to allocate staff, facility, and equipment resources to achieve the research goals.
- **Publication policy:** Individuals involved with the simulation research should publish their findings as a group within a year of completion of the funding component of the project. It is important to include the names of the team members that participated in implementing the simulation sessions in the publications.
- **Authorship rules:** Authors should be cited accurately for involvement with simulation research. Discussion and agreements about first author will be driven by the PI or Project Manager of a given research project.
- **Data collection responsibility:** The responsibility for data collection will be determined by the PI. Ultimately, it will be the responsibility of the PI to ensure that the data is being collected accurately and according to protocol. Please see section 10 for additional information.

Safety and Security

- **Emergencies**
  - *Medical:* A policy needs to state whom to contact in case of an emergency, for example, 911 or "0," and what is required in regard to documentation after the event is stabilized.
  - *Nonmedical emergency:* A statement regarding how to manage nonmedical emergencies—for example, is faculty/staff able to manage these instances? What reporting is required?
  - *AED locations:* A statement and drawing of where the AEDs are located in the simulation program.
- **Identification badges:** A statement regarding your policy on leraners, educators, guests, staff, and the like wearing identification badges within the simulation program. In some cases, access into the simulation program is only by badge.

BEEN THERE, DONE THAT: HOW CAN I CONTINUE TO IMPROVE OR SUSTAIN WHAT I HAVE ACHIEVED?

As you can see, there is much to think about when creating policies and procedures. It can be a very time-consuming, challenging, and sometimes confusing process. The following steps will assist with the development of an effective policy and procedure manual:

- Start with the existing policies from the parent institution.
- Consider using the Society manual template as a guide (http://ssih.org/membership1/ts-toolbox).
- Consider an internal and external version of your policy manual. The internal version is designed for the program staff, whereas the external should address all others.

Policies evolve as practices do. It is recommended that you reassess your policies on an annual basis to ensure they are meeting current needs. Throughout the year, new policies and procedures will be created in addition to revisions of existing ones. Version control, therefore, will be important. It is recommended that you include a version or date on each policy created and also who completed the creation or revision.

Most policy manuals tend to be lengthy and confusing. For this reason, consider dividing the manual into sections and placing each policy on its own page. This will allow for easier navigation, revisions, and control. Remember, a physical manual may not be necessary if the manual can be stored electronically. This will contribute to the "Going Green" effort and will make additions and revisions easier. Identifying a key individual to provide oversight of the policy and procedure development and reviews process will also be helpful.

SUMMARY

In summary, regardless of the size of the program's operations, policies and procedures are essential. Getting started with developing a policy and procedure manual can be a complicated process given that simulation environments offer challenging issues to those who manage and operate simulation programs and facilities. Identification and implementation of standardized policies and procedures commonly utilized within a simulation program is an efficient way to move forward, providing stability and consistency. The advantages of having formal policies and procedures cannot be underestimated. Having a foundation in place will allow for growth and expansion.

REFERENCES

Hertel, J. P., & Millis, B. J. (2002). Debriefing an education simulation. In *Using simulations to promote learning in higher education* (pp. 59–72). Sterling, VA: Stylus.

Jeffries, P. R. (2007). *Simulation in nursing education: From conceptualization to evaluation.* Washington, DC: National League for Nursing.

Kyle, R. R., & Murray, W. B. (2008). *Clinical simulation: Operations, engineering, and management.* Amsterdam, The Netherlands: Academic Press.

CHAPTER 5.3

Writing and Implementing a Strategic Plan

Gail Johnson, MS, RN, CCRN, CPHQ, CHSE and Jeanette L. Augustson, MA

ABOUT THE AUTHORS

GAIL L. JOHNSON is the Director of HealthPartners Clinical Simulation, a center that has been granted accreditation by the Society for Simulation in Healthcare (SSH), where she provides strategic and day-to-day leadership for the in situ, mobile, and simulation center based programs. She has worked in both academic and healthcare systems and has directed programs including education, quality management, risk management, and regulatory affairs. Ms. Johnson is a reviewer for SSH's accreditation program and a member of the Accreditation Council and Certification Committees. Ms. Johnson is nationally certified as a Certified Healthcare Simulation Educator (CHSE).

JEANETTE L. AUGUSTSON is the Senior Director of Education Administration for the HealthPartners Institute for Education and Research, where she provides operational oversight in support of health professional education programs, including strategic planning, finance, marketing/communications, information systems and technology, new program development, governance, and planning for organizational sustainability and advancement. She has worked in government and nonprofit organizations, developing expertise in planning, budget development, organizational development, and administrative leadership.

ABSTRACT

Strategic planning is not just for large organizations. Simulation programs also benefit from having a documented, systematic plan that outlines the process of moving forward toward achieving their mission and vision. Yet few simulation programs have a well-developed strategic plan to guide them. This chapter provides an overview of strategic planning and guidelines to add simulation program–specific goals, strategies, objectives, and tactics into an existing organizational plan. Steps to create a simulation program–specific strategic plan are outlined.

CASE EXAMPLE

Xanadu Simulation Center is a 10,000 square feet (929 m^2) center or facility within the Xanadu University Medical Center, an academic teaching hospital. Prior to the opening of this Center 2 years ago, the hospital had a one-room skills lab and two moderate-technology simulators. This area was primarily used for nursing orientation, basic life support (BLS), and advanced life support classes. After a large fund-raising initiative, and with significant financial support from Xanadu University and the Medical Center, the Simulation Center opened. Financial support included providing capital and operating expenses for 36 months. During the first 6 months of operation, 75% of the entire capital budget was spent on equipment. The Program purchased adult, pediatric, birthing, and neonatal mannequins, and the rest of the equipment was purchased at the request of hospital and university faculty. This included central line insertion task trainers, a virtual reality surgical trainer, a full-body ultrasound trainer, and a variety of other procedural task trainers. Since opening, several of these have been used only once or twice. The facility has office space, two storage rooms, three debriefing rooms/classrooms, a room dedicated for procedures, and six simulation rooms. The Program is staffed with 3.6 full-time equivalents (FTE) and a number of adjunct faculty.

Since opening, over 3,500 participants have used the Program. Most are from the nursing department, utilizing the space during their annual skills fairs. The emergency and internal medicine residents have used the procedure room to practice invasive procedures. There has been limited involvement from the medical school and college of nursing. Four to five simulation-based programs are held each month for external customers. Evaluation data demonstrates that participants enjoy the simulation experiences and debriefing, and believe they are more confident and competent after participating in their various courses.

The Program has been in operation for almost 24 months, and in your role as the Program Manager, you were asked to provide an update to the senior leadership team. During the presentation, it became evident that the simulation program lacked focus—a purpose and vision—and there was not a connection linking the Simulation Center's activities to the organization's strategic goals and initiatives. Without this connection and a lack of information showing the value of the Simulation Center to the organization, the program is at risk for budget reductions and downsizing. A decision was made to create and implement a strategic plan. You have been assigned the responsibility to make this happen. Where do you start?

INTRODUCTION

"Would you tell me, please, which way I ought to go from here?"
"That depends a good deal on where you want to get to," said the Cat.
"I don't much care where," said Alice.
"Then it doesn't matter which way you go," said the Cat.
". . . so long as I get SOMEWHERE," Alice added as an explanation.
"Oh, you're sure to do that," said the Cat, "if you only walk long enough."

(Carroll, 1865, chap. VI, Alice in Wonderland)

Much like Alice's journey, with enough effort a simulation program will go somewhere. But without a vision, it may be difficult to identify a destination. Without a strategic plan, a simulation program may be challenged with prioritization, program development, financial stability, staffing, and ensuring that adequate and appropriate simulation technologies are available. A strategic plan helps a program or organization determine which opportunities it will pursue and which it will pass by (Bower & Gilbert, 2007, p. 74).

Most health systems and academic institutions have a strategic plan. They are more common at an organizational level than a department or business unit level. If a simulation program is affiliated with a larger organization, there may be a strategic plan already developed for the overall organization or division. While the organization's plan provides direction for how the *organization* will achieve its vision, it may lack specificity that would be beneficial in guiding work at a program level.

Specific to simulation programs, the 2013 Society for Simulation in Healthcare's Accreditation Standards state that in order to be accredited, a simulation program must have a plan to accomplish its mission, and suggest this be a strategic, business, or an operational plan (SSH Council for Accreditation of Healthcare Simulation Programs, 2013, p. 3).

This chapter will provide an overview of strategic planning and guidelines to add simulation program–specific **goals**, **strategies**, and **objectives/tactics** into an organizational plan, as well as steps to create a simulation program–specific strategic plan.

THE STRATEGIC PLAN

What Is a Strategic Plan?

Strategic planning is "the process of determining what your organization intends to accomplish and how you will direct the organization and its resources toward accomplishing these goals over the coming months and years" (Barry, 2007, p. 99). Strategic planning is a systematic and coordinated process designed to ensure that the planned direction is well thought out and appropriate. A strategic plan provides the blueprint or road map for how an organization or program will accomplish its goals. It includes an assessment of internal and external environments as well as fundamental choices about:

- The program's role within the parent organization and community.
- The mission and vision the simulation program will pursue.
- Type of learners (internal, external, students, professionals, discipline/profession), who will attend.
- The kinds of programs or services that will be offered.
- Resources needed to succeed (i.e., people, expertise, relationships, facilities, mannequins, task trainers, other equipment, and money).
- The best way to combine the resources, relationships, and programming to accomplish the goals of the simulation program and parent organization (Barry, 2007).

Strategic plans are different from operational or business plans. Strategic plans are used to provide the "big picture" goals and direction over a period of several years. Historically, strategic plans were created for a 5- to 10-year period. In today's quickly changing environments, that may be too long a period, and a 2- to 3-year strategic plan may be more appropriate (Joyce & Martinez, 2007). Operational or business plans, on the other hand, are developed yearly and show how the organization or program will move toward accomplishing its strategic plan. These are narrower in focus and describe in detail how the work will be completed.

SECTION 5 • Management

Grounded in the mission and vision of the organization, an effective strategic plan will provide the simulation program with meaningful goals, strategies, objectives, and realistic **measures of success**. These elements will be described in greater detail here, with relevant examples for a simulation program.

Why Create One?

Planning and setting goals have the potential to exert a positive influence on organizational performance; organizations with strategic plans typically outperform those that do not have one in place. A clear plan and evaluation strategy contributes to accountability and accomplishing established goals (Barry, 2007). Both the process of creating a program- or department-specific strategic plan and the plan itself provide tremendous value for a simulation program. Through the planning process, key leaders, stakeholders, and simulation staff develop common assumptions and expectations. Discussions about strengths, weaknesses, opportunities, and threats (SWOT) give stakeholders an understanding of the current capabilities of the program, as well as potential needs or opportunities that could impact the program's future. Building this common understanding is an effective way of ensuring the relevance of the simulation program's mission and vision, and of garnering the support needed to advance the strategic plan.

Once completed, the strategic plan provides a critical foundation for the operation of the simulation program. It informs planning and decisions about:

- Funding and resource development
- Personnel needs
- Infrastructure development
- Collaboration and partnerships
- Professional development needs
- Provides a focus for simulation activities and prioritize usage requests.

"The process of planning not only helps keep lab faculty and staff apprised of the challenges to be faced, but it also helps to keep senior level management engaged by reason of the need for their input and approval of the plan" (Gantt, 2010, p. 308). It is easy to become so preoccupied with the day-to-day details of scheduling, developing, and facilitating simulation sessions that a program loses focus. Following a strategic plan ensures that you are moving in the desired direction, and advancing the goals that will get you there.

Strategic planning can also be used to plan for and mitigate potential or actual problems. It is a way to "resolve an interrelated set of issues or problems in an intentional, coordinated manner" (Barry, 2007, loc. 163). For example, changes in healthcare reimbursement and medical education funding may result in budget cuts from the parent organization, the increase in simulation programs in a community may increase competition and reduce external revenue, as well as other demands and challenges identified by a program. Simulation programs can use strategic planning to consider various options, including new ways to increase revenue, prioritization, exploring ways to reduce expenses, forming simulation consortiums, and influencing policy makers (Barry, 2007).

Components of the Plan

A strategic plan includes the mission statement, which is the purpose of the program or where the program is now; the vision, or where the program wants to get to; and then the strategic goals, strategies, objectives, and tactics, or how the program will get there. It will also include measures of progress or success (Figure 5.3.1).

Mission and Vision

"No wise fish would go anywhere without a porpoise."

(Carroll 1865, chap. X)

A strategic plan for a simulation program begins with the program's specific mission and vision. Even if the parent organization has an established mission/vision, a simulation program should consider creating mission and vision statements specifically for their program to provide program focus. Whether using the mission and vision of your simulation program, or the mission and vision of the parent organization, these key statements of purpose and direction are essential to the strategic planning process. A **mission** summarizes the current purpose of organization or program, and provides the reason for why a simulation program exists. Examples of mission statements include the following:

- To improve health and patient safety through simulation-based programs designed to maximize the abilities of individuals, teams, and systems (HealthPartners Clinical Simulation, 2012).

Elements of a strategic plan

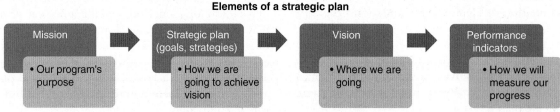

FIGURE 5.3.1 Elements of a strategic plan.

- Using simulation to improve safety, quality, and education in healthcare (Center for Medical Simulation, 2009).
- To promote health and welfare by providing quality medical education and hands-on training, and to promote and foster research in all areas of medicine for healthcare professionals (Medical Education & Research Institute, 2012).
- To accelerate nursing skill development through simulation-based learning (Fictitious Xanadu Simulation Center).

The **vision** summarizes the impact a simulation program desires to achieve. If we close our eyes and imagine the simulation program of our dreams, with the impact on participants, patients, and the healthcare system that we most desire, what would that look like in 2 years or 5 years? Vision statements are not "'what we do,' but rather 'what we will be in x years'" (Person, 2013, Loc. 683). For example:

- To be an essential partner and leader in simulation-based education and research (HealthPartners Clinical Simulation, 2012).
- MERI will be the leading hands-on medical education and training institution in the world for healthcare professionals (Medical Education & Research Institute, 2012).
- To be the regional simulation program that best prepares healthcare students and professionals to provide safe and effective care (Fictitious Xanadu Simulation Center).

Although these statements are simple and succinct, their importance to an organization or program cannot be understated: The mission directs the focus, and the vision identifies what you hope to achieve or where you want to go. Connecting the dots between these, in a thoughtful, organized manner, is the strategic plan. Besides the mission and vision statements, strategic plans typically include a description of the long-term goals and strategies, the objectives and tactics necessary to achieve them, and a way to monitor and measure progress.

Goals, Strategies, Objectives, and Tactics

A strategic plan typically includes four key elements: goals, strategies, objectives, tactics (or actions), and measures of success. These elements provide the map or direction of how a program is going to achieve its vision. Strategic plans may include other elements or use different terminology, but this framework provides a straightforward approach that will capture essential information necessary in implementing a strategic plan.

Goals

A goal reflects the priorities of the organization or simulation program in moving toward its vision. Goals should provide a meaningful description of the areas key stakeholders believe the organization must focus to advance its mission

and achieve the vision. This prioritization can be challenging; often there are many issues that stakeholders would like to address. "Strategic plans usually lack focus because organizations identify and attempt to address too many problems . . . . It all starts with prioritization of the most important issues and a commitment to direct organizational energy and resources to address them" (Zuckerman, 2006, p. 5).

Goals often reflect the themes that arise during an evaluation of the strengths, weaknesses, opportunities, and threats/challenges facing an organization. For example, if a simulation program knows that it has high satisfaction among participants but has not been able to demonstrate the impact on improving patient care, the latter may become a priority and goal for the program. If there is a problem with employee turnover, team stability may become an important goal. Funding opportunities or challenges, participation growth or decline, internal or external environmental changes, and many other factors may inform the development of goals.

It is helpful to organize goals in a framework that reflects key dimensions of the simulation program and its parent organization. It is easy to focus on only one area, like the participants/learners, at the expense of goals related to other important aspects such as internal processes and financial perspectives. The Balanced Score Card model (Kaplan & Norton, 1996) is one type of framework outlining four business perspectives or dimensions: Internal Business Process, Customer, Learning and Growth, and Financial. Utilizing these key dimensions ensures that the program is not focusing on one area at the expense of others. For example, a program that focuses only on creating exceptional learning experiences for participants and has not identified goals in other dimensions may not be operating at its full potential, and without a focus on stewardship or the financial impact, it may not be able to stay in business. This framework can be adapted to fit the focus of the business. In a healthcare organization, dimensions such as patient outcomes, patient experience, workforce, and finances may better reflect the organization's business. In a simulation program, the following framework for organizing goals may be helpful:

1. **Impact** of simulation program on patient safety, board scores, NCLEX passing rate
2. **Experience** of simulation customers or participants
3. **Internal processes** and team capacity development
4. **Finance** and stewardship

Within each of these perspectives, the program may outline one or more specific goals.

1. **Impact:** Maximize the job-readiness of nursing students graduating from Xanadu University's School of Nursing.
2. **Experience:** Increase recognition of the simulation program as a vital resource to the community, parent organization, customers, and learners.
3. **Internal processes:** Maximize staff efficiency and productive hours. Develop a research program.
4. **Finance:** Develop new revenue streams to support program development and sustainability.

Strategic plans that have one to two goals per dimension, or five to seven overarching goals if a dimension-based framework is not used, are the most efficient to manage.

Strategies and Tactics

Strategies support goals and summarize the actions an organization or simulation program will take to achieve a goal. They answer the question "How are we going to achieve this goal?" Strategies identify a general approach or method, but do not describe specific actions or projects. One or more strategies accompany each goal, addressing the major actions likely to have the greatest impact on achieving the goal. A strategy describes the "what"; tactics are how it will get the work done, who will do it, and when it will be completed.

Experience Goal: Increase recognition of the simulation program as a vital resource to stakeholders, customers, and learners.

- **Strategy 1:** Increase communication to leaders and participants about simulation program outcomes.
  - **Tactic 1:** Simulation Team will create a list of possible communication venues for electronic, print, and presentations by December 31, [Year].
  - **Tactic 2:** Director will create key speaking points regarding program outcomes by November 15, [Year].
- **Strategy 2:** Participate in organization improvement teams to promote opportunities for involving simulation-based education.
  - **Tactic 1:** Program Manager will create a list of organizational committees focused on patient safety and performance improvement.
  - **Tactic 2:** Director will identify and contact key stakeholders on those committees.

Because strategies may span 2 to 3 years, it is often helpful to break strategies down into mini-strategies—or objectives. Each objective is a component of the strategy and may help break down the strategy into key milestones. Well-written objectives are **SMART**, in that they are *s*pecific, *m*easurable, *a*ttainable, *r*elevant, and have a *t*ime frame for completion.

- **Strategy 3:** Collect and act on feedback from participants and customers to continuously improve course offerings.
  - **Objective 1:** Implement an automated evaluation process to eliminate manual data entry by the end of the second quarter (Q2).
    - **Tactic 1:** Simulation Team will evaluate the use of scannable evaluation forms versus online surveys for participant evaluations by the end of Q1.
    - **Tactic 2:** Simulation Team will determine the option that will best meet program needs by the beginning of Q2.
    - **Tactic 3:** Director will coordinate with Purchasing and the Information Technology departments to obtain and install the software program by the end of Q4.

- **Objective 2:** Update and improve core satisfaction questions and incorporate in all course evaluations by July [Year].
  - **Tactic 1:** Administrative Assistant will create a computerized evaluation template to be used for most courses by January [Year].

The goals, strategies, objectives, and tactics may be written narratively, or placed in a table.

Experience Goal: Increase recognition of the simulation program as a vital resource to stakeholders, customers, and learners (Table 5.3.1). Table 5.3.1 illustrates how strategies, objectives and tactics can be formatted into a table.

Measuring Success

So how will you know if you are accomplishing what you hope to accomplish through your strategic plan? Tracking completion of the tactics or activities outlined in your objectives is one way. **Measures** are used to evaluate the progress toward accomplishing a goal. A measure is a description of what you want to achieve and how the organization, or simulation program, is performing relative to achieving that particular goal. At least one measure of success should be developed for each goal that assists in monitoring progression toward the desired outcome (Olsen, 2012).

Measures can be focused on outcomes, quality, efficiency, or be project-based.

Experience Goal: Increase recognition of the simulation program as a vital resource to customers and learners.

- **Measure of Success 1:** Participant satisfaction consistently averages above 85%.
- **Measure of Success 2:** The percentage of simulation activities supporting organization-wide initiatives increases by 10% in year 1, 15% in year 2, and 25% in year 3.

The first measure listed has a quality focus, whereas the second measure is looking more at outcomes.

Determining what to measure can be difficult. Olsen (2012) recommends starting with what is obvious and the easiest to collect. As the plan evolves, measures can be adjusted and refined to ensure that they are meaningful. Gathering data for these measures on a monthly, quarterly,

TABLE 5.3.1			
Strategies and Tactics			
Strategy 3:	Collect and act on feedback from participants and customers to continuously improve course offerings.		
	Objective 1: Implement an automated evaluation process to eliminate manual data entry.	Who	Date
	Tactic 1: Evaluate the use of scannable evaluation forms versus online surveys for participant evaluations.	Simulation team	Q1

BOX 5.3.1

2010 HEALTHPARTNERS INSTITUTE FOR MEDICAL EDUCATION MISSION, VISION, AND GOALS

MISSION

To improve health by maximizing the abilities of people and systems to provide outstanding care.

VISION

To be an essential partner in continually improving the health of our patients and communities.

GOALS

1. Improve patient care and the health of our community (Health Dimension).
2. Support a culture of continuous learning, engagement, and excellence (People Dimension).
3. Become an essential organizational resource for improving care in clinical systems (Experience Dimension).
4. Position IME for success (Stewardship Dimension).

---

or semiannual basis, and reporting it back to the stakeholders who helped develop the plan, will help ensure that you are moving toward your vision in a meaningful, reliable manner.

Implementation

After the plan has been approved by the board of directors, executive director, or other authorized individual, it needs to be implemented. This often includes developing tactics—or determining actions needed to achieve an objective, assigning individuals, and developing a timeline. Sometimes this level of detail occurs when the goals and strategies are developed. Sometimes it occurs both during goal development as well as throughout implementation. Part of implementation also includes ensuring that any required purchases or funding needs are addressed and included in the budget for the upcoming year. After the plan is implemented, there may be organizational changes or newly recognized internal or external factors. A simulation program may need to revise its tactics, strategies, and even goals on the basis of newly identified factors.

The next sections provide two different approaches for developing a strategic plan for a simulation program. One approach, discussed in the *Novice* section, is to incorporate simulation-specific strategies, objectives, and tactics into the existing strategic plan from a parent organization or department (i.e., health system, staff development department, college of nursing, or medical school). The second, more advanced approach is to create a strategic plan including mission and vision statements that are specific to the simulation program.

HOW TO . . . FOR NOVICES

If you are developing a strategic plan for the first time, the most straightforward way to begin is to use your organization or department's strategic plan as your foundation. Your parent organization will likely have a mission, vision, and a number of strategic goals that the organization has created (Box 5.3.1). Using this method, the simulation program would identify key strategies that focus on these four goals and help move the organization closer to achieving its vision. Including simulation-specific strategies will demonstrate the value the simulation program brings to the organization. While it is not as complicated or time-consuming as creating a program-specific mission, vision, and plan, there are similar steps that should be completed: get organized, analyze the current situation, set direction, refine and approve the plan, and implement the plan (Figure 5.3.2).

Steps in the Planning Process

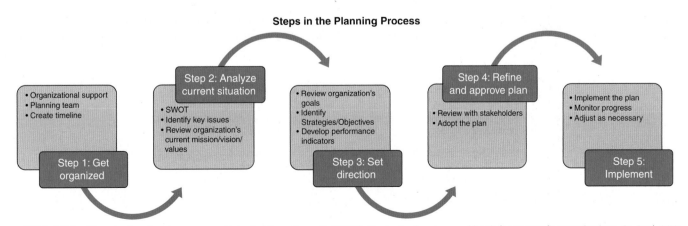

FIGURE 5.3.2 Steps in the planning process. (Adapted from Barry, B. [2007]. *Strategic planning workbook for nonprofit organizations*. St. Paul, MN: Fieldstone Alliance. [Original work published 1997], Planning Steps.)

BOX 5.3.2

QUESTIONS FOR PERFORMING A STATUS REVIEW

What goals did we achieve?
What lessons did we learn?
What challenges did we overcome?
What new customers did we acquire?

What programs/projects/courses were successful?
What didn't we accomplish, why?
What roadblocks do we continue to face? Why?
What have our customers/participants said about us?

Step 1: Get Organized

Although the time commitment is less than creating a program-specific plan, it is still beneficial to discuss your intent and the process that will be used with the individuals who provide oversight to the simulation program; this could be a board of directors or an individual. This is a great time to ask them what they see as the strengths and weaknesses of the simulation program, and their vision for its future, determine how involved they wish to be in the planning, and identify other individuals who should be involved.

In order to capture many perspectives, strategic planning work is done by a team or committee. Members should include simulation program leadership and staff, as well as key educators, participants/learners, or other individuals who are familiar with the program's offerings and processes.

Step 2: Analyze Current Situation

The next step is to critically examine the simulation program. This includes a summary of its history and current status. Questions to consider including in a status review are listed in Box 5.3.2.

The analysis also includes identifying positive and negative issues that could impact the program and affect the achievement of goals. A concise way to do this is by doing a SWOT analysis. **SWOT** stands for *s*trengths, *w*eaknesses, *o*pportunities, and *t*hreats, where strengths and weaknesses

	Positive	Negative
Internal	Strengths *What do you do well?* *What resources do you have?* *Could include, but not limited to:* • *People/simulation program staff & educators* • *Curriculum / program offerings* • *Equipment & technology, space* • *Budget* • *Participants/customers* • *Organization support*	Weaknesses *What are the existing problems?* *Could include, but not limited to:* • *Is there equipment that must be purchased in order to grow or continue to function?* • *Are there issues with the documentation process including maintenance and course records?* • *Are there staffing, equipment, space, or budget issues?* • *Is there organizational support for the program?*
External	Opportunities • *What opportunities are open to us?* • *What new initiatives is the parent organization focused on?* • *What trends can we take advantage of?* • *How can we turn strengths into opportunities?*	Threats • *What threats could harm us?* • *Who is our competition & what are they doing?* • *What threats do our weaknesses expose us to?*

FIGURE 5.3.3 A SWOT analysis.

are reflective of things within the simulation program, and opportunities and threats are external to the program (Figure 5.3.3).

The analysis helps illuminate the critical issues that should be addressed or included in the strategic plan. Barry (2007) recommends limiting the critical issues to a manageable number like four to eight.

Step 3: Set the Direction

With input from the planning team, examine the critical issues and any themes that were identified during Step 2. Look at the organization's strategic plan document to see how your program's strengths, needs, and critical issues relate to the organization's strategic plan. Are there staffing, equipment, process issues that need to be addressed? Identify simulation-specific strategies to the organization's goals. To use the example from HealthPartners, if we focus on the Health Dimension goal—improve patient care and the health of our community (Health Dimension)—one strategy could be to reduce complications associated with select procedures by incorporating a simulation-based procedural competency program. Because the plan spans several years, objectives can be year-specific. For example, Year 1: Implement an ultrasound-guided central line insertion competency program for emergency medicine residents by the end of Q2. Expand to internal medicine residents by the end of Q4. Year 2: Implement chest tube insertion competency program for applicable residents, physician assistants, nurse practitioners, and physicians new to the system by Q4. Our measures might be the number of complications from central line insertions and chest tube insertions.

Tactics may be identified during this part of the planning process, or may be identified during implementation. Tactics are the detailed action steps required to accomplish an objective or strategy. Because of the level of detail, some individuals find it more productive to create the tactics with the individuals who are going to be implementing the plan. Executives and boards of directors will typically not be interested or able to spend time on the specific action steps.

It is important to ensure your work is aligned with the goals identified in the organization's strategic plan. This alignment is important for current and future leadership support, funding support, and overall significance to the organization. In addition to creating simulation-specific strategies for the organization's goals, can simulation-based learning support any of the organization's strategies or objectives in the strategic plan? Part of the planning is to identify any enhancements or changes needed within the simulation program to support current and new strategies and objectives. Remember to focus on critical issues rather than wasting efforts on things that will not move your program toward meeting the identified goals.

Step 4: Refine and Approve the Plan

It would be beneficial to ask key leaders, stakeholders, and team members to review the draft to ensure that their input has been captured and that the strategies and measures identified are appropriate. This would also be the time to have preliminary discussions regarding resources needed to carry out the plan. After any revisions are made, the plan is reviewed with the board of directors, executive director, dean, or the individual responsible to approve budget, funding, and programmatic changes.

Step 5: Implement

If tactics, timelines, and responsible individuals were not identified in the initial planning, they must be provided in detail in the implementation phase. There may have been preliminary tactics identified, but during implementation the details come out. Tactics may be revised, deleted, and added as the plan is implemented. To maintain focus, simulation leadership and team members should review the plan on a regular basis. Progress can be monitored on a monthly, or at least quarterly, basis, and the results reported to the appropriate program champions. It may also be valuable to review the measures of success already identified by your organization for any new measures of success resulting from the contributions of simulation-based education.

As you review your plan, you might find that it is too general to really meet your needs. If this is the case, you can create a simulation-specific one. This is described in the next section.

BEEN THERE, DONE THAT: DEVELOPING A PROGRAM-SPECIFIC STRATEGIC PLAN

In the previous section, we outlined a basic set of steps that could be taken to develop a plan for a simulation program that is new to strategic planning. In this section, we add some depth to those steps for programs ready to create a more robust plan designed specifically for the simulation program. Developing such a plan, while maintaining alignment with the parent organization's mission, vision, and strategic plan, will add the greatest value for the simulation program.

Step 1: Getting Organized

As you begin developing your strategic planning process, start by ensuring that you have organizational support and buy-in from key participants. Develop a common understanding about the value the strategic plan will have for your simulation program and your goals for the process: who should be involved, how will you use the plan, with what other organizations or strategic plans should you be aligned, and so on. According to Zuckerman (2006),

> Some strategic planning efforts stray off course early on or lose momentum later because of the failure to adequately prepare the organization and its leaders for the strategic planning process. Before actually beginning strategic planning, at a minimum identify objectives, describe the planning process to be used, prepare a schedule, describe roles and responsibilities of organizational leaders, and identify the strategic planning facilitator. This information should then be communicated to affected parties clearly and consistently . . . only then should the real work begin. (2006, p. 6)

It is helpful to form a small project team, including a project leader and two or three other members, who will develop and oversee the planning process, develop documentation, draft materials for review by others, and take the next steps toward implementation. This group will be the engine driving the process forward. The project team will need to consider its own experience and capability with facilitating strategic discussions. Should you decide to work with an independent facilitator, make sure this person joins your project team and has a hand in developing the process to ensure that the outcomes of the meetings are aligned with the intent of the group.

A broader strategic planning team, representing key stakeholders, will play an important role in crafting the strategic plan. This team will provide meaningful information about the value of the simulation program, the opportunities they see, and any concerns that need to be addressed. Most importantly, as they work with you to define goals and strategies, you will be building buy-in and developing advocates for the resulting plan. "Smart process managers use participant involvement to build buy-in and consensus on whatever will result from strategic planning right from the start" (Zuckerman, 2006, p. 7). As you form this broader team, consider the following potential members:

- Leadership from your parent organization
- Funders or potential sponsors
- Customer groups
- Allies and collaborators
- Simulation team members

A final note as you are getting organized: be aware of the amount of time it will take to develop and complete your strategic planning process. It is not uncommon for the process to take 6 to 9 months, especially in complex environments with numerous stakeholders. Creating a work plan with tasks, timelines, and deliverables may help keep the process moving forward.

Step 2: Analyzing Current Situation

In the previous section, we outlined the process of conducting a SWOT analysis. This process can be enhanced by expanding your analysis to create a full **environmental scan**. An environmental scan is an examination of the current state of your program and documents the emerging issues or opportunities internal and external to your organization. A scan "helps to clearly indicate both harmful and helpful attributes, as well as external versus internal conditions affecting the decision making process" (Gantt, 2010, p. 310).

The **internal scan** should look "within" the organization for information relevant to your current focus, performance, and operations. Elements of an internal scan might include the following:

- **Customers:** Who are your current customers? How is your workload allocated among different customer types? Who will be your customers in 3 years, 5 years?
- **Outcomes:** What are you measuring? What outcomes can be documented from the past year?
- **Personnel:** What is your organizational structure? What are the roles of your team members?
- **Finances:** What are your sources of revenue? What are your annual expenses? Is your program financially stable and sustainable?
- **Current initiatives:** What are your priorities and key initiatives this year, next year?

The **external scan** should look for trends or developments outside of the program that will influence or impact how you move forward as an organization. Areas to explore may include the following:

- Developments in simulation technology
- Use of simulation-based education in your parent organization, community, and other healthcare systems
- Changes in learner needs and expectations
- Changes in healthcare in general
- Changes in training requirements for healthcare professionals
- Funding considerations
- Regulatory organization requirements

As you prepare the environmental scan for your strategic planning team, consider gathering input from stakeholders on **key issues** and summarizing it into themes. You might consider interviewing the members of the planning team individually, as well as other community members or parent organization leaders with influence related to the simulation program.

It is helpful to involve the simulation program staff and educators in this part of the process as well. As the individuals with the most daily, hands-on experience with your program, and regular interaction with your customers, they provide an invaluable perspective for shaping the program's strategic direction. They will also be instrumental in implementing the plan, and will engage in this work to a greater degree if they have a voice in developing it.

PROJECTS GALORE! SCRUMBAN: A SOLUTION TO MANAGING TOO MANY PROJECTS

Janice C. Palaganas, PhD, RN, NP
Principal Faculty, Center for Medical Simulation

Rapid growth is a concern for many simulation programs. This concern is valid because rapid growth is one of the major reasons for failures of successful businesses (Carroll & Mui, 2009; Hess, 2010; Peters & Waterman, 2006). Healthcare simulation can take many forms and meet many needs, placing a program at risk for losing its focus with too many projects competing for time, attention, and resources.

During my 5 years as a Chief Operations Officer of a Simulation Center, projects seemed to multiply every year. The projects were either developed or adopted by the team, or they were mandated or encouraged by our leadership. This led to increasingly implosive work on the department. After many minimally successful trials with different methods, for example, weekly meetings, project software, online team-based project platforms, and checklists; I continued to seek ways to manage so many projects with detailed tasks.

One day I recalled my days taking computer engineering courses and remembered a simple method my team successfully used for managing a large project that utilized multiple subprojects and tasks within the team. Computer engineers call this method "Scrum" or a "Scrum Board" (You can find many useful websites on this topic.) Of the methods I trialed, the Scrum Board seemed most effective at meeting the needs of the team while overcoming some of the problems we had encountered with other methods (e.g., some team members would forget to log in to the online platform, some items on the checklist were confusing, not everyone had the software, weekly meetings became too short, etc.). As I thought about the Scrum Board, I realized we would have to modify it for the flow of information and work in our Program. In my prior hospital management experience, I had learned the principles and practices of Lean methodology as a powerful and effective way to build and sustain continuously improving businesses and institutions. Embracing this methodology, we sought to merge a Lean-based and calendar-based framework to manage the Simulation Center's needs and goals. The final approach we adopted was called "the Sim Scrumban." Adopting the Lean methodology with Scrum Boarding is called Scrumban. Scrumban is a term used by software engineers that combines the process of "scrum" (the engineering term used for developing products in a nimble way by assigning roles in a team and task planning) and "kanban" (a Lean principle that is used for just-in-time production using methods that allow visualization of workflow).

The Sim Scrumban (Figure 1) worked. It helped us stay focused, identify barriers, move projects forward, keep the workload even without burnout, keep everyone informed, and—critical to the exploding field of simulation—say "no" to projects that were either not relevant to our mission or too overwhelming for our resources and situation.

For Sim Scrumban, we used the following:
- A large white board
- White-board or artist tape
- Small and medium post-it notes
- Post-it tabs
- Pencil, pens, and Sharpies
- Graphing paper
- Magnets
Roles in Sim Scrumban:

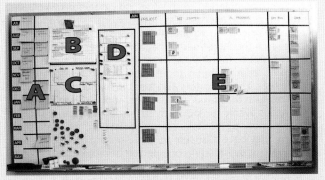

FIGURE 1 The Sim Scrumban with (**A**) The Parking Lot, (**B**) The A3, (**C**) The Burndown Chart, (**D**) The Sprint Backlog, and (**E**) The Storyboard.

- Scrum Owner—the Chief Operations Officer/Operations Director
- Scrum Master—the Project Manager
- Scrum Team—the Project Team

Key elements of the Sim Scrumban are shown in **Figure 1** and are described briefly below.

THE PARKING LOT

The Parking Lot (Figure 1A) prioritizes projects throughout the year by month. For the example shown, the team decided that, given their resources and daily activities, four total projects were feasible at a given time. Because of this, we allotted two maximum projects to be held in the parking lot per month with the knowledge that at least one project would be ongoing through multiple months and at least one project would carry over from the month prior; thus a total of four projects maximum at a given time.

THE A3

Before the implementation of a project, the project is investigated and structured into a plan that can be presented in an "A3" process format (Figure 1B). The "A3" report is a Lean technique adapted from the manufacturing field and provides a description of each project refined to a single piece of paper. The information on the A3 includes background, current conditions (needs assessment), goals, analysis performed behind the project, deliverables expected, summary of the plan and deadline, and how the project will be evaluated. The A3 provides a consistent format to outline the details of the project and keep everyone informed.

THE BURNDOWN CHART

Each project should be thoughtfully broken down into tasks. The number of tasks are tallied and projected on the Burndown Chart (Figure 1C), with a goal line to show ideal progress. The chart allows visualization of project progress by showing how many tasks have been completed over time.

THE SPRINT BACKLOG

During the planning of a project, the team agrees on the tasks that need to be completed and the order in which these tasks need to be completed. The Sprint Backlog (Figure 1D) allows visualization and order of the necessary tasks. This allows a team member to know what needs to be done before a task is started. (For our Sprint Backlog, we used Microsoft Project and printed the Gaant chart.)

THE STORYBOARD

The Storyboard (Figure 1E) is a display of the project's progress toward completion, with visual indicators for tasks, person in charge, and barriers. To monitor progress and help alleviate barriers, the Scrum Owner watches for indicators to appear in the Storyboard. The indicators also allow the Scrum Master to monitor the flow of the project and for the Scrum Team Members to flex their efforts to assist with any barriers. The indicators also assist in managing human resources such that tasks are assigned appropriately and the workload is evenly spread. Each Scrum Team Member should have a number of role tabs on the board proportionate to the time they have available to spend on projects. Role tabs, then, prevent overloading one person because that person's tabs run out during the assigning process.

In our Program, Scrum Team Members reported at weekly staff meetings. Each project report was limited to 10 minutes. The report consisted of each Scrum Team Member standing by the Storyboard and addressing three points in a rapid report:
1. What I did.
2. What I am going to do.
3. What are my obstacles, and what help do I need?
Over time, the Sim Scrumban became a source of progress and pride. Adopting this method fostered a more productive culture. Project priority, significance, processes, and progress were now understood without long, seemingly ineffective, meetings.

REFERENCES

Carroll, P. B., & Mui, C. (2009). *Billion dollar lessons: What you can learn from the most inexcusable business failures of the last 25 years*. New York, NY: Penguin Group.

Hess, E. D. (2010). *Smart growth: Building an enduring business by managing the risks of growth*. New York, NY: Columbia Business School.

Peters, T. J., & Waterman, R. H. (2006). *In search of excellence*. New York, NY: First Collins Business Essentials.

A brainstorming session with this team could be framed around the following questions:

- What are the most pressing issues facing our program today?
- What do you imagine our program will look like in 3 years?
- What partnerships will be important to achieving that vision?
- What values should guide our work as a team?

The **values** question is a different type of conversation with your team, but a powerful way to engage them in thinking about the future of your work together. Values are the core beliefs or guiding principles for how the simulation team works with its customers and with each other. Brainstorming values such as respect, integrity, excellence, teamwork, and more, and then prioritizing what is most important to the team, will help guide the work of implementing the strategic plan.

Summarizing the obtained input from key stakeholders and employees, and providing it as baseline information to the strategic planning team, will help prepare the team for productive conversations about future direction.

The final step for the project team in analyzing the current situation and preparing for the strategic planning team's work is to draft a set of **planning assumptions**. Planning assumptions are key statements that the strategic planning team will agree to as "facts" forming the basis of your discussions. On the basis of the environmental scan, and employee and stakeholder input on key issues, the planning assumptions provide a concise summary of the current status of the program and the direction in which it is pointed. Examples of planning assumptions might be:

- The simulation program is a key player in patient safety initiatives in our hospital.
- The simulation program needs to diversify its revenue streams to be sustainable.

- Simulation-based education will increasingly be relied on to fulfill student skill development and competency achievement.

These assumptions will provide a foundation for the planning team's discussions, and help them identify the focus for goals and strategies.

Step 3: Setting Direction

As you begin to develop a strategic plan with your team, keep in mind a couple of principles. First, the outcome of the process will be most effective if it is developed with a high level of engagement and consensus among the stakeholders. Without active participation, or with fractured opinions about the strategic direction, the strategic plan will have a weak foundation for implementation. Second, the process of developing a strategic plan will be iterative. It will not happen all in one retreat. It will likely happen over the course of several meetings, retreats, phone calls, or e-mails, and stretch over several months. The process will continuously take participants through a cycle of discussion, drafting, review, and fine-tuning, for each element of the plan. It may feel laborious or tedious at times, but will ensure the high level of engagement and consensus that will lead to success. The number and structure of meetings or retreats, and whether an independent facilitator is needed, will depend on the dynamics of the group.

The project team may use the following general steps to tailor a plan for the strategic planning meetings, and the work of the project team in between.

1. Develop or affirm your mission and vision statements. As stated above, because these simple but powerful statements are so critical to the organization, the need for engagement and consensus at this point in the process is fundamental. The definitions and examples provided earlier in this chapter could be provided to the strategic planning

team to initiate this conversation. Multiple discussions may be needed to arrive at a mission and vision that provide a meaningful statement of your current purpose and desired impact.

2. Develop a statement of values. Olsen (2012, LOC 2816) states, "When values and beliefs are deeply ingrained and widely shared by managers and employees, they become a way of life within the company, and they mold the company strategy." Share the values brainstormed by the simulation team, and ask the planning team to affirm what they are committed to as a simulation program.

3. Affirm the planning assumptions. Ask the planning team, "Do the proposed assumptions resonate with your understanding of our current state and desired direction?" Take the time to fine-tune them if needed.

4. On the basis of the planning assumptions and themes from discussions to date, define the goals for the next 2 to 3 years. Consider using a balanced scorecard-type framework to organize goals or ensure that you are considering all major program aspects. Make sure the goals remain broad enough that they will be applicable over multiple years. For each goal, outline the strategies that will help advance those goals, and the specific actions (objectives) that will be taken for defined periods of time. The project team can take the lead on drafting the strategies and objectives for review by the planning team. Using the examples from earlier in this chapter may be useful again. Determine how you will know whether you have achieved the goals. What are the measures of success, or performance indicators, for each goal?

Step 4: Refining and Approving the Plan

After completing the first draft of the strategic plan, Olsen (2012, LOC 6596) recommends putting the plan away for a week, and then reviewing it to determine the following:

- Does the plan connect your mission to your vision? Do all goals and strategies align with your vision and support your mission?
- Is the plan realistic? People often plan to do more than is realistic—and in a shorter time frame. Consider extending dates out farther than initially anticipated.
- Is the plan integrated? Make sure that all the elements of the plan support each other.
- Is the plan balanced? Is there balance between your dimensions or between financial, customer experience, internal processes, and others?
- Is the plan complete? Identify any holes or potential activities that are unsupported.
- Is the document clear? Will it make sense in 9 months? Consider having someone outside of the simulation program review it for clarity and consistency.

Step 5: Implementing the Plan

Completing the strategic plan will feel like a major accomplishment, but the heavy lifting comes in the implementation of the plan. As soon as the plan is completed, prepare an annual or operational plan for the upcoming year, on the basis of the strategies and objectives. As stated in the Novice section, specifying tactics for each strategy or objective, with both a due date and a person responsible, will help facilitate progress on the strategies and keep implementation on track. Determine how and when the progress and completion of the tactics in the annual plan will be monitored, identify the person responsible for coordinating these updates, and the target audience for the report. Establish the data collection needed to measure success and create a report for stakeholders that will highlight these metrics as well as progress on activities in the plan.

Despite satisfaction with the quality of their strategic plans, many healthcare organizations report a high rate of failure with implementation. Zuckerman outlines "five keys to successful implementation:

1. Communicate the plan's priorities.
2. Assign responsibilities for implementation and hold individuals accountable for progress.
3. Make sure the right people with the right skills are involved in implementation.
4. Drive the plan down into the organization so that the plan is real and meaningful to everyone.
5. Establish and use a structured progress monitoring system" (Zuckerman, 2006, p. 7).

A strategic plan will be most effective if it is reviewed regularly for relevance and alignment with the environment of the program. Even well-developed strategic plans may need to be revised after development. As objectives are completed, or new strategies emerge, it is appropriate and beneficial to update the plan.

Additionally, strategies developed for the simulation-specific plan may be able to roll up or be included in the larger organizational strategic plan. To support the program's parent organization in advancing toward its vision, you should ensure your work is aligned with the goals identified in its strategic plan. This alignment is important for current and future leadership support, funding support, and overall significance to the organization. Be sure at the end of the day you celebrate your work with the team!

SUMMARY

"Why, sometimes I've believed as many as six impossible things before breakfast."

(Carroll, 1871, chap. V)

Developing a strategic plan may seem like a lofty, impossible task. Yet with an established structure and the engagement of key planning partners, your simulation program will benefit because you are moving in the desired direction, and advancing the goals that will help achieve your program's vision. But the development is not enough. To be effective, the strategic plan should be reviewed, monitored, and updated—it is a dynamic living document, not something kept in a binder or file cabinet, but something that becomes the foundation for the simulation program's operations and success.

REFERENCES

Barry, B. (2007). *Strategic planning workbook for nonprofit organizations.* St. Paul, MN: Fieldstone Alliance. (Original work published 1997)

Bower, J., & Gilbert, C. (2007). How managers' everyday decisions create—or destroy—your company's strategy. *Harvard Business Review, 85*(2), 72–79.

Carroll, L. (1865). *Alice's adventures in wonderland* [Bookbyte digital edition for IBook]. Retrieved from BookbyteDigtal.com

Carroll, L. (1871). *Through the looking glass.* Retrieved from http://www.amazon.com/

Center for Medical Simulation. (2009). Retrieved from http://www.harvardmedsim.org/

Gantt, L. (2010). Strategic planning for skills and simulation labs in colleges of nursing. *Nursing Economics, 28*(5), 308–313.

HealthPartners Clinical Simulation. (2012). *Mission & purpose.* Retrieved from HealthPartners Clinical Simulation website: http://www.hpclinsim.com/mission–vision.html

Joyce, E., & Martinez, P. (2007). Planning and marketing for a healthy organization. In R. Patronis Jones (Ed.), *Nursing leadership and management* (pp. 223–238). Philadelphia, PA: F. A. Davis.

Kaplan, R., & Norton, D. (1996). *The balanced scorecard* [Kindle iPad version]. Retrieved from http://www.amazon.com/

Medical Education & Research Institute. (2012). *MERI overview.* Retrieved from Medical Education & Research Institute website: http://www.meri.org/about-meri/meri-overview/

Olsen, E. (2012). *Strategic planning kit for dummies.* Hoboken, NJ: John Wiley & Sons.

Person, R. (2013). *Balanced scorecards & operational dashboards with Microsoft Excel* [Kindle iPad version]. Retrieved from http://www.amazon.com/

SSH Council for Accreditation of Healthcare Simulation Programs. (2013). *Accreditation standards and measurement criteria.* Retrieved from Society for Simulation in Healthcare website: http://ssih.org/uploads/static_pages/PDFs/Accred/2013_

Zuckerman, A. (2006). Advancing the state of the art in healthcare strategic planning. *Frontiers of Health Services Management, 23*(2), 3–15.

Developing a Systematic Program Evaluation Plan

Gail Johnson, MS, RN, CCRN, CPHQ, CHSE

ABOUT THE AUTHORS

GAIL L. JOHNSON is the Director of HealthPartners Clinical Simulation, a center that has been granted accreditation by the Society for Simulation in Healthcare (SSH). She is a Reviewer for SSH's accreditation program and a member of the Accreditation Council and Certification Committee. Ms. Johnson is nationally certified as a Certified Professional in Healthcare Quality and Certified Healthcare Simulation Educator. She has a BSN, MS in Instructional and Performance Technology and is completing her PhD in Nursing, focusing on fidelity in simulation.

ABSTRACT

Many organizations are doing evaluation, but it is often limited to participant satisfaction. Expanding this to more of a systematic evaluation that includes program processes and outcomes, in tandem with the program's strategic plan, provides rich and valuable information to the program. This chapter provides an overview of some of the considerations and options when developing an evaluation plan.

CASE EXAMPLE

The leadership team at Xanadu Simulation Center, a 10,000 square feet (929 m²) facility within an academic teaching hospital, recently created a strategic plan. In addition to Simulation Center–specific goals and strategies, other strategies were created, aligning Center activities to strategic goals and initiatives of the parent organization.

Parent Organization Goal
Xanadu Medical Center's Experience goal: *Create exceptional and affordable experiences for the patients and families in our care.* Xanadu Medical Center uses patient satisfaction survey data as a measure of success. Response to one of the postdischarge survey questions, "I received education on my medications and their side effects," was lower than desired, and this became a focus for the organization.

Xanadu Simulation Center
As an alignment initiative, the Simulation Center set the following strategy: Include medication education as a critical action in at least 75% of simulation scenarios within the next 6 months. In order to evaluate this strategy, the simulation team established the following measures:

- Percentage of scenarios incorporating medication education (number of scenarios with medication education ÷ the number of scenarios).
- Rate of medication education provided by participant (number of times medication education was provided during a simulation ÷ the number of opportunities × 100).
- Organization's patient survey data regarding medication education.

A dashboard was created to monitor the percentage and rate, and this was shared with simulation staff and faculty. During monthly simulation team meetings, different aspects of the Center's evaluation plan were reviewed. This data was included in the discussion; staff were satisfied with the metrics selected. Initially, there was no medication education provided during simulations. However, over 6 months, both healthcare professionals and students started to include it as part of their discussion with the *patient* and/or *family member* during scenarios. At 6 and 12 months, a report was created for the Simulation Center's governing body and hospital leadership containing this data as well as other measures established by the program, which showed significant improvement in the identified areas. How do you think they responded?

SECTION 5 • Management

INTRODUCTION

> One of the great mistakes is to judge policies and programs by their intentions rather than their results.
>
> *Friedman, 1975*

Defining evaluation may seem like the story about the blind men and the elephant. In this Indian fable, a number of blind men are asked to describe an elephant. One felt the side and thought the elephant was like a wall, another felt the leg and thought the elephant was like a tree, yet the third felt the tail and was certain that the elephant was a rope (Saxe, 1878, p. 150). They were each correct, yet their individual interpretations did not portray the entire picture. Similarly, evaluation means different things to different people. For some, evaluation is a way to test learners' knowledge at the end of a course, for others it is a survey given to participants after a simulation, and yet others view evaluation as a way to determine the quality of a program or associated with strategic planning. Like the elephant, though, each of these conducted individually is only one aspect of evaluation. A systematic evaluation should encompass all of these and more.

There are numerous definitions of evaluation in the literature. One often cited is by Michael Scriven, a pioneer in evaluation methods and leader in evaluation theory: "Evaluation determines the merit, worth, or value of things" (Scriven, 2010, p. i). Preskill and Jones (2009, p. 7) offer "Evaluation is all about asking and answering questions that matter—about programs, processes, products, policies, and initiatives." One of the most comprehensive definitions is by Russ-Eft and Preskill (2001, p. xvii):

> Evaluation can be viewed as a catalyst and opportunity for learning—learning what works and doesn't work, learning about ourselves and the organization, and learning about how to improve what we do in the workplace. As such, it can provide new understandings and insights into our programs, processes, products, and systems. Furthermore, evaluation can provide us with the confidence with which to make decisions and take actions that ultimately help employees and organizations succeed in meeting their goals.

There are commonalities to the definitions. Evaluation is a systematic process that is purposeful and planned. It is a process that seeks to expand knowledge so informed decisions can be made about programs, processes, departments, or organizations. Through evaluation, we can gain a greater understanding of what we do and how actions impact the simulation program, parent organization, and the larger healthcare and academic communities.

THE EVALUATION PLAN

Why Create One?

Evaluating an organization's simulation program allows leadership, staff, and stakeholders to determine the success of a program and to identify potential areas for improvement.

Creating an evaluation plan provides focus and direction for implementation as well as a mechanism for reporting results. Evaluation is one component of quality management and the quality improvement process. Having a process for the evaluation of a quality improvement plan is also a requirement to meet the Society for Simulation in Healthcare's (SSH) accreditation standards. To meet the standards, a program must have a "policy for quality improvement processes and a plan for a systematic quality improvement/ performance improvement process that is not limited to assessment of learner outcomes and achievement and course evaluation by course participants" (SSH Council for Accreditation of Healthcare Simulation Programs, 2013). Evaluation plans can include measures from a strategic plan as well as operational measures that reflect day-to-day processes and activities (Addison, 2009; Jeffries & Battin, 2012; Rummler & Brache, 2013). A systematic evaluation plan includes both.

Evaluation Models

There are a number of evaluation models discussed in the literature (Parry, 2000; Russ-Eft & Preskill, 2001; Worthen, Sanders, & Fitzpatrick, 1997). Formative and summative evaluations are the focus of learner evaluation, and are discussed in another chapter (see chapter 7.3). Three different models of more global evaluation utilizing a systems perspective are presented. The first, by Kirkpatrick, focuses on learners/participants. The second, by Phillips, focuses on return on investment, and the third by Rummler, looks more at the processes, jobs, structures, and outcomes of the simulation program.

Kirkpatrick's Four-Level Evaluation Model

In 1959, Donald Kirkpatrick asserted that participants and educational programs could be evaluated at four different levels: reaction, learning, behavior, and results (Parry, 2000; Russ-Eft & Preskill, 2001; Figure 5.4.1). The first level, *Reaction*, looks at participants' reaction to the activity. Did they like it? Was the facilitator effective? Was the room comfortable? Was the content relevant? Many simulation programs already obtain this type of data by asking participants to complete a post-simulation evaluation. Level 1 evaluation data is easy to obtain and analyze. Data collection and analysis becomes more complex and costly when progressing to higher levels.

Level 2 looks at what participants learned or whether their knowledge about the topic changed as a result of the simulation activity or educational program. Learning can be assessed through pretests/posttests, direct observation, and self-assessment. However, just because a participant increased their knowledge does not guarantee that they will apply what they have learned.

Level 3 addresses changes in participants' behavior and whether they have implemented or applied what was learned during the simulation activity into their practice. Level 4 represents the impact on the organization

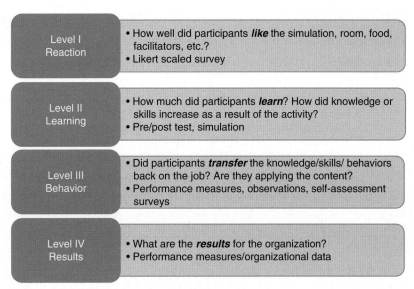

FIGURE 5.4.1 Participants and educational programs can be evaluated at four different levels: reaction, learning, behavior, and results.

(i.e., decreased infection rates, increased enrollments, increased exam score). Level 3 and 4 data can be very powerful but require more resources and are more difficult to accomplish. Because of this, it is important to be strategic when determining what will be evaluated at these levels.

For example, at the fictitious Xanadu University's College of Nursing, nursing students complete two medical-surgical clinical rotations: one at the beginning of their junior year and one during their senior year. Clinical faculty for the second rotation noted significant knowledge/skill degradation issues, and student evaluations included comments about not feeling prepared and requiring time to "relearn" things from their first clinical experience. Xanadu Simulation Center worked with the College of Nursing faculty to implement an 8-hour simulation day prior to the second medical-surgical clinical experience. Kirkpatrick's four-level evaluation process was utilized to develop the evaluation strategy.

- Level 1: Students completed a Likert-scale–based evaluation of the simulation experience and facilitator effectiveness.
- Level 2: Students completed a pre-simulation/post-simulation test designed to assess knowledge of the topics and objectives of the simulations.
- Level 3: Clinical educators observed students during their clinical rotation to ensure they had applied content from the simulation experience. Nurse preceptors completed a brief survey regarding their observations of the students.
- Level 4: Because of the staff and financial resources required to develop and implement this level of evaluation, the decision was made by executive leadership not to complete a Level 4 evaluation for this project.

Since Kirkpatrick's original work over 50 years ago, a number of other models have developed. As a result of an increasing need for education programs to demonstrate

value to an organization's financial bottom line, Jack Phillips modified Kirkpatrick's model to include an additional level, *Return on Investment* (ROI) (Phillips & Phillips, 2008a).

Phillips' Return on Investment

Phillips added a fifth level to Kirkpatrick's original work, emphasizing the importance of measuring the return on investment to the parent organization for implementing an educational activity (Phillips & Phillips, 2008a). As healthcare and education funding is reduced, many organizations need to reduce spending, resulting in greater competition between departments for their piece of the financial pie. Simulation programs may be asked to justify the value added to the parent organization for implementation or continuation of a simulation activity. This level of evaluation answers the question "does the program benefit exceed program cost?" For example, last year Xanadu Simulation Center was asked to design and implement a central line insertion competency program for all providers who insert central lines. The Plan-Do-Check-Act (PDCA) methodology was used. The content was developed along with a process to implement the competency program in one facility at a time (plan). Next, the program was rolled out for physicians and midlevel providers from one hospital (do). The program and implementation process were evaluated (check) and on the basis of the data analysis, a decision was made to roll it out to the entire five-hospital system (act). The director of the Simulation Center worked with leaders in other departments to obtain and quantify data. The Procedure Cost measures were obtained before and after implementation (Table 5.4.1).

Data reported would include the cost saved as a result of the intervention plus the ROI to the organization. In Phillips' process, attempts are made to assign a monetary value to all data. There are times when it may not be possible, and in these instances, the data can be listed as

TABLE 5.4.1

Procedure Cost Measures Obtained Before and After Implementation

Actual Procedure		Simulation Experience	
	Cost		Cost
• Number of kits/guidewires used for each procedure • Length of time on task • Number of sticks • Complications requiring additional procedures or increased length of stay • Infection rate	• Cost of each kit used • Provider salary × minutes on task • Dollar amount for increased stay, medications, or procedures related to complication of placement or infection	• Central line trainer and replacement inserts • Central line insertion kits and supplies • Faculty time (development and facilitation) • Participant time	• Cost of trainer and inserts • Cost of each kit × kits used • Faculty salary × time • Participant salary × time

On the basis of this information and the simulation expense, the return on investment was calculated using the following formula.

Return on Investment Formula

$$\text{ROI (\%)} = \frac{\text{Net program benefits [(Procedure costs before} - \text{Procedure costs after)} - \text{Program costs]}}{\text{Program costs (simulation expenses)}} \times 100$$

intangible benefits. In the central line example, reducing the number of insertion attempts (sticks) may impact patient satisfaction. Improved patient satisfaction might be an intangible benefit. Because this level of evaluation can be costly to implement in terms of time and resources, it is usually reserved for select programs or types of activities. Activities selected for ROI evaluation may be those that are "expensive, high-profile, offered to a large audience, linked to business objectives and strategy, or of interest to executive leadership" (Phillips & Phillips, 2008b, p. 8).

Organization and Processes

Many simulation programs collect participant evaluations; some may have a process for evaluating the effectiveness of the facilitator. Evaluating the participants' experience and simulation activity effectiveness is important, but like the elephant analogy, it is only one piece of the evaluation process. In a comprehensive systematic evaluation, multiple aspects of the simulation program are monitored and reviewed, analyzed, reported, and, if necessary, improved. A program is a "complex system of individuals, jobs, processes, functions, and management" (Rummler, 2004, p. 16). It may also be part of a larger health system or academic institution.

To obtain a complete picture, it is important to evaluate the simulation program outcomes and the processes and structures/functions within it (Lloyd, 2008; Rummler, 2004; Russ-Eft & Preskill, 2001). One way to do this is by evaluating aspects of the system from inputs through outputs. Rummler created the Anatomy of Performance (AOP) to illustrate the different aspects and how they work together (Figure 5.4.2).

As a complex system, many things can impact the simulation program, its functions and processes and outputs. In Figure 5.4.2, the simulation program is within the box with the heavy border. Inputs including funding, staffing, the type of simulation equipment and other technologies available, and how the program obtains supplies impact the program. It may also be impacted by environmental influences that are external to the simulation program. For example,

changes in legislation and the economy may impact medical education funding. This in turn could affect simulation programs via funding as well as potential participants. There may be a need to evaluate these inputs and identify opportunities for improvement or to capitalize on strengths. Simulation programs have two types of outputs: (1) a desired product or service, in this case creating/facilitating simulation-based activities, for customers (participants and faculty) and (2) a value-added perception by stakeholders. This could be through improved patient safety, reduction in errors, and increased successful recruitment, for example. The two are related—if participant needs are not met and course participants do not find value in the simulation experiences, stakeholders will be impacted.

In this model, there are four levels within the simulation program: the organizational level, the function level, the process level, and the job/performer level. The organizational level includes strategic planning and the relationship between the simulation program and its customers and shareholders (including the parent organization). Simulation programs also have specific functions. Xanadu Simulation Center decided that the functions are the different types of programs it provides. For example, one function is to facilitate simulations for nursing students, another is to provide procedure practice and competency assessment for medical students and residents. A third function is nursing orientation, with a fourth focusing on nursing staff development. Another function is its mobile/in situ program. Within these functions, there are specific job responsibilities, types of learners, facilitators, and equipment. Yet there are also processes that are common to all functions. Processes could include participant registration, simulation staff orientation, restocking, mannequin maintenance, and data entry. The program may choose to evaluate common aspects across all functions (process level), or aspects about one specific course, including faculty that facilitate that course (function and job levels). When a simulation program is evaluated as a multilevel system, there are opportunities to look at aspects like processes that can positively or negatively impact the outputs.

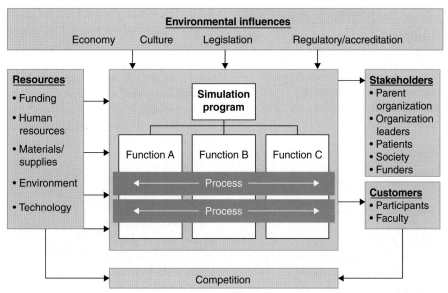

FIGURE 5.4.2 Anatomy of performance. (From Rummler, G. [2004]. *Serious performance consulting* [p. 22]. Silver Spring, MD: International Society for Performance Improvement.)

Although they vary in their approach, these models provide examples of different levels of evaluation and include an organizational impact perspective.

DEVELOPING AN EVALUATION PLAN

It is helpful for simulation programs to have a written plan that explains the evaluation process and strategy (Jeffries & Battin, 2012; Ranson, Soshi, Nash, & Ransom, 2008). Development of a successful evaluation and improvement plan is a systematic process, focusing on all areas of the simulation program. There are a number of components or steps that should be included in the written plan (Lloyd, 2008).

Develop a Measurement Philosophy

The first step is to create a purpose statement and evaluation philosophy. It may be helpful to consider the following questions: Why gather and analyze data? What are the objectives? Is it because you have been told that it is an organizational mandate or because you want to see how your program is functioning and look at ways to improve, or a combination of both? Will you be gathering data periodically for board meetings, or is analysis part of your day-to-day processes, or both? Is there some information that is used to guide and improve the simulation program operationally, and some that is part of a report, dashboard, or scorecard shared with a board of directors or executive leadership?

Accountability (Structure, Roles/Responsibilities)

Who will be accountable for writing, updating, and approving the evaluation plan?

Time Frame

A time frame for the evaluation plan should be established. This time frame includes how long the written plan is in effect as well as frequency of data gathering and reporting. Different data may be reported at different intervals. Strategic plan data may be gathered and reported quarterly, while data that is evaluated for program efficiency may be monitored more frequently.

Identify the Categories to Be Measured

The second step is to determine the categories or dimensions to be measured. Identifying categories helps ensure that the evaluation is comprehensive and not just focused on one area like participant feedback or test scores. Programs might choose the categories to be measured on the basis of the functions, processes, and organizational outcomes described in the previous section (Lloyd, 2008; Rummler, 2004; Russ-Eft & Preskill, 2001). Another way to determine categories is to use a balanced scorecard strategy (Person, 2013; Kaplan 1996).

Balanced Scorecard

Kaplan and Norton (1996) coined the term "Balanced Scorecard" to describe a monitoring and reporting strategy that looks at four dimensions or perspectives of an organization. The four categories in the balanced scorecard include customer, learning and growth, financial, and internal business process perspective. Table 5.4.2 provides examples of measures that Xanadu Simulation Center might use in their balanced scorecard.

Xanadu Simulation Center was considering implementing a comprehensive evaluation strategy. They decided to use Balanced Scorecard categories as the framework. Because it was overwhelming to think about gathering data on

TABLE 5.4.2

TABLE 5.4.2

Balanced Scorecard Example

Category	Measure
Customer	Participant satisfaction (Kirkpatrick Level 1)
Customer	Number of participants (learners)
Customer	Learning/behavior (Kirkpatrick Level 2 and/or 3)
Learning and growth (Sim Team focus)	Faculty effectiveness
Learning and growth (Sim Team focus)	Percent CHSE
Learning and growth (Sim Team focus)	Staff productivity (facilitation hours/total avail hours)
Financial	Cost per simulation activity (supplies and staff time)
Financial	Revenue growth/mix
Financial	Cost reduction/savings by reusing kits/supplies
Internal business process	Percent of interprofessional courses
Internal business process	Effectiveness of registration process
Internal business process	Equipment (mannequins, AV system) malfunction

all of the simulation activities, they decided to start small and use a PDCA cycle (see chapter 1.5). Staff chose one course to evaluate. According to the Likert-scale course evaluation data, participants ranked the course very high (5/5), and narrative comments were positive. Understandably, the simulation team was very excited. However, after reviewing financial and demographic data, the simulation staff realized that the cost for this course was very high owing to the resources required for implementation. Because of the complexity, multiple staff members were needed to facilitate and many supplies used. Although the course was well liked by participants, registration numbers remained low. Participation was lower for this course than all other simulation courses, and there had been limited growth in the number of participants in the past 2 years. For sustainability, changes needed to occur.

If only one dimension or category, such as customer satisfaction, had been evaluated, the program might not be aware of the financial or process issues. As a result, to continue offering the course would result in potential financial/budget issues, or utilizing a large number of resources for a small number of participants. Similarly, a program could focus solely on financial data and ignore participant satisfaction and impact on practice/patient care. Simulation programs are businesses, and attention must be given to the cost of implementing courses. However, it is detrimental to focus only on cost at the expense of course quality, participant satisfaction, and program efficiency.

Strategic Plan

Finally, if a strategic plan is in place, categories/dimensions may already be identified. At Xanadu Health System, the organization has four dimensions: people, experience, stewardship, and health. The Simulation Center has incorporated these dimensions into their strategic

plan. These categories are very similar to those identified in the balanced scorecard. A simulation program could choose to use the parent company's strategic plan, the simulation program's strategic plan, the balanced scorecard categories, or a combination. Xanadu Simulation Center included categories from the balanced scorecard with the dimensions from their parent company's strategic plan. Additional information on how to develop a successful strategic plan can be found in chapter 5.3.

Choosing What to Measure—Select Specific Measures

Once the categories are determined, the next step is to look at specific measures. It is important to choose measures that will impact the program, or provide information that could impact key processes and outcomes (Parry, 2000; Ranson et al., 2008). Typically one to three measures may be identified for each category. One of Xanadu Simulation Center's categories is "stewardship." Stewardship is a concept and too vague to measure directly. Instead, the program determines the aspects of stewardship that it wants to measure. To do this, Lloyd (2008) recommends that programs ask the following questions: What *aspect* of stewardship do we want to measure? What *specific measures* could we track? What *specific indicator* will we select? In this instance, the program chose to measure the percentage of revenue received from external programs. Several measures are provided in the Balanced Scorecard example (Table 5.4.2).

Prioritization Grid

There may be many things that a program wants to evaluate, monitor, or find out for purposes of improvement. Because evaluation and improvement projects do require additional resources, a program may need to limit what they can focus on and determine what to do first. One way to determine where to start is with a *Prioritization Grid*. This is a tool that many healthcare organizations use for patient care–related performance improvement (PI) processes, and is adaptable to the simulation environment as well. The team identifies potential things to evaluate or PI projects. Then, each potential improvement is analyzed and assigned points on the basis of criteria. An example of a grid and criteria is shown in Figure 5.4.3. Criteria may be customized to reflect what is important for a specific program as they make decisions.

For example, as part of its Evaluation Plan, Xanadu Simulation Center will implement two PI activities each year. For the first project, staff are deciding between their scheduling process and how they manage their video recordings. They have decided to utilize the Performance Improvement Prioritization grid to try to help them decide which one to complete first. Each staff member or evaluation team member completes a grid, assigning a score for every criterion. The total scores from team members are averaged together. The project with the highest score has first priority. For a balanced perspective, it is important to

Issue to evaluate_____

Date_____

Criterion	3 points	2 points	1 point	0 points	Score
Strategic plan	Strong relationship	Moderate relationship	Minimal relationship	No relationship	
Regulatory compliance	Required	N/A	N/A	Not required	
Patient outcome	Important improvement in patient care	Some improvement in patient care	Little improvement in patient care	No improvement in patient care	
Important to mission/vision	Very important	Important	Slightly important	Not at all important	
Problem prone	Process problems noted with high risk to success of program or staff	Process problems noted with moderate risk to success of program/staff	Process problems noted with low risk to success of program or staff	Process problems noted with no risk to success of program or staff	
High volume	Affects 100% of programs or participants	Affects 75–50% of programs or participants	Affects 50–25% of programs or participants	Affects 25–0% of programs or participants	
Productivity	Reduction of >10% work time (increased efficiency by >10%)	Reduction of <10% work time (increased efficiency by <10%)	No impact	Increase in staff/work time or decrease in efficiency	
Financial cost	No cost to implement	One time <5% cost to implement	One time 5–10% cost to implement	Ongoing cost to implement	
Financial savings	At least 10% financial savings by implementing	5–9% financial savings by implementing	<5% financial savings by implementing	No financial savings by implementing	
Customer/learner needs and expectations	Problem in this area as indicated by evaluation & complaints	Possible highly positive effect on satisfaction	Possible moderate effect on satisfaction	Minimal or no effect on satisfaction	
Total score					

FIGURE 5.4.3 Performance improvement prioritization grid. (Used with permission, HealthPartners Clinical Simulation.)

get scores from multiple people on the team. To ensure everyone is aware of all issues, someone who is knowledgeable about the potential project should present it to the team and facilitate a discussion of relevant issues prior to scoring.

Low-Hanging Fruit

Data collection and analysis can be resource-intensive in terms of time and money. However, there may be things that are easy to measure or improve and will use few resources to collect and analyze. Participant evaluations could be seen as a low-hanging fruit, especially if there is already a mechanism in place for distributing, collecting, and evaluating the data. Collecting Kirkpatrick's Level 1

evaluations (participant satisfaction data) after every simulation session or program can provide valuable data for the program. A program may have a goal that *85% of participant evaluations will average at least 4 on a 1 to 5 scale.* If participant evaluations from one simulation activity is below a 4, that could be a flag for further analysis.

Organization Initiatives

It is always beneficial to link simulation program activities to key initiatives of the parent organization. This reinforces the value-added contributions of the simulation program and may impact funding decisions. One way to do this is to include an organizational initiative as a specific measure.

TABLE 5.4.3

Xanadu Simulation Center Quality Indicators

Indicator Type/Dimension	No.	Definition	Desired Direction	Target
Stewardship	1	Revenue: % of revenue stream from external participants/groups	↑	35%
Experience	2	Participant satisfaction: % of participants that rate the value of the course/activity at least 8/10	↑	90%
Experience	3	Facilitator effectiveness: % returned DASH tools scoring ≥6	↑	80%
Experience	4	Evaluations returned: % of online evaluations completed	↑	80%
Health	5	Time to first shock: % shocks delivered in <2 minutes from in situ mock codes	↑	90%
Health	6	Impact: narrative account of how simulation experience impacted patient care/systems improvement	NA	NA
Business process	7	Manual data entry: hours per month spent manually entering evaluation data and participant data	↓	4

Regulatory and Accreditation Requirements

To meet a regulatory agency standard, Xanadu Medical Center leadership asked the simulation program to implement a simulated code and rapid response team process. Simulation staff collected data on staff performance during these simulated events. Over time, the time to recognition of event, time to correct action, and correct actions performed improved. Because of the importance to the organization, this was included as part of the simulation program's evaluation plan. Like organizational initiatives, when a simulation program collects data that shows how a regulatory or accreditation requirement is met, it is valuable to the parent organization.

Develop Operational Definitions for Each Measure

Creating definitions of what is measured, or performance indicators, provides clarity and consistency. This way, the data collection will be consistent regardless of who is collecting. An operational definition "is a description, in quantifiable terms, of what to measure and the specific steps needed to measure it consistently" (Lloyd, 2008, p. 92). It is helpful to put the indicators into a table rather than a narrative format. In addition to the definition, a target or goal should be identified. Some targets may be determined by a parent organization, by benchmarking data in the literature, or simply by reviewing prior data and determining the desired goal. Not all data needs to be quantitative.

A simulation program may wish to include key narrative statements from participants or stakeholders documenting the effect of the program and its activities on key organizational initiatives, like patient safety (Table 5.4.3).

Create a Data Collection Plan and Gather the Data

Following the identification and definition of indicators, the next step is to determine a data collection plan and then collect the data. Like the definitions, the data collection plan should be included in the overall written evaluation plan. Presenting the collection plan in a table format makes it easy to organize and review. The collection plan includes what is being measured, where the data is located, how it will be collected, and who will obtain it.

Data can be collected from multiple sources, including surveys, course records (i.e., course evaluations, performance checklists), databases, observation, individual interviews, and focus groups. The collection method should be determined on the basis of the evaluation questions. Sometimes, more than one collection method may be beneficial. Participant evaluation forms may provide preliminary information about how they value a simulation activity. This could be followed by interviews with a small randomized sample of participants to provide more detailed information about how the content from the simulation activity has been used in a clinical setting (Table 5.4.4).

TABLE 5.4.4

Xanadu Simulation Center Data Collection Plan

Indicator Type	Quality Indicator	Data Source	Collection Method	Collector
Stewardship	Revenue	Lawson report	Quarterly	Director
Experience	Participant satisfaction	Course/activity evaluations	Participants complete evaluations for at least 90% of activities (100% or CNE/CME activities)	Educator
Experience	Facilitator effectiveness	DASH tool	Twice per year for all facilitators	Director
Experience	Evaluations returned	Learning Management System (database)	Monthly	Director
Health	Time to first shock	Mock Code database	Quarterly	Educator

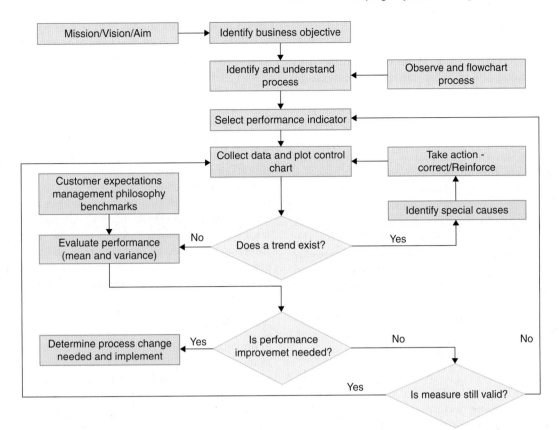

FIGURE 5.4.4 Flow of analysis. (From Jordan, G., Prevette, S., & Woodward, S. [2001]. Analyzing, reviewing, and reporting performance data. In Training Resources & Data Exchange Performance-Based Management Special Interest Group [Eds.], *The performance-based management handbook* [Vol. 5, pp. 1–76]. OakRidge, TN: Oak Ridge Institute for Science and Education.)

Analyze the Data

The collected data needs to be analyzed in order to be meaningful. Initially, the data that is collected is simply a bunch of meaningless numbers. The purpose of data analysis and review is to convert raw data into meaningful information that will increase knowledge about a program's performance. Jordan et al. (2001) recommend asking some initial questions during this phase (Figure 5.4.4):

• How does actual performance compare with a goal or standard?
• Is there a significant variance? If so, is corrective action necessary?
• Are new goals or measures necessary?
• How have existing conditions changed?

Data is often analyzed and presented in aggregate. While aggregate is important to look at trends, specific situational details that could be valuable for PI may get lost. It may be helpful to review and report trends as well as specifics.

Tools

Analysis tools can be divided into two categories (Jordan et al., 2001): tools that analyze measurement data and tools that identify root causes and design improvements. Many of these have already been described in chapter 1.5 (Table 5.4.5).

There are a number of computer programs that can assist with data analysis and reporting. Microsoft Excel is a common program and often available on personal and business computers. In addition to the basic functions (i.e., average, sum, count, standard deviation), a free add-in, the Analysis ToolPak, provides additional commands that include more advanced tools for statistical analysis such as histograms, regression, ANOVA, *t*-tests, correlation, and covariance (Person, 2013).

TABLE 5.4.5

Analysis Tools Can Be Divided into Two Categories

To Analyze the Measurement Data	To Identify Root Causes and Design Improvements
• Run chart	• Affinity diagram
• Statistical analysis	• Brainstorming
• Control chart/statistical process control	• Cause and effect/fishbone diagram
• Matrices, contingency tables	• Failure mode and effect analysis
• Flowcharts	• Histogram
• Decision trees, historical timelines	• Pareto analysis
• Scatter plots of relationships between variables	• Storyboarding
	• Gap analysis

From Jordan, G., Prevette, S., & Woodward, S. (2001). Analyzing, reviewing, and reporting performance data. In Training Resources & Data Exchange Performance-Based Management Special Interest Group (Eds.), *The performance-based management handbook* (Vol. 5, pp. 1–76). Oakridge, TN: Oak Ridge Institute for Science and Education.

REPORTING DATA

Finally, the analyzed data needs to be communicated to the team and stakeholders. This can be done verbally, in a narrative format, with tables and graphs, or in some combination. Tables and graphs can be the easiest ways to convey complex information (Russ-Eft & Preskill, 2001). Programs may choose to use a combination of reporting styles, depending on the data that is reported and the receiving audience. Information presented to a governing board may have less detail than a report shared with the simulation team. Governing boards may appreciate a one-page "big picture" executive summary overview that focuses on the strategic plan and outcomes. However, the simulation team and others involved in more day-to-day work may benefit from detailed reports. Dashboards and scorecards are reporting tools that track progress and past performance. Although often used interchangeably in practice, the two have different meanings and purposes (Pugh, 2008).

Dashboards

Dashboards, according to Pugh (2008, p. 218), "are tools that report on the ongoing performance of the critical processes that lead to organizational success rather than on the success itself." An organization's dashboard can be compared to the information provided on the dashboard of a car or in the cockpit of an airplane. Both provide important information to the driver or pilot about things that will impact their ability to achieve the desired outcome (i.e., arriving at their specific destination). A driver may monitor gauges on the car dashboard to monitor the data (fuel level, miles per gallon, speed, tire pressure) at moments in time during a trip, and performance in these areas can impact the outcome (arrival at destination). However, the gauges do not indicate whether the driver arrived on time or at all.

Dashboard data is presented in a variety of ways. Typically, they include graphs and tables presented in a manner that can be easily understood. An example of one item on a dashboard is listed below. Red, yellow, and green colors are commonly understood in the United States even without the code provided. The code provides specifics, that is,

green color equals shocks that occurred in less than 120 seconds. Still, without knowing the exact number, viewers of this table know that the ICU performed well in Q3. Using this type of visual also provides an opportunity for the simulation program to collaborate with organizational colleagues to explore why other units are not progressing or performing as expected. An initial assumption may be that the poor performance is a knowledge deficit issue. This was not correct in this particular example. During the mock codes, it was noted that mental health staff did not have a code cart/defibrillator readily available—running to obtain the defibrillator from another patient care area contributed to the delay. Patient care units with a defibrillator within their area had a faster time to first shock. The information collected and reported by the simulation program provided key information to the parent organization that affected patient care and safety (Table 5.4.6).

Scorecards

Scorecards, on the other hand, generally provide information on past performance or outcomes. Pugh (2008) compares a scorecard to a school report card. Report cards are issued after the work is completed and provide information about the work that was done. Usually, there is a gap in time between when the work was done and when the results are reported. Changes can be made that could affect future grades (outcomes), but the specific changes needed (processes) are not evident on the report card.

Although there are differences between scorecards and dashboards, in practical applications, they may not be clear-cut. As a result, organizations may include both process and outcomes measures in the same reporting document. The key is how a simulation program "uses the measures and measurement sets to align priorities and achieve desired organizational results" (Pugh, 2008, p. 219; Figure 5.4.5).

In the fictitious Xanadu Simulation Center Scorecard example, the measures are organized into five categories: stewardship, people, experience, health, and business processes. These categories were chosen to be in alignment with the four dimensions of the parent organization, Xanadu Medical Center. The Simulation Center also wanted to monitor their internal business practices

TABLE 5.4.6						
Xanadu Simulation Center Dashboard Item						
Dimension	**Objective**		**Unit**	**Q1**	**Q2**	**Q3**
Health (in situ Mock Code data)	Time to first shock ≤120 seconds		PACU			
			Med Surg 1			
			Med Surg 2			
			ICU			
			L & D			
			Pediatrics			
			Mental Health			

Fictitious data created by author.

■, ≤120 seconds; ■, <180 seconds and improving; ■, ≥180 seconds.

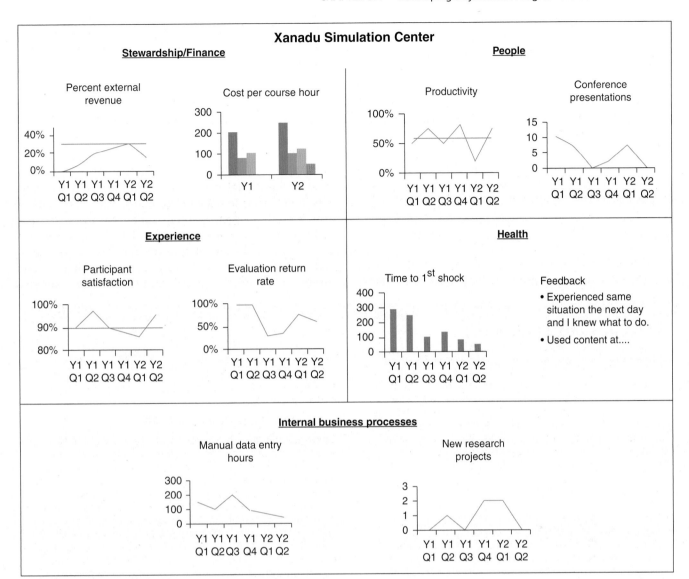

FIGURE 5.4.5   Xanadu Simulation Center.

(Kaplan & Norton, 1996), and so this fifth area was included. The goal is to organize the information in a way that is meaningful for the program and its stakeholders. While the balanced scorecard (Kaplan & Norton, 1996; Pugh, 2008) approach helps ensure that key information is presented, individual simulation programs should determine the measures and report on organizational data that fits with their program and parent organization.

Information is often collected and reported at different frequency intervals. The type of data or the individual receiving the information may determine the frequency. Numbers of participants or hours of simulation time may be an annual reporting measure, whereas facilitator effectiveness, revenue, or expenses per course may be monitored and shared more frequently. Likewise, members of the simulation team or adjunct faculty may be reviewing metrics and reports more frequently than an advisory or governing board. It is critical that simulation programs share their evaluation data with leaders within the organization and that there is a bidirectional sharing of

information. This allows the program to receive feedback on current initiatives and work together with leaders to develop new ones.

THE HOW TO ... FOR NOVICES

If you are just starting an evaluation plan, start small! It can be overwhelming to think about all of the things that could be evaluated.

Choose What to Measure

If you have developed a strategic plan, pick two key strategies and develop a metric for each strategy. If a strategic plan has not been developed yet, that is all right. Choose two areas or categories within your simulation program. The balanced scorecard described earlier provides category ideas. You could consider finance, customers, learning, or internal processes, for example.

Select Specific Measures

Determining specific measures can be difficult. It is easy to get caught up trying to find the perfect measure, only to end up 9 or 12 months later without measuring anything. Do not worry about identifying the perfect measure; just measure something. You may wish to start with data that is easily accessible. Metrics and measures are frequently modified. As you expand your evaluation strategy and become more familiar with data collection and reporting, you can fine-tune your measures. Be sure to create operational definitions and develop a data collection plan for each of the measures.

Analyze the Data and Report

Review the data and share the information with others. Create an effective report using tables, graphs, or narrative statements. Determine how often the results will be shared with the simulation team, faculty, stakeholders, and organizational leaders.

Written Evaluation Plan

Write it down! Even a small plan benefits from the formality of a written evaluation plan. This includes establishing the evaluation philosophy and individuals responsible for the collection, analysis, and dissemination of the results. Writing down the measures, definitions, and collection plan helps provide consistency and a way for the simulation team and organizational leaders to review the plan and update as necessary. After you have created two measures and are collecting data, establish a process for adding additional measures until all critical strategies are measured. Finally, develop a process to review the evaluation

---

CONSIDER THIS

PROGRAM EVALUATION PLANS
Sabrina Koh, RN, MHS(Edu), PGDip(CC), CHSE
Assistant Director, Jurong Health Simulation Centre, Singapore

Many working in the education sector are aware of the importance of program evaluation. Evaluations should be solicited not only from learners, but also from program faculty, program staff, and institutional leadership. When structured and administered appropriately, evaluations can serve as justification to initiate action or seek support for:

- Program enhancements: manpower, equipment, logistical matters
- Reviewing content delivery
- Reviewing curriculum
- Technical assistance
- Audit and/or accreditation

To ensure that our evaluations collect the appropriate information, a workgroup consisting of the Program Administrator, hospital medical affairs representative, and Simulation Program Director collaborated on developing holistic, valid program evaluation tools. When possible, all evaluation items are aligned with either local training benchmarks or institutional standards for program delivery.

EVALUATION FROM LEARNERS

Evaluations are the voices of our learners; they usually reflect accurate accounts of services rendered. We developed learner evaluation tools on the basis of Kirkpatrick's Evaluation Model to measure program effectiveness at four levels: (1) reaction, (2) learning, (3) behavior, and (4) results. Caution was taken to weigh the need for programmatic information with the burden that lengthy evaluations may place on learners.

Evaluation tools should be refined as needed. After our initial 8 months of evaluation collection, we found that some items did not elicit useful data. We refined the tool to encourage more open-ended responses and added a final question asking "*Any other comments?*" Through multiple rounds of subsequent evaluations, we observed that learners tended to skip these open-ended questions. We assumed this was either because the learner felt rushed to complete the open-ended questions or were just too tired after their simulation course. To reduce evaluation fatigue, we added commonly expected answers to these open-ended questions, giving learners the option to choose frequently given answers while retaining the ability to provide the open-ended response.

EVALUATION FROM PROGRAM STAFF

Operational and logistical support is the foundation to successful simulation programming. Recognizing the importance of staff feedback, we collect quarterly evaluation feedback from the simulation program staff (e.g., program administrator, technicians, etc.). These evaluations address program support, technical challenges, and needs for future programming. The simulation program staff evaluations are used to accurately estimate multiple aspects of Program operations, including infrastructure support, funding projections, and staffing needs. We've also found that the act of implementing staff suggestions significantly contributes to morale in our program.

EVALUATION FROM PROGRAM FACULTY

Evaluation data is also collected from the simulation program faculty to determine whether they are receiving the support necessary to facilitate curriculum delivery. Faculty evaluations collect information pertaining to simulation hardware, simulation staff support, and content of simulation curricula. Faculty evaluations are collected immediately at the end of a simulation course by way of a huddle with simulation program staff to gather impromptu feedback and points for future improvement. In addition, a formal written evaluation is also circulated quarterly for more concrete evaluation data.

EVALUATION FROM INSTITUTIONAL LEADERS

This is an attempt to measure the impact of simulation programming from the perspective of institutional leadership. Ideally, all simulation training would result in measurable clinical outcomes. While this is difficult to measure, it is still useful to understand how leadership perceives the impact of simulation and may help guide program strategy. In addition, departmental leadership feedback guides the simulation program in establishing learning "road maps" for encouraging interdepartmental collaboration.

plan—are the metrics appropriate, are they still relevant, and revise as necessary.

BEEN THERE, DONE THAT: DEVELOPING A PERFORMANCE IMPROVEMENT PLAN FOR YOUR SIMULATION PROGRAM

If you have already developed an evaluation plan, the next step is to seek out opportunities to improve your simulation program through a formal PI process or development of a PI plan.

Link to Mission, Vision, and Strategic Plan

Like a strategic plan, a PI plan should have a link to the mission and vision. It should also be integrated into the simulation program's strategic plan so that PI priorities are viewed as being as important as other organizational priorities. This ensures that there are resources allocated for planning and improvements.

Establish Authority, Roles, and Responsibilities

At the start of the PI planning process, accountability and authority are defined. Who is responsible for establishing and implementing the plan? Is there a PI committee or workgroup? Whom do they report to—a board of directors, advisory committee, president, dean? Will these individuals need to authorize or approve the plan? Even if approval is not necessary, it is important to obtain support and buy-in. Many large organizations have an organization-wide PI committee and formal plan. What will be the relationship between the simulation program's team and the larger committee?

Time Frame

PI plans typically cover a 1- to 2-year time frame. At the start of your PI program cycle, identify a number of projects that you will accomplish. Be realistic—consider the staff available, time, and resources needed. It is reasonable to plan one to two initiatives per year.

Projects

This is an opportunity to look at all aspects of your simulation program to see whether there are opportunities to improve. Where do you look? The following may provide you with a place to start.

- Program processes: Identify the processes that are most critical to the strategy or success of your simulation program and determine whether those processes are adequate.
  - Course registration
  - Evaluation
  - Scenario development
  - Medication storage, retrieval, administration
  - Facilitation
  - Equipment/Center maintenance
  - Orientation/faculty development
- Program resources/inputs
  - How are supplies obtained?
  - Job processes—are the right people in the right roles?
  - Is the environment adequate? Are environmental upgrades needed?
  - Is the technology adequate?
  - Are there funding issues?
- Data from strategic plan or other measures
- Participant and faculty feedback
- Low-hanging fruit

You may find more opportunities than time and resources available. If it is difficult to choose a project, consider letting staff or the PI team to vote using an affinity diagram or a prioritization grid may be helpful. Once an improvement opportunity has been identified, use the PDCA model described in chapter 1.5 to plan and implement changes.

Measure and Monitor Effectiveness

It is important to monitor and, if possible, measure the effectiveness of the improvement initiative. Numerical data may be collected and put into tables or graphs, or the effect may be monitored and documented in a narrative. Regardless of the method, documentation is important. Along with documenting the effectiveness of the individual improvements, consider completing a brief evaluation summary at the end of each year. This evaluation summarizes the focus of the program's PI initiatives for that year, including a summary of the PDCA cycle, outcomes, and next steps. Is there a risk of returning to the old? If so, how will you maintain the improvement?

SUMMARY

We evaluate simulation programs to ensure that the programs are headed in the intended direction and to monitor efforts in achieving the goals and objectives identified in a strategic plan. Programs should choose to evaluate things that are most critical to the success of their strategic plan. Evaluation is not a one-time process. It should be a systematic process that encompasses multiple dimensions of the program and is ongoing, continuous, and woven into the fabric of how simulation programs do business.

REFERENCES

Addison, R. H. (2009). Performance Architecture: The Art and Science of Improving Organizations. San Francisco: Pfeiffer.

Friedman, M. (Guest). (1975). *Living within our means* [Transcribed television interview]. In Heffner, R. (Host), *The Open Mind*. Video February 12, 2013, posted to Richard Heffner's Open Mind website: http://www.thirteen.org/openmind/public-affairs/living-within-our-means/494/

SECTION 5 • Management

Jeffries, P. & Battin, J. (2012). Evaluating the Strategic Plan. In *Developing Successful Health Care Education Simulation Centers* (pp. 71–84). New York: Springer Publishing Company.

Jordan, G., Prevette, S., & Woodward, S. (2001). Analyzing, reviewing, and reporting performance data. In Training Resources & Data Exchange Performance-Based Management Special Interest Group (Eds.), *The performance-based management handbook* (Vol. 5, pp. 1–76). OakRidge, TN: Oak Ridge Institute for Science and Education.

Kaplan, R., & Norton, D. (1996). *The balanced scorecard* [Kindle IPad version]. Available from Amazon.com.

Lloyd, R. (2008). Milestones in the quality measurement journey. In E. Ransom, M. Joshi, D. Nash, & S. Ransom (Eds.), *The healthcare quality book* (2nd ed., pp. 87–108). Chicago, IL: Health Administration Press.

Parry, S. (2000). *Evaluating the impact of training*. Alexandria, VA: American Society for Training & Development (ASTD).

Person, R. (2013). *Balanced Scorecards & Operational Dashboards with Microsoft Excel*. [kindle IPad version]. Available from Amazon.com.

Phillips, P. P., & Phillips, J. J. (2008a). *ROI fundamentals: Why and when to measure return on investment*. San Francisco, CA: Pfeiffer.

Phillips, P. P., & Phillips, J. J. (2008b). *ROI in action casebook*. San Francisco, CA: Pfeiffer.

Preskill, H., & Jones, N. (2009). A practical guide for engaging stakeholders in developing evaluation questions. In *FSG Social Impact Advisors* (Robert Wood Johnson Foundation Evaluation Series, pp. 3–46). Princeton, NJ: Robert Wood Johnson Foundation.

Pugh, M. (2008). Dashboards and scorecards: Tools for creating alignment. In E. J. Ranson (Ed.), *The healthcare quality book* (2nd ed., pp. 217–242). Chicago, IL: Health Administration Press.

Ranson, E., Soshi, M., Nash, D., & Ransom, S. (2008). *The Healthcare Quality Book* (2nd ed.). Chicago: Health Administration Press.

Rummler, G. (2004). *Serious performance consulting*. Silver Spring, MD: International Society for Performance Improvement.

Rummler, G. & Brache, A. (2013). Improving Performance: How to Manage the White Space on the Organization Chart. San Francisco: Jossey-Bass.

Russ-Eft, D., & Preskill, H. (2001). *Evaluation in organizations*. New York, NY: Perseus Books Group.

Saxe, J. G. (1878). *The blind men and the elephant* [Poetry of America: Selections from One Hundred American Poets From 1776 to 1876] (W. J. Linton, Ed.). Retrieved from Google Books website: http://books.google.com/books?vid=LCCN28016886&id=hdrGIl0rnhgC&pg=PR5&dq=Poetry+of+America++Saxe%22#v=onepage&q=Poetry%20of%20America%20%20Saxe%22&f=false

Scriven, M. (2010). Rethinking education methodology. *Journal of Multidisciplinary Evaluation, 6*(13), i–ii.

SSH Council for Accreditation of Healthcare Simulation Programs. (2013). *Accreditation standards and measurement criteria* [Brochure]. Retrieved from Society for Simulation in Healthcare website: http://ssih.org/uploads/static_pages/PDFs/Accred/2013_AccreditationStandards.pdf

Worthen, B., Sanders, J., & Fitzpatrick, J. (1997). Evaluation's basic purpose, uses, and conceptual distinctions. In *Program Evaluation: Alternative Approaches and Practical Guidelines* (pp. 3–24). White Plains, NY: Longman Publishers.

CHAPTER 5.5

Management of Standardized Patient Programs

Nancy Heine, RN, CANP, MSEd, and Diane Ferguson, BSN, RN

ABOUT THE AUTHORS

NANCY HEINE directs the Tom and Vi Zapara Clinical Skills Education Center at Loma Linda University School of Medicine. In 2011, the Center was granted accreditation from the Society for Simulation in Healthcare and provides over 15,000 learner/standardized patient encounters per year. Ms. Heine has participated in case development, research, and standardized patient (SP) training, including training SPs for the National Board of Medical Examiners' Clinical Skills Exam pilot project in 1995–1996. She has published several articles on SPs.

DIANE FERGUSON directs the Howard E. Butt (HEB) HEB Clinical Skills Center at the University of Texas Health Science Center in San Antonio (UTHSCSA), where she developed and implemented SP programs. Her expertise is in setting up SP programs and developing Objective Structured Clinical Exams (OSCEs). She has given numerous presentations and workshops on SP methodology. Ms. Ferguson served on the Board of Directors of the Association for Standardized Patient Educators (ASPE) for 5 years.

ABSTRACT

Simulated clinical encounters utilizing standardized patients (SPs) have evolved into a widely researched and broadly utilized education and assessment method. Utilizing this methodology effectively requires educators who are able to develop appropriate organizational structure and policies, assess program needs, manage resources, develop and maintain SP case banks, and oversee recruitment and training of SPs for a variety of educational activities. Many experienced and highly skilled individuals find themselves in the position of managing simulation or SP programs without any formal management or SP training. Simulation educators who are new to SP program management, who are managing an existing simulation program that wants to now incorporate SPs, or who want to solidify their knowledge regarding managing an SP program need to understand how to efficiently incorporate the unique aspects of the human side of simulation with the educational demands of their program or institution. In addition to the specific requirements for an SP program, this chapter will provide educational and administrative recommendations, references, and resources.

CASE EXAMPLE

You are the manager of a simulation program that serves an academic medical center. You are responsible for supporting a medical school, nursing school, and a paramedic training program. In addition, you support the hospital-based residency programs. The Center has been contacted by the deans of the respective programs and asked to incorporate **standardized patients** (SPs) into simulation scenarios. They have recently attended a quality improvement program and heard about the benefits of a formal SP program as well as interprofessional education. They are interested in working together with you to develop a program that uses SPs for purposes of education as well as assessment. While in the past you have used embedded simulated persons (ESPs) and some volunteers from the community in your simulations, you have never hired or trained a professional SP. Where do you begin? What are the strategies you can use to ensure an effective program?

INTRODUCTION AND BACKGROUND

The Standardized Patient (SP) Program Manager is one person within the institution who often has a view of clinical skills education as a continuum: across classes, across disciplines, and often across professions. This is a unique position that is an asset to administration and faculty who recognize and utilize this resource. Beyond assuming the typical managerial responsibilities associated with running a complex program, well-prepared SP Program Managers can guide faculty to achieve their vision of teaching and assessing clinical skills, especially skills that are difficult to teach with mannequins only, but are essential to caring for patients.

SIGNIFICANCE

Around the globe, there is increasing recognition of the value of the SP methodology in the education of healthcare professionals. With the increase in SP usage comes the need for individuals to manage these SP programs in ways that are efficient, effective, and evidence-based.

Integration of SPs into the curriculum requires a person with a good grasp of SP methodology to assist faculty in the development and implementation of SP activities. The role of the SP Program Manager includes facilitating the development of SP activities while ensuring they align with curricular goals. Additionally, the job includes areas of management and administration such as managing budgets, project creation, multilevel activity scheduling, personnel (SPs and SP Trainers) utilization, and in some cases, participation in strategic planning.

While SP educators (trainers) are experts at SP methodology applied to training and monitoring SPs and are ideally suited to move into a program manager role, they may be unfamiliar with the administrative duties the role requires and need significant on-the-job training in that area. On the other hand, individuals with a deep understanding of other simulation methodologies and significant administrative experience would have to become familiar with the unique aspects of SP methodology.

Traditionally, SPs have been trained for teaching and assessing clinical skills in medical and nursing school programs. The role of the SP is being expanded to include standardized family member, examinee, learner, healthcare consumer, healthcare provider, and also physical examination educator.

Managers of SP programs are facing an increasing learning curve as they are asked to provide SPs for a wider variety of roles and venues, requiring them to be able to apply educational theory across many different professions and levels of training. The qualifications and expectations of SP Program Managers are expanding to keep up with these changes.

Examples of content areas that SP Program Managers may need to understand and address are discussed in the following sections.

Patient Safety

Objective Structured Clinical Exams(OSCEs) are used to assess patient safety–related skills. A common use for SPs is in OSCE stations assessing clinical skills in specific contexts where new residents may be expected to function with minimal supervision, for example, obtaining informed consent, handoffs, identifying and managing pain, cross-cultural challenges, and recognizing and responding appropriately in deteriorating or critical patient situations (Mollo et al., 2012; Wagner & Lypson, 2009).

Continuing training and monitoring of quality of care and competence of healthcare workers is critical to maintaining patient safety. To this end, SPs have been introduced into either the actual or the simulated workplace to document the performance of important patient safety skills. For example, OSCEs utilizing SPs trained as standardized donors have been developed to assess the competency of taking a blood bank predonation health history and recording and interpreting the history (Battles et al., 2004).

SPs have been utilized to measure quality of care in actual physician practices. Trained SPs have been sent into physicians' clinics unannounced, with completion of checklists evaluating quality of care and provision of services that have been shown to lead to better outcomes of care (Peabody et al., 2000).

Interprofessional and team collaboration are vital to patient safety. Mannequins are commonly used to present emergency, critical care, and operating room scenarios, which require effective team communication. The addition of SPs, simulated family members, and simulated healthcare workers provides further challenges and opportunities for practicing and assessing team competencies, which affect patient safety.

To support all of these patient safety initiatives, the SP program and its manager must stay abreast of the rapidly changing literature in the field and the evidence that supports best practices in these programs.

Mass Casualty, Biologic and Chemical Hazard Exposure Simulations

SPs are commonly used to augment mass casualty and hazardous exposure training scenarios. SPs can give an added emotional challenge to the learner by portraying hysteria, grief, altering levels of consciousness, and acute pain. Managers of SP programs that provide this service must be skilled in communication and project management to work effectively with numerous outside agencies. The SP Program Manager is often expected to make sure the program is well prepared to handle the budget, personnel, organizational, and public relation issues associated with these endeavors.

Pediatric and Adolescent SPs

Children and adolescents have been utilized as SPs and have been trained to accurately portray a role with their real or standardized parent (Lane et al., 1999; Woodward & Gliva-McConvey, 1995). Adolescents have been trained to portray risk-taking adolescents with no evidence of adverse effects on them from their role as an SP. Guidelines for recruitment and screening of adolescents include screening the adolescent for comfort with the role, involving the adolescent's parents in the consent and discussion of the role, and using school resources in the recruitment and scheduling of SPs (Blake et al., 2006).

The use of pediatric and adolescent SPs requires the SP Program Manager to have specilaized knowledge and skills to deal with these actors and their guardians. There are also specific regulatory requirements associated with minors that need to be addressed.

Standardized "Examinees" and "Learners"

SPs are being trained as standardized examinees. In this role, SPs can be utilized in quality assurance for high-stakes examinations to test whether different SPs rate examinees similarly. Standardized applicants have been used to train interviewers in the medical school admissions process. In another role, SPs trained as standardized learners have been used to train or evaluate faculty and residents, giving feedback to learners (Pangaro et al., 1997).

Programs using SPs in these roles need to ensure they have clear policies and procedures to guide the processes. The SP Program Manager will likely be the person assigned to oversee the development of these items. Above and beyond knowing the methodology, the manager will need to be aware of the current literature on high-stakes testing as well as human resource (HR) rules and regulations that address the evaluation of faculty members.

Simulated Patient Educators

Experienced SPs who have developed expertise in physical examination, interviewing, and communication skills have been used as educators with novice learners. Other common uses of SPs in teaching physical examination are Gynecologic Teaching Associates (**GTA**s) and Male Urogenital Teaching Associates (**MUTA**s), who teach sensitive examinations on themselves, guiding and giving feedback to learners. SPs have also been taught basic ultrasound examination and are used as patient educators in teaching students ultrasound technique (Oakes et al., 2012).

Embedded Simulated Persons (Confederates)

SPs are increasingly being used to augment mannequin-based simulation scenarios, as **simulated patients**, family members, and healthcare workers.

When developing and implementing any of these or other innovative applications of SP methodology, it is important that SP Program Managers keep in mind the evidence supporting examination design, implementation, and analysis to achieve the desired outcome. Identifying and utilizing experienced local resources will make implementing a new program easier and more cost-effective.

HOW TO . . .

Defining Your Organizational Structure

Organizational structure is "the typically hierarchical arrangement of lines of authority, communications, rights and duties of an organization. Organizational structure determines how the roles, power and responsibilities are assigned, controlled, and coordinated, and how information flows between the different levels of management" (Business Dictionary, 2013).

A transparent organizational structure is essential to an SP program. Established simulation programs entering into the human side of simulation will most likely require some changes, both in organizational structure and in policies and procedures. Creating a well-defined organizational structure demonstrates to SPs, the institution, and potential clients a professional and dependable program.

The organizational structure of an SP program is usually dependent on the associated institution(s) and funding sources. University-, hospital-, and government-based programs may all have very different needs, which will affect SP program management. Some SP programs are part of a mannequin-based simulation program and some stand alone. It is important for the SP Program Manager to understand the institutional structure and the programs' place within that framework. Understanding the expectations of current and potential program stakeholders is essential, whether building a new program or expanding an established program.

Establishing an advisory board or executive committee may be helpful if starting a new program or expanding an existing one. A group of people with an understanding of simulation and knowledge of the institutional structure can be valuable to the SP Program Manager. Benefits include assisting in getting the word out to potential clients, clarifying institutional hierarchy and culture, defining the mission statement and goals of the program, setting up and approving fee schedules, referring interested parties to the program, and generally advocating for the manager and program.

While institutional organization varies widely, there are roles common to successful SP programs. These include the following:

- Clinician
- Program Manager/Director
- SP Trainer/Educator
- Administrative Support Staff
- Education Specialist/Researcher
- Psychometrician/Statistician
- Technical Specialist

Not all of these positions need to be full-time, and some of the positions can overlap in smaller venues. Many

STANDARDIZED PATIENTS IN HEALTH PROFESSIONS EDUCATION: A PROXY FOR REAL PATIENTS?

Debra Nestel, BA, PhD, FAcadMEd, CHSE-A
Board of Directors, Simulation Australia

An exciting element of standardized patient (SP) methodology is the opportunity to raise the profile of patient perspectives in health professional education programs. In particular, the role of SPs in supporting the development of patient-centeredness, cleverly articulated by several scholars (Gerteis et al., 1993; Stewart et al., 2003) as placing the patients' needs at the center of the care process—their ideas, concerns, feelings, reasons for consulting, and need for information are sought, acknowledged, and valued by clinicians and that patients are encouraged to participate in all decisions about their care to the extent they are able to and willing. This brief commentary addresses the notion of SPs as *proxies* for real patients and their role in teaching patient-centeredness, avoiding the paradox of clinicians rather than patients (or their proxies—SPs) teaching patient-centeredness (Bleakley & Bligh, 2008).

SP methodology provides a means by which *real* and *simulated* patients connect—at least at some level—to ensure real patient perspectives are offered by those who are best positioned to make such judgments. However, contemporary SP methodology often distances real patients from practices such as *scenario* or *case* development, training for role portrayal, and feedback (Nestel & Bentley, 2011; Nestel & Kneebone, 2010). Although the focus here is on scenario development, it is intended to prompt critical reflection on ways in which real patients might directly contribute to all facets of SP methodology.

Usually developed by SP educators or clinicians, scenarios are often their fictitious accounts of patient experiences, or their *interpretations* of an individual patient's experience or of a composite of real patients' experiences. So, although sometimes derived from real patients, scenarios are the SP educator's or clinician's interpretation of the patient's experience. SP educators and clinicians, by virtue of becoming a member of their profession, no longer experience healthcare as patients. That is, it is difficult to experience healthcare through the eyes of a patient after immersion in healthcare services. The personal accounts of clinicians who become patients attest to the different lenses through which the service is experienced (Jones, 2005; Klitzman, 2007; O'Brien, 2008). This is not a manipulative ploy on the part of SP educators or clinicians but the result of the important process of their own professionalization.

Without real patient involvement, much SP-based work is "a mirror for the teachers' preconceptions rather than as an authentic reflection of a patient encounter" (Nestel & Kneebone, 2010). Snow (in press), an *expert* patient observing simulation educators at work, notes, ". . . the patient voice continues to be filtered through clinicians' perspectives." She too argues that real patients, especially those with chronic illness, can be invited to participate in all phases

of simulation-based education and are perfectly positioned to teach patient-centeredness.

There are several examples of ways in which real patients can contribute to scenario development. These include inviting volunteer SPs to reflect on a recent encounter of their own in family medicine and then populating an SP scenario template (Nestel, Tierney, et al., 2008). Of course, the SPs need to agree to participate in the sharing of this information, and the scope of scenarios is limited by the experiences of the volunteers. Another approach is to interview real patients with the shared intent of crafting SP scenarios on the basis of their experiences. Capturing each patient's verbal descriptions of their ideas, concerns, need for information, and expectations addresses patient-centeredness directly (Nestel & Bentley, 2011; Nestel, Cecchini, et al., 2008; Nestel & Kneebone, 2010). Of course, this is impractical to do for all required scenarios (some real patients will be unwilling and unsuitable to participate), but it is a salutary process for all and goes some way to ensuring that SPs are proxies for real patients and not simply agents of the SP educator or clinician. Extending involvement of real patients to training SPs for role portrayal and feedback goes even further in ensuring that patient-centeredness is offered from the perspective it is purported to offer.

REFERENCES

Bleakley, A., & Bligh, J. (2008). Students learning from patients: Let's get real in medical education. *Advances in Health Sciences Education, 13*(1), 89–107.

Gerteis, M., Edgman-Levitan, S., Daley, J., & Delbanco, T. (1993). *Through the patient's eyes:* Understanding and promoting patient-centered care. San Francisco, CA: Picker Institute.

Jones, P. (2005). *Doctors as patients.* Oxford, UK: Radcliffe.

Klitzman, R. (2007). *When doctors become patients.* New York, NY: Oxford University Press.

Nestel, D., & Bentley, L. (2011). The role of patients in surgical education. In H. Fry & R. Kneebone (Eds.), *Surgical education: Theorising an emerging domain.* London: Springer.

Nestel, D., Cecchini, M., Calandrini, M., Chang, L., Dutta, R., Tierney, T., . . . Kneebone, R. (2008). Real patient involvement in role development: evaluating patient focused resources for clinical procedural skills. *Medical Teacher, 30,* 795–801.

Nestel, D., & Kneebone, R. (2010). Authentic patient perspectives in simulations for procedural and surgical skills. *Academic Medicine, 85*(5), 889–893.

Nestel, D., Tierney, T., & Kubacki, A. (2008). Creating authentic roles for simulated patients. *Medical Education, 42*(11), 1122.

O'Brien, C. (2008). *Never say die.* Sydney, Australia: HarperCollins.

Snow, R. (2014). Real patient participation in simulations. In D. Nestel & M. Bearman (Eds.), *Simulated patient methodology: Theory, evidence and practice.* Oxford, UK: Wiley Blackwell.

Stewart, M., Belle-Brown, J. B., Weston, W. W., McWhinney, I. R., McWilliam, C. L., & Freeman, T. R. (2003). *Patient-centered medicine: Transfoming the clinical method.* Oxford, UK: Radcliffe Medical Press.

successful programs have only a manager/SP trainer and administrative support. However, if research and program quality are important to the simulation program and institution, the program should have access to the other experts.

Program goals determine what roles need to be full-time and what roles might be filled with part-time or contract personnel. A brief description of the roles follows.

Clinician

A person with clinical training that is compatible with the SP program's mission. Duties may include writing SP cases, training SPs and SP educators on medical aspects of specific roles such as physical examination maneuvers, working with course faculty to develop learner level–appropriate curricula, and preparing and participating in remediation activities. This position is often a member of committees that focus on use of SPs or OSCE development. There may be one or more part-time clinicians from various disciplines, depending on the size of the program.

Manager/Director

A person with supervisory experience, particularly one who has an understanding of simulation and healthcare education, is desirable. Duties include all administrative aspects of the program such as supervising SP educators and support staff, scheduling program activities (see Appendix A—Project Request Form), handling requests to integrate SPs into the curriculum or other educational activities, managing a budget, and general project management. This person often serves on the curriculum committee and other committees that evaluate and develop curricula for the institution. This is a typically a full-time position (see Appendix B—Sample Manager Job Description).

SP Trainer

A person with experience working in an SP program is very desirable, but not necessary because there are several educator training programs available (see Appendix C—SP Trainer Educational Programs). Duties include recruiting, hiring, training, and supervising SPs. Quality assurance and performance review of SPs is usually included in this person's job description. Large programs may require more than one full-time SP trainer/educator (see Appendix D—Sample SP Trainer/Educator Job Description).

Support Staff

A person who performs administrative duties assisting the other positions in the program. Duties may include scheduling SPs for training or activities, assisting with data entry, general activity setup and breakdown, greeting learners and faculty, and setting up meetings. This is rarely a purely secretarial position, and could be full-time or part-time depending on the size of the program.

Education Specialist/Researcher

A person who assists with curriculum planning and alignment of the goals and objectives of the institution with the activities of the program. Experience in education research is helpful if the program is expected to prepare and submit studies to educational conferences. This position is often part-time or contract.

Psychometrician/Statistician

A person who can provide consultation and interpret data for setting the scoring standards of SP-related activities

and research endeavors. Other duties might include validating assessment tools such as checklists and rating scales, and developing surveys for the program and curriculum. This may be a part-time or contract position.

Technical Assistant

This person should be technologically literate to the extent of program needs. Duties may require utilizing and developing content for a learning information system, updating and maintaining computers, and interfacing with institutional information systems personnel. This could be full-time if the SP program is within a simulation program or serves a large volume of learners and activities.

Developing a Fee Schedule

Developing a fee schedule for a simulation program requires a great deal of thought and preparation. There is helpful information regarding developing center and mannequin usage fees in other chapters. The addition of SPs to a program or center will necessitate some changes to existing fee schedules, particularly to cover SP wages and SP educator time.

Program usage fees will be dependent on numerous institutional factors such as non-/for-profit status, institution-wide versus single-entity use, replacement cost versus budget supplementation, and so on. It is easy to underestimate how much time and effort goes into preparing SPs and SP activities, so seek help in establishing an initial fee schedule. Advisory boards can be helpful in this regard as can other SP educators (see ASPE SP Trainer Listserve at http://mailman13.u.washington.edu/mailman/listinfo/sp-trainer). Fee templates can be found online and from professional societies and members (see Appendix E—Sample Fee Schedule).

Line items to include in developing fee schedules are as follows:

- Hourly wage of SPs plus any benefits (include backup SPs in this calculation). Both training time and performance time should be factored into the schedule. It is a good idea to separate the two for clarity.
- SP educator/trainer time to recruit, schedule, and train the SPs.
- Technology usage and technician time to execute.
- Support staff setup and breakdown time.
- Proctor support for OSCEs or other large activities.
- Manager time (consulting, preparing reports, revising cases).
- Consultant fees—psychometrician, education specialist/researcher.
- Facility usage costs.
- Supply replacement costs.
- Material costs (paper copies, props, room supplies, DVDs, snacks).
- Travel costs (very program-dependent).

Start determining activity costs by listing the personnel that will be engaged in each project and their hourly wages or salaries. Have staff members keep a log of how much time they spend on each task for each project. Ideally, have everyone participate in this log for a year so that each activity can be evaluated for time and effort and fees justified.

A fair and understandable fee schedule is an excellent tool to use when meeting potential clients. It can be used to illustrate the amount of planning and work the program will put forth on the client's behalf. The final fee schedule should be easy to defend and openly represent the work of the program. Monitoring the program's usage, costs, and charges is important for budget analysis and reporting, and is typically the responsibility of the SP Program Manager.

Developing a Policy and Procedure Manual

A well-thought-out policy and procedure manual will help keep the SP program in line with program and institutional policies. Developing and maintaining this manual is typically the responsibility of the SP Program Manager. Samples of general simulation program policy and procedure manuals are available online and from simulation community colleagues. The focus of this section is on policies that apply specifically to SPs and SP programs.

Incorporating human simulators (SPs) adds a layer of complexity to both new and existing programs. In general, parent institution policies are sufficient to cover center safety issues, but SPs require additional protection from harm and exposure as does the institution. The SP program manual also needs to include procedures for everything from hiring SPs to how to set up for SP events.

Policies covering the following areas are important for an SP program:

- Confidentiality—Specific mention can be made about confidentiality regarding cases, other SPs, and learners. Procedures for consents should be clearly outlined.
- Management—Specific mention can be made to program scheduling, staff issues, SP responsibilities, SP use (who can, when, and costs), budget process including fee estimates, management of cases, and upkeep.
- HR policies—Specific mention can be made to pay, timekeeping, professional conduct, and performance evaluations.
- Case/scenario development—Specific mention can be made to who is responsible for case/scenario development including approval process, templates, and timelines.
- SP-specific—Specific mention can be made to video recording, cancelations, illness, no shows, inadvertent discovery of pathology, expectation for medical consultation/care (the program cannot serve in that role), incident reporting, and reporting process for learner concerns.

- Learner-specific—Specific mention can be made to video recording, honor code, reporting concerns, professional attire, and any behavioral expectations.
- Administrative—Specific mention can be made to case template, activity logistics, stocking exam rooms, ordering supplies, as well as the process for setting up and breaking down activities (who does this and how is it done).

Hiring a Standardized Patient

The job of an SP is not always easy to describe to potential recruits. Most programs use SPs in a variety of ways, from teaching physical examination skills to evaluating difficult communication skills. Roles may require the SP to portray patients who are very different from their own personalities. This adaptability requires more than memorizing a script and acting out a part. These people need to be intelligent, lifelong learners if they are to become truly valued members of the program.

The institution may dictate how SPs are to be hired, but the SP Program Manager can work with HR to develop an efficient way to process applicants. Given the specific expectations of the position, the manager may be able to negotiate a process that allows the program to determine eligibility without having the applicant go through an onerous institutional process first. There are times when a particular gender, age, ethnicity, and so on are needed for an SP role; therefore, it is important for HR to understand program needs so that they can help with the hiring process (Table 5.5.1).

There may be limitations to hiring pediatric SPs, community patients, or other specialty groups. Individuals who work as gynecological/genital/rectal examination teaching associates (GTA, MUTA) and community patients who have stable physical findings often work as independent contractors and are paid accordingly. It is best to work with your HR Department to ensure that there are no legal issues and proper procedures are followed.

Recruiting and Screening Standardized Patients

Recruitment can begin after establishing hiring policies and procedures. Deciding how to advertise for SPs often depends on how they will be used within the program. When setting up a new program, begin recruiting with the end goal in mind. If the activity requires a specific age group, gender, and so on, focus recruitment efforts toward the desired demographic. Once established, having an open application (website) process allows the program to keep a database from which to pull people who fit the desired demographic for interviewing.

Because most programs need SPs who are computer literate, having a Web-based application process is a way to be somewhat assured the applicant has computer experience. Applications should be available on institution and

TABLE 5.5.1		
SP Status Categories		
Type	**Advantages**	**Disadvantages**
Employee	For SP: • Has a stake in the institution/learners • May have access to employee benefits • Taxes removed from paycheck • Sense of security and responsibility to the institution and program For Program: • Expectations clearly outlined • Timekeeping and payment uniform	For SP and Program: • Requires more paperwork during the employment process
Contractor	For SP: • Payment in cash or check (voucher) For Program: • Specialty SPs—GTA, MUTA who contract are already trained	For Program: • May require contract developed by legal department to avoid legal issues related to employment status • Decreased control over teaching content → decreased standardization
Volunteer	For SP: • Satisfaction with volunteering For Program: • Essentially, no cost	• Difficult to standardize people who have no stake in the program and who do not want to be held to program standards • Less commitment to a schedule

program websites, which can be accessed in various ways (directly through website, via Facebook or other social media). Depending on where the SP program is located, placing advertisements in theater departments or other areas on campus may be a successful way to recruit young people. For the older demographic, well-placed advertisements in senior centers, churches, and retirement communities are good ways to find seniors who might be interested in being SPs. By far the most successful recruitment method is word of mouth from SPs who are already involved in a successful and well-run program. Once SPs know how to do their job, they are excellent recruiters because they can judge who is and who is not appropriate for the work.

Screening for appropriate applicants begins with the application itself. A brief statement pointing out the more unusual aspects of the job (role-play, video recording, wearing a patient gown, "on call" work) helps people determine whether they are right for the job before going any further. Versatility is so important for an SP that there may be applicants who could be used so seldom that it may not be worth the effort to hire them. In addition to the usual application questions, ask about body habitus (body type), illnesses, and scars that would be visible during a physical examination or might hamper their ability to take on certain roles. Be sure to add a statement that clarifies why the program needs this personal information. If the applicant is uncomfortable disclosing this information, they are probably not right for the job.

Obtain a writing sample by requesting that the applicant explain in writing why they are interested in SP work. An SP must be literate enough to give verbal and written feedback to a wide range of learners. Some communication problems may still not be evident until the applicant comes in for an interview.

In addition to screening applications, some programs bring applicants in for a group interview to observe how they interact with one another and the program staff (Cleland et al., 2009). During the interview process, you will need to discuss the applicant's feelings toward healthcare providers. Either overly negative or overly positive feelings about healthcare providers can be detrimental to learners and the program. As SPs are required to interact with a variety of individuals with different personalities and skill levels, they should be as unbiased as possible to provide a standardized performance and objective assessment.

Recruiting and screening specialty SPs such as GTAs and MUTAs requires a modified recruiting and screening process, owing to the more invasive nature of the examinations and advanced teaching requirements. The Association for Standardized Patient Educators (ASPE) GTA/MUTA special interest group (SIG) is an excellent resource for standards of practice and guidelines for recruiting, hiring, training, and performance review of GTAs and MUTAs.

Developing and Maintaining an SP Case Library

The process of developing and writing a case is discussed in another chapter (see chapter 3.4). The focus of this section is the SP Program Manager's role with regard to the **case library** (or case bank), case usage, case template, and case writing responsibilities. Programs develop and collect SP cases from both internal assignments and external sources (e.g., SP trainer listserv, ASPE, networking, MedEdPORTAL). Organizing these cases keeps them readily accessible to program users and program management. When new SP activities are under development, the program manager uses the case library to present potential cases to course faculty. These cases can be either incorporated into the curriculum or benefit case writers as a template. All cases need to be tailored to fit the level and type of learner, the competencies being assessed, and the context of performance. The evaluation tools used to rate examinees in OSCEs reflect the professional competencies desired in the profession, and as examinees seek to meet the challenge(s) of the examination, those behaviors and skills are reinforced. These behaviors have been shown to be contextual, and behaviors expected in one setting by a particular set of learners may not be the behaviors expected in different settings with different learners (Hodges, 2003). The SP Program Manager must continuously reinforce that context and applications need to be taken into consideration when developing cases or adopting cases that may have been developed for a completely different activity.

Once obtained or completed, SP cases can be organized on the basis of learner group and level, objectives and competencies they assess, chief complaint, final diagnosis, and other characteristics. For casting purposes, noting case prerequisites such as gender, ethnicity, and age assists with matching SPs to a case. Program users request cases with specific chief complaints, and communication challenges occur often enough that keeping these cases categorized by these attributes is essential. Many programs employ software that helps organize cases. In this situation, the case naming convention becomes important (even more so as the case list grows). There is no case naming standard; some programs use the "patient" name as the case name, while others use a combination of course number, year, or chief complaint to keep track of cases. Consulting other SP programs to develop a naming convention can be very helpful and is recommended if no naming convention exists or the one in use is not working.

It is generally up to the SP Program Manager to maintain the case bank and determine when sharing cases is appropriate (with author permission). The manager is also a great resource for assisting faculty in adjusting cases to meet specific programmatic and/or learner needs.

Programs should have a case template that contains all the categories of information needed in an SP case. Templates are available from simulation colleagues and associations. Provide a template when faculty want to write their own cases so that they know all the information that the SP needs to portray the case appropriately. The SP Manager should be available to review the template and the case with faculty throughout the process (Ker et al., 2005; see Appendix G—Sample Case Template).

Developing an Exam Blueprint

In the beginning stages of developing an SP-based assessment, it is useful to prepare an **examination blueprint or matrix**. An examination blueprint visually demonstrates what competencies and skills the case scenarios chosen for the activity cover. It can also point out areas that are over- or underrepresented. The blueprint can be as simple or as complex as necessary to develop an assessment that meets the course, institutional, or agency objectives. Blueprints are an excellent way to satisfy licensing, certification, and accreditation requirements by demonstrating where clinical skills are taught and tested throughout the curriculum (see Appendix H—Sample Blueprint).

Training, Monitoring, and Giving Feedback to SPs

Training

The goal of training SPs is to achieve authentic and consistent portrayal of the facts, mannerisms, and emotional characteristics of the patient case, as well as to ensure appropriate response to physical examination maneuvers. In addition, SPs are often trained to complete checklists and rating scales on the examinee's performance during the encounter, and to provide either written or verbal feedback to either the learner or the faculty, or both. Training should focus on making sure the SP accomplishes the following:

- Gives the opening statement verbatim.
- Knows the facts of the case.
- Consistently portrays the appropriate demeanor and body language.
- Responds to cues from the examinee appropriately.
- Completes checklists and rating scales accurately.
- Provides appropriate written and/or verbal feedback.
- Stays in role (character).

A standardized script ensures that multiple SPs can be trained to portray the case consistently to provide the same challenge to multiple learners. The **opening statement** is typically scripted for the SP to give verbatim, but the remainder of the information provided in the script depends on the learner's questions. There may be specific cues for SPs to give information or ask scripted questions.

For high-stakes examinations, multiple training sessions are usually necessary to ensure accuracy of portrayal and checklist completion. Experienced SPs usually require less training than newer SPs, who may need more coaching on portrayal of emotions, response to physical exam maneuvers, checklist completion, and giving feedback. If multiple SPs are to perform a case, they should be trained together for SP trainer efficiency and to standardized portrayal. A typical **training protocol** for a high-stakes exam would involve four sessions of 2 to 4 hours each, depending on the experience and number of SPs being trained:

Session 1 typically includes the following activities:

- Review case materials.
- Observe video of an experienced SP playing the role, highlighting portrayal and response to questions.
- Demonstrate simulated physical exam findings.
- Introduce checklist and guide to the checklist.
- Review schedule, general policies, and expectations with SPs.

Session 2 typically includes the following activities:

- Role-play the script with the SP trainer or clinician with feedback to the SP.
- Training on the responses to physical examination maneuvers.
- Practice with checklist and rating scale completion.
- Focus on achieving uniformity in portrayal and checklist accuracy.
- Introduce access to computer and checklist completion.

By the end of Session 2, SP trainers are encouraged to dismiss an SP from the case if they have reason to believe the SP is not going to be able to perform adequately.

Session 3 typically includes the following activities:

- Video role-play and review with all SPs for standardization of portrayal.
- SPs complete checklists and rating scales; check for accuracy of completed checklists.
- Discuss items where discrepancies in responses occur. If performance and/or checklist accuracy is poor, consider further training sessions or recasting with a different SP if problems cannot be resolved.

Session 4 typically includes the following activities:

- Perform a dress rehearsal with at least one timed run-through of the case with each SP, including checklist completion. It is beneficial to give the SP experience with both "good" and "poor" examinees to ensure that they can discriminate checklist items. A clinician or learner close to the level of the event learners is desirable to give the SP practice.
- Discuss logistics, schedule, and emergency contact information (Barrows, 2000; Furman, 2008; May, 2008; Russell et al., 2011; Wallace, 2006).

Training SPs to provide either **written or verbal feedback** to learners can be incorporated into individual training sessions, but many SP Trainers prefer to bring all the SPs for an event together for a group feedback training session. Training sessions on providing feedback typically include written materials describing principles of feedback, review of video clips with examples of effective feedback, and practice writing or giving verbal feedback. The SP's feedback should be given from the perspective of the scripted patient, on the basis of that patient's beliefs, concerns and emotions, and the interaction with the learner. Feedback should be behaviorally based, typically in the format "As Ms. Doe I felt …. when you did …." Providing a list of "feelings" SPs typically may experience is a helpful guide for SPs to formulate feedback statements (Doyle et al., n.d.; May et al., 2006).

Use of a **"Guide to the Checklist"** that describes in detail how to complete the checklist and rating scales improves **interrater reliability**. Videos can be used to demonstrate the expected sequence of questions and calibrate the emotional portrayal of the SP's character and response to physical examination maneuvers.

Using computer-based SP training programs could potentially reduce the time and cost of training multiple SPs and provide a more standardized training regimen. SPs who participated in computer-assisted training have demonstrated improved accuracy of portrayal and checklist completion over standard training (Erichetti & Boulet, 2006).

Monitoring

Trainers should monitor SPs for performance authenticity, quality of feedback provided to learners, and checklist accuracy. Monitoring and providing feedback to SPs for one out of every four performances in a high-stakes examination has been shown to improve SP checklist accuracy (Wallace et al., 1999). Structured evaluation forms like the MaSP (Maastricht Assessment of Simulated Patients) will standardize the assessment of SP performance and quality of feedback (Wind et al., 2004).

For simulation events that are administered over a prolonged period of time, **refresher training** may be needed to recalibrate SP performances. This can be done either individually or by bringing a group of SPs back together to review performances and standards. Comparison of SP scoring can reveal differences that may be due to SPs volunteering information to the examinees, misunderstanding or inaccuracy in recording checklist items, or drifting away from the original script.

Effects of Role-Play on Standardized Patients: Debriefing from the Role

In mannequin-based simulation, there is "wear and tear" on the mannequins requiring repair and replacement. In SP-based simulation, there are also some common but usually mild adverse effects of repetitive simulation. These effects are more likely to occur if the simulations are emotionally or physically demanding. The effects are typically short-lived. Minimizing these effects is an important role of the SP trainer.

Portraying **emotionally intense roles** has been associated with short-term negative psychological effects. When roles are either too close or too removed from the SP's personal experience, they may be more difficult to perform. Screening SPs for their health experiences prior to assigning roles will help to avoid an unnecessary added emotional burden. Other roles may require **physically taxing simulations** or examinations, such as ophthalmoscope exams, repeated deep abdominal exams with simulation of rebound tenderness, and breast and genital/rectal examinations. Limiting the number of examinations and providing scheduled rest breaks are ways that the SP Program Manager can reduce stress and discomfort on the SPs.

The **number of performances and time between breaks** is an important consideration for SP fatigue. The optimum number of performances in a day will vary depending on the role and the age and health of the SP. A usual guideline is 7 to 8 performances per day, and no more than 12.

Providing breaks where SPs can come out of role, relax and talk to other SPs, and enjoy light refreshments will make the work less tedious. Fatigue or boredom with repetitively portraying a role over a prolonged period of time may require recasting an SP to a different case scenario.

Providing feedback to learners requires higher levels of concentration and adds to SP stress. SPs may be concerned that they are identified by the learners as actually having the qualities of the patient they are portraying. Thus, they may prefer a chance to come out of their character role with the learner to give feedback. Coming out of role also helps SPs to put closure on an encounter and put the stress of the interaction behind them.

In general, SPs want to know whether they are doing a good job. Program Managers and Trainers should monitor SPs and give frequent feedback. This will improve SP confidence and satisfaction.

Performing in a simulation has been shown to affect **SPs' perceptions of their own health**. It may help them understand their own symptoms better or, conversely, cause them to worry more about their symptoms. Interestingly, SPs become more aware of their own doctor's clinical skills, and often become more assertive with assessing the quality of their own healthcare. It has been reported that this sometimes results in dissatisfied SPs changing doctors.

Although most of the effects of simulation on SPs are mild to moderate and transient, it is important for Program Managers and Trainers to understand the factors that may affect SPs' emotional and psychological well-being and take steps to prevent them. Trainers should meet briefly with SPs at the end of each day's performances. The SPs appreciate the opportunity to clarify their responses to the dialogue, explain the reasons for poor ratings they may have given an examinee, and to suggest modifications to the training materials on the basis of their experiences. In addition, it is important to allow the SP to "de-role," particularly after emotionally charged encounters (Boerjan et al., 2008; Bokken et al., 2004, 2006; Spencer & Dales, 2006; Wallace et al., 2002).

Maintaining Confidentiality

Confidentiality is important in OSCEs and human simulation encounters for a variety of reasons. Because SPs are performing roles that may require them to be undressed, it is important that precautions be taken to protect the SP's privacy and any videos of those encounters. Monitoring of SP performances live should be limited to only individuals who need access, especially if sensitive exams are being performed. Video review policies restrict where learners and faculty can review videos, with stipulations that videos not be viewed in public places or downloaded to computers with public access. Likewise, learner performance should be protected from view by unauthorized individuals, and learners' performances and feedback should remain confidential.

The SP policy and procedure manual should stipulate that SPs are not permitted to discuss learner performance outside of feedback sessions. Any concerns an SP has about a learner's performance should be discussed only with the appropriate SP trainers and faculty. As SPs have access to cases and examination materials that should be kept secure, it is wise to have SPs sign a consent form attesting that they will protect case material. All learners should sign consent forms indicating that they will keep information about the examination confidential. This is especially important when OSCEs are administered over a prolonged period of time.

The SP program's policy and procedure manual should address how videos will be stored, accessed, and deleted. Passwords to access reports and videos should be robust and kept secure (Barrett & Hodgson, 2011).

Dealing with Problems

Because SP activities involve humans, there is always a potential for problems to occur. While problems cannot always be avoided, it is important to have a policy for dealing with the unforeseen issue or situation. The policy should include a process for reporting problems and a process for problem resolution. Problems can range from natural disasters, power outages, and security threats to complaints of sexual harassment and suspected substance use by any of the individuals involved or interacting with the program. The SPs need to know whom to consult if they have an issue with a learner, faculty, staff, or another SP. Learners need a clear line of authority to resolve any problems they encounter. Faculty and staff need to be aware of the SP program's operating procedures, including who is to be informed if they have a concern about an SP's performance.

Performing a Postexamination Review

Often, the SP Program Manager (or Director) is surprised that examinee performance on an OSCE is lower than expected. In this case, a careful review of the examination, case, and item statistics is in order. The review may reveal problems in any of the following areas:

1. Case design—The expected sequence of the case may not have been clear, may not have matched the level of learner, or may have been too difficult to accomplish in the time provided.
2. Checklist—Items may have been ambiguous or open to interpretation (e.g., "obtained an adequate history of present illness") or the checklist may have been too long or too complicated to be completed accurately.
3. SP performance—Training, portrayal, or checklist accuracy by the SPs may have been less than what was needed.
4. Curriculum—There may be deficits in the curriculum that need to be addressed.

Sound educational practice supports having the SP Manager involved in ensuring that there are defensible pass/

fail and remediation standards, providing results to examinees and program directors in a timely manner, obtaining feedback from faculty, examinees, and SPs for quality improvement, and planning for revisions and improvements on the basis of examination results and feedback.

BEEN THERE, DONE THAT: HOW CAN I CONTINUE TO IMPROVE OR SUSTAIN WHAT I HAVE ACHIEVED?

Use Technology to Manage Your Program

A **Web-based management system** is optimal to efficiently run an SP program. There are several commercially available options that incorporate case banks, scheduling, video recording, storage and retrieval, report generation, and SP tracking. It is advisable to compare the features of each product, consider the program's needs and budget, and request a trial prior to making a commitment. Talking with users of each product will give you information on the benefits and drawbacks of the products.

Programs such as *Survey Monkey* and *Doodle* are available free, and can be used to poll SPs for their availability and to survey users for program quality review. A **website** that is accessible to potential SPs and users of your SP program can host interactive forms such as SP applications, event applications, and case development forms.

Perform Quality Improvement Continuously—Show What You Do Does Make a Difference

Periodic review of the mission statement and goals of the SP program should guide quality improvement. Perform outcome analyses, evaluate feedback, and present your accomplishments to appropriate stakeholders. Utilize a psychometrician and education specialist to analyze SP checklist accuracy, interrater reliability (for SPs and faculty raters), analyze checklist items, and review examination results.

Providing stakeholders with timely, easy-to-read reports that explain the data will provide a basis for making recommendations for changes in the curriculum, examination blueprint, cases, checklists, or rating scales. Surveying faculty, learners, and SPs periodically will highlight strengths and weaknesses of the program and provide a feedback loop for program improvement.

Network

The SP Trainers and Program Managers will benefit from the opportunities for networking provided by joining simulation associations (see Appendix I—Resources for the SP Manager), attending professional conferences, and collaborating with professionals at other institutions who have similar interests. Successful consortiums and collaborations offer the benefits of sharing cases, resources, and experience that will save time and promote innovation.

Seek Accreditation and Certification

The Society for Simulation in Healthcare (SSH) offers **accreditation** of SP programs, simulation programs or joint programs. The accreditation framework is an excellent guide for both new and experienced managers who are seeking to validate their SP programs and establish or improve the organizational structure and processes. The guidelines can demonstrate areas that need attention and reinforce efforts to seek funding or staffing for your program. Achieving accreditation can have financial benefits such as marketing and grant application advantages. The Society also offers a **certification** program for simulation educators, a process that recognizes excellence in simulation educator achievement (http://ssih.org/certification).

The ASPE offers a Core Curriculum Program to provide education on the fundamental knowledge essential for educators in the field of SP methodology (http://aspeducators.org/core-curriculum.php). The modules of this program are offered at the ASPE annual conference and as webinars. In addition, ASPE offers a Scholars Certificate Program, which promotes the advancement of SP methodology and research through scholarly endeavors by its members (http://aspeducators.org/scholars-certificate-program.php).

SUMMARY

The field of healthcare simulation is expanding rapidly. With this rapid growth comes a need for well-qualified managers who will ensure that simulation programs, irrespective of methodology used, are properly developed and maintained. Each type of simulation program has its own unique focus, demanding a slightly different skill set, but there are common principles that will guide the successful program manager. In regard to SP programs, a motivated SP or simulation educator can grow into the role of manager by taking advantage of resources that are available to enhance their skills. Doing so will help ensure the SP Program Manager is able to meet the needs of the institution, faculty, learners, and SPs, and ultimately improve patient care.

REFERENCES

Barrett, J., & Hodgson, J. (2011). Hospital simulated patient programme: A guide. *The Clinical Teacher, 8*(4), 217–221.

Barrows, H. (2000). *Training standardized patients to have physical findings.* Chicago, IL: Southern Illinois University.

Battles, J., Wilkinson, S., & Lee, S. (2004). Using standardised patients in an objective structured clinical examination as a patient safety tool. *Quality and Safety in Health Care, 13*(Suppl. 1), i46–i50.

Blake, K., Gusella, J., Greaven, S., & Wakefield, S. (2006). The risks and benefits of being a young female adolescent standardised patient. *Medical Education, 40*(1), 26–35.

Boerjan, M., Boone, F., Anthierens, S., van Weel-Baumgarten, E., & Deveugele, M. (2008). The impact of repeated simulation on health and healthcare perceptions of simulated patients. *Patient Education and Counseling, 73*(1), 22–27.

Bokken, L., van Dalen, J., & Rethans, J. (2004). Performance-related stress symptoms in simulated patients. *Medical Education, 38*(10), 1089–1094.

Bokken, L., van Dalen, J., & Rethans, J. (2006). The impact of simulation on people who act as simulated patients: a focus group study. *Medical Education, 40*, 781–786.

Business Dictionary. (2013). *Organizational structure*. Retrieved from http://www.businessdictionary.com/definition/organizational-structure.html#ixzz2OqfGFKQP

Cleland, J. A., Keiko, A., & Rethans, J. (2009). The use of simulated patients in medical education: AMEE Guide No 42. *Medical Teacher, 40*(8), 477–486.

Doyle, L., Murray, J., & Simons, D. (n.d.). *Focusing feedback on interpersonal skills: A workshop for standardized patients.* Charlottesville, VI: University of Virginia School of Medicine.

Erichetti, A., & Boulet, J. (2006). Comparing traditional and computer-based training methods for standardized patients. *Academic Medicine, 81*(10 Suppl.), S91–S94.

Furman, G. (2008). The role of standardized patient and trainer training in quality assurance for a high-stakes clinical skills examination. *The Kaohsiung Journal of Medical Sciences, 24*(12), 651–655.

Hodges, B. (2003). Validity and the OSCE. *Medical Teacher, 25*(3), 250–254.

Ker, J., Dowie, A., Dowell, J., Dewar, G., Dent, J., Ramsay, J., & Jackson, C. (2005). Twelve tips for developing and maintaining a simulated patient bank. *Medical Teacher, 27*(1), 4–9.

Lane, J., Ziv, A., & Boulet, J. (1999). A pediatric clinical skills assessment using children as standardized patients. *Archives of Pediatric and Adolescent Medicine, 153*(6), 637–644.

May, W. (2008). Training standardized patients for a high-stakes clinical performance examination in the California consortium for the assessment of clinical competence. *Kaohsiung Journal of Medical Sciences, 24*(12), 640–645.

May, W., Fisher, D., & Souder, D. (2006). *WinDix training manual for standardized patient trainers: How to give effective feedback.* Retrieved from MedEdPORTAL.

Mollo, E., Reinke, C., Nelson, C., Holena, D., Kann, B., Williams, N., . . . Kelz, R. (2012). The simulated ward: Ideal for training clinical clerks in an era of patient safety. *Journal of Surgical Research, 177*(1), e1–e6.

Oakes, J., Hamburger, M., Kruger, C., & Power, J. (2012). *Ultrasound training of standardized patients for first year introduction to clinical medicine curriculum. 11th Annual Association of Standardized Patient Educators Conference*, San Diego, CA.

Pangaro, L., Worth-Dickstein, H., Macmillan, M., Klass, D., & Shatzer, J. (1997). Performance of "standardized examinees" in a standardized-patient examination of clinical skills. *Academic Medicine, 72*(11), 1008–1011.

Peabody, J., Luck, J., & Peabody, P. (2000). Comparison of vignettes, standardized patients, and chart abstraction: a prospective validation study of 3 methods for measuring quality. *Journal of the American Medical Association, 283*(13), 1715–1722.

Russell, D., Simpson, R., & Rendel, S. (2011). Standardisation of role players for the clinical skills assessment of the MRCGP, 22. *Education for Primary Care, 22*(3), 166–170.

Spencer, J., & Dales, J. (2006). Meeting the needs of simulated patients and caring for the person behind them? *Medical Education, 40*(1), 3–5.

Wagner, D., & Lypson, M. (2009). Centralized assessment in graduate medical education: Cents and sensibilities. *Journal of Graduate Medical Education, 1*(1), 21–27.

Wallace, J., Rao, R., & Haslam, H. (2002). Simulated patients and objective structured clinical examinations: review of their use in medical education. *Advances in Psychiatric Treatment, 8*, 342–350.

Wallace, P. (2006). *Coaching standardized patients for use in the assessment of clinical competence.* New York, NY: Springer.

Wallace, P., Heine, N., Garman, K., Bartos, R., & Richards, A. (1999). Effect of varying amounts of feedback on standardized patient checklist accuracy in clinical practice examinations. *Teaching and Learning in Medicine, 11*, 148–152.

Wind, I. A., van Dalen, J., Muijtjens, A. M., & Rethans, J. (2004). Assessing simulated patients in an educational setting: the MasP (Maastricht Assessment of Simulated Patients). *Medical Education, 38*(1), 39–44.

Woodward, C., & Gliva-McConvey, G. (1995). Children as standardized patients: Initial assessment of effects. *Teaching and Learning in Medicine, 7*(3), 188–191.

Request Form for Use of the Clinical Skills Center

Thank you for your interest in using the CSC. Please fill out the form below as completely and as detailed as possible. Someone will respond to your request within 48 hours (work days) to set up a meeting with the center director.

The CSC has the following features:
- 20 clinical examination rooms with a desktop computer for SP checklist entry
- 20 laptop computers outside the examination rooms for learner postencounter exercises
- Over 80 trained standardized patients
- Various task trainers for teaching procedural skills
- Full-body mannequin simulators (SimMan)
- One-way mirror observation for live viewing by evaluators
- Digital audio/video capture

What simulation modality or modalities are you interested in using?

SPs ☐ Mannequins ☐ Task trainers ☐ <List of available trainers>

Course name/number

Learner group

Learner level

Contact person:

Name

E-mail

Phone

Type of activity:

☐ Testing ☐ Teaching ☐ Other (please describe the activity)

Preferred date of activity (please give a time frame)[*]: Enter a date.

Preferred time of activity (the CSC is open 8–5, M–F)[*]: Enter a time frame

Number of learners

Number of hours available for activity

If using SPs:

Number of SP encounters per learner

Other comments or information: Click here to enter text.

---

[*]Scheduling considerations are based on learner group (medical student activities take priority) and time available on the CSC calendar.

SP Trainer Educational Programs

ASPE Core Curriculum Program to "provide education on the core fundamental knowledge essential for educators in the field of standardized patient methodology." The modules of this program are offered at the ASPE annual conference and as Webinars

(http://aspeducators.org/core-curriculum.php).

ASPE Scholars Certificate Program to "promote the advancement of standardized patient methodology and research through scholarly endeavors by ASPE members"

(http://www.aspeducators.org/scholars-certificate-program.php).

Certificate Program in Standardized-Patient-Based Education. University of Illinois–Chicago Department of Medical Education

(http://chicago.medicine.uic.edu/grahamcpc/professional_development/certificate_program_in_teaching_and_testing_with_s/).

New York College of Osteopathic Medicine MS in Medical/Health Care Simulation Program

(http://www.nyit.edu/medicine/academics/icc/).

Southern Illinois University—"Training and Using Standardized Patients for Teaching and Assessment" workshop

(http://www.aspeducators.org/educator-opportunities.php).

APPENDIX C

Sample SP Trainer/Educator Job Description

Effective Date:	
Job Title	Standardized Patient Educator
Job Code Number	
FLSA Category	Exempt
Job Purpose	Provide administrative and technical expertise to the Standardized Patient (SP) Program by organizing and implementing SP teaching and assessment activities for use in health science center student programs. Development of training and educational materials for SPs and student groups. Monitor and document SP performances. Provide feedback to SPs quarterly regarding job performance.
Education and experience required including training, registration, and licensure	Bachelor's degree in Education, Communication, Human Resources, or related field, with 3 years of experience in the field of assignment. Should have an equivalent combination of relevant education and experience. Will consider extensive professional-level experience in lieu of educational requirement.
Knowledge, Skills, and Abilities	(1) Minimum of 3 years experience in medical field, medical education, and/or SP field. (2) Knowledge and understanding of the use of SPs in medical teaching. (3) Demonstrated ability to recruit, train, supervise, and monitor SPs or part-time employees. (4) Excellent computer, and written and oral communication skills are a must. (5) Demonstrated ability to collaborate and work within a team. (6) Record maintenance skills. (7) Ability to gather and analyze statistical data and generate reports. (8) Ability to determine training objectives. (9) Ability to interpret and assess training and development needs and to develop appropriate and creative responses. (10) Willingness and ability to travel to selected conferences/meetings and occasionally flexibility in work hours.
Supervision	Falls under the supervision of the Director of the Clinical Skills Center. Will be under the direct supervision of the senior SP educator.
Job Functions	
Number	Description
1.	Training of SPs for teaching and assessment of students: (a) Develop training material for SP cases portrayal, including checklist guides. (b) Conduct training sessions for SPs. (c) Assist with employee orientations on policies and procedures.
2.	Monitor SP performance for accuracy and appropriateness of feedback.
3.	Recruit, screen, and interview potential SPs as needed.
4.	Coordinate and supervise teaching and assessment activities involving medical students, interns, residents, physicians, and other health professions using SPs.
5.	Collaborate with senior SP Educator and Center Director to plan, develop, and implement student exercises.
6.	Participate in research and scholarly activities.
7.	Assist the Center Coordinator in maintaining SP database.
8.	Strong attention to detail, organizational skills, and the ability to work under strict deadlines in a fast-paced environment.
9.	Perform other duties as assigned.

This job description in no way states or implies that these are the only duties to be performed by the employee occupying this position. The incumbent is expected to perform other duties necessary for the effective operation of the department. Any qualifications to be considered as equivalents in lieu of stated minimums require prior approval of Human Resources.

APPENDIX D

....

Clinical Skills Center Project Request and Fee Schedule

INSTRUCTIONS:

This worksheet is designed to help you understand and estimate the costs and time involved in developing a clinical skills exercise. To begin, please complete Parts I and II and return to Diane Ferguson. If you have never worked with the Standardized Patient Program before, you may be more comfortable contacting Diane Ferguson, 567-3148, to set up an appointment to review Part III of this form.

Part I: Contact Information

Contact Name:		Dept. Name:		Dept. ID:	
E-mail:		Project ID:		Account:	
Phone:		Authorized Signature:			
			☐ E-mail Approval		

Part II: Activity Details

Section A: Description

Student Group:	☐ Medical	☐ Nursing	☐ PA	☐ Dental	☐ GME	☐ CME	☐ Other
Number of Participants:		Group Year/Level:					
Name of Exercise:							
Exercise Description (i.e., teaching vs. testing):							

Section B: Complete for Standardized Patient Activity Only			Section C: Complete for Simulation Activity Only		
Date(s):			☐ SimMan	Dates/Times:	
Time(s):			☐ Harvey	Dates/Times:	
Number of Cases:					
Time for Each Case:	(minutes)				

Part III: Project Cost Estimate

Section A: General CSC Usage Fees

Room/Center setup and cleanup fee*:		Exam Rooms	×	$15.00	×	Days		=	$0.00
Set up and use, DAVS (Digital Audio/Video System and overhead paging):				$15.00	×	Hours		=	$0.00
Set up and use, TSC (Clinical Skills Training and Evaluation software):				$20.00	×	Hours		=	$0.00
DAVS control personnel (during exercise):				$15.00	×	Hours		=	$0.00
CD creation (labor/materials):				$5.00	×	CDs		=	$0.00
DVD creation (labor/materials):				$15.00	×	DVD's		=	$0.00
Video Shared Folder— 60-Day Subscription (one-time charge):				$10.00		(1 = y, 0 = n)			$0.00
Proctor (No charge if you provide, otherwise one will be provided for you):				$30.00	×	Hours		=	$0.00
Report generation/data analysis (Hours to be determined by CSC Director):				$30.00	×	Hours		=	$0.00

Section B: Standardized Patients												$0.00
SP Training:		# SP's	×	$17.00	×		Hours				=	$0.00
SP Performance:		# SP's	×	$17.00	×		Hours	×		Days	=	$0.00
Evaluators *(additional SP's to score only)*:		# SP's	×	$17.00	×		Hours				=	$0.00
Materials:				$5.00	×		# SP's				=	$0.00
Section C: GU Labs												$0.00
		FRTA	×	$50.00	×		# of Exams				=	$0.00
		MRTA	×	$40.00	×		# of Exams				=	$0.00
GU Room & Materials Fee:		# Exam Rooms	×	$5.00	×		Days				=	$0.00
Section D: SP Trainer												$0.00
Case development *(our template, we write)*:				$50.00	×		Hours				=	$0.00
Case revision *(you write, we make usable)*:				$50.00	×		Hours				=	$0.00
(No charge for cases you write on our template with minimal to no revision/or use cases from our "bank" at no charge)												$0.00
Recruitment and scheduling:				$30.00	×		Hours				=	$0.00
SP training—the cost for the Trainer to train the SP for the role:				$30.00	×		Hours				=	$0.00
(Lesser charge may be applied if course faculty help with training)												$0.00
Section E: Simulator use												$0.00
Special procedures and part replacement costs to be determined with CSC director											=	$0.00
Section F: Miscellaneous												$0.00
Snacks for students				$2.00	×		Students				=	$0.00
Request for nontraditional/additional supplies will be determined on a case-by-case basis											=	$0.00
Grand Total											=	$0.00

*Fee that applies to all activities

APPENDIX E

Example Standardized Patient Program Policy and Procedure Table of Contents

Chapter 2	Organization Information	Effective:	June 2012
Section 2.2	Mission Statement	Revised:	
		Responsibility:	CSC Staff

MISSION

Statement The Clinical Skills Center provides state-of-the-art simulation methodology to support the development of competent and compassionate medical professionals at UTHSCSA.
- Recruit and train qualified individuals as Standardized Patients.

Supporting Statements
- Coordinate activities and programs with faculty and students to obtain/meet educational objectives.
- Maintain staff awareness of ongoing trends in simulation methodology.
- Promote the value of the Clinical Skills Center activities and programs.
- Seek potential users and new growth opportunities.
- Utilize mechanical and computer simulation units advantageous to accomplish educational goals/objectives.

ORGANIZATIONAL CHART

Statement	The Clinical Skills Center is supported by the following staff positions: • Director, Clinical Skills Center • Standardized Patient Educators (2) • CSC Coordinator • Sr. Secretary
Chart	

Chapter 4	Organizational Structure	Effective:	
Section 4.2	Contact information	Revised:	
		Responsibility:	CSC Staff

CONTACT INFORMATION

Contact

Clinical Skills Center
7703 Floyd Curl Drive MSC 7788
San Antonio, TX 78229
Main: 210-567-3101

Diane Ferguson
Director
210-567-3147
fergusond@uthscsa.edu

Nicole Manley
Center Coordinator
210-567-3148
manleyn@uthscsa.edu

Audrey Ortega
Lead SP Educator
210-567-3104
ortegaa3@uthscsa.edu

Kent Coker
SP Educator
210-567-3149
cokerk@uthscsa.edu

Frances Rizo
Senior Secretary
210-567-3101
rizof@uthscsa.edu

Chapter 4	Organizational Structure	Effective:	
Section 4.5	Job Description	Revised:	
	Director	Responsibility:	CSC Staff

THE UNIVERSITY OF TEXAS HEALTH SCIENCE CENTER AT SAN ANTONIO

JOB DESCRIPTION

Administrative and Professional

DIRECTOR OF CLINICAL SKILLS CENTER

FLSA: EXEMPT Job Code: 0746

SUMMARY

This position will be the day-to-day operations officer for the Clinical Skills Center and will manage a large volume of complex administrative and fiscal decisions. Responsibilities include development and implementation of the Clinical Assessment Program for standardized learning, and the development and coordination of a multimedia education learning center, which will include computer-based learning programs, simulation mannequins, and other learning aids for independent and small-group learning. The position will communicate with faculty and staff as well as with community-based organizations to represent UTHSCSA at various assigned committees and panels. Other responsibilities include the coordination of the Center with direction and input from faculty to develop, implement, and manage the learner instructional and assessment projects and faculty development of activities in the Center, management of activities related to administration and fiscal operations of the Center, preparation and submission of required administrative and fiscal reports, development of recommendations regarding appropriate programmatic and academic activities to be conducted at the Center, preparation and submission of grants and other outside funding applications, and supervision and guidance to assigned staff. Position will also be responsible for development and supervision of the Regional Academic Health Center program.

DUTIES

Performs a combination of the following duties:

- Supervises the planning, coordination, development, and administration of Clinical Skills Center policies and procedures.
- Manages all classified personnel activities, including hiring and terminations and supervision of employee evaluation program.
- Creates and operates all aspects of the program, including staff, equipment, and facilities.
- Oversees marketing and public relations for Center.
- Works with faculty to develop clinical scenarios and appropriate evaluation instruments.
- Works with faculty to brief classes and their teachers on SP events, evaluations, and requirements
- Develops and coordinates faculty development programs vis-à-vis Standardized Patients and areas of clinical competency.
- Collaborates with faculty, conducts and publishes educational research.
- Manages fiscal activities, including budget preparation, fiscal reports, requisitions, account management, and accounting system design.
- Prepares contracts and agreements with external organizations and assists with grant preparation.
- Represents the department within the University and with outside organizations.
- Prepares annual and periodic reports.
- Supervises the department's equipment inventory, including space utilization and office equipment.

Supervises the management and implementation of a standardized patient program for the instruction and evaluation of medical students.

Supervises the collection of valuable, reliable, and useful data on the teaching and learning process supporting clinical teaching, assessment, and curricular design.

Seeks grant opportunities for innovative initiatives in medical education.

Training and supervision of the standardized patients and the coordination of the development of all cases in conjunction with clerkship directors and other faculty.

Other duties as assigned.

EDUCATION/EXPERIENCE

Master's or Doctoral degree in education or health-related discipline with 5 years professional experience at the Master's level or 2 years at the Doctorate level, or a Bachelor's degree in a related field, with 7 years job-related business or administrative experience in an educational institution.

KNOWLEDGE, SKILLS, AND ABILITIES

Experience working with medical faculty to develop instructional programs and evaluation instruments; excellent written and oral communication skills; knowledge of medical interviewing, physical examination skills, and disease processes desirable; experience in training patient simulators for educational uses or equivalent desirable; ability to work directly with faculty during case development, evaluation, and revision process.

Ability to read and interpret professional journals, financial reports, and legal documents as necessary. Ability to write reports, business correspondence, and procedural manuals. Ability to effectively present information and respond to questions from groups of supervisors, customers, and the public. Ability to communicate technical concepts and thoughts to management. Ability to apply moderately complex mathematical equations as applicable. Ability to define problems, collect data, establish facts, and draw valid conclusions. Ability to interpret an extensive variety of technical instructions and deal with several abstract and concrete variables. Familiarity with medical terminology and/or laws, ability to work with spreadsheet and database software, and knowledge of healthcare, accounting systems, hospital human resources, and grants management.

RELATED WORK EXPERIENCE

Desirable related work experience in physician assistant training, nurse practitioner, acting/directing experience, or teaching; experience in managing projects with excellent writing and communication skills. Other: Ability to work flexible hours to administer evening and weekend workshops, courses, exams, and other meetings; basic computer literacy, familiarity with audio/video equipment would be helpful.

SUPERVISION

Received:
Work is performed under the general direction of the Associate Dean for Academic Affairs.

Given:
Provides direct and indirect supervision and management of employees in the center. Incumbent is responsible for preparing an operational budget. Additionally, is directly responsible for hiring and terminating, scheduling and assigning work, measuring performance, promoting, and determining pay.

EQUIPMENT

Personal computer and other standard office equipment.

WORKING CONDITIONS

Work is performed in an office environment.

The above statements are intended to describe the general nature and level of work performed by people assigned to this classification. They are not intended to be construed as an exhaustive list of all responsibilities, duties, and skills required of personnel so classified. Management retains the right to add or to change the duties of the position at any time.

IMPORTANT

Any qualifications to be considered as equivalents in lieu of stated minimums require prior approval of the Assistant Vice President for Human Resources.

In accordance with The University of Texas Health Science Center at San Antonio policy (HOP-Section 4.4.1), job candidates for all health science center positions must undergo a criminal background check before a job offer is made and before the candidate can begin to work.

Information resources, including data, information, technology, and software, are University resources and must be protected and used in conformance with all applicable laws and policies in accordance with 1TAC 201.13(b) Information Security Standards.

Chapter 4	Organizational Structure	Effective:	July 2010
Section 4.5	Job Descriptions	Revised:	July 21, 2010
Policy 4.5.1	**Clinical Skills Center Coordinator**	Responsibility:	CSC Staff

Position Description 9261: Management Analyst > Information Technology > Information

Technology Operations > Operations

Provide analytical support in the implementation and evaluation of departmental technology and systems, program planning and research, financial analysis, and special projects. Responsibilities include assisting with comprehensive written analysis, strategies for implementation, and system enhancements. Conducts qualitative and quantitative analysis of departmental functions and procedures by using organizational analysis and cost-benefit analysis. Conducts systems analysis, including fiscal and feasibility studies. Writes comprehensive and complex proposals/plans, including areas of cost and implementation. Conducts program and documentation evaluations and interpretation. Proposes and recommends operating alternatives for effecting uniformity and consistency across several departments that improve the operational effectiveness of the work unit. Works with other departmental personnel and external groups in analysis planning. Bachelor's degree in

Business Administration, Information Systems, or related field, with 3 years of experience in accounting, financial analysis, or related field. Under FLSA, incumbents in this position are exempt.

SCHOOL OF MEDICINE UT HEALTH SCIENCE CENTER™ SAN ANTONIO WE MAKE LIVES BETTER	The University of Texas Health Science Center at San Antonio Office of the Dean JOB DESCRIPTION

Job Title	Training Specialist (Soft title: Standardized Patient Educator)
Job Code Number	8110
FLSA Category	Exempt
Job Purpose	Provide administrative and technical expertise to the Standardized Patient (SP) Program by organizing and implementing SP teaching and assessment activities for use in health science center student programs. Development of training and educational materials for SPs and student groups. Monitor and document SP performances. Provide feedback to SPs quarterly regarding job performance.
Education and experience required, including training, registration, and licensure	Bachelor's degree in Education, Administration, Human Resources, Public Administration, or related field, with 3 years of experience in the field of assignment. Have an equivalent combination of relevant education and experience. Will consider extensive professional-level experience in lieu of educational requirement.
Knowledge, Skills, and Abilities	(1) Minimum of 4 years of experience in medical education and/or SP Training. (2) Knowledge and understanding of the use of Standardized Patients in medical teaching. (3) Demonstrated ability to recruit, train, supervise, and monitor Standardized Patients. (4) Excellent computer and written and oral communication skills are a must. (5) Demonstrated ability to collaborate and work within a team.

Job Functions	
Number	**Description**
1.	Training of SPs for teaching and assessment sessions: (a) Develop training material for SP cases portrayal, including checklist guides. (b) Conduct training sessions for SPs. (c) Assist with SP orientations on policies and procedures.
2.	Monitor SP performance for accuracy and appropriateness of feedback.
3.	Recruit, screen, and interview potential SPs as needed.
4.	Assist in administrative and technical duties for SP Programs: (a) Assist the Admin Assistant in maintaining SP database (b) Assist in all technical and logistical requirements for SP sessions.
5.	Collaborate with Center Director to plan, develop, and implement student exercises.
6.	Participate in research and scholarly activities.
7.	Perform other duties as assigned.

This job description in no way states or implies that these are the only duties to be performed by the employee occupying this position. The incumbent is expected to perform other duties necessary for the effective operation of the department. Any qualifications to be considered as equivalents in lieu of stated minimums require prior approval of Human Resources.

This job class may contain positions that are security-sensitive and thereby subject to the provisions of Texas Education Code §51.215.

Chapter 4	Organizational Structure	Effective:	
Section 4.5	Job Descriptions	Revised:	
Policy 4.5.4	**Senior Secretary**	Responsibility:	CSC Staff

SCHOOL OF MEDICINE UT HEALTH SCIENCE CENTER SAN ANTONIO	The University of Texas Health Science Center at San Antonio Office of the Dean JOB DESCRIPTION

Effective Date: 05/21/09	
Job Title	Senior Secretary (Clinical Skills Center)
Job Code Number	9041
FLSA Category	Nonexempt
Job Purpose	This is a general-level position primarily responsible for secretarial duties such as typing routine to moderately difficult documents, filing, entering data, making travel arrangements, scheduling staff meetings when requested, greeting visitors, maintaining calendars, answering phones, and opening and distributing mail. May work for nonsupervisory staff or in a secretarial pool.
Education and experience required, includingtraining, registration, and licensure	High-school diploma or GED plus 1 year of secretarial or typing and clerical experience. Secretarial vocational training may be substituted for 1 year of secretarial or typing and clerical experience.
Knowledge, Skills, and Abilities	Knowledge of personal computers and software, including word processing and spreadsheet applications. Knowledge in using calculators and other standard office equipment. Computer skills such as document formation, reformatting, editing, proofreading, storing, retrieving, and printing. Knowledge of correct grammar, spelling, and punctuation. Basic knowledge of medical and/or research terminology. Ability to communicate both verbally and in writing. Interpersonal skills, including knowledge of standard office etiquette. Work schedule flexibility: occasional early mornings, after 5.00 p.m., and weekends will be required.
Supervision	**Received:** Work is performed under general supervision. Incumbent proceeds on own initiative within policy or procedure limits established by the supervisor. Desired results are clearly defined, and work is reviewed upon completion for accuracy, quality, and completeness. New or unfamiliar situations are referred to the supervisor. **Given:** None

Job Functions	
Number	**Description**
1.	Types, proofreads, and edits documents such as manuscripts, reports, letters, forms, research articles, and other types of documents and special projects.
2.	Composes routine correspondence such as form letters, acknowledgments, and notes.
3.	Maintains office filing system.
4.	Answers all incoming calls: assists callers, routes calls to appropriate staff member, and/or takes accurate phone messages.
5.	Sorts and distributes incoming mail.
6.	Prints, copies, collates, staples, and distributes materials to staff, SPs, and students.
7.	Makes travel arrangements and reservations.
8.	Greets all incoming visitors: faculty, staff, students, and outside vendors.
9.	Maintains appointment calendar and schedules appointments.
10.	Orders, stocks, and maintains office/medical supplies or equipment.
11.	Assists with the SP Educators with the coordination of SP program activities by distributing schedules and e-mail/phone SP work schedule reminders.
12.	Assists CSC staff with prepping, setup, and breakdown of CSC activities to include materials, equipment, proctoring, and other duties as assigned.
13.	Schedules practice time for students on CSC Calendar.
14.	Prepares service request forms and catering request for the department.
15.	Laundry Service to include weekly collecting, sorting, delivery, and picking up linens.
16.	Assists the Coordinator and SP Educators with maintaining and updating CSC Activity binders and materials.
17.	Assists the Director, Coordinator, and SP Educators with maintaining and updating SP and Student data.
18.	Assists the Director, Coordinator, and SP Educators with special projects.

19.	CSC Website maintenance and updates.
20.	Performs other duties as assigned.

This job description in no way states or implies that these are the only duties to be performed by the employee occupying this position. The incumbent is expected to perform other duties necessary for the effective operation of the department. Any qualifications to be considered as equivalents in lieu of stated minimums require prior approval of Human Resources.

This job class may contain positions that are security-sensitive and thereby subject to the provisions of Texas Education Code §51.215.

Expectation/Overview of Policies for Front Desk

- Lunch between 11:00 a.m. and 1:00 p.m. Adjustments will be made to lunch schedule on the basis of business needs for front desk support—that is, if an activity starts at 12:30 p.m., will be required to be at desk at 12:30 p.m.
- 1 hour for lunch or 30 minutes and two 15-minute breaks.
- Cannot work over 40 hours per week without prior approval.
- Work schedule is 8:00 a.m. to 5:00 p.m. Will receive advance notice by Diane Ferguson if needed outside of these hours. All adjustments to work schedule must be requested and approved in advance with Diane Ferguson. Will not be able to take vacation hours during first 6 months of employment without prior approval (UTHSCSA policy). Personal leave hours can be used, but prior approval is required.
- At lunch time, put up "out to lunch" sign at desk—must not take lunch at desk.

Chapter 4	Administration and Organization	Effective:	July 2010
Section 4.6	Staff Recruitment	Revised:	July 21, 2010
Policy 4.6.1	**Staff Recruitment**	Responsibility:	CSC Staff

TO:		Dr. A		Dr. D
		Dr. B		Dr. E
		Dr. C		
FROM:		Michael Black		
DATE:		October 29, 2008		
SUBJECT:		Pre-Approval Process to Recruit Non-Faculty New and/or Replacement Positions		

Effective this date and until further notice, a new procedure for hiring *non-faculty* new and/or replacement positions has been put in place. All *non-faculty* positions irrespective of the funding source must have pre-approval prior to the establishment of a job posting and recruitment strategy.

Challenging economic times and events in our nation require institutions such as ours to re-assess costs, revenues, reduce expenses, and evaluate how work can be better accomplished while increasing organizational effectiveness and efficiencies.

Sour resource stewardship is a key responsibility of every Health Science Center leader. In support of these activities, the Deans have agreed to establish a procedure for requesting approval for the hiring of *non-faculty* new and/or replacement positions, irrespective of the planned funding source(s). The Vice Presidents initiated this policy in November of 2007. This is how the procedure works:

1. When a new and/or replacement position is identified for recruitment, hiring supervisors contact their HR Consultant in the Office of Human Resources (OHR). Various strategies are explored to indentify the most cost effective solution. If that solution is to recruit for the new position or replacement, the hiring supervisor completes a Request for Approval to Recruit (attached.) This form can be found, completed on line and printed for signatures at http://www.uthscsa.edu/hr/pdfs/req_app_recruit.pdf.
2. Once completed, the Request is forwarded to the Dean and/or his or her designee, who must be a Senior Leader, for approval/disapproval.
3. If approved, the Request is forwarded to OHR. The hiring authority is contacted and the job posted.
4. If not approved, the Request is returned to the hiring authority, at which time he or she are encouraged to re-contact the HR Consultant to explore other remedies.

This procedure is to be followed under the following circumstances:

- Neet to recruit for a new and/or replacement position
- Position reclassifications resulting in a salary increase

PLEASE NOTE: This procedure *does not* apply to:

- faculty recruitments
- current job openings posted prior to the date of this memo

This procedure is not intended to substitute or replace other internal school/research/clinical/business unit processes. Please do not hesitate to contact me or Mary Maher should you have any questions with respect to this change of procedure.

Chapter 4	Clinical Skills Center: SP	Effective:	July 2010
Section 4.1	Pay Rate	Revised:	July 21, 2010
Policy 4.1.1	**Pay Rate**	Responsibility:	CSC Staff

PATIENT PAY RATE

Statement	The Clinical Skills Center pay rate policy for the following positions: • GU Patient • Standardized Patient • New Hire Standardized Patient

Pay Rate	• GU Female Patient
	  • Breast and Pelvic Exam
	    • $50 per student
	    • $50 per preceptor—only paid for one preceptor per day
	  • Breast only Exam (with no pelvic exam)
	    • $25 per student
	    • Not paid for preceptor breast examination
	• GU Male Patient
	  • $40 per student
	  • $40 per preceptor—only paid for one preceptor per day
	• Standardized Patient (SP)
	  • Training: $15 per hour
	  • Performance: $15 per hour
	• New Hire Standardized Patient
	  • Training: $15 per hour—training hours are not paid to a new hire SP until their first performance is completed, within 30 days.
	  • Performance: $15 per hour

Chapter 4	Clinical Skills Center: SP	Effective:	July 2010
Section 4.2	Timekeeping/Timesheets	Revised:	July 21, 2010
Policy 4.2.1	**Timekeeping/Timesheets**	Responsibility:	Nicole Manley

TIMEKEEPING/TIMESHEETS

Statement	The Clinical Skills Center timekeeping policy: Exempt staff positions turn in monthly timesheets to the Medical Dean's office administration—generated by the Medical Dean's office administration: • Director, Clinical Skills Center • CSC Coordinator • SP Educators • Senior Secretary Nonexempt staff positions turn in: • Weekly timesheet to Director • Weekly timesheet to Medical Dean's office • Monthly timesheet to Medical Dean's office

Signing In/ Out on Session Timesheet Log	Hourly positions (Standardized Patients) will be required and responsible for signing in/out following the guidelines below:
	
	• Sign in/out on activity sign-in sheet prepared by SP Educator.
	• Must sign in with schedule start time along with initialing next to entry and no sooner. If the SP arrives before schedule time, they may complete log but CANNOT write arrival time, but can only write schedule start time.
	  • Example: If the schedule start time is 12:30 p.m. and the SP arrives at SP lounge at 11:45 a.m., then must write 12:30 p.m. on log.
	• When the SP arrives past schedule start time, they are required to write the ACTUAL arrival time.
	  • Example: If the schedule start time is 12:30 p.m. and the SP arrives at 12:35 p.m., then the SP is required to write 12:35 p.m. on log.
	• Must sign out with actual sign-out time along with signing name next to entry.
	• Timekeeping will be reported following guidelines below:
	  • Time will be reported in 15-minute increments.
	  • Minutes will be rounded down/up to the nearest 15-minute increment.
	    • ≤7 rounded down and ≥8 rounded up
	      • :00–:07 = :00
	      • :08–17 = :15
	      • :18–:37 = :30
	      • :38–:47 = :45
	      • :48–1:00 = 1:00
	    • Examples:
	      • SP logs in at 12:32 p.m.—will be rounded down to 12:30 p.m. SP logs in at 12:38 p.m. will be rounded up to 12:45 p.m.
	      • SP logs out at 1:37 p.m. will be rounded down to 1:30 p.m. SP logs out at 1:38 p.m. will be rounded up to 1:45 p.m.

| Hourly Payroll Report and Administration | Hourly employee payroll will be processed as follows:
• SP Educators/Sr. Secretary will prepare sign-in log sheets.
• SP Educator will make any corrections as needed, including an explanation of corrections on log.
  • Example: SP writes the incorrect time or does not sign out.
• SP Educator will give all logs to Sr. Secretary to complete calculations.
• Sr. Secretary enters hours to be paid on CSC payroll spreadsheet (located at CSC Shared Drive) and use payroll calculator to determine the number of hours to be paid. Calculator accounts for rounding up/down on the basis of procedures above.
• Sr. Secretary will then provide CSC coordinator with the report by payroll deadline.
• CSC coordinator will audit the report and enter hours to be paid into UTHSCSA timekeeping system.
• Reports and all sign-in logs will be maintained in binder and kept by Sr. Secretary for reference. |

APPENDIX F

Sample SP Case Template

H-E-B- CLINICAL SKILLS CENTER

UT HEALTH SCIENCE CENTER™

SAN ANTONIO

SP Case

Learner Group:

Learner Level:

Course number:

Case name:

Author

6/7/2014

<u>General guidelines for use</u>

Case objectives and competencies to be evaluated must be included.

If the case is not problem/symptom-based, feel free to delete the "symptom" boxes and use the description text box.

You may delete any of the sections that do not apply.

The SP portrayal is always enhanced with more information rather than less.

Attach any related articles or insert hyperlinks for educational purposes if it will clarify your vision.

STANDARDIZED PATIENT CASE

Learner and Level:	Formative or Summative:
Time with SP:	Time for checklist, PEQ, a/o feedback:

Chief Complaint/Presenting Problem:	
Actual Diagnosis (if applies):	
Author(s):	
Case Objectives: (Should be clear and measurable)	(Please include what competency(s) is to be evaluated, e.g., Communication skills, History taking, etc. as well as course or other objectives.)
Patient name:	
Patient demographics:	
Who will evaluate this encounter?	SP only (SP plays role and then evaluates examinee) SP and faculty Faculty only SP observer (watches the encounter and scores in real time)
Will the learner get verbal feedback from the SP?	

SP RECRUITMENT GUIDE

Age (range):
Gender:
Race/ethnicity (understand that we may not have all ethnicities at the age you need):
Approximate height, weight, general stature, physical condition (please do not get too specific; short/tall, over/underweight, in good shape, etc.):
Should any real medical conditions rule out an SP (previous appendectomy, for instance)?
Other important role information:

STANDARDIZED PATIENT SCRIPT

Chief Complaint/Presenting Problem:	
Patient Name/demographics:	
Case Setting:	E.g., Clinic, ED, hospital
Type of Encounter:	E.g., new patient, follow-up, emergent
OPENING STATEMENT (SP to volunteer):	

HISTORY OF PRESENT ILLNESS

CHIEF COMPLAINT:	
Onset:	
Location:	
Duration:	
Severity:	
Character/radiation:	
Timing/frequency:	
What makes it better:	
What makes it worse:	
Associated symptoms:	(You can expand the X description below)

Associated symptom X:	
Onset:	
Location:	
Duration:	
Severity:	
Character/radiation:	

Timing/frequency:	
What makes it better:	
What makes it worse:	
Associated symptoms:	

Associated symptom X:	
Onset:	
Location:	
Duration:	
Severity:	
Character/radiation:	
Timing/frequency:	
What makes it better:	
What makes it worse:	
Associated symptoms:	

DESCRIPTION OF SP ROLE

Case purpose:	(E.g., DBN, evaluation of teaching or counseling, etc.)
Problem:	(Why is the SP in the room?)
SP role and expectation(s):	(Description of the case, what the SP should do, how they should act, what they should ask/answer)

OTHER RELEVANT/IMPORTANT INFORMATION:

Past medical/surgical history:	
Current medications: (Include OTC and routine; length of use; reason for taking, etc.)	
Family history:	Parents: Siblings:

HEALTH MAINTAINENCE AND PREVENTION

Allergies:	
Health Screening: Men: >50 Women: <45, >45	
Exercise:	
Sleep:	
Diet:	
Weight change:	
Tobacco/Alcohol/Drug use:	
Sexual history/activity:	

SOCIAL HISTORY

Occupation:	Environmental exposure?
Relationship status:	
Children:	
Stressors:	
Cultural/Spiritual issues:	
Safety issues:	

PHYSICAL CHARACTERISTICS/EXAM

SP General Appearance:	(Gown vs. professional dress, well groomed vs. unkempt)
SP Body Language/Mood/Affect:	
Pertinent Physical findings: The student has to perform the exam and perform it correctly to get this information.	(SP must be able to simulate—such as pain—tell the SP exactly how to describe the finding OR the PE information can be included with the postencounter exercise)

SP Prop(s) (anything to improve realism—bag of pill bottles, moulage, etc.):	
Special supplies or other props needed in the exam room for this case:	(Male prostate model, X-ray, etc.)

SP or Observer Checklist:

Please let me know if you need an example. We have an interpersonal/communication skills checklist and a PE checklist that we prefer you use because the SPs are trained specifically to them already.

SCENARIO

(Pre-encounter information for learner)	
CC:	
Setting:	
Vital signs:	BP P R T
Notes:	
Student assignment:	**15 minutes with patient:** Take a history and perform a physical exam relative to the patient's chief complaint(s).
	10 minutes for write-up: Answer the postencounter questions on the computer.

APPENDIX G

SAMPLE BLUEPRINT

OSCE Matrix: MS3 IM Clerkship skills performance evaluation						
Cases Competencies	Case 1	Case 2	Case 3	Case 4	Case 5	
Data gathering, counseling[1] (What should they do?)	HPI and review of lab results	CV exam				
Documentation[2] (What should they note?)	Assessment and Plan	Dx Workup				
Interpersonal & Communication Skills[3] (What should they say?)	Acknowledge pt. fear	Recognize acute situation				
Professionalism[4] (How should they behave?)	Respect pt. decision	Maintain calm in stressful situation				

[1] **Data gathering skills** that result in efficient but detailed information gathering/sharing and appropriate choice of physical examination maneuvers.

[2] **Documentation skills** that effectively convey the essence of the interview/examination while relaying critical information and next steps to other healthcare providers.

[3] **Interpersonal and communication skills** that result in effective information exchange and teaming with patients, their families, and other health professionals.

[4] **Professionalism** as manifested through a commitment to carrying out professional responsibilities, adherence to ethical principles, and sensitivity to a diverse patient population.

Adapted from: Bingham, M. H. A., Quinn, D. C., Richardson, M. G., Miles, P. V., Gabbe, S. G. (2005). Using a healthcare matrix to assess patient care in terms of aims for improvement and core competencies. *Journal on Quality and Patient Safety, 31*(2), 98–105.

APPENDIX H

RESOURCES FOR THE SP MANAGER

Association of American Medical Colleges: https://www.aamc.org/

Group on Information Resources (GIR): Simulation in Academic Medicine Special Interest Group

Association of Medical Education in Europe: http://amee.org/

Association of Standardized Patient Educators: http://www.aspeducators.org/

Association for the Study of Medical Education (in Europe) (ASME): www.asme.org.uk

Best Evidence Medical and Health Professional Education: www.bemecollaboration.org

California Simulation Alliance (CSA): www.californiasimulationalliance.org

Foundation for Advancement of International Medical Education and Research: http://www.faimer.org/

International Nursing Association for Clinical Simulation and Learning: https://inacsl.org/

MedEdCentral: http://www.amee.org/index.asp?pg=29

MedEdPORTAL: www.mededportal.org

Society in Europe for Simulation Applied to Medicine (SESAM): http://www.sesam-web.org/

Society for Simulation in Healthcare: http://ssih.org/

The Simulation Studio: http://www.meetup.com/The-SP-Studio/member/18563871/

To learn about or brush up on business affairs, healthcare, and science, look for free massive open online courses (MOOCs) such as https://www.coursera.org/ and https://www.udacity.com/.

CHAPTER 5.6

Simulation Alliances, Networks, and Collaboratives

Juli C. Maxworthy, DNP, MSN, MBA, RN, CNL, CPHQ, CPPS, CHSE and KT Waxman, DNP, MBA, RN, CNL, CENP

ABOUT THE AUTHORS

JULI C. MAXWORTHY is the former Director of the Simulation Center at Holy Names University and currently serves as the Chair of the Simulation Committee at the University of San Francisco Dr. Maxworthy is a registered nurse with a strong critical care clinical background and has advanced degrees in nursing administration, business, quality, and patient safety. She is currently the Vice Chair for the Society for Simulation in Healthcare (SSH) Accreditation Council and has been a Reviewer of simulation programs since 2010. Her last clinical role was that of Vice President of Quality/Patient Safety and Risk.

KT WAXMAN Assistant Professor and Chair, Healthcare Leadership and Innovations Department at University of San Francisco School of Nursing and Health Professions. She is also Director of the masters in Healthcare Simulation Program. She is the Director of the California Simulation Alliance through the California Institute for Nursing and Healthcare. KT served as co-chair for the 2013 International Meeting on Simulation in Healthcare (IMSH) and is a member of the oversight, publication and leadership committees for the SSH.

ABSTRACT

Simulation programs around the world are similar, yet unique. They all share a common goal of educating healthcare workers in a manner that ultimately enhances patient outcomes. These programs can be expensive to implement and sustain. Working with others in a collaborative way can streamline processes, maximize the use of resources, and help faculty avoid reinventing the wheel. Collaboration on a global basis opens up opportunities for teams to share resources, leverage individual research strengths, and apply or test theories and ideas across a broad range of environments. In this chapter, multiple models of alliances, networks, and collaboratives at the regional, state, national, and international level will be described as well as tools to provide a framework for success in developing an alliance.

CASE EXAMPLE

Laura, the newly appointed a manager of the local simulation program, has just relocated to Shufflerville and is unfamiliar with the community. As an experienced leader in this community, you know there are several choices she can make in regard to maximizing her simulation program. She can apply lessons she has learned from her previous place of employment and hope that doing so is effective. You know this approach does not always work well.

As a passionate supporter of the use of simulation in education of healthcare professionals, you have a vested interest in Laura's success. You have deep roots in the local simulation community and decide to call her and offer your assistance. Before making the call, you stop, ponder, and decide to make a list of actions you will recommend to Laura. The number one item on the list is to join the regional simulation network. What rationale will you give her for doing so?

INTRODUCTION AND BACKGROUND

Ultimately, regardless of the educational focus, bringing groups together to achieve common goals is what we need to do to improve the overall quality of educational programming in our communities. As communities of interest evolve, the needs of those involved change. Being connected through different formal and informal mechanisms facilitates growth and positive change. These interactions among individuals and groups can range in form

SECTION 5 • Management

423

from simple communication to formal organizational structures.

Groups typically coalesce around a common goal, purpose, or need and can be very useful to the region they serve. In the simulation community, common goals include enhancing the quality of simulation-based education, creating efficient methods of operating a simulation program, or learning to leverage limited resources. Groups could be interested in sharing equipment, space, scenarios, faculty, or staff. The possibilities for collaboration in simulation are endless.

There are several terms that are frequently used when describing forms of collaborative working between two or more organizations. In the simulation literature, these terms include alliance, consortium, coalition, network, and collaborative. There are subtle linguistic distinctions inherent in terms that are often neglected, but they do exist. For example:

Alliance is a term used to describe a purposeful relationship between organizations. Typically, they are developed in a more formal manner and are focused on a particular mission or issue. Alliances are often formed as a means to develop or influence policy.

Coalitions are a form of an alliance of organizations where the organization may have diverse missions but they seek to gain benefits that might not be achieved separately.

Collaboratives typically involve the exchange of information, a willingness to alter individual activities to accomplish a common good, sharing of resources, and expanding capacity of those in the group.

Consortia (consortiums) have the same goal as coalitions—to gain benefits they would not otherwise achieve—but typically, the organizations have a common mission.

Networks are typically loosely structured and allow for making connections and the voluntary sharing of ideas and, potentially, resource.

For purposes of generalizing in this chapter, the overarching phrase of alliances, networks, and collaboratives will be used. Regardless of the term used for the resultant group, when simulation stakeholders work together, organizations and individuals benefit from being able to share knowledge, financial and educational resources, and ideas to train large numbers of students and professionals, as well as provide training for simulation educators (Jeffries & Battin, 2012). By bringing multiple academia and service organizations together with other stakeholders, resources can be consolidated, and effective partnerships can emerge. Collaboration can begin internal to the organization, bringing interprofessional groups together to create scenarios, and agree on learning objectives and overall simulation strategies. This is a good first step to gain organizational buy-in, which can lead to success.

Bringing leaders together to develop strategies, partnerships, and coordinate resources is key to leveraging

assets across a particular geographic area (Eder-Van Hook, 2004). Collaborative efforts among simulation programs have been in existence for as long as there have been programs. However, formalizing these efforts over large geographic areas is a recent phenomenon.

SIGNIFICANCE

It is critical in this time of rapid healthcare change that individuals and groups work together for the betterment of those they serve. As healthcare simulation is a relatively new industry with specific content and expertise required, the importance of developing connections with others who have similar interests cannot be stressed enough. There are a variety of published models and tools that exist that can assist in designing an effective and efficient entity for collaboration among groups. The Agency for Healthcare Research and Quality (AHRQ, 2013) has developed a toolkit for community quality collaboratives that works well for potential simulation alliances. These tools work off the premise that an alliance has specific life stages. These stages include vision, growth, establishment, extension, and rebooting. Figure 5.6.1 depicts the life cycle of an alliance.

The growth of simulation programs throughout the world is due in large part to the collaborative nature of the work and the efforts of simulation groups to work together to achieve common goals. Simulation programs that do not connect with the resources that can be found within their community of interest often struggle unnecessarily.

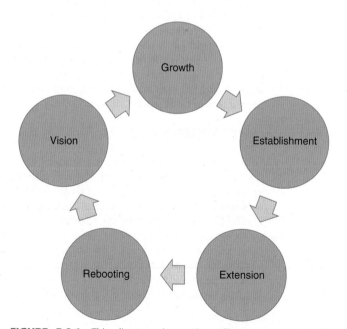

FIGURE 5.6.1 This diagram shows the different stages, including vision, growth, establishment, extension, and rebooting. (From Agency for Healthcare Research and Quality. [2013]. *Sustainability for community quality collaboratives. An overview of the art & science of building staying power.* Retrieved from http://www.ahrq.gov/legacy/qual/value/suscqcollab1.htm#managing)

TABLE 5.6.1

Sample Questions for a Regional or Statewide Needs Assessment

1. Do you have a simulation program at your institution?
2. Are you from a school or hospital or other?
3. What type of simulators do you use?
   a. Laerdal
   b. CAE/Meti
   c. Gaumard
   d. Standardized patients
   e. Other
4. Where did you obtain your simulation scenarios?
   a. Wrote our own
   b. Purchased from a vendor
   c. Purchased from publisher
   d. NLN
   e. CSA
   f. Other
5. Do you have dedicated space for your simulation lab?
6. If yes, what is the square footage?
7. Do you have dedicated faculty for your simulation program?
8. Have your faculty been trained in simulation?
9. If yes, where were they trained?
10. If yes, how many FTEs?
11. Would you be interested in collaborating with others in your region who are conducting simulations?
12. Would you be interested in meeting in person once a month with others with common interests?
13. Would you be willing to host a meeting at your facility?
14. What do you see as the top three needs of a regional collaborative?
    a. Research
    b. Space sharing
    c. Equipment sharing
    d. Scenario development
    e. Best practice identification and sharing
    f. Policy and procedure development
    g. Other

To meet the needs of the community, regardless of the structure of the group, the group should complete a needs assessment (see Table 5.6.1 for an example of a Needs Assessment survey). After the stakeholders have been clearly identified, successful simulation groups report that they developed an initial survey and sent it to stakeholders for input. These surveys provided the necessary information about the available resources, people, equipment, and needs within their community. By leveraging these resources, successful simulation alliances, networks, and collaboratives have been able to provide additional educational courses to meet the needs of the community.

Many simulation programs are now working together as integrated systems. Learners from different professional disciplines are therefore able to gain experience in learning as part of an interprofessional team. These interprofessional educational experiences provide the means by which those from different areas of healthcare can learn to appreciate the strengths and contributions others bring to patient outcomes.

An additional benefit of working together is that these organized groups can collect information such as a directory of simulation sites and faculty, types of equipment at each site, scenarios, and so on.

EXAMPLES OF REGIONAL ALLIANCES, NETWORKS, AND COLLABORATIVES

Throughout the world, simulation alliances, networks, and collaboratives have been developed to assist those new and experienced in the field connect in ways that provide optimal experiences for their learners. The following examples demonstrate how successful alliances, networks, and collaboratives were born and sustained.

California, USA

The Bay Area Simulation Collaborative

The Bay Area Simulation Collaborative (BASC) was launched in 2006 and encompassed the counties surrounding the San Francisco Bay Area in California, USA. The project received start-up funding from the Gordon and Betty Moore Foundation (GBMF) and is managed by the California Institute for Nursing & Health Care (CINHC). Three specific objectives guide the work of this group (Waxman & Telles, 2009).

1. To develop a faculty development program for the 35 schools of nursing and 65 hospitals in the Bay Area.
2. To develop an evidence-based scenario template and write scenarios together to share among the community.
3. To conduct a research study on simulation.

This successful collaboration of schools and hospitals was the first formalized urban simulation group in the country. It has served as a demonstration model for other collaboratives in the state, country, and around the world.

The California Simulation Alliance

Leveraging the success of the BASC, the California Simulation Alliance (CSA) was developed in 2008 as a virtual alliance to benefit all healthcare simulation users in California. Led by the CINHC, the purpose of the CSA is to "enhance and foster the development of simulation as a modality for transforming the education of nurses and other healthcare professionals" (CSA, n.d.). The overarching framework for the alliance includes a governance structure, core committees serving the state, and interfaces with seven regional collaboratives that engage local communities in networking and fostering shared partnerships.

The seven regional collaboratives are the Rural Northern Area Simulation Collaborative (RNASC); the Capital Area Simulation Collaborative (CASC); the BASC; the Central Valley Simulation Collaborative (CVSC); the Southern California Simulation Collaborative (SCSC), which was funded by Kaiser Permanente Community Benefits Program replicating the work of the BASC; and the San Diego Simulation

Collaborative (SDSC), partially funded by the Employment Development Department through the State of California.

The CSA strives to be a cohesive voice for simulation in nursing and healthcare education in California. It does this through interorganizational research, dissemination of information on simulation to stakeholders, and providing a vehicle for creating a common language for facilitating the advancement and expansion of simulation programs and methods.

Additionally, the Alliance provides a source for best practice identification and a forum for information sharing including leadership for faculty development and in the coordination of a range of novice to expert classes for emerging simulation faculty. Subscribers to the CSA also benefit from access to resources for equipment/vendor pricing agreements, and a repository of scenarios, which have been validated and tested.

Integrating simulation into academic and service curricula serving multidisciplinary teams and transforming learning is essential to the success of simulation programs. The CSA shares best practice models for successful curriculum integration, holds workshops on this process, and provides consultation to hospitals for the integration of simulation into their patient safety programs to meet priority patient safety imperatives.

Since launching the CSA in 2008, initial grant-funded investments have been leveraged to expand the resources available. Significant progress has been made in setting up and providing key programs as a foundation for simulation users in academic and service settings across California. The CSA built a faculty development program using Benner's Novice to Expert model. To date, that program has identified and trained 16 individuals as CSA faculty, providing an average of 12 classes each year conducted in various locations across the state. Over 2,000 faculty, clinical educators, and providers have been trained through attending one or more of these faculty development classes.

Specialized simulation programs were identified and prepared as Apprentice Sites to provide individualized coaching and mentoring of emerging simulation faculty. Thus far, 16 individuals have completed the Apprentice program. The curriculum for this program was obtained from SimHealth Consultants in Oregon and adopted by each site. Two Apprentice Sites were identified in northern California: the Center for Advanced Pediatric and Perinatal Education (CAPE) at Stanford, and Samuel Merritt University, an interprofessional healthcare university. Two were identified in southern California: Providence Little Company of Mary Medical Center in Torrance, and Loma Linda University in Loma Linda, a medical and nursing school in an academic medical center.

Over 75 evidence-based simulation scenarios have been developed and made available for use as one of the CSA subscriber benefits. Scenarios include general med/surg, pediatrics, OB, critical care, first responders, LGBTQ, home care and leadership. A newsletter is prepared and sent out every other month to 3,000 contacts on the CSA list serve. A website was launched in 2011 (https://www .californiasimulationalliance.org). Initially hosted for 3 years by Education Management Solutions (EMS), the site has a dedicated section for each of the seven collaboratives. The website is hosted by EMS as an in-kind contribution to the CSA. The website also includes the simulation course calendar and provides links to key simulation resources.

Outcomes from the initial work of the CSA now serve as a framework for more focused development. With the provision of targeted resources, implementation of new educational programs and projects in collaboration with the established network of simulation programs with the provision of targeted resources will strengthen the advancement of simulation programs across both service and academic settings. In the next phase of development, CSA is well positioned to leverage prior grant-funded programs and resources by providing leadership in the coordination and extension of needed program areas. Specific objectives and activities have been identified as priorities for new funding (Waxman et al., 2011).

Oregon, USA

The Oregon Simulation Alliance

One of the first organized alliances/collaboratives in the USA, established in 2002, the Oregon Simulation Alliance (OSA) is an independent organization, with formal by-laws, policies, and procedures. It is a unique public-private, multisector, multidisciplinary, not-for-profit organization (a 501c3 corporation). The OSA was started as an initiative from the governor's office to improve the healthcare delivery and increase the number of healthcare providers with the use of medical simulation technology. The mission of the OSA is to "ensure quality patient care for all Oregonians through the use of simulation technology and practice to help healthcare workers to be more confident, competent and compassionate in providing patient care" (Oregon Simulation Alliance, 2013). The vision for the group is "the OSA envisions an efficient statewide network of simulation technology resources, information and training systems" (Oregon Simulation Alliance, 2013). The work of the OSA has been a model for many other programs.

Indiana, USA

The Southeast Indiana Simulation Consortium

The Southeast Indiana Simulation Consortium was formed in 2008 as part of a regional grant and program called Economic Opportunities for 2015 (Jeffries & Battin, 2012). The region consists of 10 counties in a predominantly rural section of Indiana. The three main goals of the simulation consortium are the following:

1. Develop the infrastructure for the use of simulation methodology in the education system.
2. Increase the capacity of nursing graduates in the region.
3. Provide coordination through the development of a regional healthcare network of partners.

Tennessee, USA

The Tennessee Simulation Alliance

The Tennessee Simulation Alliance (TNSA) was formed in 2009. This was a result of an initiative focused on building capacity through collaboration from a Robert Wood Johnson Partners Investing in Nursing (PIN) grant. In partnership with the Tennessee Center for Nursing, a needs assessment was conducted in 2007, sending a survey to all nursing schools in Tennessee (Hallmark, 2013). The survey asked about types of simulation equipment, numbers of faculty with expertise in simulation, concerns about integrating simulation into curriculum, and interest in establishing a simulation alliance. Meetings were held with key stakeholders, and it was identified that there was definite interest in forming an alliance. Support came from vendors and others, and the first TNSA meeting was held in 2009. The board consists of an interprofessional group.

Hawaii, USA

The Hawaii Statewide Simulation Collaborative

The Hawaii Statewide Simulation Collaborative was formed in 2010 and includes academic, practice, and industry partners. Prior to developing the collaborative, a survey was distributed to schools and hospitals in the state to identify the top priorities in simulation. The top priorities identified were as follows:

1. Sharing best practice
2. Simulation facilitator development
3. Curriculum development
4. Research

The structure of this collaborative includes a steering committee, core operational team, and three committees (Wong, 2013).

Florida, USA

The Florida Healthcare Simulation Alliance

In February 2012, the Blue Cross and Blue Shield of Florida Foundation (BCBSF) awarded the Florida Center for Nursing (FCN) a grant to establish the Florida Healthcare Simulation Alliance (FHSA). The FHSA builds on a successful PIN's Future grant awarded to the FCN to examine the state of simulation programs in nursing education in Florida.

The Alliance is coordinating and expanding the use of all forms of simulation in academic settings, healthcare institutions, and agencies across the state to advance healthcare education and to foster patient safety. All levels of healthcare education as well as the simulation and training industry are involved in regional and statewide activities and collaborations. The Alliance is committed to including undergraduate and graduate medical education, nursing and allied health education, and professional staff development in hospitals and other healthcare settings.

Because of the geography and population distribution of Florida, as well as the large number of locations using simulation, the Alliance is building a state model of eight regional collaboratives. The membership of the collaboratives will form the core of the FHSA's Stakeholders Council. A Steering Committee of the Stakeholders Council has been formed with representatives from each region. This committee provides FHSA staff advice and guidance for the development of useful services and activities. In addition to the eight regional collaboratives, FHSA is developing special interest groups, as well as statewide services and programs (FHSA, 2013).

Victoria, Australia

The Victorian Simulation Alliance

The Victorian Simulation Alliance (VSA) was established in August 2010 in response to a perceived need within the state to support educators in the rapidly developing area of healthcare simulation. Working in close collaboration with the CSA, the VSA was modeled on the successful BASC and CSA established through the CINHC (VSA, 2013). The VSA provides a "community of practice," which brings together and supports educators involved in implementing simulation-based teaching and learning in undergraduate, postgraduate, vocational, and ongoing health professional education. Its mission is to "create an environment that fosters collegiality, collaboration, networking and sharing among those engaged in health professional simulation-based education and research" (VSA, 2013).

It aims to reduce the isolation of educators operating in regional and remote areas of the state by providing a platform for communication and networking. The membership is multidisciplinary and spread across universities, vocational education and training, and healthcare providers. It also aims to support the ongoing development and implementation of simulation within health professional education across regional and metropolitan Victoria by:

- Creating a cohesive voice and a common language
- Facilitating ongoing professional development and education
- Information dissemination
- Best practice identification
- Scenario development and sharing
- Fostering collaboration and partnerships
- Facilitating interorganizational research
- Standard and policy setting
- Identifying opportunities and lobbying for funding
- Linking internationally

This multidisciplinary statewide community of practice connects and supports educators from different education sectors and both public and private healthcare providers. The VSA has contributed actively to setting the strategic direction of simulation in their state. While there are aspects that are unique to each alliance (CSA and VSA), they share a number of goals, and from the outset of their

SECTION 5 • Management

RESEARCH NETWORKS

Adam Cheng, MD, FRCPC, FAAP, and Marc Auerbach, MD, MSc, FAAP
Co-Chairs, INSPIRE (International Network for Simulation Based Pediatric Innovation Research and Education)

The field of healthcare simulation has grown rapidly in the past couple of decades, both as an educational intervention (Cheng et al., 2013; Donoghue et al., 2009; Geis et al., 2011) and as the environment for research (Hunt et al., 2009; Weinger, 2010). Recent articles have described important attributes of simulation research (McGaghie et al., 2010) and the types of research studies that should be conducted to advance the science of simulation (Cook, 2010). Although the quantity of simulation-based research (SBR) is on the rise, the quality is highly variable (Cook et al., 2011; McGaghie et al., 2012). In a recent systematic review of simulation-based educational research, 22.5% of studies had a randomized controlled study design, 15.1% were multicenter studies, and only 5.3% reported patient and/or healthcare outcomes (Cook et al., 2011). What can be done to help advance the quality of SBR on an international level?

In the field of healthcare research, the establishment of research networks has helped to advance clinical care by producing high-quality research that directly influences patient care and outcomes. The establishment of these national or international networks has various benefits, including but not limited to: (a) the ability to recruit from multiple centers, thus increasing the available pool of subjects; (b) the inclusion of multiple centers increases generalizability of findings; (c) network members provide a rich source of expertise and experience to draw from; (d) a mix of novice and more experienced investigators allows for structured mentorship opportunities and development of the "next generation" of researchers; (e) the ability to coordinate research activities on the basis of a common research agenda; and (f) the enhanced ability to secure grant funding for research projects (Cheng et al., 2011).[10] Within the simulation community, the International Network for Simulation-based Pediatric Innovation, Research and Education (INSPIRE) has been successful in becoming an active and productive international research collaborative that is currently engaged in various single and multicenter SBR trials.

INSPIRE is currently the world's largest SBR network, comprising over 100 academic institutions and 500 members from 25 countries around the world. The mission of the network is to improve the delivery of medical care to acutely ill children by conducting SBR to answer questions pertaining to resuscitation, technical skills, behavioral skills, debriefing, patient safety, and simulation-based education. To achieve this goal, the network conducted a series of consensus-building activities to establish a common research agenda. These activities resulted in the development of seven key research themes, each with specific research aims: (a) Debriefing; (b) Teamwork and Communication; (c) Procedural and Psychomotor Skills; (d) Technology; (e) Acute Care and Resuscitation; (f) Human Factors; and (g) Patient Safety. Currently, the network has over 35 active research projects spanning all seven themes. To support these projects, a structured research process with dedicated resources is offered by the network, thus helping to ensure that project ideas are brought to fruition, and that ongoing projects are brought to completion and publication. The resources provided to support research include (a) an online project submission process with coordinated feedback (www.inspiresim.com); (b) biannual network meetings at international simulation conferences with project working groups and expert consultations; (c) grant writing support and review; (d) research networking and matching process to identify content experts; (e) website for research coordination and communication; and (f) manuscript oversight to enable publication. Through networking and collaboration, INSPIRE has provided a venue for novice and experienced simulation researchers to gather, share thoughts, and collectively advance the field by conducting high-quality, impactful SBR. The combined efforts of INSPIRE membership have helped researchers capitalize on the benefits of effective collaboration, and in doing so assist in overcoming some of the common challenges inherent in SBR. Collaborations of this kind in other specialties and/or professions will be critical in establishing a solid foundation for the sustained growth and proliferation of SBR on the international level.

REFERENCES

Cheng, A., Hunt, E., Donoghue, A., Nelson, K., LeFlore, J., Anderson, J., . . . Nadkarni, V. (for the EXPRESS Pediatric Simulation Collaborative). (2011). EXPRESS—Examining Pediatric Resuscitation Education using Simulation and Scripting: The birth of an international pediatric simulation research collaborative—From concept to reality. *Simulation in Healthcare*, 6(1), 34–41.

Cheng, A., Hunt, E. A., Donoghue, A., Nelson-McMillan, K., Nishisaki, A., Leflore, J., . . . Nadkarni, V. M. (2013). Examining pediatric resuscitation education using simulation and scripting (EXPRESS): A multi-center, randomized-controlled trial. *JAMA Pediatrics*, 167(6), 528–536.

Cook, D. A. (2010). One drop at a time: Research to advance the science of simulation. *Simulation in Healthcare*, 5(1), 1–4.

Cook, D. A., Hatala, R., Brydges, R., Zendejas, B., Szostek, J. H., Wang, A. T., . . . Hamstra, S. J. (2011). Technology-enhanced simulation for health professions education: A systematic review and meta-analysis. *JAMA: the Journal of the American Medical Association*, 3306, 978–988.

Donoghue, A. J., Durbin, D. R., Nadel, F. M., Stryjewski, G. R., Kost, S. I., & Nadkarni, V. M. (2009). Effect of high-fidelity simulation on Pediatric Advanced Life Support training in pediatric house staff: a randomized trial. *Pediatric Emergency Care*, 25(3), 139–144.

Geis, G. L., Pio, B., Pendergrass, T. L., Moyer, M. R., & Patterson, M. D. (2011). Simulation to assess the safety of new healthcare teams and new facilities. *Simulation in Healthcare*, 6(3), 125–133.

Hunt, E. A., Vera, K., Diener-West, M., Nelson, K. L., Shaffner, D. H., & Pronovost, P. J. (2009). Delays and errors in cardiopulmonary resuscitation and defibrillation by pediatric residents during simulated cardiopulmonary arrests. *Resuscitation*, 80(7), 819–825.

McGaghie, W. C., Issenberg, S. B., Cohen, E. R., Barsuk, J. H., & Wayne, D. B. (2012). Translational educational research: A necessity for effective health-care improvement. *Chest*, 142(5), 1097–1103.

McGaghie, W. C., Issenberg, S. B., Petrusa, E. R., & Scalese, R. J. (2010). A critical review of simulation-based medical education research: 2003–2009. *Medical Education*, 44(1), 50–63.

Weinger, M. B. (2010). The pharmacology of simulation: A conceptual framework to inform progress in simulation research. *Simulation in Healthcare*, 5(1), 8–15.

relationship, both alliances worked toward the creation of a platform that would formally link and support their activities (English, 2013).

GLOBAL ALLIANCES

Trans-Pacific Alliance

While the concept of forming an international community of practice may have appeared daunting 20 years ago, advances in technology, communication, and travel provide the ability for individuals and organizations today to connect easily, despite geographical distance. International collaboration assists health professional education to keep pace with changes in simulation technology by taking advantage of the collective knowledge of faculty from different countries and education contexts. Hovancsek et al. (2009) cite the benefit of having "another set of lenses," which contributed valuable insights and a richness to their National League for Nursing (NLN) project involving the development of Web-based resources aimed at faculty development.

Collaboration on a global basis opens up opportunities for research teams to share resources, leverage individual research strengths, and apply and test theories and ideas across a broad range of environments. In 2012, the Trans-Pacific Alliance was formally launched between VSA and CSA. The expressed purpose of the Alliance was to leverage the strengths of each organization and set the stage for future resource sharing and collaboration. The Alliance has provided a vehicle for connecting the Research Committees of the CSA and VSA and established a platform for the identification and coordination of international research activity and the lobbying of funding.

Working cooperatively will help to ensure the sustainability of simulation-based education, helping to mitigate the relatively high costs associated with this form of training through the sharing of resources and expertise. Through the Alliance, the CSA and VSA have gained direct access to the education resources within each Alliance, including a large range of validated scenarios. Operating within a paradigm of inclusiveness, the Alliance has the potential to link other existing state and national alliances in the future.

Both organizations describe similar initiatives:

- Establishing effective and sustainable communication processes
- The sourcing and provision of simulation education and training
- Scenario development, validation and sharing, research and development

These combined efforts will ultimately speed up the translation of the latest evidence to the members of the global partnership so that it can be implemented at a much faster rate than if the organizations were operating independently.

HOW DO WE GET STARTED?

After reading about successful alliances, many may wonder how they too may either start or join a collaborative endeavor. The easiest starting point is with the Internet by doing a word search for your geographic area and the terms "simulation alliance" or "collaborative." If that effort yields a positive result, reach out to the organization or individual and find out what is happening and how you can become involved. If you do not find anything via the Internet, the next step would be to inquire with other local simulation programs to determine what is available. After you have contacted several programs in your area, if you determine there is nothing available, you may want to consider starting an alliance.

If you are interested in finding others who are working in the simulation field, one of the best places to start is to attend simulation based conferences and network with others who are interested in expanding the field. There are usually sessions at these meetings on how to successfully build alliances/collaboratives. Joining professional simulation associations is another way to connect to others who may be interested in joining forces. You might be surprised at the number of groups that are geographically close to your site that you can work on developing an alliance/collaboration.

As noted in the examples provided earlier, funding is a key factor in successfully launching an alliance. There are potential private or public funding sources that can be utilized to obtain seed money for the endeavor. It is important early in the development phase of the project to determine whether funding can be obtained as it will make a difference as to the scope of the work that can be accomplished. Many funders have expectations that there will be a plan in place for sustaining the work once their funding comes to an end. Therefore, it is critical to incorporate such sustainability plans into submissions to potential funders.

As with any group, it is important to ensure the members of the alliance are participating at a level such that forward progress can be seen. If this does not happen, the work will stagnate, and individuals will disengage from the project. Ensuring that regularly scheduled meetings actually are held and are not cancelled will assist in moving the agenda of the group forward. Rotation of leadership is a means by which continual growth can occur. Frequent in-person meetings with topics of interest being presented is also a means to keep membership engaged.

There are many ways a group can use the activities and questions developed by AHRQ in its life cycle model to keep members engaged (Table 5.6.2). As with any project, the culture in which the work is to be performed needs to be taken into consideration. When dealing with multiple sites with multiple agendas, it helps to use a consensus model to keep moving forward.

SECTION 5 • Management

TABLE 5.6.2			
AHRQ's Life Cycle Phases Along with a Listing of Common Activities, Key Questions to Ask, and Desired Outcomes			
Phase	**Common Activities**	**Key Questions**	**Desired Outcomes**
Vision	Defining goals Assessing market forces Recruiting leaders Securing initial funding	What are we trying to accomplish? Who will help us get there?	Clear goals High energy and engagement Initial funding
Growth	Demonstrating value Recruiting members Building strategic plans Leveraging and extending funding	How will we get there? What do our stakeholders expect?	Early "wins"—producing recognizable value Road map for growth Committed membership
Establishment	Institutionalizing value Executing plans Retaining members Building infrastructure	Are we on track and delivering value? How do we sustain commitment and success?	Recognition as a leader and trusted source Sustainable business plan Reliable funding
Extension	Delivering recognized value Assessing results; benchmarking Adjusting plans and structure	What is working or not working? How has the market shifted?	Continued demonstration of value and recognition New perspectives New or renewed funding
At times, organizations are challenged by events and circumstances that force significant regrouping and changes, which may be unplanned or outside of a typical life cycle.			
Rebooting	Responding to significant shifts or negative events	What went wrong? How will we adjust and continue?	Renewed vision Practical plan of action Retaining critical leaders, members, and funding

SOCIAL MEDIA

Utilizing social media can be an effective way for groups to meet, form, communicate, and stay engaged. Several simulation alliances, networks, and collaboratives have Facebook or Linkedin pages to recruit new members, communicate with existing members, and announce activities or special events.

BEEN THERE, DONE THAT: HOW CAN I CONTINUE TO IMPROVE OR SUSTAIN WHAT I HAVE ACHIEVED?

Sustaining Your Alliance

Once the alliance or collaborative has been established, a plan for sustainability needs to be developed. This needs to be discussed with key stakeholders early in the process. Questions such as whether the alliance should become a nonprofit (501c3) or for-profit need to be considered. Additionally, a decision needs to be made about where the alliance will be housed. Will it be housed in a school, hospital, workforce center, or will it be virtual? Will a website be created? How will it be marketed?

Funding is a key consideration to move forward once the alliance has been established. Some ways to obtain funding to keep the alliance viable are as follows:

- Subscription or membership fees
- Hosting conferences
- Creating curriculum for courses to be offered, and charging a fee
- Donations from industry partners, foundations, or private donors
  - Working with vendors is important but focus on partnerships and strategy.
  - Be careful not to be perceived as only partnering with one particular vendor
  - Private donations can be obtained from interested parties. Foundations in hospitals are often untapped resources.
- Grants
  - Grant funding is possible for planning grants, program development, faculty training, and research, but you will most likely not find a grant funder for sustainability. Specificity is critical for grant funders. Some only fund equipment, some personnel, and many focus on program development with key outcomes tied to patient safety.

Regardless of the funding source, it is essential to creating a business plan for your alliance. Often, with initial grant funding or donations, a budget can be created for that distinct time period, but budgeting beyond that point is essential for long-term success. A 3-year budget should be created to determine how much revenue is needed to offset any expenses. If you do not have the skills needed to create a plan, it is best to work with an expert in this field to help you create a realistic and sustainable business plan. See chapters 4.2, 4.4, and 4.7 for information on budgeting, creating a business plan, and obtaining grant funding, respectively.

STEM AND SIM

Tom Lemaster, RN, MSN, MEd, Paramedic
Board of Directors, Society for Simulation in Healthcare

Science, Technology, Engineering, and Mathematics (STEM) for high-school students has come to represent a national effort to attract capable students to consider careers that are dependent on developing a strong math and science foundation prior to entering higher education. In addition to formal educational programs, the spirit and intent of STEM curricula has been picked up by the industries whose futures depend on a well-educated technical workforce for virtually all aspects of using and maintaining future technology-based tools and for the engineering and design of new products. Recently, many professional organizations have joined in the national STEM effort to attract, motivate, and help junior and senior high-school students prepare for technical and scientific careers by providing access to their professional conferences and exhibitions that provide exposure of their domain-specific use of science and technology that would appeal to student interests.

Students' interest in health and medical careers often depend on their study in related biological sciences, images portrayed in televised medical programs, and/or family encouragement. By its very nature and purpose, simulation changes the dynamics of healthcare education and training and allows students to become immersed in hands-on patient care. Supervised junior and senior high-school students can experience doing medical procedures without risk, using simulation just as students in college-level programs do. With the advances in healthcare simulation, medical procedures can be performed and learned at least as well as learning to fly in a flight simulator. As a world leader in the advocacy and improvement of simulation as a means for healthcare and medical training, the Society of Simulation in Healthcare (SSH) has sponsored two significant STEM-related opportunities for young students at their annual international meeting, first in Orlando and then in San Francisco.

Student opportunities begin with interactive time on the exhibit hall floor to visit the many vendors participating at the conference. The simulation technology itself exposes students to a wide range of modeling and simulation research, development, engineering, and operational careers related to the development of new simulation capability.

Students also have the opportunity to discuss careers in healthcare and other related medical fields by pairing them with educators. This provides immersive hands-on experience, actually doing things, under the supervision of the industry experts.

During the STEM program, the students are divided into smaller groups and provided the opportunity to participate in simulation scenarios. The scenarios are led by educators associated with the simulation industry vendors. Students are given an opportunity to debrief as with all simulation experiences.

In addition to the interaction with simulation experts, during the 2014 IMSH meeting, STEM students saw presentations from the 2013 National microMedic competition. The contest was hosted and sponsored by the US Army Telemedicine and Advanced Technology Research Center (TATRC), Carnegie Mellon Entertainment Technology Center, and Parallax Inc.

Contest entrants were challenged to use microcontroller and sensor systems to create medical applications and products for possible use in the healthcare industry, medical simulation training, and the battlefield. The contest was judged by representatives of US Army, Carnegie Mellon University, and from the greater scientific community. The experience concluded with a large group debriefing session, with simulation experts attending the meeting.

The students who participated in this STEM experience found the exposure stimulating and enlightening. Strategically, the Society has an interest in helping to ensure that simulation takes a much more visible place in medical education, and working to avoid healthcare consumers' fears associated with the transformation of medical education, including a significantly increased dependence on simulation as a training medium. Exposure of students and their parents to hands-on experience with simulators could play a significant role in cautiously introducing healthcare consumers to the simulation environments before reliance on simulation becomes highly variable to the general public in much the same way aviation flight simulators replaced hours of real flight time with severe public backlash, which is a risk for healthcare simulation at this stage in its adoption as a training alternative. Commercial manufacturers of healthcare simulation products should be most interested in this potential benefit from investing in STEM education activities.

SECTION 5 • Management

SUMMARY

Alliances, networks, and collaboratives are important at a regional, statewide, national, and global level when there is a shared common vision and the participants agree on specific goals and objectives they want to achieve. These cooperative working groups should not be limited to one discipline, although many begin in one discipline or another. Enabling all disciplines to participate reflects simulation as the truly interprofessional teaching modality it is.

Beginning anything new can be daunting. Be aware that there are many who have blazed the trail and are willing to assist, and usually all it takes is an e-mail to find someone who has done this work before.

Alliances, networks, and collaborations are like other relationships: they require frequent nurturing to ensure their continued growth. The ultimate benefit of simulation is to improve patient outcomes. By working together, simulation groups can achieve goals they could not have achieved alone and thus improve the preparation of those who may one day take care of us.

REFERENCES

Agency for Healthcare Research and Quality. (2013). *Sustainability for community quality collaboratives. An overview of the art & science of building staying power.* Retrieved from http://www.ahrq.gov/legacy/qual/value/suscqcollab1.htm#managing

California Simulation Alliance. (n.d.). Retrieved from www.california-simulationalliance.org

Eder-Van Hook, J. (2004). *Building a national agenda for simulation-based medical education.* Washington, DC: Advanced Initiatives in Medical Simulation.

English, L. (2013). *Creating a statewide simulation network: hear from the experts.* Paper presented at the International Meeting on Simulation in Healthcare, Orlando, FL.

Florida Healthcare Simulation Alliance. (2013). *What is the FHSA?* Retrieved from http://www.floridahealthsimalliance.org/About/WhatistheFHSA.aspx

Hovancsek, M., Jeffries, P. R., Escudero, E., Foulds, B. J., Husebo, E., Iwamoto, Y., . . . Wang, A. (2009). Creating simulation communities of practice: An international perspective. *Nursing Education Perspectives, 30*(2), 121–125.

Jeffries, P., & Battin, J. (2012). *Developing successful health care education simulation centers: the consortium model.* New York, NY: Springer.

Oregon Simulation Alliance. (2013). *About the OSA.* Retrieved from http://oregonsimulation.com/about/

Victoria Simulation Alliance. (2013). *About the VSA.* Retrieved from http://www.vicsim.org/index.php?option=com_content&view=article&id=1&Itemid=2

Waxman, K., Nichols, A., O'Leary-Kelley, C., & Miller, M. (2011). The evolution of a statewide network: the Bay Area Simulation Collaborative. *Simulation in Health Care, 6*(6), 345–351.

Waxman, K., & Telles, C. (2009). The use of Benner's framework in high-fidelity simulation faculty development: The Bay Area Simulation Collaborative Model. *Clinical Simulation in Nursing, 5*(6), e231–e235.

SECTION 6

Environmental Design

CHAPTER 6.1

Building a Simulation Center: Key Design Strategies and Considerations

Michael A. Seropian, MD, FRCPC, Guillaume Alinier, PhD, MPhys, PgCert, SFHEA, CPhys, MInstP, MIPEM, Ismaël Hssain, MD, MSc (MEd), Bonnie J. Driggers, RN, MS, MPA, Brian C. Brost, MD, Thomas A. Dongilli, AT, and Michael C. Lauber, FAIA

ABOUT THE AUTHORS

MICHAEL A. SEROPIAN is a Professor of Anesthesiology & Pediatrics at Oregon Health & Science University. He has 19 years of experience in simulation education development and training. He has developed/designed many simulation facilities and has been instrumental in developing multiple simulation collaboratives and ventures. He is the Director of Anesthesia Simulation Service, has published extensively, and trained hundreds of individuals across professions in the use of simulation-based methods. He is a past president of the Society for Simulation in Healthcare (SSH).

GUILLAUME ALINIER is a Simulation Training and Research Manager, Hamad Medical Corporation Ambulance Service, Doha, Qatar. In addition, is a professor of Simulation in Healthcare Education and National Teaching Fellow at the University of Hertfordshire, School of Health and Social Work, Hatfield, UK, and a Visiting Fellow, Northumbria University, Faculty of Health and Life Sciences, Newcastle, UK. He serves on several SSH and INACSL committees, is widely published, and provides philanthropic advice on simulation design around the world.

ISMAËL HSSAIN is an emergency physician at Mulhouse General Hospital, France. He is the Teaching Director of the Center for Emergency Medical Services Education and mobile simulation unit in the region. Dr. Hssain is Medical Director of the US-based National Association of Emergency Medical Technicians (NAEMT) *Advanced Medical Life Support (AMLS)* course in France. He has been instrumental in running several simulation instructor courses for emergency physicians at international conferences.

BONNIE DRIGGERS is Professor Emeritus at the Oregon Health & Science University (OHSU). Bonnie served as the Director of Clinical Teaching Systems and Programs for the OHSU School of Nursing and Co-Director of the OHSU Simulation and Clinical Learning Center for several years. Currently, Ms. Driggers provides consultation in the areas of simulation education, program development, implementation, and facility design. She serves on several Society for Simulation in Healthcare (SSH) Committees including the SSH Board of Directors and Executive Committee.

BRIAN C. BROST is a Professor of Maternal Fetal Medicine at Mayo Clinic. He is Operations Director at their Multidisciplinary Simulation Center. His love for simulation started with developing task trainers for amniocentesis, in utero transfusion and stenting, CVS, cervical cerclage, twin-twin transfusion laser therapy, Cesarean delivery, and for circumcision. His proudest accomplishment includes developing a long-standing 2-week preclinical training program for interns in OB/Gyn and Family Medicine at Mayo and now for international training programs.

THOMAS A. DONGILLI, Director of Operations at the Peter M. Winter Institute for Simulation, Education, and Research (WISER) at the University of Pittsburgh and the University of Pittsburgh Medical Center (UPMC) has extensive experience in facility design and implementation. Mr. Dongilli has authored book chapters on simulation center design and management, co-chaired the 2014 International Meeting on Simulation in Healthcare (IMSH 2014), and led the efforts in creating the first SSH Policy and Procedure Manual for Simulation Centers.

MICHAEL C. LAUBER is President of Ellenzweig, an architectural design firm in Cambridge, Massachusetts. His 35 years of experience includes the design of numerous educational facilities for Medicine, Nursing, Pharmacy, and Allied Health. This work has included programming and design of 18 simulation centers, including facilities for Michigan State University, Brown University, and

Case Western Reserve University. Michael holds a Master of Architecture from Harvard University and a Bachelor of Arts from Cornell University.

ABSTRACT

Development of a healthcare simulation facility is complex and multifaceted. The task requires the design (form) to serve the education, research, and assessment needs (function) of the simulation program. Form must meet function. There is no "one-size-fits-all" solution. A deliberate process that accounts for the multiple steps and parties involved will likely yield a facility that will meet the mission of the program. These steps involve planning as well as highly technical expertise. Involving parties with experience will help mitigate risk related to developing a facility that falls short of expectations and need. A good understanding of a program's mission, its curricular needs, learner and faculty skill, and budgetary constraints are foundational elements in developing a well-informed facility. It is important to appreciate that the facility is more than walls but rather hallways that determine the flow, rooms and adjacencies that create educational isolation, room types that serve both the simulation activity itself and the operational aspects to support that activity pre-, intra-, and postsimulation. Equipment selection and audiovisual design play an equally important role in function. While the process, especially in cases of large facilities, can be overwhelming, understanding the process will increase the likelihood that the facility will meet functional needs.

CASE EXAMPLE

You have been given space in a new building that is being built for a variety of stakeholders. The building is 200,000 square feet (18,580 m^2) and the simulation center will be no greater than 20,000 square feet (1,858 m^2). You and your team would like to develop a simulation facility that meets the interprofessional needs of your institution while embracing best-accepted design principles. How should you go about planning and designing this new space? Who should be involved in the design phase? How detailed do the initial plans need to be? Are there design considerations that will impact the ability of the simulation program to achieve its mission and vision?

INTRODUCTION

> Although facilities must be adequate to meet the goals and objectives of the Program, the defining characteristic of an accredited program is the work it does, not the physical structure.

Worldwide, the number of healthcare simulation centers and in situ training initiatives has rapidly increased since the turn of the century (Weinstock et al., 2005). Several government initiatives are strongly promoting and supporting simulation in the context of healthcare to ensure competent clinicians and promote patient safety (Alinier & Platt, 2013). The Society for Simulation in Healthcare's (SSH) glossary of terms for accreditation defines a simulation center as "an entity with dedicated infrastructure and personnel where simulation courses are conducted. A center may support several Simulation Programs" (SSH, 2012). To be accredited, the Society states that a program must have ". . . appropriate areas for activities such as education, technology storage, and debriefing, and appropriate separation of simulation and actual patient care materials" (SSH, 2012). Depending on the group of learners and training focus, the equipment, technology, and layout may differ greatly. There are many circumstances in which a dedicated simulation facility is not an absolute requirement to run a simulation program.

Designing a clinical simulation center is not a straightforward exercise as there is no "one-size-fits-all" solution

and desired attributes and features evolve over time. The objectives of training conducted in *facility-based* simulation are at times different from the objectives of *in situ* simulation (see chapter 2.2). This chapter will primarily focus on *facility-based* simulation. Designing and building a simulation center to serve the training needs of an institution or organization can be an intimidating responsibility. A common initial struggle is determining where to start. This chapter provides information useful in designing a simulation center that best meets the needs of an institution and provides the flexibility to adapt to future educational needs.

All space is not equal. Successful implementation of simulation-based education, training, assessment, and research requires space that is thoughtfully designed. Healthcare education facility design is trending toward areas that support smaller-group work, with active and interactive learning in highly flexible spaces. The space should balance efficiency and efficacy while adhering to accepted architectural and educational concepts and theories. Programs use this space to meet their programmatic and institutional needs and, therefore, must be structured to allow educationally sound activities to reliably occur. Form must meet function. Ultimately, the space should engage the learner in an immersive experience. The environment (people and room) and the equipment contribute to a learner's engagement. Unfortunately and too often, the simulation facility design precedes thoughtful consideration of what stakeholders seek to achieve within the location.

There are currently few written peer-reviewed resources that specifically address simulation facility design considerations. Existing centers often only have *some* elements of best-understood practice. In this sense, visiting or learning about other centers is important to understand what was successful and what they would change. It is equally important to understand their context. What are they trying to achieve in their facility and does that apply to your program's goals? If they are meeting some of your envisioned goals, having the ability to determine what is still needed can truly allow the site to provide the optimal learning experience.

The design process can involve many people that represent a variety of skillsets. Stakeholders (learners, educators, executives, etc.), simulationists, architects, engineers, and information technology (IT) engineers are but a few of the groups involved. Having individuals on your team that have experience and skill in the design of a simulation facility can be extremely helpful and should be utilized whenever possible. All members of the group should have the same objective: to produce a space that translates a program's vision into a usable physical form.

In light of the rapid evolution of simulation as well as other paradigm shifts like interprofessional education and practice, most simulation programs *will not have all the answers to some important questions as the design process progresses*. Using available information to inform functional need is important. Educated and deliberate forecasting will decrease the risk of designing a center with compromised function. There are many emerging mitigation strategies such as the design of flexible space that can be morphed into a variety of configurations to meet future needs. Visiting other established centers and developing relationships with key personnel will provide valuable insight into what works and what does not. No single center represents best practice. Learning from each other is critical. The individuals involved must discriminate what seems attractive to the eye versus what is functionally superior. A center that has a big "wow" effective may be functionally crippled.

This chapter will present a variety of important concepts that will apply to any facility, irrespective of size and shape. It is laid out in a manner to succinctly address a variety of important topic areas with respect to simulation facility design.

- What types of rooms are typically seen in a simulation center?
- Who would you expect to be involved in the design of a simulation facility?
- What is the typical process for design and development of a simulation facility?
- What equipment is relevant to the purpose of the designed simulation facility?
- What quick tips and pearls of wisdom exist in the design and development of simulation facilities?

FORM MEETS FUNCTION— IMPORTANT INITIAL STEPS

The relationship between form and function ultimately relates to more than the position of walls, windows, and doors and is not always intuitively obvious. Simulation center designers should seek the ideal intersection of a clinical, theatrical, and educational environment.

When thinking about how to design a simulation facility, there are two common initial approaches: make it like the hospital or make it like another simulation center—both have an initial significant advantage and both also have multiple disadvantages that are explored here. In the first approach, a new simulation center could look like a current clinic, unit, or hospital space. After all, wouldn't you want the training space to be an exact replica of the actual clinical environment? Clinics and hospitals were designed to maximize patient–provider interactions and flow; seldom do these sites consider the environmental principles needed to maximize pedagogical training. Simulation centers can have very diverse types of clinical situations and simulation events running in close proximity to each other. Evaluating how the simulation center staff, learners and participants, and teachers/facilitators can potentially interact is crucial to minimize distraction and maximize the training/interaction as learner and faculty time is a precious resource.

Alternatively, the floor plan from another successful simulation program can be copied and recreated. This approach seems the most expeditious to rapidly opening a facility, but bypasses several important steps that may fail to meet institution-specific needs. You may build a beautiful space that is entirely inappropriate to the educational, training, and assessment needs of your institution. When comparing and contrasting one center's design to another, you must consider (at minimum) the following:

- Mission, vision, goals, and purpose
- Type and number of learners
- Experience of the simulation faculty/educators
- Personnel and financial resources

Defining Functional Needs

Successful programs have identified several key factors important for designing a vibrant healthcare simulation center. Developing a clear *mission* and *vision* is an essential but often delayed or even overlooked component in the early stages of simulation center planning and design. The mission and vision should guide the functional needs of your facility.

A mission statement should clearly describe what you do, who you serve, and why/how you propose to do it. Mission statements articulate the simulation center's purpose for both internal and external members of an organization or institution. A readily apparent mission statement provides a foundation for the next steps in your strategic planning. A vision statement sets a direction for your business planning by clearly describing "where do we want to go as a unit" or "what do we want to look like as the simulation center moves forward." The vision statement should provide a clear direction for the staff of the simulation center, but does not say how to achieve this goal. (For more information on how to properly formulate mission and vision statements, see chapter 5.3.)

To develop a clear mission and vision statement for your center requires a needs assessment (see chapter 5.1 on performing a needs assessment), including an investigation of who the stakeholders for your institution are and their simulation-based needs to guide you to a successful facility design. In most simplistic terms, a stakeholder is a person, department, institution, or organization that can have a potential interest in your project. Stakeholders include persons or entities both inside and outside your proposed simulation center who have something to gain (or lose) by successful execution and completion of your simulation facility and its curricular offerings and thus may facilitate, alter, or even prevent its completion (see chapter 4.5). It is important to identify all key stakeholders to optimize your educational/training/research space by clearly understanding their expectations, and determining their requirements and needs.

A subset of stakeholders will determine the curricular needs for the new simulation center, which is another critical component to the simulation space design. Educational stakeholders may include the institution executives, simulation center staff, and also learners/participants. Stakeholder development of the simulation-based expectations and needed curriculum will help define the placement, quantity, and type of rooms. Curricular need will also directly influence the flow of facility users and the infrastructure required to meet their needs. Facility flow issues will be more complex if the facility is a mixed-use facility for students and practitioners. A well-developed initial curriculum will define the quantity of learners, the learning objectives, the educational strategies, and evaluation needs. All of these influence design directly. While we describe the need to understand and incorporate curricular needs, it is not uncommon in this early phase of simulation to not have a well-defined curriculum. This certainly increases the risk related to the design process.

National or international regulatory bodies may dictate some aspects of healthcare simulation center design and equipment. For example, in 2012, the French Higher Healthcare Authority published a national report that includes guidelines for simulation programs with a tiered system (three levels) to classify simulation centers. The system takes into account the number of simulation and debriefing rooms, among many other factors such as staffing, learner population, and activities (Haute Autorité de Santé, 2012). As one approaches center design, it will be important to understand the regulatory implications within the region in which the center will be functioning.

Delays or inability to open a center can occur if the proper regulatory agencies are not involved. Depending on where your simulation center is located (e.g., hospital, clinic, or free-standing) will determine the regulatory agencies with which you will need to coordinate.

While much of what has been mentioned will help determine the capacity and functional needs that will drive how you design and equip your simulation center, the available budget must also be considered. Mission, vision, and stakeholder needs must all take into account the reality of budgetary constraints. Budgets are either determined by the design (not recommended) or are defined beforehand (recommended). The intrinsic goal should be to have realistic planning and design that are in alignment with functional needs and budget. An imbalance between budget and need will only lead to disappointment.

FORM MEETS FUNCTION—ROOMS AND SPACES

Depending on the size and intent, a simulation facility may have many different rooms and spaces. In this section, we will cover the key rooms that should be considered. Spaces and rooms such as lounges, locker rooms, and reception areas will not be covered in this chapter. These general rooms can be space-consuming and are often sacrificed for more functional education space. Findings from a needs assessment and activity flow studies can guide the placement of these spaces. While there are rooms common to most simulation facilities, it is not only the type of rooms that make for an effective learning environment, but also the relationship of rooms to each other (adjacencies), the flow of learners in the environment, the ratio between certain types of rooms, and the reflection of the stated need of programs through deliberate space-program verification.

A successful simulation facility must include the needed control infrastructure, dedicated supply and support space to properly reflect the size of the program needs, and relationships to and with other rooms. Additional infrastructure to support simulation and skills training with medication rooms, soiled utility, and space for specialized servers that will service the simulation program are also necessary. The example plan in this chapter for a 20,000 square feet (1,858 m^2) interprofessional space has multipurpose and flexible space that can be utilized for skills training, lectures, and small-group work. If your space is smaller or larger than this, the concepts for planning and design considerations will be similar.

The high-fidelity clinical simulation rooms need not be labeled by function (e.g., critical care or labor and delivery) as each room can achieve this functionality through the flexible use of the appropriate equipment and sufficient storage. Instead, they may be labeled as a smaller- and a larger-sized simulation room. The larger simulation

TABLE 6.1.1

Sample Room Types and Sizes

Room Type	Size in Approximate Square Feet (m²)
Debriefing room	350 (32.3)
Clinical simulation control room	200 (18.6)
Clinical rooms	
Regular (e.g., medical-surgical unit)	275 (25.5)
Large (e.g., operating room)	500 (46.4)
Storage	10%–20% of net assignable square feet/meters
AV/IT closet	300 (27.9)
Office	
One-person	120 (11.2)
Two-person	180 (16.8)
Four-person	250 (22.2)
Medication room	100 (9.3)
Multipurpose room	500–1,500 (46.5–139.4)
Support/supply/prep room	400–1,000 (37.2–92.9)
Standardized patient (SP) room	120–150 (11.2–13.9)
SP control room	100 (9.3)
Faculty monitor room	Depends on number of SP rooms
SP prep room	300–1,000 (27.9–92.9)
Bed skills lab	1,800 (167.2)

room can accommodate simulations that require more space for equipment and people (e.g., operating rooms and labor and delivery rooms) and for multiple patient scenarios, while the smaller room may accommodate a simple medical-surgical setup.

It is important to note from the start that not all simulation facilities following best known practice will have all of the rooms noted in the information that follows (Table 6.1.1). They are likely to provide the functions described for the rooms either in an individual room or combined with other rooms to fit the space and purpose of the space. The actual number of rooms will be determined in the space-programming phase once one understands what needs to occur in the facility and for how many learners.

Clinical Simulation Room Types

The rooms may be configured for a specific purpose or may be designed flexibly as a variety of clinical rooms, including the possibility of a two-patient solution. These include but are not limited to intensive care unit room, operating room, labor and delivery room, emergency department room, outpatient settings, and medical-surgical rooms to name a few. The equipment present in the room at the time of the simulation will determine the room's configuration. The rooms are commonly equipped with cameras, ceiling speakers, microphones, and local inputs to capture content that will be stored in a central server and available for replay or simultaneous capture to conference space or debrief rooms. Data, telephone, power, headwall(s), gases (oxygen, air), vacuum, sink(s), and diagnostic sets are commonly available at each bed location as well as other appropriate areas to support flexibility. Each bed location may also accommodate a patient monitor. The rooms also typically include a computer with display for retrieval of information and simulation patient data. While the simulation rooms are similar to clinical rooms, they are often not exact replicas, as what is needed to immerse the learner/participant is not always the same as what is needed to provide care. It is important to remember that the primary purpose of clinical simulation rooms is to provide education rather than provide clinical care (Figure 6.1.1).

Clinical Simulation Control Room

The clinical simulation control room primarily facilitates the successful implementation of an active simulation scenario. Faculty and simulation technicians have the ability to control and direct simulations through the control room features. This includes but is not limited to mannequin-based, hybrid, and standardized patient (SP)-based simulation. The control room allows for indirect observation of a scenario through audiovisual (AV) technology and may also have direct visualization through a one-way-glass solution. Control of simulators, cameras, microphones, and capture capabilities are a central feature of this room. Educators and simulation operators/technicians will additionally have the ability to direct

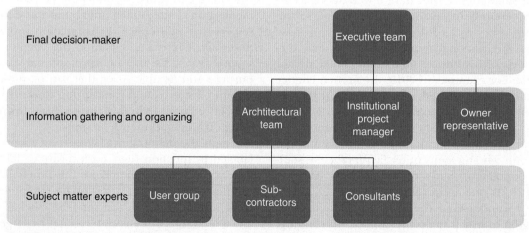

FIGURE 6.1.1   Simplified project organizational structure example.

live voice interactions between the mannequins and learners. The control room is key to the fiction contract established with learners (Dieckmann et al., 2007) so they do not see the backstage work involved in running a scenario. Control rooms vary in size depending upon the number of clinical simulation rooms controlled as well as other factors. Most important to consider is who needs to be in the room, what equipment will be there, and what size do you need to ensure adequate flow of personnel/faculty. A control room controlling one simulation room may vary from 60 to 200 square feet (5.6 to 18.6 m^2). This will increase when a single control room is designed to manage more than one simulation room.

An important ratio to consider is between simulation rooms and control rooms and is dependent upon simulation control philosophy as well as physical space constraints. Ratios can extend from 1:1 to 1:12 and beyond. While a ratio of 1:1 may seem ideal, that ratio may have significant operational, educational, and staffing implications owing to physical separation of activities. This can become an issue in larger centers. Conversely, shared spaces have challenges associated with them such as heat, noise levels, and flow control.

Debriefing Room

Debriefing is an essential part of simulation-based learning. Debriefing rooms are designed to encourage active group-based learning and may be used for real-time broadcast of simulation scenarios as well as playback of archived material during the debriefing process. As such, as with all rooms in a simulation center, design with flexibility in mind (Bradley & Postlethwaite, 2003). Often, they are configured as a small conference room with modular tables and comfortable chairs to support conversation primarily after simulations have occurred. Typical size for a debrief room varies; 350 square feet (32.5 m^2) is usually adequate to hold 10 to 15 people. It is not uncommon for people to undersize the debrief rooms, thereby causing a programmatic limitation for their educators and learners. Preferably, the rooms will be located close to clinical simulation rooms or SP environments to allow for minimal interruption as learners transition from the clinical simulation to the debriefing rooms. In addition, the debriefing rooms should have a whiteboard or smart-board technology.

The ratio of debriefing to simulation rooms is an important consideration and is dependent upon the debriefing philosophy of the organization, whether the space is to be used for multiple purposes, and the actual space available. A 1:1 ratio is ideal as it allows for all debriefing to occur away from the clinical simulation area should the course require such. Many facilities do not have this luxury and may opt for a lower ratio. This will of course have implications on capacity to do certain types of simulation concurrently.

Multipurpose Classroom

Multipurpose classrooms can be flexibly configured for a variety of teaching and learning approaches; lecture-based learning (theater-style seating), desk-based learning, group-based learning, team-based learning, and station-based learning are a few examples.

Multipurpose rooms may also be configured with perimeter services (gases, data, and power), stretchers or exam tables, and center table(s) with perimeter chairs around the table. Curtains may be used to separate each bed location.

These rooms can be used to train cognitive, behavioral, and technical skills. Multipurpose space should be considered when an activity does not require the same setup for each session and when utilization is not high enough to warrant a specific single-purpose use. Multipurpose rooms allow greater flexibility for scheduling and sharing space. For example, a medium-sized multipurpose room may be utilized for a lecture-based learning with theater-style seating for 50 learners on Day 1 of a course, for group learning with 8 tables for 6 to 8 people on Day 2, and for station-based learning on Day 3 where the learners rotate through multiple skill stations. Multipurpose rooms vary in size and may include the option for a mobile partition to increase the flexibility even further.

Standardized Patient Environment

Standardized patient simulation involves the use of individuals trained to portray patients and family members for the purpose of student learning. The SP environment is a microsystem in itself. There is no single best-design solution as people experiment with a variety of configurations that separate operations from education (i.e., front-stage vs. backstage). This environment is often used for high-stakes evaluations and must be designed accordingly. Ideally, an SP learning environment may include some or all of the following:

- SP patient room
- SP control room
- SP preparation, waiting, changing, and meeting space
- Faculty/educator monitor and observation room
- Storage/preparation room
- Medication room
- Debrief/multipurpose room(s)
- Kitchen area
- Soiled utility

Note: Not all of these areas will be described in this section; most have been described elsewhere.

SP Patient Room

SP-based rooms are typically designed to replicate an outpatient examination (medical) room with an exam table, chairs for the provider, patient, and patient family. The room may be configured in a variety of other ways to meet the needs of the program. Typical sizes vary from 100 to 350 square feet (9 to 32.5 m^2). Rooms may be configured with access to electronic medical records and digital resources.

SECTION 6 • Environmental Design

These rooms are typically equipped with cameras, ceiling speakers, microphones, and local inputs to capture content that will be stored in a central server and available through an AV capture or learning management systems for replay, evaluation, and/or live broadcast to conference space or debrief rooms.

SP Control Room

The primary purpose of the SP control room is for faculty and/or simulation technician operators to coordinate, record, and facilitate SP encounters and learner flow. The room provides the educator or technician access to AV control devices and/or learning management systems. The space should be at minimum large enough for equipment, seating, counter or storage space, and displays.

SP Preparation Room

SP environments may include SP preparation areas to prepare and train the SP for the encounter. In addition, the area includes space for changing into the appropriate attire for the simulation as well as space for waiting, training, and presimulation discussion with faculty and/or simulations scenario operators. The space is usually configured with small lockers, a bathroom, and modular table(s) with chairs for conferencing and refreshments. In certain regions, strict gender separation may be required.

Offices, Office Support, Audiovisual Server Room, and Mechanical Spaces

Offices

Offices for faculty, technicians, and support staff are best included near the area they support. Some may debate this point and suggest that offices be located centrally. This is a philosophical issue with no one opinion being entirely correct. It is useful to have some office space that is near the area that they support. Office space varies in size depending upon the number of individuals in the space. Beyond offices for permanent personnel who reside at the facility, one must also consider office hoteling (e.g., a room with work cubicles) options for individuals with more casual or intermittent use of the facility. This space may be configured with cubicles or a variety of other counter configurations to house nonpermanent personnel. Additional space should be allocated for office support functions such as copying, printing, and other administrative support functions.

Audiovisual and Data Server Room

Server rooms are necessary to support the wide array of simulation, AV, video teleconferencing, learning management, and simulation-specific equipment/systems. The room houses electronics and servers that manage the high volume of data collected (AV and data). Server rooms vary in size depending on the size of the center and sophistication/complexity of the AV systems. These rooms have specific HVAC (heating, ventilation, air conditioning)

requirements to ensure proper heat dissipation, power delivery, and access for easy repair. Special caution is warranted here in that this server room may house equipment that is quite different from that in typical server rooms. Standard institutional specifications for this type of room many not apply. It is important to check with appropriate regulatory agencies to ensure that you conform to their specifications.

Mechanical, Electrical, and Plumbing

All buildings have space assigned to them for mechanical components and functions. This includes ducts, elevators, and electrical grids to name a few. The engineering and architectural team should ensure that the mechanical, electrical, and plumbing (MEP) (liquid and gases) meet the functional needs and code requirements of the facility. Innocent placement of an elevator in the wrong place can create all sorts of flow problems. Additionally, elevator size should be considered to ensure that medical and simulation equipment can be transported with ease.

Having the capacity to supply medical gases, compressed air, and vacuum are increasingly necessary for simulation-based learning. Space may be required for oxygen tanks and compressors to supply medical oxygen and air if there is no availability to pipe it into the space. Compressors and vacuum units will have specific requirements relating to noise isolation, plumbing, and power. Some cost-effective options include headwalls that are equipped with their own compressors to assist with realism.

Supply/Preparation/Storage Rooms

Supply/preparation and storage rooms serve a support function for the facility with respect to consumable supplies, simulation equipment, medical equipment, office equipment, and storage and preparation of items needed for simulation-based encounters. Theses areas are variable in size and location and are critical for effective operation of the facility (Passiment et al., 2011). Depending on the size of the facility, one or more rooms may be required. What is important is to ensure that the rooms are relatively proximal to the areas they supply. As the room functions to act as a storage, preparation, and supply area, it is important to consider sinks and other required utilities to support the center (e.g., washer/dryer). The storage solutions vary in cost and efficiency. There is no single "best" solution. It is important to outline what will be placed in the room and have the architect design it to ensure all will fit. For example, beds and stretchers have a very different footprint than an intravenous (IV) pole or a box of IV fluids. Fixed storage solutions (e.g., fixed shelves) versus mobile solutions (e.g., mobile wire shelves) is an important consideration as each have their advantages and disadvantages.

In the literature, there is no clear evidence for the absolute amount of storage space required in a simulation facility. The most important consideration is that most people complain they do not have enough of it. The common benchmark of 10% to 25% of net assignable square feet can serve as a guide. Planning for and laying out the equipment and supplies intended for storage will allow for a much more precise figure. The underestimation of storage requirements is one of the top, if not the top complaint that users have.

As stated previously, laying things out with the design team will confirm your storage needs. Beyond discrete rooms, it is important to remember that storage space can be creatively incorporated into a variety of locations such as hallways and simulation rooms. This will not only off-load the burden form the storage rooms but may also aid with operations and proximity of supplies. Including power in storage solutions for equipment that requires recharging is another example of creativity that will save you time and space. When deciding to have a storage closet inside a specific training room, it is always worth considering whether it should also be accessible from the "other side of the wall" or in a common storage room in case the equipment may be required in another location while a class is taking place in that particular room. When designing these solutions, acoustic isolation is also an important consideration as different structures such as walls, doors, and windows have different acoustic properties.

Medication Rooms

Medication rooms store and dispense specific medications and supplies that support simulation scenarios in the clinical simulation rooms and SP patient rooms. Learners access medications for their scenarios from this space, allowing video-capture of the medication retrieval and preparation process. Computerized medication/supply dispensing systems may be included in these rooms. Note that the use of real or "faux" medications requires careful attention to safety and regulatory requirements.

Specialized Simulation Skills Labs

A variety of specialized simulation labs may be included in a simulation facility depending on the specific needs of the program. Their primary intent is to provide a venue for deliberate practice of specific skills and procedures while also allowing for flexibility (where possible). We will describe a few examples of those typically seen in simulation facilities. Note that many professions including nursing, allied health, and medicine all use some form of skills lab.

- Perimeter bed skills lab, common in nursing and some allied health professions, vary in size depending on the number of beds in the room. A 12-bed solution may require 2,000 square feet (185.8 m^2) to accommodate the beds and a center seating and table area. These rooms are often configured with perimeter medical-surgical beds and with center table(s) with perimeter chairs around the table(s). The table and chairs in the center of the room allow for small-group learning, lectures, and skills demonstrations in addition to activity at each bedside. These rooms may be equipped with cameras, ceiling speakers, microphones, and local inputs to capture content that will be stored in a central server.

Additionally, the rooms will have appropriately sized display and/or smart-board technology to play back or broadcast content from remote or local sources. Each bed location should also accommodate a patient monitor and computer with display.
- Procedural training environments may include rooms with table and chairs or more sophisticated virtual reality (VR) equipment. The primary intent of the lab is to allow learners to practice technical, cognitive, and procedural skills on a variety of media. This may include biologic tissue or synthetic materials. In the case of biologic tissue, the lab will need to accommodate for additional requirements including appropriate flooring, refrigeration units, sinks, as well as biohazard disposal. The rooms are similar in flexibility to what has been described for multipurpose rooms in terms of furnishings. VR surgical and procedural trainers as well as "box" trainers have their own specifications that may require wall mounting of displays versus simply rolling in an all-inclusive unit.
- Cadaveric and animal surgical labs have special requirements and are not simply a room but rather a constellation of rooms that are required to manage and host the learner encounters, cadavers, and/or animals. Abattoirs, prep areas, refrigeration rooms, and biohazard disposal areas are just a few of the required rooms to meet the requirements. In some countries, animal-based labs must follow strict procedures. The specifics of these spaces are beyond the scope of this chapter but if they apply to your potential space, collaboration with experts to ensure regulatory compliance may be necessary.

Home Environment and Other Specialty Areas

There are many versions in recreating a home environment. Some centers literally build mini-apartments with stairs to replicate the nuances of first responders navigating difficult environments, to more basic areas that include a kitchenette, seating area, and perhaps a bed. Functionally, they all serve a similar purpose—to recreate the home environment so that home health professionals and first responders can simulate encounters in a nonclinical environment such as the home.

Beyond the home environment, pharmacy (hospital and community) simulation rooms are emerging. These spaces are intended to replicate the flow and procedures generally encountered in the real setting. A hospital pharmacy area may include a faux sterile hood as well as medication-dispensing units versus a community pharmacy that may include a prescription counter, medication, and supply shelves as well as a "consult" room for individual consultation or immunizations and assessment.

The allied health specialties in particular have considerable experience in the use of simulation. Radiography laboratories, dental simulation labs, and first responder environments are a few examples. These environments share the same characteristics as others in that the space is either flexible to represent a variety of environments (e.g., disaster environment) or it may be fixed because of the physical footprint of the equipment (e.g., dental procedural simulation). Depending on the purpose of the facility, the actual learner population served, the simulation modalities utilized, and the staffing model, the rooms that constitute the center may vary greatly in number and types (Nel, 2010).

In Situ (Point-of-Care) Simulation

In situ simulation may be defined as "Simulation-based testing or educational interventions that occur in a real environment as opposed to a simulated one" (SSH, 2012). It relies on supplementing the local resources of the work environment with educational know-how and simulation technology (Møller et al., 2012).

Many simulation programs that have an affiliation with a clinical partner have the capacity to take equipment from the facility to the actual clinical area for in situ or point-of-care simulation. Depending on the type of simulation planned, in situ simulation may leverage the equipment and resources of the clinical environment itself. This simplifies the need to bring supplies and increases the environmental fidelity of the space—because it is the real thing Hssain, Alinier, Souaiby (2013). The simulation team only needs to bring simulation and AV equipment to support the encounter. In many cases however, the simulation equipment may have to be stored in the hospital environment itself. This can be problematic in overcrowded clinical environments. Any storage solution must consider security and safety. To meet regulatory requirements in certain countries, the team may also be required to bring their own supplies that are explicitly labeled "not for human use." The implication of using a native clinical environment for training is that training supplies and equipment could be confused with actual patient care equipment/supplies. This poses a safety hazard that must be mitigated (Table 6.1.1).

FORM MEETS FUNCTION—THE PROJECT TEAM AND PHASES

Prior to construction, the planning and design process typically comprises several distinct steps involving members of the institutional team working in conjunction with the architectural/consultant team. A project vision statement, which outlines the overall goals and mission of the facility and a project budget, should be well developed and well established. The following is an abbreviated review of key elements that describe the project team and phases.

Project Team

A simulation center project typically involves a fairly wide variety of participants, reflecting the various user groups that will utilize the center as well as, sometimes, consultants are required to address all of the various technical design

aspects of the project (Table 6.1.2). In all cases, the more experienced the group is in simulation and simulation facility design, the lower the risks to the project. The project team in simulation facility design varies by the size and the nature of the space involved. In the case of in situ simulation where no specific design is required, then the team may simply involve those people who plan to use the space. While the in situ space is physically set, the equipment and other needs such as AV and IT will need to be arranged to meet the objectives of the simulation-related encounter.

When physical renovation or new construction is involved, many more people with specific skill sets will be involved. The space must meet not only the needs of the institution but also the regulatory and code requirements. If an institution is fortunate to have individuals with substantive skills in simulation, then those individuals should be considered as valuable resources. The key characteristics of individuals involved as simulation subject matter experts goes beyond simply understanding simulation. Subject matter experts must understand core concepts of fidelity, equipment use, spatial and flow considerations, and operations. In the absence of such expertise, consultants can often play a valuable role in ensuring that the right questions are asked and that the key elements of the project are addressed (Table 6.1.2, Figure 6.1.1).

Project Phases

Phase I—Space Programming

This initial phase establishes the basic components of the simulation facility—the spaces that will make up the center. The outcome of this phase will be a list of spaces (with descriptive narrative), with associated areas, plus adjacency diagrams depicting idealized layout relationships. The program document gives the architect the guidelines for layout work in subsequent phases.

Also important in this phase is establishing the requirements of the AV and IT systems throughout the center, because these requirements form a key part of the project program.

The programming phase may also include development of a very conceptual layout and then development of an associated cost estimate so that all parties can be sure that the space program—and the associated size of the actual simulation facility itself—are in line with budgetary parameters.

On the owner side, this phase will typically involve the Steering Committee and the complete set of users, to ensure that all project requirements are documented.

If a consultant is being used, this phase will involve the simulation center consultant, the architect, the building engineers, and the AV/IT consultant.

The activities in this phase involve intensive meetings between the owner team and the architectural team working to develop the space program and technical requirements. This process usually involves at *minimum* two sets of meetings: one to discuss the basic requirements, the second to allow the architectural team to present the draft space program to the constituent groups.

TABLE 6.1.2

Suggested Design Team Members and Function

Group/Individual	Partial Functional Description
Architect	Provides architectural consultation, expertise, and design. The architect works with the various project groups to lead the project from conceptual planning and design, through to construction and eventual completion of the project. They leverage their specific knowledge of design to translate the vision of the stakeholder into actual form, while integrating the various technical details required of such a technologically advanced facility.
Owner representative	This may be a person or group of people who often represent the financial stakeholders of the facility. This representative may be an executive or their designee. It is not uncommon, however, for an owner to hire a firm to function as their representative to ensure that the interests of the owner are addressed and that the project remains on budget and on time.
Institutional simulation subject matter leaders	If the institution is fortunate to have people with simulation proficiency or expertise, then these individuals can play a key role in informing the process with respect to the application (simulation) and requirements for successful simulation. They are the subject matter experts (SME) in simulation. They should ensure that the vision for the facility is properly translated by the design team into function and form.
Simulation design consultants	If meaningful simulation expertise does not exist within the institution, the utilization of a simulation design consultant can help directly impact the planning stages of a project. Simulation design consultants can act as surrogates for the role of owner's simulation expert if such expertise does not already exist within the institution. They often bring a wealth of information from a broader context. They should ensure that the vision for the facility is properly translated by the design team into function and form.
Project manager	This individual keeps things on time and on budget. The project manager interfaces with most groups and may at times find they may have to juggle conflicting budgetary, time, and stakeholder needs. The project manager can either be someone within the institution's employee resources or they may be a firm selected as a consultant to provide the services of project management. Note that there may be several project managers—architectural project manager, institutional facilities project manager, and so on. They all should ensure that the vision for the facility is properly translated by the design team into function and form.
IT and AV designers or consultants	This may be an in-house or external resource that serves to ensure that the proper AV and IT systems are in place to serve the needs of the equipment and the end users. They should ensure that the vision for the facility, from an AV/IT context, is properly translated by the design team into function and form.
Construction contractor	Once designs and permits are obtained/issued, the contractor builds the facility. Having the construction contractor involved early is important to ensure that they are in alignment with some of the unique aspects related to a simulation facility. There are nuances (e.g., electrical and plumbing) that veer from common practice in traditional buildings.
Educator—user group	This group represents individuals who will inform the process with respect to the curricular, political, and quantitative requirements for the facility. These individuals may or may not be simulation educators, but will be those that utilize the space once completed. Their input and participation in the planning and design process is critical to the success of the project.
Facilities management	Depending on the institution, representatives from facilities management are often involved to ensure that the project runs smoothly and follows institutional requirements. They are in essence owner-representatives but with particular focus on the process, project management, and construction. These individuals may replace, or compliment, the project managers noted earlier in this table.
Executive decision group	In medium to larger projects, an executive decision group is often formed to deal with financial and important design questions. Ultimately it is this group that makes all final decisions. A well-formed group will delegate certain decisions to trusted stakeholders.
Equipment planners	These individuals may come from the institution or may be hired. They specialize in specifying, sourcing, and procuring equipment required for a project. In this case, that would include simulation and medical equipment. The specifications should be developed in conjunction with a variety of groups in this table.
Engineers	Engineers are a vital part of the team. They are responsible for essential design elements that include but not limited to plumbing, gas services, HVAC, electrical, lighting, and acoustics.
Institutional project core group	This group typically is made up of a combination of individuals that include simulation experts (if present), faculty/educators, IT, and administration. The key function of this group is to be the point group for contractors and vendors to communicate with as the process proceeds. This group has the responsibility of communicating with other relevant groups to ensure that key decisions are thoughtful and representative. This group typically does not have any fiscal authority.
Vendors	Once the equipment tendering and selection process has been completed, simulation equipment manufacturers can be engaged in the design process. Their input in ensuring the proper integration of their solutions, products, and systems is very important to a successful outcome.

Note: The descriptions are intended to provide basic context of individual roles. The actual job descriptions are much more complex and will vary by location and project. The most relevant issue is to appreciate that the teams involved must be well choreographed and in sync.

The term stakeholder has not been included in the table as it represents many things and may have different meanings in different institutions and organizational structures. Stakeholders may refer to the actual participant, faculty, and financial decision maker(s), to name a few.

Adapted from Seropian, M., & Lavey, R. (2010). Design considerations for healthcare simulation programs. *Society for Simulation in Healthcare*, 5(6), 338–345.

SECTION 6 • Environmental Design

Phase II—Schematic Design

After the approval of the space program and the budget, the implementation team can proceed to the design phases of the project, where the detailed layout of the center is established on the basis of the space-programming document.

In the Schematic Design phase, the overall layout of the simulation facility is established. This usually involves development of a number of layout options by the planning team, and review of these options with the owner team. After a few meetings, a final layout is established and that plan forms the basis of subsequent work.

This phase will also involve the development of the exterior design concept of the building (if it is a stand-alone facility) as well as development of preliminary engineering systems design, including HVAC, electrical, plumbing, structural, as well as IT/AV. Initial discussions regarding sustainable design also commence in this stage, setting sustainable goals for the project with follow-up required in subsequent phases.

At the end of this phase, the schematic design documents are customarily submitted to a cost estimator for development of a schematic cost estimate. If the estimate comes in above the budget, the entire project team will come together to develop a strategy to reduce cost—either by reducing project size, reducing the cost of specific project systems, or some combination of both. Participants in this phase usually include, on the owner's side, the executive decision group and a user committee, to provide feedback on the evolving schematic design documents.

On the architectural side, the entire project team will participate, and will provide system descriptions for cost-estimating purposes. The architectural team will be looking to the Steering Committee for formal approval of the Schematic Design documents and cost estimate, to make sure there is agreement on scope and project concepts prior to proceeding into the next design phase.

Phase III—Design Development

This phase involves the "development and refinement" of the design established in the Schematic Design phase. The floor plans are drawn at a larger scale, and much more detail is added. Three-dimensional views of interior space are developed, to allow the design team to advance the design of the walls, ceilings, and floor treatment, and to allow the owner group to understand the actual appearance of the center. Room data sheets and elevation drawings are key elements of this phase.

This phase will establish a more detailed design approach to all of the systems involved in the center, from architectural floor plans, wall and ceiling treatments, lighting design, location of major equipment, building engineering systems (e.g., power and ventilation), and IT and AV systems. On the owner side, the executive decision group will continue to provide oversight of the evolving project. A user group will continue to provide detailed input on the whole variety of design issues.

On the architectural side, this phase will again involve the full team, and will likely involve consultation with the vendors of the software integration systems, and the simulation equipment manufacturers. Depending on which software package is selected, that vendor may actually develop the detailed AV and IT requirements and systems design.

At the end of this phase, the complete Design Development documents are submitted to a cost estimator for pricing. Again, if there is any discrepancy between cost estimate and budget, the entire team will come together to work out a solution. Similar to Schematic Design, the architectural team will look to the owner for formal approval of the submitted documents and estimate.

Phase IV—Construction Documents

This final design phase involves the full, detailed documentation of all aspects of the project; the contractor for construction will use these documents. This is typically the longest of the three design phases, as it requires adequate time to document in great detail all of the project requirements.

The owner team will periodically review the evolving project details, usually involving a somewhat smaller user group. This review will typically involve discussion of very detailed questions, such as exact placement of wall-mounted equipment, design of storage shelving, and so on.

At the end of this phase, the owner may do a thorough, formal review of the final construction documents and provide a very detailed list of comments for discussion and action by the architectural team. However, much of this review likely has occurred at the end of the Schematic Design and Design Development phases.

During this phase, the owner team will attend to other aspects of the facility operation, such as selecting (and eventually purchasing) items that will not be provided by the general contractor, including movable furniture, loose equipment such as exam tables and hospital beds, specialized pieces of equipment, mannequins, and simulation software. It is important that this process proceeds in tandem with the schedule for completion of construction so that all aspects of the project are ready at the same time.

Phase V—Construction

The construction contractor (builder) of the project will usually be selected by bidding or by negotiation; in the latter case, the builder may become involved much earlier in the project, sometimes in the Schematic Design phase or even earlier. The early participation of the builder can provide valuable input as to cost, schedule, and constructability.

During construction, the owner team is generally reduced to one or two facilities' staff and one or two user representatives. While the facilities' staff responds to construction issues and authorizes payments, the user representative will be called on to address a continuing stream of detailed questions that arise in any construction project.

The full architectural team will remain involved, usually represented on-site by a single person for each firm, but with the entire design team involved to retain oversight and respond to issues during construction.

A particularly important player in this phase is the AV/IT designer, who will carefully monitor the installation of AV and IT infrastructure and eventually of the AV and IT systems components themselves. Representatives of some of the key vendors will also become heavily involved.

This will include for instance representatives of a simulation software company or other simulation equipment manufacturer/vendor. If the AV systems are provided through the software vendor, which often happens, then this vendor will also be a key player in this phase. The coordination among these project participants during construction is essential to a successful outcome.

Phase VI—Post Construction and Commissioning

After the general construction is complete, work is not done. Before occupancy, all of the facility systems need to be tested to make sure they are all working correctly, and working successfully in tandem. This includes the HVAC and electrical systems, IT, and of course all of the various AV equipment and software integration components that are at the heart of the day-to-day operations of the center. Adequate time needs to be allotted for this activity. It may take several weeks to months to work through this commissioning process.

FORM MEETS FUNCTION— TIMELINE, DELIVERABLES, AND COMMUNICATION

Timelines and Deliverables

Regardless of the size and complexity of the project, timelines and deliverables are important. A timeline refers to the time it will take for a specific task to be accomplished. The task should result in a *measurable* deliverable. Each task may in itself have a series of subtasks and subdeliverables. This is further complicated in that different tasks may actually be dependent on each other. That is to say that one task must be completed before the next can begin, while there are other tasks that do not have dependencies and can be performed in parallel.

Timelines and deliverables are of little value if they do not have a responsible party or individual (owner) attached to them and accountability. Proper documentation of a well-worded, precise deliverable and expected milestones can save a project time, money, and risk. An easy way to remember this concept is the acronym TOADD.

- **T**imeline
- **O**wner
- **A**ccountability
- **D**eliverables (with associated milestones)
- **D**ocumentation

Following the **TOADD** principle not only improves organization but also improves communication. While communication is complex in healthcare, it is equally complex in construction and design with significant safety implications. An effective communication strategy should be established from the outset with clearly delineated lines of communication. Rigorous adherence to these principles

must be respected and acknowledged. Communication protocols should not be purely linear but should incorporate strategies that provide cross-checks and loop-backs to reduce the risk of errors and omissions. Communicating in a language that is understandable and relevant to the person(s) receiving it is important.

Designating one responsible party for communication from each group described in Table 6.1.2 is a common strategy. The person should be selected on the basis of expertise, organization, reliability, and role within the group. Funneling communication through an unskilled individual can lead to negative results. Written communication should be clear, concise, and not buried in long streams of prose. While this seems like common sense, it is frequently not followed.

Depending on the sophistication and experience of the team members, protocol-driven forms may be used for communication. For example, a form to request a change may include the following (Figure 6.1.2):

- Date
- Requester's name and role
- Request to (name or entity)
- Purpose
- Change requested
- Current state
- Reason for change
- Financial impact
- Expected date of response

FORM MEETS FUNCTION— EQUIPMENT CONSIDERATIONS

As stated before, a simulation facility can have multiple functions including education, research, and assessment. The equipment in the facility includes medical, simulation, technical (including AV and computers), general furnishings, and consumables. Educators will see a course they need to give, while those on the side of operations will consider what is needed to operationalize it (Figures 6.1.3 and 6.1.4). The process of identifying equipment for your simulation center can be very time-consuming. If not done correctly, it can also compromise the educational objectives of the training programs. There is a fine balance of considering the needs of your stakeholders related to course development, the operationalization of the courses, and the acquisition of equipment to match and assist with obtaining these objectives. Whether purchasing equipment or taking donations, you should always consider the courses you plan to offer and how this equipment will contribute to the objectives being met. Many centers fall into the trap of being pressured to purchase equipment first, build the center, and then look at what courses they should consider. This methodology could contribute to inappropriate purchases or worse, the purchase of the wrong equipment and equipment that remains unused.

Time Units

Description	1	2	3	4	5	6	7	8	9	10	11	12
Identify stakeholders/Mission/Vision	◄►											
Identify/Select/Convene design team	◄——►											
Commissioning phase		◄——►										
Space programming			◄——►									
Schematic design and detailed design				◄——►								
Construction documents & Permits					◄———►							
Construction							◄—————————►					
Equipment identification & purchase			◄———————————————►									
AV/IT				◄———————————————►								
Identify curricular and volume needs	◄———————►											
Sign-off/Hand-over												◄►

FIGURE 6.1.2 Sample timeline.

Didactic and group learning	Give lecture
	Observe recorded video of performances (debriefing software and hardware from above)
	Teach with simulators
	Observe simulation
	Record educational sessions
Simulation Practice Sessions	Operate simulator and patient monitor
	Teach content
	Debrief with video
	Record video of performances
Assessment	Listen and view live to simulation room
	Communicate with simulation room as educator or voice of the patient
	Record simulation session

FIGURE 6.1.3 A course through the eyes of an educator.

Classroom or Debriefing Room	Computer with PowerPoint installed.
	Display with associated input source to show curricular content
	Microphone and speakers
	Inter or intranet connectivity
Simulation Room	Simulator, medical and associated equipment
	Display with associated input source to show curricular content
	Computer for display or EHR
	Cameras, microphones, and recording capabilities for review and reflection
	Inter or intranet connectivity
Simulation Room	Cameras, microphones, and recording capabilities for review and reflection
	Simulator, medical and associated equipment
	Computer for running simulator
	Inter or intranet connectivity

FIGURE 6.1.4 A course through the eyes of operations.

As part of the initial stakeholder analysis, you will want to understand how courses will be taught and what environments will be needed. The identification of environments is important to equipment acquisition. As an example, if you plan on having an anesthesia course in an operating room setting, you may need to purchase an anesthesia machine, operating room table, IV poles, and other equipment and supplies specific to an operating room setting. Understanding the course objectives will also assist with the identification of equipment needs. While making these decisions, you should ask yourself, "Do I need this piece of equipment to help me meet my course objectives or is this something that just adds to the ambience of the room setup?" This will allow you to refine your equipment requirements to the "must haves," "like to have," and "nice to have."

Basic Furnishings, Finishes, and Flooring

Irrespective of the size and sophistication, simulation facilities require basic furnishing such as desks, tables, chairs, and counters. Well-thought-out furnishing selection and finishes will impact flexibility and function. Modular versus fixed furnishings are a good example of this. Additional considerations include the following:

- Whiteboards or smart-board technology placement.
- Sufficient counter space should exist to account for workspace, or computers and other equipment that will require a resting surface.
- Other basic furnishings such as sinks, towel dispensers, soap/hand gel dispensers, and storage systems are important to consider.

- Flooring that is durable and resistant to moisture and heavy use. Some facilities will use raised flooring for additional flexibility (e.g., to run cabling); however, this is extremely costly.
- The center should be inviting to the learner, educator, and other staff. Finishes should consider this while being durable and practical.
- Window coverings should not only be aesthetically pleasing but be practical to help educators and learners meet their objectives.

Medical Equipment and Simulation Equipment

Early in the design process, you will want to identify the medical equipment required to meet programmatic functional needs. Beyond meeting the educational, assessment, or research needs of the simulation program, medical and simulation equipment informs the design process. Design elements that need to be considered include the following:

- Sizing (dimensions) and space allocation and storage needs for equipment and supplies
- Electrical, plumbing, and structural requirements to support equipment
- IT requirements of equipment

The facility must support the equipment within it. Doors must be wide enough to accommodate different pieces and sizes of equipment, hallways should be designed to accommodate for equipment turn radius, the electrical system must support the power draw of not just one piece of equipment but all, and the ventilation must account for volatile gases or enriched oxygen. This list of considerations is long and detailed. The point, however, is that the architects, engineers, and other vendors must understand what equipment will be used and how.

Medical equipment in a simulation facility will vary by center. Table 6.1.3 provides a list of some medical equipment that a simulation facility may need to acquire. In some cases, the medical equipment needs will be very specific (e.g., a specific IV pump) and in others more general (e.g., any medical-surgical bed). The equipment can be purchased at a variety of stages depending on budget and need. Matching equipment to an affiliated health center or other clinical environment may provide advantages related to training, purchasing power, and donation.

As a general rule, when purchasing simulation equipment, it is important to first know your stakeholders, know their courses, and then purchase the simulation equipment accordingly. Simulation equipment, as is the case for medical equipment, should facilitate a defined educational/research strategy for training and/or assessment. There are many types of simulation equipment to consider. They include the following:

- Patient simulators/mannequins of various sexes, ages, and levels of technical features
- Physical task and procedural trainers
- VR task and procedural trainers
- Anatomical models
- Computer/screen-based simulators

A detailed description of these categories is beyond the scope of this chapter; however, an equipment purchasing strategy is important to develop early in the design process.

Technical Equipment (Audiovisual and Information Technology)

IT and AV equipment are becoming important parts of many simulation facilities. One should take into consideration how the simulation facility will operate, how courses will be taught, what assessment needs exist, and how technology can assist with these efforts. Not having the right technology will compromise your course flow, learning objectives, and assessment capabilities.

The IT needs of a simulation facility move beyond simply having access to Internet or intranet systems. Systems may be required to support AV broadcasts, playback and recording needs, as well as the low-voltage or IT needs of the simulation systems themselves. The selection of appropriate cameras and microphones for broadcasting, processing/editing, recording, or playback is increasingly complex. Table 6.1.4 describes some key considerations. Cameras and microphones should be able to provide good-quality audio and visual experiences for the learners and educators. However, audio and video quality is only as good as the speakers and display that are used. A common pitfall is undersizing displays or using less-expensive projectors with poor image quality and lower lumens.

Many commercially available AV systems leverage software packages that manage and display the AV content. These packages are hybrid learning and AV management systems. Ease of use and reliability of these systems has greatly improved and should be a key consideration in purchasing. There are also a number of stand-alone simulation and SP center calendar management, facilities management, and learning management systems on the market that can assist with the tasks of day-to-day operations, course or case creation, and data management. This software and hardware can range in price, technical requirements, and features (Table 6.1.4).

Digital and analog systems have pros and cons. Digital systems have the potential to be of higher quality. However, this is not always the case. Equating digital with quality is a mistake. Digital systems are likely to be more flexible and upgradable. Budget, quality, and future needs will ultimately determine what system is most applicable. The different systems will have impact on cabling, power, and heat dissipation (ventilation). Compatibility should also be one of the factors you should consider when making your AV/IT purchases. You should ensure that the AV and or IT equipment is compatible with the simulation equipment you are purchasing or already own. You will also want to ensure that the AV/IT equipment is compatible with your organization's IT systems. Some equipment will not work on some networks owing to bandwidth and firewall issues.

AV systems and servers can be local (e.g., control room) or placed in a separate location. Depending on the complexity of your system and the size of your facility, either may apply. In either case, sufficient space must be allocated

TABLE 6.1.3	
Examples of Medical Equipment	
Patient beds	Defibrillators
IV poles	IV pumps
Exam lights	Wheelchairs
Overbed tables	Stretchers
Anesthesia machines	Booms
Ventilators	Headwalls
Crash carts	Patient lifts

TABLE 6.1.4	
Audio/Video Considerations	
Camera and microphone placement to capture needed content	Broadcast, monitoring, playback, and recording capabilities
Camera type (fixed vs. movable)	Audio speaker requirements for content and paging needs
Camera mounting—ceiling, wall, or on a track	Microphones—fixed, directional, or portable
Relation of microphones to ventilation system	Ease of use of system
Reliability of the system	Internal/external simulation data transmission

for these systems. The design team, AV vendor, and IT department will need to help to determine how much space and its location. Additionally, the allocated space may have specific ventilation and cooling requirements to ensure that the equipment does not overheat and is maintained to manufacturer specification.

FORM MEETS FUNCTION— ADDITIONAL CONSIDERATIONS UNIQUE TO SIMULATION

As stated in the introduction, a simulation facility is an odd marriage of a clinical, theatrical, and educational environment. As such, there are some additional important characteristics to consider that may be foreign to the architects as well as the MEP contractors.

Facility Systems

The design team will outline and define rooms, power, and cabling to support basic building functions such as HVAC, telephone, data, and plumbing. While this may seem obvious, there may be specific code and institutional needs related to this.

Cabling

There are a variety of solutions to provide pathways for cabling, power, and other simulation-related equipment. Raised floors, floor channels, or in-wall solutions all have pluses and minuses when considering cost, flexibility, and acoustics. The project team should consider each option and do a cost-benefit analysis to achieve the functional need related to the space at the best price point.

Acoustics

Sounds in a simulation center can be very disruptive and interfere with training or testing. Whether it is noise from the outside, noise from other simulation rooms, or people talking in the hallway, it can compromise your learning environment. The size, shape, furnishings, doors, and flooring of a room all impact sound transmission. Walls should be constructed of materials that prevent unwanted transmission of sound. Where possible, walls should go from floor to ceiling slab. Many facilities are built with hung/drop ceilings and wallboard that extends only to the edge of the hung tiles. This creates a perfect and unwanted sound transmission space within the ceiling. Certain rooms may create more noise than others and therefore each room type must be considered individually. If budget permits, an acoustic engineer can solve many of the issues related to unwanted sound transmission.

Many facilities use mobile partitions or wall divider systems to increase room flexibility. It is important to consider the acoustic quality of the dividers as they vary. The noise rating of the divider should be specified prior to purchase. Once a divider system has been specified, the structural requirements to physically support and house the system must be taken into consideration by the design team.

Shared spaces offer many benefits. Sound isolation is not one of them. Whether it is a large skills lab or a shared control room, the transmission of sound of unrelated activity can be disruptive and problematic. The use of walls, furnishings, and technology (e.g., headsets) may provide a viable mitigation solution. It is important to ensure that the design team understands how the room is to be used and can identify potential acoustic issues related to the space.

In addition to physical design issues related to acoustics, placement and location of AV equipment is important to consider as well. Placing microphones next to a vent will result in noise generated by airflow that will interfere with audio quality. Similarly, vents should be sized appropriately to a low-noise-level specification.

Gases

Clinical simulation spaces often require gases and vacuum to support the simulations and other activities in the center. The gases may include oxygen, air, nitrous oxide, and carbon dioxide. It is important to determine how these gases are to be used, as there are multiple design implications.

- If the gases are to be used on human beings (e.g., a face mask delivering oxygen to an SP), then specific code requirements will apply in many jurisdictions. The cost of medical-grade gases and plumbing is far greater than nonmedical grade.
- The use of pure oxygen in a confined space can increase the ambient oxygen concentration considerably and therefore pose an explosive/fire hazard. In this circumstance, ventilation would need to be designed to ensure that ambient oxygen concentration remains below a specific level.
- The use of compressed air in lieu of oxygen is a reasonable solution. This solution, however, must take into account equipment that requires the use of pure oxygen (e.g., modern ventilators). The more modern systems will alarm if less than 100% oxygen is detected and will need to be decommissioned and altered to disable this feature. The manifold (cover plate) will also need to be labeled "not for clinical use or human use" to avoid safety errors from occurring.
- Oxygen, air, and vacuum may originate locally or be plumbed in from adjacent facilities (e.g., health system). In the former case, design consideration must be given to house compressors, vacuum units, and gas cylinders.
- Appropriate and well-placed gas regulators and shutoff valves and systems should be in place, which are often required for safety and regulatory reasons (Figure 6.1.5). Additional shutoff valves/systems in control rooms will also give operators the ability to easily emulate a critical gas failure (Figure 6.1.6).

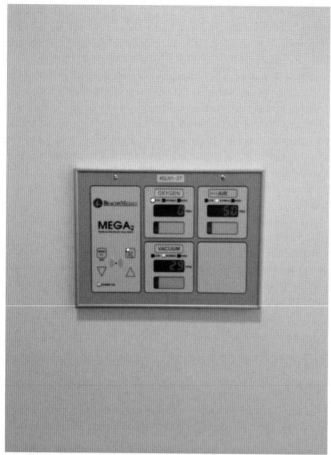

FIGURE 6.1.5 Gas alarm panel with shutoff valves in the corridor. (Photo: University of Hertfordshire, Hertfordshire Intensive Care and Emergency Simulation Center.)

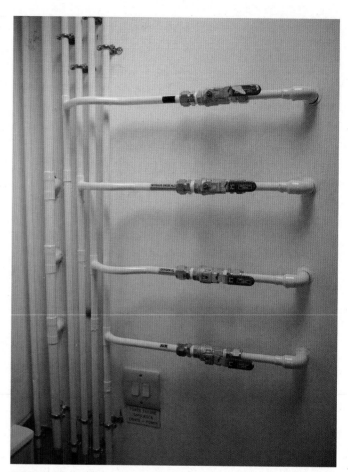

FIGURE 6.1.6 Control room, gas shutoff valves, and master switch for power and lighting in the simulation room. (Photo: University of Hertfordshire, Hertfordshire Intensive Care and Emergency Simulation Center.)

Heating, Ventilation, and Air Conditioning

The HVAC system not only provides comfort to the building occupants, but also ensures that equipment is maintained to manufacturer specification. Room temperature is a function of many things. The number of people in a room as well as the presence of heat-generating equipment will contribute to a room's temperature. If possible, each room should have its own ambient temperature control. Vents and other mechanical items associated with the HVAC system should be placed in such a way as to not impede core facility functions. New HVAC technology has had a positive impact of design and sound issues typically associated with HVAC. Technologies like "chilled beams," where the beams would be water-cooled or heated from a centralized unit, have led to a drastic reduction of sound generation. As with other engineering considerations, it is suggested that you meet with your engineering team to discuss the best methods and equipment to help meet the simulation center's operational needs.

Electrical and Lighting

Educational spaces have specific needs and requirements in addition to "normal" electrical considerations for any building. Identifying the likely final location of equipment will assist the design/construction team with placement of power outlets, lights, and switches.

Power

Sufficient power to run and maintain the facility is important. A list of the power requirements related to equipment to be housed in the facility allow the engineers to determine optimal power delivery systems. Electrical engineers do not simply determine the location of outlets but the amount of power available within specific zones. Outlets should be placed in proximity to anticipated areas of need. They may be located in the ceiling, wall, or floor. This powers lights, equipment, and other important infrastructure. Many centers request that clinical rooms emulate real environments by giving the appearance of having normal and emergency power outlets. While the electrical design of such a system is not the same as for a hospital, it must be designed in a manner to simulate primary, secondary, and total power failures WHILE still maintaining power to key pieces of equipment (e.g., mannequin or camera). All this needs to be controlled from a specific location such as the control room (figure 6.1.6). Similar considerations apply to lighting during a power failure. Specific code requirements may preclude simulating a complete power failure.

Lighting

The quality, location, type, and temperature of lighting are important. This does not only apply to the lights themselves, but also to the use of appropriate shades in rooms where windows are present. The temperature and quality of light in a room will impact camera-capture quality as well as display quality. The appropriate placement and use of light switches and dimming is important. Certain rooms may require zone lighting to provide optimal viewing of content on displays. Other rooms may have special characteristics that prevent transmission of light from one room to another. Specifically, rooms that use "one-way glass" will need to accommodate for the likelihood of unwanted light transmission to the room being observed. This will occur when the lighting from a room is sufficient to overcome the "one-way" properties of the glass. Keep in mind that the source of light may not only be traditional lights but may also originate from computer displays, ambient outdoor light, or any device that emits light. Appropriate use of blackout shades and other strategies is important to address this real issue.

QUICK TIPS, PEARLS, AND COMMON PITFALLS

Equipment and Resources

- If your center is part of a medical center or is hospital-based, talk with the maintenance department. You may be surprised at the equipment they have and their willingness to refurbish it for your center. There may be patient beds, wheelchairs, or stretchers that may not be fit for real patients any longer, but may be able to be repaired and utilized within your center.
- Talk with your facility's planners. These groups will have a detailed knowledge of construction and renovations. You may be able to obtain equipment such as headwalls and exam lights from units that are being remodeled.
- A quick trip to your institution's warehouse may be very beneficial when looking for surpluses of medical and office equipment. It is also beneficial to establish a communication plan with someone in your warehouse. This will allow you to create a "wish list" that you can share with them and have them contact you when something becomes available.
- Decide whether actual medical equipment or supplies are necessary for the simulation (buy the model currently in use by your hospital) or if a prop is sufficient.
- Establish a relationship with your purchasing department. Have a member of your simulation center on the hospital supply acquisition team. They can often get new equipment at a significant cost reduction or even donated for educational purposes.

As an example, if the hospital is purchasing 25 new defibrillators, perhaps they would also purchase one for your simulation center or include a requirement in the purchasing agreement that the vendor provide a unit for teaching use. The cost when purchased in bulk is much cheaper. Because you will be required to teach courses that may utilize this equipment, you will need the most current version for your center. You should reach out to your purchasing department to help them understand what you are trying to do and see whether they can be of any assistance to you.

Design Pearls

- Visit simulation programs early to understand the different approaches to simulation facility design, paying attention to flow, flexibility, adjacencies, operational efficiencies, ratios of simulation rooms to control rooms and simulation rooms to debrief space. Ask the sites what would they design differently if they could. Ask them whether the design meets their current needs and the needs of the future. If not, why not? Look for equipment in the hallways and ask why it is there.
- Consider creating distinct learning zones. Creating highly effective learning environments requires negotiating functional requirements with a less tangible, but still essential, understanding of how best to facilitate the movement of people, different learning methodologies, educational modalities, and public and private space. Flexible design maximizes utilization and future programmatic need. Carefully planned adjacencies define flow patterns that support optimal learning and efficiency. These objectives can be achieved by creating three distinct learning zones for high-fidelity clinical simulation, SP-based simulation, and skill and procedural training.
- Define a standard for ratios between control rooms and simulation rooms and simulation rooms and debrief rooms. Deviate from the standard purposefully as the ratio will impact more than just a single room but also adjacencies and flow.
- Consider establishing a goal for storage for each simulation area 10% to 25% of net assignable square footage to create flexibility.
- Consider a "Simulation Apartment" concept where learning is "isolated" from interruptions by having the simulation room, control room, consumables, medications, and debrief spaces relatively adjacent to one another. This allows for educational isolation as well as efficiency in operations.
- Mobile partition walls create spaces with size flexibility, especially for multipurpose rooms. They are also expensive and have specific support structure requirements.

- Select furniture that supports flexibility—tables that fold and roll with ease, chairs that stack onto rolling units.
- Ensure that the rooms you design are sized to accommodate the typical learner load.
- Stay away from labeling rooms with too much specificity unless the rooms are solely intended for that purpose. A room labeled as an ICU can take a life of its own and make the space nonflexible. Moreover, defining a room tends to incentivize individuals to purchase equipment that adds little to the simulation.
- This is your space; design it to fit your stakeholders' needs.
- Mock up the rooms prior to building to make sure they will meet your needs and to evaluate the flow of equipment into and out of the room.
- A clear and nonthreatening entrance to your simulation space is always a great beginning for your learners and educators.
- If you think you have enough storage, you are likely wrong; list the equipment to be stored and lay it out.

Project Team and Process Pearls

- A Project Shepherd—On the owner side, it is extremely helpful to designate a single individual as the point person for the project throughout its duration. Sometimes referred to as the "Project Shepherd," this individual helps maintain the focus on the original mission and goals of the project and serves as the clearinghouse for all owner correspondence, and in so doing provides clear direction to the team. This may be the project manager or may simply be a champion who acts as a resource for the project team.
- Project Management—Though this has been mentioned before, it warrants another mention. A successful simulation center project requires the full and careful coordination of a large number of technical systems and the people who design and install them. There is ample opportunity for miscommunication, so make sure that this coordination happens.
- Avoid interpreting documents such as architectural floor plans or elevations unless familiar with their use.
- Force those communicating with you to explain and document the function related to concepts on technical lists or drawings. Rather than just list 20 pieces of AV equipment, the vendor should list the equipment and document what function the equipment will provide that is relevant to the user.
- Avoid the temptation of circumventing communication protocols.

- If you note that communication is not effective, make your concerns know and document.
- Have frequent coordination meetings between relevant groups to ensure everyone is on the same page.
- Trust but confirm and verify. When so many people/groups are involved, mistakes and assumptions will be inevitable.
- Stick to your timeline and deliverables. Not doing so can cause problems for others and sets the precedent that it is OK to be late.
- Do not be shy to say you do not understand something, especially technical materials/subjects.
- Commissioning—Do not underestimate the time needed to commission (test) all of the various technical systems; the simulation facility is NOT simply ready to go when the contractor is done.
- Unless you have specific room layout requirements over an extended period of time, consider making your rooms small, medium, and large "stages" that can meet the needs of multiple learner group types.
- Consider the comfort and needs of your simulation staff in your facility design. Lounges, changing rooms, and cafeterias are important for those that work in a fixed building. They are often sacrificed for educational or operational space.

Common Pitfalls

- Not enough storage . . . not enough storage . . . not enough storage!
- Inability to move large equipment through doors or around corners—make certain your doors are wide enough to accommodate the equipment you plan to use.
- No clear mission or vision, failure to clearly establish the support of key stakeholders, and no clear governance or business plan. Without a clear mission/vision, it is difficult to sell your new program to initiate collaboration and buy-in, develop a business and governance plan, obtain initial and ongoing funding stream, and subsequent faculty and learner training necessary for successful center initiation and ultimate sustainability of your program.
- Inadequate faculty training programs.
- No clear flow segregating participants from SPs from simulation center staff.
- Poor acoustic capture and isolation.
- No planning for future growth and expansion.
- No vetting equipment needs to match institutional direction.
- Inadequate debriefing space necessitating debriefing in simulation rooms.
- Poor communication resulting in error and omissions.
- Visiting other simulation centers to see how their space works and assuming what you see is best practice.

CHALLENGES FOR SIMULATION IN LATIN AMERICA

Augusto Scalabrini-Neto, MD, PhD
President, Brazilian Association for Simulation in Healthcare

Latin America, considered from Mexico to Chile and Argentina, is a large continent, with about 21 different countries. Despite the common language (Spanish for most of the countries) and Iberic heritage, each one has its own cultural and economic characteristics. Some reached an advanced degree of development, both cultural and economic, while others are still struggling. Even inside the same country, there are many regional discrepancies, from both the cultural and the economic points of view. This patchwork makes the generalization of concepts and analyses very difficult.

We also have to consider that even the wealthiest Latin American countries do not have a per capita gross internal product close to the United States and Europe. So, the money spent on education, and in particular medical education, does not match what is spent in more-developed nations.

The formal Latin American educational system is the traditional European model. Many Universities base their courses in formal lectures, in big conference rooms, and the distance between teacher and student is large. Furthermore, a large number of undergraduate medical schools are focused on the admission tests for medical residencies, considering the students' performance best according to the number of students admitted to residency programs. Thus, the focus is not on competencies or skills, but on passing a terminal, isolated test.

Some Latin American countries are now starting to implement interprofessional education (IPE), but this concept is still new to Latin America. Thus far, education has been profession-specific and students never trained together. To change these paradigms is a significant challenge.

First, from the economic point of view, to implement a simulation center can be very challenging. The cost of simulation equipment can be high, and many institutions do not have a budget adequate to purchase these devices. Thus, low-cost simulation is essential for the development of the method. New alternatives must be found to make simulation economically viable to everywhere.

Traditional Latin American teachers do not adapt easily to active teaching models. It is a problem for them to feel exposed, and resistance is created under the argument "I have always taught this way, and it has always worked." Thus, implementing a new teaching methodology such as simulation can be very hard, and training faculty becomes another challenge. Fortunately, the younger faculty are much more open to new techniques and technology. Training efforts, therefore, are being placed on them.

Colombia was the first country in Latin America to adopt simulation-based education. For regional reasons, simulation started there first. In Columbia, the Asociación Colombiana de Simulación Clínica is a traditional and strong simulation society, which had its first meeting in 2011. Simulation is widely used among this group.

Brazil was next, and in 2010 the Brazilian Association for Simulation in Healthcare (ABRASSIM) was founded. This organization currently has more than 300 members. Simulation is spreading all over the country, and the number of simulation centers is increasing rapidly. Chile and Mexico had a similar experience with simulation, establishing the Sociedad Chilena de Simulacion Clinica y Seguridad del Paciente (SOCHISIM) and Asociación Mexicana de Simulación Clinica (AMESIC) in 2011. All these countries have faculty development programs with national and international courses, and research is growing fast.

Other countries such as Argentina, Bolivia, Costa Rica, Honduras, Ecuador, Peru, and Panama are starting their societies, reflecting the increasing interest of these nations in simulation. Most of the Latin American simulation centers are linked to Universities, but hospitals are starting to develop them as well. Because of this relationship, most centers are dedicated to undergraduate courses, especially medicine. Skills training centers are the most common model, but high-technology simulation is becoming more present.

This is an overview of the challenges of simulation in Latin America today. Much has been done, and the technique is gaining more and more importance. However, there is much still to be done, especially as developing countries strive to implement their programs and to create low-cost simulation solutions.

Thanks to Dr. Juan Manuel Fraga for his kind suggestions and data.

WHAT CAN I DO TO GET STARTED TODAY BEFORE MY SIMULATION FACILITY IS READY? WHAT ELEMENTS OF MY SIMULATION PROGRAM CAN I DEVELOP PRIOR TO GETTING THE KEYS?

The core concept to appreciate is that a simulation PROGRAM leverages space to achieve its goals. Preparing your *program* to be ready for opening day is important. The SSH accreditation guidelines are a resource for this process (SSH, 2012). The goal should be to be as high functioning as possible on Day 1. While all may not apply, the following elements should be considered:

- Write a mission and vision statement if not already done.
- Establish your simulation program governance and organizational structure.
- Engage executive leadership early in the simulation program.
- Hire your personnel on the basis of existing demands and anticipated demands. If a director (or similar) has not been hired, then prioritize this.
- Develop a business plan and budget.
- Establish a commissioning plan for the new facility.
- Develop metrics and processes to evaluate what the program does.
- Develop policies, procedures, and guidelines for core areas such as confidentiality, scheduling, and equipment use to name a few.
- Identify and develop your educators and faculty.
- Prepare materials about your center for your institution and the community.

BEEN THERE, DONE THAT: WHAT CAN A CENTER THAT ALREADY EXISTS DO TO CONTRIBUTE TO THE DEVELOPMENT OF FUTURE SITES?

It is much easier to accommodate changes in your layout design before building than to remodel or reconfigure your space at a later date. Traveling to a variety of different simulation centers through the US and/or world is well worth the time. We each should share (as an unwritten obligation) to aid others in other's quest to optimize their learning space and budget.

As you use your new simulation center, any shortcomings in your facility design will quickly become apparent. Some of these can be easily fixed and others may require a sizable remodel. Talk with other centers and see whether they had similar issues and what solutions they were able to implement. As you find limitations, or more importantly, solutions, share them with others in the simulation community. While remodeling is inevitable to some degree over time, successfully designed centers will need to expand as they become more successful. Anticipate growth in your initial plan and project designs. While we take whatever space allocated for education, use your stakeholders to help vision for a future where growth will be a necessity—and expansion will follow.

Rarely do successful hospital or clinic environments remain static through long periods of time. The same holds true for simulation or educational spaces. New approaches or recent technology will sometimes lead to difficulties in readily adapting your current space to new or novel techniques. Sharing your experiences and innovations through online communities, publications, or conferences will be appreciated by all in our small, but actively growing community. Sharing verbally with each other is important, but does not have the degree of impact as is seen with publication. Support our education and simulation journals by disseminating your work in a written form.

SUMMARY

A simulation facility can be as simple as a room or as complex as a clinical environment. Understanding your mission, vision, and who you will serve should guide the process. Understanding the types of rooms that are typically found in a simulation facility will help you define the required spaces. A useful analogy is that of a theater—what does the front-stage look like (simulation room or classroom) and what does the backstage (e.g., control room) need to support a successful encounter on the front stage? The architectural team in collaboration with the user/owner team must agree to design a flexible facility that will allow form to meet functional need. The design process is complex even in the simplest of facilities. Trying to overdesign a center is costly and does not always lead to the best functional result for your target audience. Learn from others and reach out for pearls. Enjoy your new center!

REFERENCES

Alinier, G., & Platt, A. (2013). International overview of high-level simulation education initiatives in relation to critical care. *Nursing in Critical Care, 19*(1), 42–49.

Bradley, P., & Postlethwaite, K. (2003). Setting up a clinical skills learning facility. *Medical Education, 37*(1), 6–13.

Dieckmann, P., Gaba, D., & Rall, M. (2007). Deepening the theoretical foundations of patient simulation as social practice. *Simulation in Healthcare, 2*(3), 183–193.

Haute Autorité De Santé. (2012). *Guide de bonnes pratiques en matière de simulation en santé.* Retrieved from http://www.has-sante.fr/portail/jcms/c_1355008/guide-bonnes-pratiques-simulation-sante-guide

Hssain I., Alinier, G., Souaiby, N. (2013). In-situ simulation: a different approach to patient safety through immersive training. *Mediterr J Emerg Med, 15,*17–28.

Møller, T. P., Østergaard, D., & Lippert, A. (2012). Facts and fiction—Training in centres or in situ. *Trends in Anaesthesia and Critical Care, 2*(4), 174–179.

Nel, P.W. (2010). The use of an advanced simulation training facility to enhance clinical psychology trainees' learning experiences. *Psychol Learn Teach, 9*(2), 65–72.

Passiment, M., Sacks, H., & Huang, G. C. (2011). *Medical simulation in medical education: results of an AAMC survey* (pp. 1–44). Washington, DC: Association of American Medical Colleges.

Seropian, M., & Lavey, R. (2010). Design considerations for Healthcare Simulation Facilities. *Simulation in Healthcare, 5*(6), 338–345.

Society for Simulation in Healthcare. (2012). *Society for simulation in healthcare's accreditation of healthcare simulation programs.* Retrieved from Society for Simulation in Healthcare website: http://ssih.org/accreditation-of-healthcare-simulation-programs

Weinstock, P. H., Kappus, L. J., Kleinman, M. E., Grenier, B., Hickey, P., & Burns, J. P. (2005). Toward a new paradigm in hospital-based pediatric education: The development of an onsite simulator program. *Pediatric Critical Care Medicine, 6*(6), 635–641.

CHAPTER 6.2

Space: Potential Locations to Conduct Full-Scale Simulation-Based Education

Guillaume Alinier, PhD, MPhys, PgCert, SFHEA, CPhys, MInstP, MIPEM, Fernando Bello, PhD, Ashwin A. Kalbag, MBBS, DA, MD, FFARCSI, FRCA and Roger L. Kneebone, PhD, FRCS, FRCGP

ABOUT THE AUTHORS

GUILLAUME ALINIER's career started in 2000 at the University of Hertfordshire, UK, where he was involved in assessment, simulation-based education, and faculty development, as well as designing and running the large multiprofessional simulation center, a hub of knowledge development and collaboration for over 10,000 students, professionals, and visitors annually. He has been involved in projects in relation to interprofessional simulation, conducts workshops, helps develop simulation centers internationally, and regularly contributes to journal publications and book chapters. Prof. Alinier currently leads research and simulation projects at Hamad Medical Corporation Ambulance Service in Qatar.

FERNANDO BELLO is a Reader in Surgical Graphics & Computing in the Department of Surgery and Cancer at Imperial College London, UK. His main research interests are in medical virtual environments and modeling and simulation, including development of patient-specific simulation; e-learning applications for a number of surgical procedures; and exploring the integration of simulation and context. He has published widely in technological, as well as medical and educational journals.

ASHWIN A. KALBAG is a consultant in Anaesthesia and pain management at Charing Cross Hospital in London, which is part of Imperial College NHS Trust. He takes a keen interest in training and education and has been appointed as college tutor by the Royal College of Anaesthetists in the UK. He also is a confidential trainee advisor for the Imperial School of Anaesthesia. Dr. Kalbag has a keen interest in medical simulation and has held the position of Honorary Simulation Fellow at the University of Hertfordshire (UK) clinical simulation centre and helped devise scenarios and run simulation sessions for medical trainees.

ROGER L. KNEEBONE is Professor of Surgical Education at Imperial College London, UK. He has a clinical background, having trained and practiced both as a general surgeon and as a family physician. He has a wide range of research interests, with a particular focus on innovative approaches to contextualized simulation and interdisciplinary practice. Roger has an international profile, publishes widely, and reviews for many international journals.

Conflict of Interest: *Fernando Bello* is a founding shareholder and nonexecutive director of Convincis Ltd. but receives no payment for his involvement. *Roger Kneebone* is a founding shareholder of Convincis Ltd. but receives no payment for his involvement.

Acknowlegment: Roger Kneebone and Fernando Bello would like to thank the Distributed Simulation team and the London Deanery STeLI project for funding the DS development and research.

ABSTRACT

Simulation can be done for system testing, orientation, and, more commonly at the present time in healthcare, for educational purposes. Choosing where and how to set up a space to be used for any type of simulation-based activity, whether it is for educational or operational purposes, is an important decision with potentially long-term consequences. Several key factors will be explored in this chapter alongside consideration of the various options available. This will be considered in line with anticipated usage in terms of participant volume, type(s) of activity(ies), anticipated growth, the breadth and depth of the technology currently available, and the implementation of innovative ideas. There is not any proven best solution at the moment, but this knowledge gap certainly provides a great opportunity, especially if the variables thought to affect learning outcomes or transfer of learning to the clinical area can be controlled. This chapter is complementary to other chapters in this book and will also address key questions in relation to identifying, obtaining, and configuring the space best suited to establishing a simulation program, or simply facilitating simulation-based learning activities on the basis of needs, circumstances, and resources. This chapter will help readers, whether they are beginners or seasoned simulationists/educators/technicians/technologists/managers/directors, decide what might be their best option(s) for consideration in terms of possible locations and setups, judge the potential impact on their simulation program in terms of expected advantages and drawbacks, and hopefully make the right decision on the basis of their circumstances.

CASE EXAMPLE

You are in charge of setting up a simulation program and have been given the opportunity to consider several options as to where these could be delivered. You can either set up a new center, refurbish an existing facility, or facilitate simulation-based educational sessions on a temporary or permanent basis in the clinical environment. In all cases, the aim will be for you to come with the best solution to conduct full-scale simulated healthcare professional interactions and patient care scenarios taking in consideration your actual needs and resources, and very importantly, the expected outcome. Ranging from in situ clinical or prehospital care areas, to the repurposing of existing facilities, depending on the intended aim(s) and objectives, the possibilities are potentially vast and hence require careful consideration.

INTRODUCTION AND BACKGROUND

Simulation in its various modalities is now widely used in healthcare education. Owing to the complexity of the technology used in the early days of the field, simulation making use of full-body patient simulators traditionally took place in dedicated rooms or simulation centers where considerable effort was made to mimic the real working environment (Abrahamson & Wallace, 1980). Unencumbered by cables and wires (due to Wi-Fi), portable simulation programs enabled by modern technology mitigate several limitations of more traditional (nonportable) simulation and introduce new approaches to healthcare education and research (Kobayashi et al., 2008).

High-fidelity full-scale simulation is increasingly utilized to test systems or protocols and to orient new staff to an environment. In a purely educational context, full-scale simulation relies on either bringing the learners to a specific location or taking the educators and the tools of the trade (simulators and audiovisual [AV] system) that may be required to the learners in their usual working environment. In both cases, a space has to be either permanently or temporarily dedicated to the learning experience (Figure 6.2.1). That space may need to be adapted so the intended objectives of the simulated experience can be addressed in an optimal way. A dictionary will define "space" as the boundless three-dimensional (3D) extent in which an object exists and events occur, having relative position and direction. In the context of healthcare simulation, it can either mean the space designed to conduct simulated clinical events, or the space needed for group discussions or debriefing following a simulated act, or indeed simulation of events in the space where they normally happen, that is, "in situ simulation."

These educational opportunities open up a large number of options to consider, ranging from solely running in

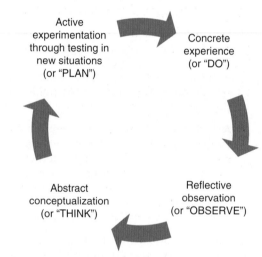

FIGURE 6.2.1 Kolb's circle of experiential learning (Kolb, 1984).

situ simulation sessions in any location required, to reconfiguring a small or large space for simulation-based educational activities on a permanent or temporary basis, which may significantly influence the technology adopted, and the time and monetary investment allocated for the physical alterations made to this space or environment. The other potential consideration is designing from scratch a completely dedicated simulation center, which is discussed in chapter 6.1.

SIGNIFICANCE

The educational environment, which consists of the spatial entity, as well as the conditions in which a particular activity is carried out, has a significant impact on the assimilation and retention of knowledge, along with the learning that occurs. As such, the space where one may decide to facilitate simulation-based educational activities needs to be considered in the light of a variety of factors that will ultimately affect the success of the program. Making the right decision is often about achieving the right balance, compromising if and where it is most appropriate to do so. Unfortunately, as for many other things, there is no "one-size-fits-all" solution that can be solely put forward in this chapter, because individual circumstances can vary greatly, ruling out certain possibilities and imposing other constraints.

THEMES

The Simulation Space as a Macroentity

Carefully choosing the location of a simulation facility is an important decision because it is a factor that may significantly influence how much usage will be made of such a facility. The potential options are numerous and include the following:

- A stand-alone facility (e.g., private commercial facility)
- A facility on a university campus
- A facility part of a wider healthcare campus
- A mobile facility or solution
- A clinical room used by real patients (in situ)

Each of the above presents advantages and drawbacks that need to be considered with great rigor and according to the individual circumstances and objectives. Combined with this, a key contributor to the effective utilization of a simulation facility in terms of ease of access by clinicians or students is its steering by a multidisciplinary committee whose leaders have received training in simulation education and debriefing (Weinstock et al., 2005). The location matters considerably as ease of access by learners may significantly impact on the usage, especially if it is not compulsory. The exact location of a simulation facility may strongly influence the type of learners who will use it. As such, an on-site simulation training facility situated close to operating theaters may be falsely or rightly perceived as being a facility dedicated to anesthesia training. On the other hand, if it is located near a more generic patient care area or training facility, it may more easily encourage interprofessional learning and collaboration (Meek, 2008). A simulation center located on a university campus may have difficulties running programs for qualified healthcare practitioners, while a center in a hospital building may impose strict limitations to the number of sessions scheduled for undergraduate students. In both instances, careful thought also needs to be given to potential future expansion and anticipated changes in the focus of the simulation programs or even the technology.

The notion of a mobile facility or solution implies a means of portability of the equipment required to conduct simulation sessions. Such an approach is normally implemented for very good reasons, whether these are economical or practical, but is certainly not inferior to other solutions. For example, in the UK, a bus has been equipped to function as a mobile clinical skills laboratory that moves from hospital to hospital in the busy city of London, offering the required training to nursing and medical students on-site so they do not have to waste time traveling back to the university's skills center (Nicol et al., 2007). The equipment that is usually required to be moved around to run simulation sessions includes an AV system and a patient simulator. Examples of portable simulation solutions that have proven to be highly successful and made use of fully equipped simulation carts have been described in detail by Weinstock et al. (2009) and Calhoun et al. (2011). Strictly speaking, if no observers are present and there is no need to record the scenario, there is no requirement for an AV system. Similarly, if the scenario only requires a standardized patient and no patient simulator, then the equipment required may only include some scenario-specific items and some needed moulage supplies. A portable simulation solution lends itself to being used anywhere: a teaching laboratory temporarily set up as a simulation room, a public space, or an actual clinical room. The latter suggested location links directly to in situ simulation, which will be discussed in "In Situ Simulation Space" section below, while an example of the former will be presented in "Innovative Portable Simulated Clinical Environment—Distributed Simulation" section.

Kobayashi et al. (2008) compared center-based ("standard") simulation with simulation conducted in other locations from a research and educational perspective, with consideration of ease of access for learners, cost, opportunity for interdisciplinary training, benefits, and challenges. The proposed classification includes standard simulation and "portable simulation," which comprises "mobile" (including progressive when the patient transitions through different settings), "off-site" simulation, away from the clinical environment, and "in situ" or "on-site" simulation (Kobayashi et al., 2008). Although this provides valuable information, a more rigorous approach would be for a single institution with a large population of learners to conduct an objective study looking at the impact on the participants' learning of the various potential locations, defining a set of skills to be trained, measurable learning outcomes, and looking at various simulation modalities, each consistently facilitated by the same educators.

The Simulation Space as a Microentity

The space to run a simulation program should also be considered at the microsystem level, irrespective of where it is actually hosted, as discussed in the previous section of this chapter. The physical space chosen to run simulation training should be conducive to learning. In some cases, there may be periods of time in a session that may be run in an atmosphere that may not be perceived as being conducive to learning. In such cases, a scenario might be run in a chaotic atmosphere with ambient noise and (planned/scripted) disruptions. In contrast, the debriefing of such a learning experience should always occur in the best possible environment to ensure that learners' attention is

SECTION 6 • Environmental Design

totally focused on discussing aspects of the scenario in an orderly and constructive manner.

The special layout aspect is also of importance in the context of a scenario. From an ergonomics perspective and to enable transfer of learning between a simulated environment and the clinical context, the two spaces need to be similar. This relates to the theory of **situated learning** (Lave & Wenger, 1991), whereby an environment provides vital cues and reminders to clinicians, thus playing an important role in triggering visual recall followed by actions in the care they provide to patients. As such, the positioning of pieces of medical equipment, a scrub sink, or medical gases may prompt their potential use to participant trainees in a more systematic manner than if they had to literally think about it and request for that element to be made available. An exception where no identical reproduction of an existing clinical setup is required would be when the objective of the simulation exercise is to test or do research about various setups in order to maximize efficiency, productivity, patient safety, or other aspects that would enhance clinical practice or service delivery. In such a case, one may be more adventurous as to the space design, the layout of pieces of furniture, or the ergonomics of medical services, breaking conventional rules to investigate alternative solutions that may prove more effective. This may refer to the systems testing aspects of an innovative clinical facility, for example.

When considering simulation space as an educational venue, it can be designed in various ways depending on space availability, needs, the intended type of simulation activity offered, and the potential use of that space for other activities (Alinier, 2008a, 2008b; Brost et al., 2008).

In Situ Simulation Space

In situ simulation is a distinct form of simulation. It can be defined as "simulations that occur in the actual clinical environment regardless of whether the participants are participating during the course of caring for actual patients" (Henriksen et al., 2008). The actual real-life clinical environment is a particularly attractive space to deliver simulation-based education for institutions with financial and physical space limitations, as it is possible to implement a simulation program using minimal permanent space (Calhoun et al., 2011), though there are a range of logistical challenges to ensure access and availability. For institutions that are just beginning to develop simulation programs, in situ simulation offers an opportunity to begin to expose clinical personnel (educators and providers) to simulation, while a dedicated simulation center is being constructed. In such circumstances, one requires more than an existing patient care area on a temporary basis. Simulation programs without a dedicated center require a dedicated storage space for the training equipment, especially as it is fairly specialized, expensive to maintain, and can be easily damaged.

Simulation in a real working environment achieves higher levels of realism (Henriksen et al., 2008) and promotes memory recall as per situated learning theory (Lave & Wenger, 1991), and hence can be considered as the key advantage of in situ simulation. Experiences recreated in simulation laboratories may accomplish this to some degree, but as in situ, training is more closely aligned with the actual "work" of the healthcare provider, and there is an anticipated higher likelihood that the learning will be more successfully assimilated. The actual workday can be used, which means that on-duty clinical providers can be involved. This alleviates the need to schedule healthcare workers on nonclinical days, pay overtime, or schedule additional providers to "backfill" the clinical unit while one team is off the unit for training. It also provides an opportunity to review at frequent intervals the skills related to high-risk or infrequent events. Frequent reinforcement of the skills needed for these types of scenarios will likely result in better retention. However, this enhanced efficiency must be balanced by the necessity of conducting in situ simulations for all shifts, not just the day shift, to achieve competency for the entire provider team.

Implementing simulation training in an unoccupied treatment room, patient room, operating room, or emergency bay provides a number of opportunities to begin to realize the benefits of simulation. It is likely that the most valuable benefits of in situ simulation are related to the identification of latent hazards, knowledge gaps, and opportunities for clinical teams to rehearse infrequent and/or high-risk clinical scenarios (Hssain et al., 2013). Realistic, but intentional equipment malfunctions, deliberate errors (especially common errors), missing information, or even the simultaneous introduction of more than one simulated patient reflect a naturalistic approach. Facilitating healthcare providers or institutional chiefs to experience or witness simulation-based educational sessions may help further the development and funding of simulation programs.

In situ simulation is a fairly common practice in hospitals either because it is proving more economical than building a dedicated training facility, the hospital may not have the space necessary to build a center, or because it may be judged the most appropriate setting to provide training. It is important to realize that in situ simulation also presents a number of disadvantages (Calhoun et al., 2011; Patterson et al., 2008). Commonly cited drawbacks of doing hospital-based in situ simulation include potential interruptions and cancellation of sessions to deal with real emergencies and surges in patient volume, possible risk of mixing patient use and educational resources (equipment, training drugs), space temporarily not usable for real patient care, infection control issues, noise (from the surrounding environment or generated by the training session), potential issues with permission to video-record the learning event in a patient care area, time to set up the venue (equipment, patient simulator, and AV equipment) and test the equipment, and the risk of causing anxiety to real patients who may see the commotion potentially created by the simulated event. While measures do exist to prevent some of these limitations, they are often always omnipresent.

The units that often derive the greatest benefits from in situ simulations are—at baseline—high-acuity, high-census areas. These include critical care units, operating rooms, and emergency departments (EDs), all of which are areas that are subject to large surges of patients and seasonal variations in census and acuity. The facilitation of in situ simulation sessions should stress the system, but those conducting the simulations also need to be sensitive to the system stressors already in place. This might mean that the simulation team consults with the charge nurse and/or physician prior to conducting an in situ simulation during a particularly busy time (Henriksen et al., 2008). It is sometimes preferable to organize "small doses" of training by limiting the length of the scenarios and the debriefings—so clinical care in the unit is not negatively impacted upon—and to organize in situ simulation sessions during expected downtimes such as early mornings or late afternoons. Healthcare providers involved in in situ simulation sessions might be under the impression (rightly or wrongly) that during that time patient care is being delayed or neglected. This also raises a different debate in itself owing to cultural or political obstacles whereby in situ simulation may simply be perceived as totally inappropriate. Some healthcare providers may even express concerns that in situ simulation might be perceived as either disruptive or intimidating to patients and their families.

Just-in-Time Simulation Space

Just-in-time simulation differs from in situ simulation in the sense that it is for the planned rehearsal of a specific procedure just before it is performed with a real patient. The practice of this type of simulation approach is still in its infancy. The simulation experience is recreated for training purposes before a real clinical case on the basis of known information about a particular patient. This is particularly relevant to the area of surgery where real patient data acquired through an MRI or CT scan can be uploaded onto a virtual reality simulator, allowing the surgeon to practice the surgery in advance of the actual surgery. This requires a dedicated storage area for this particular training equipment, which, if large enough, could also be used by the surgeon as a room in which to rehearse his clinical cases without disruption.

In the case of extremely complex medical interventions, such as the separation of conjoined twins, just-in-time training can go well beyond the surgical procedure and also involve an in situ rehearsal with the complete operating team. This type of simulation exercise helps all members of the multiprofessional clinical team practice complex cases and fully realize their role and expected input during a complex procedure. It can be repeated to simulate varying physiological responses from the patient(s) so the team can prepare itself to respond to such situations.

Innovative Portable Simulated Clinical Environment—Distributed Simulation

Portable simulation aims to facilitate the bringing of simulation-based training to the learners. Such approaches typically provide mannequin-based training in mobile facilities (Paige et al., 2009). While this type of simulations may address the availability and accessibility shortcomings of static simulation centers by taking place close to participants' clinical environment, they tend to lack flexibility and thus may not respond to the educational needs of a given clinical team.

Recently, Kneebone et al. (2010) introduced the concept of **Distributed Simulation** (DS). The aim of DS is to provide accessible, portable, and self-contained immersive simulation for training and assessment. By doing so, it sets out to strike a balance between the realism of the clinical setting and the functionality of the simulation center. Underpinning the DS concept is a belief that simulation should provide an approach to learning that is generally accessible, that can become part of the normal range of educational facilities, and that can be tailored to the needs of individual groups.

A vast majority of immersive simulation activity aims to reproduce real clinical environments as closely as possible. However, it is recognized that fidelity is only one of several factors affecting the educational effectiveness of a simulation encounter, and trying to reproduce all the elements of a real clinical environment can incur high costs. A key feature of DS is that it seeks to optimize the level of fidelity by, instead of faithfully *reproducing* all aspects of a clinical setting, *selecting and recreating* only those salient features that provide key cues that engage participants and achieve educational outcomes. This process of "selective abstraction" is rooted on the "circles of focus" model (Kneebone, 2010), which describes the concentric nature of participants' selective perception, awareness, and attention to the different elements that make up a clinical setting within a simulation. Rigorous and extensive observations of real settings are followed by in-depth discussions between clinicians, design engineers, and psychologists to identify key components constituting a particular simulation setting, the emphasis being on simulation *function*, rather than *structure*.

The resulting specifications of DS include the following (Kneebone et al., 2010):

- A self-contained immersive environment that can be closed off from its surroundings, allowing any available space to be converted into a convincing "clinical" setting for the duration of the simulation.
- Minimum necessary cues (visual, auditory, and kinesthetic) to recreate a realistic "clinical" environment (including clinical equipment and sounds).
- Key requirements of static simulation centers (for observing, recording, playback, and debriefing) in a simple, user-friendly format.
- Practical, lightweight, and easily transportable components that can be erected quickly by a minimal team.
- The flexibility to recreate a range of clinical settings according to individual requirements.

The DS system consists of two main parts: the simulation environment and the AV control room. This is analogous to a traditional static simulation facility, but with the already mentioned advantages of portability, flexibility, and ease of access. The key elements of the DS simulation environment are a self-contained, enclosable space; vital items of equipment represented through pull-up backdrops; and a lightweight, custom-designed operating lamp. The self-contained, enclosable space is provided by a 360-degree inflatable structure that can be erected in 3 minutes with minimum effort (Figure 6.2.2A), and that can effectively block participants away from the surrounding environment, creating a boundary in clinical training that establishes the context for education and professional practice. When deflated, the structure folds into a bag the size of a family tent.

The pull-up backdrops used inside the inflatable enclosure are printed with high-resolution graphics of clinical equipment, such as trolleys, instrument cupboards, anesthetic machine, and so on (Figure 6.2.2B). They can effectively recreate key components within the clinical space at minimum cost and may be tailored to the requirements of a specific simulation.

A tripod-mounted, portable operating lamp represents another crucial component of the DS simulation environment (Figure 6.2.2A, C). The lamp is molded from lightweight plastic and uses low-voltage LEDs. Although considerably smaller and lighter than a standard operating lamp, its circular shape, adjustable position, and multiple bright lights adequately recreates an actual operating lamp in both appearance and function. A video camera and microphone integrated in the central handle provide quality recording of the interactions in the operative field.

The DS simulation environment has a footprint of 5 by 4 m and a height of 2 m. It can be easily set up by two people in under an hour, and packed down in less than 30 minutes. All key components can be transported in the boot of a small car. Figure 6.2.3 shows a complete DS surgical simulation environment. A key counterpart to a simulation environment is a control room from which the simulation can be observed and managed without disruption (Meek, 2008). DS provides a portable AV control room that may be located remotely from the simulation. It consists of wireless cameras, a laptop computer, lightweight speakers, and bespoke recording and playback software (Figure 6.2.4). The wireless cameras complement the video camera integrated in the DS lamp. They are high-definition, portable, lightweight cameras with integrated microphones that can be positioned within the DS enclosure to offer a wide range of different views to satisfy individual learning and teaching needs, through recording of team interaction and team performance. Detailed observation of various clinical areas highlighted the importance of adequate audio cues. These are recreated in the DS simulation environment through small loudspeakers hidden within the inflatable structure. Playback of a variety of clinical sounds (e.g., heart monitor, ventilator, clinical background noise) may be controlled from the laptop computer in the portable AV control room (Figure 6.2.4).

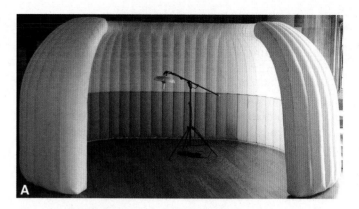

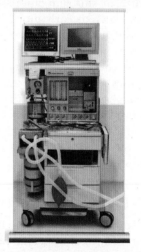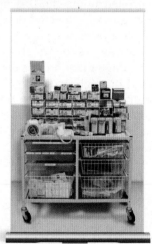

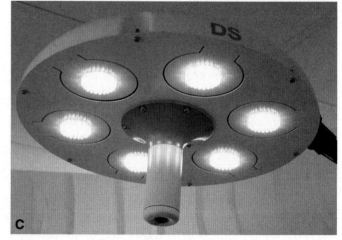

FIGURE 6.2.2 A. DS inflatable structure and lamp. **B.** DS pull-up backdrops. **C.** DS operating lamp.

Figure 6.2.5 shows various possible configurations of the DS simulation environment that combine a mixture of bespoke simulated equipment and props, with standard, off-the-shelf models, real clinical equipment and simulated patients.

Educational Technology Considerations

There is a wide array of technology now available to support learning and teaching activities in healthcare (Alinier, 2011), including interactive white boards (Glover et

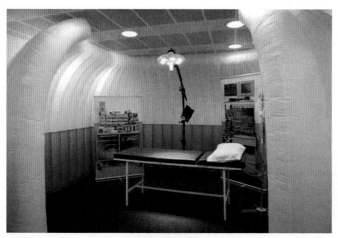

FIGURE 6.2.3 DS surgical simulation environment.

al., 2005), personal response systems (Jensen et al., 2009), and other more specialized pieces of equipment such as virtual reality simulators designed for a specific procedure (Chin & Forbes, 2008). Some of these can be more or less portable, while others need to remain where they have been set up to prevent damage or because they require access to specific services or a very accurate calibration to work properly (i.e., stereoscopic projectors to achieve 3D effect).

It is generally preferable to opt for technology that is mobile rather than being forced to make a room too specialized because of the installation of fixed assets. There are, however, instances when a facility has to be designed around a particular piece of technology owing to the need for a specific room configuration (Bridge et al., 2007) or access to specific services.

Irrespective of the investment made in the purchase of educational technology or configuration of the environment, it does not essentially guarantee educational effectiveness. An educational tool is only ever as good as the teacher using it (Satish & Streufert, 2002; Weinstock et al., 2009).

THE HOW TO . . .

. . . Obtain What You Want?

Having ascertained what the best solution is to achieve a specific goal, a proposal presenting the case should be made for a specific solution. This should only be done once all options have been objectively considered and ruled out for valid reasons. The proposal can include a rigorous SWOT (Strengths-Weaknesses-Opportunities-Threats) analysis of the various options considered to justify the choice made. The preferred and most appropriate solution should be presented with strong and valid arguments so it is more likely to be accepted and receive institutional support. This should include expected benefits such as return on investment, improvement in services, and, ultimately, expected enhancement of patient care services and patient safety.

. . . Ensure the Right Decision Is Made Regarding the Choice for a Future Simulation Space?

As the number of simulation programs has tremendously increased around the world over the last decade, it is highly likely that other people with the same dilemma, similar constraints, and comparable circumstances have already tested at least one of the options under consideration. Simulation equipment vendors are usually a very good source of information as they are likely to know customers who have been in a similar situation and will be receptive to queries from fellow simulation users. They will be able to share their experience and make further recommendations on the basis of their insight of having had to make similar decisions regarding the selection of the best possible simulation space for their program(s). Another resource is the many healthcare simulation consortiums that exist throughout the world. You can also ask questions on the discussion boards on the Society for Simulation in Healthcare (SSH) website.

. . . Decide on How Much Space You Actually Need?

In order to determine the amount of space required to deliver a simulation program, it is necessary to first establish the type of clinical environment and equipment required, the total number of learners that need to receive the training, the number of participants per session, their availability, and the human resources available to facilitate the training. This will help develop a draft schedule and even determine whether sessions need to be run in parallel in different areas or rooms. The type of simulation equipment selected and simulation activities intended will also impact on the size of the space required. Scenarios involving participants from several professions and disciplines require more space than uniprofessional scenarios.

BEEN THERE, DONE THAT: HOW CAN I CONTINUE TO IMPROVE OR SUSTAIN WHAT I HAVE ACHIEVED?

Having established a simulation program is a great achievement in itself, but efforts need to be maintained so the activities and resources remain current and meet the ever-evolving demands of healthcare practice. A simulation center, a mobile, portable or in situ program, and the staff involved in their operation and delivery of educational sessions need to be maintained up to date on several fronts. Technology, equipment, and procedures constantly evolve and so should the educational programs and the teaching approach used (Alinier, 2007).

SECTION 6 • Environmental Design

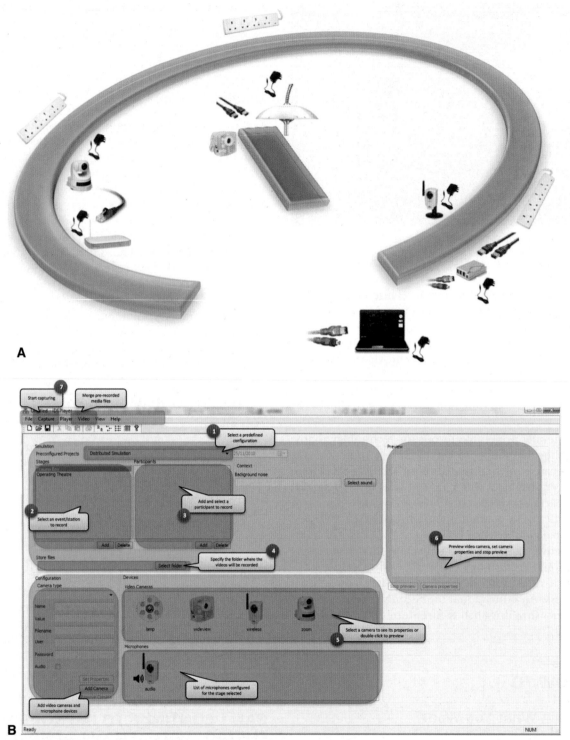

FIGURE 6.2.4 **A.** DS portable AV control room components. **B.** DS AV software interface.

A way of remaining current with a vision of improving what has been achieved is by staying in contact with the wider simulation community. Being actively engaged with other professionals in the relevant specialties and other simulation educators helps remaining up to date and opens opportunities for collaboration. Well beyond sustaining a current portfolio of activities, collaboration can often be linked to innovative research that furthers knowledge in a domain of practice. The research

opportunities in simulation-based education are still vast (Dieckmann et al., 2011). Investigations around the effect of the environment and actual configuration within which simulation-based training is facilitated and how it actually transfers to actual clinical practice are still highly relevant. They can be used to better inform the design of simulation facilities or indeed to explore whether other spaces are more effective from both educational and financial terms.

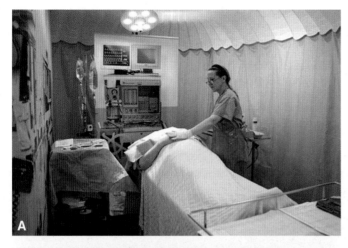
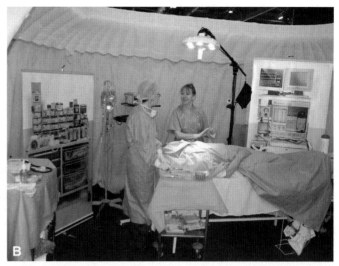
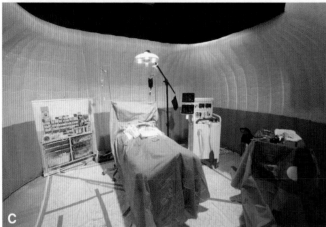
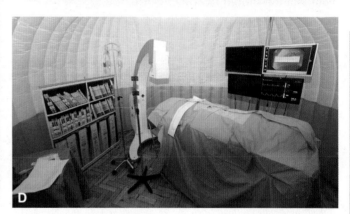
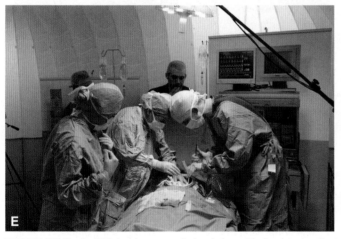
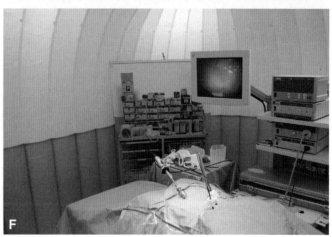

FIGURE 6.2.5 **A.** DS intensive care unit simulation with simulated patient. **B.** DS elective surgery simulation with simulated patient. **C.** DS surgical simulation environment with simulated anesthetic machine. **D.** DS angiography/angioplasty simulated environment with simulated C-arm. **E.** DS emergency surgery simulation with high-fidelity prosthetic model. **F.** DS laparoscopic surgery simulation environment with real laparoscopic stack and box trainer.

SUMMARY

Space can be considered in different ways. With regards to simulation-based education, it could be a permanent physical location within a larger entity or it could be a temporary setup such as in the case of in situ or mobile simulation. Irrespective of how it is considered and of the educational modality used, space is a key element of simulation-based education as it is where the learning occurs. This learning might involve complex thinking processes that are directly affected by the environment, which may be too distractive if inappropriate or, on the contrary, enhance the assimilation of skills and knowledge if it is highly suitable. Other factors, such as the location of a training venue, impact on operational aspects linked to utilization and potential for future expansion. These need to be carefully considered to ensure the success of simulation-based educational initiatives within an institution or a wider area. Another important aspect to consider is that irrespective of where simulation is conducted, it can only be as effective as the facilitation approach utilized by the educators involved.

Considering the space from a layout and equipment point of view requires also careful consideration so that it is fit for purpose. It is also important to keep in mind that utilization may change over time, hence it is advisable not to make simulation-dedicated space overspecialized with permanent fixtures unless absolutely necessary. Simulation should strengthen clinical practice by being tailor-made for learners to attain specific educational goals as well; simulation must be widely accessible to learners to fully address their training needs, which include time and geographical constraints. Also, simulation design and implementation should be cost-effective.

REFERENCES

Abrahamson, S., & Wallace, P. (1980). Using computer-controlled interactive manikins in medical education. *Medical Teacher*, 2(1), 25–31.

Alinier, G. (2007). A typology of educationally focused medical simulation tools. *Medical Teacher*, 29(8), e243–e250.

Alinier, G. (2008a). All-in-one room schoolhouse: Clinical simulation stage, control, debrief, and utilities all within a single room. In R. R. Kyle & W. B. Murray (Eds.), *Clinical simulation: Operations, engineering, and management* (1st ed., pp. 239–242). San Diego, CA: Academic Press.

Alinier, G. (2008b). The patient simulator suite: A single dedicated clinical simulator stage surrounded by dedicated control, observing/debriefing, utility, and office rooms. In R. R. Kyle & W. B. Murray (Eds.), *Clinical simulation: Operations, engineering, and management* (1st ed., pp. 261–265). San Diego, CA: Academic Press.

Alinier, G. (2011). Simulation technology in healthcare education. In A. Lazakidou & I. El Emary (Eds.), *Learning oriented technologies, devices and networks* (pp. 69–89). Ankara, TK: Lap Publishing.

Bridge, P., Appleyard, R. M., Ward, J. W., Philips, R., & Beavis, A. W. (2007). The development and evaluation of a virtual radiotherapy treatment machine using an immersive visualization environment. *Computers & Education*, 49(2), 481–494.

Brost, B., Thiemann, K., Belda, T., & Dunn, W. F. (2008). Creation of structure-function relationships in the design of a simulation center. In R. R. Kyle & W. B. Murray (Eds.), *Clinical simulation: Operations, engineering, and management* (1st ed., pp. 185–199). San Diego, CA: Academic Press.

Calhoun, A. W., Boone, M. C., Peterson, E. B., Boland, K. A., & Montgomery, V. L. (2011). Integrated in-situ simulation using redirected faculty educational time to minimize costs: A feasibility study. *Simulation in Healthcare*, 6(6), 337–344.

Chin, M. W., & Forbes, G. M. (2008). Should simulator use become mandatory in endoscopy training? *Journal of Gastroenterology & Hepatology*, 23(7), 996–997.

Dieckmann, P., Phero, J. C., Issenberg, S. B., Kardong-Edgren, S., Ostergaard, D., & Ringsted, C. (2011). The first Research Consensus Summit of the Society for Simulation in Healthcare: Conduction and a synthesis of the results. *Simulation in Healthcare*, 6(Suppl), S1–S9.

Glover, D., Miller, D., Averis, D., & Door, V. (2005). The interactive whiteboard: A literature survey. *Technology, Pedagogy and Education*, 14(2), 155–170.

Henriksen, K., Battles, J. B., Keyes, M. A., & Grady, M. L. (2008). *Advances in patient safety: New directions and alternative approaches. Vol. 3. Performance and tools (AHRQ Publication No. 08-0034-3)*. Rockville, MD. Agency for Healthcare Research and Quality.

Hssain, I., Alinier, G., & Souaiby, N. (2013). In-situ simulation: A different approach to patient safety through immersive training. *Mediterranean Journal of Emergency Medicine*, 15, 17–28.

Jensen, R., Meyer, L., & Sternberger, C. (2009). Three technological enhancements in nursing education: Informatics instruction, personal response systems, and human patient simulation. *Nurse Education in Practice*, 9, 86–90.

Kneebone, R. (2010). Simulation, safety and surgery. *Quality Safety Health Care*, 19(Suppl. 3), 47–52.

Kneebone, R., Arora, S., King, D., Bello, F., Sevdalis, N., Kassab, E., ... Nestel, D. (2010). Distributed simulation—Accessible immersive training. *Medical Teacher*, 32(1), 65–70.

Kobayashi, L., Patterson, M. D., Overly, F. L., Shapiro, M. J., Williams, K. A., & Jay, G. D. (2008). Educational and research implications of portable human patient simulation in acute care medicine. *Academic Emergency Medicine*, 15(11), 1166–1174.

Kolb, D. (1984). *Experiential learning: Experience as the source of learning and development*. Englewood Cliffs, NJ: Prentice Hall.

Lave, J., & Wenger, E. (1991). *Situated learning: Legitimate peripheral participation*. Cambridge, UK: Cambridge University Press.

Meek, T. (2008). Anaesthetic simulators: Making the most of your purchase. *Current Anaesthesia & Critical Care*, 19, 354–360.

Nicol, M., Warren, A., & Connolly, J. (2007). Development of a clinical skills bus: Making simulation mobile. *International Journal of Clinical Skills*, 1, 101–113.

Paige, J. T., Kozmenko, V., Yang, T., Paragi Gururaja, R., Hilton, C. W., Cohn, I., Jr., & Chauvin, S. W. (2009). High-fidelity, simulation-based, interdisciplinary operating room team training at the point of care. *Surgery*, 145(2), 138–146.

Patterson, M. D., Blike, G. T., & Nadkarni, V. M. (2008). In situ simulation: Challenges and results. In K. Henriksen, J. B. Battles, M. A. Keyes, & M. L. Grady (Eds.), *New directions and alternative approaches: Vol. 3. Performance and tools* (AHRQ Publication No. 08-0034-3, pp. 1–18). Rockville, MD: Agency for Healthcare Research and Quality.

Satish, U., & Streufert, S. (2002). Value of a cognitive simulation in medicine: Towards optimizing decision making performance of healthcare personnel. *Quality & Safety in Health Care*, 11(2), 163–167.

Weinstock, P. H., Kappus, L. J., Kleinman, M. E., Grenier, B., Hickey, P., & Burns, J. P. (2005). Toward a new paradigm in hospital-based pediatric education: The development of an onsite simulator program. *Pediatric Critical Care Medicine*, 6(6), 635–641.

Weinstock, P. H., Kappus, L. J., Garden, A., & Burns, J. P. (2009). Simulation at the point of care: Reduced-cost, in situ training via a mobile cart. *Pediatric Critical Care Medicine*, 10(2), 176–181.

CHAPTER 6.3

Technical Infrastructure

Brian Moores, and Amar P. Patel, MS, NREMT-P, CFC

ABOUT THE AUTHORS

BRIAN MOORES is an experienced healthcare audiovisual and network technology design consultant. Mr. Moore has designed the audiovisual and network systems design for the UCSF Teaching & Learning Center, Loma Linda University Centennial Simulation Center, as well as New York's Memorial Sloan-Kettering Center for Image-Guided Interventional and Minimally Invasive Therapy. Mr. Moores studied Telecommunications Systems.

AMAR P. PATEL is responsible for integrating technology-based educational programs to include human patient simulation, healthcare gaming, and hybrid education. He has provided consultative services in the establishment of countless simulation programs across the country to include the development of audiovisual systems that directly tie technology to simulation. Amar is a contributing writer to *Carolina Fire EMS Journal* and has published articles on simulation center design and the ever-changing technical infrastructure needs for simulation centers.

ABSTRACT

At the heart of the simulation center design is the technical infrastructure. Establishing the needs of the program and determining how to best integrate the technology will allow a center to meet their mission and vision by providing an education of high quality and flexibility. Although the technical needs of a program are often one of the last items considered, the complex nature of healthcare simulation technology warrants further discussions and decisions early on. A list of what is desired in the center will help shape the overall scope of the technical needs. Utilizing a Technical Specification Worksheet, a simulation center can lay out what they need and how it can be integrated into their overall design plan. The key to designing a successful technical infrastructure is to look at the overall educational scope of the center, add what a committee has tasked for the center, and who is responsible for teaching within it. The complex nature of understanding how the technical needs integrate with the practical ones can be done with some independent research and guidance.

CASE EXAMPLE

Karen Smith, director of education for ABC University, has been asked to establish a simulation center for their nursing school, medical school, and the local hospital where their students train. The university has experience integrating technology into their educational program but never utilized high-technology simulation. Although Karen's staff is ready to assist her with designing a center, they are concerned about their expectations as the project moves forward. Karen is familiar with using computer-based methods for learning but has limited experience with camera system operations, recording, and troubleshooting. She has never had to integrate a simulator into the audiovisual system let alone attempt to troubleshoot it if something goes wrong. An oversight committee was established by the program dean, which included members of each of the schools and the hospital that will utilize this new center. A final simulation center architectural design (Appendix A) was agreed upon and will be used as the foundation for the next step. The committee requested that Karen reach out to other simulation programs and attempt to understand the technical infrastructure needs of both a new building and a renovated space. They are looking for flexibility in how the audiovisual system and the simulators will function within the space but are unsure of what that would involve both logistically and technically. Karen put together a list of needs, on the basis of the committee's input, and has been asked to report back her findings. She will have to do her own research in addition to presenting potential cost/benefits to the administrative board responsible for funding this project (Appendix B).

SECTION 6 • Environmental Design

INTRODUCTION AND BACKGROUND

The complex nature of designing a simulation center does not only involve the physical infrastructure but must include the technical aspects as well. A designer and the faculty tasked with teaching within it must consider the technical needs of the space early on. So much of simulation can be accomplished using low technology with little to no technology. The challenge becomes when a center is intending to create a high immersive environment that requires a large amount of technology to help them accomplish that. The choices you make early on in a project can either hurt or help you. It is important to consider all of the options and understand what features you may be giving up. As (a) an educator, (b) a technician, or (c) the program manager, you must consider the technical needs of the center at present and in the future.

SIGNIFICANCE

The technical nature of designing a center can be an overwhelming task for one person. The need to understand how each piece interacts with the other is the reason why it is important to lay out all of the different possibilities. For these authors, this has become a vital way for them to share their own personal and professional experiences to help others learn from their successes and mistakes. The constant changes in technology and the need to understand how a center can grow, by planning ahead, is likely to be part of the initial technical design phase. We currently live in an ever-changing environment where we have seen the progression from wired to wireless communication devices and the complexity of these devices increasing as the need arises. Although it can also be one of the most expensive, it is the authors' hope that they can help you decide the needs of the students and the program.

Systematic Overview

This chapter has been designed to focus on the technical needs of a simulation center design. Because there are a lot of systems to choose from, it is extremely important that you pick the system that meets the needs of your students and your program. The case study will utilize Karen's experience as she begins to lay out a technical design of ABC University Simulation Center. Karen's experience is being used as an example to illustrate how many different aspects a simulation center must consider before making a final decision. For this particular case example, the final direction that has been chosen should not be considered the only option or the best option. This option was based on Karen's curriculum and Technical Specification Worksheet that will both be discussed in greater detail later on in this chapter. The hope is that this chapter will create an open dialogue and sharing of information, early on, with your Information Technology (IT) teams and **audiovisual (AV) designers**.

The chapter will begin by discussing a technical specification worksheet, the importance of knowing the program's current and future curriculum, and space **pathways**. They will discuss in great detail the technical aspects of simulation center design and end with the future design concepts that should be considered for those aspiring to stay ahead of the technology curve (Ross, 2012). With so much to consider, it is important to take the time to understand the concepts presented in this chapter and ask the right questions to ensure you have the right technology with both your budget and needs in mind.

METHODS

Technical Specification Worksheet

The Technical Specification Worksheet (Appendix C) provides a wide variety of questions that each designer and simulation expert should consider as they begin to work through the technical needs of the center. Having a reference tool available for you to utilize will help ensure that you are asking the right questions as you solicit information from not only your administrative board, key stakeholders, faculty, and potential vendors, but are thinking through the true design needs and issues that may result early on. As shown in Appendix C, this three-page document provides questions regarding simulation, video, and audio devices; the recording system; the paging system; the intercom system; control rooms and control systems; support and operational requirements; and training. The hope is that you utilize this worksheet to guide you through the technical consideration of your center.

The presented case study will utilize this tool to show you how Karen determines the needs of ABC University Simulation Center. The answers to questions posed in this worksheet will change depending on the initial and long-term focus of her program. You must remember that there are a variety of answers depending on how the curriculum is currently set up and may change depending on how she integrates simulation into the educational program.

Curriculum

Having a basic understanding of the curriculum is vital in the development of not only the physical space, but also the technical needs of the simulation center (Kyle & Murray, 2008). The needs of the center are truly established during the initial design phase, as much of the physical space requirement will need to be adjusted to account for the AV systems and simulation technology. Having a basic understanding of what a simulation center hopes to accomplish in the first 5 years can help you work through the Technical Specification Worksheet.

As experts in education, we often have difficulty connecting the needs of the program with the established curriculum. As technical designers, we understand how to provide educators with what they need but lack the expertise in integrating the simulation technology. The core of any good design understands the needs of the student and the educator by utilizing the curriculum. The curriculum is the key to creating a solid, technically efficient, and effective system.

An in-depth review the Technical Specification Worksheet should act as a guide for Karen to work through matching her programmatic needs to the technical needs. As a simulation center designer, you must take into account that the needs of the center will evolve with time. In addition to utilizing the Technical Specification Worksheet and a layout of the program curriculum, it is imperative that you ask the right questions early on in the process. The right questions are based on the Technical Specification Worksheet.

Karen's Curriculum

Karen has been tasked with investigating the technical needs for her new 3,500 square feet (325.2 m^2) simulation center. The center will be the home to students from the school of (a) medicine, (b) nursing, (c) pharmacy, and (d) the College of Allied Health. In addition to new healthcare providers, Karen's program will be responsible for providing simulation-based education to two hospitals that have partnered and provided funding to the program. With such a wide variety of students and experience levels, the committee decided to include clinical simulation, standardized patient, and skills training rooms. They decided to integrate a total of five simulators and a wide variety of skills trainers. The chosen simulators were a combination of wired pediatric and wireless adults. They requested that she choose an AV system that offers her the greatest versatility allowing for remote viewers to see the simulation experience and students to be able to see their own performance at a later date. Karen noted that she would like the system be standardized across the center because initial staffing will be limited and some technologically inexperienced staff members, from their partner organizations, will be teaching. Furthermore, the administrative board outlined the need for a security system to protect the center's assets at all hours. With having limited experience in integrating the technology, they asked that she try to find comparable programs to investigate their overall physical design and technical infrastructure.

In essence, Karen will be tasked with initial and ongoing medical education for 2,000 students annually. Although the curriculum largely focuses on initial task-based skills early on, many of the students will quickly move to the standardized patient and simulation suites as their education progresses. For ongoing medical education, Karen is still looking to understand their needs outside of mock codes. She developed a plan to provide critical care and emergency room education but is waiting to conduct a need analysis until the final capabilities of the center has been determined by the administrative board. Karen will begin her investigation having the core curriculum designed and anticipate having to make design and curriculum changes as she learns more about the technical needs of her center.

The Investigation

Over the past 3 months, Karen visited countless centers attempting to understand how they designed their AV system and integrated simulation technology into these systems. Although her investigation provided her with a tremendous amount of information, it brought to light many issues she had not previously considered. As requested by the administrative board, Karen will be presenting her findings and recommendations for final review and approval.

Infrastructure Design Philosophy

In the course of Karen's investigation, she came to a very important conclusion early on. She discovered that there are generally two distinct infrastructure philosophies currently in simulation center design. The first design utilizes a wired coaxial-cabled system, while the second utilizes an **Internet Protocol** (IP) data network.

A wired coaxial-cabled system consists of a series of point-to-point cables and associated pathways and is considered to be the most common infrastructure design. At its core, this is analog technology and is based on the premise of viewing and capturing real-time video. Early on, Karen discovered that this type of system is typical of **legacy analog security systems**. Although power requirements do vary, cameras can be powered either locally or from rack-mounted power supplies. Analog systems can reside on a **shared data network** pathway; it is not uncommon for the direction of the pathways to diverge, which creates additional pathways and coordination issues. In interviewing simulation center AV designers, Karen discovered that it was harder to retrofit an existing space with this type of infrastructure because there is not much flexibility for cable placement. The distinct advantage for an analog system was the ability for coaxial-based cabling systems to provide longer cable runs than network-based systems.

While visiting a new simulation center in the Midwest, Karen discovered a second type of infrastructure, which is based on an IP data network and may have both wired and wireless technologies. She was intrigued to learn more about this technology and how well it worked in both small and large spaces. Karen discovered that this type of infrastructure could provide one distinct advantage when compared to the analog point-to-point infrastructure. It allows for power to be distributed over data cables and therefore dramatically reduces the amount of power receptacles required in the design. The other major advantage is the ability to (a) distribute camera, (b) physiological monitoring, and (c) audio signals from any location through this network. However, where there are advantages in using a point-to-point IP data network infrastructure, there are also limitations. One of the primary disadvantages to this type of system is the need to utilize devices called **encoders** and **decoders** to process the audio and video signals. This process would incur time delays that would create a **nonlinear non-real-time** experience. Karen found that this would not be a problem if the staff and students were not observing through a window and an online video stream at the same time. In essence, this does present a problem if real-time viewing is mixed with the non-real-time viewing. She heard that it would be difficult to concentrate and operate mannequins under these conditions. Puzzled as to which direction she should choose, she now has enough information to determine whether she needs a real-time or a non-real-time system for observation of the simulation experiences.

Space Planning and Pathways

Following a review of the University's simulation design committee report, Karen decided to host a meeting that would help everyone determine how much space would be needed for each type of room. Early on, the administrative board outlined the basic curriculum and provided Karen with the general direction of the center. In discussing how to work through the technical design, with other simulation centers, she decided this would be the logical time for space planning to begin.

Space planning is the most important first step in the design process to ensure that the planned curriculum and simulation center's educational directives will be met. Throughout her investigation, Karen was repeatedly advised that the curriculum drives how the AV and space requirements will be defined. Furthermore, making these decisions early on can impact how well staff will be able to facilitate simulation experiences within the space.

In two of the centers Karen visited, she liked seeing how flexible and multipurpose the simulation rooms were. These rooms could be used as intensive care units, operating rooms, or emergency room bays just by utilizing the headwalls and the associated AV connectivity in different configurations. During her tour, she was informed that during the space-planning phase of the project, the design team and simulation center faculty had discussed various room configurations. Furthermore, they evaluated the impact the space had on the defined curriculum and anticipated AV technology needs. The design team took the time to ensure that the layout of the center and chosen AV system matched the needs of the program before the center was built.

In many design projects, the curriculum and technology are afterthoughts. Space allocation is decided before the curriculum and the simulation experiences are planned. Karen found that the primary reason this happens is because of tight budgets, concerns over design and construction scheduling, and the desire to simply complete the project quickly. Many projects are driven by real costs associated with budget constraints and funding. It is always prudent to look carefully at the overall expected

capabilities of the simulation center and take into consideration how the curriculum and technology will fit rather than trying to make them fit after the physical space layout has been decided. The overall floor plan of a simulation center can have a fair amount of flexibility as long as architectural requirements and building code compliance are maintained. From others that have made similar mistakes, Karen learned that it was imperative that the simulation faculty be involved early on in the planning process.

Although there are vast differences in the types of technology Karen considered integrating into the center, she found that establishing pathway requirements was dependent on which type of technology the administrative board selected for the simulation center. An analog point-to-point-type system will allow for cable runs up to 600 feet (182.9 m) to occur (BICSI, 2009), whereas an IP network system is restricted to maximum cable runs of 290 feet (88.4 m; BICSI, 2009). Furthermore, wireless network systems will still require placement of wired access points within the system and are also restricted to the maximum cable distance of 290 feet. In further discussing her options with a number of AV designers, Karen discovered that it is important to have all cable pathways far away from electrical motors, HVAC (heating, ventilation, air conditioning) motors, medical imaging systems, and other electronic devices that may generate any type of electrical magnetic interference (BICSI & InfoComm International, 2006). A good rule of thumb is to run analog video cables and network data cables at a minimum of 12 inches (30.5 cm) away from each other. This distance will ensure that there is no induced noise or static on lines that have been designated for core AV system functionality.

Simulation Workflow and Design Impact

During a conversation with a colleague at a simulation center she was visiting, Karen was advised to ensure that she had a good understanding of anticipated simulation workflow and how it would impact the design of her center. It was strongly emphasized that not coordinating the workflow with the design would result in work-arounds. Furthermore, this would cause distinct challenges with program efficiency and capacity. It is true that with a certain amount of creativity, any space can accommodate most scenarios. But, the fundamental idea of building a new facility or renovating an existing space is to create a more efficient use of the space and the technology to optimize simulation realism, student testing, and the students' educational experience.

If portability and mobile scenarios are to be an important aspect of the simulation center, then the workflow must move easily from space to space or even off-site with very limited constraints and obstructions. This translates into the necessity for an extremely flexible infrastructure design with the ability to reconfigure the spaces very quickly. Wireless technology best fits this type of workflow. The very nature of ad hoc wireless network systems allows for multiple devices to join the network anywhere and at any time as long as there is coverage and adequate bandwidth.

In situations where there is a fixed space designated for simulation, it is extremely important to have all of the technical tools needed to conduct the simulation experience available in each of the rooms. This will help improve program efficiency and ensure that time is not wasted looking for any of the devices needed to start or stop a scenario. If a room will be designated primarily as a task training room, then the task trainers, their associated simulation components, and AV connectivity must be accessible in the space. Thinking about even the smallest components that may delay the start of a simulation experience will help to create a fluid workflow.

One of the highlights during Karen's visit of other centers was seeing how many television monitors and projectors were mounted throughout these centers. Karen found that AV designers like to distribute wall-mounted video displays such as large-screen-format LCD or LED monitors judiciously around a simulation center. This allows for greater flexibility for the simulation specialists to create scenario locations for showing physiological monitoring of human patient simulators. It also allows for another location to play back the simulation experience during a debriefing session (Ross, 2012). In essence, you are able to create a very open-ended workflow that increases program productivity and efficiency. This open-ended workflow allows for a specialist to set up for either a simulation experience or debriefing session at the same time because the tools are all already in place.

Systems Design and Equipment Specifications

In most AV simulation center design projects, there will be a formal system design that may include a set of AV drawings, specifications, and an equipment list or bill of materials. Karen asked the director of the AV and IT staff during her visits to tell her about their process from initial system design conception to final implementation. This is what she discovered.

Karen found that if the project were new construction, then there would be an AV design consultant on the architect's design team. This consultant will typically have experience in AV technology design planning, acoustics, and architectural space planning for simulation centers. If the project involves renovating an existing space, then there may not be an AV design consultant on the architect's design team. The scope of the project will depict the types of members available on these respective teams. Karen discovered that in some cases, many of these experts collaborating on the project are individuals from within the organization. They are typically members of the simulation center, internal AV or IT, and the architect/general contractor.

In a new design project, there are usually several phases that take place during the architectural planning/construction process. They are generally as follows:

- **Schematic Design**—Preliminary space planning and design layouts.
- **Design Development**—Infrastructure and initial building services design layouts. This will include engineering, equipment, and furnishings. It is typically the initial design plans and specifications phase.
- **Construction Documentation**—Final designs for all building services, furniture/fixtures, and architectural/engineering plans for trades and services that would go to bid. The final design specifications are created.
- **Construction Administration**—Project management of the actual construction process and associated trades during installation.

The AV design of a simulation project follows these phases:

- **Schematic Design**—Preliminary AV simulation space layouts and considerations, and cost estimate summary or AV project budget.
- **Design Development**—AV and network infrastructure pathways design drawings and heat/power load calculations for AV equipment. General AV equipment locations are determined.
- **Construction Documentation**—Final AV design plans, narrative performance specification, and equipment list issued for AV contractors to bid.
- **Construction Administration**—Project management of the actual construction process and AV contractor during installation.

Although renovation projects may follow a similar phase timeline as new construction projects, Karen found that there could be a shorter timeline and phases to completion of the construction depending on the overall scope of the project. If the institution is acting as the design team, it will be extremely important to reach out to the simulation vendors to obtain any implementation advice they are willing to offer. In many cases, they can provide design assistance during the project. As you seek advice, it is important to remember that vendor-directed system design assistance may limit the capabilities of your center. Specifically, simulation vendors may push the design toward their own simulator capabilities, making it more difficult for you to integrate other technology later on. Furthermore, this may prohibit the center's ability to expand in the future.

The AV design documentation that is usually created during a simulation AV project consists of a set of AV drawings. These drawings show the architectural device locations for all of the AV systems components, as well as all of the related pathways and infrastructure. A full AV design package would consist of AV facility plans, AV electrical drawings, systems drawings, a narrative description of the project, and an equipment list or bill of materials that need to be purchased for the project.

The AV facility plans will show all of the technical infrastructure devices on the floor plans as well as the building elevations. These facility drawings can provide Karen and the administrative board with a good understanding of each of the rooms and their relationship to the AV devices and overall programmatic workflow.

In addition to the AV facility plans, a set of AV electrical drawings will be provided. These drawings will show the actual infrastructure. This will include conduit, cable tray, junction boxes, and pathways. They will also show AV electrical requirements such as power receptacles and their associated mounting heights. The AV electrical drawings are intended to be coordinated with the electrical engineer's drawings so that a complete set of electrical drawings can be generated for the project.

The final set of AV drawings is system diagrams. These drawings will illustrate in detail how each of the systems are interconnected and how this connectivity is distributed in the pathways and the infrastructure of the spaces. These drawings are also referred to as "single-line drawings."

In addition to the AV (a) facility, (b) electrical, and (c) system diagram, an AV specification will be provided. This specification typically follows the Construction Specification Institute (CSI) format and will include the installation practice and specifics, working conditions, bidding terms where applicable, and a narrative functional description of the systems, spaces, and their performance requirements.

The final component of the AV design documentation is the equipment list or bill of materials. This document is usually done in a spreadsheet format. It will indicate the required equipment and the quantities needed to make up the AV system. In some cases, accepted substitutes or alternate equipment will be listed. The equipment list may include cameras, video and audio switchers, microphones, speakers, display devices, and recording devices.

If an institution opts to design the simulation center with resources from within the institution, it is always recommended that they create a basis of design document. A basis of design documents combines elements of the schematic and design development phases with a basic system specification. In other words, it is a road map of the anticipated simulation project with some design detail and direction. It will allow for the ability to get a preliminary cost estimate and a sense of what will actually be required to build the AV system. It is also important to seek a design professional to review the documentation to ensure that the direction matches the need and is within the established budget. The basis of design can be presented to an AV contractor who may be able to finish the final details on the design documentation and do the installation. This can be a very cost-effective approach. It is dependent on the qualifications and past project history of the AV contractor.

The final design approach is to hire a design build firm to design and implement the AV technology of the simulation center. In this type of project, the design build firm will provide a turnkey solution. In some instances, an institution may require the design and build to be complete by separate organizations. In many cases, the overall project costs of a design build firm may be less than that of an AV design consultant and the subsequent bidding/award process. If a single company is completing all aspects of the AV technology, the outcome may be a well-coordinated integration because one firm is designing and installing the entire system. In this type of project, the design build firm will generate all documentation to correspond with the various design and construction phases of the project.

THEMES

Karen has noted while investigating the potential designs and types of AV systems that would fit the needs of ABC University Simulation Center. With so many options to choose from, Karen decided to see what items were most commonly mentioned throughout her visit to other programs. For her, the primary goal is to determine where she can get the greatest functionality of the space with the lowest impact to the overall budget of the project.

As Karen put together her initial impressions from visiting other centers, she also decided to put together a Room Function Table (Appendix D), which outlined how the administrative board and she would like to see each room be utilized. Her table illustrates where technology will be utilized and how they envision the space be allocated at any given point. Although overwhelmed with this task, Karen does feel that she will be able to accomplish what has been requested of her with some guidance and support of other simulation centers.

The overwhelming theme that was discussed by many different programs during her visits was to think into the future. She found that there is still a mixed batch of simulation technology, and while there are numerous options available, it is important to have an idea of what type of simulation technology you will be integrating and what are your requirements. Much of the industry is moving toward wireless technology where the simulator, infrastructure, and AV system are capable of being run and managed wirelessly. Karen found more and more centers being able to wirelessly control both their simulators and their learning management system from any location without having to allocate an actual control room space. The integration of a wireless AV system does require Karen to involve IT early on in the project. But, on the basis of the experience of other programs, she believes it will help her and her teams expand the overall capabilities of the simulation center.

During Karen's visits to other centers, a simulation specialist did bring up the need to determine early on whether you are going to have a separate control room for each clinical simulation room, centralized control room, or no formal control room. The ABC University drawings (Appendix A) do show control rooms operating more than one space, and although this does save the overall cost in running AV systems, it does bring up concerns with the overall utilization, sound isolation, and functionality. A number of simulation directors have expressed their own concern with each of these types of spaces receiving a mixed set of reviews, and most expressed concerns with sound issues, cost, and flexibility in all of these designs. Systematically, integrating AV into these types of designs had become a cost barrier for two of the centers Karen visited. The key takeaway from this part of the visit was to plan ahead and consider what will actually be happening in the space in order to plan for how to integrate a functional AV system regardless of the final control room chosen.

THE HOW TO . . .

Having had time to review the most notable themes discovered during her visit to numerous simulation centers around the country, Karen decided to begin to work with an AV designer on developing an assumption table. An assumption table (Appendix B) is a comprehensive list of video, audio, control, and recording equipment needed in any room where a need for technology has been identified. Karen presented her room function table (Appendix D) to the AV designer who worked closely with her to put together this assumption table. This table is an important step in determining how the AV system would be laid out and what the overall cost of the AV section of the project would be.

Assumption Tables

On the basis of Karen's Room Function Table, the appropriate next step is to review the Assumption Table that would be created and presented by an AV designer. It is not unusual for a simulation center to request three different proposals focusing on low-, midrange-, and high-cost AV designs. In essence, the center is looking for three different proposals from AV designers that offer them a design that ranges from a Fiat to a Ferrari. The key is to not only see the different costs associated with an AV design, but to learn about the equipment and the design setup. At the end of the day, once the system is installed, it will be the faculty responsible for troubleshooting an AV system. Although a good installer is always available to troubleshoot, Karen learned that you have to have an expert on-site because a problem can result in class delays. The Assumption Table can also serve as a means to determine which experts need to be part of the AV system discussion.

BEEN THERE, DONE THAT

Although Karen took an optimal approach at how she designed the technical infrastructure of ABC University Simulation Center, her approach is not always something commonly seen. The authors wish to share their own experience in what they have seen occur in other centers across the country in hopes that each of you learn from these lessons. These lessons are in no particular order and

illustrate the complexities involved in putting together a solid AV system.

Improving the center after the technical infrastructure has been designed and installed can only occur in a number of different ways. Most commonly occurring is how centers simply find the solution and integrate that piece of technology into an existing design. A rework of the entire design can be costly and suboptimal but is always a possibility. Sustaining the technical infrastructure involves a coordinated effort between the organization's internal technical resources, the simulation center, and, if allowed, the installer. Having an individual maintain the technical infrastructure that has never designed, built, or installed it can be more challenging than one would imagine. The installers understand how the system works and are able to troubleshoot even the most complex of problems. Those tasked with managing the system with limited experience in the design and install will have a significant learning curve. Furthermore, there could be added expense as they "brush up" on how and why the system was installed in its current form. For this reason, it is important to maintain a working relationship with the designer and installer, and obtain a set of as-built AV drawings. This can help you overcome even the largest of problems.

During the building design phase, it is important to have your IT and AV designers on-site. They will be able to provide the simulation center staff with their personal and professional experience as the overall design is drafted. Because the center is not like most educational and hospital environments, it is important to let the designers know what you hope to accomplish. One of the most common oversights that have been seen is the failure to mention where microphones will be placed. It is important to let the designers know that you will place microphones in the ceiling and that you will need to have the best audio signal available for recording. This will ensure that the designers take sound absorption and insulation into consideration as well as avoid placing items that may unnecessarily vibrate above those ceiling spaces.

As the complexity of the design grows, the simulation centers seem to keep forgetting to involve all of the staff that will ultimately be running and supporting the systems day in and day out. There are details and nuances to the technical aspects of a simulation center that are sometimes overlooked by senior leadership. It is common for the major stakeholders and senior leadership of an institution to make design and budget decisions after evaluating the input they receive from the technical staff. There may be misinterpretation and misunderstandings of some of the technical requests, and this can translate into a potential problem and later become a significant gap. It is a good practice to create an internal programming report with input from all simulation staff including AV, IT, and nursing and educational personnel so that you can compile a list of all of the requirements. Furthermore, it is important to schedule a follow-up review with the entire team to validate the report. At the conclusion of the team meeting, you should then schedule a design meeting that can accommodate all of the key people for the right meetings.

Creating very flexible simulation spaces is an important process with today's ever-evolving audiovisual technologies. The design process has become more focused on how a space can be configured to allow as many different types of rooms or scenarios as possible. The idea is that a space does not have to have a purpose to be built. In essence, you are creating a simulation space without walls, giving it the greatest flexibility possible. An open environment allows for simulation specialists to quickly reconfigure it for the next simulation experience.

Similar to developing an open-concept center, we have to pay close attention to designing an AV system that allows for the continuum of care. The continuum of care is one of today's most discussed and requested simulation methodologies and environments. It allows for realistic team-based simulations that accurately depict real-world clinical workflows and processes. Continuum of care scenarios are extremely effective in teaching departmental handoffs and patient transfer scenarios. Control capabilities and logic of continuum of care scenarios need to be well thought out to accommodate the complexity of these types of AV systems.

Lastly, to ensure that we are capturing those complex scenarios that may involve multiple departments in many different environments, it is important for us to consider integrating the appropriate type of lighting. Lightsout infrared camera systems are becoming an excellent teaching tool for "disaster-after-the-generator-goes-out" scenarios. This technique allows for the recording of healthcare workers working in a totally dark environment only with flashlights. In today's world, many of us have experienced this real-world scenario first-hand.

SUMMARY

Future of Simulation Lab Design

The AV technology world is evolving at an exponential pace. It is almost certain that the next generation of simulation systems will be entirely wireless. System flexibility and reduced infrastructure costs will be the driving force for these new systems. The ability to create ad hoc scenarios and real-time continuum of care sessions will become standard in the majority of medical simulation programs. Furthermore, the wireless technology will allow centers to move freely between spaces without worrying about cable length constraints or physical connection/interface locations. Ultimately, this will provide a rich environment for creating highly realistic simulations.

A new converged wireless pathway will supplant the current design trend in consolidated, shared cabling pathways. The next-generation wireless access points will be able to handle multiple high-bandwidth streams/channels from telemetry devices, information systems servers, IP telephony, and video/audio streams with an extremely reliable quality of service. This will provide an experience that will be as consistent as last-generation cabled solutions.

As IT systems such as Electronic Health Record (EHR) or Electronic Medical Record (EMR) become the center of most patient care and treatment documentation, it will be essential for these systems to become integrated into the next-generation medical and nursing school simulation scenarios. As multimodality care systems replace the current single-modality systems, there will be the need to visualize several systems on the same display simultaneously. This will further drive the capabilities of handheld mobile devices to capture, stream, and document scenario data and subsequently display it on any wall, boom, or arm-mounted large-screen display at any place and at any time.

Planning a future-proof hybrid infrastructure is essential for creating successful simulation systems that will be productive for several years. Although conventional thought is that the technology needs to be replaced every 5 years, sometimes the technology itself requires architectural and environmental considerations. High-capacity wireless systems need to be free from highly reflective metal ceilings, walls, electromagnetic interference, and duct systems. This creates a new pathway consideration that is much more complicated than establishing a point-to-point cable pathway. There is also the problem of future wireless technology systems overlapping with existing ones. This will become more of a problem as the Internet service providers implement long-distance cellular systems that can blanket an urban environment with 10-fold the capacity of today's systems. Although this is not far in the future, many telecommunications industry experts believe that this technology may be in use by 2014 in several parts of the US.

Creating the technical infrastructure of a simulation center is no easy task. It involves patience and the ability to seek out experts in technical infrastructure design. The design will change as the complexity of the needs is realized and simulators begin to be integrated into the AV system. For any program to be successful in meeting their needs, they must have a curriculum, seek guidance, visit other programs, and be involved in the design process from design to installation. With support, you can have a center that will not only meet the needs of your center today, but also be sophisticated enough to meets the needs of your program in the future.

REFERENCES

BICSI. (2009). *Telecommunications distribution methods manual* (12th ed.). Tampa, FL: Author.

BICSI & InfoComm International. (2006). *AV design reference manual* (1st ed.). Fairfax, VA: Author.

Kyle, R. R., & Murray, W. B. (2008). *Clinical simulation: Operations, engineering, and management.* New York, NY: Elsevier.

Ross, K. (2012, November). Practice makes perfect, planning considerations for medical simulation centers. *Health Facilities Management.* Retrieved from https://www.ecri.org/Documents/Reprints/Practice_Makes_Perfect_Planning_Considerations_for_Medical_Simulation_Centers(Health_Facilities_Management).pdf

APPENDIX A

ABC University Simulation Center Design with AV System Integration

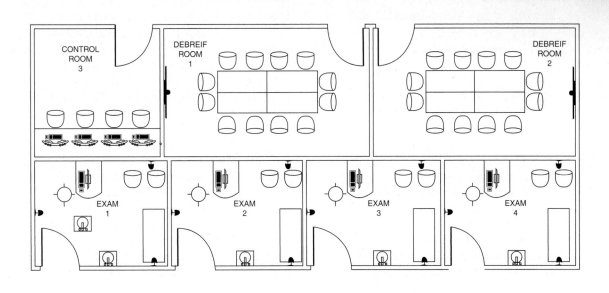

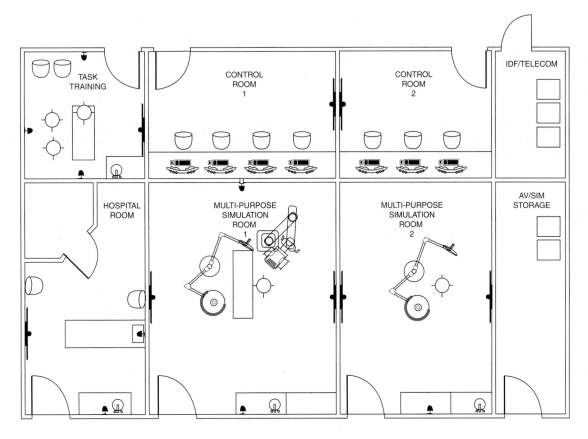

APPENDIX B

ABC University Simulation Center: Functionality Assumption Tables

Exam Room Nos. 1, 2, 3, 4

Video	(3) P/Z/T wall-mounted video cameras
	(1) Wall-mounted DVI/HDMI input plate
Audio	(1) Ceiling-mounted loudspeaker for sound reinforcement
	(1) Ceiling-mounted microphone
Control	Centralized control from control room only
Recording	Centralized recording from control room only

Task Training

Video	(4) P/Z/T wall-mounted video cameras
	(1) Video connection at retractable column
	(1) Wall-mounted 60-inch (152.4 cm) LCD/LED monitor
Audio	(1) Ceiling-mounted microphone
Control	Centralized control from control room only
Recording	Centralized recording from control room only
Physiological Monitoring	(1) Headwall-mounted VGA/DVI input

Hospital Room

Video	(3) P/Z/T wall-mounted video cameras
	(1) Wall-mounted 60-inch LCD/LED monitor
Audio	(1) Ceiling-mounted microphone
Control	Centralized control from control room only
Recording	Centralized recording from control room only
Physiological Monitoring	(1) Headwall-mounted VGA/DVI input

Multipurpose Room No. 1

Video	(4) P/Z/T wall-mounted video cameras
	(2) Wall-mounted 60-inch LCD/LED monitor
	(1) Spring arm–mounted 24-inch (61 cm) surgical monitor
Audio	(2) Ceiling-mounted, linear-phase array microphones
Control	Centralized control from control room only
Recording	Centralized recording from control room only
Physiological Monitoring	(1) Boom-mounted VGA/DVI input
	(1) Headwall-mounted VGA/DVI input

Multipurpose Room No. 2

Video	(4) P/Z/T wall-mounted video cameras
	(2) Wall-mounted 60-inch LCD/LED monitor
Audio	(2) Ceiling-mounted, linear-phase array microphones
Control	Centralized control from control room only
Recording	Centralized recording from control room only
Physiological Monitoring	(2) Headwall-mounted VGA/DVI input

Control Room No. 1

Video	(1) Wall-mounted 60-inch LCD/LED monitor
	(2) Video recorder computers
Audio	(2) Ceiling-mounted loudspeakers
	(2) Desk-mounted push-to-talk microphones
	(2) Headphone stations
Control	(2) 21-inch (53.3 cm) touch-screen touch panels
Recording	Centralized recording servers in AV Storage

Control Room No. 2

Video	(1) Wall-mounted 60-inch LCD/LED monitor
	(2) Video recorder computers
Audio	(2) Ceiling-mounted loudspeakers
	(2) Desk-mounted push-to-talk microphones
	(2) Headphone stations
Control	(2) 21-inch touch-screen touch panels
Recording	Centralized recording servers in AV Storage

Control Room No. 3

Video	(1) Wall-mounted 60-inch LCD/LED monitor
	(4) Video recorder computers
Audio	(2) Ceiling-mounted loudspeakers
	(4) Desk-mounted push-to-talk microphones
	(4) Headphone stations
Control	(4) 21-inch touch-screen touch panels
Recording	Centralized recording servers in AV Storage

Debrief Room No. 1

Video	(1) P/Z/T wall-mounted camera
	(1) Wall-mounted 60-inch LCD/LED monitor
	(1) TV connection outlet
Audio	(2) Ceiling-mounted loudspeakers
	(2) Ceiling-mounted microphones
Control	(1) iPad for control
Recording	Centralized recording from control room only

Debrief Room No. 2

Video	(1) P/Z/T wall-mounted camera
	(1) Wall-mounted 60-inch LCD/LED monitor
	(1) TV connection outlet
Audio	(2) Ceiling-mounted loudspeakers
	(2) Ceiling-mounted microphones
Control	(1) iPad for control
Recording	Centralized recording from control room only

AV/SIM Storage

Video	(3) Video switchers
	(3) Multiwindow camera processors
Audio	(1) Audio matrix mixer
	(8) Wireless microphones
Control	(1) AV control processor
Misc.	(2) AV equipment racks
Recording	(1) 16-TB AV storage server

APPENDIX C

Technical Specification Worksheet

Simulation Devices

How many rooms will require high-technology mannequins? _____

How many mannequins need to be utilized simultaneously? _____

Will the mannequins be wired or wireless? _____

How many wired? How many wireless? _____

Will there be a requirement for labor and delivery, mother and child simulations/mannequins? _____

Where will the physiological monitor connectivity for the mannequins be located in each room if wired? _____

Will there be a requirement for medical gases and suction? If so, which rooms and locations in the room? _____

Where will the mannequins and ancillary equipment be stored? _____

Video Devices

How many rooms will require video cameras? _____

Will the cameras be wall-mounted or ceiling-mounted? _____

What type cameras? Pan/tilt/zoom or fixed? _____

How many of each type in each type room? _____

Which rooms will require LCD/LED monitors? _____

Will the monitors be ceiling- or wall-mounted? _____

What are the required sizes of the monitors? _____

Audio Devices

How many rooms will require audio recording with microphones? _____

Will the microphones be wireless or ceiling-mounted? _____

How many microphones will be required in each space? _____

Will the playback in each space be from integral LCD/LED monitor speakers or ceiling speakers? _____

Recording System

How many simulation scenarios/cases will need to be recorded simultaneously? _____

Will the recording device have removable media/ on-board or network storage? _____

How much recorded material (GB) will need to be stored and for how long? _____

Will the recordings/files be accessible to faculty and staff via the network with proper rights and security? _____

Paging System

What spaces will require paging? _____

What spaces can the pages originate from? _____

Will the pages be initiated from desktop microphones and or handheld microphones? _____

Will there be ceiling-mounted paging speakers or wall-mounted speakers? _____

Intercom System

What spaces will require an intercom? _____

Will the intercom be via phone headset or fixed wall system? _____

Will cell phones or Vocera-type systems need to be integrated into the system? _____

Control Room and Control System

Will the majority of the AV equipment be located in the control room(s) or AV Closet/IDF? _____

Will there be a requirement for headphones for each operator in the control room(s)? _____

Will the voice of the mannequins originate from a desktop microphone in the control room? _____

Will the operators utilize a touch-screen touch panel for controlling the simulation scenarios? _____

Will there be Web-based control so that the system may be controlled from any location? _____
How many cameras need to be viewed in the control room(s) simultaneously? _____

Support and Operational Requirements

Who will support the simulation center for AV? Mannequins? _____
How many staff members will be required or available to operate the simulation center? _____

Will the system be required to create continuum of care scenarios from room to room? _____

Will the AV vendor/integrator have remote access for troubleshooting and system repair/reboot? _____

How fast of a response will be required by the AV integrator for on-site service of major problems? _____

Training

How much training time will be required for simulation staff? Will there be separate training for techs? _____
Will there be a requirement for a system manual and online help support? _____

Simulation Center Room Function Matrix

Room Name	Audio			Video				Other		Simulation	Control			Support	
	Playback	Recording	Monitoring	Large Screen Display	Local Computer Input	Video Camera	Manequin Vitals Display	Intercom	Paging	Record Vitals Patient Data	Touch Panel	Web Based	BYOD Control	AV Equipment Racks	Simulation Server Racks
Exam Room 1	█	█	█		█	█		█	█			█			
Exam Room 2	█	█	█		█	█		█	█			█			
Exam Room 3	█	█	█		█	█		█	█			█			
Exam Room 3	█	█	█		█	█		█	█			█	█		
Task Training	█	█	█	█	█	█	█	█	█	█	█	█			
Hospital Room		█		█	█	█	█	█	█	█	█	█			
Multi-Purpose Sim 1	█	█	█	█	█	█	█	█	█	█	█	█			
Multi-Purpose Sim 2	█	█	█	█	█	█	█	█	█	█	█	█			
Control Room 1	█		█	█	█	█		█	█		█	█			
Control Room 2	█		█	█	█	█		█	█		█	█			
Control Room 3	█		█	█	█	█		█	█		█	█			
Debrief 1	█	█	█	█	█	█		█	█		█	█			
Debrief 2	█	█	█	█	█	█		█	█		█	█			
IDF/Telecom								█	█						█
AV/Sim Storage								█	█					█	█
Corridors		█	█			█			█						

CHAPTER 6.4

Transitioning to a New Center

H. Michael Young, BBS, MDiv, and Morgan A. Scherwitz, MSN, RN

ABOUT THE AUTHORS

H. MICHAEL YOUNG is a Simulation Technology Specialist who works for the Center for Instructional Innovation, Tarleton State University's academic IT division. Michael provides full-time technical and operational support to the Department of Nursing's *Center for Clinical Simulation & Competency*. Mr. Young is an active member of Society for Simulation in Healthcare (SSH), Chairman for Certified Healthcare Simulation Operation Specialist (CHSOS) certification subcommittee, a former member of the SSH Board of Directors, and a regular contributor to International Nurses Association for Clinical Simulation and Learning (INACSL) forums.

MORGAN A. SCHERWITZ has worked as the nursing laboratory manager for the past 5 years at Tarleton State University. Ms. Scherwitz was previously a labor and delivery nurse and graduated with her Masters of Nursing in education with a deep desire for educating future nurses. In collaboration with her colleagues, Ms. Miller transitioned her program to a new center and has distinguished the lab as its own center, capable of generating self-sustaining revenue.

ABSTRACT

One of the most challenging situations any simulation program may face is moving to a new space. While the excitement of getting a new building or space stands at the forefront and paves the way, those who go through the move look back with different, more experienced eyes. Many centers start off with very little space, or space that is less than ideal for simulation-based training. When funding and opportunity finally present themselves, many are eager to move forward. It is an exciting time but fraught with many challenges. While there are many methods for transition, this chapter seeks to provide suggestions that could help guide other simulation staff through a transition from one simulation center to another, maximizing effort and minimizing risks associated with a move.

CASE EXAMPLE

ABC University Medical Center has had a simulation center for over 2 years. The simulation center occupies a part of the hospital previously inhabited by the hyperbaric unit. The staff comprises 1.5 full-time employees who work at least 5 days a week, providing quality simulation experiences for hospital staff. Because of a lack of space within the center, many of the simulation sessions are performed *in situ*. The administrative team of the university has been working for the past year to build a proper simulation center. Transition planning must begin immediately to ensure a smooth transition.

INTRODUCTION

In the life of a simulation program, there is rarely a more exciting time or a more stressful one than when transitioning from an older facility to a new one. The purpose of this chapter is to provide suggestions for those simulation programs that will be transitioning to a new dedicated space. These transitions often do not allow the simulation program to function at the new and the old facilities simultaneously. Typically, simulation programs do not have the luxury of using both spaces while in transition; when the new facility opens, the old facility must close or be evacuated for preparation of another space. Having equipment fully functional in two locations is not usually an option or even a reasonable expectation.

Planning starts while the program is in its current facility (academic building, leased property, partner facilities, etc).—If the issues are not addressed early on there is the possibility that others will become involved with different objectives. In an academic program, department administrators and university leadership will all be putting pressure on the simulation program leadership regarding

479

access to the building (the timeline to availability etc.). However, such a schedule is somewhat unpredictable depending on when construction or renovation actually begins. Additionally, the schedule will be impacted by a myriad of variables throughout the entire project that will likely interfere with completion target dates. It will be important to communicate the unpredictable nature of construction, renovation, and transition to inquiring parties that insist on establishing their own schedules.

"WHERE DO I BEGIN?"

When should planning for the transition begin? The process should begin as soon as dedicated space has been approved and regardless of the amount of lead time for planning for the transition, few are ready for the challenge. The more time spent in planning the logistics of the transition, the greater the chances for success, and the fewer frustrations all will have. The first step in preparing for the transition is to appoint or recruit a transition planning team. The team might be made up of a few members in the beginning, but should grow as the planning continues and more key people are identified. The initial mission of the committee will be to define the critical issues and priorities early. For example:

- What courses/events will be interrupted? How long?
- What technologies will be off-line in transition? How long?
- Any servers to be moved?
- Will there be network availability in transition?
- Who will begin the inventory of the capital equipment?
- What will be moved to new facilities? What will not?

Once these priorities have been identified, recruit or appoint "gatekeepers." Unless a staff member's time can be dedicated to the transition, assigning one person to be gatekeeper may be overwhelming, especially if it is a large program with a large inventory. Consider the different types of capital inventory, and whether it is going to be moved to the new facilities, reassigned to other departments, or placed in surplus.

RECRUIT VENDORS TO SECURE, MOVE, AND SET UP LEASED EQUIPMENT

Workgroup copiers and printers and other technologies can be heavy and relatively fragile. Early in the planning phase, the transition team would be wise to secure the assistance of the vendors to help secure, move, and set up equipment on behalf of the simulation program. Whether the vendors agree to do this as a free service or with a fee attached, the value of recruiting their assistance should not be overlooked. Nevertheless, a vendor can be motivated

to agree to such an arrangement as a matter of customer service, and with incentives that include the hope of additional sales. Aside from office equipment, manufacturers of other assets (e.g simulators) will sometimes happily move the larger items purchased from them. This distributes the workload to experts who know how to safely move those technologies most critical to a simulation center's mission. Provide vendors with a move-in schedule, establish contingencies, and prioritize accordingly. As schedules are adjusted toward the end of the building project, keep vendors apprised of changes in the timeline. Keep a list of vendor contacts and alert them every time a change affects the move-in plans. Assign one transition team member to maintain communication with vendors who have agreed to participate in the move.

SCHEDULE REGULAR TRANSITION TEAM MEETINGS

Time and care must be taken when planning a move of a simulation center. Equipment is costly and must be handled with care. Investing time into planning the move of a simulation center will reduce stress. The size of the center will have to be considered when planning for a move, however, no matter the size of the center, it is prudent to begin planning as early as possible. As soon as key individuals are aware that an impending move is occurring, planning needs to begin.

Early in the initial planning phase, meetings should be held at least monthly, with assignments, action items, and due dates distributed among the team members. Clear communication and concerted efforts are critical during the entire transition phase. Expectations of individuals and teamwork should be addressed with agreement amongst the transition team members. Establishing a master calendar that is open and accessible to the team will be important to ensure a clear understanding of all aspects related to the move (Table 6.4.1 and Figure 6.4.1). The calendar should include static and variable events with the caveat that team members should accept that calendar events will likely change throughout the new building timeline. Nevertheless, keep the calendar up to date as new information becomes available from contractors. Transition team leadership should be included in milestone meetings with the architect and contractors. Administrators do not always remember to share what they learn in such meetings with the transition planning team. Having a representative (such as the chairperson of the transition team) at the meeting helps keep everyone informed. What may not be important to an administrator or contractor may be of great interest to the transition team orchestrating a timely move.

Persons will need to be enlisted to the transition team on the basis of their ability to fill key roles. This may be the simulation manager, laboratory assistants, information technology (IT) support, and administrators. Keeping the team small will help keep the group on task. As

TABLE 6.4.1

Calendar Checklist

1. Move officially announced
2. Organize basic team
   - Meet monthly
3. Priorities and objectives established
4. Assess inventory
5. Discard unused items
6. Establish budget
7. Team evolution
   - Include gatekeepers
   - Meet more frequently
8. Contact vendors
9. Order new supplies
10. Determine integration of old and new equipment
11. Establish timeline including dates and times
12. Identify logistical gaps
    - Add members as needed
13. Evaluate workload for faculty/staff
14. Recruit volunteers
15. Hire/recruit movers
16. Firm up calendar events
    - Vendor availability
    - Equipment delivery
    - Official move-in date
    - Mover availability
17. Establish labeling system
18. Map out staging areas
19. Map out storage areas
20. Pack rarely used items as early as possible
21. Disassemble all equipment in old space
22. Pack all equipment and supplies prior to move
23. In new space, set up shelves, storage, and beds
24. New supplies received
25. Move equipment
    - Account for each item as it is received in the new center
26. Assemble and test equipment

the plans for the transition evolve, the team may evolve as well. There may be a need to add ad hoc members for smaller, well-defined tasks. For example, adding individuals who are willing to pack or manage the staging process at the new facility will be of use to the team. Planning may include persons outside of leadership positions. Those who will be directly impacted by the move or who will play key roles in the moving process should be active in the planning process.

Priorities should be established early. This will allow the team to achieve their overarching goal of a successful move. Consider what courses or events will be interrupted. The length of the interruption during the move must be accounted and the program schedule adjusted accordingly. This should be a creative process in which ideas are formulated for alternatives to simulation and lab space. Lab time may be front-loaded in the semester or pushed to the end of the semester depending on the scheduled date for the transition. Be flexible in your thinking process and

in the schedule for the upcoming courses to best accommodate all the changes the center will be facing. Even the best-laid plans may require minor changes to accomplish the task at hand. Open and frequent communication with educators/staff using the lab is essential so the move does not interfere or halt the progression of scheduled courses. Planning a move during a semester break is best if your schedule allows this opportunity.

ASSESSING INVENTORY

Begin assessing the inventory of the facility. This includes equipment in storage or items rarely used. It is prudent to discard unused equipment if it not going to be used in the future. This will reduce the amount of equipment that must be transported to the new facility and decrease the workload. Check your institution's policies regarding discarded items. For example, a university system may require discarded equipment to be sent to a central location to be auctioned or reallocated.

Items that continue to be used for scheduled simulation sessions should be packed and transported after their use has concluded. On the receiving side, items in highest demand must be unpacked first. Consider what equipment will be needed to get the simulation center up and running. This equipment should be given priority in the move.

As mentioned previously, the transition planning team may evolve at this juncture to include persons who will function as gatekeepers in different locations of the new center or type of inventory. For instance, a person may be assigned to be the overseer of the simulators, while another person may manage consumables. Dividing the equipment among the team allows the task to not overwhelm any one person. Keep in mind that although there may be multiple gatekeepers, having a single project manager over the entire move is crucial to ensure the appropriate flow of materials and to troubleshoot problems. The transition team leader will have a greater understanding of all the working pieces and can circumvent issues as they arise. The transition team leader will additionally ensure that items are not lost during the move or misplaced.

The transition team leader can direct the meetings and ensure that each member of the team understands pertinent details such as the official move date. The final meetings prior to the move should center on identifying and closing gaps in logistics as they are detected. The group must be flexible and creative to overcome the obstacles. Adding team members who are able to assist with the logistical challenges is one method of overcoming this hurdle.

Logistical problems may become evident as the team moves through this process. Issues that may surface include transportation for the materials, financing for the movers, and recruiting enough persons to assist with the move. Doorways or elevators may not be large enough to accommodate large items such as beds or storage units.

Calendar Event	Date Set	In Progress	Completed	Notes
1. Move officially announced				
2. Organize basic team • Meet monthly				
3. Priorities and objectives established				
4. Assess inventory				
5. Discard unused items				
6. Establish budget				
7. Team evolution • Include gatekeepers • Meet more frequently				
8. Contact vendors				
9. Order new supplies				
10. Determine integration of old and new equipment				
11. Establish time line including dates and times				
12. Identify logistical gaps • Add members as needed				
13. Evaluate workload for faculty/staff				
14. Recruit volunteers				
15. Hire/recruit movers				
16. Firm up calendar events • Vendor availability • Equipment delivery • Official move in date • Mover availability				
17. Establish labeling system				
18. Map out staging areas				
19. Map out storage areas				
20. Pack rarely used items as early as possible				
21. Disassemble all equipment in old space				
22. Pack all equipment and supplies prior to move				
23. In new space, setup shelves, storage and beds				
24. New supplies received				
25. Move equipment • Account for each item as it is received in the new center				
26. Assemble and test equipment				

FIGURE 6.4.1 Calendar event log.

This could potentially halt the move or cause damage to items as the movers attempt to move large items through small openings. Consider an alternative exit or methods to disassemble large equipment to smaller components to allow them to be moved without damage.

The transition team leader should assign a team member to oversee the tasks as they are identified within the group. Additionally, dates and time frames should be established by the group for each task. Consider the order in which events must occur and create a calendar of events that is kept in a central location accessible to all for editing.

Typically, faculty and staff will continue to have their regular workload in addition to any move-related tasks. Evaluate staff workloads to determine whether some tasks can be reassigned to free up key staff to assist with the logistics of the move. Persons from other departments may be willing to volunteer to assist with the moving process.

Faculty and staff cannot be expected to move large equipment. Possible injury and loss of time for the injured team member would only create new challenges. Team members would be put to better use by being assigned to manage the movers and accounting for the materials and equipment that are being moved. A university likely has a department devoted to facilities management who can assist with moving equipment; usually this entails interdepartmental billing to cover the expenses involved.

Contacting vendors to move equipment such as headwall units and simulators is prudent even if a fee is attached because the vendor will have the expertise to properly install the equipment in the new facility. Items that are part of the infrastructure of the old building such as headwall units and compressors will necessitate plumbers and electricians. Universities may have departments dedicated to providing these services. A stand-alone center may have to contract these services or use staff with expertise in these areas. Consider these costs when developing the budget.

Investing time into organizing, labeling, and packing boxes is essential and will reduce the workload of unpacking. Like items should be packed with like items. Each box should be clearly labeled to include a detailed description of the contents. Color coding labels on the boxes is one method of organizing the move. A "green" label may alert the movers or team members to deliver a box to the control room or a "yellow" label could be used to identify the items in the box, such as computer parts. Whatever method the team chooses to label and identify the boxes, it is essential to disseminate this information to all involved persons to avoid confusion. Should an item be needed prior to the move or prior to boxes being unpacked at the new facility, it can be easily located. The label should include the location where the box is to be delivered, enabling movers to deliver the item to the appropriate location.

While packing, determine what items will be used daily and what items are rarely used and need to be stored—this will need to be established by the team prior to the move. The items should be placed in the correct box with other items going to the same location and then the box must be labeled with the appropriate delivery location.

It may be necessary to label where a box originated from; however, take care that the movers do not confuse the location of origination with the delivery location. It is prudent to only list the location of origination if it is essential knowledge to assist in the move. For instance, simulator parts may be kept in your storage room and also in the simulation lab. Listing the location of origination may assist you when attempting to identify items after the move.

A central receiving location at the new facility should be established. At this location, boxes can be accounted for and the project manager can direct movers to the correct location. This location will act as a staging ground to keep the move running forward. Unfortunately, harried and exhausted movers may not spend the needed time delivering boxes to the correct location at the new facility. The movers may focus on moving items from one building to another, with little care that it has arrived in the correct space. Keep in mind, costs may increase if movers have to haul boxes throughout a large building rather than dropping off items at one central location.

It will then become the team's responsibility to transport the boxes to the correct location. Appropriate moving equipment such as a dolly (hand truck) and carts should be supplied to the team members in an effort to reduce possible injury, and expedite the task at hand.

Determine how new equipment and old equipment may integrate. For instance, can portable compressors for the simulators be stored outside the new lab because the new facility has built-in compressors? If the new control room has new computers, what should be done with the laptops that came with the simulator? Such decisions should be made before the move to make the best use of space. The sooner the new space is up and working without having to navigate through boxes of items not immediately needed, the sooner the simulation program can resume.

DELIVERY AND SETUP

Upon the arrival of new and existing equipment, a team member (or multiple team members) must be designated to ensure that the equipment is powered up and configured so it is ready to be used. This includes equipment disassembled for the move. For example, simulators require that all computers, cords, peripherals, and means of data communication be configured, calibrated, and tested to ensure that they are still in good working order after the ordeal of the move. It is possible that items become damaged in the process of disassembly and transportation.

In an effort to reduce the amount of items to be moved, newly purchased consumables should be delivered to the new facility. This can be arranged at the time of the order by requesting delivery closer to the determined move-in date. Remember, these items will not be labeled like the other boxes. One option is to have the transition team leader on-site during delivery so appropriate labels or clear direction can be provided. To avoid confusion, delivery of newly purchased items should not be scheduled on the same day as the move. The transition team leader or designated team member can direct the delivery person to place items in a specified location. Another option is to have all items delivered to the central receiving location in the building and then the team members can move the equipment to the proper place at a later time. Universities and large hospital centers may have a central receiving department where deliveries must be made. In any case, it is unwise to complete delivery to the new building if shelves for the storage of supplies have not been delivered or assembled yet.

It is necessary to integrate the existing consumables with the new consumables. Placing consumables in one location verses having many locations throughout the building will reduce costs and also ease the stress of inventorying all consumables. Create a plan for where items will be stored. For example, simulator parts will be placed in your control room cabinets and consumables in the storage room.

Create a plan of organizing the storage room. Determine the amount of space for storage on carts, bins, cabinets, or shelving units and begin to plan out where certain items will be placed. Create a drawing of the storage room floor plan, outlining where certain items will be placed. This will ensure that those tasked with unpacking will place items in the correct location. This will also reduce the amount of time spent having to reorganize items after being unpacked.

Building a sequential timeline in which events must occur is essential. For instance, beds must be in the new facility before mannequins can be put into service. Shelves must be assembled prior to items being unpacked and stored. As in any move, issues are likely to surface. The vendor for the beds may not be able to deliver until after the official move date. The team must be creative and find ways to work around these issues, such as storing mannequins on tables or desks until beds are delivered.

ROLE EVOLUTION

Who will be managing the inventory in the new facility? As your program changes and grows, so too will staffing assignments. At the opening of the new facility, chances are that staffing will remain the same until equilibrium occurs and all faculty, staff, and administrators find their place in the new environment. Changes in floor plans will inevitably result in reexamination of how resources will be managed, how spaces are scheduled and staffed. The degree to which such changes occur will depend on the size and scope of the simulation program and how the budget adapts to the new environment. Begin realigning roles throughout the transition period. This does not mean that promotions get finalized or titles get changed prior to the move. Change can be a motivator for any program, but it can also be a challenge because with a new building often come new technologies and new responsibilities.

Clarifying role changes early in the process of transition will give simulation team members a sense of hope, and can help motivate them to take on the new challenges knowing that their role will improve and align with the new floor plan and technologies. Having team members focus on only part of the changes will make stress more manageable and improve team dynamics if open communication is maintained. The transition team needs to be kept informed about administrative decisions regarding role responsibilities, and gatekeepers are recruited or appointed to coordinate and communicate how current and future inventories are managed during the move.

TECHNICAL CONSIDERATIONS OF A MOVE

Most simulation programs rely on one or more central servers and the network that connects workstations with the data stored on them. Servers are not just important for storing and accessing electronic files, but fulfill many other tasks associated specifically with simulation. If the move is to a different building on the same campus, chances are the servers will remain in the same data center. However, some specialized servers may still need to be moved—such as those that manage the audiovisual (AV) and scheduling system for the center. Protecting the data on these servers needs to be coordinated with the institution's IT department. If a simulation center is fortunate enough to have its own IT staff, include these specialists on the transition team. Decisions made in isolation of those with special knowledge and skills are poorly considered, regardless of the specialty.

Simulation technologies have evolved tremendously over the last decade or so. This evolution has been enabled by two different drivers: the ubiquity of wireless access points and other mobile platforms as well as the refinement of simulation technique. So, both technology and technique have a symbiotic relationship. Consequently, moving from one facility to another is complicated by the dependence on a technological infrastructure outside of the simulators themselves.

As an educator or administrator, understanding these technologies is not as important as seeking out the appropriate expertise to reduce downtime and improve the success of the move (See chapter 6.1 for more information regarding the design elements to consider when building a new facility.)

When moving into a new but existing building, the infrastructure will need to be assessed to ensure it is compatible with the equipment you are bringing. Such an assessment will include electrical and technological readiness. If leasing the new facilities, will the lessor allow alterations? Do local building codes require approval of such modifications? If alterations are permitted, will the lessee be required to return the building back to its original condition upon moving out?

As discussed earlier, ideally the move would be done during a break, but for simulation programs that are contracted with or partnered with area hospitals and clinics (and perhaps others), interim breaks are not always scheduled as they are in academia. In such a case, all parties must be informed when the program will not be able to service the hospital education program. It goes without saying that much marketing needs to be done with such partners so that everyone knows the moving schedule. If the program has a contract with a client that must be honored, much negotiation should be done before either party is found in breach of the contract.

Before moving into the new space, the data network needs to be working and cable wall plates available where equipment reliant on network access will be used. For example, moving or installing a new server should not be preceded by the network for which it will communicate with other network devices. Know where all of the network and electrical outlets are and plan locations of equipment prior to the move.

There are two primary uses of servers in most simulation programs: user authentication and data/file storage. While there are other functions that can be performed by servers, it is difficult to operate a simulation program without authentication and file storage functions. Who is responsible for maintaining user authentication? Are you moving across campus or across town? If across town, authentication cannot easily be supported by your institution, so setting up a local authentication server will be necessary so that users can have a common login across all computers they use in the simulation program. That said, if moving across campus to a new building, having a network infrastructure in the new building that has not been connected to the main campus falls short of full functionality.

If users have assigned credentials for logging into computers in your old space, will they be using the same credentials for logging into the new building? Again, if moving across campus, chances are the center will continue to use the same authentication server; if across town, chances are the new building will need an authentication server of its own.

There are other solutions for enabling access to the authentication server of the original site to work in the new one, but this depends on the continued relationship of the simulation program with the original hosting institution. Communication is extremely important early in the transition process so financial planning and appropriate steps are taken to ensure that both learners and employees can access their files and other network resources upon move-in.

WHAT'S IN THE BOX?

More valuable than the server hardware and technological infrastructure of a building are the electronic files collected over time within a simulation program. Electronic files include information that have been created for proposals, policies and procedures, correspondence, research projects, and reference material. The most dynamic kinds of information are stored in structured databases, or software that supports the organization of data in tables, allowing queries to be run to build reports and subsets of information. Structured data can be as simple as a spreadsheet or as complex as a server-based relational database system. Data can be used to assess a simulation program's effectiveness and its ability to meet criteria and defined objectives. When planning to move to new facilities, one would be wise not to overlook the various kinds of electronic information that has been collected and stored in a number of files within the organization.

- Simulation videos, bookmarks, assessments, checklists, and so on.
- Inventory records, including electronic invoices, correspondence, and so on.
- Files in progress on staff computers and server shares.
- Programmed scenarios, rubrics, setup worksheets.
- Software licensing information.
- Financial records.
- Administrative/organization policies and procedure documents.
- Warranty information/records, service agreements, maintenance records.
- E-mail correspondence.

Consider the individuals who serve as data gatekeepers within the simulation program: managers, technicians, coordinators, educators, directors, and program leaders. Individuals who save any electronic information using the organization computers and servers become gatekeepers when only they have access to that information. In a perfect world, such information is saved to a central server, which is backed up off-site, but few simulation programs have the resources or expertise to maintain such systems and processes. If such a system does not exist in the initial planning phase of the move, it would be extremely wise to begin to centralize all data, and ensure it gets duplicated outside of the old and new buildings. Again, your institution's IT department may be able to help you, but it would be beneficial to also seek outside council regarding your options. Depending on the volume of data (size in drive space: kilobytes, megabytes, gigabytes, terabytes, etc.), inexpensive Web-based solutions exist, and competition is high in this industry, so cost per megabyte is affordable and sustainable.

In a broader sense, there are only two types of electronic files: (1) static or fixed information often used for reference or documentation only and (2) dynamic or ever-evolving data that resides in tables that rarely are reduced in size and more likely being added upon on a regular basis. In either case, consider the implications if these electronic files should catastrophically disappear. Dynamic data recorded in a file or system of files, whether you are adding or subtracting information, is often included in a single place, such as a database. If the database becomes damaged or destroyed, repair is difficult, and in some cases impossible without entering the information again. An example of static forms of information is represented by word processing documents that were created and retained for historical purposes. If one item is lost, the other documents may not be damaged at all. However, of the two types of files, dynamic is a preferred way of storing repetitive variables (records), of which research and reports can be derived.

Up to the day of transition, documents and databases should be backed up incrementally, and on the final day prior to move-in, a full backup should be done. An incremental backup only duplicates data that has changed since the last full backup. Many organizations have learned the hard way that it is necessary to have more than an incremental backup file that only has the most recent changes of any file or database. All other content is lost. A full backup contains all files—new and old, with recent and old changes.

Speaking to your IT department or a consultant about how to ensure the backup is complete and is validated helps to ensure that the data you had at the old site is the same data you have when the new center opens. If the simulation program does not have its own IT specialist, this process will be much more challenging, and becomes more important to contract with a reputable consultant.

BEEN THERE, DONE THAT

Audiovisual Simulation Considerations

Many simulation programs use proprietary AV systems that integrate with the various simulator models. Moving the AV equipment and reconnecting them to cameras, microphones, and servers in the new facility requires special attention to details. For example, the AV system uses a database to record the names and locations, the type of camera, and means of connecting to the server. Chances are the floor plan will be different. The vendor will present the simulation program with a quote for making the move, which, most likely, will include moving the equipment racks, cameras, microphones, and so on. Explore the cost of moving equipment, the loss of income of not being able to use the equipment for clients, and so on. Consider also updating old equipment to be compliant with current and evolving standards. Compare the cost of updating now with the cost of waiting. Many programs take the opportunity to upgrade from an older, less efficient system to

a new system altogether. Making such a purchase during the transition could be more convenient and help reduce downtime. However, learning the new system will require time as well. If a new system is purchased, at least two full-time employees should attend the core training before the move so the transition will be smoother. Educator buy-in of new technologies may be slow; training and orientation for the educators may alleviate resistance to change.

In addition to the AV system transition, seek the advice from your simulator's experienced customer service representative. Especially if new simulators are purchased in lieu of the move, consider how these new simulators might interface (or not) with the new building's infrastructure. Many simulator manufacturers are moving to wireless communication, so if there has been no installation of the appropriate wireless access points or routers, reaching the simulator from a control room may be difficult, if not impossible.

Team Dynamics Considerations

Work station or office locations may differ in the new center. Often new centers are larger than previous centers. Physical separations and distance may change the dynamics of the team. It may also effect interpersonal relationships since communication and interaction may be less frequent than before (Palaganas, 2011).

SUMMARY

While exciting, the transition from old to new is not easy. Discussing floor plans, placement of doors, and even the purchase of new furniture and technologies dominate the interest of many in the throes of change. However, the devil is truly in the details. As with any change, there will be growing pains and the likelihood for successful transition increases with careful planning.

REFERENCES

Palaganas, J.C. (2011). How to Maintain the Success of Your Simulation Center: Policies, Procedures, and Project Pull. *Center for Simulation and Research: 2011 Regional Simulation Conference: Creating a Culture of Change.*

SECTION 7

Educational Development

CHAPTER 7.1

Assessing Learning Needs

Rebecca Wilson, PhD, RN, CHSE, and Debra Hagler, PhD, RN, ACNS-BC, CNE, CHSE, ANEF, FAAN

ABOUT THE AUTHORS

REBECCA WILSON is the Director of Interprofessional Education in Health Sciences at the University of Utah, with responsibility for providing direction and oversight for the interprofessional education program for health professions students. In her previous position, Dr. Wilson was a nursing education specialist in the Multidisciplinary Simulation Center at Mayo Clinic in Arizona. She has designed and developed a variety of simulation-based education activities, taught simulation faculty development courses, and mentored new faculty.

DEBRA HAGLER is a Clinical Professor in the College of Nursing & Health Innovation and the Coordinator for Teaching Excellence, Health Solutions at Arizona State University. She teaches courses for interdisciplinary staff and higher education faculty development, and for prelicensure through doctoral-level students. Dr. Hagler has conducted funded research on integration of educational simulation and on competency testing through simulation.

ABSTRACT

Stakeholder needs and available resources are important factors for the simulation educator to consider when planning educational programs. Educators should assess learning needs in a systematic process using multiple sources of data. In academic settings, learner assessment may be conducted on the individual, cohort, or curricular level. In service settings, learner assessment may be conducted on the individual, unit, role, site, or organizational level. Distinguishing the differences between learning needs and other types of performance needs helps to focus educational programs and use scarce resources efficiently.

CASE EXAMPLE

Carla, the clinical educator at a 250-bed community hospital, has been working in this role for 6 months when she is asked to put on a course to address patient falls. She quickly responded to the request for an education program by expending time, resources, and creativity in developing a great patient scenario and debriefing plan. And yet, the education received mixed reviews and had minimal impact on performance. Organizationally, there is concern that funding such resource-intensive education may not be wise. What might the educator do in the future to respond to requests for specific educational programs? Could starting with a learning needs assessment increase the chances of hitting the educational mark and making a difference in the learners' performance?

INTRODUCTION AND BACKGROUND

In the service setting (aka practice setting, clinical setting), a common source of requests for educational programing is the manager who identifies a performance problem or requests an in-service education session not directly connected to a learning goal. An educational offering can be developed to meet the manager's expressed need, but may not provide a lasting solution to the problem. This approach can be compared to providing requested treatment for a patient before conducting a physical assessment and history (Muller & Roberts, 2010).

In the academic setting, establishing a new course or degree program without carefully considering learner needs in the light of available programs, technology, and resources has the potential to waste time and money from both the learner's and the school's perspectives.

Regardless of the setting, the purpose of conducting a learning assessment in any setting is to establish evidence for planning a high-value educational intervention. A systematic process of data collection from multiple sources has been shown to guide effective instructional design (Iqbal & Khan, 2011; Stetar, 2005).

SIGNIFICANCE

Learning needs in academic settings are most often defined around a preset curriculum, or course of study. A curriculum has been defined as a plan made for guiding learning (Glatthorn et al., 2006). Learning needs in academic settings are generally identified in advance on the basis of desired program completion outcomes for the expected learners, and then plans are adjusted on the basis of the characteristics of learners who actually enroll. The process of academic advising helps learners identify educational programs for which they are prepared or could become prepared. This is a different starting point than designing learning activities to improve the performance of healthcare providers who are already employed. Although it is uncommon to designate educational programs in clinical settings as curricula, a new graduate orientation program, residency, or ongoing staff development program is a workplace curriculum created to address the learning needs of the employees or the healthcare providers involved.

Curricular design begins with identification of the educational program's purpose and relationship to the mission and vision of the organization (Iwasiw et al., 2009). Early on, stakeholders within and outside the organization should be involved in identifying program goals. For instance, if the purpose of the program is to provide a route for an agency's staff members to earn a credential that is needed for a new healthcare service, stakeholders would include the organization's administrators over the area and related areas, providers who will use that service or refer patients, regulatory agencies that manage that professional group, target patient populations, and possibly others. Reaching clarity early in the planning process on the purposes for the educational program from the perspective of different stakeholders and, if there are divergent opinions, whose purposes take precedence will help prevent disappointments and project failures. After the overall purposes and goals are clear, agreeing on specific program completion outcomes promotes accountability for educators and learners, for example what should the providers or students who complete the program be able to do when the program is complete? In addition to formally assessing learning needs during curriculum design or revision, gaps in achievement between the program outcomes and the present curriculum can appear at any time. Gaps may be related to changes in external factors such as new regulations or standards in the workplace or on internal factors such as educators whose teaching is not consistent with the intended curriculum (Keating, 2010). When outcome measures such as licensing or certification exam pass rates fall or employers of graduates identify gaps in the graduates' readiness to assume professional roles, then educators are already overdue to make a careful formal assessment of where the curriculum is not supporting the expected outcomes.

PERFORMANCE ANALYSIS: THE BIGGER PICTURE

Simulation-based education is resource-intensive and costly (Lapkin & Levett-Jones, 2011). Administrators expect that resources expended for teaching-learning make an impact on employee and team performance that in turn increases clinical and organizational effectiveness (Tobey, 2005). Conducting an up-front analysis of needs is becoming more pervasive as employee learning is viewed as part of the overall strategic plan (Iqbal & Khan, 2011).

The likelihood that an educational effort will achieve the expectation of cost-effective impact can be maximized by conducting a performance analysis. A performance analysis paints a broad picture of the desired organizational outcomes and compares the outcomes to current performance data (Rossett, 2009). The purpose of a performance analysis is to identify discrepancies (gaps) between actual and ideal performance as well as assess organizational readiness to capitalize on new opportunities (Brown, 2002). In addition, the performance analysis will analyze the basis of the performance gap and guide the selection of interventions (Stetar, 2005). Performance analysis frequently uncovers both learning and nonlearning needs. This distinction is important to the success of the interventions, which often encompass both educational activities and organizational changes to support performance (Iqbal & Khan, 2011; Rossett, 2009).

The process of performance analysis can be divided into diagnostic and recommendation phases. During the diagnostic phase, the educator works to describe gaps in performance as well as uncovering factors that are contributing to the gap. During the recommendation phase, the educator makes targeted recommendations directly linked to the identified gaps.

The initial activity in the diagnostic phase involves defining ideal performance and gathering data about current performance: comparison of these two states allows the identification of discrepancies (gaps) in performance (Iqbal & Khan, 2011). The second activity involves finding the factors that are leading to the gap. Rarely is there a single cause for less than ideal performance. Performance is influenced by a multitude of drivers and barriers including internal motivation and environmental factors (Rossett, 2009). Pertinent questions for the educator to ask to help identify these drivers and barriers include what types of performance are rewarded and what obstacles are in the way of desired performance.

Mager and Pipe (1984) created a flow diagram to guide a more comprehensive analysis of performance problems and uncover both learning and nonlearning (performance management) needs. In this analysis, a learning need is uncovered when there is a skill or knowledge deficit identified. The defining question being, "Could employees do it if their lives depended on it?" If the answer is yes, then additional information alone is not the solution to the identified gap. In this case, a learning-based intervention without other management structure will have little influence on improving performance.

A learning need is said to exist when gaps are identified in knowledge or skill that are required for acceptable performance. At this point, an in-depth learning **needs assessment** is undertaken to guide the design, delivery, and evaluation of a proposed educational intervention. Rossett (2009) summarized the distinction between performance analysis and training needs assessment in this way: "Performance analysis guarantees doing the right things, training needs assessment is about doing those right things right" (chap. 1, para. 7).

PERFORMING A LEARNING NEEDS ASSESSMENT

A learning needs assessment is a systematic process of collecting data from a variety of sources to guide training design (Iqbal & Khan, 2011). The focus of the learning needs assessment is twofold. The first is on the gaps in knowledge, skill, or application of knowledge and skills; the second is on what the learners need in the learning environment (Tobey, 2005). The primary outcome of the learning needs assessment is a planned educational intervention that provides high value for the organization (Iqbal & Khan, 2011; Stetar, 2005). The data gathered regarding current and desired skill level also forms the basis for evaluating the effectiveness of the intervention (Tobey, 2005).

Ideally, a learning needs assessment begins proactively with the educator scanning both the organization and external horizon for opportunities, followed by making the business case for addressing the training needs that are identified (Tobey, 2005). Often, the learning needs assessment begins in response to a request for training. In that case, scanning and making the business case take place in a reactive manner. Once the gaps in knowledge or skills important to the organization are identified, the learning need is investigated in further detail through data collection and analysis. Finally, recommendations can be made. The five steps in the Learning Needs Assessment are outlined below.

Step 1. Environmental/Organizational Scanning

Environmental scanning involves looking at the world outside the organization for forces that impact the needed capabilities of healthcare workers. These concerns may be as broad as the impact of globalization, disaster preparedness economics, and workforce demographics (Andre & Barnes, 2010), or more directly related to the provision of healthcare such as pending legislation, current regulations, and broad concerns of the healthcare community such as access, quality, and patient safety (Forbes & Hickey, 2009). Additional forces considered in the academic setting include changes in affordability and access for current and future learners (Andre & Barnes, 2010).

Published professional standards for each discipline provide a beginning set of competencies to include in plans for those learners. Recommendations from professional bodies such as the Institute of Medicine and the Carnegie Institute often carry such weight as to reach the level of a national policy.

Organizational scanning requires investigation of institutional/organizational vision, mission, values, and philosophy (Iwasiw et al., 2009; Tobey, 2005). Knowledge of the organization's strategic plans will assist the educator in identifying not only current needs, but also projecting future performance needs for healthcare providers (Brown & Green, 2011).

Step 2. Identifying the Business Need

For educators working in academia, aligning with the business need focuses on the social expectations of education in preparing members of the healthcare workforce (Iwasiw et al., 2009). Aligning education with identified social needs as well as the institution's mission and philosophy is important in making the case for new curricula.

Educators who work in the service setting must often make a strong case for how planned education will actually assist the organization in meeting its mission and organizational goals. The goal of this portion of the needs assessment is to quantify the effects of the performance gaps on the organization's ability to meet its goals (Stetar, 2005).

Step 3. Identifying Potential Curriculum

The ideal approach to performing a learning needs assessment begins with the activity steps above. In reality, in service settings, the process often begins with incoming requests for education based on a manager's perception that employees are not doing what they are supposed to be doing (Mager & Pipe, 1984; Tobey, 2005). This is a crucial moment of decision for the educator who can simply respond to the request or dig deeper to ensure that the perceived gap reflects a true educational need.

Performance problems are not the only source of a perceived need that is used as justification for a new curriculum. A new organizational initiative may require enhanced staff knowledge and skills, sparking a deeper investigation into projected learning needs. Regardless of its genesis, once the decision has been made to embark on a learning needs assessment, the educator needs to create a data collection and analysis plan.

Step 4. Data Collection

The desired outcome of data collection is to gain a clearer picture of the nature of the problem or opportunity (Brown, 2002). The focus is on identifying gaps between the learner's current performance and expected performance; this holds true for students and experienced clinicians. Educators should start with a strong data collection plan that first considers what types of information are necessary in a broad picture, and then constraining the plan on the basis of context to avoid prematurely closing off choices (Tobey, 2005). The educator must plan to collect data that clarifies performance expectations, identifies the current (or theorized) general learning needs, and determines the needs of the potential learners. Each of these is explored in more detail below.

Performance expectations.

They are commonly defined as what the person should be doing (Iqbal & Khan, 2011). Defining these expectations often involves a job or task analysis. A job or task analysis is a method that details the requirements for a job including the tasks to be performed, the conditions for performance, how often the tasks are to be done and when, as well as the quantity and quality of work required. In addition, the analysis determines the skills and knowledge required to perform each task along with where and how the knowledge and skills can be best acquired (Brown, 2002).

Learning needs.

They are specifically the knowledge, skills, and attitudes required to meet performance expectations that the learners (whether employees or students) do not currently possess. These needs are the gap between actual and desired performance. As in Performance Analysis, it may be difficult to separate learning needs from nonlearning needs. Remember Mager and Pipe's (1984) suggestion regarding investigating whether or not employees could do the task if they were required. If the answer is no, due to lack of knowledge or skills, there is a learning need. If the answer is yes, then further investigation of nonlearning needs is warranted. In academic settings, faculty often must make assumptions regarding the gaps that will exist for learners and then adjust the curriculum to meet specific needs as they become evident (Glatthorn et al., 2006).

Learner needs.

Analyzing and addressing the needs of learners can increase motivation to learn (Iqbal & Khan, 2011). In the service setting, it is important to know the learner's position within the organization, attitude toward the targeted job performance, and whether the education is voluntary or mandatory. In addition, it is advisable to consider the learner's current level of knowledge and skills, previous experiences with education, and learning preferences (Tobey, 2005). Ideally, this is known during the planning process, but an early reassessment and adjustment of the curriculum may be necessary.

Data Sources

Tobey (2005) defines four stages of data collection: validating the business need, defining the performance expectations, uncovering detailed learning needs, and assessing learner needs. Each of these stages requires different sources for data collection.

In order to get the best data, it is important to target a cross section of employees or learners (Brown, 2002). The best source for clarifying the business need is with organizational leaders, including program deans or administrators. Performance expectation data, related to what the learner needs to do on the job, is best acquired from managers, subject matter experts, and those who have already demonstrated the desired performance. This often takes the form of a job or task analysis, a procedure that provides information about the content, or tasks that will form the basis of instruction and evaluation (Brown & Green, 2011). Information on learning needs comes from subject matter experts or high performers and the learners themselves. Subject matter experts are a source for identifying the knowledge and skills required to perform well in a specific position. The data collected on knowledge may encompass both the content and the structure of that content. Skills are often interpreted by a process analysis, which may take the form of steps on a flowchart.

In the academic setting, data may also be acquired through a practice analysis or through a review of credentialing or licensing requirements (Iwasiw et al., 2009). Current job performers are the best source for understanding existing levels of knowledge, skills, and ultimately performance; this same group can provide data on environmental factors that either support or present barriers to desired performance. Existing data such as previous performance evaluations may also contribute to the analysis.

A myriad of factors influence readiness to learn. Current providers or students are the primary sources for identifying the learners' needs in terms of the learning context (Tobey, 2005). During data collection, it is important to capture at least some general traits such as age, culture, prior knowledge and attitudes toward the topic, and the method of training. Consider the range of learners—those who may be challenged, the average learner, and the high achiever. This data may be summarized in a chart or by creating a fictitious learner profile of the average learner (Brown & Green, 2011).

Methods and Tools

Educators have a wide variety of methods and tools to obtain the needed information about learners, each with their own strengths and weaknesses. When possible, it is best to acquire both **quantitative** and **qualitative data** to paint a more complete picture (Brown, 2002). The most common methods/tools used by educators are surveys, interviews, observation, assessments, and document reviews (Brown, 2002; Tobey, 2005).

Surveys are beneficial in gathering data from a larger number of people in a short time period. The utility of surveys is limited by the potential for selection bias because data is obtained only from those motivated to respond. Data obtained may not be valid if respondents select answers without reading the questions, and even when respondents are conscientious, poorly worded questions can be confusing. It is beneficial to have members of the target audience review questions for clarity prior to survey distribution.

Interviews can be used to get more in-depth, qualitative data around a particular topic. The interview may be highly structured or may be semistructured to allow exploration of items that arise from the discussion. The interview may center on a topic, such as what knowledge and skills are needed to effectively perform during patient resuscitation. Alternatively, the interview may take the form of a critical incident review, where the interviewee is asked to describe a time when they performed well or were not satisfied with their performance (Tobey, 2005). Preparation prior to conducting the interview is crucial to making this time-intensive method as efficient as possible.

Focus groups can be useful for exploring staff members' views and opinions of performance issues and learning needs. Holding focus groups on important initiatives is a way of encouraging employee involvement and drawing on their knowledge of work processes for early planning. A focus group of up to 10 persons can be scheduled to discuss needs in the overall organization or around a specific topic. Larger groups make it difficult for everyone to speak. Generally, an experienced neutral person from another part of the organization facilitates the discussion by raising questions, clarifying, summarizing, and making notes. The session might be recorded (with the permission of the participants) to capture all the key ideas. Focus group members should not be quoted by name in written notes or reports (Cook, 2005).

Observation and assessments are similar in that both entail watching a person or team performing a task. Observation typically involves an expert performer accomplishing the task in question and is often followed by an interview to further clarify what was observed. Assessments involve observing current performers to more objectively identify gaps. Often, the assessment tool is created from the results of observing expert performance, and the tasks may be performed in a specific place (such as a simulation program). Assessments often create anxiety in the learner. This can then affect performance. Therefore, creating a psychologically safe environment is important to gathering accurate assessment data. The inherent weakness in this method is the validity and reliability of the assessment, based on the difficulties of creating a tool that measures critical elements by multiple raters.

Document review consists of collecting data from relevant existing files. This may be aggregate data from standardized testing or licensing boards, employee performance reviews, patient health records, or policy and procedure manuals as examples.

Data Analysis

Data analysis is the objective review of information that has been collected. This may be done when all the data is collected, or analysis of data from one source may be used to inform data collection from others. In this phase of the learning needs analysis, the emphasis is on description rather than interpretation (Tobey, 2005). Quantitative data is often summarized by descriptive statistics, whereas qualitative data is examined for recurring themes as well as differences among participants. It is often beneficial to periodically share the data with the requestor to validate accuracy, and at times it may be wise to share data and interpretations with members of the target audience (Brown & Green, 2011).

Step 5. Make Recommendations

Depending on your role, you will be sharing your recommendations regarding training needs and possibly about nonlearning needs uncovered in the analysis. These recommendations are based on interpretations of the data within context (Tobey, 2005). Training recommendations include areas of emphasis, objectives, learning activities, learning environment, and target audience.

CONSIDER THIS

HOW TO INTEGRATE SIMULATION INTO PRELICENSURE CURRICULUM

Soledad Armijo, R MD, EdD
Director Centro de Simulación Clínica y Escuela de Medicina, Universidad Diego Portales, Santiago, Chile

A systematic approach for integrating simulation into prelicensure programs may be guided by Harden's concepts of curricular planning (Harden, 1986) and Kotter's eight-step change model. The Centro de Simulación Clínica y Escuela de Medicina utilized Harden's six curricular components to develop a proposal for integrating simulation into prelicensure programs.

The first curriculum component involves learning outcomes. Simulation considerations based on this component include the following:
a. Outcomes selected should be better elicited using simulation compared to traditional strategies.
b. Educators should define verifiable outcomes, considering initial, intermediate, and final levels of achievement, related to a general core competencies model for each professional field (Boyd et al., 1996; Frank & Danoff, 2007; Schwarz & Wojtczak, 2002; Spielman et al., 2005).
c. Outcomes should be based on individual knowledge, skills, and attitudes.

d. Outcomes should incorporate interprofessional competencies (Barr et al., 2005), and Barr competencies (common, complementary, and collaborative; Interprofessional Education Collaborative Expert Panel, 2011).

The second curriculum component involves teaching and learning methods. Simulation considerations based on this component include the following:
a. Methods should be more learner-centered than educator-centered.
b. The approach should be problem-based.
c. Curriculum should be systematic and planned, and not opportunistic.
d. Simulated experiences should be sequentially inserted to reinforce tasks and skills necessary for promoting the learner to higher levels of training.

The third curriculum component involves educational strategies. Simulation considerations based on this component include the following:

a. The simulation modality, equipment, and materials should be matched to the desired objectives.
b. Feedback should be provided in debriefing.

The fourth curriculum component involves the context for the learning. Simulation considerations based on this component include the following:

a. The simulated environment should be as realistic as possible.
b. The environment should have a level of realism that will engage the learners.

The fifth curriculum component involves the learning environment. Simulation considerations based on this component include the following:

a. The environment should be positive and confidential where learners feel comfortable to make mistakes and learn about errors.
b. Feedback should be effectively provided to promote positive and desirable development (Archer, 2010).

The sixth curriculum component involves the assessment procedures. Simulation considerations based on this component include the following:

a. It is essential that assessments accurately measure the desired learning outcomes.
b. Formative and summative assessment could be used in simulation.
c. Formative assessment in procedural training programs could be designed in a mastery learning approach (Wayne et al., 2006).
d. Objective structured clinical examinations (OSCEs) are valuable instruments to certify terminal competencies in a summative approach.

Implementation of the curriculum was based on John Kotter's eight-step model for leading large-scale changes.

Kotter's Step 1: Establish a sense of urgency

The current curriculum was analyzed and a strengths, weaknesses, opportunities, and threats (SWOT) analysis was performed. The findings were communicated with leadership and, to establish a sense of urgency, the focus was on trends in healthcare education and the effects of simulation on patient safety. It was stressed that a simulation-based, student-centered approach would promote teamwork skills highly desirable in today's healthcare workforce.

Kotter's Step 2: Create a guiding coalition

To lead the change effort, a visioning leadership team was assembled. This team met with authorities, educators, and key stakeholders of the program. The visioning leadership team worked to ensure an efficient and sustainable simulation infrastructure. This team also played a key role in strategic hiring of simulation staff.

Kotter's Step 3: Develop a vision and a strategy

The visioning leadership team engaged in a strategic planning process (see chapter 5.3). In addition to developing a vision and mission for the simulation program, the team developed a strategy for implementation on the basis of six curricular components and McLaughlin's eight steps for scenario design (McLaughlin et al., 2008).

Kotter's Step 4: Communicate the vision for change

The vision for simulation was communicated at multiple institutional leadership meetings. In addition, e-mail was utilized to communicate the vision to a broad group of faculty.

Kotter's Step 5: Empower broad-based action

An administrative workforce was established to ensure an actionable plan for simulation. Motivated and energetic faculty were recruited to participate in simulation faculty development opportunities. Key faculty members were identified to communicate the simulation vision to stakeholders across different schools. The vision was also broadly repeated via institutional courses, conferences, mailing, and Web resources.

Kotter's Step 6: Generate short-term wins

Short-term wins were achieved in the areas of faculty development, simulation program design, and equipment acquisition. Deliberate effort was made to celebrate success for each of these short-term wins. Stakeholders and leaders were briefed on success in a variety of meetings, and a Web site was developed to recognize team members for their contribution. Students were recruited to become agents of change, proposing new ideas that ultimately resulted in the initiation of a junior educator program.

Kotter's Step 7: Never let up, consolidate gains, and produce more change

As initial simulation courses were delivered, the core simulation staff continued to recruit additional simulation faculty and identify new courses/programs for simulation integration. As simulation faculty were developed, they were encouraged to develop additional simulation courses and curricula, which led to exponential growth of simulation activity. Though simulation integration was first aimed at the prelicensure curriculum, soon simulation grew to be included in other postgraduate and continuing education programs.

Kotter's Step 8: Incorporate changes into culture

To ensure sustained change, general guidelines and processes were developed for program activity and course development. Processes that were institutionalized include confidentiality agreements, fiction contracts, Debriefing Assessment for Simulation in Healthcare (DASH) assessments, Anaesthetists' Non-Technical Skills (ANTS) surveys, and SIMS surveys. Surveys were evaluated for improvement opportunities. Scholarly activity was encouraged to share experience with the larger international simulation community.

By utilizing Harden's concepts for curriculum planning and Kotter's strategies for change, a high-quality simulation program can be effectively integrated into an existing curriculum. As with most change initiatives, the process may be challenging but it delivers rewards on the level of faculty, students, and ultimately, patients.

REFERENCES

Archer, J. C. (2010). State of the science in health professional education: Effective feedback. *Medical Education,* 44(1), 101–108.

Barr, H., Koppel, I., Reeves, S., Hammick, M., & Freeth, D. (2005). *Effective interprofessional education: Argument, assumption and evidence.* Oxford, UK: Blackwell.

Boyd, M. A., Gerrow, J. D., Chambers, D. W., & Henderson, B. J. (1996). Competencies for dental licensure in Canada. *Journal of Dental Education,* 60(10), 842–846.

Frank, J. R., & Danoff, D. (2007). The CanMEDS initiative: Implementing an outcomes-based framework of physician competencies. *Medical Teacher,* 29(7), 642–647. doi:10.1080/01421590701746983

Harden, R. M. (1986). Ten questions to ask when planning a course or curriculum. *Medical Education,* 20(4), 356–365.

(continued)

CONSIDER THIS

HOW TO INTEGRATE SIMULATION INTO PRELICENSURE CURRICULUM *(continued)*

Interprofessional Education Collaborative Expert Panel. (2011). *Core competencies for interprofessional collaborative practice: Report of an expert panel* (Interprofessional Education Collaborative). Retrieved from http://www.aacn.nche.edu/education-resources/IPECReport.pdf

Kotter, J. P. (1995, March–April). Leading change: Why transformation efforts fail. *Harvard Business Review,* 59–67.

Kotter, J. P. (1996). *Leading change.* Boston, MA: Harvard Business School Press.

McLaughlin, S., Fitch, M. T., Goyal, D. G., Hayden, E., Kauh, C. Y., Laack, T. A., ... Gordon, J. A. (2008). Simulation in graduate medical education 2008: A review for emergency medicine (SAEM Technology in Medical Education Committee and the Simulation Interest Group). *Academic Emergency Medicine,* 15(11), 1117–1129.

Schwarz, M. R., & Wojtczak, A. (2002). Global minimum essential requirements: A road towards competence-oriented medical education. *Medical Teacher,* 24(2), 125–129.

Spielman, A. I., Fulmer, T., Eisenberg, E. S., & Alfano, M. C. (2005). Dentistry, nursing, and medicine: A comparison of core competencies. *Journal of Dental Education,* 69(11), 1257–1271.

Wayne, D., Butter, J., Sidall, V., Fudala, M. J., Wade, L. D., Feinglass, J., & McGaghie, W. C. (2006). Mastery learning of advanced cardiac life support skills by internal medicine residents using simulation technology and deliberate practice. *Journal of General Internal Medicine,* 21(3), 251–256.

SUGGESTED READINGS

Armijo, S., Muñoz, P., & Las Heras, J. (2012). *Leadership strategies to develop an undergraduate clinical simulation center.* Paper presented at Centro de Simulación Clínica y Facultad de Medicina Universidad Diego Portales, AMEE Conference, Lyon, France.

Grant, J. (2010). Principles of curriculum design. In T. Swanwick (Ed.), *Understanding medical education: Evidence, theory and practice.* Chichester, UK: Wiley-Blackwell.

Hafferty, F. (1998). Beyond curriculum reform: Confronting medicine's hidden curriculum. *Academic Medicine,* 73, 403–407.

Kotter, J., & Rathgeber, H. (2006). *Our iceberg is melting.* New York, NY: St. Martin's.

Peyton, J. W. R. (1998). *Teaching and learning in medical practice.* Rickmansworth, UK: Manticore Europe.

Waxman, K. T., & Telles, C. L. (2009). The use of Benner's framework in high-fidelity simulation faculty development: The Bay Area Simulation Collaborative model. *Clinical Simulation in Nursing,* 5(6), e231–e235.

BEEN THERE, DONE THAT: HOW CAN I CONTINUE TO IMPROVE OR SUSTAIN WHAT I HAVE ACHIEVED?

Overcoming Barriers

The most commonly stated barriers to conducting thorough learning needs assessment are lack of time and money. Another significant barrier is a premature decision that education or training is the solution to the problem. Approaches to overcoming these barriers to conducting learning needs assessment are not exclusive to this endeavor. It is important to get buy-in of area managers, who may not be familiar with the purpose or the process, particularly if they have already decided that education is the answer. Providing information regarding the increased likelihood of developing effective training based on data can help you sell the importance of a needs assessment (Brown & Green, 2011). Once access is granted, moving forward in a systematic and timely fashion will increase stakeholder trust (Muller & Roberts, 2010). Sharing progress and data at strategic points along the way will help to validate the process and to ensure that recommendations do not come as a complete surprise.

If training has already been mandated, the educator can incorporate a brief learning and learner needs assessment during the prebriefing phase of a simulation learning session. This is a time to quickly assess current knowledge and learner attitudes toward the learning session. In contrast to a typical classroom setting, the educator in simulation learning observes performance to identify gaps, which is a very powerful learning needs assessment tool. The information gathered during the simulation and debriefing may be used to inform further instruction and may uncover information regarding barriers to performance experienced in the practice setting.

Dealing with Nonlearning Needs

Information and education will not solve every problem. To be an effective simulation educator or manager, it is essential to develop the skills necessary to determine whether a problem is related to a knowledge or skill deficit or a problem of will, or something else entirely. Motivation is a complex concept as applied to both learning and performance (Brophy, 2010). Perhaps there is a perceived form of punishment (such as having to stay after the shift) or a lack of reward (no one seems to notice anyway) for correctly doing the task, or there is a reward for not doing it/doing it incorrectly (such as having more time for something else or saving money on supplies). In such cases, learning about how to do the skill is not the answer, or not the whole answer. In other cases, the education needed is so extensive and expensive that it would be more feasible to redesign or reassign the task (Stetar, 2005).

Performance can also be affected by factors unrelated to knowledge or expertise. If needed supplies are not available, or staffing is limited, it may not be possible for employees to follow the established protocol. The educator can serve as an advocate in these situations by identifying when performance problems are unlikely to be solved by additional education or by education alone. Barriers to effective performance might require innovations such as providing sinks in proximity to the work area or keeping supplies stocked for ready use. Performance issues may require leaders to establish consequences and follow through consistently.

SUMMARY

Learning needs assessments are critical to creating effective instruction. This is especially true when the instruction will be delivered using simulation. Data regarding the performance gaps; knowledge, skills, and attitudes important to performance; and learner needs form the basis of this assessment. The simulation educator must become skilled in acquiring data from a variety of sources and through different methods. Doing so will strengthen the validity of the educator's assessment. The data must be analyzed objectively and then interpreted through the context of organizational or institutional needs to arrive at recommendations. The success of the simulation educator's analysis of learning needs can be evaluated along the way by sharing data with managers, subject matter experts, and members of the target audience as well as a summative evaluation based on the effectiveness of the educational intervention ultimately provided.

REFERENCES

Andre, K., & Barnes, L. (2010). Creating a 21st century nursing work force: Designing a bachelor of nursing program in response to the health reform agenda. *Nurse Education Today*, 30(3), 258–263.

Brophy, J. (2010). *Motivating students to learn* (3rd ed.). Abingdon, UK: Routledge.

Brown, A., & Green, T. D. (2011). *The essentials of instructional design: Connecting fundamental principles with process and practice* (2nd ed.). Boston, MA: Pearson Education.

Brown, J. (2002). Training needs assessment: A must for developing an effective training program. *Public Personnel Management*, 31(4), 569–578.

Cook, S. (2005, October). Focus groups: How to use them effectively in learning needs analysis. *Training Journal*, 24–26.

Forbes, M. O., & Hickey, M. T. (2009). Curriculum reform in baccalaureate nursing education: Review of the literature. *International Journal of Nursing Scholarship*, 6(1), 1–16. doi:10.2202/1548-923X.1797

Glatthorn, A. A., Boschee, F., & Whitehead, B. M. (2006). *Curriculum leadership: Development and implementation*. Thousand Oaks, CA: SAGE.

Iqbal, M. Z., & Khan, R. A. (2011). The growing concept and uses of training needs assessment: A review with proposed model. *Journal of European Industrial Training*, 35(5), 439–466. doi:10-1108/0309059111138017

Iwasiw, C., Goldenberg, D., & Andrusyszyn, M. (2009). *Curriculum development in nursing education* (2nd ed.). Sudbury, MA: Jones and Bartlett.

Keating, S. (2010). *Curriculum development and evaluation in nursing* (2nd ed.). Danvers, MA: Springer.

Lapkin, S., & Levett-Jones, T. (2011). A cost-utility analysis of medium vs. high-fidelity human patient simulation manikins in nursing education. *Journal of Clinical Nursing*, 20(23–24), 3543–3552. doi:10.1111/j.1365-2702.2011.03843.x

Mager, R., & Pipe, P. (1984). *Analyzing performance problems* (2nd ed.). Belmont, CA: Lake.

Muller, N., & Roberts, V. (2010). Seven cures to skipping the needs assessment. *T+D*, 64(3), 32–34.

Rossett, A. (2009). *First things fast: A handbook for performance analysis* (2nd ed.). San Francisco, CA: John Wiley & Sons.

Stetar, B. (2005, March). Training: It's not always the answer. *Quality Progress*, 38, 44–49.

Tobey, D. (2005). *Needs assessment basics*. Alexandria, VA: ASTD Press.

CHAPTER 7.2

Common Theories in Healthcare Simulation

J. Bradley Morrison, PhD, and Cathy Deckers, RN, MSN, EdD

ABOUT THE AUTHORS

J. BRADLEY MORRISON is Associate Professor of Management at the Brandeis International Business School and a faculty member at the Center for Medical Simulation in Boston, MA. His research focuses on the challenges of human performance in dynamically complex environments, such as operating rooms, labor and delivery suites, and emergency departments. He uses the tools of system dynamics to study phenomena such as dynamic problem solving, coping and resilience in the emergency department, and crisis resource management.

CATHY DECKERS has spent her professional career focusing on education and operations management in both the service and academic arenas. She has extensive experience in group dynamics, facilitation, and teamwork and has served in a number of executive roles related to organizational design and development, strategic planning, regulatory compliance, and quality management. Currently, she works for CAE Healthcare as a consultant responsible for Nurse Residency implementation and project management using high-fidelity simulation at hospital sites.

ABSTRACT

The ability of high-fidelity simulation to create contextually meaningful experiences that can promote psychomotor skill development, clinical decision making, and emotional engagement to improve healthcare professional practice makes it a valuable learning tool. Using simulation with intentionality to produce targeted outcomes from the learning experience is imperative given the time and resource intensity of this methodology. Educational theory helps achieve this goal by providing the rationale and frameworks of practice that are necessary to produce standardized outcomes. This chapter reviews some of the foundational and more commonplace educational theories related to simulation practice. It is not intended as a comprehensive literature review, nor is it an attempt to integrate existing theories to develop a grand theory of learning through simulation. Rather, the intent is to provide access to relevant bits of theory to encourage simulation educators to use in practice.

CASE EXAMPLE

Using a simulation-based learning experience takes considerable time and resource that is oftentimes seen by educators and administrators alike as outside the norm for a learning activity. As the Director of the Simulation Program at the University for Health Sciences, you are charged with creating the value proposition for the use of simulation as a learning tool that can deliver a targeted return on investment. You know that your ability to create a rational proposal is paramount to the continued use of simulation in educational practice for both the academic and service settings you serve. As you strive to improve the ability to deliver the expected outcomes of the simulation experience, you wonder how you can use theory to streamline and support the educator's practice.

INTRODUCTION AND BACKGROUND

Basic theory and empirical research from a variety of disciplines have the potential to usefully inform the design, execution, and debriefing of healthcare simulation experiences for the training and development of adult learners. Relevant research can be found in disciplines as wide ranging as neuroscience, physiology, psychology and social psychology, developmental theory, learning theory, organizational behavior, judgment and decision making, theater arts, linguistics, and many others. There has been much work exemplifying and suggesting that theories (specifically those that have studied the subtleties of adult learning through experience) have a direct bearing on many of the educational design choices that simulation educators are tasked to make (Jeffries, 2005). Indeed, it was Kurt Lewin, often considered one of the fathers of experiential learning, who said, "there is nothing so practical as a good theory" (Schein, 1996, p. 28).

The purpose of this chapter is to provide a high-level introduction to some common theories that simulation educators can draw upon to help with a more thoughtful approach to the various decisions and tasks required to successfully design, implement, and deliver a simulation program for healthcare professionals. The theories presented here were chosen because of their useful connections to healthcare simulation, and the chapter describes their main features in a summary fashion. This chapter is not intended as a comprehensive literature review, nor is it an attempt to integrate existing theories or develop any grand theory of learning through simulation. Rather, it is to make relevant bits of theory easily accessible to simulation educators through the summaries in this chapter.

Streams of theories that provide foundational concepts for creating a learning environment using simulation serve as an organizing framework for this chapter. The chapter begins with a summary of pertinent work in learning theory by Dewey, Lewin, and Piaget, providing a clear understanding of how learning occurs through the dynamic interaction and collaboration between learners and experts. These learning theories are predicated on the belief that the relationships between context, meaning, identity, and practice result in expertise development that is transferable into professional practice. The following section describes how Malcolm Knowles built on those foundations to develop a model of andragogy—a model that focuses on how adults learn (as opposed to children) and has served to propel the field of simulation. The basic tenets of his theory are related to the importance of the individual's historical experience and motivation and how these two factors texture the learning environment. The model of andragogy also speaks to the role of the "teacher" as more of a facilitator, an important aspect of simulation-based learning. Next is a description of David Kolb's experiential learning model (ELM) that highlights the importance of learning as cyclical and evolving through practice. Sections on reflective practice and situated learning as theoretical practice are described throughout the majority of theories presented within this chapter, yet have also been included within the foundational theory stream. Additional theoretical frameworks related to decision making and situation awareness (SA) have been included to provide understanding of some of the simulation work being done within the patient safety and human factors realms.

FOUNDATIONAL THEORY IN EXPERIENTIAL LEARNING: DEWEY, LEWIN, AND PIAGET

John Dewey, perhaps the most influential educational theorist of the 20th century, called attention in 1938 to a growing conflict between the then traditional education and a more progressive approach that he called "the new education," saying "there is an intimate and necessary relation between the processes of actual experience and education" (Dewey, 1938, pp. 19–20). Experiential methods of education include mentorships, internships, work/study programs, cooperative education, studio arts, laboratory studies, and field projects, as well as computer simulation games and healthcare simulation. The distinctive characteristic is that "the learner is directly in touch with the realities being studied . . . rather than merely thinking about . . . or only considering the possibility of doing something with it" (Keeton & Tate, 1978, p. 2). Perhaps the most basic point in Dewey's philosophy is simply that regardless of what we do or do not do as educators to manage it, people do indeed learn through their experiences. This notion then leads to a way of thinking that there could be great value to being intentional about what those experiences are and what learners learn. It also spawned great interest in how learners, especially adult learners, learn.

Kurt Lewin, often called the founder of American social psychology, developed social science field theory and a methodology of action research that over the next few decades became the cornerstone for most organizational development efforts (Lewin, 1947, 1951). His work with groups to develop training in leadership and group dynamics led to the fortuitous discovery of the "T-group" (training group) as the staff of the training session somewhat reluctantly allowed the participants to participate in their evening summary and analysis of the day. The "T-group" provided an active dialogue between the researcher-observer, trainer, and the trainee about how to interpret the actions and results of the day, a dialogue that yielded great value as the trainees ultimately were learning about themselves from themselves. Ronald Lippitt, one of Lewin's colleagues in those sessions describes the discovery of the T-groups: "The evening session from then on became the significant learning experience of the day, with the focus on actual behavioral events and with active dialogue about differences of interpretation and observation of the events by those who had participated in them" (Lippitt, 1949, as cited in Kolb, 1984). Lewin and his colleagues had made the discovery "that learning is best facilitated in an environment where there was a dialectic tension and conflict between immediate, concrete experience and analytic detachment," a point of view that clearly underscores the importance of experience followed by debriefing to enhance learning through experience (Kolb, 1984, p. 9). Further work led to recognizing the importance of a spirit of inquiry, expanded consciousness and choice, and authenticity in relationships (Schein & Bennis, 1965). Following this seminal work, educators in this stream of theorists developed structured exercises, simulations, role-plays, and other methods in which a simulated situation was designed to create personal experiences for learners that would initiate their own process of inquiry and understanding.

Sean Piaget studied cognitive development processes with an interest in intelligence and how it develops. Piaget noticed that children at different ages had qualitatively different ways of arriving at wrong answers to questions. These age-related regularities led him to the powerful conclusion that intelligence is shaped by experience. Action is key. Cognitive development stages move from an enactive stage to an iconic stage to stages of concrete and formal operations. This work provided a scientific foundation for a theory of instruction founded on tailoring curricula to the needs of learners on the basis of their age or stage of cognitive development. Piaget's work focused on learners' representations of knowledge, and the curricula developed in this stream became experience-based. In particular, children were learning not only the content but also about the process of discovering knowledge. Piaget's stages of cognitive development ended in adolescence, but other researchers have suggested that the developmental process extends into adulthood (Kohlberg, 1969; Kolb, 1984; Kurtines & Greif, 1974).

The foundational work of Dewey, Lewin, and Piaget was extremely influential in the development of theories of learning, knowledge, and education over the next several decades. Their influence is especially evident in theories of andragogy (adult learning) that Malcolm Knowles developed and experiential learning that David Kolb developed.

FROM PEDAGOGY TO ANDRAGOGY

Participants in healthcare simulations are almost exclusively adults, so it is important to consider the distinct characteristics of adults as learners. Most formal educational institutions in modern Western society were designed and developed on the basis of a model for educating children and youth, a model often called "pedagogy," which means literally the art and science of teaching children (Knowles, 1996). However, adults learn differently than younger students. A considerable body of research and theory about the adult as learner has developed, starting with Lindeman's proposition that adults should be actively involved in choices about what, how, and when they learn rather than passively following the direction of the teacher whose primary methodology is transmission techniques (Lindeman, 1926). Lindeman wrote that the purpose of adult education "is to discover the meaning of experience; a quest of the mind which digs down to the roots of the preconceptions which formulate our conduct" (Lindeman, 1925, p. 3 as cited in Brookfield, 1984). He introduced into the English language the term "andragogy," which means the art and science of teaching adults (Taylor & Kroth, 2009). Scholars continued for several decades to study effective methods for educating adults, but it was Malcolm Knowles who presented a unified theory of andragogy, popularized the term, and described its implications for education in practice (Knowles, 1970).

In his early work, Knowles summarized four key assumptions about adult learners, to which he added two more over the next several decades. Those assumptions have been embraced by many in simulation and relate to the adult's: (1) need to know, (2) self-concept, (3) experience, (4) readiness to learn, (5) orientation to learning, and (6) motivation (Knowles, 1990).

Adults need to know why they should learn something. Adults invest time and energy understanding the cost and benefits of learning something and the risks of not learning it. Adults want to know "what's in it for them" and how they can apply new knowledge or skills to some problem or opportunity that is relevant to them. Knowles suggested that ideally the educator will make a case for the need to know through real or simulated experiences in which the learner experiences the benefits of knowing or the costs of not knowing (Knowles, 1996). In contrast to pedagogy, it is important to include adults in the choices about what they learn.

Adults have a deep need to be self-directing. As people mature, they move from a self-concept of dependence on others to one of independence or self-directedness. Adults take responsibility for their own decisions, including those about what, when, and how they learn and develop. They live with the consequences of their decisions. Having reached maturity, adults may even resist situations in which others are imposing their will (Taylor & Kroth, 2009). Because most adults have been educated in a system that was based largely on dependency on a teacher, often when these adults are put again into a structured learning environment, they revert to their conditioning as students with dependency on the teacher. But, this creates a conflict with their self-concept that often manifests as withdrawal from the learning process (Knowles, 1996). Educators can help learners transition to seeing themselves as self-directed learners by creating and maintaining a collaborative learning environment that fosters mutual respect.

Adults have a greater volume and different quality of experience than youth. Adults have accumulated a vast stock of experience that can serve as a resource for learning. This experience is greater in both magnitude and variety than that of the younger learner. Groups of adults will have even more heterogeneous experiences. An adult's experience must be respected and valued, otherwise adult learners will experience this as rejection. Given this experience, adults have much to contribute to discussions, and there is much to be gained from methods that tap into the accumulated experience "such as simulation exercises and field experiences, that provide learners with experiences from which they can learn by analyzing them" (Knowles, 1996, p. 256). Experience can also be an impediment because of habits of thought and less openness to new ideas.

Adults become ready to learn when they experience in their life situation a need to know or be able to do in order to perform more effectively and satisfyingly. This is a stark contrast with the pedagogical model that assumes learners are ready to know when they are told so by their instructor. For adults, readiness depends on what they need to know for the life situations they are currently facing. Adults are ready to learn those things that will help them cope more effectively (Knowles, 1980).

Adults enter into a learning experience with a task-centered orientation to learning. Whereas in the pedagogical model learning is subject-centered, the andragogical model emphasizes a task-centered (or problem-centered or life-centered) orientation. When adults perceive that something will help them perform tasks or solve problems they are confronting, they are motivated to learn (Knowles, 1990).

Adults are motivated to learn by both extrinsic and intrinsic motivators. The most potent motivators for adults appear to be internal pressures, such as the desire to maintain or enhance self-esteem, achieve a better quality of life, enjoy increased job satisfaction, broaden job responsibilities, and experience greater self-actualization. The pedagogical model assumes that youth are primarily motivated by extrinsic factors such as pressure from adults, grades, certificates, and so on. Adults seek learning because of external motivators (e.g., wages, promotions, working conditions, perquisites) as well, but internal motivators seem to be more potent (Knowles, 1990).

EXPERIENTIAL LEARNING

Drawing on the foundational work of Dewey, Lewin, and Piaget, David Kolb, together with Ronald Fry, developed a model of **experiential learning** that has gained widespread popularity among educators and theorists (Kolb & Fry, 1975). Kolb offered a perspective on learning that combines experience, perception, cognition, and behavior. Kolb's perspective conceptualized learning as a continuous process grounded in experience. He emphasized that the process of learning creates knowledge through the *transformation* of experience. The theory was an explanation of "how people learn from experience and process that experience in different ways to generate understanding" (Cox, 2006, p. 200).

The core of ELM is the notion that learning is cyclical and encompasses four stages: (1) concrete experience,

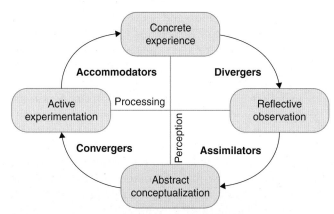

FIGURE 7.2.1   Kolb's experiential learning model.

(2) reflective observation, (3) abstract conceptualization, and (4) active experimentation (Figure 7.2.1). Although the learning process can begin with any of the four stages, many descriptions begin with concrete experience. Concrete experience might come from a variety of contexts, such as field work, laboratory work, classroom exercises, "real-world" experience, role-plays, simulations, and others. The key is that a person carries out a particular action or behavior and sees the results of the action or behavior. This stage (concrete experience) is both concrete and active. The learner then has an opportunity to reflect on and understand the action and effect. If the same action were taken again under similar circumstances, it should be possible for the learner to anticipate the effect. This stage (reflective observation) is concrete (focused on a specific action or behavior) and reflective. In the third stage, the learner aims to understand the general or abstract principles that govern the action and effect. This stage (abstract conceptualization) is abstract and reflective. The fourth stage is to plan and execute a (possibly new) course of action. This stage (active experimentation) is active and abstract.

On the basis of this model, Kolb also recognized that individuals differ in their preferences and strengths in the learning processes involved in each stage and used this insight to develop a typology of learning styles (Kolb, 1984). He identified two dialectically distinct modes of grasping experience and two dialectically distinct modes of transforming experience that map closely to the two dimensions underlying the four-stage model of experiential learning. He proposed four distinct styles of learning roughly corresponding to the "corners" in the four-stage cycle. For the "diverging" style, concrete experience and reflective observation are dominant. Divergers are good at viewing concrete situations from many points of view. They are likely to prefer working in groups and receiving personalized feedback. For the "assimilating" style, abstract conceptualization and reflective observation are dominant. Assimilators are strong at viewing a wide range of information and putting it into a concise and logical form. They are likely to prefer reading and lecture, exploring analytical models, and having time to think. For the "converging" style, abstract conceptualization and active experimentation are the dominant learning-style abilities. Convergers are best at finding practical uses for ideas and theories. They are likely to prefer experiments, simulations, laboratory work, and practical applications. For the "accommodating" style, concrete experience and active experimentation are dominant. They are quite good at learning from hands-on experience. They are likely to prefer working with others, setting goals, doing field work, and testing out different approaches to get a project done. The key point is that there are indeed differences in how people learn, and educators need to take these styles into account in their design and delivery of learning curricula (Kolb & Kolb, 2005).

For simulation educators, Kolb's experiential learning theory has important implications. Most fundamentally, it provides justification and legitimacy for the use of simulation in learning curricula. More generally, it underscores the importance of including a diverse range of methods in a curriculum. It makes explicit the need for reflection, which simulation educators usually stimulate through the use of skillful debriefings. But the theory implies that we need to go further and ensure that each of the four stages is addressed (Clark et al., 2010). Simulation cases can provide a concrete experience. Debriefings can trigger reflective observation. Debriefings should also include moving from the concrete and specific to more abstract or generalizable principles in an abstract conceptualization stage. Inquiry about how simulation experiences are relevant for other settings (e.g., a learner's department, institution, or practice) would foster such conceptualization. Active experimentation should be encouraged, for example by asking about what a learner would do differently or even by repetition of an identical or similar simulation scenario. Creating opportunities for anticipatory thinking allows for expertise building that is not necessarily defined within the simulation scenario, but is created through the distributed learning within the group setting. This can be accomplished during the briefing prior to simulation through the development of a plan of care or concept map that creates a shared mental model for the group. During the simulation activity, reflective inquiry can be promoted through the use of crew resource management principles that encourage participants to work together as a team by creating opportunities for cross-checking their teamwork toward the shared goal that was developed at briefing. Finally, note that simulation educators too learn through experience. Every simulation and debriefing is a concrete experience that offers an opportunity for reflection, abstraction, and planning for experimentation for the educator as well.

REFLECTIVE PRACTICE: SIMULATION

The practice of caring for humans is not an exact science. Healthcare practitioners continuously use their experiences to improve their skills. Reflective practice is one of the tools commonly used to do this. It is widely agreed that the reflective process results in a change in behavior because of learning (Dewey, 1933; Nielsen et al., 2007; Schon, 1991). Research supports the idea that an understanding of professional knowledge (particularly in the healthcare field) is primarily developed through practice and the systematic analysis of experience known as reflection (Gould, 1996). Reflective practice highlights the artistry of professional practice by placing an emphasis on integrating theory and practice through a process of tailoring the theoretical knowledge to fit the specific circumstances found in clinical practice rather than holding to a rigid and technical application of theory to practice (Dewey, 1933; Schon, 1991).

Defining reflective practice has been a challenge throughout the years and among the various healthcare professions. Ruth-Sahd (2003), after a comprehensive review of the nursing literature, defines reflection as "a means of self examination that reviews past practice with the intent of improving practice and understanding of self" (p. 488). She adds that it is a "creative, non-linear, imaginative process" (p. 488). Thompson and Pascal, from Australia, add that reflective learning is related to learning from experience and has four characteristics: (1) a two-way interactive blending of theory and practice to seek integration (e.g., debriefing process that seeks to highlight the rationale behind actions that are taken during the simulation through a conversation between participants and including the expert facilitator when necessary); (2) active learning that seeks to validate knowledge, skills, and attitudes through participation in the learning to develop confidence (e.g., simulation practice using psychomotor skills to insert a chest tube, or obtain a patient history, or console a grieving patient); (3) participative learning where meaning is created and determined jointly between learner and teacher as a result of the experience (e.g., use of facilitation skills to explore the learner's thought processes related to the experience not necessarily the stated outcome of the simulation); and lastly (4) evaluative inquiry of personal bias and the status quo (e.g., using a postsimulation journal to understand how one's personal bias or way of doing business influenced how decisions were made during a simulation or how cues were observed or missed; Thompson & Pascal, 2012).

Schon (1991), expanding upon Dewey's previous work (experiential methods in education), describes a two-part model of reflection that outlines different activities for each type of reflection. Reflection-in-action is described as the intuitive process that takes place during care activities that reflects tacit knowledge and the professional artistry of competence—when thought and action are integrally linked (Schon, 1987). *Reflection-on-action* is the retrospective conscious process that occurs to understand past action related to their personal construct of reality (e.g., bias, experience, and knowledge) with the intent of improving future practice. Each type of reflection has been identified as an important way to improve clinical practice and learning. Perhaps a significant aspect of reflection that is missing from Schon's initial work is something Thompson and Pascal (2012) identify as *reflection-for-action*. Reflection-for-action identifies future strategies for clinical practice derived by understanding the conflict between values and practice, intent and action, and patient need versus caregiver need (Kim, 1999). This refers to the process of planning and thinking about what is to come that has in some circles been identified as anticipatory planning (Benner et al., 1999; Endsley et al., 2003). This type of planning draws upon the professional knowledge of the participant and allows for the individualization of the intervention to meet the specific needs of the problem taking into account the resources available within the environment.

A critical element of reflective practice involves the practitioner's ability to use the discovery to inform future practice so as to avoid routine or habitualized actions where little thought or analysis takes place before action (Argyris & Schon, 1974). **Critical reflective practice** is more than just a review of learning that has taken place or the emotions that one has felt. Critical reflective practice strives to understand and create new meaning through the analysis of actions and values and their influence within the practice setting. This type of reflection can then create a synthesis for future practice for the professional.

Reflective practice techniques work well with simulation learning. Reflection-on-practice is a key factor in the development and improvement of clinical reasoning and decision making (Tanner, 2006). The focus of reflection can be used to highlight the specific cues, patterns, inferences, and information that were required to make decisions during the simulation practice. Understanding how to break complex tasks into basic elements allows the practitioner to develop specific strategies for the situations that are encountered. Reflective practice within simulation learning should be cultivated as a deliberate practice to enhance the meaningfulness of the simulated learning event. This may take the form of a guided experience by an expert practitioner or could simply be a cohesive team's self-exploration of practice.

Reflection can be utilized during the many phases of simulation practice to enhance the learning process. Reflection-on-action is frequently done in the form of debriefing following simulation experiences. Another use of critical reflection can be done in the form of a prebriefing. Prebriefing prior to the start of simulation explores the use of reflection-for-action in an attempt to provide a shared mental model for the team prior to performance in the simulated learning event. Error recovery, a specific instructional strategy that focuses on error detection and error mitigation, can be explored through reflective practice either pre- or postsimulation (Dror, 2011). When using this technique, the focus of reflection would be on the error detection, shifting the attention away from the protocol or procedure and focusing the reflection on the ability to generate error recovery actions through the

contextualized performance (Dror, 2011). These are just a few of the ways and places that reflective practice can be incorporated with simulation-based learning.

SITUATED LEARNING THEORY: LEGITIMATE PERIPHERAL PARTICIPATION

Situated learning theory is based on the premise that learning is an outcome of a process that occurs within an activity, is situated within a sociocultural environment, and is distributed across time, people, and tools (Brown, 1992; Lave & Wenger, 1991). It is predicated upon the belief that knowing and context cannot be separated from each other (Barab & Hay, 2000), and learning is dependent upon and created within the practice environment (Benner, 1984; Lave, 1993). All things contributing to that moment occur and become the means for understanding and dealing with future situations (Lave & Wenger, 1991). Communities of practice support the transition of identity and learning through **legitimate peripheral participation.** Meaning and understanding are a dynamic exchange between individuals, community, and the environment in which novices experiment to build knowledge and play at crafting their identity (Lave & Wenger, 1991). Understanding is not an isolated experience but part of a broader context of relationships, and the development of a skilled identity in practice is formed as a result of these multiple interactions (Lave & Wenger, 1991). The dynamics of the feedback loop move knowledge from an abstract concept to a personalized knowing that deepens with experience, whether in real practice or simulated environment.

Traditional healthcare learning utilizes an apprenticeship model, representing a sociocultural learning methodology, characterized by novice enculturation in conjunction with an experienced expert that results in active engagement with the practice. The learner transforms through the practice and gains knowledge and **expertise** through experience with the context, tools, and social practices he/she has encountered. The expert practitioner guides the learning by providing contextual guidance, feedback, and relevant clinical experiences to assist the novice to develop expertise by interacting within the culture. Knowledge is both socially constructed and mediated. Meaning and understanding are negotiated between the dynamic exchange between individuals, community, and the environment and are part of the richness of the practice (Benner, 1984; Lave & Wenger, 1991). There is a level of "experimentation" that exists while the learner builds knowledge and identity while moving from the periphery to central. This type of learning is not a linear application of theory to practice. It is complex and requires individualization and modification of knowledge to meet specific situations and respond to the specific context (Benner, 1984, 1991; Kim, 1999; Schon, 1991).

SECTION 7 • Educational Development

Pedagogies of contextualization, such as high-technology simulation, allow learners to practice clinical skills within a dynamically changing environment to determine the specifics of "what," "how," and "when" interventions should occur (Benner et al., 2010). The context of the setting including the environment, time pressure, and high-stake outcomes transforms the learning process from mere knowledge to individualized application of practice.

The simulation environment is important in this context of learning because "activities, tasks, functions and understandings do not exist in isolation; they are part of broader systems of relations in which they have meaning" (Lave & Wenger, 1991, p. 53). The realism of artifacts is important to the learning process and is commonly referred to as "suspension of disbelief" within simulation circles. For optimal learning to occur, there needs to be a continuity of experience and consistency between the learning environment and target environment where future performance is expected as the goal. Learners respond positively to the accuracy of clinical artifacts, up to and including the contextual storyline used to formulate the simulated clinical experience. These concepts must be kept in mind when designing simulation-based learning events.

In today's healthcare environment where healthcare educators are under intense pressure to produce caregivers that can adapt quickly to the fast-paced environment, simulation is recognized as an important tool to bridge the practice gaps and provide individuals with standardized learning environments to accelerate assimilation into their healthcare role. Having the ability to "practice" before performing allows the learner to gain clarity about the multifaceted factors that are important in caring for patients. Research has indicated that the role of observer during a simulated learning event, as legitimate peripheral practice, results in learning (Jeffries, 2005).

Legitimate peripheral participation through simulation practice is a valid process for building new interprofessional communities of practice (Lave & Wenger, 1991). The use of simulation can assist in breaking down the insular boundaries of clinical identities, by engaging multiple clinical services together in the practice of delivering patient care. Engaging different professional identities to work together by bolstering communication, knowledge, and skills practiced together rather than in silos allows for the reexamination and redefining of both the boundaries of the **community of practice** and how the community itself is defined and identified (Johansson, 2006). This intersection of interprofessional communities facilitates a new level of collaboration as the boundaries of the community shift through the engagement together, ultimately leading to delivery of higher quality of care. The process of jointly designing simulation practice events as an interdisciplinary team creates an environment where individuals can come together to explore new meanings for building interprofessional communities of practice.

Simulation education has the opportunity to provide healthcare training that improves the critical thinking skills and expertise of practitioners. Situated learning theory provides a framework for designing these learning opportunities that accounts for the complex relationship between the practice and the practitioners and how learning occurs within a professional practice setting. Providing contextual fidelity in the process, environment, and artifacts used during the simulated event can help provide learning opportunities to bridge the gaps that are currently present in the traditional apprenticeship model of training. If properly designed, the simulated learning events can be a useful tool to prepare our healthcare professions for the complexity that will be encountered in healthcare environments.

FRAMEWORKS FOR SIMULATION EDUCATORS

Simulation educators need to give consideration to what, not just how, learners learn. Pamela **Jeffries' simulation model** suggests that the design of the simulated learning experience is paramount to the delivery of desired outcomes (Jeffries, 2005). She further suggests that there is a multitude of factors to consider within this design. The discussion in this section will focus on the design characteristics of objectives and the link to learning/knowledge outcomes.

Bloom's taxonomy was created in 1956 to serve as a foundational language about learning goals. Within the taxonomy, three domains of learning were identified: cognitive, psychomotor, and affective (Bloom et al., 1956). Within healthcare, we often describe these domains as knowledge, skills, and attitudes. Bloom's taxonomy provided definitions for the cognitive domain of learning and provided a hierarchical order from simple to complex and from concrete to abstract. These definitions described the phenomenon of learning and are commonly used today to determine course and/or curriculum objectives, activities, and assessments for teaching (Krathwohl, 2002). Bloom's taxonomy has been readily adopted within the healthcare education realm as a guideline for preparing learning objectives and assessment tools.

Bloom's taxonomy was revised and updated in 2001 by Anderson, Krathwohl, and others to reflect a more active 21st century framework. The revision changed Bloom's original hierarchy to Remembering, Understanding, Applying, Analyzing, Evaluating, and Creating (Anderson et al., 2001; Figure 7.2.2). The categories of Understanding through Creating are considered to be the most valuable outcomes indicating a transfer of learning into meaningful practice rather than just the promotion of retention and recalling of information (Mayer, 2002). The reorganization of the taxonomy adds another dimension of knowledge known as Metacognitive Knowledge to capture the transition of knowledge application. Metacognition has been defined as the awareness and understanding of one's own thought process (Merriam-Webster Online, 2013).

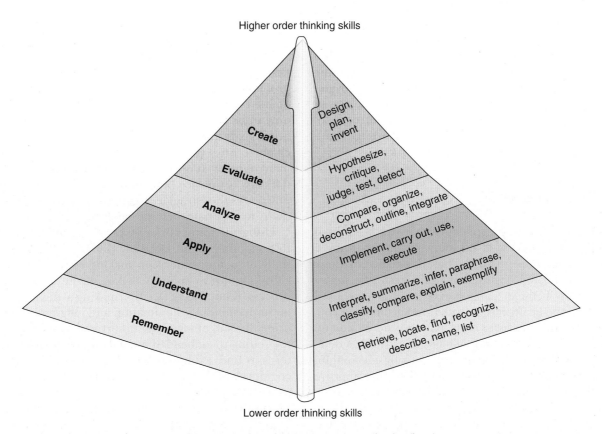

Representation of Bloom's taxonomy (revised)

FIGURE 7.2.2   Bloom's taxonomy. (Source: http://www.learnnc.org/lp/media/misc/2008/blooms_new.png)

Flavell's classic article on metacognition outlines three distinct types of metacognitive knowledge (Flavell, 1979):

1. Strategic knowledge: the knowledge of general strategies for learning. This knowledge focuses on processes that assist with knowledge use or the "what and how."
2. Cognitive task knowledge: the knowledge about different cognitive tasks and their difficulty levels. This reflects the learner's ability to discriminately choose the appropriate process and prioritize when it is utilized to fit the specific situation.
3. Self-knowledge: the knowledge of one's strengths and weaknesses. Self- efficacy and motivation are closely related concepts that are included in this type of knowing. Accuracy of self-perception is the goal here to promote expertise development and new knowledge construction (Pintrich & Schunk, 2002).

Simulation as a tool for learning lends itself to training objectives that reflect the higher-order categories. Moreover, simulation has the ability to create learning exercises that can simultaneously integrate the knowledge, skills, and attitude domains during a learning activity. It is important that simulation educators are aware of the responsibility for this design and spend sufficient time planning the learning experience. Jeffries indicates that planning

activities include creating objectives for the experience, providing guidelines for the role performance, and outlining the outcome expectancies (Jeffries, 2005).

The International Nursing Association for Clinical Simulation and Learning (INACSL), with the assistance of an advisory board of simulation experts within the professional community, has developed INACSL Standards for Simulation, 2013—a set of standards that represent a set of foundational best practices to guide the practice of teaching with simulation (Boese et al., 2013; Decker et al., 2013; Franklin et al., 2013; Gloe et al., 2013; Lioce et al., 2013; Meakim et al., 2013). These standards address the minimal components of simulation practice, provide terminology definitions, and include rationale, outcomes, criteria, and guidelines for teaching with simulation. The standards address the process of simulation, outlining "must have" components such as professional integrity, participant objectives, facilitation methods, facilitator responsibilities, debriefing, and assessment/evaluation measures. The INACSL standards of simulation best practice support the basic tenets of the Jeffries simulation model and outline the minimal components of simulation practice.

Simulation as a learning experience provides the learner with a vast array of resources, data, and tools to analyze and assemble into working goals for care of the patient. The ability to mimic time pressure and competing priorities during this process augments decision-making skill building that is necessary for gaining expertise. Educators must be cognizant that teaching with simulation is a resource-intense proposition and should strive to be good stewards of this resource. It is the design of the learning experience that guides knowledge synthesis and provides value for that resource allocation. There must always be an ability to measure the specific benefits and outcomes of the simulation training. The tools and standards that have been described here can assist with that process.

DECISION MAKING

Simulation is a learning experience that can be utilized to highlight the process of decision making by giving a contextual environment for deliberate practice of these skills. The simulated environment can create the necessary ambiguity between data observed and goals chosen to challenge the healthcare provider under time and consequence pressure to assist with expertise development. Research in the aviation and military industries has demonstrated that participation in contextually meaningful experiences helps develop assessment skills that improve the participant's ability to understand current and project future needs to guide practice actions (Endsley, 1997; Means et al., 1993). The development of expertise has been identified as being centrally important to preparing a healthcare worker for today's practice setting where the fast pace and focus on error reduction is key.

While the traditional view of decision making as a logical and progressive process has application during the learning phases of professional practice, it does not explain the intuitive decision making that takes place in healthcare settings. Naturalistic Decision making (NDM) can be utilized to describe this dynamic and adaptive process. NDM research has a long history in the aviation and military domains. These domains have done extensive research to understand what goes into decision making and have utilized that knowledge to create decision-centered training. This type of training focuses on development of SA, pattern and cue matching, mental model construction, and utilization of cognitive feedback to improve performance specific to contextual situations. Additionally, designers of monitoring equipment have been interested in using this type of research to optimize the Human Computer Interaction (HCI) interface to promote optimal decision making.

Zsambok defines NDM as: "how experienced people, working as individuals or groups in dynamic, uncertain, and often fast-paced environments, identify and assess their situation, make decisions, and take actions whose consequences are meaningful to them and to the larger organization in which they operate" (Zsambok, 1997, p. 5). NDM focuses on time spent trying to understand the situation rather than generating a set of options to choose from. NDM focuses more energy on the assessment of the situation to come to complete understanding rather than generating a set of options for solutions using a rationale

and conscious process. This is a process of decision making that is noted as part of expert practice.

Orasanu and Connolly identified eight characteristics consistent with an NDM environment: ill-structured problems, uncertain/dynamic environments, shifting/ill-defined and/or competing goals, action/feedback loops, time stress and high stakes, multiple players, and organizational goals and norms (Orasanu & Connolly, 1993). These characteristics certainly describe the healthcare environment of today. It is exactly these characteristics that create difficulty for novice practitioners for the first few years of practice as they struggle to gain the practice expertise necessary to negotiate their way safely for patient care delivery.

Using the framework of NDM as a guide, Gary Klein's Recognition-Primed Decision (RPD) model focuses centrally on adaptive decision making as behavior that specifically utilizes expertise as part of the decision-making process (Klein, 1993). Decision making in this model hinges on understanding the situation and judging its familiarity using the skill of matching observed characteristics within the setting to embedded mental models of normative patterns to find a solution. This happens tacitly rather than cognitively and improves the speed of the decision-making process. Key elements of this model are the ambiguity or incompleteness of situation understanding, time pressure, high-stake consequences, and expertise/tacit knowledge (Drillings & Serfaty, 1997; Klein, 1993). The RPD model supports that expertise leads directly to accurate decision making with no deterioration of performance under time pressure and no need to contrast/compare decision choices (Endsley, 1995; Klein, 1993; Lipshitz, 1997).

Understanding the differences between how a novice makes sense of the practice setting to make decisions compared to how an expert does so is helpful to be able to design learning experiences that will build expertise in decision making. Expert decision making requires the ability to develop a situational understanding of the world through matching patterns and taking action (Bogner, 1997; Dreyfus, 1997; Schraagen, 1997). Research shows that experts spend the majority of decision-making time in the assessment and classification of a situation rather than in conscious development of structured courses of action, making SA a key feature in dictating the success of real-world decisions (Endsley et al., 2003). Expert practitioners have SA skills that allow them to recognize and determine the significance of cues and patterns within the practice setting more rapidly than the novice, thus leading to more effective decision making (Klein, 2000; Lipshitz & Shaul, 1997; Orasanu & Connolly, 1993). As expertise develops through experience with individualized situations that are not exactly as before or like the norm, decision making becomes a rapid process of matching cues, taking action, and evaluating outcomes. This process is part of the RPD model and is defined as mental simulation. These mental simulations are usually the first and only option considered to solve the problem and generally result in high-quality outcomes (Kaempf et al., 1996; Klein et al., 1995; Stokes et al., 1997).

SIMULATION THEORIES

Pamela B. Andreatta, EdD, MFA, MA
President, Society for Simulation in Healthcare (2015)

The uses of simulation in advance of "real" applications are long-standing. Whether preparation in an applied context is not feasible (e.g., space walks, hazardous material cleanup, mass casualty disasters, etc.), too costly, or inefficient, simulation methodologies have historically provided the best alternative to the true context. We have used simulation-based methods for healthcare education long before the introduction of the computer-driven models we use today. The roots of these instructional practices lay within the theoretical foundations of why the apprenticeship model of clinical instruction works in the first place: experiential learning establishes the requisite contextual and situational factors that are essential for performance in complex environments.

The foundation of experiential learning theory is that experience plays a central role in a cycle of learning: a learner has an experience, the experience promotes observation and reflection, the observation and reflection transform the experience into abstractions, the abstractions are actively tested by the learner, which leads to further experiences. Learning experiences may be formal or informal, directed or flexible, derived from standards or organic in nature. The common component of all experiential learning environments is the active engagement of the learner toward assembling, analyzing, and synthesizing perceptual cues stemming from the instructional context.

In conjunction with experiential learning theory, deliberate practice theory establishes the underpinnings for the processes by which humans achieve expert performance. Deliberate practice theory proposes that deep expertise is developed through highly motivated learners engaging in concentrated repetitive practice on well-defined objectives, and deliberatively reflecting about their experiences to learn from them. Social cognitive theory postulates that learning optimally takes place in groups with the support of peers, facilitators, and others in contextually accurate settings. In this view, the learner is part of a complex system of practice, and learning is constantly occurring through interaction with peers, educators, senior clinicians, patients, and the physical environment. Learners are able to work together and independently, while gathering information about how others address problems, derive solutions, develop or apply techniques, and so on. Here, experience itself is part of a broader social, political, and cultural landscape, where patterns that we take for granted shape every aspect of the way we learn. These interactions encourage learners to develop a deeper understanding of the content than might be possible through individualized study alone. Additionally, healthcare is a highly social profession in which professionals must be able to work collaboratively toward understanding and solving problems.

Foundationally, simulation-based learning environments are just that: learning environments. Therefore, it could be argued that any aspect of the simulation-based learning construct could be tied to any of the multiple theories about how humans learn and acquire expertise. However, the value of simulation to healthcare education is that it provides an experiential learning construct that facilitates the type of deliberate practice and peer interaction essential for developing proficient clinicians. This is unfeasible in the real healthcare context given the associated implications for patients. To that extent, understanding the factors that experientially contribute to performance in the true environment is essential to creating effective simulation-based instruction.

BEEN THERE, DONE THAT: HOW CAN I CONTINUE TO IMPROVE OR SUSTAIN WHAT I HAVE ACHIEVED?

Situation Awareness theory, developed by Mica Endsley in 1997, is an important part of the RPD theory and has been a focus of training within the aviation and military realms for decades to improve accuracy and expertise of novice practitioners. SA is defined by a domain-specific goal and is context specific: changing as the environment changes. Endsley defined three different levels of SA:

1. Level 1 SA—Perception: collection of data within the environment.
2. Level 2 SA—Comprehension: synthesis of disjointed data points in light of a goal to create understanding.
3. Level 3 SA—Projection: the ability to project future actions on the basis of understood meaning (Endsley, 1997).

Decision making in the SA model is guided by the development of goals, which provides the impetus for choosing the appropriate mental model to use. The mental model that is chosen guides the practitioner to prioritize what types of data to pay attention to and which to minimize in order to achieve the goal. The mental model also allows for what type of data would be predictive to indicate that there was a potential problem. This SA decision-making process requires a continuous reprioritization of data that is based on matching with the "normal" schema. SA is known to be negatively impacted by factors such as stress, workload, complexity, and automation. The immersive and contextual features of high-fidelity simulation (HFS) incorporate these realities into the practice situation, allowing for a more realistic experience that enhances expertise development. Focus on the participant's ability to identify factors that negatively impact their decision-making capability can be a key learning outcome of HFS, making it a valuable learning tool.

Naturalistic decision skills training moves away from merely using policies and procedures as the foundation for teaching and suggests that efforts should be focused in the areas of SA, pattern matching, cue learning, typical versus anomaly, mental model development, and managing uncertainty and time pressure (Klein, 2000). Research in aviation has documented that decision-making skills can be trained and that proficiency can be improved by enhancing SA through simulation practice (Kaempf & Orasanu, 1997; Means & Gott, 1988; Robertson & Endsley, 1995; Roth, 1997).

The goal in utilizing NDM principles to improve training suggests that the instructor role should support processes that accelerate proficiency in cue and pattern recognition. In order to provide deliberate practice in SA, the instructor must utilize specific techniques such as goal-directed task analysis, crew resource management principles, and guided reflection techniques to support the development of patterns for improved schema storage in long-term memory. Well-indexed and stored schema lead to reduced decision-making time and improved quality in contextually stressed situations, creating adaptive, resilient, and risk-taking practitioners (Cannon-Bowers & Bell, 1997). Simulation training objectives should be focused on mental simulation, SA, knowledge organization, cue/strategy feedback, and reflective practice to enhance decision-making capability. HFS, if designed with purposeful intent, can meet these requirements.

SUMMARY

It is widely agreed that simulation will not take the place of human patient care, yet it does provide a realistic alternative to care that allows for experiential practice to accelerate the development of expertise (Gordon et al., 1999; Issenberg et al., 2005). The ability to allow the learner to engage in the professional role using the tools of the profession to creatively problem-solve differentiates a simulation learning experience from that of role-play (Lowenstein, 2007). The simulation environment creates valuable action feedback loops that are uniquely tied to the choices of the decision maker, and this process actively builds decision-making expertise, making simulation a good fit for training NDM (Means et al., 1993). The point of simulation is not just to frontload the practitioner with experience and a place to practice, but to maximize that experience to facilitate the decision-making capability of a seasoned practitioner without requiring many years of practice.

Linking theory and established tools/methods to the learning experience is key to promoting the science of simulation-based learning. Utilizing theory to create contextually meaningful experiences that promote psychomotor skill development, clinical decision making, and emotional engagement is what makes simulation such a powerful learning tool.

REFERENCES

Anderson, L. W., Krathwohl, D. R., Airasian, P. W., Cruikshank, K. A., Mayer, R. E., Pintrich, P. R., . . . Whittrock, M. C. (2001). *A taxonomy for learning, teaching, and assessing: A revision of Bloom's taxonomy of educational objectives.* New York, NY: Longman.

Argyris, C., & Schon, D. A. (1974). *Theory in practice: Increasing professional effectiveness.* London, England: Jossey Bass.

Barab, S. A., & Hay, K. E. (2000). Doing science at the elbows of experts: Issues related to the science apprenticeship camp. *Journal of Research in Science Teaching,* 38(2), 70–102.

Benner, P. (1984). *From novice to expert: Excellence and power in clinical nursing practice.* Menlo Park, CA: Addison-Wesley.

Benner, P. (1991). The role of experience, narrative, and community in skilled ethical comportment. *Advances in Nursing Science,* 14(2), 1–21.

Benner, P., Hooper-Kyriakidis, P., & Stannard, D. (1999). *Clinical wisdom and interventions in critical care: A thinking-in-action approach.* Philadelphia, PA: Saunders.

Benner, P., Sutphen, M., Leonard, V., & Day, L. (2010). *Educating nurses: A call for radical transformation.* San Francisco, CA: Jossey-Bass.

Bloom, B. S., Engelhart, M. D., Furst, E. J., Hill, W. H., & Krathwohl, D. R. (1956). *Taxonomy of educational objectives: The classification of educational goals. Handbook 1: Cognitive domain.* New York, NY: David McKay.

Boese, T., Cato, M., Gonzalez, L., Jones, A., Kennedy, K., Reese, C., . . . Borum, J. C. (2013). Standards of best practice: Simulation standard V: Facilitator. *Clinical Simulation in Nursing,* 9(6S), S22–S25.

Bogner, M. S. (1997). Naturalistic decision-making in health care. In C. E. Zsambok & G. Klein (Eds.), *Naturalistic decision-making* (pp. 61–69). Mahwah, NJ: Lawrence Erlbaum Associates.

Brookfield, S. (1984). The contribution of Eduard Linderman to the development of theory and philosophy in adult education. *Adult Education Quarterly,* 34(4), 185–196.

Brown, A. L. (1992). Design experiments: Theoretical and methodological challenges in creating complex interventions in classroom settings. *Journal of Learning Sciences,* 2, 141–178.

Cannon-Bowers, J. A., & Bell, H. H. (1997). Training decision makers for complex environments: Implications of the naturalistic decision making perspective. In C. E. Zsambok & G. Klein (Eds.), *Naturalistic decision-making* (pp. 91–98). Mahwah, NJ: Lawrence Erlbaum Associates.

Clark, R. W., Threeton, M. D., & Ewing, J. C. (2010). The potential of experiential learning models and practices in career and technical education & career and technical teacher education. *Journal of Career and Technical Education,* 25(2), 46–62.

Cox, E. (2006). An adult learning approach to coaching. In D. R. Stober & A. M. Grant (Eds.), *Evidence based coaching handbook: Putting best practices to work for your clients.* Hoboken, NJ: Wiley.

Decker, S., Fey, M., Sideras, S., Caballero, S., Rockstraw, L. R., Boese, T., . . . Borum, J. C. (2013). Standards of best practice: Simulation standard VI: The debriefing process. *Clinical Simulation in Nursing,* 9(6S), S27–S29.

Dewey, J. (1933). *How we think: A restatement of the relation of reflective thinking to the educative process.* Boston, MA: D.C. Health.

Dewey, J. (1938). *Experience and education.* New York, NY: Kappa Delta Pi/Touchstone.

Dreyfus, H. (1997). Intuitive, deliberative, and calculative models of expert performance. In C. E. Zsambok & G. Klein (Eds.), *Naturalistic decision-making* (pp. 17–28). Mahwah, NJ: Lawrence Erlbaum Associates.

Drillings, M., & Serfaty, D. (1997). Naturalistic decision-making in command and control. In C. E. Zsambok & G. Klein (Eds.), *Naturalistic decision-making* (pp. 71–80). Mahwah, NJ: Lawrence Erlbaum Associates.

Dror, I. (2011). A novel approach to minimize error in the medical domain: Cognitive neuroscientific insights into training. *Medical Teacher,* 33(1), 34–38.

Endsley, M. R. (1995). Situation awareness in dynamic human decision-making: Theory. *Human Factors,* 37, 32–64.

Endsley, M. R. (1997). The role of situation awareness in naturalistic decision-making. In C. E. Zsambok & G. Klein (Eds.), *Naturalistic decision-making* (pp. 269–284). Mahwah, NJ: Lawrence Erlbaum Associates.

Endsley, M. R., Bolte, B., & Jones, D. G. (2003). *Designing for situation awareness: An approach to user centered design.* Boca Raton, FL: CRC Press.

Flavell, J. (1979). Metacognition and cognitive monitoring: A new area of cognitive-developmental inquiry. *American Psychologist,* 34, 906–911.

Franklin, A. E., Boese, T., Gloe, D., Lioce, L., Decker, S., Sando, C. R., . . . Borum, J. C. (2013). Standards of best practice: Simulation standard IV: Facilitation. *Clinical Simulation in Nursing*, 9(6S), S19–S21.

Gloe, D., Sando, C. R., Franklin, A. E., Boese, T., Decker, S., Lioce, L., . . . Borum, J. C. (2013). Standards of best practice: Simulation standard II: Professional integrity of participant(s). *Clinical Simulation in Nursing*, 9(6S), S12–S14.

Gordon, M. S., Issenberg, S. B., Mayer, J. W., & Felner, J. M. (1999). Learning outcomes for simulation education in medicine. *Medical Teacher*, 21(1), 32–36.

Gould, N. (1996). Introduction: Social work education and the "crisis of the professions." In N. Gould & I. Taylor (Eds.), *Reflective learning for social work*. Aldershot, England: Arena.

Issenberg, S. B., McGaghie, W. C., Petrusa, E. R., Gordon, D. L., & Scalese, R. J. (2005). Features and uses of high-fidelity medical simulations that lead to effective learning: A BEME systematic review. *Medical Teacher*, 27(1), 10–28.

Jeffries, P. R. (2005). A framework for designing, implementing, and evaluating simulations used as teaching strategies in nursing. *Nursing Education Perspectives*, 26(2), 96–103.

Johansson, F. (2006). *The Medici Effect*. Boston, MA: Harvard Business School Press.

Kaempf, G., Klein, G., Thordsen, M. L., & Wolf, S. (1996). Decision-making in complex command-and-control environments. *Human Factors*, 38(2), 220–231.

Kaempf, G. L., & Orasanu, J. (1997). Current and future applications of naturalistic decision-making. In C. E. Zsambok & G. Klein (Eds.), *Naturalistic decision-making* (pp. 81–90). Mahwah, NJ: Lawrence Erlbaum Associates.

Keeton, M., & Tate, P. (Eds.). (1978). *Learning by experience—What, why, how*. San Francisco, CA: Jossey-Bass.

Kim, H. S. (1999). Critical reflective inquiry for knowledge development in nursing practice. *Journal of Advanced Nursing*, 29(5), 1205–1212.

Klein, G. (1993). A recognition primed decision (RPD) model of rapid decision-making. In G. Klein, J. Orasanu, & R. Calderwood (Eds.), *Decision-making in action: Models and methods* (pp. 138–147). Norwood, NJ: Ablex.

Klein, G. (2000). Analysis of situation awareness from critical incident reports. In M. R. Endsley & D. J. Garland (Eds.), *Situation awareness analysis and measurement* (pp. 51–71). Mahwah, NJ: Lawrence Erlbaum Associates.

Klein, G., Wolf, S., Militello, L., & Zsambok, C. (1995). Characteristics of skilled option generation in chess. *Organizational Behavior and Human Decision Processes*, 62(1), 63–69.

Knowles, M. S. (1970). *The modern practice of adult education: Andragogy versus pedagogy*. New York, NY: Association Press.

Knowles, M. S. (1980). *The modern practice of adult education: From pedagogy to andragogy* (Rev. & updated). Englewood Cliffs, NJ: Prentice Hall.

Knowles, M. S. (1990). *The adult learner: A neglected species* (Rev. ed.). Houston, US: Gulf Publishing Company.

Knowles, M. S. (1996). Adult learning. In R. L. Craig (Ed.), *ASTD training & development hand book: A guide to human resource development* (4th ed., pp. 253–265). New York, NY: McGraw Hill.

Kohlberg, L. (1969). Stage and sequence: The cognitive-developmental approach to socialization. In D. A. Goslin (Ed.), *Handbook of socialization theory and research*. Chicago, IL: Rand McNally.

Kolb, A. Y., & Kolb, D. A. (2005). Learning styles and learning spaces: Enhancing experiential learning in higher education. *Academy of Management Learning & Education*, 4(2), 193–212.

Kolb, D. A. (1984). *Experiential learning: Experience as the source of learning and development*. Upper Saddle River, NJ: Prentice Hall.

Kolb, D. A., & Fry, R. (1975). Toward an applied theory of experiential learning. In C. Cooper (Ed.), *Theories of group process*. London, England: John Wiley.

Krathwohl, D. R. (2002). A revision of Bloom's taxonomy: An overview. *Theory into Practice*, 41(4), 212–218.

Kurtines, W., & Greif, E. B. (1974). The development of moral thought: Review and evaluation of Kohlberg's approach. *Psychological Bulletin*, 81, 8.

Lave, J. (1993). Situating learning in communities of practice. In L. B. Resnick, J. M. Levine, & S. D. Teasley (Eds.), *Perspectives on socially shared cognition* (pp. 17–36). Washington, DC: American Psychological Association.

Lave, J., & Wenger, E. (1991). *Situated learning: Legitimate peripheral participation*. New York, NY: Cambridge University Press.

Lewin, K. (1947). Group decision and social change. In T. N. Newcomb & E. L. Hartley (Eds.), *Readings in social psychology*. Troy, MO: Holt, Rinehart & Winston.

Lewin, K. (1951). *Field theory in social science*. New York, NY: Harper and Row.

Lindeman, E. C. (1925). *What is adult education?* New York, NY: Columbia University, Butler Library Lindeman Archive.

Lindeman, E. C. (1926). *The meaning of adult education*. New York, NY: New Republic.

Lioce, L., Reed, C. C., Lemon, D., King, M. A., Martinez, P. A., Franklin, A. E., . . . Borum, J. C. (2013). Standards of best practice: Simulation standard III: Participant objectives. *Clinical Simulation in Nursing*, 9(6S), S15–S18.

Lippitt, R. (1949). *Training in community relations*. New York, NY: Harper & Row.

Lipshitz, R. (1997). Naturalistic decision-making perspectives on decision errors. In C. E. Zsambok & G. Klein (Eds.), *Naturalistic decision-making* (pp. 3–16). Mahwah, NJ: Lawrence Erlbaum Associates.

Lipshitz, R., & Shaul, B. (1997). Schemata and mental models in recognition primed decision-making. In C. E. Zsambok & G. Klein (Eds.), *Naturalistic decision-making* (pp. 293–304). Mahwah, NJ: Lawrence Erlbaum Associates.

Lowenstein, A. J. (2007). Role-play. In M. J. Bradshaw & A. J. Lowenstein (Eds.), *Fuszard's innovative teaching strategies in nursing and health related professions* (pp. 173–185). Sudbury, MA: Jones & Bartlett.

Mayer, R. E. (2002). Rote versus meaningful learning. *Theory into Practice*, 41(4), 226–232.

Meakim, C., Boese, T., Decker, S., Franklin, A. E., Gloe, D., Lioce, L., . . . Borum, J. C. (2013). Standards of best practice: Simulation standard I: Terminology. *Clinical Simulation in Nursing*, 9(6S), S3–S11.

Means, B., & Gott, S. (1988). Cognitive task analysis as a basis for tutor development: Articulating abstract knowledge representations. In J. Psotka, L. D. Massey, & S. A. Mutter (Eds.), *Intelligent tutoring systems: Lessons learned* (pp. 35–57). Mahwah, NJ: Lawrence Erlbaum Associates.

Means, B., Salas, E., Crandall, B., & Jacobs, T. O. (1993). Training decision makers for the real world. In G. Klein, J. Orasanu, & R. Calderwood (Eds.), *Decision-making in action: Models and methods* (pp. 306–326). Norwood, NJ: Ablex.

Nielsen, A., Stragnell, S., & Jester, P. (2007). Guide for reflection using the clinical judgment model. *Journal of Nursing Education*, 46, 513–516.

Orasanu, J., & Connolly, T. (1993). The reinvention of decision-making. In G. Klein, J. Orasanu, & R. Calderwood (Eds.), *Decision-making in action: Models and methods* (pp. 3–20). Norwood, NJ: Ablex.

Pintrich, P. R., & Schunk, D. H. (2002). *Motivation in education: Theory, research, and applications*. Upper Saddle River, NJ: Merrill Prentice-Hall.

Robertson, M. M., & Endsley, M. R. (1995). The role of crew resource management (CRM) in achieving team situation awareness in aviation settings. In R. Fuller, N. Johnston, & N. McDonald (Eds.), *Human factors in aviation operations* (pp. 281–286). Hants, England: Avebury Aviation.

Roth, E. M. (1997). Analysis of decision-making in nuclear power plan emergencies: An investigation of aided decision-making. In C. E. Zsambok & G. Klein (Eds.), *Naturalistic decision-making* (pp. 175–192). Mahwah, NJ: Lawrence Erlbaum Associates.

Ruth-Sahd, L. A. (2003). Reflective practice: A critical analysis of data-based studies and implications for nursing education. *Journal of Nursing Education*, 42, 488–497.

Schein, E. H. (1996). Kurt Lewin in the classroom, in the field, and in change theory: Notes toward a model of managed learning. *Systems Practice*, 9(1), 27–47.

Schein, E. H., & Bennis, W. (1965). *Personal and organizational change through group methods* (2nd ed.). New York, NY: John Wiley.

SECTION 7 • Educational Development

Schon, D. A. (1987). *Educating the reflective practitioner.* New York, NY: Jossey-Bass.

Schon, D. A. (1991). *The reflective practitioner* (2nd ed.). New York, NY: Basic Books.

Schraagen, J. M. (1997). Discovering requirements for a naval damage control decision support system. In C. E. Zsambok & G. Klein (Eds.), *Naturalistic decision-making* (pp. 227–232). Mahwah, NJ: Lawrence Erlbaum Associates.

Stokes, A. F., Kemper, K., & Kite, K. (1997). Aeronautical decision-making, cue recognition, and expertise under time pressure. In C. E. Zsambok & G. Klein (Eds.), *Naturalistic decision-making* (pp. 183–196). Mahwah, NJ: Lawrence Erlbaum Associates.

Tanner, C. A. (2006). Thinking like a nurse: A research-based model of clinical judgment in nursing. *Journal of Nursing Education, 45*(6), 204–211.

Taylor, B., & Kroth, M. (2009). Andragogy's transition into the future: Meta-analysis of andragogy and its search for a measurable instrument. *Journal of Adult Education, 38*(1), 1–11.

Thompson, N., & Pascal, J. (2012). Developing critically reflective practice. *Reflective Practice: International and Multidisciplinary Perspectives, 13*(2), 311–325.

Zsambok, C. E. (1997). Naturalistic decision-making: Where are we now. In C. E. Zsambok & G. Klein (Eds.), *Naturalistic decision-making* (pp. 3–16). Mahwah, NJ: Lawrence Erlbaum Associates.

CHAPTER 7.3

Assessment in Healthcare Simulation

Wendy Anson, PhD, CHSE

ABOUT THE AUTHOR

WENDY ANSON is a Research Analyst for educational psychology and technology at MedStar Health's Simulation, Training & Education Laboratory (SiTEL). She is also a member of the SSH Accreditation Committee and has presented on assessment, tool rating, and competencies in healthcare simulation. Dr. Anson has served as a consultant for the National Center for Research on Evaluation, Standards & Student Testing, as well as other university organizations. She received the Annenberg Multimedia Scholar fellowship for a communication tool and was awarded a US patent for an online assessment tool that she developed.

Acknowledgments: The author would like to express tremendous gratitude to Rachel Yudkowsky, MD, MHPE, Associate Professor in the Department of Medical Education at the University of Illinois at Chicago College of Medicine and Director of the Dr. Allen L. and Mary L. Graham Clinical Performance Center, who graciously gave her time and expertise to look over multiple drafts and provide vital, timely feedback and input. The chapter could not have been done without her. The author would also like to thank USC professor Harold F. O'Neil, Jr., PhD for his teachings, Dr. Elizabeth Sinz who contributed helpful suggestions to the manuscript, and editor Dr. Janice C. Palaganas who consistently offered thoughtful, pertinent, judicious, and invaluable feedback throughout on content and organization.

ABSTRACT

Peer-reviewed studies using healthcare simulators have shown reliable, reproducible data for assessing students within varied specialties and learning levels. Simulation as a methodology has become a focus in the assessment of procedural, clinical decision making, behavioral, and communication skills of health professionals and teams. Simulation is being used more and more to demonstrate that learning has occurred in an environment wherein emphasis has moved to observed evidence of "competencies." This chapter outlines technical, trainee, trainer, and tool components of simulation-based assessment.

CASE EXAMPLE

Sara, a Simulation Educator, works in a multilevel, multispecialty simulation center used by a variety of medical schools and hospitals for training of their medical students, residents, fellows, and RNs. A program director in a surgical specialty new to her center asked her for a central venous catheter (CVC) placement simulation assessment tool for a simulation exercise. The program director wants reportable outcomes. Understanding the complexity of assessment, Sara seeks out research help and has found that there are no psychometricians at her institution.

INTRODUCTION

Outcomes-based education has become a focus in healthcare profession education, and there has been an increasing need to provide evidence that learning has occurred (Scalese & Issenberg, 2008). Healthcare simulation (HCS), integrated into the larger healthcare education curriculum, is currently being used to provide this evidence, specifically with a focus on observed evidence of competencies. According to McGaghie et al. (1978),

"competence includes a broad range of knowledge, attitudes and observable patterns of behavior which together account for the ability to deliver a specified professional service" (p. 19).

Within the context of observing behaviors, there are two general types of assessment: "formative" (assessing learning during the teaching process or path, e.g., quizzes, question and answer, or in class discussion) and "summative" (assessment or testing of learning at the end of course/program, e.g., high-stakes testing or pass/fail grading; Scalese &

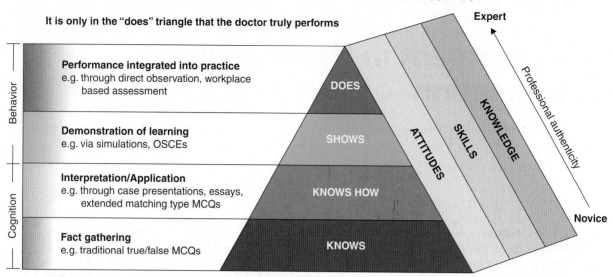

FIGURE 7.3.1   Miller's Pyramid of Competence. (Based on work by Miller, G. E. [1990]. The assessment of clinical skills/competence/performance. *Academic Medicine, 65*(9 Suppl), S63–S67. Adapted by Drs. R. Mehay & R. Burns, UK, January 2009.)

Issenberg, 2008). Learners are observed, and then given feedback on their performances. There are two varieties of simulation feedback—formative and summative. Performance feedback during the simulation itself and discussions during postsimulation debriefing often serve as formative assessment. Formative assessment in a medical simulation setting is frequently understood as the four-step model presented by Rudolph et al. (2008): (1) note salient performance gaps related to predetermined objectives, (2) provide feedback describing the gap, (3) investigate the basis for the gap by exploring the frames and emotions contributing to the current performance level, and (4) help close the performance gap through discussion or targeted instruction about principles and skills relevant to performance. Alternatively, the purpose of "summative assessment" is to collect, analyze, and summarize data that is then provided to decision makers in the organization or institution so that they can decide on the competence of the learners, for example, pass or fail (Smith & Ragan, 1999). While formative assessment serves to inform the learner and the educator how to achieve learning for that learner or learner group, summative assessment serves to inform the educator whether or not the learner is competent to pass a course or level of competence. It is often referred to as "high-stakes" testing since the consequences of not passing a summative assessment are often significant, for example passing or failing a course, completing or failing a program, losing employment, or not being hired. This chapter focuses on the summative assessment of competencies using simulation and elucidates the use of simulation in providing valid and reliable outcomes on learner performance in a given domain or multiple domains.

Summative assessment often follows a set of predetermined criteria that, if met, demonstrates a level of competence. The use of simulation allows assessment of higher levels of competence. In Miller's Pyramid of Competence (Figure 7.3.1), the lowest "knows" stage level of the pyramid (e.g., "what is a central venous line?") can be assessed using simple knowledge tests, for example multiple-choice questions (MCQs). The "knows how" stage (e.g., "this is what needs to be done to insert a central venous catheter") can be assessed using MCQs, patient management problems, or essay questions. The "shows" or "does" competency level is problematic in the clinical environment—not only for ethical reasons of having learners demonstrate on real people for competency evaluation, but because assessment in that context would not be reliable due to multiple variables and challenges. For example, the number and types of real-world cases that occur in the clinic are unpredictable, and so it cannot be assumed that each student would be presented with the same number and types of cases within their set clinical rotation. For this reason, clinical rotations or time spent in a clinical environment are not reliable measures of competence. HCS can be structured to assess an individual or team at all levels of competence, including the "shows" levels.

Outcomes related to education have focused on competencies or skills, and more recently on robust credentialing (e.g., milestones, accreditation, or certification standards). Credentialed healthcare providers are also increasingly being required to demonstrate that they meet acceptable standards for continued practice through recredentialing or regular assessment of competencies (e.g., Maintenance of Certification [MOC]). More and more certification and MOC programs are mandating simulation assessment as part of the process (e.g., MOCA, NRP, FLS). Peer-reviewed studies using healthcare simulators have shown the modality to provide reliable, reproducible data (Boulet & Murray, 2010). Simulation as an assessment methodology can also provide reliability through consistent testing environment, a selection of tasks that align with students' expected level of expertise, an environment focused on evaluation of student performance rather than patient needs, and technology to represent, archive, and often compute performance outcomes with increased accuracy and objectivity. At the same time, a variety of considerations influence simulation assessment potential to embody a rigorous, viable methodology for the testing of healthcare providers and students. This chapter will explore the following five areas of simulation-based assessment:

1. Learner aspects (e.g., pre- and postlicensure)
2. Assessor aspects (e.g., simulationists and raters)
3. Programmatic aspects (e.g., program needs and resources)
4. Simulation modalities (e.g., standardized patients [SPs] or mannequin-based simulation [MBS])
5. Assessment tools

The last two areas (numbers 4 and 5) are combined into one section. In this section, considerations and examples of appropriate assessment tool use are described within each simulation platform category. It is noted that the purpose of the chapter is to increase awareness of the complexity of simulation-based assessment; speaking to comprehensive local programmatic and psychometric considerations within a full-scale, multilayered healthcare assessment program is beyond the current scope.

LEARNERS

Individuals being assessed can be delineated as either prelicensure (e.g., undergraduate or graduate student at university) or postlicensure (e.g., licensed practicing provider). Most prelicensure assessment activities coincide with programmatic curriculum necessary to pass to be granted a degree by the program, while most postlicensure assessment activities correspond to hospital or unit practice competencies, policies, or procedures. The stakes are typically high in summative assessment despite the learner level—for example, the prelicensure student may not pass a course or graduate the program if (s)he fails an assessment and the postlicensure provider may lose his/her job or a portion of the job if (s)he fails an assessment. Because of the high-stakes nature of summative assessment, individuals involved with assessment are obligated to develop a fair simulation with every possible opportunity for fair assessment (Joint Committee on Fair Testing Practices in Education, 2004). This requires involvement with educators, researchers, and assessors who have a deep understanding of the learner group being assessed.

EXPERT'S CORNER

A CLEAR MESSAGE EMERGES FROM THE NLN HIGH-STAKES ASSESSMENT PROJECT

Mary Anne Rizzolo, EdD, RN, FAAN, ANEF
Board of Directors, Society for Simulation in Healthcare

Fair evaluation of student performance in the clinical area is a very weak link in the assessment of nursing students. Creating a fair testing environment with patients whose conditions can change at any moment in an often chaotic healthcare setting is a near-impossible task. Furthermore, many faculty are underprepared for their evaluator role. Not all faculty have been educated in assessment methods, and unintentional biases emerge when switching from the role of teacher to evaluator (Stroud et al., 2011). These are just some of the factors that led me to propose a project to explore the feasibility of using high-technology simulation to assess prelicensure students in schools of nursing. The project was funded by Laerdal Medical in 2010. It was designed to be a feasibility study and the basic questions were these: Can high-technology simulations provide a fair, valid, and reliable method for summative assessment? How hard is it to do? What are the biggest challenges? The project is ongoing with expected completion in the fall of 2014. An overview of the project and some findings to date provide the foundation and context for the concluding message.

OVERVIEW OF PROJECT

The project began with a Think Tank of esteemed individuals* who shared their expertise and wisdom and recommended scenarios to assess students at the end of their program. Dr. Pamela Jeffries then assembled a team of expert simulation authors to design the simulations while the evaluation team, comprising Drs. Marilyn Oermann and Suzan Kardong-Edgren, examined evaluation tools and planned the training of raters. The scenarios were piloted and refined, and then schools of nursing across the country ran the scenarios and sent video recordings of student performances. Raters, chosen on the basis of their expertise in both simulation and evaluation, scored the videos at two different points in time, and inter- and intrarater reliability statistics were generated. In the final phase, now in progress, the authors of the scenarios are scoring the video recordings, and then discussing the rationales for their scores to come to consensus on scoring criteria. The final scoring criteria will be given to the raters who will once again score the videos twice, and inter- and intrarater reliability scores will be calculated.

DESIGN AND IMPLEMENTATION ISSUES

We found that substantial time was required to design, develop, and pilot the scenarios, each with three parallel forms, but the task is achievable. The differences in designing scenarios for teaching versus assessment, and other lessons learned from this aspect of the process have been reported by the authors who created the simulations (Willhaus et al., 2014). Standardizing the implementation of the scenarios by different individuals at multiple sites was also a challenge, but can be handled by standardizing the testing environment and implementing rigorous training sessions for facilitators. Other suggestions on design and implementation issues are included in my chapter in *Clinical Simulations in Nursing Education: Advanced Concepts, Trends, and Opportunities* (Rizzolo, 2014).

TOOLS

Testing existing tools or developing new ones to use for scoring a simulation is a much bigger challenge and will require

(continued)

A CLEAR MESSAGE EMERGES FROM THE NLN HIGH-STAKES ASSESSMENT PROJECT *(continued)*

considerable research. Different tools or a combination of tools are required to measure different competencies of students at various points in the curriculum. Tools intended to evaluate higher-level learning, such as clinical judgment and reasoning, are extremely difficult to norm. Our study worked with one tool and found that the biggest challenge was gaining consensus on the criteria to use for scoring. For example, if the tool item is "collects appropriate assessment data" and there are four pieces of data that should be obtained, how do you score a student who only completes three assessments when the tool's scoring mechanism only permits a met or not met option? Resolving issues like this would be the challenge for any tool selected. A manuscript on the norming process used in this study is in development.

THE CLEAR MESSAGE

Watching simulation authors and raters all with a passion for simulation and fair evaluation practices, struggle with the norming process has provided me with new respect for the difficulty of this task. More importantly, it has opened my eyes to the varied expectations of faculty regarding clinical performance of students. For me, the clear message that has emerged from this study is that there is an urgent need for faculty to engage in deliberative conversations to clarify behaviors/expectations of students at the end of each course and at the end of the program. An exercise in creating a simulation exam can be a great stimulus to push for these conversations to occur. If it does, we will make giant strides, not only in improving our assessment practices, but also in resolving the huge discrepancy between faculty and employers regarding essential competencies of new graduates (Berkow et al., 2008).

Our current methods of evaluating the clinical practice competencies of students are woefully inadequate. While many challenges remain for using simulation as a method of summative assessment, I applaud the path taken by brave faculty (Wolf et al., 2011) and encourage others to follow their lead and help us fill in the potholes in the long, difficult road toward more fair, reliable, and valid assessment practices.

*S. Barry Issenberg, MD, Pamela R. Jeffries, PhD, RN, FAAN, ANEF, Kathie Lasater, EdD, RN, ANEF, Carrie B. Lenburg, EdD, RN, FAAN, ANEF, M. Bridget Nettleton, PhD, RN, Marilyn H. Oermann, PhD, RN, FAAN, ANEF, Mary Anne Rizzolo, EdD, RN, FAAN, ANEF, Theresa M. (Terry) Valiga, EdD, RN, FAAN, ANEF, Linda Wilson, PhD, RN, CPAN, CAPA, BC, CNE.

REFERENCES

Berkow, S., Virkstis, K., Stewart, J., & Conway, L. (2008). Assessing new graduate nurse performance. *Journal of Nursing Administration, 38*(11), 468–474.

Rizzolo, M. A. (2014). Developing and using simulation for high stakes assessment. In P. R. Jeffries (Ed.), *Clinical simulations in nursing education: Advanced concepts, trends, and opportunities* (Chap. 9). Washington, DC: National League for Nursing.

Stroud, L., Herold, J., Tomlinson, G., & Cavalcanti, R. B. (2011). Who you know or what you know? Effect of examiner familiarity with residents on OSCE scores. *Academic Medicine, 86*(10 Suppl.), S8–S11.

Willhaus, J., Burleson, G., Palaganas, J., & Jeffries, P. (2014). Authoring simulations for high-stakes student evaluation. *Clinical Simulation in Nursing, 10*(4), e177–e182.

Wolf, L., Dion, K., Lamoureaux, E., Kenny, C., Curnin, M., Hogan, M. A., . . . Cunningham, H. (2011). Using simulated clinical scenarios to evaluate student performance. *Nurse Educator, 36*(3), 128–134.

Acceptable passing standards for summative evaluation differ according to the learner level and may be constructive or absolute. Prelicensure student assessment is often constructive. For example, a finishing resident is judged to be competent or not via "static or pass/fail dichotomous ratings of competence," which are modified for novice residents early in training and at each level toward full competency in that skill (Holmboe & Hawkins, 2008). Program directors become responsible for framing accreditation competencies into the program and throughout the levels, often following a mastery learning model. In mastery learning, testing is used to gauge unit completion at a preset minimum passing standard (Kulik et al., 1990). Advancement to the next educational unit depends on a given measured achievement at or above the mastery standard (or there is continued practice until the mastery standard is reached), to ensure achievement of all educational objectives with the least amount of outcome variation (McGaghie et al., 2010). McGaghie et al. (2010) explain that mastery learning has seven complementary features:

1. Baseline (i.e., diagnostic) testing.
2. Clear learning objectives, sequenced as units ordered by increasing difficulty.
3. Engagement in educational activities (e.g., skills practice, data interpretation, reading) that are focused on reaching the objectives.

4. Establishment of a minimum passing standard (e.g., test score, checklist score) for each educational unit.
5. Formative testing to gauge unit completion at a preset minimum passing mastery standard.
6. Advancement to the next educational unit given measured achievement at or above the mastery standard.
7. Continued practice or study on an educational unit until the mastery standard is reached.

Because the goal of many postlicensure assessment programs is to bring all clinicians to an acceptable level of performance and not to rank-order them, only absolute performance standards are appropriate. Therefore, it is necessary to set reference standards for a defined performance measure (Lammers et al., 2008).

With respect to learner level, the process of standard setting should ensure that cut score setting (determination of competency score) is not arbitrary, but is reasonable, defensible, and fair. Absolute standards reflect a certain level of mastery. Most assessments set out to confirm that a domain of knowledge or skill has been mastered. A passing score should be determined through a systematic, reproducible, and unbiased process by a group of content experts for that learner group and level (Yudkowsky 2009).

Summative assessment simulations often require more resources (e.g., faculty time, simulation staff, equipment) than written examination or educational simulations. When choosing to use HCS, educators must first determine whether or not HCS is the most appropriate assessment tool for the competency level (e.g., Miller's Pyramid) being assessed. Simulations should be developed and criteria chosen appropriate to the level of the learner. Dry runs (practice run-throughs) of the simulation with learners from the target group are necessary to determine appropriateness and fairness of the simulation-based assessment.

BIAS FOUND IN HEALTHCARE SIMULATION
Janice C. Palaganas, PhD, RN, NP
Author, Researcher, Assessor, and Assessor Trainer for the National League for Nursing High-Stakes Assessment Multi-Site Research Study

When developing or analyzing assessment activities, biases described in research, assessment, and education literature are often considered, and measures are taken to screen for such biases. There are different sources of bias that are described in research literature (e.g., threats to internal, external, construct, and statistical conclusion validity). A goal in constructing an assessment test is to create a test in which inferences made by assessors of a learner's competence or skill level is accurate (or valid) and the assessment platform is seemingly as real as possible to the event or skill being assessed. This accuracy can be undermined by bias. Some common research, assessment, and education biases and a description of each are listed briefly in Table 1. Like any assessment activity, these biases occur often in simulation assessment. There is extensive research behind each of these biases that are beyond the focus of this textbox and chapter. In addition to research and education bias, there is also simulation bias that is often overlooked in simulation-based assessment. This chapter will focus briefly here on these types of simulation biases commonly observed in simulation-based assessment.

FAMILIARITY EFFECTS
Learners previously exposed to simulations have a familiarity with simulation that can allow them to anticipate or miss many assessment items, causing a familiarity effect. Learners who are familiar with simulation may be more comfortable in the assessment and may perform better than those learners who are not. Paradoxically, learners familiar with simulation may also demonstrate simulation habits in the assessment that may harm their scores. Some common familiarity effects include the following:
• **Modality Familiarity Effect.** Learners influenced by this bias will perform physical assessments on the modality within its limitations. For example, if a mannequin was being used, the learner may know where to feel a pulse and easily distinguish mannequin breath sounds through the mechanical overlay in comparison with another learner not influenced by this bias. Similarly, if a standardized patient was used, a learner familiar with this modality may more readily physically assess the patient, or if a virtual simulator was used, a learner familiar with this modality may be more facile with the haptic equipment. Another presentation of the

TABLE 1

Common Biases Seen in Simulation-Based Assessment

Bias in Literature	How It May Appear in Simulation	Additional Resources
Design bias	When the simulation was not structured or screened to control for internal (does not allow for observation of the item) and external (the item being assessed does not fit the simulation or learner group) validity.	Cook and Campbell (1979)
Assessor's bias	Untrained assessor rates lower or higher, may know some learners and grade differently, may not have the adequate experience or knowledge to assess the skill. This is also known as "experimentor bias" or "investigator bias." Also presents in the trained assessor as a "rater drift," where the assessor over time drifts toward their expectation despite adjustments made during rater training.	Fernandez-Ballesteros (2003); see "Assessors" section
Procedural bias	Learners feel psychologically unsafe in being assessed or in the simulation environment.	Cook and Campbell (1979)
Halo effect	When the assessor is positively influenced by his/her impression of a learner (physical appearance, reputation, personality). Reverse-halo effect is when the assessor is negatively influenced by learner factors.	Nisbett and Wilson (1977)
Inference distortion	When one group of learners (from different profession, learned from a different professor, different school) learned something different, used a different learning method, or did not learn the item being assessed.	Popham (2012)
Demographic bias	Gender, racial, socioeconomic, profession bias.	Popham (2012)
Simulation Bias	**How It May Appear in Simulation**	**Additional Resources**
Familiarity effect	Includes modality familiarity effect, simulated resource familiarity effect, trained simulation habit effect, informed effect, and hypothesis-guessed simulation	See Familiarity Effects
New-to-simulation effect	Includes pauses, delays, laughing, and other awkward behavior of a learner new to simulation during a simulation.	See New-to-Simulation Effects
Simulation external validity	When two or more simulations assessing a skill or set of skills differs. This may appear through the facilitation skills of the ESP or scenario director.	See Simulation External Validity

(continued)

CONSIDER THIS

BIAS FOUND IN HEALTHCARE SIMULATION *(continued)*

modality familiarity effect is a willing dismissal of any technological glitches, including the simulation monitor.

- **Simulated Resource Familiarity Effect.** The learner familiar with simulated resources may access embedded simulated providers more readily, interviewing them extensively throughout the simulation, as well as immediately accessing other resources such as code team, other team members, charge nurse, or attending physician.
- **Trained Simulation Habit Effect.** Learners develop simulation habits that stem from undergoing many simulations at a previous simulation program. These habits may positively or negatively bias assessment activities. Trained simulation habits are often difficult to assess because some learners may have learned the habit in clinical practice, whereas for others they may be natural habits. Some habits often noted as positive during assessment include washing hands immediately before and after patient contact, use of gloves, and communicating out loud so that the scenario facilitators are able to hear the learner's thoughts and needs. Other trained simulation habits include making inquiries to the scenario facilitators behind the camera or window (e.g., attempting to engage with a facilitator via microphones in the room who might answer their questions via speakers, also known as "voice of God").
- **Informed Effect.** As an assessment simulation repeats with learners over time, there is a possibility that a previous learner may have informed a current learner on the cases being simulated or any other aspect of the simulation-based assessment that may allow the current learner to anticipate events or skills to perform. Learner ethics and code of conduct may be questioned in this case. Frequently, because the simulation interacts with learner actions and the informed learner may not have the same actions as the informant learner, the scenario may progress differently than what was previously informed.
- **Hypothesis-Guessed Simulation.** Some learners are familiar with the flexibility of simulation, often psychologically engrossed with a previous simulation case, and may steer the simulation in the direction of a diagnosis or finding that they self-select during a simulation. In research, the bias "hypothesis guessing" occurs when a subject's performance is influenced by their knowledge of findings that they expect to gather (Cook & Campbell, 1979). For example, a learner may state out loud that there is a foreign object in the airway when there is not and progress through the simulation as though the case was an airway obstruction. This learner may have done this because of something he saw in the airway, likely attributed to the simulator, or because he was anticipating this scenario. Regardless of the reason, simulation is a flexible method. Learners are familiar with this flexibility and do not feel the limitations of the case, steering the simulation down a self-determined path. This bias may be redirected

through the facilitation of an embedded simulated provider.

NEW-TO-SIMULATION EFFECTS

Learners new to simulation are often distracted by the unfamiliar environment, equipment, process, or modality (e.g., mannequin, standardized patient, virtual simulator, etc.). This may create pauses or delays in performance. The unfamiliar simulation may impede on a learner's fiction contract (see Experts' Corner: Helping Learners "Buy in" to Simulation), allowing awkward behaviors such as laughing or appearing frozen. The learner not familiar with a modality may be reluctant to physically touch the modality or do what (s)he would do in a real-life setting. This may create false-negative results when being assessed in a simulated environment.

THE PROBLEM WITH SIMULATION EXTERNAL VALIDITY

External validity in the setting of simulation is the consistency of a simulation that could be generalized to other simulation programs. If a learner were to be assessed on the same skill or set of skills at different sites or different days with different simulation facilitators, the learner should, in fair assessment, achieve the same assessment scores. Simulation programs organically form as a result of needs and resources, especially human resources. The differing nature of simulation programs is its own threat to simulation external validity. Because simulation programs differ from site to site, including those within organizations, it is extremely difficult to standardize a simulation. Cues may be given at one site or in one simulation, where it is not given (or at the same degree) as another. There may also be **Facilitator Bias** where a simulation is facilitated more smoothly by experienced embedded simulated participants or by the scenario director who can anticipate events and has the experience to interact more immediately with the learners' actions. Equipment may also differ, with one or more potentially subtracting or adding to the realism of the case. Assessment scores may differ from one site to another site or one simulation with certain simulation staff to another simulation with other simulation staff. One way to help overcome these problems with external validity and replication is to provide example videos of how the simulation should look and be conducted.

REFERENCES

Cook, T. D., & Campbell, D. T. (1979). *Quasi-experimentation: Design & analysis issues for field settings.* Chicago, IL: Rand McNally.

Fernandez-Ballesteros, R. (Ed.). (2003). *Encyclopedia of psychological assessment.* Thousand Oaks, CA: SAGE.

Nisbett, R. E., & Wilson, T. D. (1977). The halo effect: Evidence for unconscious alteration of judgments. *Journal of Personality and Social Psychology,* 35(4), 250–256.

Popham, W. J. (2012). *Assessment bias: How to banish it.* Boston, MA: Pearson.

ASSESSORS

The selection of appropriately qualified and fair assessors (or people who perform the assessment through observation and an assessment tool, also known as "raters") and the training of assessors is a critical component of fair and consistent assessment. A process should be developed to match

the characteristics of the assessment with the qualifications of assessors by virtue of their experience and education. Once qualified assessors are selected, a systematic training program must be implemented (Feldman et al. 2012; see Table 7.3.2, below). Dry runs (practice run-through of the simulation prior to the exercise) are key in the process of training assessors. Reference copies of the relevant assessment tool, the scenario progression, policies regarding the activity, the assessor evaluation rating tool, and fellow assessor files should be made available for all assessors at the appropriate times.

How to Train Assessors

Holmboe and Hawkins describe two types of accuracy measures in rating: the first kind are decisions whether the behavior did or did not occur (checklists). The other type involves "judgmental measures," where the assessor must apply a judgment involving accuracy when providing a rating: accuracy in whether a learner has attained a level of performance (criterion accuracy), accuracy in distinguishing among learners (normative accuracy), and accuracy in discriminating between a performance or competence dimension (stereotype accuracy; Holmboe & Hawkins, 2008). Observational assessment of learners in clinical settings, and, by extension, to simulation settings, can fall prey to subjectivity, false impressions, ageism, racism, sexism, and misinterpretation (McGaghie et al., 2009). In Performance Dimension Training (PDT), raters receive expected performance standards for each level of performance. Assessors receive "Frame of Reference" training where they define "satisfactory" performance (the anchor point) and practice evaluating. Assessors need to reach agreement on common nomenclature for the desired expectations of interest, and agree on the relative importance of the different components of the behavior being assessed (Holmboe & Hawkins, 2008).

Assessor errors include halo, leniency, severity, central tendency, and idiosyncratic rating and are described in Table 7.3.1 (Downing, 2003). In addition, Feldman et al. (2012) list and define rater training components in Table 7.3.2.

Once the assessors are trained, Feldman et al. (2012) explain how to assess the reliability of raters' scores. They describe two primary methods for assessing the reliability of the Simulation-Based Training ratings as a whole:

1. Agreement is the most simple and most common. Agreement tells you whether or not your raters picked exactly the same score for a particular behavior.

2. Correlations tell you whether or not your raters followed similar patterns, but not whether they agreed exactly.

Assessor training should occur with use of the rating method with which the assessor will rate learners—whether it is a live simulation or video. The mean of the passing score for each item is determined, with the passing score for the case being the simple average of passing scores for all items. The researcher or educator directing the assessment program should seek to understand any differences in ratings of the same case and find ways to create consistency between assessors; this may include elimination of a rater who consistently scores too high or too low relative to the other assessors. Assessor performance should be routinely (annually at minimum) evaluated to ensure inter-rater reliability (consistency across assessors) and to evaluate individual assessor competence.

PROGRAMMATIC ASPECTS

Assessment requires as optimally controlled an environment as possible to ensure consistent cases for learners and assessors, and requires the facilities, simulation staffing, and technology to support this level of standardization. The facilities and technology should also be appropriate to the individual or teams being assessed.

Dry runs are recommended to highlight potential inconsistencies between simulations. The assessment should begin with a standardized orientation of the learner to the environment and assessment tools, followed by implementation of the standardized simulation.

Assessment does not end after the activity. Adequate technical and research support is needed for the appropriate analysis of data. Just as the assessors should be appropriately qualified, so should the human factors, psychometric, and statistical support. Most institutions (educational and hospital) have resources and departments accessible for support. Because of the high-stakes implications in summative assessment, a process and secure plan must be developed, implemented, and maintained to ensure confidentiality, data, and test security.

SECTION 7 • Educational Development

TABLE 7.3.1

Assessor Bias Errors

Rater Error	Description	Consequence
Central tendency	Avoiding extreme positive or negative ratings.	Reduces ability to discriminate performance.
Halo error	All ratings based on one very positive or negative observation.	Positively or negatively skewed ratings.
Primacy/recency effect	All ratings based on observations made early or late in the scenario.	Positively or negatively skewed ratings.
Contrast effect	Ratings are made relative to performance of previous group.	Positively skewed ratings when prior group performed very poorly, negatively skewed ratings when prior group performed very well.
Potential effect	Ratings based on perceptions of future potential.	Usually positively skewed ratings.
Similar-to-me effect	Ratings based on degree of similarity to the rater.	Tendency to rate people who resemble themselves higher.
Stereotype effect	Ratings based on group inclusion rather than individual differences.	Positively or negatively biased ratings for some groups.

TABLE 7.3.2

Feldman et al.'s How to Train a Rater Checklist

Feldman et al.'s "How-to" Rater Training Curriculum Components
- *How* to Assess Reliability
- **Over Time**
  Same observer scores the same video-taped scenario at two different points in time
- **Across Multiple Raters**
  Two different observers score the same scenario
  In real time
  Video
- **Percent Agreement**
  Agreements/(agreements + disagreements)
  Number of times observers agree
  Number of opportunities to agree
  Tasks:
  1. Pair up with a buddy.
  2. Use the measurement tool that both you and your buddy used during previous exercise.
  3. Compute inter-rater agreement using the ratings you did in the previous exercise (p. 9).
  4. Debrief to entire group.
     a. What teamwork dimensions did you use for this exercise?
     b. What was your inter-rater agreement?
     c. What were the challenges?
- Courtesy of Rosen, Types of Rater Training
- **Rater Error Training (RET)**
  Focuses on *avoiding* rater errors and biases.
- **Performance Dimension Training (PDT)**
  Focuses on *defining* skill dimension.
- **Frame of Reference Training (FOR)**
  Focuses on *discriminating* between skill levels.
- Rater Error Training
- Reduces occurrence of rating errors.
- Refine and Realign
- Raters discuss where and why they disagreed.
- Goal is to come to consensus on how to rate behavior using observed examples.
- Rating "rules" can be generated to help in addition to the rating guide.
- Rating skills are refined and realigned to common criterion.
- Normative Reference Strategy
- Rating standards and rules are developed through a consensus process between a group of raters.
- Reliability and validity are assessed by comparing ratings across raters and dimensions.
- Accuracy, sensitivity, and reliability are relative to the group of raters.
- Raters refine and realign until adequate level of reliability is reached.
- Criterion Reference Strategy
- Rating standards and rules are developed using an expert set of raters and set of examples.
- Reliability and validity are assessed by comparing raters to expert ratings using standard set of example scenarios.
- Accuracy, sensitivity, and reliability are relative to an expert set of "gold standard" ratings.
- Raters refine and realign until adequate reliability is found with expert ratings.
- Comparing Strategies

- Reliability and Rater Turnover
- Quality Monitoring and Improvement
- QMI should be a continuous process.
- Has implications for effectiveness of training, planning, and performance improvement.
- Key PointsRaters should be knowledgeable about the task being rated, but experts are more resistant to training to external criterion.
- Raters with similar backgrounds rate more similarly.
- Expert and novice raters have been shown to rate with adequate levels of reliability with effective rater training.
- Consider external factors such as availability, buy-in, and potential biases.

Feldman, M., Lazzara, E., Vanderbilt, A., & DiazGranados, D. (2012). Rater training to support high-stakes simulation-based assessments. *Journal of Continuing Education in the Health Professions*, *32*(4), 279–286.

ASSESSMENT TOOLS

There are generally two types of assessment tools with which learners are observed and graded: checklists and global rating scales. These are used to assess procedural skills, critical decision making, team skills, and communication. Assessment tools are typically scored in the following way:

- **Checklists:** items are scored dichotomously (e.g., done or not done).

- **Weighted Checklists:** items judged to be more critical to a successful procedure are assigned higher point values.
- **Rating Scales:** each item is assigned points on a scale.

Assessment tool development is highly complex. For example, when developing an assessment test or tool, the assessment group or tool developers need to determine what the passing score is, also known as the "test cut score" (Yudkowsky, 2009). This cut score and standard setting is determined by content experts. In a contrasting group procedure for standard setting, five or more assessors with content expertise are selected to divide the scores into categories such as pass/fail. The assessors must have a full understanding and be in agreement about the scope and dimension of all behaviors expected in each performance category for that learner level. The cut point demarcates the boundaries between those performance categories on the exam score distributions (Yudkowsky et al., 2009). In the "Angoff Standard-Setting Procedure," judgments are carried out at the item level. On a scale of 0 to 1.0, each assessor answers independently, "what is the probability that one borderline score will accomplish this item correctly?" (Yudkowsky et al., 2009, p. 133). Divergent ratings might then be discussed and assessors have the opportunity to modify their judgments if they wish.

A process should be developed for the selection of appropriate assessment tools, specifically to ensure that the tool selected is appropriate, reliable, valid, and fits well with the testing conditions and requirements. The creation of a tool that is valid and reliable often can take years of expert psychometric and statistical support. For this reason, educators and researchers with time constraints for their simulation education delivery are encouraged to reference existing valid and reliable tools published in the literature. These tools are typically developed and vetted for a specific research purpose at a specific institution, so the challenge faced by adopting or adapting published tools might be that while the tool is a good fit for its developed purpose, it may not be an adequate fit for another assessment focus at another institution. Challenging factors include the following:

- The tool was tested on a specific group of learners in a specific circumstance that may not be similar or apply to another assessor's learners or circumstances.
- The tool was designed for healthcare providers who are coming into the simulation with a different level or amount of knowledge and expertise than those students of another assessor.
- The tool was designed to "test out" credentialed healthcare providers, not teach healthcare students.

Many programs are not familiar with the best practices requirement for validity and reliability and choose homegrown tools without any history of testing for validity (the tool is accurately measuring the intended variable) and reliability (the items are clear enough to establish a general consistency with each item across assessors). Some programs that are familiar with the need for valid and reliable tools often adapt published tools and change items on the adopted published tool to better fit their assessment need. However, when tools are tested for validity and reliability, the test comprises a holistic analysis, meaning that any change made to an existing tool threatens and discredits the validity and reliability of that tool.

The process of selecting a site-specific institutional simulation assessment can be guided with the Assessment Tool Selection Template presented in this section (Table 7.3.3). This Assessment Tool Selection Template addresses the necessary considerations mentioned throughout this chapter, linking the specific objectives, learners, learning goals, and learning needs to the particular institutional performance goal. As an example, the opening case study will be revisited and addressed using this template.

Steps to using this framework as a guide:

1. First, together with your faculty, fill out who, what, which, and why. This determines the learner levels and specialties, learning goals, and the institutional and/or curricular need.
2. Now, fill in your ideal performances and which measures would indicate passing of that measure.
3. From this, you can decide the appropriate simulation environment and modality.
4. Finally, perform a peer-reviewed literature search, and select the appropriate assessment tool to use or plan to develop.

Once an assessment tool is chosen, assessors must be trained (see "Assessors" section above). This training establishes a level of inter-rater reliability (concordance in scores between assessors). During assessor training, assessors may adjust expectations of items to be in concordance with other assessors. Over time, this adjustment may "drift" toward their initial expectations. Because of this, repeated reevaluation of inter-rater reliability is needed.

SIMULATION MODALITIES AND ASSESSMENT TOOLS

Assessment is traditionally done in domains of measurable skills from history taking, physical examination, procedural performance, clinical decision making, and patient management to such areas as teamwork, cultural competence, and professionalism. The ACGME Toolbox of Assessment Methods suggests that HCSs are most appropriate for evaluations of those outcomes that require trainees to "show how" they are competent to perform (Scalese & Issenberg, 2008).

One attractive benefit in using HCS for assessment is that it can provide a consistent platform for rater observation of learner performance. Instruments for simulation evaluation are increasingly reliable with some promising validity (Kardong-Edgren et al., 2010).

Learners are tested with these checklists or rating scales in a variety of simulation "scenarios" in one or another of

TABLE 7.3.3		
Assessment Tool Selection Template		
Consideration	**Example**	**Fill in as Appropriate**
WHO gets the simulation?		
Professions and levels	**Surgical PG Y-1 to PGY-2**	
	Surgical Physician Assistant Students	
	Critical Care Nurse Practitioner Students	
WHAT is the learning goal?	**CVC Placement**	
WHICH CVC placement will you teach? ... because?	**US-guided IJ CVC placement** because: American Society of Anesthesiologists Task Force recommendation	
WHY (the need in your environment is)? -Institutional -Curricular -Both	**US-guided is safest for patient population:** previous complications, underlying vascular anomalies, limited access sites for attempts, difficult to identify surface landmarks, inexperienced operators **Both** Pine Hospital reports mechanical errors; pneumothorax, artery punctures; learner levels have been assessed "not up to standard" during live IJ CVC placement	
Ideal Performances	**Perform US-guided IJ CVC insertion with no mechanical errors in under 15 minutes**	
By which Passing Measures?	a. Learners must make fewer than three needle passes b. Learners must demonstrate successful location and cannulation of vein on first try—no artery attempts	
Which Simulation Modality(s) are the most appropriate for these performance measures?	**Partial Task Trainer (PTT)** 1. Blue Phantom anthropomorphic simulation US training model, Advanced Medical Technologies, LLC 2. central venous access head neck and upper torso simulation model, Advanced Medical Technologies, LLC	
Choose Assessment tool type and tool	**Checklist** **Pine Hospital US IJ CVC Simulation Placement Checklist (Author, Year)**	

"Example column" based in part on Evans et al. (2010).

the simulation modalities. Testing of team, communication, cognitive, or psychomotor skills best takes place in the simulation modality appropriate to that skill domain. A key principle of Simulation-Based Education (SBE) is that educational goals must dictate decisions about the acquisition and use of simulation technology (McGaghie et al., 2010). In HCS-based assessment, assessments might be grouped into five major modalities: partial task trainers, SPs, hybrid, mannequin-based, and virtual reality (VR). These modalities are described below with example assessment tools appropriate or common to each modality.

Partial Task Trainers

Static simulators that reproduce anatomic regions and/or clinical task events provide education and assessment in basic procedural skills such as intravenous line insertion, suturing, intubation, and lumbar puncture (Scalese & Issenberg, 2008). Partial task trainers mimic body parts or regions (e.g., the arms, pelvis, or torso). These trainers are scaled from infant to adult sizes. They range technically from simulated skin with "blood"-filled veins to moving organs with appropriate vasculature viewable on ultrasound machines. These trainers also differ by specialty (e.g., for surgical skills, multilayered pads are used with cutdown procedures, cyst removal, subcuticular suturing, and knot tying; for anesthesia, there are airway trainers;

for obstetrics and urology, there are birthing trainers, and simulators of the pelvis/perineum). There are also computerized task trainers such as a cardiopulmonary patient simulator with blood pressure, arterial, venous, and precordial pulses as well as heart and lung sounds synchronized to simulate 30 different cardiac conditions (Scalese & Issenberg, 2008).

Simulation Assessment Tools for Partial Task Trainers

There are two common assessment tools used for partial task trainers: the checklist and the rating scale.

1. **Technical dichotomous checklist, individual** Checklist items are statements or questions that reflect concrete, observable behaviors that can be scored dichotomously as "done" or "not done." An example of this is the "Objective Structured Assessment for Technical Skills" (OSATS) by Martin et al. (1997). Specifically, in Figure 7.3.2, the *Control of Hemorrhage Checklist below*, each OSATS technical dichotomous checklist comprises a list of items to be checked "done" or "not done".

2. **Global rating scale** The rating scale is used to demonstrate how well the individual performed a procedure or action in

| | | | RESIDENT STICKER | STATION 4 CONTROL OF HAEMORRHAGE |

| RESIDENT STICKER | STATION 4 CONTROL OF HAEMORRHAGE |

INSTRUCTIONS TO CANDIDATES

You have just identified a stab wound to the inferior vena cava. Control the haemorrhage and repair the vessel.

Start Time:

CHECKLIST

ITEM	Not Done/ Done Incorrectly	Done Correctly
CONTROL OF HEMORRHAGE		
1. Applies pressure to stop bleeding <u>first</u>	0	1
2. Asks assistant to suction field	0	1
3. Inspects injury by carefully releasing the IVC	0	1
4. Ensures all equipment needed for repair is at hand before starting	0	1
5. Control of bleeding point (use deBakey forceps /Satinsky clamp or prox/distal pressure)	0	1
REPAIR		
6. Select appropriate suture (4.0/5.0/6.0 polypropylene)	0	1
7. Select appropriate needle driver (vascular)	0	1
8. Select appropriate forceps (de Bakey)	0	1
9. Needle loaded 1/2–2/3 from tip 90% of time	0	1

FIGURE 7.3.2 Example of technical dichotomous checklist rating of individual, *OSATS Control of Hemorrhage Checklist.* (Reprinted with permission from Martin, J., Regehr, G., Reznick, R., Macrae, H., Murnaghan, J., Hutchison, C., & Brown, M. [1997]. Objective structured assessment of technical skill (OSATS) for surgical residents. *British Journal of Surgery, 84*(2), 273–278.)

a static setting (e.g., how well the physical therapist provided information on cardiac rehabilitation or how well respiratory therapist handled ventilator). Rating scales rate the item along a spectrum of response options. The items on this type of tool often presents as numeral points, assessing aspects of a skill commonly measured on a 3-, 4-, 5-, or 7-point scale (also known as Likert scale after the psychologist Likert who studied the use of numeral point items to create a simple sum) (Figure 7.3.3).

3. **Technical Behaviorally Anchored Rating Scale (BARS), individual**

Because scales can lead to subjective judgment, behaviorally anchored items are often provided for the rating options to theoretically improve consensus among raters. This is called a "Behaviorally Anchored Rating Scale." For example, the OSATS

"Technical Domain-Specific rating scale with behavioral anchors" (Martin et al., 1997) includes a number of items all assessing aspects of operative skill and the anchoring of points 1, 3, and 5 on the 5-point scale by behavioral descriptors (Figure 7.3.4). The OSATS technical rating scale is used to demonstrate how well the individual performed a procedure or action in a static setting, for example operatively controlled and repaired a hemorrhage in terms of "respect for tissue," "time and motion," "instrument handling." Rating scales rate the item along a spectrum of response options, usually no more than 7 (Yudowsky, Downing, & Tekian, 2009). Because scales can lead to subjective judgment, behaviorally anchored items are provided for the rating options and therefore improve consensus among raters. Kim et al. (2009) note that rating scales, in indicating

Directions: Circle the number that most closely corresponds to your observations of the employee. Do this on at least two different occasions.

Scale: 1 = Poor   2 = Below average   3 = Average   4 = Above average   5 = Excellent

Knowledge of work:	1	2	3	4	5
Clinical skills:	1	2	3	4	5
Communication skills:	1	2	3	4	5
Concern for patient safety:	1	2	3	4	5
Concern for team:	1	2	3	4	5
Overall quality of work:	1	2	3	4	5

Total:

FIGURE 7.3.3   Example of nontechnical Global Rating Scale, rating of individual, *End-of-Year Global Rating Employee Assessment Scale.*

how well the action was performed and not simply that it was "done or not done," is best for reporting levels of expertise (see Figure 7.3.4). (Note: Use of this tool for partial task training assumes that there will be an assessment of fine-grained skills with tissue, e.g., surgical suturing with a beef tongue.)

Standardized Patients

An SP is

a person who has been carefully coached to simulate an actual patient so accurately that the simulation cannot be detected by a skilled clinician. In performing the simulation, the simulated patient presents the "gestalt" of the patient being simulated; not just the history, but the body language, the physical findings and the emotional and personality characteristics as well. (Barrows & Abrahamson, 1964; see chapter 3.3)

SPs are trained to provide a consistent account of their condition, answer a range of questions about themselves, and can portray people from a variety of cultures, ethnicities, and/or those with communication problems and/or specific mental or physical conditions. The SP is trained to provide standardized answers and behaviors so that a group of students can be reliably tested. SPs are to be distinguished from "Embedded Simulated Persons" (ESPs)

in mannequin simulation. ESPs are embedded acting participants leveraged to facilitate the learners through objectives in the simulation (see chapter 3.3). SPs are also trained to evaluate the healthcare students' skills in history taking, physical exam, clinical reasoning, and ability to take part in a challenging conversation, as well as general communication skills on the basis of a checklist of items. The SP proceeds through the interaction with the student and then scores the student on the basis of their observations (McLaughlin et al., 2006). SP simulations are used exclusively (without task trainers or other simulation modalities) in many medical, graduate nursing, and physician assistant schools as Objective Structured Clinical Examinations (OSCE). OSCEs are also used in board exams such as the USMLE in the US and MCC in Canada.

Simulation Assessment Tools for SPs

Below are examples of scales used in SP simulations that are designed to be rated by the SPs themselves, as well as scales that are designed to be rated by faculty (Figure 7.3.5, Tables 7.3.4 and 7.3.5).

Hybrid Simulation (Mixed Modality)

"Hybrid" simulations use multiple modalities to achieve the objective of the assessment. For example, an SP can

Please rate the candidate's performance on the following scale:

	1	2	3	4	5
Respect for tissue	Frequently used unnecessary force on tissue or caused damage by inappropriate use of instruments		Careful handling of tissue but occasionally caused inadvertent damage.		Consistently handled tissues appropriately with minimal damage.
Time and motion	Many unnecessary moves		Efficient time/motion but some unnecessary moves.		Economy of movement and maximum efficiency
Instrument handling	Repeatedly makes tentative or awkward moves with instruments.		Competent use of instruments although occasionally appeared stiff or awkward.		Fluid moves with instruments and no awkwardness.
Knowledge of instruments	Frequently asked for the wrong instrument or used on inappropriate instrument.		Knew the names of most instruments and used appropriate instrument for the task.		Obviously familiar with the instruments required and their names.
Use of assistants	Consistently placed assistants poorly or failed to use accidents.		Good use of assistants most of the time.		Strategically used assistant to the best advantage at all times.
Flow of operation and forward planning	Frequently stopped operating or needed to discuss next move.		Demonstrated ability for forward planning with steady progression of operative procedure.		Obviously planned course of operation with effortless flow from one move to the next.
Knowledge of specific procedure	Deficient knowledge. Needed specific instruction at most operative steps.		Knew all important aspects of the operation.		Demonstrated familiarity with all aspects of the operation.

Overall, on this task, should this candidate: ☐ **Pass**   ☐ **Fail?**

FIGURE 7.3.4 Example of technical, Behaviorally Anchored Rating Scale, rating of individual, *OSATS*. (Reprinted with permission from Martin, J., Regehr, G., Reznick, R., Macrae, H., Murnaghan, J., Hutchison, C., & Brown, M. [1997]. Objective structured assessment of technical skill (OSATS) for surgical residents. *British Journal of Surgery, 84*(2), 273–278.)

SECTION 7 • Educational Development

	Strongly agree 1	Agree 2	Neutral 3	Disagree 4	Disagree strongly 5
a. Rapport and relationship building—an overarching skill Rating _____					
b. Opens the discussion Rating _____					
c. Gathers information Rating _____					
d. Understands patient's perspective Rating _____					
e. Shares information Rating _____					
f. Reaches agreement on problems and plans Rating _____					
g. Provides closure Rating _____					
h. Addresses family interviewing skills Rating _____					

FIGURE 7.3.5 Example of nontechnical Likert scale, rating of individual, individual to be rated by faculty, *Kalamazoo Communication Rating Scale*. (Reprinted with permission from Makoul, G. [2001]. Essential elements of communication in medical encounters: The Kalamazoo consensus statement. *Academic Medicine, 76*(4), 390–393.)

TABLE 7.3.4

Example of Nontechnical Likert Scale, Rating of Individual; Individual to Be Rated by SP: UIC CIS Scale, 2006

Please Rate Your Agreement with Each Item	Rating
I felt you greeted me warmly upon entering the room.	( ) Strongly disagree ( ) Disagree ( ) Neutral ( ) Agree ( ) Strongly agree ( ) Not applicable
I felt you were friendly throughout the encounter. You were never crabby or rude to me.	( ) Strongly disagree ( ) Disagree ( ) Neutral ( ) Agree ( ) Strongly agree ( ) Not applicable
I felt that you treated me like we were on the same level. You never "talked down" to me or treated me like a child.	( ) Strongly disagree ( ) Disagree ( ) Neutral ( ) Agree ( ) Strongly agree ( ) Not applicable
I felt you let me tell my story and were careful to not interrupt me while I was speaking.	( ) Strongly disagree ( ) Disagree ( ) Neutral ( ) Agree ( ) Strongly agree ( ) Not applicable
I felt you showed interest in me as a "person." You never acted bored or ignored what I had to say.	( ) Strongly disagree ( ) Disagree ( ) Neutral ( ) Agree ( ) Strongly agree ( ) Not applicable
I felt you were patient when I asked questions.	( ) Strongly disagree ( ) Disagree ( ) Neutral ( ) Agree ( ) Strongly agree ( ) Not applicable
I felt the resident displayed a positive attitude during the verbal feedback session.	( ) Strongly disagree ( ) Disagree ( ) Neutral ( ) Agree ( ) Strongly agree ( ) Not applicable

Reprinted with permission from Yudkowsky, R., Downing, S. M., & Sandlow, L. J. (2006). Developing an institution-based assessment of resident communication and interpersonal skills. *Academic Medicine, 81*, 1115–1122.

TABLE 7.3.5

Example of Nontechnical Rating BARS; Individual to Be Rated by SP, RUCIS Scale, 2009

UIC CIS 2009 (RUCIS)

Please choose the option that best describes how you feel toward the resident's communication skills. Some items also have a "not applicable" option. Select this option when the context of the case does not allow you to observe that aspect of the resident's performance.

1. **Friendly communication**
   ( ) You did not greet me, or greeted me perfunctorily, or communicated with me rudely during the encounter.
   ( ) Your greeting and/or behavior during the encounter was generally polite but impersonal or distant.
   ( ) You greeted me warmly and communicated with me in a friendly, personal manner throughout the encounter.
   ( ) Your greeting and overall communication were friendly and compassionate. Overall, you created an exceptionally warm and friendly environment that made me feel comfortable to tell you all of my problems.

2. **Respectful treatment**
   ( ) You showed an obvious sign of disrespect during the encounter. For example: You treated me as an inferior.
   ( ) You did not show disrespect to me. However, I observed some signs of condescending behavior. Although I believe it was unintentional, it made me feel that I was not at the same level with you.
   ( ) You gave several indications of respecting me. If there was a physical exam, this includes draping me appropriately.
   ( ) You were exceptionally respectful throughout the encounter. Your verbal and nonverbal communication showed respect for my privacy, my opinions, my rights, and/or my socioeconomic status, etc.

3. **Listening to my story**
   ( ) You rarely gave me any opportunity to tell my story and/or frequently interrupted me while I was talking, not allowing me to finish what I said. Sometimes I felt you were not paying attention (e.g., you asked for information that I already provided).
   ( ) You let me tell my story without interruption, or only interrupted appropriately and respectfully. You seemed to pay attention to my story and responded to what I said appropriately.
   ( ) You allowed me to tell my story without inappropriate interruption, responded appropriately to what I said, and asked thoughtful questions to encourage me to tell more of my story.
   ( ) You were an exceptional listener. You encouraged me to tell my story and checked your understanding by restating important points.

4. **Honest communication**
   ( ) You did not seem truthful and frank. I felt that there might be something that you were trying to hide from me.
   ( ) You did not seem to hide any critical information from me.
   ( ) You explained the facts of the situation without trivializing negative information or possibilities (e.g., side effects, complications, failure rates).
   ( ) You were exceptionally frank and honest. You fully explained the positive and negative aspects of my condition. You openly acknowledged your own lack of knowledge or uncertainty, and things you would have to consult with others. When appropriate, you also suggested I seek a second opinion.
   ( ) **Not applicable.** There was no information for the clinician to provide.

5. **Interest in me as a person**
   ( ) You never showed interest in me as a person. You only focused on the disease or medical issue.
   ( ) In addition to talking about my medical issue, you spent some time getting to know me as a person.
   ( ) You spent some time exploring how my medical issue affects my personal or social life.

Reprinted with permission from Iramaneerat, C., Myford, C. M., Yudkowsky, R., & Lowenstein, T. (2009). Evaluating the effectiveness of rating instruments for a communication skills assessment of medical residents. *Advances in Health Sciences Education, 14*, 575–594.

be used in conjunction with partial task trainers and mannequins (Kneebone et al., 2005).

Nontechnical scale with Likert evaluation. Kneebone et al.'s (2006) "Integrated Procedural Performance Instrument (IPPI)" is used, where the assessment combines SPs with partial task trainers and medical equipment (Figure 7.3.6).

Mannequin-Based Simulation

Complex clinical events such as team responses to simulated hospital emergencies require use of lifelike full-body mannequins that have computer-driven physiological features (e.g., heart rate, blood pressure) and ability for the performance of procedures that are invasive or traumatic (e.g., IV insertion, chest compressions). With staff facilitation or programming, these mannequins can respond to physical interventions, react appropriately, and record clinical events in real time (McGaghie et al., 2010).

Mannequin simulators comprise the functionality and programming to represent a wide range of pathophysiology and to respond dynamically to user actions. Many MBS are used in crisis management skills because they can be programmed with a wide range of responses and can adapt to emergencies. For example, an MBS may simulate blood pressure, multiple peripheral arterial pulses, breath and heart sounds, muscle twitches from nerve simulation, papillary reflexes, salivation, lacrimation, and bleeding from several anatomic sites (Scalese & Issenberg, 2008). In MBS, vital signs can be displayed in real time; it can respond to the administration of multiple medications and procedures, including intubation and ventilation, chest compressions, and defibrillation; needle or tube thoracostomy and arterial and venous cannulation. Many mannequin simulators have built-in preprogrammed patient profiles and can simulate scenarios involving those patients, and can also be customized. Owing to its peripheral pulses with oxygen saturation and electrocardiographic and other monitoring capabilities for evaluation of advanced cardiac and moulage, it can teach and assess trauma skills. Some mannequins can assess some adult and neonate obstetric skills including delivery and postpartum care. MBS can be

NB F2 completion refers to the end of the second year of the Foundation Programme.

Assessor: candidate:

A.

		Below expectations for F2 completion	Borderline for F2 completion	Meets expectations of F2 completion	Above expectations for F2 completion		Unable to comment
1	Introduction/establish rapport	1	2	3	4	5	6	7
2	Explanation of intervention including patient's consent to proceed	1	2	3	4	5	6	7
3	Assessment of patient's needs before procedure	1	2	3	4	5	6	7
4	Preparation for procedure	1	2	3	4	5	6	7
5	Technical performance of procedure	1	2	3	4	5	6	7
6	Maintenance of asepsis	1	2	3	4	5	6	7
7	Awareness of patient's needs during procedure	1	2	3	4	5	6	7
8	Closure of the procedure including explanation of follow-up care	1	2	3	4	5	6	7
9	Clinical safety	1	2	3	4	5	6	7
10	Professionalism	1	2	3	4	5	6	7
11	Overall ability to perform the procedure (including technical and professional skills)	1	2	3	4	5	6	7

B. How would you rate the candidate's performance (circle one)

        Incompetent   Borderline   Competent

C.

Demonstrated strengths	Areas for development

FIGURE 7.3.6 Example of technical and nontechnical Likert scale rating, rating of individual, *IPPI*. (Reprinted with permission from Kneebone, R. L., Kidd, J., Nestel, D., Barnet, A., Lo, B., King, R., … Brown, R. [2005]. Blurring the boundaries: Scenario-based simulation in a clinical setting. *Medical Education*, *39*(6), 580–587

engineered to simulate a wide variety of settings, complications, patients, and patient events.

Some procedural and case-specific checklists have been developed for evaluation of crises where specific solutions or "best actions" have been identified by expert analysis and are recognizable in the simulation (Kim et al., 2009). Yudkowsky (2009) notes that checklists are used to convert the examinee's behavior during the observed performance into a number that can be used for scoring. The MBS

modality with its range of real-time reactions is an appropriate modality in which to test whether or not a trainee has chosen the "best action" in response to a patient event.

Simulation Assessment Tools for MBS

Below are examples of assessment tools used in MBS.

Weighted technical checklist, individual: Weighted checklist items may be used to identify the items of "key importance

Doctor actions	P	D_1	D_2	Weight
1. Assess airway	1.00	–	–	1
2. Assess breathing – respiratory rate and O_2 saturation	0.88	0.31	0.34	1
3. Assess circulation – blood pressure and heart rate	0.88	0.42	0.40	1
4. Establish level of consciousness	1.00	–	–	1
5. Expose the patient	0.77	0.55	0.33	1
6. Above four issues in less than 1 minute	0.17	0.63	0.62	2
7. Establish need for IV access	1.00	–	–	1
8. Initiate fluid replacement	0.99	0.11	0.21	2
9. Provide appropriate fluid replacement	0.86	0.30	0.35	3
10. Determine need for type and cross	0.50	0.31	0.11	4
11. Proper sequencing of survey	0.42	0.70	0.69	3
12. All of the above in less than 3 minutes	0.17	0.60	0.51	3
13. Premorbid history ⋮ penicillin anaphylaxis	0.25	0.22	0.14	1
14. Examination of lower extremity – circulatory exam	0.55	0.35	0.14	1
15. Examination of lower extremity – neurological exam	0.52	0.43	0.13	1
16. Determine need for x-ray	0.81	0.26	0.08	1
17. Determine and implement immobilization of left leg	0.23	0.47	0.30	1
18. Provide analgesia	0.45	0.22	0.17	1

FIGURE 7.3.7 Example of weighted technical checklist, rating of individual, *Trauma-haemorrhagic hypotension secondary to long bone fracture.* (Reprinted with permission from Murray, D., Boulet, J., Ziv, A., Woodhouse, J., Kras, J., & McAllister, J. [2002]. An acute care skills evaluation for graduating medical students: A pilot study using clinical simulation. *Medical Education*, 36(9), 833–841.)

CHECKLIST

ACTION	YES (2 points)	With prompting (1 point)	NO (0 points)
PROBLEM SOLVING			
Prompt ABC assessment			
Implements concurrent management approach (4 points)			
SITUATIONAL AWARENESS			
Avoids fixation error (4 points)			
Re-assesses and re-evaluates situation (4 points)			
RESOURCE UTILIZATION			
Calls for help when indicated			
Delegates and directs appropriately			
LEADERSHIP			
Maintains calm demeanor			
Acts decisively and maintains control of crisis			
Maintains global perspective			
COMMUNICATION			
Communicates clearly and concisely			
Closes the loop and uses names			
Listens to team input			
TOTAL SCORE (30 points)			

FIGURE 7.3.8 Example of Mannequin-based, nontechnical multipoint scale, rating of the individual within a team, *The Ottawa CRM Checklist.* (Reprinted with permission from Kim, J., Neilipovitz, D., Cardinal, P., & Chiu, M. [2009]. A comparison of global rating scale and checklist scores in the validation of an evaluation tool to assess performance in the resuscitation of critically ill patients during simulated emergencies [abbreviated as "CRM simulator study IB"]. *Simulation in Healthcare*, 4(1), 6–16.)

Resident #:   Scenario #:

Staff #:   Date :

APPENDIX 1 - OTTAWA CRISIS RESOURCE MANAGEMENT (CRM) GLOBAL RATING SCALE

EVALUATION CRITERIA:

This evaluation scale is directed towards assessing competence in crisis management (CM) skills and care of critically ill patients. The standard of competence has been set at the senior resident level, i.e., the third-year resident who has had prior ICU experience, and through experience as a senior housestaff physician, has previous experience in managing crises. As there exists a requisite base of medical knowledge required to effectively manage crises, this will also be evaluated. However, the focus of evaluation will be on crisis management skills. The skills listed below comprise essential aspects of crisis management. In the simulator case scenario sessions, performance in each of these areas will be assessed, in addition to the amount of prompting or guidance required during the case scenario sessions.

The following criteria will be evaluated:

LEADERSHIP SKILLS
Stays calm and in control during crisis
Prompt and firm decision-making
Maintains global perspective ("Big picture")

SITUATIONAL AWARENESS
Avoids fixation error
Reassesses and re-evaluates situation constantly
Anticipates likely events

COMMUNICATION SKILLS
Communicates clearly and concisely
Uses directed verbal/non-verbal communication
Listens to team input

PROBLEM SOLVING
Organized and efficient problem solving approach (ABC's)
Quick in implementation (Concurrent management)
Considers alternatives during crisis

RESOURCE UTILIZATION
Calls for help appropriately
Utilizes resources at hand appropriately
Prioritizes tasks appropriately

OVERALL

Resident #: _____

Staff : _____

Date: _____

Time: _____

FIGURE 7.3.9 Example of nontechnical Global Rating Scale, rating of the individual within a team, *Ottawa Crisis Resource Management (CRM) Global Rating Scale*. (Reprinted with permission from Kim, J., Neilipovitz, D., Cardinal, P., & Chiu, M. [2009]. A comparison of global rating scale and checklist scores in the validation of an evaluation tool to assess performance in the resuscitation of critically ill patients during simulated emergencies [abbreviated as "CRM simulator study IB"]. *Simulation in Healthcare, 4*(1), 6–16.)

OVERALL PERFORMANCE

1	2	3	4	5	6	7
Novice; all CM skills require significant improvement		Advanced novice; many CM skills require moderate improvement		Competent; most CM skills require minor improvement		Clearly superior; few, if any CM skills that only require minor improvement

I. LEADERSHIP SKILLS

1	2	3	4	5	6	7
Loses calm and control for most of crisis; unable to make firm decisions; cannot maintain global perspective		Loses calm/control frequently during crisis; delays in making firm decisions (or with cueing); rarely maintains global perspective		Stays calm and in control for most of crisis; makes firm decisions with little delay; usually maintains global perspective		Remains calm and in control for entire crisis; makes prompt and firm decisions without delay; always maintains global perspective

II. PROBLEM SOLVING SKILLS

1	2	3	4	5	6	7
Cannot implement ABC's assessment without direct cues; uses sequential management despite cues; fails to consider any alternative in crisis		Incomplete or slow ABC assessment; mostly uses sequential management approach unless cues; gives little consideration to alternatives		Satisfactory ABC assessment; without cues; mostly uses concurrent management approach with only minimal cueing; considers some alternatives in crisis		Thorough yet quick ABC without cues; always uses concurrent management approach; considers most likely alternatives in crisis

FIGURE 7.3.9 (continued)

III. SITUATIONAL AWARENESS SKILLS

1	2	3	4	5	6	7
Becomes fixated easily despite repeated cues; fails to reassess and re-evaluate situation despite repeated cues; fails to anticipate likely events		Avoids fixation error only with cueing; rarely reassesses and re-evaluates situation without cues; rarely anticipates likely events		Usuallly avoids fixation error with minimal cueing; reassesses re-evaluates situation frequently with minimal cues; usually anticipates likely events		Avoids any fixation error without cues; constantly reassesses and re-evaluates situation without cues; constantly anticipates likely events

IV. RESOURCE UTILIZATION SKILLS

1	2	3	4	5	6	7
Unable to use resources and staff effectively; does not prioritize tasks or ask for help when required despite cues		Able to use resources with minimal effectiveness; only prioritizes tasks or asks for help when required with cues		Able to use resources with moderate effectiveness; able to prioritize tasks and/or ask for help with minimal cues		Clearly able to use resources to maximal effectiveness; sets clear task priority and asks for help early with no cues

V. COMMUNICATION SKILLS

1	2	3	4	5	6	7
Does not communicate with staff; does not acknowledge staff communication, never uses directed verbal/non-verbal communication		Communicates occasionally with staff, but unclear and vague; occasionally listens to but rarely interacts with staff; rarely uses directed verbal/non- verbal communication		Communicates with staff clearly and concisely most of time; listens to staff feedback; usually uses directed verbal/non-verbal communication		Communicates clearly and concisely at all times. encourages input and listens to staff feedback; consistently uses directed verbal/non-verbal communication

FIGURE 7.3.9 (continued)

in defining clinical performances." These analytic items were found by Murray et al. (2002) to discriminate between low- and high-ability performers (Figure 7.3.7).

Emergent situations are characterized by dynamic, changing conditions over time depending on mannequin-environmental or team-initiated actions and interactions. Hence, it is difficult to have a single "best action" or specific remedy that can be checked off on a checklist of emergencies that commonly occur in the ICU or ER (e.g., respirator failure, shock, etc.; Kim et al., 2009). Common nontechnical skills assessed via MBS include communication, teamwork, leadership, and decision making (Yule et al., 2006).

Nontechnical skills multipoint scale for individual rated as part of team: Crisis resource management (CRM) are nontechnical skills used to keep patients safe in medical emergencies. The Ottawa CRM Checklist assesses CRM using a multipoint scale assessing individuals as part of a team (Figure 7.3.8).

Nontechnical skills Global Rating Scale for individuals rated as part of team: The Ottawa CRM Global Rating Scale assesses the individual within the team (Figure 7.3.9).

Nontechnical skills rating scale rating teams as teams: The State Obstetric and Pediatric Research Collaboration (STORC) Clinical Teamwork Scale measures teamwork in the clinical setting using a global scale (Figure 7.3.10).

VR Simulation

Simulation assessment on the VR simulator allows examinees to perform required techniques on virtual patients or simulate a wide variety of procedures from intravenous cannulation to laparoscopic cholecystectomy and endoscopic methods (McGaghie et al., 2010). The most common use of VR simulators is for evaluation of competence in performing procedures including nonoperative invasive techniques and surgeries. McGaghie et al. (2010) note that these techniques require both psychomotor and perceptual skills that are different from traditional open approaches because the practitioner must perform complex invasive procedures on the basis of indirect and limited viewing of 2D images representing the 3D task. The learner may need to overcome reduced depth perception and poor-quality imaging with some simulated displays—manipulate delicate instruments at a distance from the operative site, with consequent limitations on tactile feedback and compensate for a conflict between proprioception and visual feedback. These weaknesses can be addressed in many ways within the VR modality. Haptic touch and pressure feedback technology can convey the feel of the procedure. Simulators with haptic sensors can capture and record trainee "touch" in terms of location and depth of pressure at specific anatomical sites. McGaghie et al. (2010) caution that much more work is needed in "reliability estimation" of haptic data. VR simulators are now in use to educate surgeons, medical subspecialists, clinical and advanced nurses, and other

professions in complex procedures that are too dangerous to practice on live patients (McGaghie et al., 2010).

Serious gaming is another type of VR simulation where evaluation of other management and communication skills for individual teams in a virtual environment (e.g., emergency department, trauma bay, delivery room, or community setting) may occur. Remote and simultaneous assessment of multiple participants caring for virtual patients in a computer-generated environment is also possible (Scalese & Issenberg, 2008).

In addition to their current perceptual and psychomotor functionalities, one of the greatest benefits for VR and serious games simulation modality assessment may lie in their "metarealistic" capabilities. Because digital technology can probe subcutaneously, and dynamically show, for example, multiple layers of the skin and organs, requisite knowledge in both quantifiable behaviors and principle-based actions can be tested. An example is an understanding of how to correctly align the patient's head and maneuver the needle during an ultrasound-guided internal jugular central venous catheter placement (US-guided IJ). The procedure of keeping the patient's head at the correct angle and visualizing the distance between the midpoint of the internal jugular and the lateral border of the carotid artery operationalizes the underlying principle that this zone represents the area of nonoverlap between the internal jugular and carotid artery. Through VR functionality, the trainee can dynamically visualize that, relative to this zone, the margin of safety decreases and the percentage overlap increases from 29% to 42% to 72% as the head is turned to the contralateral side form 0 (neutral) to 45 and 90 (Troianos et al., 2011). The serious game/VR modality allows the player to pierce the skin at the correct angle, set the head angle, and see through to and navigate around the vein and artery to be sure that the head angle is compatible with these key anatomic areas, which are in turn visible and able to be manipulated. In this way, the player can demonstrate that he/she has a command of the concepts and principles of US-guided IJ needle insertion and can then go on to demonstrate the psychomotor skills within the partial trainer or MBS exercise.

Simulation Assessment Tools for Virtual Trainers

Standardized assessment metrics are often built into the technology by the vendor and can be generated by computerized reports.

Sources of Evidence-Based or Best Practices Simulation Assessment Tools

Table 7.3.6 summarizes the types of checklists and rating scales relevant to simulation assessment as described in the previous section. In addition to peer-reviewed literature, other sources of assessment tools can be found through

CTS - Clinical Teamwork Scale™ (Global)

Please note: **Not relevant**- The task was not applicable to the scenario.

Overall	Not Relevant	Unacceptable	Poor			Average			Good			Perfect
1. How would you rate teamwork during this delivery/emergency?	☐	0	1	2	3	4	5	6	7	8	9	10

Communication	Not Relevant	Unacceptable	Poor			Average			Good			Perfect
Overall Communication Rating:	☐	0	1	2	3	4	5	6	7	8	9	10
1. Orient new members (SBAR)	☐	0	1	2	3	4	5	6	7	8	9	10
2. Transparent thinking	☐	0	1	2	3	4	5	6	7	8	9	10
3. Directed communication	☐	0	1	2	3	4	5	6	7	8	9	10
4. Closed loop communication	☐	0	1	2	3	4	5	6	7	8	9	10

Situational Awareness	Not Relevant	Unacceptable	Poor			Average			Good			Perfect
Overall Situational Awareness Rating:	☐	0	1	2	3	4	5	6	7	8	9	10
1. Resource allocation	☐	0	1	2	3	4	5	6	7	8	9	10
2. Target fixation	☐ Yes	☐ No										

Decision Making	Not Relevant	Unacceptable	Poor			Average			Good			Perfect
Overall Decision Making Rating:	☐	0	1	2	3	4	5	6	7	8	9	10
1. Prioritize	☐	0	1	2	3	4	5	6	7	8	9	10

Role Responsibility	Not Relevant	Unacceptable	Poor			Average			Good			Perfect
Overall Role Responsibility (Leader/Helper) Rating:	☐	0	1	2	3	4	5	6	7	8	9	10
1. Role clarity	☐	0	1	2	3	4	5	6	7	8	9	10
2. Perform as a leader/helper	☐	0	1	2	3	4	5	6	7	8	9	10

Other	Not Relevant	Unacceptable	Poor			Average			Good			Perfect
1. Patient friendly	☐	0	1	2	3	4	5	6	7	8	9	10

Additional Notes (Anything regarding individual performance, assertion of position, etc?):

_____

On-Site Reviewer   *Print Name*   *Sign*   *Date*

The CTS-Clinical Teamwork Scale™ was developed by the STORC OB Safety Initiative Team (www.storc.org) through support of the Agency for Healthcare Research and Quality (1 U18 HS015800-02). Guise J-M, Deering S, Kanki B, Osterweil P, Li H, Mori T, Lowe N. STORC OB Safety Initiative: Development and Validation of the Clinical Teamwork Scale to Evaluate Teamwork. Simulation in Healthcare, 3 (4): 217-223, 2008

FIGURE 7.3.10   Example of nontechnical Likert scale rating of the team as a team. (The CTS Clinical Teamwork Scale was developed by STORC OB Safety Initiative Team, [www.storc.org] through support of the Agency for Healthcare Research and Quality [I U18 HS015800-02]). (Guise, J.-M., Deering, S., Kanki, B., Osterwall, P., Li, H., Mori, T., & Lowe, N. [2008]. STORC OB safety initiative: Development and validation of the clinical teamwork scale to evaluate teamwork. *Simulation in Healthcare, 3*(4), 217–223.)

TABLE 7.3.6

Healthcare Simulation Technical and Nontechnical Checklist and Rating Scale Assessment Tools

	Checklists		Rating Scales		
	Dichotomous	Weighted	Likert	Behaviorally Anchored Rating Scales (BARS)	Multipoint
Technical/Individual	E.g., Operative Structured Assessment of Technical Skills	E.g., the Israeli Board of Anesthesiology Examination Committee	E.g., Global Rating Index for Technical Skills (GRITS)	E.g., OSATS Global Rating of Technical Performance	E.g., Checklist of Expected Actions, Department of Obstetrics and Gynecology, SUMC
Technical/Team	E.g., OTAS (Observational Teamwork Assessment of Surgery) checklist				E.g., Pediatric Resuscitation Team Training Checklist Falcone et al.
Nontechnical/Individual			E.g., Kalamazoo Doctor-Patient Communication Rating Scale; IPPI	E.g., Calgary-Cambridge Observation Tool	
Nontechnical/Individual within a team		E.g., BARS Teamwork Scale, Wright et al.	E.g., OTAS (Observational Teamwork Assessment of Surgery) Likert, Crew Resource Management; E.g., NOTECCHS, Crew Resource Management	E.g., Ottawa GRS	E.g., Ottawa CRM checklist
Non technical/ Team as a whole		E.g., CATS Communication & Teamwork Skills Assessment	E.g., TEAM (Team Emergency Assessment Measure)E.g., Anesthetists' Non-technical Skills (ANTS) System; Crew Resource Management	TAS (Teamwork Assessment Scales)	E.g., STORC Clinical Teamwork Scale

HIGH-STAKES SIMULATION AND PHYSICIAN ASSESSMENT

Adam I. Levine, MD
Director, Mount Sinai Human Emulation, Education, and Evaluation Lab for Patient Safety (HELPS) Center

The term "High-Stakes Simulation" is generally reserved to imply simulation-based activities where one's performance has grave or significant consequences on life or livelihood. From someone who has devoted a significant amount of effort to developing, conducting, and reporting on our simulation-based assessment and retraining program, I actually think the term is used too infrequently. Quite frankly, I consider all the simulations I facilitate to be *high-stakes*; simulation is too resource-intensive to be anything less. As educators, we owe it to our learners to make every simulation *high-stakes* for their sake and the sake of their future patients. If, as simulation educators, we weren't convinced of the absolute virtue of simulation, then why would any of us devote so much time and energy to an educational modality that, at times, only impacts a relatively small number of learners? Surely there are more economical ways to educate, but, as they say, "you get what you pay for."

In 1994, I began the simulation program at Mount Sinai. I considered all our simulations to be *high-stakes* but also felt strongly that the simulated environment should not be used for assessment. Even so, the use of standardized patients was on the rise. Their use rapidly morphed from educational "experiences" for our medical students to objective structured clinical examinations (OSCEs). Student enthusiasm also morphed; they were no longer thrilled about going to the Morschand Center (the standardized patient center at Mount Sinai, memorialized in the infamous Seinfeld episode where Jerry asks Kramer "do all schools use these?" and Kramer replies "only the good ones"). Although I was encouraged to assess student performance in simulation and was invited to sit on committees for developing simulation assessment tools, I avoided these like the plague. I had no interest in my *high-stakes* simulation sessions becoming as unpopular as the OSCEs.

To this day, I have fended off suggestions to assess students in my simulation center. I have, however, embraced the concept of assessing residents, fellows, and practicing anesthesiologists in the simulated environment. After all, any attempt to educate a learner must include some degree of judgment of their performance to debrief them constructively and change future behavior. Over time, it became apparent to me that resident performance in simulation correlated well with clinical performance. This realization was later put to use when I was asked to develop simulations for the purpose of assessing a physician whose competency was being questioned; we were to determine whether this physician was "remediateable." Now I know people look at simulation for assessment as if they were facing a firing squad, but it couldn't be any worse than the "traditional" tools used to assess this physician (e.g., multiple-choice and oral examinations), which he failed abysmally. However, once in the simulated operating room, this physician performed admirably and convinced not only me, but also a committee assembled by the New York State Society of Anesthesiologists that he was indeed a candidate for remediation. People are impressed to learn that not only can simulation be a very powerful tool to assess performance, but in this very early example helped salvage a physician's career. Now, 20 years later, we have developed a vibrant simulation-based reentry program for anesthesiologists. The CARE (Clinical Anesthesia RE-Entry) Program, which includes both simulation-based assessment and clinical retraining, is a much needed service for anesthesiologists who have been out of practice for a variety of reasons. Not all anesthesiologists that present for the CARE Program finish successfully and, we believe, society is a little safer for it.

Do I think everyone should dive in and embrace these *high-stakes* activities in their simulation program? Probably not, especially considering the significant impact of a failed remediation. Obviously no one would think that this activity is any thing less than *high-stakes*, but then again nothing in simulation should be anything less.

---

professional organizations (e.g., AORN, ACS, SSH) and agency regulations and mandates (e.g., Joint Commission).

SUMMARY

Assessment development and implementation is a complex activity. Fairness and accuracy require careful attention to learner (pre- and postlicensure), tool (simulation modality), assessor, and programmatic components. For this reason, institutional simulation programs are encouraged to access institutional statistical and psychometric support, as well as content experts in the areas of the subject matter case at hand and of assessment itself. Validating assessment tools and testing for their reliability is also a complex process, often requiring over a year of study, analysis, and refinement. For this reason, many educators and researchers choose to reference the peer-reviewed literature for exemplary studies wherein tools were developed. Assessor

training is key to best practices simulation assessment. Clear focus on these factors can lead to defensible, reportable outcomes for healthcare performance assessments.

REFERENCES

Barrows, H., & Abrahamson, S. (1964). The programmed patient: A technique for appraising student performance in clinical neurology. *Academic Medicine, 39*(8), 802–805.

Boulet, J. R., & Murray, D. J. (2010, April). Simulation-based assessment in anesthesiology: Requirements for practical implementation. *Anesthesiology, 112*(4), 1041–1052.

Downing, S. M. (2003). Validity: On the meaningful interpretation of assessment data. *Medical Education, 37*, 830–837.

Evans, L., Dodge, M., Shah, T., Kaplan, L., Siegel, M., Moore, C., … D'Onofrio, G. (2010). Simulation training in central venous catheter insertion: Improved performance in clinical practice. *Academic Medicine, 85*(9), 1462–1469.

Feldman, M., Lazzara, E., Vanderbilt, A., & DiazGranados, D. (2012). Rater training to support high-stakes simulation-based assessments. *Journal of Continuing Education in the Health Professions, 32*(4), 279–286.

Joint Committee on Fair Testing Practices in Education. (2004). *Code of fair testing practices in education.* Washington, DC: American Psychological Association. Retrieved from http://apa.org/science/programs/testing/fair-code.aspx

Kardong-Edgren, S., Adamson, K., & Fitzgerald, C. (2010). A review of currently published evaluation instruments for human patient simulation. *Clinical Simulation in Nursing, 6*(1), 25–35.

Kim, J., Neilipovitz, D., Cardinal, P., & Chiu, M. (2009). A comparison of global rating scale and checklist scores in the validation of an evaluation tool to assess performance in the resuscitation of critically ill patients during simulated emergencies (abbreviated as "CRM simulator study IB."). *Simulation Healthcare, 4*(1), 6–16.

Kneebone, R. L., Kidd, J., Nestel, D., Barnet, A., Lo, B., King, R., … Brown, R. (2005). Blurring the boundaries: Scenario-based simulation in a clinical setting. *Medical Education, 39*(6), 580–587.

Kneebone, R., Nestel, D., Yadolllah, F., Brown, R., Nolan, C., Durack, J., … Darzi, A. (2006). Assessing procedural skills in context: Exploring the feasibility of an integrated procedural performance instrument (IPPI). *Medical Education, 40*(11), 1105–1114.

Kulik, C., Kulik, J., & Bangert-Drowns, R. (1990). Effectiveness of mastery learning programs: A meta-analysis. *Review of Educational Research, 60*(2), 265–306.

Lammers, R. L., Davenport, M., Korley, F., Griswold-Theodorson, S., Fitch, M. T., Narang, A., … Robey, W. C. (2008). Teaching and assessing procedural skills using simulation: Metrics and methodology. *Academic Emergency Medicine: Official Journal of the Society for Academic Emergency Medicine, 15*(11), 1079–1087.

Martin, J., Regehr, G., Reznick, R., Macrae, H. K., Murnaghan, J., Hutchison, C., & Brown, M. (1997). Objective structured assessment of technical skill (OSATS) for surgical residents. *British Journal of Surgery, 84*(2), 273–278.

McGaghie, W., Butter, J., & Kaye, M. (2009). Observational assessment. In S. M. Downing & R. Yudkowsky (Eds.), *Assessment in health professions education* (pp. 185–215). New York, NY: Routledge.

McGaghie, W. C., Issenberg, S. B., Petrusa, E. R., & Scalese, R. J. (2010). A critical review of simulation-based medical education research: 2003–2009. *Medical Education, 44*(1), 50–63. doi:10.1111/j.1365-2923.2009.03547.x

McGaghie, W., Miller, G., Sajid, A., & Telder, T. (1978). *Competency-based curriculum development in medical education an introduction.* Geneva, Switzerland: World Health Organization.

McLaughlin, K., Gregor, G., Jones, A., & Coderre, S. (2006). Can standardized patients replace physicians as OSCE examiners? *BMC Medical Education, 6*, 1472–6920.

Murray, D., Boulet, J., Ziv, A., Woodhouse, J., Kras, J., & McAllister, J. (2002). An acute care skills evaluation for graduating medical students: A pilot study using clinical simulation. *Medical Education, 36*(9), 833–841. Retrieved from http://www.ncbi.nlm.nih.gov/pubmed/12354246

Rudolph, J. W., Simon, R., Raemer, D. B., & Eppich, W. J. (2008). Debriefing as formative assessment: Closing performance gaps in medical education. *Academic Emergency Medicine, 15*, 1010–1016.

Scalese, R., & Issenberg, S. B. (2008). Simulation-based assessment. In E. S. Holmboe & R. E. Hawkins (Eds.), *Practical guide to the evaluation of clinical competence* (pp. 179–200). Philadelphia, PA: Mosby-Elsevier.

Smith, P., & Ragan, J. (1999). *Instructional design.* New York, NY: John Wiley & Sons.

Troianos, C., Hartman, G., Glas, K., Skubas, N., Eberhardt, R., Walaker, J., & Reeves, S. (2011). Guidelines for performing ultrasound guided vascular cannulation: Recommendations of the American Society of Echocardiography and the Society of Cardiovascular Anesthesiologists. *Journal of the American Society of Echocardiography, 24*, 1291–1318.

Yudkowsky, R. (2009) Performance Tests. In S.M. Downing & R. Yudkowsky (Eds.), *Assessment in health professions education* (pp. 217–243). New York, NY: Routledge.

Yudkowsky, R., Downing, S. M., & Tekian, A. (2009). Standard setting. In S. M. Downing & R. Yudkowsky (Eds.), *Assessment in health professions education* (pp. 119–148). New York, NY: Routledge.

Yule, S., Flin, R., Paterson-Brown, S., & Maran, N. (2006). Non-technical skills for surgeons in the operating room: A review of the literature. *Surgery, 139*(2), 140–149.

SECTION 7 • Educational Development

CHAPTER 7.4

Continuing Medical Education

Jason Zigmont, PhD. CHSE-A, Angie Wade, MPH, CCRC, Leslie A. Lynch, and Leslie Coonfare, MBA, BSN, RN-BC

ABOUT THE AUTHORS

JASON ZIGMONT is the System Director of Learning Innovation for OhioHealth. Dr. Zigmont oversees simulation and experiential learning including CME for a health system that includes 8 hospitals and 42 care sites. He serves on SSH's Education committee, which is responsible for all CME for the Society and heads the subcommittee on preparation for the CHSE. He holds a PhD in Adult Learning specifically focused on Experiential Learning, and is a nationally registered Paramedic.

ANGIE WADE is a Learning Outcomes Manager for OhioHealth. In this role, she works with educators and simulationists to develop curriculum, implement educational programs, measure for outcomes, and provide analysis. Her expertise involves program evaluation, health education, research, and statistical analysis. Additionally, she has led the evaluation for several national and state-level evidence-based programs. She has presented at various National Conferences with emphasis on measuring outcomes, and has received multiple prestigious research awards.

LESLIE A. LYNCH is Administrative Director of the OhioHealth Continuing Medical Education (CME) Program. She has been involved in CME for over 25 years, and has achieved full accreditation from every survey. Leslie has presented at the Ohio State Medical Association's annual conference for state-accredited CME providers and presented a poster on the case example at the Alliance for Continued Education for Healthcare Professionals' (ACEHP) annual conference.

LESLIE COONFARE is the System Director of Learning for OhioHealth in Columbus, Ohio. In this role, she oversees clinical and nonclinical education including nursing continuing education for a health system with 8 hospitals and 42 care sites. Leslie is certified in nursing professional development by the American Nurses Credentialing Center, and has presented at various National Conferences on nursing leadership development. She received her Masters in Business Administration from Baldwin Wallace University.

Acknowledgments: OhioHealth Center for Medical Education & Innovation (CME&I)

ABSTRACT

This chapter provides an overview of the processes associated with granting credit for continuing education provided to physicians and nurses. The chapter is designed to highlight key components that simulation programs should consider when thinking about becoming an approved provider of continuing education for health professionals.

CASE EXAMPLE

Program Director Dr. Laura Berry was asked to provide continuing medical education (CME) credit for a course that the simulation program plans to offer. During the last Simulation Program Steering Committee meeting, the committee decided that granting CME regularly would be one way to encourage practicing healthcare providers to attend patient safety programs that will be given at the simulation center. Until this point, the simulation program has not offered continuing education credit for any of its simulation courses. Dr. Berry is looking to better understand the processes for granting CME and wonders where she could start.

INTRODUCTION, BACKGROUND, AND SIGNIFICANCE

Most healthcare disciplines require completion of a certain number and type of approved continuing education (CE) credits to remain licensed. Hospitals, health systems, and other organizations such as simulation programs can become accredited to grant CE credit for various professional disciplines. While only continuing medical education (CME) for physician and CE for nurses will be outlined here, there are many other types of CE targeted at other health-related disciplines such as pharmacy, physical therapy, and athletic training.

As healthcare providers can have a difficult time completing their required CE owing to time constraints, cost, availability, etc., offering approved CE credit can be a means of attracting a larger audience to the simulation program's courses.

To become an approved or accredited provider of CE, a **program** must meet specific criteria set forth by the various accreditation bodies. These criteria are typically embedded in an extensive accreditation process. Accredited providers may provide credit to those that attend and participate in approved eligible courses. Within these courses, various educational formats such as simulation can be used as long as they are appropriate for the setting, objectives, and desired results of the activity.

To assure high-quality educational programs, accredited providers who wish to provide CME or CE are required to follow a standardized process for program development. Typically this includes the following steps: 1) the rationale for the educational intervention (the needs assessment), 2) how it was determined must be documented and, 3) kept in mind as planning proceeds. Completion of a gap analysis between current practice and what is considered best practice also needs to be documented. The needs assessment and gap analysis is often driven by hospital leadership, staff, or through information provided in reporting (i.e., hospital score cards, patient safety data). Once the need has been identified, educational staff works with identified experts in the field to plan and schedule the intervention. Standardized tools are used to conduct a thorough needs assessment and gap analysis, identify objectives of the intervention, and determine the desired **outcome**. Ideally, innovative and creative planning processes are used in the interventional design, incorporating adult learning theories, behavior change methodology, and experiential learning (i.e., simulation). Additionally, **evaluation** must be carefully planned to ensure appropriate measures of the intervention at all stages. Though these requirements must be met, there is flexibility in how programs comply with them.

Increasingly, CE has been embracing adult learning principles and interaction through simulation. This move away from the traditional lecture format is occurring as focus is placed on changing behaviors and practices. Simulation is a way to do both with positive evaluation results from the participants as well. The processes required to offer CME and CE can also provide structure and documentation to simulation interventions.

CONTINUING MEDICAL EDUCATION

Organizations must be approved to be providers of CME to grant CME credit for educational activities. This accreditation is awarded by the **Accreditation Council for Continuing Medical Education** (ACCME, 2013 a-e) or ACCME-accredited state medical societies. State medical societies must meet the accreditation criteria for their own educational activities, and are also granted the ability to appoint providers at the state level. Additionally, some simulation programs have partnered with accredited CME providers through formal relationships such as joint providership to start offering CME as they build toward their own accreditation. With regards to CME, the accredited organization providing the CME credit is referred to as the '**provider**,' individual educational interventions are referred to as 'activities,' and all activities from one CME provider make up a 'program.'

There are several types of accreditation that must be approved directly by ACCME or by their state's medical society:

1. *ACCME Accreditation (National level):* There are specific requirements that must be met and documented to obtain accreditation (ACCME, 2013). These can be found on the ACCME website www.accme.org. In order to become accredited by the ACCME at the national level, 30% of the learners must be from outside the region (i.e., home state and contiguous states). If the audience is from the local region only, accreditation should be sought by the state medical society (ACCME, 2013). Accreditation is achieved through an application (self-study) and a site visit or review of activity files, as well as paying the applicable fees. Annual reports (number of activities by type, number of physician/nonphysician attendees, number of credit hours granted, income and expenses) and annual fees are also required.
2. *State Medical Society Accreditation:* Each state provides state guidelines for accreditation. The state guidelines are usually based closely on the ACCME standards.
3. *Joint Providership:* A nonaccredited organization can also work with an accredited organization to provide credit for an activity. This is known as joint providership. The CME provider is responsible for ensuring that all requirements are met but can merely oversee the activity from a management standpoint. Some providers charge for this service. For smaller simulation programs, this may provide a good option to offer credit without a large infrastructure needed to obtain accreditation.
4. *Organizational Accreditation:* Organizational accreditation combines physician, nurse, and pharmacist

credit. Details regarding eligibility can be found at the ACCME website under Joint Accreditation (ACCME, 2013). Organizations must demonstrate that 25% of the education provided in the last 12 months is "designed by and for the entire healthcare team" versus one discipline or another. This process is more detailed but may be very beneficial for simulation programs within a healthcare system intending to provide team training and draw a national audience.

5. *Individual Activity Accreditation*: A provider may seek credit for some disciplines by applying for individual **activity accreditation** versus accreditation as an organization. Some examples include physical therapists, athletic trainers, and pharmacists. Additionally, there are specialty credits available for podiatrists, family practitioners, psychologists, and so on; application, fees, and, in some cases, organizational accreditation are required. In other cases, the organization may already be accredited and very simple paperwork needs to be completed to apply for credit. Once the target audience is determined, the process for applicable credit should be researched.

ACCME Accreditation Process

The typical ACCME accreditation process for a new applicant takes 12 to 18 months. The first steps in the accreditation process are as follows:

1. A preapplication process to determine eligibility
2. A self-study to explain and demonstrate how the requirements are met (ACCME, 2013)
3. An "Evidence of Performance in Practice" review (activity files)
4. An initial interview process

Many resources are available on the ACCME website (http://www.accme.org) that describe the requirements, provide examples, questions and answers, and so on. The criteria for compliance are discussed in the next section, CME Criteria for Compliance.

Multiple tools and resources are available to assist with the accreditation process. Various websites, CME support services, and consultants can serve as valuable sources of information. Examples include the following:

- ACCME website (www.accme.org)
- Planning documents and applications
- **Alliance for Continuing Education in the Health Professions (ACEHP)** website www.acehp.org
- Sample resources (i.e., planning documents, **disclosure forms**, etc.) can be accessed on the authors' website www.ohcme.com

ACCME Criteria for Compliance (ACCME, 2013)

Every approved provider must have a CME mission statement. Mission statements vary greatly in length and content depending upon the individual providers. At a minimum, they include the following:

- Purpose of the CME Program
- Target audience
- Content, types of activities (i.e., simulation, courses, regularly scheduled series, enduring materials online)
- Expected results in terms of the educational outcomes that will be measured

For a simulation program, the CME mission statement should mirror the simulation mission statement or be very closely related.

Providers should evaluate CME activity against their mission statement to determine whether the proposed activities fall within the identified scope. This includes directly sponsored activities, as well as joint providership requests from nonaccredited organizations.

Whether as a provider or a joint sponsor, organizations applying for ACCME accreditation must describe and document how the need for the content is determined. Documentation can take many forms, such as patient safety data, process improvement or quality data measures, peer review patterns, or electronic medical record reports. Ideally, the mechanism used to identify the need can also be used to measure the outcome following the educational intervention. The applying organization should maintain documentation of educational needs for all CME activity.

CME Activity Planning

A performance or knowledge gap should be documented for all CME activity. A thorough gap analysis requires a team approach to meet the CME requirements for integrating educational design with content expertise. The documentation should include a description of the following:

- The current state of the target audience (i.e., how they currently practice or manage the problem)
  - Budget/Financial: **Commercial Support**, grants, **vendors**, secure resources, registration fees
  - Event planning, e.g. food, location
  - Documentation: COIs, Disclosure forms
  - Technology needs
- A description of best practice (i.e., what they need to do differently)
  - Facilitation
  - Format for learners
  - Data collection/surveys
  - Address barriers
- What needs to be taught to the learners to change from current to best practice (**Figure 7.4.1**)
  - Educational design format
  - What needs to be taught to change
  - Barriers to address/change
  - Outcomes and measurement methods
  - Expert content

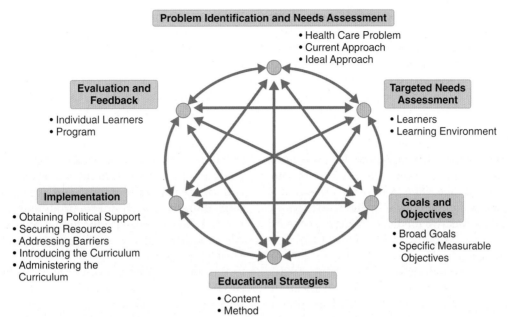

FIGURE 7.4.1 Educational activity planning cycle. (From Kern, D. E., Thomas, P. A., Howard, D. M., & Bass, E. B. [1998]. *Curriculum development for medical education: A six-step approach.* Baltimore, MD: Johns Hopkins Press.)

At a minimum, identifying the need/gap, planning, and analysis of the intervention should be a collaborative effort between the CME provider, simulationist, and the content expert. If the resources exist, experts in educational design and outcome measurements should also be included. Additional tools for use in identifying, planning, and implementing CME activity can be found on the Ohio-Health website (www.ohcme.com).

Information gathered through the gap analysis should be translated into the course objectives (see chapter 8.1). Objectives should be written in a way that focuses not just on skills but ultimately on care outcomes. Objectives should be analyzed to determine whether they relate to the following:

- Knowledge—Does the learner know *what* to do?
- Competence—Does the learner know *how* to do or apply it?
- Performance—Does the learner actually *do* it?

This helps significantly in determining the most appropriate design or format in the next step of the CME accreditation requirements.

Once the learner objectives are established and necessary content to narrow the gaps are identified, the next step is to consider the most effective method of teaching to move the learner from current to best practice. The implied meaning by the CME requirements is that simply transmitting knowledge is no longer sufficient. The intent of CME is to affect a measurable change, so keeping the reason and the goals of the educational offering in mind is critical to proper planning of the activity. This means that you need to demonstrate outcomes from your program. The benefit of describing the outcomes is the ability to demonstrate value to the organization. Providing demonstrated value can increase institutional support (i.e., resources, acknowledgment).

Often, the main goal of a requested CME activity is to disseminate information or increase awareness on a topic. This is no longer an acceptable justification for providing CME credit. Simulation is an asset to CME providers that are trying to transform their educational culture from solely didactics to a combination of perspectives and formats that engage the adult learner and produce required, measurable, and meaningful outcomes (Zigmont et al., 2011b). If it is determined that competence or performance change is the goal, then simulation may be the best format to deliver the content. Historically, CME has largely been associated with increased or improved knowledge (such as measured by a pre-/post-test) and, thus, commonly took the form of a didactic lecture. Proponents of simulation may be met with resistance when encouraging this format owing to the ingrained culture that begins in medical school (Curtis et al., 2012; McGaghie et al., 2009). This is where simulation and applying adult learning theory can partner with CME to produce an outcome that demonstrates its value to all stakeholders (Curtis et al., 2012; Zigmont et al., 2011).

Educational planning must include identification of the target audience. This is not only important for determining the content, but there are also factors to consider on the basis of the discipline, specialty, setting (i.e., inpatient, outpatient), and other characteristics of the target audience. There may be learning styles, cultures, teams, and other differences to consider when designing the activity to impact a needed change (McGaghie et al., 2009; Zigmont et al., 2011). On the basis of the target audience, there may be multiple applications needed to obtain discipline-specific CE credit. Each will have its own deadline and documentation requirement related to the scope of the targeted learners.

The ACCME Accreditation most recent criterion 6 states, "The provider develops activities/educational interventions in the context of desirable physician attributes (e.g., Institute of Medicine (IOM) competencies, Accreditation Council for Graduate Medical Education (ACGME) Competencies)" (ACCME, 2013). The majority of these sources overlap in intent, but the object is to identify and document which competencies the learning will address or potentially improve.

Identified competencies include patient care, medical knowledge, practice-based learning and improvement, interpersonal and communication skills, professionalism, and system-based practice. The American Osteopathic Association's (AOA) competencies include osteopathic philosophy and manipulative medicine (American Board of Medical Specialties [ABMS], 2013; AOA, 2013). It is possible that physicians will eventually have to demonstrate learning in every competency (Davis et al., 1999). This has implications for maintenance of certification, which is an emerging area for both CME and simulation involvement.

Reviewing competencies in detail may reveal additional areas to consider for CME activity. The competencies can also assist in identifying some of the difficulties learners might have when attempting to implement the change education suggests they make. For example, the "Patient Care and Procedural Skills" competency by the American Board of Medical Specialties (ABMS) specifies that care provided should be "compassionate, appropriate and effective treatment for health problems and to promote health" (ABMS, 2013). If a CME activity is to support this competency but only addresses "appropriate and effective treatment," the provider consider including additional activity to ensure that 'promotion of health' is included.

Standards for Commercial Support

The ACCME's Standards for Commercial Support (SCS) (ACCME, 2013) help providers and planners to ensure balance and objectivity in CME presentations such that commercial entities do not have control of the content. Providers need to be sure that educational interventions for which they grant credit are unbiased, based on scientific evidence, and promote improvement in healthcare, and not a **commercial interest**.

A program offering CME must ensure that anyone involved in planning or able to affect the content (including the selected faculty and even their spouses) must disclose any financial relationship with any commercial interest that may be perceived as a conflict of interest (COI). These relationships and the type of relationship (i.e., research funding, honoraria, stock holder) must be provided to the audience prior to the activity. Should anyone able to affect the content have a potential COI, providers are required to have a mechanism in place to resolve the conflict. This requirement is often met by the review of presentations by a nonbiased individual. A disclosure should be required from reviewers as well.

Most commonly, disclosure forms are created by providers that request the information to meet these standards. However, there are now electronic mechanisms available to assist with this as well. In addition, providers typically supply the information regarding what has been disclosed (which must be done even if there is no potential COI) either on slides, in conference materials, and/or verbally during introduction. Regardless of the mechanism used, it must be documented in the file along with the signed disclosure forms.

There are many more details to these requirements, including but not limited to the management of funding received, payment of honoraria and expenses, and ensuring separation of education from promotion (i.e., vendor support). When receiving educational grants from commercial supporters, the provider, planner, and the supporter must sign a letter of agreement. Other examples, as well as the remaining details of the SCS can be found on the ACCME website (www.accme.org) and on the OhioHealth website (www.ohcme.com).

Measuring Outcomes

An essential element of the planning process in any simulation-based CME activity involves identification of the desired outcomes and how best to measure them. This should include pre-thought into the design and collection of data, as well as the plan for analysis and dissemination of information (e.g., reporting, publication). Too often, this is an area overlooked and underplanned; thus, many great interventions lack evidence of the impact that was made. Measurement of impact should be done for both the individual activities as well as the entire program. Key factors to consider when planning the analysis of activities and overall programs include the following:

1. *Promoting Improvements in Healthcare*—Successful interventions and activities can make a prominent impact in healthcare. Identifying these changes can be challenging if careful consideration is not put into the planning and identification of outcomes and how to measure them. Educational interventions using simulation can provide opportunities to measure competence and performance more accurately than typical CME activities (i.e., didactic lecture) and should be considered prior to implementation. Effective measurement can serve as a catalyst to improve programs and interventions by integrating lessons from findings of what works and what does not.

2. *Analyzing Changes in Learners*—Analyzing changes in learners can prove challenging if the desire is to move beyond uninformative information such as happiness index, "how does that make you feel?" However, many programs fail to analyze the changes and impact on practice. Programs often focus measurement on knowledge gained versus competence, performance, and/or patient outcomes. Therefore, it is important to carefully select measurement tools that go beyond measuring

knowledge. Assessment tools need to measure the actual impact these interventions have on changing learners' practices, which in turn will make analysis more meaningful (ACCME, 2013).

3. *Selecting Appropriate Measures/Assessment Tools*—Maintenance of CME accreditation requires some level of analysis and outcome measurement, specifically measuring competence, performance, and patient outcomes (ACCME, 2013). Most accredited CME providers have developed tools to analyze the educational interventions on the basis of these principles. Further research has been done in the area of psychometrics developing standardized questions and surveys pertaining to specific behaviors, attitudes, skills, knowledge, ability, achievement, etc. Utilizing proven standardized measures provides the most reliable survey data because of the less subjective nature. The following key terms have been identified by the ACCME accrediting organization to aid in the understanding and effective measurement: competence, performance, and outcomes (ACCME, 2013).

Competence—Knowledge put into action by the learner.

Performance—A measure of the actual "practice of the learner" or evidence of performance *in practice.*

Outcomes—There are various types of outcomes: patient outcomes, research outcomes, executive/clinical staff outcomes, administrative outcomes; those are the consequences in the system, in your stakeholder, in the place of application of your performance. These are measured to determine the impact of the educational intervention (Table 7.4.1).

It is important that outcome measurements are customized to the activity, and are in place prior to beginning the activity. Various types of data can be used in analyzing the educational interventions and program as a whole. These include the following:

- Self-reported data: surveys (pre-, post-, and follow-up intervention)
- Observational data

TABLE 7.4.1

Case Example Methods and Outcomes

Training Format	Learner Outcomes		
	Knowledge	Competence	Performance
Didactic Training	Knowledge	Competence	Performance
Goal: Educate all prior to installation of new anesthesia machines and patient monitors.	✕		
Physicians (41)			
Anesthesiologists			
Residents			
Nonphysicians/Techs (32)			
Anesthesia Technicians			
Biomedical Technicians			
CRNAs			
Perfusionists			
Simulated Training	Knowledge	Competence	Performance
Goal: Provide "hands-on" experience to all clinical staff to help familiarize them with new equipment and advanced technology before "going live."		✕	
Objective: Simulation training participants should be more confident in their ability to:			
Prepare staff using new equipment for rapid response to potential complications.		✕	✕
Troubleshoot anesthesia machines and patient monitor alarms.		✕	✕
Utilize knowledge of the new equipment capabilities.		✕	✕
Perform a daily checkout on the anesthesia machines and patient monitor.		✕	✕
Properly use the anesthetic gas analysis.		✕	✕
Set alarm limits and parameters on the anesthesia machine.		✕	✕
Set alarm limits for the patient monitor.		✕	✕
Training Outcomes	Knowledge	Competence	Performance
A smoother transition at "go live"			✕
CME credits received for participation			✕
Improved patient safety through the implementation of new technology			✕
Reduced rates for physician malpractice insurance			✕
Reduced training days			✕
Troubleshooting			✕

*Total required to be trained, $n = 43$.

- Organizational data: patient charts, electronic records, administrative/provider data
- Public Health data: health status measures, epidemiological data

It is important to identify measures that effectively provide information about the impact made by the educational intervention. Additionally, outcome results can provide valuable information that can be effectively applied to improve future activities, and are a necessary component to maintaining compliance for CME (**Table 7.4.2**).

TABLE 7.4.2

TIPS AND CHALLENGES

Challenges	Advice
Audience size	Smaller groups • Use smaller groups to your advantage (i.e., simulation). Larger groups • Audience response systems. • Breakout/skill stations. • Involve champions to help "market."
CME credit	• Involve CME in entire process. • Request credit early.
OME "lingo"	• Define in layman's terms.
Changing culture from didactic to interactive	• Demonstrate value and results from the activities you can do. • Work with simulationists to develop content.
Documentation	• Conflict of Interest forms. • Disclosure forms. • Final Report—document final outcome(s), descriptive information. • Needs Assessment—provides a "gap analysis" and proposed problem/gap in service. This document should be used to help identify the outcome(s). • Outcomes Assessment. • Planning Document.
Financial support	• Apply for grants. • CME fees for registrants. • Display fees from vendors. • Involve CME as early as possible as certain things can negate credit. • Philanthropy.
Identifying and measuring outcomes	• Design outcome measurement prior to implementation. • Document final outcomes. • Pre/postmeasurement. • Use Needs Assessment to identify the outcome.
Marketing	• "Early Bird" incentives. • Catering/food provided. • Media materials—brochures, e-blasts, posters, postcards, Web site, advertisement at CME conferences/symposiums. • Online registration option.
Staff	• Awareness of resources available. • Cross-train CME and simulation staff. • Train staff to "be the expert."

Program Evaluation and Reporting

Successful program evaluation requires both analyses of the activities and their outcomes, as well as the process. Ideally, program evaluation should address whether the program is fulfilling the mission, meeting the goals or performance measures, producing the desired impact/results, making the greatest possible impact, and making the most efficient use of funds and resources. The ACCME (2013) has provided the following criteria, although continually changing, that provides a solid foundation for program evaluation and improvement:

- Criterion 11—The provider analyzes changes in learners (competence, performance, or patient outcomes) achieved as a result of the overall program's activities/educational interventions (**Table 7.4.3**).
- Criterion 12—The provider gathers data or information and conducts a program-based analysis on the degree to which the CME mission of the provider has been met through the conduct of CME activities/educational interventions.
- Criterion 13—The provider identifies, plans, and implements the needed or desired changes in the overall program (e.g., planners, teachers, infrastructure, methods, resources, facilities, interventions) that are required to improve on the ability to meet the CME mission.
- Criterion 14—The provider demonstrates that identified program changes or improvements, that are required to improve on the provider's ability to meet the CME mission, are underway or completed.
- Criterion 15—The provider demonstrates that the impacts of program improvements, that are required to improve on the provider's ability to meet the CME mission, are measured.

Once programmatic data is analyzed and reviewed, a provider is required to determine any necessary changes to the program, implement recommend strategies, and evaluate the success of the strategies in an ongoing process improvement format.

NURSING CONTINUING EDUCATION

In order to provide approved CE for nurses, an organization must become an approved provider through an agency such as the American Nurses Credentialing Center (ANCC) (www.aacn.org). An **approved provider unit** has the authority to plan, implement, and evaluate its own CE activities during the 3-year approval period.

CE in nursing consists of planned, organized learning experiences designed to improve the following: knowledge, skills, and attitudes of nurses in the areas of practice, education, theory development, research, and administration. CE outcomes should be focused on improving the health of the public and the nurse's pursuit of professional career goals.

TABLE 7.4.3					
Analyzing Changes in Learners					
	Process	**Description**	**Educational Format**	**Measurement: Source of Data**	**Disadvantages**
Learner outcome levels	Knowledge	Participant knows what to do	Didactic lecture, online video (LMS), informational	Pre- and posttests/assessments of knowledge (same questions)	Self-reported data (subjective)
	Competence	Participant knows how to do what the CME activity intended them to do	Simulation, skills workshop, standardized patients, role-play, case-based scenarios	Observation in setting	Self-reported data, intention to change (subjective)
	Performance	Participant does what the CME activity intended them to be able to do in their practices	Simulation, skills workshops	Observation of performance in patient care setting, medical records, patient charts, databases; self-reported change	Self-report of performance (subjective)
Other outcomes	Patient health	Changes in patient health due to educational activity/ changes in practice	NA	Patient health data. Epidemiological data, patient records, insurance data, registries (i.e., incidence/ prevalence data), etc.	HIPPA, data entry/collection methods may vary, missing or duplicate data, covariates
	Community health	Changes in population health due to educational activity/ changes in practice	NA	Population health data: CMS data, CDC, MMRW, Health Departments, Insurance, Organizations, etc.	Aggregate data, data entry/collection methods may vary, missing or duplicate data

References: Moore, D. E., Jr., Green, J. S., & Gallis, H. A. (2009).

Approved provider units must meet the following criteria:

1. Have a clearly defined department that is administratively and operationally responsible for continuing nursing education.
2. Have Nurse Planner(s) who meet(s) qualifications of:
   a. Minimum of Bachelor of Science in Nursing (BSN)
   b. Knowledge of adult learning, ANCC Accreditation criteria, and Board of Nursing rules
3. Not have a relationship with a commercial entity that produces, markets, resells, or distributes a product used on or by patients.

SIMILARITIES AND DIFFERENCES BETWEEN NURSING CE AND CME

Similarities and differences exist between Nursing CE and CME. The educational activity planning cycle is similar for both **provider units**, with program outcomes focused on improving patient care. Both Nursing CE and CME have the ability to award contact hours for **provider-directed, learner-paced activities** and **learner-directed, learner-paced activities**. Nursing CE and CME both award one contact hour of CE for every 60 minutes of programming.

The primary difference between Nursing CE and CME are the requirements/criteria of the accreditation approver. Nursing CE requires a **Primary Nurse Planner** to be responsible for the Approved Provider Unit, with a minimum of a BSN. Planners submitting a *provider-directed* or *learner-directed* activity form for approval must have a minimum of a BSN and meet ANCC and Board of Nursing criteria.

APPLYING FOR CREDIT

The application process for CME credit varies by organization and program type. Some criteria relate to the overall CME Program versus individual activities and are thus not pertinent to the application for credit for specific activities (i.e., mission statement, program analysis). Organizations will need to identify the desired target audience(s), research requirements and fees, and determine the available budget and priorities before deciding which type of credit to offer.

Many healthcare professionals, in addition to physicians, can apply CME credit to their own CE requirements. For example, depending on board of nursing rules, nurses may be able to use CME credit for licensure renewal; however, nurses with specialty-specific certification through ANCC may only use 37.5 hours of the required 75 CE hours from medical education (CME)-approved hours (American Nurses Association, 2010).

BEEN THERE, DONE THAT: HOW CAN I CONTINUE TO IMPROVE OR SUSTAIN WHAT I HAVE ACHIEVED?

Many organizations offering CME or CE are going beyond the standard provider status, making efforts to not only sustain the current programs they have, but taking the next steps in improving the quality of educational activities provided.

The ACCME offers an opportunity for providers to receive Accreditation with Commendation (ACCME, 2013).

ACCME Commendation Criteria

The former criteria 16 to 22 (ACME, 2013) was recommended for those seeking accreditation with commendation. Similar standards still apply (see ACME website for most current requirements):

- Criterion 16—Compliance requires that the CME provider play a role in the improvement of practice. The CME entity should be able to demonstrate a presence, influence, or contributory role in changing practice in some way within the organization's improvement processes. Examples involving simulation could be the improvement of a hands-on skill or procedure, or learning a new skill or procedure identified by the medical staff office for credentialing purposes. Simulation with CME could also demonstrate change in dealing with a difficult patient or managing a patient. The example provided at the beginning of this chapter would also qualify. Regardless of the type of intervention, the key is to include some type of assessment (i.e., pre-/post-assessment) to measure a change due to the intervention activity. This assessment could be in support of a quality improvement initiative where data is already available for use as an assessment. A learner's ability to perform a procedure, process, or patient interaction could be assessed and documented by an observer(s) before and after the activity. An organization might also demonstrate collaboration between CME and process improvement groups. There are multiple opportunities with CME and simulation to improve practice, but to comply with Criterion 16, CME must be part of the organization's processes and documentation must be available to confirm compliance.
- Criterion 17—The ACCME would like CME providers to supplement the educational activities they provide with additional tools to support the content and increase the potential for change. Their website lists many examples and states that even though some of these strategies may be considered educational, the idea is that information and tools be provided in addition to the accredited activities.
- Criterion 18—This criterion asks CME providers to look beyond the needs assessment and gap analysis of their own learners and consider what else might be affecting the issue that the education is attempting to address.
- Criterion 19—This criterion requires providers to respond to information they collected in needs assessments and gap analyses that indicates actual or potential barriers to learning. Identification of such barriers can be challenging given the wide variation in medical practices, hospitals, institutions, and so on. It is important that barriers to

change are identified and considered in the development of CME content as well as in outcome measurement.
- Criterion 20—The ACCME is looking for providers to demonstrate active engagement in collaborative and cooperative projects. This criterion is intended to encourage providers to reach beyond their planning committees to involve organizations that can help them with the two prior criteria and break down the barriers that might be blocking success. Providers often interpret this criterion to mean that they need to participate in joint providership; however, the ACCME says it does not consider simply having a joint providership, in and of itself, evidence of compliance with this standard. If the joint providership is a by-product of a larger collaboration and if this larger collaboration is substantive, then it could provide evidence of compliance with the standard.
- Criterion 21—In order to comply with this requirement, a CME provider must show that CME is integrated into their organization/system's quality improvement structure. Examples of this might include CME as a standing agenda item at various committee meetings, CME or simulation mentioned as a resource in the organization's quality improvement plan, or quality improvement committee and CME committee having joint membership.
- Criterion 22—In this criterion, ACCME requires that the CME provider be in a position to influence their activities. This can be accomplished in many ways (see ACCME website for suggestions).

A provider must comply with all these criteria to receive accreditation with commendation. These criteria are primarily about collaboration between CME and the rest of the organization or outside organizations. To earn commendation, a provider must demonstrate that they involve additional stakeholders when appropriate and not plan education with their input only. A provider might work with other departments within the same organization to plan education, or for instance, they may work with the American Heart Association to provide a CME activity.

SUMMARY

A CME or CE program should strive to provide high-quality educational interventions that advance the knowledge, competence, and performance of healthcare professionals to improve the health of the patients/public being served. Becoming accredited or maintaining accreditation provides many benefits for not only physicians and nurses, but other clinical staff as well. Interprofessional collaboration to develop team training and including adult learning principles, exemplified in simulation, should also be a goal. Obtaining CE is a necessary component of maintaining licensure for clinical staff, accreditation bodies are looking for innovation and adult learning methods, and the healthcare industry has many quality and safety initiatives to implement. This is an environment ripe for simulation and CE.

Updated Information

At the time of publication, the ACCME had reviewed criteria and implemented multiple changes in an attempt to "simplify and evolve the accreditation process." The updated ACCME Criteria can be found at http://www.accme.org/sites/default/files/626_20140225_Accreditation_Requirements_Document_0.pdf.

REFERENCES

Accreditation Council for Continuing Medical Education. (2013a). *The accreditation requirements of the Accreditation Council for Continuing Medical Education (ACCME): Standards for commercial support.* Retrieved from http://www.accme.org/sites/default/files/626_Accreditation_Requirements_Document_20120924.pdf

Accreditation Council for Continuing Medical Education. (2013b). *CME providers: Accreditation criteria.* Retrieved from http://www.accme.org/requirements/accreditation-requirements-cme-providers/accreditation-criteria

Accreditation Council for Continuing Medical Education. (2013c). *CME providers: Criterion 20.* Retrieved from http://www.accme.org/requirements/accreditation-requirements-cme-providers/criteria/criterion-20

Accreditation Council for Continuing Medical Education. (2013d). *CME providers: First-time applicants.* Retrieved from http://www.accme.org/cme-providers/first-time-applicant/determining-your-eligibility

Accreditation Council for Continuing Medical Education. (2013e). *CME providers: Joint accreditation.* Retrieved from www.accme.org/cme-providers/joint-accreditation

Accreditation Council for Continuing Medical Education. (2013f). *Murray Kopelow: Engagement CME environment exploring criteria 18, 19 and 20.* Retrieved from http://www.accme.org/education-and-support/video/faq/engagement-cme-environment-exploring-criteria-18-19-and-20

American Board of Medical Specialties. (2013). *MOC competencies and criteria.* Retrieved from http://www.abms.org/maintenance_of_certification/MOC_competencies.aspx

American Nurses Association. (2010). *Nursing professional development: Scope and standards of practice* (#NPD-20 ed.). Silver Springs, MD: Author.

American Osteopathic Association. (2013). Retrieved from http://www.osteopathic.org/inside-aoa/development/continuing-medical-education/Pages/default.aspx

Curtis, M. T., DiazGranados, D., & Feldman, M. (2012). Judicious use of simulation technology in continuing medical education. *The Journal of Continuing Education in the Health Professions, 32*(4), 255–260.

Davis, D., O'Brien, M. A., Freemantle, N., Wolf, F. M., Mazmanian, P., & Taylor-Vaisey, A. (1999). Impact of formal continuing medical education: Do conferences, workshops, rounds, and other traditional continuing education activities change physician behavior or health care outcomes? *JAMA: The Journal of the American Medical Association, 282*(9), 867–874.

McGaghie, W. C., Siddall, V. J., Mazmanian, P. E., & Myers, J. (2009). Lessons for continuing medical education from simulation research in undergraduate and graduate medical education: Effectiveness of continuing medical education: American College of Chest Physicians Evidence-Based Educational Guidelines. *Chest, 135*(3 Suppl.), 62s–68s.

Moore, D. E. Jr, Green J. S., & Gallis, H. A. (2009). Achieving desired results and improved outcomes: integrating planning and assessment throughout learning activities. *The Journal of Continuing Education in the Health Professions, 29*(1),1–15.

Zigmont, J. J., Kappus, L. J., & Sudikoff, S. N. (2011a). The 3D model of debriefing: Defusing, discovering, and deepening. *Seminars in Perinatology, 35*(2), 52–58.

Zigmont, J. J., Kappus, L. J., & Sudikoff, S. N. (2011b). Theoretical foundations of learning through simulation. *Seminars in Perinatology, 35*(2), 47–51.

SUGGESTED READINGS

Accreditation Council for Continuing Medical Education. (2009). *What's the difference between "knowledge," "competence," "performance" and "patient outcomes"?* Retrieved from http://www.accme.org/ask-accme/whatsdifference-between-knowledge-competence-performance-and-patientoutcomes

Boyers, P. J., Lynch, L., Stewart, W., Stobbe, B., & Winfield, S. (2010). Anesthesia training in new technology.

Castanelli, D. J. (2009). The rise of simulation in technical skills teaching and the implications for training novices in anaesthesia. *Anaesthesia and Intensive Care, 37*(6), 903–910.

Chang, C. H. (2013). Medical simulation is needed in anesthesia training to achieve patient's safety. *Korean Journal of Anesthesiology, 64*(3), 204–211.

OhioHealth. (n.d.). *Center for learning, CME & I.* Retrieved from www.ohcme.com

Ohio Nurses Association. (n.d.). Retrieved from www.nursing.ohio.gov

Ohio Nurses Association. (2012–2013). *Continuing education provider manual.* Retrieved from http://www.ohnurses.org/education/Teach/approved-providers/provider-manual-and-forms/2012-2013ONAProviderManualRevised.pdf

Olympio, M., Reinke, B., & Abramovich, A. (2006). Challenges ahead in technology training: A report on the training initiative of the Committee on Technology. *APSF Newsletter,* 43–48.

Ross, A. J., Kodate, N., Anderson, J. E., Thomas, L., & Jaye, P. (2012). Review of simulation studies in anaesthesia journals, 2001–2010: Mapping and content analysis. *British Journal of Anaesthesia, 109*(1), 99–109.

Simplification and evolution [Press release]. (2013). Retrieved from http://accme.org/requirements/accreditation-requirements-cme-providers/simplification-and-evolution

SECTION 8

Faculty Development

CHAPTER 8.1

Educator Training and Simulation Methodology Courses

Jason Zigmont, PhD, CHSE-A, Nichole Oocumma, PhD (ABD), BSDH, MA, CHES, CHSE, Demian Szyld, MD, EdM, and José M. Maestre, MD, PhD

ABOUT THE AUTORS

JASON ZIGMONT, System Director of Learning Innovation, for OhioHealth in Columbus, Ohio, oversees simulation and experiential learning including CME for a health system that includes 8 hospitals and 42 care sites. He serves on the Society for Simulation in Healthcare's Education committee and heads the subcommittee on preparation for the Certified Healthcare Simulation Educator. He holds a PhD in Adult Learning, specifically focused on Experiential Learning, and is a nationally registered Paramedic.

NICHOLE OOCUMMA, Experiential Learning Outcomes Manager, for OhioHealth in Columbus, Ohio, is responsible for the design, development, and management of system initiatives and programs. She has 20 years of experience in curriculum development, specifically in medical education and public health. In this role, she is responsible for faculty development, facilitating learning through simulation and bedside teaching, and designing and measuring outcomes that demonstrate a system value.

DEMIAN SZYLD, Associate Medical Director, New York Simulation Center for the Health Sciences (NYSIM), codirects faculty and program development, research, and center management at the simulation center of New York University Langone Medical Center and the City University of New York (CUNY). A faculty member of the Institute for Medical Simulation, he teaches faculty development courses in the USA, Spain, Colombia, and other Latin American countries. Additionally, he serves as the Vice-Chair of the Society for Simulation in Healthcare Affiliations Committee.

JOSÉ M. MAESTRE serves as the Education Director at *Hospital virtual Valdecilla* in Santander, Spain. In this role, he promotes interprofessional team training using simulation and instructor development. Other affiliations include anesthesiologist and member of the Simulation Working Party of the Anesthesia and Critical Care Spanish Society; Director of the Spanish Simulation Instructor Courses at the Center for Medical Simulation, Boston, MA; and Harvard Macy Scholar at the Program for Educators in Health Professions.

Acknowledgments: The authors dedicate this chapter to their families and mentors.

ABSTRACT

A growing number of healthcare organizations around the globe are using healthcare simulation. It offers opportunities to help individuals become excellent providers and learn how to be more effective when working in teams. The challenge for the professionals dedicated to the use of simulation as a teaching method is to create learning experiences that promote reflective practice and significant behavioral change that result in measurable outcomes. Apart from content knowledge, the education, skills, and behaviors essential for teaching healthcare professionals through experiential learning lie beyond common clinical background and training. Instead, they come from the fields of adult learning, education, psychology, organizational behavior, and management. This chapter provides general guidance for different levels of development and a comprehensive theoretical foundation for those who want to start or advance their role as educators or managers of simulation centers. These principles and framework are offered as a practical and applicable example and guide based on the background and experience of the authors and peer-reviewed literature.

CASE EXAMPLE

Anna has been hired to serve as the Education Director of a recently opened simulation center. It is the result of a merger of three different educational institutions that have been using simulation as a teaching tool. There is already an extensive cadre of seasoned faculty with different perspectives on the use of experiential learning, and several novice instructors willing to start working in the brand new state-of-the-art facilities. The Board wants Anna to unify the curriculum and the instructional design, and start a quality improvement program for all simulation activities. Some members of the Board have expressed concern that most of the courses are aimed at a single discipline. "They work in silos. We need an interprofessional focus," stated the Executive Director.

Anna soon realized that the type of educational background and formal training varied widely amongst faculty members. Some have become certified instructors in specific clinical areas. They have completed courses that mainly use standardized patients to train participants, and have adopted a similar model in their own activities. Most of the surgical faculty, very experienced clinical experts in their fields, believe that practice with task trainers and virtual reality facilitate mastery, and are mainly focused on psychomotor skills training. Only a few have attended formal courses on education in healthcare.

The simulationists who use mannequins to teach clinical decision making and teamwork have varied backgrounds. Some have attended external courses that teach the use of simulation in education, and others have attended short courses organized at their home institutions. Anna had met many who had signed up for seminars, workshops, or attended national and international simulation conferences. The novices have mainly followed an apprenticeship model of education, and have collaborated in different activities along the way. They are all using different debriefing styles. Simulation technicians have followed a similar pathway. Simulation at the Nursing and Medical Schools is flourishing. Students normally train alone, and there is still a tendency to separate preclinical and clinical content. Integration of simulation with clerkships at the University and with clinical rotations in the Residency programs is still in its infancy.

After her initial assessment, Anna is ready to formulate a blueprint for a faculty development program. She asks herself, "What are the needs of faculty prior to teaching with simulation? Should I write a policy describing training requirements at our sim center? How do I motivate faculty and promote interprofessional cooperation from the beginning? Should I train simulation technicians too? How do I ensure engaging/safe learning experiences for all participants?"

INTRODUCTION, BACKGROUND, AND SIGNIFICANCE

Faculty development is a critical component of any healthcare simulation program. With skilled educators who are comfortable with and capable of teaching with simulation technology, healthcare simulation programs can efficiently and effectively achieve meaningful learning and improved outcomes.

Faculty development programs for healthcare **simulation educators** can be formal (courses) or informal (apprenticeship). Faculty can access formal courses at the institution where they teach or may join a regional, national, or international course such as those offered at society meetings, hotels and resorts, or simulation centers. In addition to taking courses and learning from experience, educators can further develop by creating a faculty development program or joining peer groups or communities of practice. In this setting, educators might observe **simulation sessions** and give feedback or **debrief**.

This chapter proposes a comprehensive framework that describes a long-term process to implement, assess, and manage simulation-based educational activities. This pathway is not static, and will evolve over time with deliberate practice and feedback, along with advancements in the field.

HOW TO DESIGN FACULTY DEVELOPMENT PROGRAMS FOR HEALTHCARE SIMULATION EDUCATORS

Designing faculty development programs for healthcare simulation educators should follow standard curriculum design principles. Kern et al. (1998) outline six steps to curriculum design:

1. Problem Identification and General Needs Assessment
2. Needs Analysis of Targeted Learners
3. Goals and Specific Measurable Objectives
4. Educational Strategies
5. Implementation
6. Evaluation and Feedback

Step 1: Problem Identification and General Needs Assessment

Problem identification and general needs assessment is presented in the case example, as it identifies the problem of educator training for healthcare simulation and begins the general needs assessment process (see chapter 7.1 for more information on performing a needs assessment).

Step 2: Needs Analysis of Targeted Learners

Simulation allows participants to experience complex clinical situations in an interactive manner. The environment plays an important role in replicating substantial aspects of the actual clinical work. It can recreate emotional responses similar to real-life situations. It values and provides a time and space to reflect on performance. This unique learning environment poses many challenges and barriers to success for faculty accustomed to teaching in more traditional settings.

Within the broad field of healthcare simulation, spanning screen-based simulators, partial task trainers, animal models, cadavers, programs with **standardized patients**, and immersive simulations with mannequins, educators should understand and appropriately employ relevant learning theories, select and manage technology, create or select relevant clinical cases and scenarios, give learners actionable feedback, encourage reflection, and facilitate transfer of knowledge. Given the broad skill set and multiple domains, healthcare simulation educators are often trained to different levels with different core concepts.

The Society for Simulation in Healthcare (SSH) has developed a voluntary process for Certification of Healthcare Simulation Educators. It validates the knowledge, skills, and abilities essential to qualified individuals who are instructors or managers of simulation educational interventions. It identifies and standardizes best practices, and indicates a level of competence and educational expertise. There are two levels of certification: Certified Healthcare

---

TABLE 8.1.1

Examples of Advanced Educational Concepts and Skills for Mastery Learning

- Learning styles
- Activating passive learners!
- Upset participants
- Learner-developed simulations
- Teaching procedural skills
- Breaking bad news
- Difficult conversations
- Advanced debriefing strategies (e.g., guided team self-correction)
- Conducting simulations in the clinical setting
- Exploring, diagnosing, and closing performance gaps
- Metacognition
- Collaborating and negotiating

Simulation Educator (CHSE) and CHSE-Advanced (see chapter 1.4 for more information on certification).

In accordance with novice to expert theory (Dreyfus & Dreyfus, 1980) and the SSH Committee for Certification of Healthcare Simulation Educators, this section focuses on three levels of educator development—entry, basic, and advanced—that define the levels of competence and educational expertise in the area of healthcare simulation education (Table 8.1.1). Knowledge of these levels and competencies benefits learners, educators, health administrators, funders, and patients by ensuring standards in simulation education.

Simulation technicians often provide support and training to simulation educators in areas of equipment, programming, as well as use of simulation and technology. Therefore, development of these individuals is also a focus in this section (see chapters in sections 3 and 6 for more

---

EXPERT'S CORNER

AN UNCONVENTIONAL JOURNEY TO HEALTHCARE SIMULATION
Don Combs, PhD
Board of Directors, Society for Simulation in Healthcare

Forty years ago, I entered the doctoral program in political science at the University of North Carolina (UNC)-Chapel Hill. My intent was to explore conflict, conflict resolution, and public policy analysis, which at that time was a newly emerging specialization. The focus of political science itself is often stated as the understanding of *who gets what when and why* and, on the basis of that understanding, *how things can be made better*.

Around the time I arrived in Chapel Hill, the Robert Wood Johnson Foundation made its first national grant award of several million dollars to establish healthcare practices in rural areas of the United States. The National Office for this program was based at UNC. Through an unusual set of interactions with faculty, I was hired to be a "participant observer" in what became known as the Rural Practice Project (RPP). I was charged to write contemporaneous notes about the development and implementation of the RPP. For the following 4 years, I worked to document the establishment of 12 new rural health centers across the nation. I was hired as

the Administrator responsible for standing up the last funded center in Surry County, Virginia. This health center development experience became the fodder for my dissertation and gave me 3 years of real-world working experience, which in turned qualified me for a "practitioner" faculty position in public administration at Old Dominion University (ODU).

While teaching at ODU, I became involved in the Area Health Education Center (AHEC) program, a long-running federal program for primary care in medically underserved areas. My AHEC work led to connections with leadership at Eastern Virginia Medical School (EVMS). I was recruited to join the EVMS Senior Management to focus on governmental relations, strategic planning, and program development. In my 30 years at EVMS, I have been fortunate to be involved in both local and national efforts to improve education, to adapt new technologies, and to travel and collaborate with colleagues around the world.

My experience has provided many opportunities to identify the challenges confronting contemporary healthcare—patient safety, quality outcomes, initial and continuing competence of practitioners, effective incorporation of new technologies, effective teamwork, and increasingly, explicit performance metrics. I have witnessed efforts to respond to these challenges in rural Botswana, central Bulgaria, Nepal, Montana, Virginia, Hong Kong, Singapore, and scores of other healthcare settings. As someone interested in improving healthcare, I am always searching for technologies and applications that can help us do better. And, in the last 25 years, this increasingly has pointed to the role of healthcare simulation.

In 1996, I was asked to chair the annual meeting of the Association of Academic Health Centers, and developed a program around the theme "The Digital Decade." The point was to help the leaders of the nation's academic health centers understand the tsunami of change that was headed their way as computers became faster, software became both better and easier to use, visualization capabilities were enhanced, and rapid prototyping took hold. We had demonstrations of early mannequins, task trainers, and epidemiological simulations as part of the agenda.

Following that AAHC meeting, I became an advocate for the expanded use of simulation in medical and health professions education and in healthcare practice. I began to regularly attend conferences such as Medicine Meets Virtual Reality (MMVR), the International Meeting on Simulation in Healthcare (IMSH), and a variety of related technology-oriented meetings around the world. I also began to focus on identifying resources for EVMS' simulation programs and was able, in 2011, to move into a new 25,000 square feet (2,322.5 m^2) center housing standardized patients, task trainers, mannequins, and an immersive lab. Our major teaching healthcare system provided an endowment for the center, and we continue to actively seek commercial partners for the development of new programming.

My current involvements with medical simulation include overseeing the Sentara Center for Simulation and Immersive Learning and the National Center for Collaboration in Medical Modeling and Simulation at EVMS. I serve on the Society for Simulation in Healthcare's Board of Directors and as Chair of its Public Affairs and Government Relations Committee, as well as on the Policy Board of the National Modeling and Simulation Coalition. These roles emerged as a result of what has been an unconventional career, at least insofar as I am not a clinician or a simulation practitioner. On the other hand, the continuing focus on understanding who gets what when and why and the implementation of policies that can make things better, a broad exposure to healthcare education and practice settings worldwide, and an abiding interest in emerging technologies and their effective incorporation into healthcare practice is perhaps not as unconventional a professional journey as it at first might seem. This is the case for many educators entering healthcare simulation.

information about specific knowledge and competencies needed by simulation technicians).

Entry-Level/Novice Simulation Educators

Background and Experience

Entry-level simulation educators are new to simulation or have limited experience. In a prelicensure health professions education context, they might be practicing healthcare professionals who serve as clinical or adjunct instructors. Owing to program requirements, they might be asked to teach with simulation between one and a few times per semester. They do not have formal training in simulation education and may not have any formal training in education. They usually rely on educational strategies that they have developed in other settings such as classrooms, wards, and their own training. In some contexts, although novice at simulation education, they might have significant experience in another domain. In this case, they might be well suited to serve as content experts and assist during debriefing. Some entry-level faculty develop expertise in a single domain; for example, they may teach the American Heart Association's Pediatric Advanced Life Support (PALS) on a weekly basis. Nonetheless, these gains do not translate to other courses or topics.

Competencies

Entry-level simulation educators rely on course directors and other healthcare simulation educators to establish a context for learning. They must maintain a psychologically safe learning environment throughout the educational process but are not necessarily expected to help establish it. It is expected that they will teach to the curriculum, meet the objectives set forth by course directors, and employ scenarios and curricula that are created by others (content leaders), published in peer-reviewed literature, or that are commercially available. They are novice managers of simulation technology, capable of teaching with partial task trainers that are inanimate and using scenarios that are not complex without improvising (see Consider This). The feedback and evaluation they provide is not likely to be standardized. As they do not steer far from the teaching plan, they cannot tailor the learning experience to the learners. They can work well with a more advanced simulation instructor such as a healthcare simulation educator who can set the tone and pace and lead the simulation session. Teaching knowledge and understanding comes easily, but teaching how to apply that knowledge may not be within reach of the entry-level educator (Binstadt et al., 2007). Their students may have improved confidence levels and have acquired new knowledge and skills following the simulation.

Healthcare Simulation Educators—Basic Level

Background and Experience

Healthcare simulation educators at the basic level are more experienced instructors. They strive to achieve proficiency to early expert levels of expertise through formal training and experience at the design and implementation levels of the curriculum and frequently have formal training in simulation education. Healthcare simulation educators might teach often (more than once per month) and at a high level, and therefore they have improved their skills as they have been exposed to challenging situations. They may have taught many different types of courses with different levels of learners. They have taught in different domains such as clinical knowledge, teamwork, patient safety, and psychomotor or procedural skills. Simulation education is their preferred teaching modality. They are flexible as they teach to the curriculum and use multiple methods because they see the larger picture.

Competencies

At this level, simulation faculty can establish and maintain a context for learning. They introduce learners to the simulation environment in a way that is conducive to learning and can teach independently or with a content expert or more novice instructor. They can teach different topics and scenarios at a high level, including different types of learners. They can employ multiple technologies, including sophisticated simulators and complex simulations with multiple patients and embedded simulation personnel. They can create their own teaching scenarios and debriefing guides. They have a structured approach to debriefing but can deviate from it at times to meet a particular learner's needs. Feedback is of high quality: specific, actionable, and constructive. They use video effectively, when it is available, to illustrate a point rather than to shame learners or replay long segments without a definite purpose. If the curriculum has set a standard, the healthcare simulation educator at this level is prepared to teach to this standard and help learners reach it. Key features at this level are the ability to collaborate with others, to give and receive feedback, to engage in deliberate planning, to follow routines, and to have a broader view of the simulations. For example, healthcare simulation educators understand the value of a particular simulation session in the context of the entire curriculum and can therefore adjust the focus onto one objective and come back to others in another session. Most importantly, these educators teach complex cognitive processes, including application and synthesis of knowledge. Their students gain new understanding through transformative experience and reflection.

Healthcare Simulation Educators—Advanced Level

Background and Experience

Experts in simulation education, the advanced healthcare simulation educators have been immersed in the healthcare simulation environment for many years, designing, implementing, and evaluating simulation programs across domains. They select curricula and scenarios and design new ones. They lead simulation programs, coach other faculty, and work on improving their own practice. Many have done research in simulation and have leadership positions locally, regionally, and internationally through specialty societies or other organizations. They have taken basic and advanced courses for simulation instructors and adapted strategies from other domains. Frequently, they teach in simulation instructor courses and promote faculty development in other formal and informal ways. They have mastered the competencies of beginners and proficient educators and consistently deliver high-quality, transformative courses. They are experts and masters of the technology and the technique.

Competencies

Advanced healthcare simulation educators consistently perform at a high level in all domains of simulation education. A particular feature is that they can reliably help learners of all levels, including other faculty and themselves, to reflect on and improve their performance across domains, including helping other faculty improve their teaching abilities and effectiveness. A critical competency of advanced educators is that they can reconsider established practices in the field and challenge them, experimenting in formal and informal ways. Additionally, they develop and implement faculty development initiatives to improve learning outcomes for all learners, not just those they reach directly.

EXPERT'S CORNER

WHY SCENARIO FACILITATORS SHOULD NOT BE NOVICE
Janice C. Palaganas, PhD, RN, NP
Director, Institute for Medical Simulation; Principal Faculty, Center for Medical Simulation; Past Director, SSH Accreditation and Certification

One of the advantages of healthcare simulation is the ability to interact with learners in a way where the patient outcomes are related to their actions and interventions. Supporting this advantage, there needs to be a level of experience and expertise behind the mirror. Often, a learner or group of learners will engage in a simulation in an unanticipated way. Because of this, the faculty directing the simulation must be ready to promptly respond to unanticipated actions in a way that is realistic for the patient care event—whether it is patient signals, verbal response, cueing an embedded simulated provider or family how to respond, or stopping the simulation as a safety intervention. If novice or faculty without experience in this area are directing the simulation, training is necessary on how to facilitate the simulation and the event, as well as the multiple outcomes that may occur. Some ways to overcome this challenge are to develop scenarios with deep thought and planning around if's and then's (if the learners do this, then this will happen) and to validate the scenario with multiple target learners as a means to train facilitators without clinical experience around the event simulated.

Healthcare Simulation Technician

Background and Experience

Healthcare simulation technicians come from healthcare and technical backgrounds. Many simulation centers employ prehospital providers such as emergency medical technicians or paramedics, nurses, students, information technology professionals, actors or standardized patients, laypeople, and teachers as simulation technicians. They provide technology and teaching assistance for simulation-based activities.

Competencies

Simulation technicians are responsible for creating and maintaining the learning environment at the physical level. They support educators by preparing the classrooms and clinical spaces, collecting and maintaining the inventory and supplies, operating and maintaining the simulation equipment, and, in many cases, by acting and performing other duties within the simulation scenario. They must develop interpersonal skills and technical language to interact with students, staff, faculty, and other personnel. They must follow policies and at times create them. Some may manage other individuals. As in the clinical environment, teamwork and flexibility are of paramount importance.

Step 3: Goals and Specifically Measurable Objectives for Faculty Development

This section provides an overview of what training at each level should consist of, with a detailed list of goals, **target mental models**, and skills for each level of training. This section does not provide a comprehensive list of objectives for each level. Rather, the focus on goals, target mental models, and skills allows faculty development directors to tailor both their educational program and assessment methods to meet the specific needs of their programs.

A note about target mental models, also known as frames: a target mental model reflects a set of goals, knowledge, assumptions, and so on that helps educators to predict and interpret the situations they will most likely face at their level of development (Zigmont et al., 2011b). The challenge is to help the trainee to identify their current mental model so that the learning experience facilitates reaching the target. Although assessment methods are available, this chapter focuses on the individual being able to use and test the new mental models and skills in practice rather than solely passing an assessment.

Faculty Development of Entry-Level Educators

Goals

The goal of entry-level faculty development is to take simulation neophytes and introduce them to what simulation is, when to use simulation, and when not to use simulation. The target audience is those individuals who are interfacing with your simulation educators. They may be subject matter experts and/or individuals who are "testing out" simulation for use within their own courses.

Target Mental Models and Skills

Simulation is a method of education, not a piece of equipment. It is somewhat natural for those new to simulation to think about the equipment as a tool and a set of features. Their first questions are often, what can it do, what scenarios do you have, and how do you get all of that technology to work? They may have had experience with simulation or at least have used a mannequin to learn cardio-pulmonary resuscitation (CPR). If their focus is on the equipment, the first step is to help them change their focus on the simulator and start thinking about simulation as an educational methodology.

The easiest way to facilitate the reconsideration of their mental model is to immerse them in a simulated experience. Their first experience must allow learners to gain an understanding of both the simulation itself and of the debriefing process. Ideally, the immersion would be in a simulation that uses both simulators, such as high-technology mannequins, and standardized patients (SPs) or embedded simulated persons (ESPs). It is very important to provide an effective debriefing process after this experience, as learners will often need to process their thoughts as educators in addition to discussing the medical content of the scenario. The facilitator may therefore be required to "debrief the debriefing" to help the learner understand everything that occurred.

Simulation equipment includes multiple methodologies, including skills trainers, mannequins, SPs, virtual reality, and real-life experiences (Wang, 2011). When an educator is new to simulation, all of the equipment and technology can be daunting. The goal of the entry-level program is to expose the novice educator to the potential options and explain how simulation staff can help in choosing the right methodology.

A good way to give entry-level faculty exposure to the equipment and the environment is to give them a standard tour of the simulation center. The tour should include some hands-on experience with the equipment, as well as an opportunity to meet some of the staff and, preferably, some of the SPs.

Entry-level faculty development is designed both to provide an opportunity to learn about the methodology of simulation and to promote the simulation program. Part of entry-level training should be providing guidance as to when simulation should and should not be used, on the basis of the center's mission statement, requirements, or other guiding principles. Of particular importance is the precept that simulation should be used to improve patient outcomes and facilitate organizational change (del Moral & Maestre, 2013). Such guidelines will help prevent educators from using simulation without first thinking about why or from coming to the simulation center only to "play with the toys." Increased exposure to the theory and practice of simulation may build interest in the use of the simulation center.

A key skill for the entry-level simulation educator is to learn how to work with the staff before, during, and after a simulation. This knowledge includes a basic understanding of what each staff member does and what type of information they may share. For example, when working with technical staff, they may provide patient vitals or history, as appropriate. Additionally, when working within a debriefing, the entry-level simulation educator should understand the core tenets of debriefing. Although an entry-level course cannot completely prepare novices to work with the simulation staff, it should provide a common language and guidelines for further interaction.

Assessment

Directly observing entry-level faculty operate equipment and conduct simulation sessions can yield valuable information but is resource-intensive. Other assessment options may include knowledge testing, student evaluation survey data, and self-report.

Faculty Development of Healthcare Simulation Educators—Basic Level

Goals

The goal of healthcare simulation educator faculty development is to provide the faculty with the knowledge, mental models, and skills to design, implement, and manage simulation-based educational interventions independently. As this group represents the core of educators, they should be well schooled in the principles, practice, and methodology that apply to simulation-based education. This section uses the CHSE-Basic educational blueprint as the framework for outlining essential knowledge and skills (see chapter 1.4 for the full blueprint). This framework provides a good starting point for all simulation educator faculty development programs, and can be adapted and expanded, as appropriate, for any specific program. The CHSE blueprint is broken into five domains:

    I. Display Professional Values and Capabilities
    II. Demonstrate Knowledge of Simulation Principles, Practice, and Methodology
    III. Educate and Assess Learners Using Simulation
    IV. Manage Overall Simulation Resources and Environments
    V. Engage in Scholarly Activities.

Target Mental Models and Skills

Simulation educators must display a high level of professional values and capabilities. Simulation educators often assume a leadership role and mentor entry-level educators. Simulation educators should therefore be constantly looking for ways to integrate simulation into new programs and work with content experts to improve outcomes. Additionally, simulation educators should understand that they serve a diverse group of learners.

There is a difference between education and summative assessment and there should be a clear delineation. Simulation is currently being used for both education (formative assessment) and **summative assessment**. Simulation educators should distinguish between **formative assessment** (*for* learning) and summative or high-stakes assessment (*of* learning). The challenge for a simulation educator is choosing the appropriate type of assessment and understanding the differing learning environments involved in each type of assessment. Ideally, simulation education should be done separately from summative assessments to ensure psychological safety. Unfortunately, simulation may be used as a punishment to show that students are failing. It is the simulation educator's responsibility to ensure that students are not scarred by their simulation experiences.

There are principles and theories that underpin the utilization of simulation as an educational tool. Simulation has underpinnings in adult learning, education, psychology, organizational behavior, and management. There is no way for the simulation educator to understand all of the principles and theories behind simulation, but it should be a lifelong learning effort to grow in these areas. Faculty development should reflect the principles and theories utilized most at the facility. For example, the author's centers utilize the Theoretical Foundations of Learning Through Simulation (Zigmont et al., 2011b) along with the 3D Model of Debriefing: Defusing, Discovering and Deepening (Zigmont et al., 2011a) as its guiding theory and principles. These principles are used as a common language and backed up by broader theories of experiential learning (Kolb, 1984) and deliberate practice (Ericsson & Charness, 1994). Whatever theories or principles are adopted should be used throughout the program and should guide the program evaluation (see chapter 7.2 for more information on educational theories used in simulation programs).

Simulation is one component of a curriculum, and curriculum development is more than just one simulation. A single scenario can kick-start a program, but it takes an entire curriculum to improve educational outcomes. There are multiple curriculum models; one being utilized frequently in simulation (and a focus of the SSH Education Committee) is Kern's Six Step Model of Curriculum Development (Kern et al., 1998). Simulation educators should understand the curriculum development process, as they will often be helping others with curriculum development.

Feedback and debriefing is at the core of simulation. Without feedback and debriefing, a simulation becomes just one more experience (Cantrell, 2008; Van Heukelom et al., 2010). Each learning experience should be debriefed and feedback given as soon as possible after the simulation. Simulation educators should understand the role of feedback and debriefing as part of the reflective process after an experience (see chapter 8.2 for more on the practice feedback and debriefing).

The environment and location of a simulation are important. For each simulation, the simulation educator should decide whether it is best to learn as an individual, team, or system, and then decide where the best place for that learning should be. In some situations, such as intact trauma resuscitation teams, it may be beneficial for the training to be provided in situ to achieve a more authentic learning environment.

Simulation takes many resources, and they should be managed appropriately. Simulation is a time- and money-intensive method of education, and therefore should be used to achieve the highest possible impact. The cost of running a simulation includes not only the simulator but also the staff, space, and medical equipment. Simulation educators should be aware of each methodology, the costs, and limitations. Simulation educators should help others to select the least expensive simulation that will achieve the educational objectives.

Designing a simulation is more than just picking a case. Simulation educators should understand how to pick the correct modality and case(s) to achieve the identified learning objectives. Thus, educators should fit the cases/modality to the learning objectives rather than the other way around. For example, rather than starting with "let's do a code," the simulation educator might start with the learning objective of improving critical thinking skills and focus on when or when not to call a code. The simulation educator must also always keep up on new modalities and be constantly learning so that the right resources are used for the right application. Simulation educators should work with the rest of the team to help create and plan simulations and, in some cases, even help program simulations.

Simulations require a team of people and resources. Simulation educators may be formally or informally in charge of the simulation team for any particular course. They may have to recruit, orient, and/or train SPs, technicians, and content experts. It may be challenging to motivate, put together, and lead a whole interprofessional team, so healthcare simulation educators may have to work with an advanced educator to mentor the team. It is the simulation educator's responsibility to make sure the team is ready for the activity.

Preparation is the key to success. It is not unusual for something to go differently than planned in a simulation. It is helpful for simulation educators to pilot the case and develop materials for both learners and the simulation team. Learners will need the appropriate instructions, equipment, and environment. Piloting the case will tell the simulation educator where potential pitfalls are and what changes should be completed before the course begins.

Orientation and briefings set the tone. Simulation educators should ensure that learners are oriented to the equipment, environment, and expectations. Simulation educators should teach learners how to interact with the simulator and the environment, including any ground rules. Simulation educators should pay particular attention to creating a psychologically safe environment for learning. If learners are being assessed, the simulation educator should set appropriate expectations and limitations (Forsythe, 2009).

Conducting a simulation means more than just telling the mannequin what to do. Any simulation educator quickly learns that the students are not familiar with the script and that the simulation may go astray. The simulation educator should manage personnel and equipment during the class to react quickly to both planned and unplanned events. Additionally, the simulation educator should know when to stop a simulation, especially when it is way off track (Dieckmann et al., 2010).

Learner evaluation is not a test but a way to find and remedy gaps in learning. In addition to understanding the difference between formative and summative assessment, a core skill of a simulation educator is the ability to identify the learner's performance gaps and use them to facilitate debriefing. It is the responsibility of the simulation educator to provide feedback that leads to the learning objectives of the curriculum.

Program evaluation is ongoing and never ending. All simulation educators should make a commitment to ongoing program evaluation and improvement. Program evaluation can come from self, peer, and learner evaluation. It is the responsibility of the simulation educator to seek this feedback and to use it to improve the simulated cases and the overall curriculum, in addition to their own performance and that of the other simulation team members (Elfrink et al., 2009).

Simulation resources and environments must be appropriately managed. Simulation educators should understand their role and the policies of the simulation center. Depending on the organization, the educator may have more or less responsibility for the actual operations of simulators. They need to understand how the technology works, including simulator features, medical equipment, and room setup. Additionally, they should understand how to use video capture/debriefing, if available, and the policies surrounding video recording.

Scholarly activities should be integrated throughout the educational program. Simulation educators should have a solid grasp of the literature related to the use of simulation in health professions education as well as how to produce their own scholarly work. Simulation educators should see participating in professional development as a core responsibility, including keeping up to date and disseminating their data through presentations and publications.

Assessment

Faculty development consists of more than taking a single course. It requires constant mentoring and attention. The CHSE-Basic is a formal assessment program for those who have 2 years of experience in simulation (see chapter 1.4 for more information). Within a faculty development program, there is a responsibility to ensure that simulation educators are embracing lifelong learning and constantly striving to enhance their knowledge and skills.

Faculty Development of Healthcare Simulation Educators—Advanced Level

Goals

The goal of advanced-level simulation educators is to develop as individuals who can create faculty development programs, mentor others in education, and perform learner assessment, program evaluation, and research. Advanced simulation educators are leaders in their local centers as well as regionally, nationally, and internationally.

Target Mental Models and Skills

Advanced simulation educators are mentors of other educators. Advanced educators teach faculty development courses at all levels and also act as mentors during and after individual simulation courses, both formally and informally. Therefore, advanced educators should have both a well-rounded knowledge base and experience in all areas of simulation. They do not necessarily know everything about simulation, but they should know where to get the knowledge and experience needed, reaching outside their organization if necessary.

Learner assessment comes with risks and must be managed. Advanced educators understand not only all areas of assessment but also the positive and negative impact that assessment may have. They should be consulted about and play an active part in any high-stakes assessment using simulation, including maintenance of certification or licensure. Advanced educators may be arbiters when learners disagree with formal assessments and may help educators understand assessments and their impact. Additionally, advanced educators may need to create policies and procedures to guide assessments.

Advanced educators often provide oversight over a series of programs and/or a center. The advanced educator evaluates the simulation team as a whole and identifies gaps. The evaluation data can then be used to develop future faculty development programs and to provide individual feedback. Program evaluation at the advanced level also includes evaluating whether the programs are making best use of the available resources.

Simulation and research should go hand in hand. Advanced simulation educators understand that educational research is a way to both publish results and provide rigor to programs. Research provides ways to justify program expenditures and secure future resources both internally and externally. The advanced educator often acts as a senior author, mentoring educators, the simulation team, and learners on research and research methods. As part of their own development and to serve as a resource for the entire team,

advanced-level educators make conscious efforts to stay abreast of evolving simulation education research.

Deliberate practice is needed for continuous improvement. Advanced simulation educators must constantly improve their own skills and knowledge. Advanced educators often film their own debriefings to share with other advanced educators for feedback. They serve as peer reviewers at a regional, national, and international level.

Promoting simulation is a responsibility of the advanced educator. The advanced educator should be an advocate for simulation at the local, regional, and national levels. Advanced educators should present at multiple venues to help promote simulation as a learning methodology. Advanced educators often serve as consultants for new programs both internally and externally.

Assessment

Assessment of the advanced-level simulation educator includes peer review, portfolio assessments, and review of academic productivity. There is no one method that will be valid for assessing an advanced educator (for the CHSE-Advanced assessment process, see chapter 1.4).

Professional Development of Simulation Technicians

Goals

The goal of simulation technician professional development is to create technicians who understand the educational process and how to interact with simulation educators. The goal is not to turn technicians into educators but to help them work as part of the simulation team. Professional development for technicians will vary widely, depending on their background.

Target Mental Models

It is helpful to program scenarios, but sometimes it is necessary to improvise. There seem to be two schools of thought for creating scenarios: program everything or program nothing. The technician should work with the educator to determine what should be programmed and scripted rather than just improvised. Scenarios that need to be highly standardized (such as Objective Structured Clinical Examinations) should be tightly scripted. Although scenarios may be programmed, the technician should also be able to work with the educator when things go wrong and adapt to circumstances as they arise, including when the learners and/or the equipment behave differently than expected.

The goal of any simulation is to achieve certain learning objectives. Technicians should help educators to achieve their objectives and end the scenario when the objectives are met or when the simulation is so off script that the objectives will never be met. Each scenario should be designed around the objectives, not the other way around. Technicians should also help educators to select the best simulator that will help them reach their objectives.

Less is more. There can be a natural tendency for the simulation technician to want to do more and push the limits of the simulation. Technicians may want to include moulage (see chapter 8.3), advanced features, and other enhancements. The technician should work with the educator, and use the least technology and fewest features needed to achieve the learning objectives.

Technicians should understand the clinical components of the simulation. Technicians must be able to react when given feedback from the educator or the content expert. They do not necessarily need to know all of the physiology or the effects of every drug, but they should know how to make the simulator react when appropriate. Additionally, the simulation technician may often be the "voice" of the patient, so they should know what questions will be asked and how to answer.

Simulation takes a team. The simulation technician is a key member of the team. Technicians should know their role along with the role of the educator, content expert, and other members of the team. They should understand how they interact with the team and how to provide consultative help to the rest of the team. The educator may not understand everything about the simulators, and it is the technician's job to bridge that gap.

Skills and Assessment

It is beyond the scope of this chapter to outline the specific technical skills that a simulation technician needs or how to evaluate simulation technicians. See sections 3 and 6 for a detailed treatment of these topics.

Step 4: Educational Strategies for Faculty Development

Planning the Personal Blueprint

Educators should be encouraged to create a personal learning plan for attaining their professional goals and objectives. The plan should be realistic and possible to achieve with available resources. The faculty development program should offer activities that consider the diverse needs of faculty members. As Rosenthal and Stanberry (2011) noted, "In addition to differences in their professional focus, faculty members differ on the basis of rank, length of service, sex, under-represented minority status, and family situation (e.g., having young children or elderly parents)" (p. 693).

Engaging in Reflective Practice: Developing Expertise

Purpose

The ultimate goal of reflective professional development is not solely knowledge acquisition, but improved performance through behavioral change (Osterman & Kottkamp, 1993).

Deliberate Practice

Expertise cannot be accounted for by an accumulation of knowledge and extensive professional experience, as noted by Ericsson (2008):

> After some limited training and experience…an individual's performance is adapted to the typical situational demands and is increasingly automated, and they lose conscious control over aspects of their behavior and are no longer able to make specific intentional adjustments…. When performance has reached this level of automaticity and effortless execution, additional experience will not improve the accuracy of behavior nor refine the structure of the mediating mechanisms, and consequently, the amount of accumulated experience will not be related to higher levels of performance. (pp. 989–991)

Thus, it is necessary to reveal and reproduce the mechanisms underlying superior performance. In this regard, the representative skills and behaviors that capture the essence of expertise in simulation-based education have been described above in the different levels of faculty development. They can be identified and taught to all learners under controlled and standardized conditions.

The meta-analysis of the simulation-based medical education literature by McGaghie et al. (2011) found that conditions where practice has been uniformly associated with significant improvements in performance include motivated individuals; well-defined learning objectives; ample opportunities for focused, repetitive practice; appropriate level of difficulty; rigorous, reliable measurements that provide informative feedback that promotes monitoring and gradual refinements of performance; and more deliberate practice that allows advancement to the next skill or behavior. They state, "The goal of [deliberate practice] is constant skill improvement, not just skill maintenance" (p. 707). They further note that a growing body of evidence shows that the comparative effectiveness of simulation-based medical education with deliberate practice "is a much more powerful predictor of professional accomplishment" (p. 707) than traditional education.

Reflective Practice

Reflective practice as an educational strategy in professional development as articulated by Osterman and Kottkamp (1993) begins with the task of creating awareness in action—making the unconscious conscious. "To gain a new level of insight…the reflective practitioner assumes a dual stance, being, on one hand, the actor in a drama and, on the other hand, the critic who sits in the audience watching and analyzing the entire performance" (p. 19). This perspective on their own practice allows individuals to lay bare the adjustments they need to make to improve as educators (Osterman & Kottkamp, 1993).

Reflective practice and feedback are the catalysts that drive the experiential learning cycle described by Kolb (1984). This cycle posits that learning begins with a concrete experience that "is the basis for observation and reflection. These observations are assimilated into a theory from which new implications for actions can be deduced. These implications or hypotheses then serve as guides in acting to create new experiences" (p. 21).

Professional development programs are thus crucibles of experiential learning. Faculty come to the program with a multitude of concrete experiences. They draw on prior experience as well as the new experiences offered by the program to begin the cycle of reflective learning, "a dialogue of thinking and doing" (Schön, 1987, p. 31) through which the educator becomes more skillful.

Feedback

Faculty development programs must provide educators with high-quality feedback on their performance. Despite the desire to improve, learners commonly lack awareness of what new actions or adjustments are needed to achieve success (Osterman & Kottkamp, 1993).

Feedback can provide the insight necessary to identify areas of improvement. Nevertheless, there may be a reluctance to give critical feedback, for fear of harming the relationship with the recipient. The "Debriefing with Good Judgment" approach described by Rudolph et al. (2006) provides an excellent model for giving high-quality, actionable feedback. This method of giving feedback opens a dialogue between the instructor and the learner in which the instructor shares observations and judgments while also eliciting the learner's mental models and understanding of the situation. Feedback is given in a context of psychological safety and without bias against the learner's attitude or abilities. There are other methods for debriefing that can be matched to a specific course or session to support the learning objectives (see chapter 8.2 for more information on feedback and debriefing).

Developing Proficiency and Mastery

Simulation educators can engage in mastery learning using a Personalized System of Instruction (Keller, 1968). It is typically divided into small, thematically coherent modules with outcome-based objectives, which determine the overall competencies expected of learners at completion of the program. Learning occurs by direct experience and feedback, and also by observing and imitating others, "including various forms of imitation, some of which occur automatically and unconsciously, as well as conscious deliberate, modeling" (Kihlstrom, 2013, The Importance of Teaching Earnestly section). Some examples of advanced educational concepts and skills for mastery learning in a healthcare simulation faculty development program are given in Table 8.1.1.

Step 5: Implementation

Establishing Professional Networks and Supporting a Culture of Teaching

The director of the faculty development program can oversee the institutional fit, time, and resources needed to cultivate sustainable and valuable networking relationships, and evaluate the effect on individual career outcomes. Programs can advocate for support and rewards for the time-intensive collaborative efforts of their faculty members, for example, through promotion of a culture of teaching so that it is recognized as much as clinical research. Programs can also promote institutional funding for research in the field of healthcare simulation and encourage institutions to create policies to protect the time necessary to engage in faculty development activities (Ramani, 2006).

Selecting Continuing Education and Continuing Medical Education Activities

A continuing education program can meet specific learning needs by providing Continuing Education and Continuing Medical Education activities. There can be a balance between internal and external programs. Some centers design and implement their own faculty development courses, and others have collaborated or contracted with other established organizations to provide these services.

Step 6: Evaluation and Feedback

Preparing for Certification and Accreditation

Formalized mechanisms for providing feedback to faculty members about their instructional progress are of critical importance and value. The simulation program as a whole may also seek accreditation. In addition to creating the CHSE, SSH has also developed an accreditation process for simulation programs focused on healthcare that will include standards for teaching/education.

BEEN THERE, DONE THAT: HOW CAN I CONTINUE TO IMPROVE OR SUSTAIN WHAT I HAVE ACHIEVED?

Designing a Faculty Development Process for Going Above and Beyond

The Education Director in the opening case example soon realized that after an educator has taken courses to learn the foundations and applications of simulation in healthcare, and has organized simulation activities, it might seem that the faculty development program has succeeded in teaching the instructor how to use simulation as a teaching tool effectively. Nonetheless, the Education Director may wonder, how much have the students learned in the simulations? What kinds of evidence should instructors seek and accept as tangible proof of teaching performance?

To answer these questions, a faculty development program should encourage activities focused on continuous reflective practice. While reflective practice might take place in any situation, it may not, because of time constraints and production pressure, in modern healthcare organizations. An effective faculty development program should promote a process that establishes formal and planned learning opportunities.

Trained and highly motivated faculty members are the most valuable resource of a simulation center, and promoting and facilitating their career advancement will improve the program value and outcomes, as well as faculty satisfaction and retention. Implementing a supervised training period will ensure that the instructors adopt effective and safe educational techniques before they embark on independent practice. When learning professionals work in concert with their key partners, it demonstrates the institutional value of working as a team to accomplish the overall mission.

Leadership should also be cultivated in the faculty development program. As Brown and Posner (2001) observed, leaders should create "a climate of openness, safety, and trust...[provide] learning activities that encourage the exploration of alternative personal perspectives...[promote] critical reflection...provide opportunities for assessment and feedback...[and allow]...the time necessary for...personal exploration" (p. 278).

SUMMARY

Faculty development programs are especially important in healthcare simulation centers because the simulation instructors who come to simulation from domains outside education often lack training in pedagogy or adult learning. Simulation instructors must be familiar with the theories and strategies used in education to be effective.

Faculty development programs need a curriculum. The model curriculum described in this chapter is based on Kern's six steps of curriculum design. The educational strategies advocated in the curriculum are grounded in experiential learning theory and peer-reviewed literature. The strategies used to instruct simulation faculty reflect the same methods that they will use to train the learners in their own simulation centers.

There are many resources available to the Education Director who is running a faculty development program. Professional networks, continuing education courses, onsite and away, and conferences can all assist the Education Director in creating an environment of continuous professional improvement.

REFERENCES

Binstadt, E. S., Walls, R. M., White, B. A., Nadel, E. S., Takayesu, J. K., Barker, T. D., ... Pozner, C. N. (2007). A comprehensive medical simulation education curriculum for emergency medicine residents. *Annals of Emergency Medicine, 49*(4), 495–504, 504.e1–504.e11. doi:10.1016/j.annemergmed.2006.08.023

Brown, L. M., & Posner, B. Z. (2001). Exploring the relationship between learning and leadership. *Leadership & Organization Development Journal, 22*(6), 274–280. doi:10.1108/01437730110403204

Cantrell, M. A. (2008). The importance of debriefing in clinical simulations. *Clinical Simulation in Nursing, 4*(2), e19–e23. doi:10.1016/j.ecns.2008.06.006

del Moral, I., & Maestre, J. M. (2013). A view on the practical application of simulation in professional education. *Trends in Anaesthesia and Critical Care, 3*(3), 146–151. doi:10.1016/j.tacc.2013.03.007

Dieckmann, P., Lippert, A., Glavin, R., & Rall, M. (2010). When things do not go as expected: scenario life savers. *Simulation in Healthcare: Journal of the Society for Simulation in Healthcare, 5*(4), 219–225. doi:10.1097/SIH.0b013e3181e77f74

Dreyfus, S. E., & Dreyfus, H. L. (1980). *A five-stage model of the mental activities involved in directed skill acquisition.* Berkeley, CA: Operations Research Center, University of California.

Elfrink, V. L., Nininger, J., Rohig, L., & Lee, J. (2009). The case for group planning in human patient simulation. *Nursing Education Perspectives, 30*(2), 83–86.

Ericsson, K. A. (2008). Deliberate practice and acquisition of expert performance: A general overview. *Academic Emergency Medicine: Official Journal of the Society for Academic Emergency Medicine, 15*(11), 988–994. doi:10.1111/j.1553-2712.2008.00227.x

Ericsson, K. A., & Charness, N. (1994). Expert performance: Its structure and acquisition. *American Psychologist, 49*(8), 725–747. doi:10.1037/0003-066X.49.8.725

Forsythe, L. (2009). Action research, simulation, team communication, and bringing the tacit into voice society for simulation in healthcare. *Simulation in Healthcare: Journal of the Society for Simulation in Healthcare, 4*(3), 143–148. doi:10.1097/SIH.0b013e3181986814

Keller, F. S. (1968). Good-bye, teacher .... *Journal of Applied Behavior Analysis, 1*(1), 79–89. doi:10.1901/jaba.1968.1-79

Kern, D. E., Thomas, P. A., Howard, D. M., & Bass, E. B. (1998). *Curriculum development for medical education: A six-step approach.* Baltimore, MD: Johns Hopkins University Press.

Kihlstrom, J. F. (2013). *How students learn—And how we can help them.* Retrieved from http://socrates.berkeley.edu/~kihlstrm/GSI_2011.htm

Kolb, D. A. (1984). *Experiential learning: Experience as the source of learning and development* (Vol. 1). Englewood Cliffs, NJ: Prentice-Hall.

McGaghie, W. C., Issenberg, S. B., Cohen, E. R., Barsuk, J. H., & Wayne, D. B. (2011). Does simulation-based medical education with deliberate practice yield better results than traditional clinical education? A meta-analytic comparative review of the evidence. *Academic Medicine: Journal of the Association of American Medical Colleges, 86*(6), 706–711. doi:10.1097/ACM.0b013e318217e119

Osterman, K. F., & Kottkamp, R. B. (1993). *Reflective practice for educators: Improving schooling through professional development.* Newbury Park, CA: Corwin Press.

Ramani, S. (2006). Twelve tips to promote excellence in medical teaching. *Medical Teacher, 28*(1), 19–23. doi:10.1080/01421590500441786

Rosenthal, S. L., & Stanberry, L. R. (2011). A framework for faculty development. *The Journal of Pediatrics, 158*(5), 693–694.e2. doi:10.1016/j.jpeds.2011.01.009

Rudolph, J. W., Simon, R., Dufresne, R. L., & Raemer, D. B. (2006). There's no such thing as "nonjudgmental" debriefing: A theory and method for debriefing with good judgment. *Simulation in Healthcare: Journal of the Society for Simulation in Healthcare, 1*(1), 49–55.

Schön, D. (1987) Educating the Reflective Practitioner, San Francisco: Jossey-Bass.

Van Heukelom, J. N., Begaz, T., & Treat, R. (2010). Comparison of postsimulation debriefing versus in-simulation debriefing in medical simulation. *Simulation in Healthcare: Journal of the Society for Simulation in Healthcare, 5*(2), 91–97. doi:10.1097/SIH.0b013e3181be0d17

Wang, E. E. (2011). Simulation and adult learning. *Disease-a-Month, 57*(11), 664–678. doi:10.1016/j.disamonth.2011.08.017

Zigmont, J. J., Kappus, L. J., & Sudikoff, S. N. (2011a). The 3D model of debriefing: defusing, discovering, and deepening. *Seminars in Perinatology, 35*(2), 52–58. doi:10.1053/j.semperi.2011.01.003

Zigmont, J. J., Kappus, L. J., & Sudikoff, S. N. (2011b). Theoretical foundations of learning through simulation. *Seminars in Perinatology, 35*(2), 47–51. doi:10.1053/j.semperi.2011.01.002

SECTION 8 • Faculty Development

CHAPTER 8.2

Debriefing

Keith E. Littlewood, MD, and Demian Szyld, MD, EdM

ABOUT THE AUTHORS

KEITH E. LITTLEWOOD practices clinically in the areas of cardiothoracic and transplant anesthesiology. His interests and responsibilities within education range from oversight of medical simulation and standardized patient programs to curriculum development and evaluation to educational research programs. The Clinical Performance Education Center at the University of Virginia serves a full range of healthcare providers in terms of level, profession, and discipline. Keith's areas of particular interest within simulation include translational simulation research and the application of emerging theory from education and psychology in the quest to understand and improve simulation education. He is politically active in the areas of patient safety and healthcare access.

DEMIAN SZYLD was trained as an Emergency Physician and completed a Simulation Education Fellowship. With an interprofessional team, he codirects faculty and program development, research, and the center's management at the New York Simulation Center for the Health Sciences (NYSIM), the simulation center of New York University Langone Medical Center, and the City University of New York (CUNY). He is a Faculty member of the Institute for Medical Simulation of the Center for Medical Simulation in Boston and teaches faculty development courses in the USA, Spain, Colombia, and other Latin American countries. He serves as the Vice-Chair of the Affiliations Committee of the Society for Simulation in Healthcare (SSH). He practices Emergency Medicine at Bellevue Hospital Center in Manhattan.

Declaration of Interest: Keith E. Littlewood has received support from Pfizer Pharmaceutical and the Josiah Macy Foundation for the development and investigation of interprofessional education programs in medical simulation.

ABSTRACT

Debriefing is a crucial component of essentially any simulation experience intended to help participants change the way they think and practice. The basic tenets of debriefing are linked with important aspects of adult learning theory and fit well within the current movement toward **learner-centered active learning.** The discussion here will first briefly address the educational theory that underpins debriefing in simulation, consider the common goals of all debriefings, and define practical issues for including debriefing in curriculum design. The focus will then shift to more advanced concepts of debriefing, including the description and applications of different strategies for debriefing in common use. The important topic of assessment of debriefing for the purposes of faculty development and quality improvement will be reviewed with a description of current practice. A topic that will arise periodically in this discussion is the general applicability of simulation to essentially all clinical education settings. The debriefing skills learned and perfected in simulation sessions provide the healthcare educator with a powerful tool that can be used throughout their clinical educational practice.

CASE EXAMPLE

The medical simulation program at Allodynia University has been generally successful. In a few short years, the number and breadth of learners has grown dramatically and the simulation sessions are typically well received by participants and faculty alike. However, the medical director and operations director have become concerned by findings of their quality improvement reviews. Debriefing sessions have been sometimes eliminated or truncated, appear to be widely inconsistent between faculty members, and do not necessarily achieve many of the defined goals and objectives of the experiences.

The directors proceed to discuss these issues with selected members of their faculty and are alarmed at their findings. Some of the interviews reveal a sense that the debriefing is of limited value or intimidating and unpleasant for learners. Other faculty say that they have found the time allotted for debriefing is really better used to give a mini-lecture on the patient's problem(s). Still other faculty note that they find the most efficient approach is to step away from the simulator for a moment and discuss any questions that the learners have before moving to the next scenario. Most faculty indicate that they do not have a good idea of what the real goals of the debriefing sessions really are or should be.

The directors now realize that they have a faculty with very uneven investment in debriefing and limited understanding of its real purpose and no familiarity with best practices. The center itself does not have adequate assessments, policy, or procedures in place to ensure achievement of defined standards and educational quality improvement. The directors realize that in the rush to production, faculty development has not provided an adequate understanding of the educational basis, value, and best practice of debriefing. They are now faced with the challenge of proving to faculty that debriefing is important, to provide faculty with the tools to become good facilitators of debriefing, and to measure the quality and impact of debriefing.

INTRODUCTION

Debriefing has been a cornerstone of simulation education in healthcare from its earliest days. Simulation educators now continue to place great emphasis upon debriefing. This is apparent from any number of indicators, including the design of simulation centers with investments of space and technology, the development of curriculum with the allocation of faculty and learner time, and the requirements of accrediting and certifying bodies regarding debriefing. Debriefing is thus ubiquitous in the world of healthcare simulation, something that most educators may have simply accepted without critical consideration. There are, however, at least two important reasons to reflect upon the role of debriefing within simulation education. The first is that debriefing demands huge resources in the already resource-intensive simulation environment. Faculty and learner time, specialized learning spaces, **faculty development**, and advanced audiovisual equipment with technical support all come to mind as part of the investments required for debriefing. It is incumbent upon directors of simulation programs to consider first the necessity, and secondly the cost-effectiveness of debriefing. Further, if faculty are to be trained and held to standards in debriefing, it is important that the data and rationale for its use be part of faculty development and that there be explicit standards available to evaluate quality. In this way, debriefing becomes a shared, valued cornerstone of simulation education. A second reason for rigorously considering debriefing is to assess its potential for transfer to other educational encounters, both within and outside of the immersive simulation environment. If debriefing allows educators to better facilitate learning in the clinical setting, lecture hall, and other settings, then faculty development and practice in the simulation center has the potential to improve learning beyond simulation events (e.g., practice and patient safety). With these issues in mind, this chapter first briefly reviews the history and applications of debriefing in other fields and considers debriefing within the context of adult learning theory.

History

Debriefings are generally agreed to have arisen from the military, and to have served several purposes in that context. The earliest reasons for debriefing were the simple collection of information from troops who had completed an action so as to assess tactical success, discuss lessons learned for future missions, reinforce the protection of sensitive information, and to generate archival data. Early on, it was also noticed that personnel seemed to gain some emotional benefit from these discussions. Later, **critical incident stress debriefing (CISD)** arose with the hope of providing emergency service providers with psychological support following stressful and traumatic experiences. Discussion of the structure and processes of such sessions provide important historical considerations for the simulation educator (Dyregrov, 1997). Interestingly, this aspect of debriefing has come full circle with the current use of structured debriefings to help military personnel transition from the stressors of combat to civilian life (Fillion et al., 2002; MacDonald, 2003).

A different type of debriefing is found in the literature of psychology research that may be of particular interest to the educational researcher. Participants in psychology studies may be intentionally misled about the purpose of the experiment and/or placed in situations that could be emotionally traumatic. Several high-profile studies gave rise to controversy about the limits of ethical research and the responsibilities of the researchers to subjects (Milgram, 1963). Currently, ethical practice requires that research design provide a mechanism to support participants and inform them of such deceit (Sharpe & Faye, 2009). A debriefing session is typically used in this situation to "de-hoax" the experience and to address trauma that may have been suffered, or could be subsequently suffered, by the participant. Simulation educators should be aware of this standard and practice when intentional misrepresentations are used in educational research. Up to this point, then, debriefings had served multiple purposes that most often were directed no more than tangentially toward an improved educational or training effectiveness.

The educational debriefing historically most familiar to healthcare educators arose in aviation. Debriefing in aviation has a long-standing linkage with debriefing in healthcare simulation. Over three decades ago, pioneers in human patient simulation looked to cockpit resource management (CRM; Cooper et al., 1980), and later crew resource management, in developing exercises in the management of simulated clinical crises (Howard et al., 1992). This led to the creation of anesthesia crisis resource management (ACRM), which has been more recently adopted and adapted by other specialties and disciplines. Debriefing was described as an integral part of this earliest work in crisis management and team training (albeit discipline-specific team training) and so it remains. During these decades, line of flight training (LOFT) has evolved within aviation and is a mainstay of commercial airlines. The National Aeronautics and Space Administration summarized these practices in a technical memorandum that demonstrated the continued linkage between simulation debriefing in aviation and medicine (Dismukes et al., 1997).

The Theoretical Contexts of Debriefing

The goal of this section is to discuss debriefing within the contexts of strategies, philosophies, or theory commonly referenced in simulation education. Healthcare simulation educators have a wide variety of backgrounds. Clinicians, in particular, may typically have limited formal exposure to educational theory. They may have a working knowledge of pieces of theory that they have learned from their own initiative through self-study, workshops, and faculty development. They may have then implemented it in their own practice with institutional colleagues and within institutional norms. This kind of educational heterogeneity is widespread in healthcare. An obvious example is one of the "gold standards" of active learning, problem-based learning, that demonstrates a striking lack of standardization (Smits et al., 2002). The ambitious goal of the following brief discussion, then, will be to touch upon debriefing through the lens of a few educational perspectives commonly used in healthcare. The reader can thus choose familiar threads and consider the role of debriefing within familiar context(s). This is intended to create a starting point for the discussion of different debriefing methodologies. A full treatment of the theories mentioned below is clearly beyond the scope of this discussion, but references are provided for further review by the interested reader. In the broadest sense, most of our discussion will regard theories that fall into the paradigms of (1) **behaviorism**, (2) cognitivism, and (3) constructivism.

Behaviorists look upon the learner as a passive "clean slate" or vessel that responds to or is filled by environmental stimuli. Effectively structured reinforcement and/or punishment increase the likelihood of desired behaviors. Learning, therefore, is achieved (and demonstrated) simply by a change in the behavior of the learner. There is little or no need to consider internal mental states or consciousness within most of these theories. Many simulation educators probably would not think of their educational practices as relying upon behaviorism. It is true that simulation experiences, and the debriefing in particular, are often designed to promote deep learning in adults. But the classic works of Pavlov and Skinner, and the transitional work toward cognitivism by Tolman and Bandura, may still be relevant in some simulation and debriefing experiences. A defining question is whether there are educational encounters in which the important outcome is a reinforced, successful behavior and the participant's understanding and values are, at most, secondary. An example might be teaching basic life support to a layperson. The physiology and data supporting newer protocols with circulation-airway-breathing sequencing may be referred to, but it is not expected that the participant will particularly change their worldview or synthesize new knowledge or demonstrate deep understanding. The important outcome is the ability to reliably implement a simple algorithm in a crisis that most people will never see. Another example might be the placement of a central venous catheter in a task trainer with the demonstration of aseptic technique for the purposes of credentialing. While the importance of line-associated infections and the anatomy of the central circulation will be reviewed, the participant is essentially demonstrating a competency. The feedback of technique corrections and eventual credentialing are used to reinforce the behavior of following a checklist during routine procedures. The debriefings here take the form of direct feedback on well-defined correct and incorrect behaviors, with likely suggestions or requirements for improvement. The plus-delta technique described later may serve as a very efficient method of allowing high throughput by minimally trained mentors for such activities. This type of educational encounter is mid-level in terms of Bloom's taxonomy or Miller's pyramid. Regardless of level, such training is very important in terms of public health and represents a core mission for many centers.

Cognitive psychology attempts, in part, to understand processes that occur with learning and the development of expertise. In many ways, the learner is viewed as a processor of information. Pioneers such as Chomsky, through his work in linguistics, argued that behaviorism could not explain phenomena of knowledge creation and application such as generative grammar. Clinical educators are often drawn to the metaphor of the mind as a computer with incoming information, algorithmic processing, structured storage of routines that become refined and automated (and thus markedly more efficient), and resultant output in the form of ways of thinking and practicing. **Cognitive load theory** is particularly relevant to simulation education. This model concerns, in part, severe limitations of **working memory** in actively managing new and unique elements of data and environment (Plass et al., 2012). The development of expertise is actually the ability to put together multiple elements in a **schema** that can be handled singly and thus improve capacity. An everyday example includes the confusion of a novice in the face of overwhelming and seemingly unrelated stimuli that includes hypotension, tachycardia, and a history of decreased intake and fluid losses. With more experience, this constellation will become an interrelated schema separate from other input and will be identified as a hypovolemic patient who requires fluid resuscitation. With further development, the diagnosis and early treatment will become automatic, and cognitive work will be directed toward considerations of deviations from expected presentation, responses to management, and longer-term diagnostic and treatment strategies. This development of schema can occur only with repetition, early reinforcement of successful schema (and modification or rejection of those that are less successful), and eventual automatic implementation of repeatedly successful schemata. This model is logical and probably self-evident to many simulation educators. In the literature, it is described as **Deliberate Practice** (Ericsson, 2008; Ericsson et al., 1993). Expert performance requires four elements: motivation, a defined goal, feedback, and opportunity for repetitive practice. Within the context of debriefing, this model is helpful in considering those techniques in which observation of actions is used as a vehicle of inquiry to understand participants' internal schema or **frames**. Given that working memory is fixed, the key difference between experts and novices is the number and complexity of schemata they have available.

Discussion now centers on understanding and ways of thinking and practicing rather than simply judging an action or behavior as correct or incorrect. The arguments for the importance of this distinction will be useful in the discussion of advocacy-inquiry debriefing. **Instructional scaffolding** is another concept relevant to simulation education. First described by Bruner (1960) and expanded by others, scaffolding is the provision of learners with a framework understandable to the novice that is later progressively removed as new understanding and technical skills are developed (Vygotsky, 1978). Vygotsky's work in this area can be considered a confluence of cognitive and social constructivist thinking (see below). It describes scaffolding as built upon the prior knowledge of learners, initially within a social context and with the help of "more knowledgeable others," be they teachers, peers, or representations of others' knowledge. With attainment of expertise, this scaffolding is no longer required. As learners progress in simulation, we can think of reducing the scaffolding, allowing them more independent, less prompted practice.

Constructivism is an educational paradigm that maintains that learning is an active, social, and fundamentally constructive process. New information and experience is linked to relevant prior knowledge that has been reactivated and will be revised and/or reinforced. The learner then develops new hypotheses that are tested and negotiated through social interactions in the learning environment. Here, again, the learner is not an empty vessel, but brings prior experiences, cultural views, and individual motivations to the educational experience. The **experiential learning cycle** of Kolb (1984) builds upon these concepts and has gained popularity in the simulation community as a helpful model that links cognition and reflection, experience and behavior. Four stages are described that represent the steps of learning (Figure 8.2.1). This pathway to meaningful change includes reflective observation as one of four critical stages. In this context, reflection refers to the consideration of the actions of others and/or oneself. The relevance of reflection to debriefing is obvious and includes discussion of actions and at times reviewing video recordings. Another important consideration may be less apparent; while learners are presumed to experience each of these stages to some extent, Kolb's theory postulates that individuals have propensity and preference for different permutations of the perception and processing axes as noted by the trapezoid labels in Figure 8.2.1. Simulation participants who predominate as divergers and assimilators have already incorporated reflection in learning. Accommodators and convergers lie on the other side of the processing spectrum, tending toward active experimentation to test and understand perception. It is unlikely

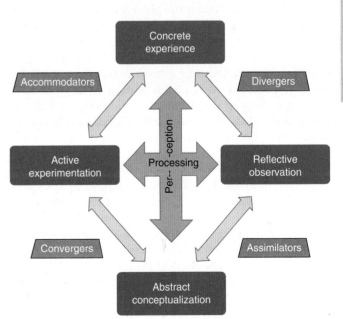

FIGURE 8.2.1 Representation of Kolb's Experiential Learning Cycle showing axes of perception and processing that define learning style as described in the text. Includes bidirectional paths between perception and processing nodes. (Modified from Kolb, D. A. [1984]. *Experiential learning: Experience as the source of learning and development.* Englewood Cliffs, NJ: Prentice-Hall.)

that participants in a debriefing will have had a formal evaluation of their learning style. Still, the variance in the learning styles of simulation participants is worthy of consideration when there are apparent differences in comfort level and facility of group members with the debriefing experience. Unlike many other educational techniques (lectures, books, podcasts, writing papers, team-based learning, problem-based learning, e-learning, etc.), combining simulation (concrete experience) with debriefing (reflective observation) allows educators to reach groups of learners that contain accommodators and convergers in their preferred fashion.

DEBRIEFING IN HEALTHCARE SIMULATION

Components and Progression of Debriefings

Regardless of setting or technique, most debriefings can be thought of as having core components and following a few necessary steps or phases. The commonly accepted elements of a debriefing include (1) the debriefer, (2) the participant(s), (3) the experience to be considered, (4) the impact of the experience, (5) recollections, (6) report, and (7) time (Lederman, 1992). In this case, of course, the experience in question is the simulation scenario itself. The impact of the experience typically includes emotional motivation to consider the scenario experience within the context of previous experiences and usual practice. The recollection and reporting of the experience is particularly relevant in understanding the perceptions and position of the participants. The time of the debriefings considered here usually occurs immediately after a simulation scenario. Many experts in healthcare simulation agree that educators should devote at minimum equal time debriefing and generally recommend a ratio of two to three debriefing time to one simulation time (e.g., 15-minute simulation with a 30- to 45-minute debriefing). It is noteworthy that there are other time frames in which reflections occur over the longer period of a defined experience (e.g., a clinical rotation or semester course) or time period (e.g., internship) with individual or mentored debriefing. These longer time frames have seldom been described in conjunction with simulation. They are, however, in keeping with the concept of longer-term oscillation between deeply established, comfortable ways of thinking and practicing versus substantively new understanding (Meyer & Land, 2005). The increased and longitudinal exposure to simulation during education and training may provide opportunity for this type of reflection. In any case, there is evidence that debriefing should follow the simulation rather than occur within the scenario (Van Heukelom et al., 2010).

The physical setting of the debriefing relates to the goal of creating a collegial and safe environment that is usually quiet, comfortable, and private. Successful debriefing in the same space as the scenario has been described (Senger et al., 2012). However, for simulated case scenarios, a dedicated space separate from the simulation bay is more typically used. Participants include those who are actually involved in the scenario, but may also include faculty or participants who were observing remotely. Audiovisual equipment capable of replaying important segments of the scenario is often helpful, although supporting data is conflicting (Savoldelli et al., 2006; Scherer et al., 2003). Nonhierarchal cues, such as all participants seated about a table or in a circle, helps support an atmosphere of mutual respect and parity. A multipurpose space being used for debriefing is presented as an example in Figure 8.2.2.

It is important to remember that the debriefing is considered by most to be an integral part of the simulation experience. The introduction to the session (prebrief) affects the quality of learning and student actions during the simulation, as well as the debriefing. Although occurring postsimulation, the debriefing is rooted in the design of the simulation and the learning objectives; the unique aspects of the simulation itself is a result and is threaded into the debriefing.

It is worthwhile to consider the typical progression of a debriefing session. Several authors have described the steps or phases that occur in the natural course of most debriefings. A popular conceptualization is referenced (Gardner, 2013; Rudolph et al., 2008) and summarized in Table 8.2.1. Although originally presented for a particular debriefing technique, these phases can be generalized.

The first is the **reactions phase**, a phase full of the emotion and energy remaining from the scenario itself. This phase must be managed carefully to maintain the emotional investment of the participant while allowing the energy level to be refocused into the deeper discussion of events in the next phase. The participant will often be self-critical and uncertain about his or her performance. An environment of support and respect must be unambiguously demonstrated with careful, active listening and

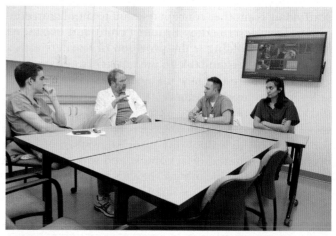

FIGURE 8.2.2 A simple, multiuse space used for debriefing with basic furniture and audiovisual playback capability.

TABLE 8.2.1

Common Phases of Debriefings, with Important Components and Considerations

Phases of Debriefing

Primary Purpose	Characteristics
Reactions	• Clear the air. • Review the facts to eliminate basic misunderstandings and technical distractions. • Appreciate issues important to participants for immediate clarification or later discussion. • Reinforce supportive environment with respect and genuine interest in the participant's experience and perceptions.
Analysis	• Further explore the experience as it relates to learning goals. • Generate new understandings through discussion, deliberation, and teaching. • Generalize the specific experience to broader considerations of thinking and practice.
Summary	• Consider interconnectedness of debriefing issues with one another and real-world thinking and practice. • Revisit points that were not treated in depth but deemed to be of high importance. • Review points of debriefing that have generated and/or may promote new understanding.

Adapted from Gardner, R. (2013). Introduction to debriefing. *Seminars in Perinatology*, *37*(3), 166–174; Rudolph, J. W., Simon, R., Raemer, D. B., & Eppich, W. J. (2008). Debriefing as formative assessment: Closing performance gaps in medical education. *Academic Emergency Medicine*, *15*(11), 1010–1016. Retrieved from http://dx.doi.org/10.1111/j.1553-2712.2008.00248.x

consideration. Additionally, participants will often be focused on issues such as proper drug doses, fidelity of the simulation, and precise steps of an algorithm. It will be difficult to move forward until these concerns are addressed in some way. Common strategies include a simple statement of fact (e.g., "It is recommended that dantrolene be reconstituted with warmed sterile water"), redirection (e.g., "I agree that the breath sounds may have been difficult to interpret, but it may be worthwhile to discuss what you would do with such a patient who is wheezing"), or marking or "sign post" indicating the desire for more in-depth discussion and a plan that it will be discussed in the analysis phase (e.g., "The issue that you just raised seems like something that we should look at more closely once we have had a chance to address a few of these other issues"). While participants may be focused on technical and superficial issues, the debriefing facilitator should listen for the deeper challenges of the scenario by listening to the stated and implied learner issues during this phase. These issues should be considered for later discussion to maintain participant investment. The novice debriefer may feel frustrated that no real progress is being made during this phase and thus be tempted to skip or abbreviate this phase. The reaction phase, however, represents processes that can be guided but that cannot be rushed. The participants will need time to "decompress" and move from their initial emotional state of scattered specifics to focused, genuine discussion and reflection on practice.

The **analysis phase** involves the hard work of considering the events as variously experienced by participants not only at face value, but for their implications in daily practice. This phase allows the opportunity to generalize the specifics of the scenario to the generalities of everyday healthcare. With these generalizations, participants can validate some aspects of their own practice and consider changes for improvement in others, thus preparing for transfer. The particulars of different techniques in reaching these goals will be discussed later within the context of those techniques.

The usual goals for the **summary phase** are noted in Table 8.2.1. This segment can serve multiple purposes, as needed. First, there are practical considerations. For example, time management of debriefings can be extremely challenging for the novice. These challenges include efficient shepherding of a group through the reactions phase without hurrying the processes therein, and choosing and/or validating a limited number of topics in the analysis phase to allow deeper discussion. Even with more experience, facilitators may elect to dig down into a topic that has generated important sustained discussion and find themselves short of time for other intended discussion. This means that the summary phase may be needed, in part, for "catching up" with topics or issues that were not fully treated in the analysis phase. This approach does not allow for careful reflection, but does make sure that important issues (e.g., appropriate alternatives to central venous cannulation in a crisis) are not left unaddressed. "Unfinished business" may be more effectively approached with prioritization and framework, for example, recommending further reading (e.g., "Current recommendations in mass casualty incidents include the use of laryngeal mask airways for providers who are not highly experienced in airway management. Our own institution has adopted these guidelines and they can be found in the emergency preparedness binder"). Such practicalities aside, there are few commonly stated goals for the debriefing summary phase. This is an opportunity to recapitulate important concepts from the debriefing with clarifications and consensus in the group's understanding. Structured summation can also lead to the extraction of key action items that will allow participants to operationalize new ways of practicing in the future. The facilitator should also look for participant opportunities to understand what they have discussed and reconsidered in new contexts. This previously unappreciated interconnectedness leads to both stronger anchoring in prior knowledge and to the creation or refinement of advanced schemata (Meyer & Land, 2005; van Merrienboer & Sweller, 2010). For this reason, some debriefing strategies encourage the learners to produce the summary rather than the educator.

Debriefing Strategies

There are a variety of debriefing strategies used by simulation educators, some of which will be discussed in detail below. Before that discussion, however, two important points should be addressed. First, regardless of the technique, the fundamental goals of the debriefing are to create a safe environment and facilitate a discussion that allows scenario participants to purposively reflect upon what they have experienced. Depending upon the educational model invoked, this reflection can be thought of as amplifying the successes and failures of the session, clarifying the critical elements of the experience, and/or catalyzing new understandings and practices within the participant. The second point is that there is no compelling evidence that supports a single technique as superior for all situations. This presents a challenge to the novice in considering which technique of debriefing to adopt and eventually master. Circumstances will dictate the first debriefing method(s) of most simulation educators. The initial exposure may be from a local simulation center mentor, the experience of a faculty development session, dedicated training in debriefing, or from the literature. Development is likely to start within the culture of the particular simulation team of one's institution. This should not be of concern to the novice. Accomplished debriefers have often started with one technique, gravitated toward another or others, and ended up being facile with several, including a personalized hybrid, in many cases. Others find the technique sooner or later that best suits their educational practice and develop proficiency predominately within that technique. The best advice and reassurance may be that regardless of the technique, any thoughtful debriefing is offering the learner an educational opportunity otherwise missed. The eventual development of expertise will come with practice, good mentorship, and, to no small extent, exploring new methods. In these ways, our practice as educators and debriefers mirrors our development as healthcare professionals. We gain knowledge and structure from mentors and then refine our own evidence-based styles that are effective and context-appropriate.

METHODS

Several popular debriefing methods (Table 8.2.2) will first be compared and contrasted. Attention will then be focused upon practical aspects of debriefing including curriculum development, logistics, faculty development, and quality improvement.

The **plus-delta** technique is considered an adaptation from flight crew debriefing. The methodology is straightforward. Typically, three columns are created on a device viewable by the group such as an erasable board or electronic display. During the debriefing, the first column is progressively filled in with actions of individuals and/or the team. The second column is labeled "plus" and describes the positive or effective characteristics of the actions, while the third column will list opportunities for improvement in the future for these actions ("delta" for change). Plus-delta is a reliable debriefing method with

TABLE 8.2.2	
Four Commonly Described Debriefing Methods	
Medical Simulation Debriefing: Commonly Described Approaches	
Approach	**Comments**
Plus-Δ ("plus-delta")	Straightforward method defines successful actions and results (plus) or needing improvement in some way (delta).
GAS (gather, analyze, summarize)	Highly structured technique intended to provide standardization for national education and training program.
4Es (events, emotions, empathy, explanation)	Adopted from sociology education with emphasis on understanding events, the emotions therein, and reaching an explanation and plan for future experiences.
Advocacy with inquiry Debriefing with good judgment	An observation is paired with the debriefer's point of view and followed by a genuine inquiry to understand the current frame of reference of the participant so that both future actions and frames can be improved or sustained.

a few obvious advantages over other approaches. One of the more important of these is that it is an easy method to master with minimal training in its most basic form. Participants new to simulation can also quickly and comfortably master their role. They are not faced with the deeper and potentially threatening explorations of behaviors typical of other methods. Some facilitators use this method exclusively and successfully, and almost all facilitators use plus-delta in some situations. One of the strengths of plus-delta is its adaptability over a range of experiences and circumstances. For example, plus-delta can be used after a complex team experience, but is also suitable for a simple "checklist" review of competency demonstration of technical skills. A common pitfall to avoid when using this method is vague statements or descriptions. "Good communication" is not as useful as "used clear language when requesting equipment," for example. Additionally, plus-delta can be used in a typical debriefing setting with audiovisual support and a structured schedule, but can also be used effectively at the bedside for short sessions with rapid turnover and a technical focus. Plus-delta can also be helpful when the summary phase needs to cover or recap important points that were not fully addressed in the analysis phase quickly, as previously discussed. Finally, this method can yield a written record of the analysis and discussion. For example, when applied to clinical settings, it is important to document and act on system-level issues such as missing equipment or faulty communication systems so that errors are not repeated.

The *GAS* method of debriefing is particularly notable for its development and specific deployment. An acronym for Gather, Analyze, and Summarize, GAS is a debriefing method developed for American Heart Association training in consultation with a university simulation center (Cheng et al., 2012). The technique was intended

THREE LEGS OF A SUCCESSFUL TEAMWORK PROGRAM

Robert Simon, EdD
Education Director, Center for Medical Simulation

My 25+ years of experience with high-performance, high-stakes teams in aviation and healthcare has led me to think that a successful teamwork program resembles a three-legged stool (Figure 1).

First, leadership feels that it's important to take a seat on the stool. Once leadership views teamwork as an effective method for improving effectiveness and safety, a program is set to start. Careful planning for introducing, organizing, and reinforcing the three legs takes time, thoughtfulness, and commitment.

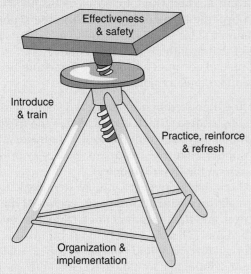

FIGURE 1 Three legged stool concept

The first leg is to introduce and train the organization in teamwork concepts and methods. Here, a common teamwork language is established and practiced. Leadership expresses its support and plans. Educators are an interdisciplinary team composed of opinion leaders in the organization. The Educator team combines didactic and experiential approaches to instruction as they train *all* members of the organization. Importantly, the Educator team models effective teamwork behaviors while working and encourages others to do likewise.

The second leg is to organize and implement the teamwork system. It is clear to all members that teamwork has taken a prominent spot in all organizational endeavors, especially when it comes to high-level performance and for patient safety. Team members are able to identify themselves as part of a team, plan and replan, debrief, distribute workload, cross-monitor, maintain situation awareness, and so on. Similarly, employee evaluations, quality improvement/quality assurance teams, Morbidity and Mortality conferences, incident reports, rounding, and so on all include teamwork considerations.

The third leg comprises opportunities to practice, reinforce, and refresh. Teamwork is reinforced in the second leg every day. The third leg is different because it is a program of formal, scheduled simulation and training. Team simulations with team debriefings are a routine part of this leg.

Airlines throughout the world have adopted the three-legged stool. Healthcare organizations desiring to leverage the power of teamwork to improve performance and safety will do the same. It won't be easy or inexpensive, but it will most certainly be worth it.

to be learner-centered, standardized across facilitators, participants, and sessions, and to promote self-reflection to improve understanding, practice, and future learning. **GAS debriefing** follows the stages detailed earlier—those of reaction, analysis, and summary. The debriefing is highly structured in content and timing. In the "gather" phase, participants provide their perspectives of the session. The facilitator's role during this phase is to ask guiding questions that promote the sharing of participants' observations, even while noting and organizing important points for the next phase. During the "analyze" phase, the facilitator leads a review of the events, looking at objective data initially. Participants and facilitator then consider actual performance compared to expected performance, the so-called performance gap. Discussion then moves to an understanding of actions by considering their basis. This important step is common to other debriefing techniques. The pivotal concept shared by some debriefing techniques is that actions can indicate the reasoning and motivation behind the participant's action (Rudolph, Simon, Dufresne, & Raemer, 2006). The roles of parameters ranging from emotion, assumptions, and beliefs to knowledge and situational awareness

are considered. In the summary phase, participants articulate the key points that they intend to use in their practice improvement.

The **4Es debriefing** technique is rooted in reports by sociology educators of class-size simulation and debriefing in the 1990s. The name itself refers to the stages of this debriefing method, namely (1) Events, (2) Emotions, (3) Empathy, and (4) Explanation (Petranek et al., 1992). During the events phase, participants describe the experience from their perspectives. Even for the large number of learners involved, the importance of allowing all who wished to speak to be heard was emphasized. Further, the facilitator(s) sought to elicit the particular experiences of participants directly involved in "a particular interaction that was meaningful." The emotions phase of debriefing focuses upon the feelings of the participants during the simulation. The responsibility of the facilitator(s) is to create "a social atmosphere where all emotions and ideas are respected," a familiar charge in current debriefing strategies. The next stage is intended to harness the information and emotional energy built up to this point, now turned to empathy for the viewpoint of others. So, rather than considering the experience through the lens of expected performance or prior experience, participants are asked to consider the perceptions and feelings of others. Empathy for other participants was a fundamental goal for the sociology educators who developed the 4Es technique. These original descriptions have been translated to healthcare simulation scenario debriefing. For present-day simulation debriefing, empathy is modified to consider the challenges and efforts of individuals and teams in the scenario and to supportively discuss performance. Finally, in the explanations phase, the important lessons of the scenario are identified, clarified, and reviewed.

There has been some confusion in the simulation literature regarding the history of the 4Es debriefing method arising predominately from incorrect citations and an implication that the 4Es were derived from the "6Es" or "7Es" by the same primary author. In point of fact, the 4Es method was used for full-class oral debriefings as described above. A later development was the written debriefing, in this case a journal kept by students during a sociology course. For this work, the two additional Es are "Everyday" (relationship of the simulation to everyday behaviors) and "Employment" (reflections on practical applications from the simulation actually instituted into behaviors outside of the simulation exercises). These technical details are less important than the reason for progression to written reflection. In an article that is essentially rumination upon this experience (and often erroneously cited as a description of 4Es debriefing), Petranek declared as a principle of his simulation practice maturation: "Playing a simulation or a game is the adolescent step in learning, whereas oral debriefing is the young adult stage and written debriefing is the older adult stage of learning" (Petranek, 1994). Healthcare simulation debriefing has not adopted written debriefing on any large scale, but such experience in other disciplines deserves consideration. It is not uncommon for nursing students to write reflections or "write-ups" after simulation sessions. In current educational practice, widely available technology provides an opportunity for mentors and participants to maintain electronic reflections over several experiences and time. Whether this represents a more advanced stage of adult learning in simulation will require future investigation.

Advocacy-inquiry and **debriefing with good judgment** will be discussed together because the latter fundamentally incorporates the former but they are sometimes mentioned as separate techniques. Debriefing with good judgment has been described as having three fundamental components (Rudolph et al., 2006). The first is a model based in cognitive psychology that seeks to understand the actions of participants as based within their **mental models** (termed by the authors as frames and also called schemata or reference frames, among other terms, in the literature). While actions can be observed, frames are the bundled elements of prior and proven experiences and observations that are used to make sense of the clinical challenge faced in the scenario. Thus, frames lead to learners' actions. The second element is a declared attitude ("stance") in the debriefing

of genuine curiosity about the basis of action within participant frames, all within a supportive setting rather than a facilitative or socratic "nonjudgmental" or a harsh, critical "judgmental" stance. The critical balance here is that the curiosity is explored, in part, with frank, evaluative judgments of performance, yielding the name *debriefing with good judgment*. Specifically, this process represents the third element, the method of investigation called advocacy-inquiry. This way of communicating during a debriefing is based on an advocacy and an inquiry. The advocacy is two-pronged: (1) an observation is made and (2) a point of view is expressed. This is followed by the inquiry, where a question leading to a frame is made. To paraphrase the creators of this method (Rudolph et al, 2006), the facilitator posits a hypothesis based upon her/his observations (and own frames and biases) in the advocacy and then welcomes testing of that hypothesis through inquiry.

Example of advocacy and inquiry that could be used to explore the trainee's frames:

1. "Joe, I noticed that you didn't use epinephrine (observation) which is indicated as the treatment for anaphylaxis (point of view)." (advocacy) "I wonder what your treatment strategy or priorities were at the time?" (inquiry)
2. "I saw that Florence took a few steps back, looked at all three patients within 45 seconds of their arrival, and then recommended taking the one in bed A to CT scan. (observation) I think this was premature, as a fluid bolus trial, repeat vital signs, and a little time would have helped the whole team have a clearer view of how to prioritize—the patient in bed A needed to go to the OR, whereas the one in bed B with the pelvic fracture would have benefitted from early CT followed by angiography and embolization. (point of view) What was running through your (to the whole team) mind as you were evaluating these trauma patients?" (inquiry)

The naming of this technique as "good judgment" emphasizes its position between the purely judgmental assessment that would merely indicate the facilitator's opinion that an error was made ("Epinephrine must be given in all cases of anaphylaxis and you did not. That is why the patient did poorly") and the nonconfrontational use of simple observations ("What was the blood pressure when you chose phenylephrine?"). Good-judgment proponents believe that judgmental statements clearly deliver the assessment of the facilitator, but that the facilitator will gain no insight into the frames of understanding within the participant and risks damaging the teacher–learner relationship if they appear uninterested, harsh, or both. Without this insight, there is limited opportunity for discussion of the need and means of genuine change and educators risk spending time on the wrong thing, for example, assuming a performance gap is due to knowledge deficit rather than skills in prioritizing or managing stress during crisis. At the other end of the spectrum, simple observations do not address either the underlying issues of why actions were taken or the mentor's perception of performance. The participant will then have uncertainty in making sense of the simulation experience and its take-home lessons.

A fundamental aspect of debriefing with good judgment is to discover and explore the cognitive schemata that have led to decisions and action with the goal of sustaining good performance (appreciative inquiry) or improving poor performance (critical inquiry). The facilitator cannot, a priori, understand why a participant has chosen any particular action—sometimes trainees themselves do not know initially. With the tacit understanding that the participant is doing his/her best, it is implicit that the ways of thinking and practicing demonstrated in the scenario made sense as the best considered choice at that time and in that situation. It is the task of the facilitator to genuinely inquire into the participant's frames of reference and to help the participant reflect upon what part(s) of those frames led to successful and unsuccessful actions. Finally, these reconsiderations of previously stored behaviors are summarized and taken as ways of improving performance in future patient management. To reiterate, change is sought not just in future actions, but, more fundamentally, in the frames of the participant. Figure 8.2.3 is a variation of diagrams often used to illustrate this process, additionally including cognitive components within the participant's frame.

BEEN THERE, DONE THAT: HOW CAN I CONTINUE TO IMPROVE OR SUSTAIN WHAT I HAVE ACHIEVED?

Having discussed the basis and goals of debriefing with this strategy, it is also necessary to consider the challenges. The creators mentioned in their early work that "Most medical educators are able to reliably demonstrate competence after approximately 2 days of lecture and practice; expertise appears to require considerably longer to develop" (Rudolph et al., 2006). Such commitments of time and delayed proficiency may be difficult for busy clinicians and other educators, especially the faculty member who facilitates only occasionally. Additionally, simulation programs must consider the faculty development requirements in time, expertise, and opportunity cost compared to any perceived benefits of this method of debriefing.

Measuring and Maintaining Quality in Debriefing

As noted earlier, debriefing has played a long-standing and valued role in healthcare simulation. The assessment of the quality of debriefing sessions is a more recent development. There are obvious challenges in this endeavor. There are a wide variety of debriefing techniques used, and there is further variation of those techniques among programs and individuals. Given the heterogeneity of

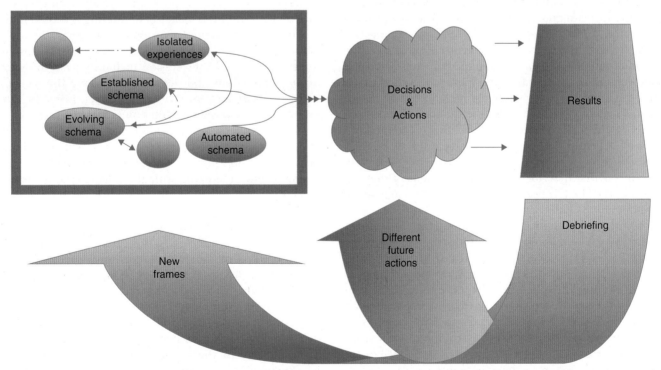

FIGURE 8.2.3 Representation of the participant's frame (rectangle) driving decisions and actions and, ultimately, results. Debriefing, in turn, considers these observable phenomena in seeking to understand the underlying frames with the intent of modifying future actions and creating new frames of reference.

learners and educational missions, this variation is neither a surprise nor a failing. There is no current standard of debriefing practice that could meet the needs of all programs. Quality measurement would thus require either an instrument that works across techniques or, alternatively, instruments individualized to debriefing strategies. The more fundamental challenge is posed in a simple question: What is to be measured? When considered in the educational "tool-bench to bedside" analogy to translational research (Littlewood, 2011), the universal goal of healthcare simulation is to improve the well-being of patients. Data are emerging that simulation does have an impact on meaningful patient outcomes (Cook et al., 2011). But separating the quality of a debriefing and its impact on patients is a daunting challenge. It is logical to attempt measurement of surrogate markers. Two examples of such instruments have been recently described. The Debriefing Assessment for Simulation in Healthcare (DASH; Brett-Fleegler et al., 2012) is an instrument with scoring rubrics for facilitators and participants, as well as observers not part of the debriefing. There are six areas (elements) of assessment. The first concerns the establishment of the environment through orientation to learning objectives, the immersion environment and equipment, and commitment to respect. This emphasizes the foundations of successful debriefing in setting the stage for the session. Other elements concern the maintenance of an engaging and safe environment, the organization of the debriefing, and whether meaningful discussion was promoted. Finally, the identification and discussion of performance gaps and the development of strategies to narrow those gaps are evaluated. The simulation group that created the strategy of debriefing with good judgment, the Center for Medical Simulation (CMS), developed the DASH instrument. It is available at http://www.harvardmedsim.org/debriefing-assesment-simulation-healthcare.php. It is not surprising that principles of observation and inquiry, as well as examining the frames of participants, are included in this assessment. This emphasis does raise the question of how well DASH would perform across all debriefing techniques.

The Objective Structured Assessment of Debriefing (OSAD; Arora et al., 2012) is another recently described tool. It was first described for the assessment of debriefings in surgical education and training. Logistical goals of development included applicability to simulation and clinical settings and minimal time requirement (5 minutes) by the rater. The authors set out to develop an evidence-based methodology that would be tested for validity and reliability. The design was based upon review of the literature in multiple disciplines and expert opinion. The tool that was eventually developed has considerable domain overlap with DASH. Considerations include creation of a safe and engaging environment, exploration of learner reactions, reasoning, and effectiveness, and strategies for improvement based upon the experience.

Methods of assessing debriefing quality such as these provide simulation programs with a tool for educational quality improvement. The development of standardized, widely accepted instruments will also promote important research. The most obvious utility in this regard is to provide an assessment of debriefing quality within the designed experimental variation of variables such as facilitator experience, technology utilization, and setting. Another such benefit is to provide evidence of debriefing standardization and quality during the conduct of research projects.

HOW TO PROMOTE SUCCESSFUL DEBRIEFING

There is no single blueprint for simulation programs to develop debriefing programs. Educational mission(s), learners, faculty, resources, current level of development, and educational philosophies are a few of the many parameters that should be considered. There are, however, several decision points that both individual educators and programs will face by design or by default in their development. Several questions are posed below to provide proactive considerations.

Where does the debriefing process start? Debriefing, implicitly or explicitly, is really a part of the educational experience from its inception. Debriefing should be a part of the curriculum development process. Attaining the educational goals and objectives of a scenario will rely upon elucidation and reflection during debriefing. This means that the amount of time devoted to debriefing and the number of elements expected in the debriefing must be feasible for repeated performances. It has already been discussed that on the day of the scenario, debriefing is rooted in the creation of an engaging environment as early as the orientation. Faculty can help keep learners oriented by describing the structure of the session including what to expect during simulations and debriefings. During the scenario itself, the facilitator must observe, collect, prioritize, and prepare the various discussion points that arise. These will be unique to each group in their particulars. One of the marks of a well-crafted scenario is that it will consistently produce decision points and actions that provide debriefing substrate in keeping with the educational goals and objectives.

Which technique should I choose? As mentioned in the introduction to debriefing strategies, there are multiple considerations in addressing this question. From a theoretical standpoint, the different techniques have different strengths. As discussed, one may be learned more quickly than another. The plus-delta technique, for example, requires little training and allows rapid deployment. It is by design focused on actions and behaviors and is relatively superficial. Other techniques seek to understand the reasoning of the participant to promote improved performance in the future, which is particularly important in curricula that stress critical thinking and clinical reasoning. Debriefing with good judgment is a commonly described technique of this type. Sometimes, the type of debriefing will be mandated in some way. GAS debriefing was discussed as an example of a prescribed debriefing technique in the interest of standardization. Another example might be in research projects with certain elements required in the debriefing. To reiterate an earlier point, the particular technique chosen by the novice may well be a matter of circumstance. Most simulation educators try a variety of techniques in their careers and eventually gravitate toward some individualized version of their preferred method. As debriefers are exposed to different courses, educators, and institutions, and as simulation-based healthcare education grows, debriefers will be familiar with these techniques and will likely be exposed to other debriefing techniques. As mentioned, a very common criterion for selecting a debriefing technique is to subscribe to the one used most prevalently in one's home institution (see chapter 8.1).

How do I debrief a "failed" simulation? A simulation session can fail to meet expectations in a variety of ways. If the healthcare providers are unable to meet reasonable expectations, then the debriefing can proceed as usual and may improve future patient care. Participants are likely to be acutely aware of their failings. Debriefing calls for balance between respect of the individual and direct observations of performance; "critique the behaviors, not the people" is a useful standard. For the participant with extensive debriefing experience, the integrity of the process should be already accepted. In the unfortunate situation of a participant relatively inexperienced with simulation and debriefing, great care must be taken to be supportive for the sake of the experience at hand, as well as those in the future. In the final analysis, it is the responsibility of the facilitator to help the participant improve. Integrity requires that substandard performances be addressed so that educators do not implicitly approve or give credence to wrong actions even if they are not the primary goal of the exercise.

Another type of failure can occur when a device does not behave as expected. A mannequin can abruptly malfunction with no sign of life or grossly abnormal vital signs and appearance. This is a situation that must be first handled in the scenario itself, but that has implications for the debriefing, and it requires that the debriefer be facile. For example, when the "simulator dies," the facilitator may decide to divert to an arrest response. The debriefing would then change from its original goals and objectives to consideration of the resuscitation effort. Alternatively, the simulation may be aborted or restarted to preserve the educational integrity and ensure reaching learning goals.

What if a participant will not engage? This is an issue that many faculty worry about but that is gratifyingly rare. However, with more mandated appearances in the simulation program (e.g., increasing curricular involvement, insurance incentives, maintenance of certification requirements, etc.), participant resistance could become more frequent. Learners may have difficulty engaging during the simulation or during the debriefing. During the simulation, an embedded simulation person (ESP) or actor/confederate can try to engage the participant directly. Faculty can also call on the telephone into the room so as to engage the participant by tasking them directly. During the debriefing, the participants may exhibit behaviors that erode the immersive environment ranging from realism complaints ("I would have checked the oxygen in a *real* patient") to outright attacks on the experience ("I have to be here but there is no good reason"). Within the debriefing, less extreme behaviors can often be redirected with questions, for example, "When you have had a clinical situation with these issues, how have you handled them?" (as opposed to "Well, what would you do with a real patient?"). Many programs also attempt to avoid nonengagement by overtly stating a contract of mutual respect and participation at the beginning of a session. Most participants respond to a reference to this stated or implied agreement, especially in the setting of a highly professional program. Other options include speaking to the individual privately at the end of the session or calling on them by name and being explicit about their participation. At some point, however, it must be remembered that the experiences of the other learners are being disrupted. The option of removing a participant would be considered by most educators as regrettable and severe. This is something that has never been done at many programs. However, if other measures fail, the uncooperative participant must be made aware in no-nonsense terms that their continued behavior will require removal.

How do I become an expert? Most educators will be first exposed to debriefing within their own programs. Further development can be sought in a variety of ways. Several simulation programs have educational offerings that include or are devoted to debriefing. Many professional societies offer workshops with a specialty or discipline specificity. The most important key to expertise is experience, especially mentored experience initially. This mentored experience raises the issue of "debriefing the debriefer." Such experiences, often informal, allow the developing faculty members to reap the same benefits of guided recollection and reflection in developing improved skills in debriefing that simulation participants gain from debriefing of their simulation experiences. No one can be an expert facilitator without experience and, regardless of faculty development and mentoring, must take the lead and then "solo" at some point. It is important to remember that any opportunity, even if inelegant, to reflect upon an experience and consider how to improve is a valuable educational experience. In summary, reflection, peer feedback, coaching, and repetitive practice—the same elements that lead to clinical expertise—are ways to improve and sustain debriefing skills.

How do I maintain expertise? Just as practice is the key to improvement, it is core to maintenance and refinement of expertise in debriefing. Again, exploring new techniques is an opportunity to expand one's repertoire as well as challenging current practice. Some of the programs that offer introductory training in debriefing also offer advanced experiences that may provide a broader view of debriefing, more in-depth training, and/or ways to teach and evaluate debriefing for program faculty. Additionally, the literature now contains frequent reports of new developments and data in debriefing covered in further depth in chapter 8.1.

NEW CHALLENGES AND FUTURE DIRECTIONS FOR EXPERTS

Simulation education in general and debriefing practice in particular are developing so quickly that it would be difficult to predict future practice. There are, however, ongoing important initiatives and challenges that will shape the development of debriefing.

Quality improvement is a cornerstone of sustainability in any simulation program. If the debriefing is truly considered to be a critical aspect of simulation education, then quality improvement should surely focus on this area. The challenges of assessing debriefers and debriefings, each unique by nature, and the recent development of instruments to answer these challenges were discussed previously. These tools, combined with current audiovisual technologies, allow debriefings to be evaluated objectively and with apparent reliability.

Interprofessional education (IPE) may be one of the most important uses of simulation education in healthcare. The great irony of the touted potential for team training, of course, is that most simulation teams have been single-discipline and specialty groups, with any interprofessional roles enacted by ESPs. The challenges and failings of interprofessional simulation have been described (Masiello, 2012). Data are now emerging that properly conducted programs can change team performance (Pemberton et al., 2013). There is a paucity of literature regarding interprofessional debriefing in clinical settings (Salas et al., 2008) and even less to be found in the setting of simulation. It seems self-evident that the importance of a psychologically safe environment would be even more important in the interprofessional setting to improve open communication and genuine sharing of emotions and frames. Other reasonable strategies would be to ensure inclusion of facilitators from participating disciplines and specialties. This serves the purposes of both perceived advocacy and support for learners and the availability of increased professional expertise. The creation and deployment of interprofessional scenarios, including debriefing, requires an educational interprofessional practice (Tullmann et al., 2013) analogous to clinical interprofessional practice with many of the same challenges and competencies.

Improvement of clinical education is an obvious target of the debriefing expert. There are some reports of postevent debriefing in the clinical setting, particularly in the resuscitation literature (Couper & Perkins, 2013; Mullan et al., 2013). All of the benefits of debriefing that apply to simulation education should be expected to apply to clinical situations as well. Faculty who learn to debrief well have developed a skill that can serve trainees and colleagues (and patients) outside the physical walls of the simulation center. When clinical faculty come to value debriefing as a powerful educational experience, there should be a greater penetration of debriefing into everyday educational practice. Simulation educators are uniquely positioned to provide the expertise, faculty development, and mentoring to accelerate this process.

Research questions in simulation debriefing are myriad. The importance of debriefing, the role of prebriefing, the efficacy of different debriefing methods, the possible role of longer-term reflections, and how to train debriefers are all important questions in debriefing. A cursory look at a current issue of a simulation journal shows interesting and important work such as the investigation of how debriefers can reach deeper cognitive levels and how culture influences debriefing outcomes (Chung et al., 2013). Again, if we as a community of simulation educators believe that debriefing is central to effectiveness, then investigation and development in debriefing is paramount.

SUMMARY

There is a long-standing and half-serious adage among seasoned simulation educators that simulation scenarios are just an excuse to do a debriefing. This does reflect the truth that the simulation debriefing represents a precious moment in education and training. A successful simulation recreates the emotional energy of clinical situations and challenges the cognitive capacity of participants—it is the concrete experience. There is a malleability born of this emotional state and the scrutiny of self, peers, and mentors that allows individuals to genuinely consider their performance and reconsider the bases of actions for future improvement. This is fundamental change at the highest level because it affects what the practitioner actually does every day.

Successful simulation debriefings, regardless of the particular technique selected, require the provision of a supportive and psychologically safe environment. The vulnerability of participants in the simulation scenario extends to the debriefing period. Learners trust their peers and facilitators to be professional and objective. In this sense, the successful debriefing begins as soon as a participant is introduced to the culture of a simulation program. Part of this culture is the contract, stated or implied, that all individuals involved are respected as dedicated, capable, and intelligent practitioners who are doing their best and are seeking to become better.

Debriefing plays a critical role in healthcare simulation. This role is supported by historical experience and educational theory. Continued improvement in simulation education requires excellence in debriefing practice through the continued refinement of best practices, faculty development, and investigation. Faculty development and assessment in debriefing are challenging. Basic debriefing skills can be gained relatively quickly, but take years to refine. It is time to develop ways of "teaching the teachers" with greater efficiency and to provide continuing mentorship in the form of educational quality improvement. The debriefing skills developed in simulation should not be limited to the simulation program. With proper training, faculty can apply these skills to the clinical setting with all of the benefits inherent in simulation debriefing. The simulation community is in a position to improve clinical education. Just as participants take the lessons learned from simulation to the improved care of patients, faculty can take debriefing to the clinical setting for improved educational practice.

REFERENCES

Arora, S., Ahmed, M., Paige, J., Nestel, D., Runnacles, J., Hull, L., ... Sevdalis, N. (2012). Objective structured assessment of debriefing: Bringing science to the art of debriefing in surgery [Research support, non-U.S. Gov't review]. *Annals of Surgery, 256*(6), 982–988. http://dx.doi.org/10.1097/SLA.0b013e3182610c91

Brett-Fleegler, M., Rudolph, J., Eppich, W., Monuteaux, M., Fleegler, E., Cheng, A., & Simon, R. (2012). Debriefing assessment for simulation in healthcare: Development and psychometric properties [Validation studies]. *Simulation in Healthcare: The Journal of the Society for Medical Simulation, 7*(5), 288–294. http://dx.doi.org/10.1097/SIH.0b013e3182620228

Bruner, J. S. (1960). *The Process of education.* Cambridge, MA: Harvard University Press.

Cheng, A., Rodgers, D. L., van der Jagt, E., Eppich, W., & O'Donnell, J. (2012). Evolution of the Pediatric Advanced Life Support course: Enhanced learning with a new debriefing tool and web-based module for Pediatric Advanced Life Support instructors [Research support, non-U.S. Gov't review]. *Pediatric Critical Care Medicine, 13*(5), 589–595.

Chung, H. S., Dieckmann, P., & Issenberg, S. B. (2013). It is time to consider cultural differences in debriefing. *Simulation in Healthcare: The Journal of the Society for Medical Simulation, 8*(3), 166–170. http://dx.doi.org/10.1097/SIH.1090b1013e318291d318299ef

Cook, D. A., Hatala, R., Brydges, R., Zendejas, B., Szostek, J. H., Wang, A. T., ... Hamstra, S. J. (2011). Technology-enhanced simulation for health professions education: A systematic review and meta-analysis [Meta-analysis research support, non-U.S. Gov't review]. *JAMA: the Journal of the American Medical Association, 306*(9), 978–988.

Cooper, G. E., White, M. D., & Lauber, J. K. (1980). *Resource management on the flightdeck: Proceedings of a NASA/industry workshop* (NASA CP-2120). Moffett Field, CA: NASA-Ames Research Center.

Couper, K., & Perkins, G. D. (2013). Debriefing after resuscitation. *Current Opinion in Critical Care, 19*(3), 188–194. http://dx.doi.org/10.1097/MCC.0b013e32835f58aa

Dismukes, R. K., Jobe, K. K., & McDonnell, L. K. (1997). *LOFT debriefings: An analysis of instructor techniques and crew participation* (NASA Technical Memorandum 110442 DOT/FAA/AR-96/126). Retrieved from http://ipv6.faa.gov/training_testing/training/aqp/library/media/Final_LOFT_TM.pdf

Dyregrov, A. (1997). The process in psychological debriefings [Comparative study]. *Journal of Traumatic Stress, 10*(4), 589–605.

Ericsson, K. A. (2008). Deliberate practice and acquisition of expert. *Academic Emergency Medicine*, 988–994. http://dx.doi.org/10.1111/j.1553-2712.2008.00227.x

Ericsson, K. A., Krampe, R. T., & Tesch-romer, C. (1993). The role of deliberate practice in the acquisition of expert performance. *Psychological Review, 100*(3), 363–406.

Fillion, J. S., Clements, P. T., Averill, J. B., & Vigil, G. J. (2002). Talking as a primary method of peer defusing for military personnel exposed to combat trauma [Review]. *Journal of Psychosocial Nursing & Mental Health Services, 40*(8), 40–49.

Gardner, R. (2013). Introduction to debriefing. *Seminars in Perinatology, 37*(3), 166–174.

Howard, S. K., Gaba, D. M., Fish, K. J., Yang, G., & Sarnquist, F. H. (1992). Anesthesia crisis resource management training: teaching anesthesiologists to handle critical incidents [Research support, non-U.S. Gov't research support, U.S. Gov't, non-P.H.S.]. *Aviation Space & Environmental Medicine, 63*(9), 763–770.

Kolb, D. A. (1984). *Experiential learning: Experience as the source of learning and development.* Englewood Cliffs, NJ: Prentice-Hall.

Lederman, L. C. (1992). Debriefing: Toward a systematic assessment of theory and practice. *Simulation & Gaming, 23*(2), 145–160. http://dx.doi.org/10.1177/1046878192232003

Littlewood, K. E. (2011). High fidelity simulation as a research tool [Review]. *Best Practice & Research. Clinical Anaesthesiology, 25*(4), 473–487.

MacDonald, C. M. (2003). Evaluation of stress debriefing interventions with military populations [Review]. *Military Medicine, 168*(12), 961–968.

Masiello, I. (2012). Why simulation-based team training has not been used effectively and what can be done about it. *Advances in Health Sciences Education, 17*(2), 279–288. http://dx.doi.org/10.1007/s10459-011-9281-8

Meyer, J. F., & Land, R. (2005). Threshold concepts and troublesome knowledge (2): Epistemological considerations and a conceptual framework for teaching and learning. *Higher Education, 49*(3), 373–388. http://dx.doi.org/10.1007/s10734-004-6779-5

Milgram, S. (1963). Behavioral study of obedience. *Journal of Abnormal and Social Psychology, 67*(4), 371–378.

Mullan, P. C., Wuestner, E., Kerr, T. D., Christopher, D. P., & Patel, B. (2013). Implementation of an in situ qualitative debriefing tool for resuscitations. *Resuscitation, 84*(7), 946–951. http://dx.doi.org/10.1016/j.resuscitation.2012.12.005

Pemberton, J., Rambaran, M., & Cameron, B. H. (2013). Evaluating the long-term impact of the trauma team training course in Guyana: An explanatory mixed-methods approach. *American Journal of Surgery, 205*(2), 119–124. http://dx.doi.org/10.1016/j.amjsurg.2012.08.004

Petranek, C. (1994). A maturation in experiential learning: Principles of simulation and gaming. *Simulation & Gaming, 25*(4), 513–523.

Petranek, C., Corey, S., & Black, R. (1992). Three levels of learning in simulations: Participating, debriefing, and journal writing. *Simulation & Gaming, 23*, 174–185.

Plass, J., Moreno, R., & Brunken, R. (Eds.). (2012). *Cognitive load theory.* Cambridge, England: Cambridge University Press.

Rudolph, J. W., Simon, R., Dufresne, R. L., & Raemer, D. B. (2006). There's no such thing as "nonjudgmental" debriefing: A theory and method for debriefing with good judgment [Research support, non-U.S. Gov't research support, U.S. Gov't, non-P.H.S.]. *Simulation in Healthcare: The Journal of the Society for Medical Simulation, 1*(1), 49–55.

Salas, E., Klein, C., King, H., Salisbury, M., Augenstein, J. S., Birnbach, D. J., ... Upshaw, C. (2008). Debriefing medical teams: 12 evidence-based best practices and tips [Research support, U.S. Gov't, non-P.H.S.]. *Joint Commission Journal on Quality & Patient Safety, 34*(9), 518–527.

Savoldelli, G. L., Naik, V. N., Park, J., Joo, H. S., Chow, R., & Hamstra, S. J. (2006). Value of debriefing during simulated crisis management: Oral versus video-assisted oral feedback [Comparative study randomized controlled trial research support, non-U.S. Gov't]. *Anesthesiology, 105*(2), 279–285.

Scherer, L. A., Chang, M. C., Meredith, J. W., & Battistella, F. D. (2003). Videotape review leads to rapid and sustained learning [Comparative study evaluation studies]. *American Journal of Surgery, 185*(6), 516–520.

Senger, B., Stapleton, L., & Gorski, M. S. (2012). A hospital and university partnership model for simulation education. *Clinical Simulation in Nursing, 8*(9), e477–e482. http://dx.doi.org/10.1016/j.ecns.2011.09.002

Sharpe, D., & Faye, C. (2009). A second look at debriefing practices: Madness in our method? *Ethics & Behavior, 19*(5), 432–447. http://dx.doi.org/10.1080/10508420903035455

Smits, P. B. A., Verbeek, J. H. A. M., & de Buisonje, C. D. (2002). Problem based learning in continuing medical education: A review of controlled evaluation studies [Meta-analysis research support, non-U.S. Gov't]. *BMJ (Clinical Research Ed.), 324*(7330), 153–156.

Tullmann, D. F., Shilling, A. M., Goeke, L. H., Wright, E. B., & Littlewood, K. E. (2013). Recreating simulation scenarios for interprofessional education: An example of educational interprofessional practice. *Journal of Interprofessional Care, 27*(5), 426–428. http://dx.doi.org/10.3109/13561820.2013.790880

Van Heukelom, J. N., Begaz, T., & Treat, R. (2010). Comparison of post-simulation debriefing versus in-simulation debriefing in medical simulation [Comparative study]. *Simulation in Healthcare: The Journal of the Society for Medical Simulation, 5*(2), 91–97. http://dx.doi.org/10.1097/SIH.0b013e3181be0d17

Van Merrienboer, J. J. G., & Sweller, J. (2010). Cognitive load theory in health professional education: Design principles and strategies [Review]. *Medical Education, 44*(1), 85–93. http://dx.doi.org/10.1111/j.1365-2923.2009.03498.x

Vygotsky, L. S. (1978). *Mind in society: The development of higher mental processes.* Cambridge, MA: Harvard University Press.

CHAPTER 8.3

Realism and Moulage

Rebekah Damazo, RN, CPNP, CHSE-A, MSN, and Sherry D. Fox, RN, PhD, CHSE

> How well a simulation replicates or represents "reality" is a core question in all fields that use simulation.
>
> —*Dieckmann et al., 2007*

ABOUT THE AUTHORS

REBEKAH DAMAZO is the director and cofounder of the Rural Northern California Clinical Simulation Center in Chico, California, and Professor of Nursing at California State University, Chico. Ms. Damazo is widely known for her excellence in the development of theatrical moulage for use in patient simulation. She has offered numerous moulage training courses and workshops throughout the world and has authored a moulage handbook.

SHERRY D. FOX is the financial director and cofounder of the Rural Northern California Clinical Simulation Center in Chico, California, and Professor of Nursing at California State University, Chico. The Center offers regular training courses, moulage books, and moulage kits for simulation educators. Dr. Fox assists with moulage workshops and presentations.

ABSTRACT

Simulation is a technique that uses guided experiences to evoke or replicate substantial aspects of the real world (Gabba, 2007). Perception of realism in simulation cases can have a tremendous influence on student experiences and ultimately impact learning (Nanji et al., 2013). The art of moulage can provide simple and inexpensive cues to build into simulation scenarios, without dramatically increasing the workload of educator or technician. Adding moulage to human patient simulations can set the stage for meeting the objectives of the scenario, provide meaningful clues to the patient condition, support decision making, improve differential diagnosis, and provide realistic training situations that use multiple senses and provide stress inoculation. Beginning and advanced simulation teams can enhance their scenarios with simple and cost-effective methods to increase realism and fidelity, which will enhance learning outcomes and student satisfaction.

This chapter will describe the uses of moulage and considerations for achieving the right level of realism. Basic supplies, resources, and techniques will also be presented.

CASE EXAMPLE

The simulation team has come together to discuss the development of a case scenario focused on recognition of the signs of child abuse. As they discuss the learning objectives with the content expert, they debate how to create realistic clues that should alert the caregiver to the potential for abuse. How subtle should the signs be? What is the appropriate level of moulage to use to achieve the desired level of fidelity? After much discussion, the team agrees that providing an outline of an imprint of a hand on the child's back would be an appropriate diagnostic clue for this group of learners. The handprint on the child's (mannequin) back is a clue that he/she did not sustain his/her injuries in a fall as reported in the scenario history (Figure 8.3.1).

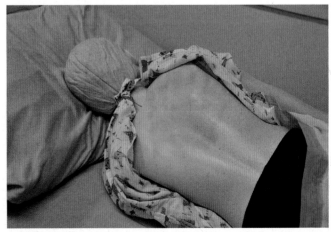

FIGURE 8.3.1 Moulage can provide meaningful clues.

INTRODUCTION AND BACKGROUND

Moulage has been used for centuries as an art to depict illness and injury (Worm et al., 2007). Moulage, from the French meaning casting or molding, is often defined as the "art" of creating mock injuries. Moulage has been used for centuries to help clinicians recognize and diagnose seldom seen illnesses (Joshi, 2010). The natural picture of disease—left untreated—can be seen in medical museums with detailed moulage models and figures (Worm et al., 2007). More than a century ago, the Greeks developed a three-dimensional wax figure to teach physicians how to diagnose syphilis in its various stages as well as other forms of infectious disease with skin manifestations, such as smallpox (Joshi et al., 2010; Worm et al., 2007). While severe manifestations of many infectious diseases have disappeared with sophisticated antibiotic therapy, we are seeing some diseases reemerge as new threats. Today, many clinicians may never have seen the clinical presentation of once common diseases such as varicella or rubeola. Owing to waning immunization vigilance, these diseases are reemerging as threats and are sometimes overlooked in the differential diagnosis. Therefore, in recent years, disease outbreaks have found clinicians going back to the museums and galleries to become reacquainted with rare disease presentations not commonly seen (Worm et al., 2007).

Medical history is full of molds and casts of disease that were created so that the study of human anatomy did not solely depend on the dissection of bodies. Moulage was even used as a public health deterrent to show individuals the stages of syphilis hoping to avert the disease. Even after more than a century, many of the wax models remain lifelike with accurate rendering of skin diseases, reflecting close collaboration between the artist and the physician (Joshi et al., 2010).

Moulage is a natural fit with simulation as technicians and clinicians collaborate to develop high-fidelity (as close to reality as possible) simulation scenarios. Moulage has been shown to be an effective teaching resource to provide students with a clear picture of a specific clinical situation as well as for student assessment. Basic assessment courses as well as advanced courses such as those used for training early recognition and emergency response teams can be enhanced through the use of realistic moulage. Notice how in Figure 8.3.2 the victim is staged to provide a clear clinical picture of the situation. First responders are able to make quick assessments and take appropriate actions during training exercises as a result of moulage reality.

It is often said "A picture is worth a thousand words." This is especially true in the health sciences. Effective moulage can greatly enhance the learning outcomes for simulation. Students become more immersed in the realism of the simulation and can move quickly to solutions, without having to suspend disbelief. The need for explanations is minimized, a sense of urgency is created, and students are more likely to act quickly on their assessments.

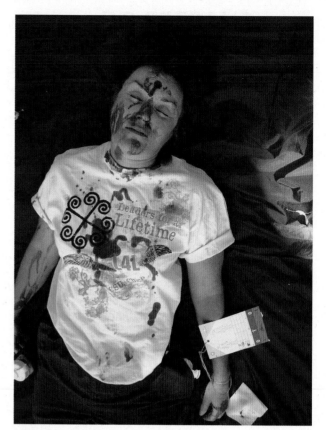

FIGURE 8.3.2 Moulage helps stage a campus shooting drill.

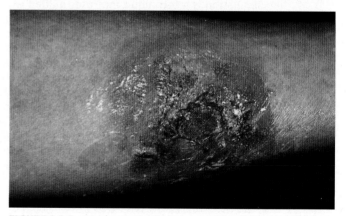

FIGURE 8.3.3 Moulage can assist in representing subtle wound features.

Adding low-cost, simple moulage techniques are within the capability of both novice and advanced simulation personnel (Figure 8.3.3).

SIGNIFICANCE

Many novices to simulation note the labor-intensive nature of developing scenarios, programming mannequins, and implementing the simulation experience. Without a context for using moulage, taking additional time to increase the realism or **fidelity** of scenarios may seem to simply add work and not purpose. When moulage is used appropriately with simulation scenario design, it has the ability to:

1. **Set the stage for scenario objectives:** Objectives should be the basis of all scenario development. Moulage can nudge the student toward understanding objectives as they relate to the case scenario. For example, an intravenous infiltrate can be placed on the mannequin and support the need for regular patient assessment.
2. **Enhance assessment opportunities:** Well-placed wounds or stage blood can prompt the student to explore diagnostic options.
3. **Provide meaningful clues to the patient condition:** Sweat, cyanosis, or edema can provide information to the student that will allow for proper diagnosis and treatment (Mould et al., 2011).
4. **Support decision making:** Moulage techniques can guide the student to the proper treatment decision and build confidence and provide the opportunity for self-assessment (Tofil et al., 2009).
5. **Improve differential diagnosis:** Moulage can assist the student in determining the right diagnostic pathway (Lee et al., 2003).
6. **Create realistic training situations:** Realism has been shown to increase students' ability to perform well under pressure (Potter, 2008; Saiboon et al., 2011; Scott et al., 2010).
7. **Engage all senses in the learning experience :** Odors can provide strong and unique clues. It is possible to create the smell of infection or vomit or blood. Nanji et al. (2013) used an electrosurgical unit applied to bovine muscle tissue to create the smells common in an operating room. It should be noted that there were no statistical differences in the perception of reality among participating students. Using commercially available odors can create the smells associated with various infections. These odors provide clues to support student findings and actions.
8. **Provide stress inoculation:** Exposing students to traumatic events such as burns or traumatic injuries can provide a strong visual representation of how a trauma patient actually looks as well as "the unpleasant interventions that may be used to care for the patient" (Hollis, 2002). Exposure to these experiences in the simulated environment helps to prepare clinicians for the impact in the field.

Effective moulage can greatly enhance the simulation experience, helping to achieve objectives, without overshadowing the simulation. Moulage techniques can be relatively simple, cost-effective, and easy to apply. For example, a simulation educator may use a wig on a mannequin to provide gender or age clues. In some cases, these clues can be enhanced with simple additions, such as fake eyelashes or actual wrinkles. Notice the improved reality in Figures 8.3.4 and 8.3.5.

Because skin lesions are primarily three-dimensional, subtle details may go unnoticed (Krishna, 2011). Even with the advent of high-resolution photography, sometimes the clinician is unable to translate the images to diagnostic ability. Figure 8.3.3 shows how moulage can assist in representing subtle wound features. As another example, diaphoresis can be an important clue for many disease conditions. Figure 8.3.6 shows how this can be accomplished in a simple manner with a premade "sweat" formula.

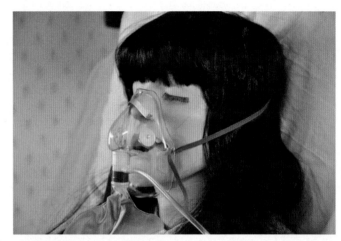

FIGURE 8.3.4 Improved reality.

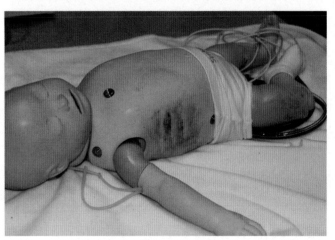

FIGURE 8.3.5 Improved reality.

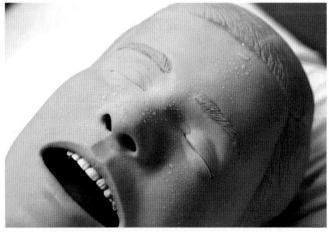

FIGURE 8.3.6 An example of a simplified moulage scene.

SECTION 8 • Faculty Development

In all cases, simulation educators should strive to achieve balance to avoid making the simulation about the moulage instead of having moulage provide cues that guide students to reach the desired learning outcomes (Damazo, 2012).

GUIDELINES FOR SUCCESSFUL MOULAGE

1. **Start with a well-planned scenario.** The case background and history should provide initial diagnostic information and set the student up for success. The moulage should work with the scenario to guide the student to the objectives and not simply be a creative "add-on."

   Remember, moulage is NOT the end; it is the means to the end. Extensive moulage can sometimes steal the scene and distract participants rather than guide them through the course objectives. It is important, therefore, that the simulation educator makes sure that the moulage provides necessary authentic details but does not take over the case.

2. **Work with the physiology of the mannequin.** The blue lips created with moulage may provide the visual clue of cyanosis, but the scenario's clinical picture will be enhanced with a low SpO_2 reading and perhaps a mannequin that is wheezing.

3. **Plan enough time for setup and cleanup.** Discussions and decisions about how the moulage will be used in the scenario should be part of designing the scenario and developing the teaching plan. This will ensure that adequate time is included for both staging and cleanup. If elaborate moulage is planned, be sure to include the moulage timing as part of the teaching plan.

TIPS FOR USING MOULAGE WITH HUMAN PATIENT SIMULATORS

Simulators are expensive and sensitive educational tools with complex computerized functions. Never forget that you are "dressing up" an elaborate electronic system (Damazo, 2012).

1. **Always follow manufacturers' guidelines** to avoid the risk of voiding manufacturers' warranties. When in doubt, it is best to test the moulage on an inconspicuous area of the mannequin or on a test skin piece (such as a neck skin) that is not attached to the simulator. All mannequins have been designed to create reality, but some parts of the mannequins are harder and more stain-resistant than other parts and therefore less subject to damage from potions or products (Figure 8.3.7).

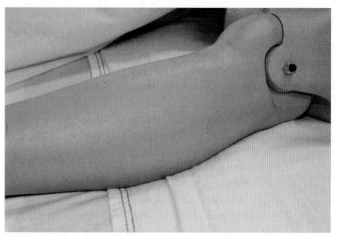

FIGURE 8.3.7 Some parts of the mannequins are harder than other parts and less subject to damage from potions or products.

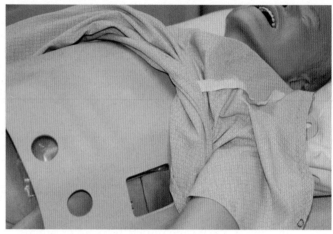

FIGURE 8.3.8 Design scenarios to minimize contact with the more porous and vulnerable parts of your mannequins.

Where possible, design scenarios that minimize contact with the more porous and vulnerable parts (Figure 8.3.8) of your mannequins. Remember to use a barrier between the mannequin and any substance that may stain or damage it. Products used to simulate red blood are notorious for seeping into the soft skin of the mannequin and can only be removed with difficulty.

2. **Never place or use liquids near electronic parts.** Always avoid using liquids or gels (they can melt) near electronic parts (Figure 8.3.9).

3. **Keep a stock of reusable wounds on hand to save prep time.** Many commercial products are durable if handled gently and refrigerated between uses.

4. **Do not leave makeup in place for extended lengths of time.** The mannequin-manufacturing companies have struggled to create a porous, lifelike feel to the mannequin skin. This skin is subject to chemical reactions with makeup or products that may be applied as moulage. Always clean up immediately after the case is complete to minimize the risk of chemical reactions.

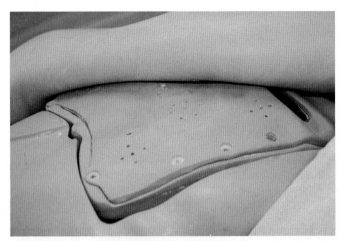

FIGURE 8.3.9 Always avoid using liquids or gels (which may melt) near electronic parts.

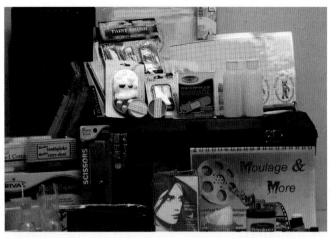

FIGURE 8.3.10 A common moulage kit configuration.

TIPS FOR USING MOULAGE WITH LIVE ACTORS (STANDARDIZED PATIENTS)

When using moulage or theatrical makeup with live actors, it is important to remember that individuals may be subject to reactions from some theatrical products.

1. **Some products used in moulage can cause rashes or irritation.** Before applying any product or moulage, always ask about allergies or skin sensitivities. Some individuals may also be sensitive to smells or sounds that occur in the lab.
2. **Have cream-based makeup removers and lotions on hand.** Caution is required to ensure that the actor does not have any adverse outcomes from participation. When working with older actors, remember that their skin is often thin and sensitive, so use caution.
3. **Some of the materials used may stain clothing.** Keep a store of clothes or costumes you can offer the actors to avoid damage to their personal items. Always warn actors, if it is possible, that their clothes may be damaged.

CREATING A MOULAGE KIT

A moulage kit is a helpful tool. By having all the makeup, tools, and materials available in one kit, the simulation educator can save time. There are numerous fully assembled moulage kits available from commercial sources. A moulage kit is typically purchased as a kit or it is a personal accumulation of tools and materials that are used frequently in simulation scenarios. Figure 8.3.10 shows a common kit configuration.

Cleanup products can also be included with the kit to allow for easy removal of moulage. Several authors have provided information on how to construct a kit

(Damazo, 2012; Hindman, 1988; Lindsey, 2003). As part of its efforts in emergency preparedness training, the Federal Emergency Management Agency (FEMA, n.d.) has developed a list of some common items to include in a moulage kit. These include the following:

- Makeup (various colors)—be sure to test before applying on mannequin
- Cotton balls
- Sterile gauze pads
- Glycerin
- Palette knife
- Brushes (various types)
- Tongue depressors
- Sponges (stipple, gauze, makeup)
- Mixing palette
- Effects gels (blood, clear, flesh-colored)
- Effects gel applicator
- Stage blood (premixed and powder mixes)
- Scissors
- Utility knife
- Plastic wrap
- Liquid starch
- Pocket comb
- Rubbing alcohol
- Petroleum jelly
- Liquid adhesive and adhesive remover
- Empty mixing bottles
- Flesh putty (various colors)
- Premade prosthetics (various injuries such as blisters, burnt skin, bone fractures, open wounds)

MOULAGE MATERIALS

There are numerous commonly available materials that can be used to create realistic scenes using moulage techniques. The materials range from common household products to food to sophisticated molding and modeling products using special effects gels, latex, or specialized polymers. The simulation educator or technician who is interested in becoming a moulage expert may explore some of the many products available or take a course to learn how to use the materials.

Figures 8.3.11 and 8.3.12 show how a bruise can be created using basic eye shadow colors and then aged and positioned to provide diagnostic clues. Theatrical supply houses are also great sources for most of the molding or gel materials you may need. Typically, they also offer training in the use of these products. Figures 8.3.13 to 8.3.17 show how realistic some of these materials make the simulation scene.

MOULAGE AND DISASTER PLANNING

Injury simulation and moulage play key roles in disaster preparedness (Atlas et al., 2005; Auer, 2004; Scott et al., 2010). For disaster scenarios, moulage can range from

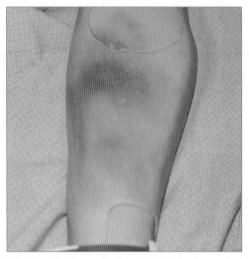

FIGURE 8.3.11 A bruise can be created using basic eye shadow colors and then aged and positioned to provide diagnostic clues.

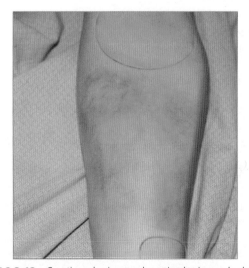

FIGURE 8.3.12 Creating a bruise on a leg using basic eye shadow colors and then aging and positioning to provide diagnostic clues.

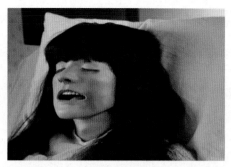

FIGURE 8.3.13 Creating a facial bruise using basic eye shadow colors and then aging and positioning to provide diagnostic clues.

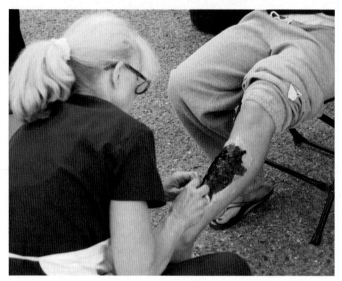

FIGURE 8.3.14 Layering moulage materials to create burn effect on a live actor.

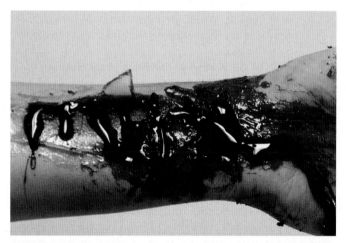

FIGURE 8.3.15 Applying gel effects material and rubberized glass pieces to create injury.

spraying "blood" on victims to development of intricate wounds and burns for specific disaster drills, such as chemical spills. No existing mass casualty triage system has been scientifically scrutinized or validated to provide a standardized approach. The Centers for Disease Control attempted

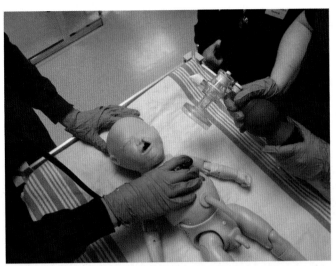

FIGURE 8.3.16   A facial mask made out of moulage materials can enhance scenario fidelity.

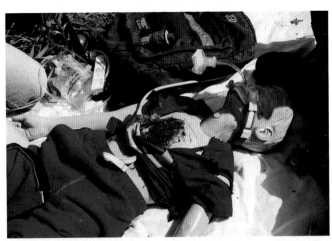

FIGURE 8.3.17   Using combined simple and complex techniques to set up a disaster scene.

to create a disaster triage system. For training purposes, this system includes well-scripted victims and detailed moulage directions and can serve as a starting point for disaster planning agencies (Cone et al., 2009).

As with all scenarios, a disaster scenario requires specific objectives and well-thought-out staging of victims, and moulage that makes sense and provides clues to support learning outcomes. Injury simulation plays an important role in disaster training.

BEEN THERE, DONE THAT: HOW CAN I CONTINUE TO IMPROVE OR SUSTAIN WHAT I HAVE ACHIEVED?

As with any artistic endeavor, continued study and practice improves performance. By obtaining feedback from learners, especially those who are practicing clinicians, simulation educators can refine their art and improve learning that occurs in simulation experiences. In addition, accessing information from manufacturers and networking with other simulation educators will provide a wealth of innovative methods to expand and refine your repertoire of moulaging techniques.

SUMMARY

Moulage is a tool that can help reinforce learning. There are many choices—from elaborate theatrical makeups, masks, and effects to simple changes—that can help reinforce or provide cues to improve convincing aspects of simulation fidelity. Accomplishing more convincing fidelity can help the learner achieve the expected outcomes while respecting instructor time, supplies, and resources.

SECTION 8 • Faculty Development

EXPERT'S CORNER

HELPING LEARNERS "BUY IN" TO SIMULATION

Jenny W. Rudolph, Phd,[1-3] Cate McIntosh, MBBS, FANZCA,[4,5] Robert Simon, EdD,[1-3] and Daniel B. Raemer, PhD,[1-3]
[1]Center for Medical Simulation, USA; [2]Massachusetts General Hospital, USA; [3]Harvard Medical School, USA; [4]Hunter New England Skills and Simulation Centre, Australia; [5]John Hunter Hospital, Australia

There was such an adrenaline rush in the room ... everyone felt it. We all just helped the patient who just crashed and were able to resuscitate him. It was really close, but the team made some key decisions that helped.

It was just so hard to get past the plastic skin ... it was so hard and cold ... and the fact that it never moved in the bed. None of my patients are that still and I couldn't get the thought out of my head that this is just a dummy.

What feels real to one person may not feel real to another. When people think of what makes simulation real, they usually think of the things they interact with—the simulator, the props, and the people acting out the role of providers. We invite you into this "Expert's Corner" to explore the hidden psychological side that makes things feel real enough for your learners to "buy in" to simulation.

"Buying into" a simulation is challenging; we ask participants to act *as if* things are real (Dieckmann et al., 2007). For this reason, we instructors are dependent on learners; the simulation is likely to flop if they don't play an active role, taking care of the "patient" to the best of their ability. That means that we have to work to earn their engagement, not assume it. There are two hidden psychological parts to this: (1) We have to do something unusual for many instructors—reveal that we are interdependent with them to create a good learning experience, and (2) like a novelist or playwright, we have to create a fictional environment engaging enough to draw them in (Dieckmann et al., 2007; Eco,1994).

Fortunately, German simulation expert Peter Dieckmann blazed a trail for us to do this: Create a shared agreement

(continued)

with learners about their participation called a "fiction contract" (Dieckmann et al., 2007).

The "fiction contract" (Dieckmann et al., 2007) is a verbal agreement between instructors and learners about what we owe each other and should expect of each other to have a good simulation session or course.

A collaboratively created fiction contract is just one of the key "ingredients" to consider when developing your simulation program. In addition, there are other factors that we won't explore in this piece such as motivation for participating in a simulation, or the level of leadership support for simulation in the participant's organization. These factors will also influence the degree to which our participants "buy in."

To create a fiction contract, at the beginning of a simulation session, we instructors state that we have done our best to make the simulation look as real as possible, but acknowledge the limits (e.g., the mannequin patient's skin color does not change; breath sounds can only be heard in specific locations on the chest; invasive procedures cannot be performed on standardized patients). We then share that we are interdependent with the learners to make the learning experience as engaging as possible. We ask for their commitment to "meet us halfway" and do what they can to act as if everything is real (Dieckmann et al., 2007). We clarify that the quality of the learning experience depends on two interdependent factors: what we instructors have done to make it as realistic as possible, and their willingness to participate as fully as possible.

As simulation developers, what this means for us is that we need to have a thorough understanding of the important components of the task or situation being simulated so that we make sure important "cues" are included. In addition, it is our responsibility to understand who our learners are. Different learners require different learning conditions, and what may result in high engagement for experienced clinicians will be overwhelming and confusing for more junior learners.

Working to create this simple agreement with learners to act as if things are real is important because it impacts learners' willingness to engage even when they question the realism of the simulation.

How can this fiction contract influence learners' willingness to engage? First it is necessary to understand how learners perceive the simulation that influences that engagement (Figure 1). Dieckmann and colleagues argue that healthcare simulations have three kinds of fidelity, where fidelity describes how closely the simulator and/or the simulation resembles the "real thing." "Fidelity" is an often vaguely defined term, with multiple types and definitions proposed in the literature. Importantly, it is a multidimensional construct and not a binary "high" or "low" notion. Several authors of this article have adapted Dieckmann et al.'s terminology (Nanji et al., 2013; Rudolph et al., 2007) and continue the loose categorization of fidelity into three types. *Physical fidelity* is the degree to which the simulation approximates the visual, tactile, auditory, and olfactory nature of the situation or task being simulated. *Conceptual fidelity* is the degree to which the simulation progresses plausibly given the causal factors involved. If the patient's physiological, pharmacological, responses make sense for a given intervention, or if standardized patients' or embedded simulated providers' emotional reactions make sense given participants' actions, this is conceptual fidelity. *Emotional/experiential fidelity* is the degree to which the simulation creates feelings in learners that they would expect in a comparable

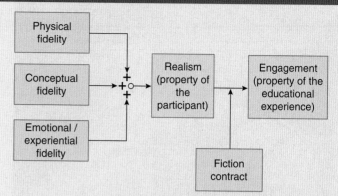

FIGURE 1 The three kinds of fidelity combine to influence how realism is perceived by individuals in a simulation.

real-world situation. When the simulation evolves to produce stress, relief, time pressure, or joy, these are examples of emotional/experiential fidelity (see Figure 1).

The three kinds of fidelity combine to influence how realism is perceived by individuals in a simulation. Perceptions of realism differ among participants even though all experience the same simulation fidelity. Importantly then, realism is subjective, that is, it is experienced and perceived by the learner, whereas fidelity is an objective property of the simulation.

Thus, it is not only the visible, obvious aspects of simulation fidelity that influence whether our learners engage, it is also their individual subjective perception of realism that is important. This subjective perception varies in ways we can't always predict.

The quality of the fiction contract, we suggest, is an important factor that may influence how, if, or to what degree learners are willing to actively engage in the simulation. The quality of the fiction contract influences learners' willingness to engage despite perceived lapses in realism. If done well, learners are more likely to feel we are treating them fairly and with respect, and therefore try to participate, even in the face of perceived realism lapses.

In contrast, unilaterally dictating to learners how they should feel about the simulation is not a high-quality fiction contract. If learners are told they *must* "suspend disbelief" and play along if they are to do well, learners may get defensive or disengage by finding fault with the simulation. Instead, by articulating our interdependence with learners by asking them to meet us halfway in creating a meaningful learning session, we can help learners engage in simulated events. By recognizing that we and the learners need each other to create a good learning experience, the fiction contract catalyzes engagement, even when fidelity and perceived realism are far from perfect.

REFERENCES

Dieckmann, P., Gaba, D., & Rall, M. (2007). Deepening the theoretical foundations of patient simulation as social practice. *Simulation in Healthcare: The Journal of the Society for Medical Simulation, 2*(3), 183–193.

Eco, U. (1994). *Six walks in the fictional woods.* Cambridge, MA: Harvard University Press.

Nanji, K. C., Baca, K., & Raemer, D. B. (2013). The effect of an olfactory and visual cue on realism and engagement in a health care simulation experience. *Simulation in Healthcare: The Journal of the Society for Medical Simulation, 8*(3), 143–147.

Rudolph, J. W., Simon, R., & Raemer, D. B. (2007). Which reality matters? Questions on the road to high engagement in healthcare simulation. *Simulation in Healthcare: The Journal of the Society for Medical Simulation, 2*(3), 161–163.

REFERENCES

Atlas, R., Clover, R., Carrico, R., Wesley, G., Thompson, M., & McKinney, W. (2005). Recognizing biothreat diseases: Realistic training using standardized patients and patient simulators. *Journal of Public Health Management & Practice, 11*(6), S143–S146.

Auer, C. (2004). Not as bad as it looks. *Bulletin of the Atomic Scientists, 60*(5), 8.

Cone, D., Serra, J., Burns, K., MacMillan, D., Kurland, L., & Van Gelder, C. (2009). Pilot test of the SALT mass casualty triage system. *Prehospital Emergency Care, 13*(4), 536–540. doi:10.1080/10903120802706252

Damazo, R. (2012). *Moulage and more: Theatrical tricks and amazing tools to create simulation reality.* Chico, CA: Printed at California State University.

Dieckmann, P., Gaba, D., & Rall, M. (2007). Deepening the theoretical foundations of patient simulation as social practice. *Simulation in Healthcare, 2*(3), 183–193. doi:10.1097/SIH.0b013e3180f637f5

Federal Emergency Management Agency. (n.d.). *HSEEP vol. IV. Moulage kit.* Retrieved from https://hseep.dhs.gov/hseep_vols/viewResults.aspx?qsearch='moulage'

Gabba, D. M. (2007). The future vision of simulation in healthcare. *Simulation in Healthcare, 2*(2), 126–135. doi:10.1097/10.S14.0000 258411.32212.32

Hindman, D. (1988). Moulage: Setting up a basic kit. *JEN: Journal of Emergency Nursing, 14*(5), 316–317.

Hollis, C. (2002). Multidisciplinary mock trauma code: Targeting drinking and driving in the high school population. *Journal of Emergency Nursing, 28*(6), 559–561.

Joshi, R. (2010). Moulages in dermatology-venereology. *Indian Journal of Dermatology, Venereology & Leprology, 76*(4), 434–438. doi:10.4103/0378-6323.66579

Joshi, R., D'Costa, G., & Kura, M. (2010). Moulages of J. J. Hospital. *Indian Journal of Dermatology, Venereology & Leprology, 76*(5), 583–588. doi:10.4103/0378-6323.69088

Krishna, S. (2011). Modern moulage. *Indian Journal of Dermatology, Venereology & Leprology, 77*(1), 64. doi:10.4103/0378-6323.74987

Lee, S. K., Pardo, M., Gaba, D., Sowb, Y., Dicker, R., Straus, E., . . . Knudson, M. M. (2003). Trauma assessment training with a patient simulator: A prospective, randomized study. *The Journal of Trauma, 55*(4), 651–657.

Lindsey, J. (2003). Moulage magic! Injury simulations so real they'll amaze you. *JEMS: Journal of Emergency Medical Services, 28*(3), 122.

Mould, J., White, H., & Gallagher, R. (2011). Evaluation of a critical care simulation series for undergraduate nursing students. *Contemporary Nurse: A Journal for the Australian Nursing Profession, 38*(1/2), 180–190.

Nanji, K. C., Baca, K., & Raemer, D. (2013). The effect of an olfactory and visual cue on realism and engagement in a health care simulation experience. *Simulation in Healthcare, 8*(3), 143–147.

Potter, B. (2008). Using moulage to enhance emergency care skills. *Athletic Therapy Today, 13*(4), 11–14.

Saiboon, I., Jaafar, M., Harunarashid, H., & Jamal, S. (2011). The effectiveness of simulation based medical education in teaching concepts of major incident response. *Procedia—Social and Behavioral Sciences, 18*, 372–378.

Scott, L., Carson, D., & Greenwell, B. (2010). Disaster 101: A novel approach to disaster medicine training for health professionals. *The Journal of Emergency Medicine, 39*(2), 220–226.

Tofil, N., White, M., Manzella, B., McGill, D., & Zinkan, L. (2009). Initiation of a pediatric mock code program at a children's hospital. *Medical Teacher, 31*, 3241–3247. doi:10.1080/01421590802637974

Worm, A., Hadjivassiliou, M., & Katsambas, A. (2007). The Greek moulages: A picture of skin diseases in former times. *Journal of the European Academy of Dermatology & Venereology, 21*(4), 515–519. doi:10.1111/j.1468-3083.2006.02018.x

CHAPTER 8.4

Expecting the Unexpected: Contingency Planning for Healthcare Simulation

Cecilia Canales, MPH, and Yue Ming Huang, EdD, MHS

ABOUT THE AUTHORS

CECILIA CANALES began working in simulation at the UCLA Simulation Center as a technician where she developed contingency planning trainings and procedures for dealing with unexpected situations, simulation center moves, and creating new simulation centers. In 2010, she became the Director of Operations and Curriculum Development at the UC Irvine Medical Education Simulation Center, where she helped to develop a new simulation center and training program with the lessons of contingency planning in mind.

YUE MING HUANG is Adjunct Associate Professor of Anesthesiology and Director of Education & Operations at the UCLA Simulation Center. She oversees the administration and development of simulation programs, instructor training and evaluation, and research collaborations. With 14 years of experience including serving as a cochair for the Operations Track at the International Meeting for Simulation in Healthcare and planning for the expansion of the UCLA Simulation Center, she has witnessed the importance of contingency plans.

ABSTRACT

Contingency planning, or planning for what could go wrong, is a necessary part of any program that relies heavily on technology and people. Regardless of the time and effort put into preparing for a simulation session, inevitably there are unforeseen events that can delay, disrupt, or discombobulate a well-planned simulation training activity. Whether the situation is logistical nightmares, scenario glitches, equipment malfunction, learner obstacles, or embedded simulated persons (ESPs) who do not act as expected, even the best-planned sessions often require last-minute adjustments, trouble-shooting, and disaster management. As facilitators and simulation operators, we are expected to react to all possible situations seamlessly so as to not take away the learning experience. While simulation specialists often need to improvise and "go with the flow" as part of the normal business of running simulation sessions, just "winging it" is neither sufficient nor efficient in handling all problems. A systematic and organized approach for contingency planning should be part of every simulation program's standard operations. This chapter will focus on some specific areas to consider, common problems to anticipate, and potential strategies for a sustainable process of mitigating disaster.

CASE EXAMPLE

It has been weeks of planning in the works: multiple iterations of clinical scenario revisions to ensure that the goals and objectives of the simulation session are educationally sound and logistically feasible; scenario programming changes; moulage, supplies, and equipment preparation; even piloting and revising the script with current students. The scenario you have worked so hard to bring to life is finally ready for prime time. You have your session and students scheduled. The ESPs are on cue and the scenario begins to unfold beautifully. As you get ready to head into the most critical portion of the scenario, you notice that the vital signs are not reacting as expected. You quickly survey your desktop, and glancing at your screen you notice that the mannequin has lost connection with the computer controls. You try to keep the scenario flowing while trying to reconnect, but it is taking too long and the students and ESPs are getting confused because their interventions are not working as expected. *Do you stop the scenario? Can you get it to reconnect quickly? If it does reconnect, do you try to finish the same scenario? How much of the technical difficulties do you divulge? What contingency plans do you have for times when things do not go as expected? Surely this is not the first time the mannequin has lost connectivity.*

INTRODUCTION

Developing a contingency plan involves making decisions in advance about the management of human and financial resources, coordination and communications procedures, and being aware of a range of technical and logistical responses . . . Time spent in contingency planning equals time saved when a disaster occurs.

—*International Federation of Red Cross and Red Crescent Societies, 2012*

Contingency plans are emergency plans to ensure rapid, organized, and effective conduct of rescue operations to minimize impact on the affected stakeholders. In most organizations, contingency plans are in place for dealing with natural disasters or catastrophic accidents. However, **contingency planning** is not only for major disasters; it also applies to and is a necessary component of any successful educational program, particularly when there is high reliance on technology and people. In cases of natural disasters, people's lives are at stake. In education, catastrophic consequences are less frequent; although lives are not lost when a course does not go as intended, learning opportunities may be lost and program sustainability may be affected. These losses in time, reputation, and resources are important enough to warrant a "Plan B."

In simulation-based education and training, regardless of the amount of work and effort one puts into development, programming, and preparations, at some point something unexpected will occur. It is in the nature of daily operations. Facilitation and operation of simulation-based education will inevitably result in failures in the system that very well could impact the quality of educational sessions. It does not matter what type of simulator one uses, what sophisticated audiovisual integration or home-grown system is in place—eventually things will go awry.

The question is, are simulation programs prepared to handle potential failures without missing a beat and negatively affecting learners? Is there a contingency plan for adverse events that one could predictably expect or reasonably anticipate? Many simulation experts can "wing it" through improvisation on the spot and get by in the heat of some technical difficulty, or as a last resort accept the misfortune and apologize for the unintentional occurrences. However, experience indicates that mishaps could occur more than once, and each person may deal with them differently. The solutions and ideas that have been tested and proven to work need to be documented and shared, or the value of learning from experience is lost.

Simulation facilitators and operators rely on technology, equipment, ESPs, staff, educators, and participants to work in unison for a successful educational session. When any of these are misaligned or not optimally functioning, even the best-planned educational session could be derailed. Thus, the ability to anticipate problems and expect the unexpected is especially important in simulation-based education due to high reliance on technology and a desire to create realistic environments for learning. There are emergency evacuation plans for earthquake, fire, and other disasters. There needs to be a simulation disaster plan as well.

Educators are constantly barraged with factors that threaten the quality of simulation sessions. Problems could occur at any stage of simulation curriculum development and implementation. At the first conceptualization level, learning objectives should drive any educational activity, but often various constraints limit what we can do and an ideal session becomes one compromised by inadequate resources. Planning a simulation activity opens up a multitude of areas where things could go wrong and until the activity is implemented, it is difficult to anticipate all the possible scenarios for contingencies. Depending on circumstances and resources, contingency plans may vary between sites.

Effective contingency planning is more than just the advance preparation of written instructions that may be found in an operating procedures manual. A contingency plan is a live document that involves the practice of identifying resources as well as a streamlined method for communication and decision making during unexpected events. The goal is to manage problems in the shortest possible time without affecting educational gains. It is crisis resource management behind a dynamic simulation stage.

Very little has been written about contingency planning for simulation-based education. Tips on operations and administration of simulation programs refer to developing contingencies and propose questions for consideration (Huang & Dongilli, 2008; Stillsmoking & Murray, 2008). Troubleshooting guides for specific equipment are available but are often very technical and difficult to understand. Dieckmann et al. (2010) proposes a set of useful scenario "lifesavers" that could be used to redirect learners to minimize interruptions in the flow of the scenario. These could help restore the scenario to its intended progression ("within" the scenario) or change the original course of the scenario ("outside" the scenario) to match the unexpected actions in a logical way.

This chapter divides the discussion into three topic areas for contingency planning: technology, people, and things beyond your control. Outlined are examples of how quick roles and small changes within a scenario can be made seamlessly to offset failures in the system. These lessons are based on a combined 20 years of experience working in simulation operations, administration, education, and research. In each section, consider the following questions: "What is going to happen? What are we going to do about it? What can we do ahead of time to be prepared?" Those new to simulation should focus on preparation and prevention, as well as developing efficient processes. Advanced users could add to their repertoire of skills by considering further refinement, adaptation, and improvement of their contingency plans.

TECHNOLOGY

Technology is perhaps the most obvious culprit of a simulation program that frequently requires troubleshooting. Both an asset and a liability, technology is inherent in the world of simulation and has a huge impact on the success of our programs. Simulation programs range from single room to complex, high-tech, multimillion-dollar facilities with state-of-the-art capacities. Yet, even the most basic and simple program includes some level of integration of simulators, clinical equipment, and audiovisual equipment. As simulators become more advanced, and facilitators find more ways to distribute experiential exercises to the learners, there is greater dependence on technology to deliver educational sessions. Thus, it is critical to examine and plan for contingencies related to failures in technology.

Technology encompasses everything related to simulators, clinical equipment, and the intricate simulation program facility network. Potential problems could include the following:

1. Simulator hardware malfunction
2. Simulator software and programming errors
3. Clinical equipment malfunction
4. Audiovisual equipment issues
5. Wireless connectivity issues
6. Multimedia integration problems

Table 8.4.1 summarizes examples of technology-related problems and some possible contingency plans. When after troubleshooting the technology the problem is still unresolved, there are contingency alternatives that could save the day, including the following:

1. Stay the course of the scenario by going along with the unexpected changes.
   - Use an embedded simulated person (ESP) to relay messages while remaining in character (e.g., the embedded simulated nurse states, "We have been having some technical problems with our monitors all day long. Let me take the vital signs manually").
   - Announce the technical difficulty during orientation or via paging system ("We apologize that we are encountering a technical difficulty with the simulator today. For the purpose of this scenario, please assume that chest rise is visible by the CO_2 tracing").
   - Discuss during debriefing—make it a learning point ("What would you do if in real life the equipment failed on you?").
2. Change the scenario
   - If the scenario was supposed to be a difficult airway scenario, but the laryngospasm and pharyngeal obstruction did not activate and the participant intubates the simulator without any problems, turn it into an anaphylaxis or bronchospasm case instead.

- If simulator failure is known before session, choose scenarios that would not be affected by equipment malfunction and/or tell participants during orientation that a certain piece of equipment is not available or working that day (see Table 8.4.1).

PEOPLE

People are the greatest strength and resource to a simulation program. People can also be the biggest barrier to effectively implementing a simulation scenario. All the human resources, the personalities and experiences that educators, facilitators, learners, ESPs, and staff bring with them come into play on the simulation stage. There is great synergy if properly aligned but could be a nightmare to manage if diverging opinions, expectations, and feelings are not properly addressed. Potential problems to consider are the following:

1. Staff—training, out sick, or otherwise unavailable
2. Educators—training, late, or cancellation
3. Embedded Simulated Persons—training, off cue, or improper improvisation
4. Learners—difficult, aggressive, sensitive, distracted, no show, or late arrivals
5. Unexpected visitors—impromptu tours for important visitors, interruptions

One of the most common reasons that scenarios do not progress as expected is the unpredictable nature of human behaviors. People are the cornerstone of both the problems and the solutions. People can misbehave, intentionally or unintentionally. For various reasons, humans err and may not function at their best, even with the best intentions. Unexpected events could be participants who make up their own scenarios (for instance pretending something is done without actually doing it), ESPs that are too helpful and detract from learning objectives, or facilitators who are uncomfortable with simulation and resort to using the simulator as a backdrop to start lecturing.

Troubleshooting personnel issues may be even more difficult than troubleshooting technology, as feelings are involved and relationships can be at stake. However, everyone needs to be on the same page regarding the flow and expectations of the educational session. When everything is going smoothly, everyone is usually happy. When things go awry, high stress makes humans react in ways that may not be ideal, so it is important to manage people during these high-stress events and communicate effectively to mitigate distress.

Aside from proper training, the best way to avoid personnel problems is to make sure that everyone has the same expectations. Proper orientation and piloting of educational sessions with everyone who will be involved in the actual implementation will help identify areas of confusion. The concepts of teamwork and communication

TABLE 8.4.1

Technology Problems and Contingencies

Example Problem	Contingency Plan
Simulator Hardware Malfunction	
Birthing simulator does not release baby (baby is stuck inside).	If baby is critical to scenario development, simulate delivery and bring in a second baby to be used in the scenario. If baby is not critical to scenario development, simulate delivery and quickly give "baby" wrapped in blankets to other ESPs.
Compressor stops working.	Connect the mannequin to an alternate air source. If an alternate source is not available, run the scenario as "low-technology" simulation or with ESPs providing cues on pulses and chest rise.
During surgical airway procedure, the participant goes through the back of the trachea causing a leak.	For the current scenario, when critical actions are met, end the scenario. If damage occurred early in the training day and there are more scenarios planned, repair the damage by taping or gluing together the trachea to get through the rest of the day. Prevent this from happening in the first place by having the ESP stop the participant if they do an incorrect procedure that could damage the simulator.
Heart, lung, or bowel speakers malfunction.	Have the ESP let the participant know what they are hearing.
Lungs rip or have a leak and you are unable to positive-pressure-ventilate.	Turn on spontaneous breathing if the simulator has separate mechanism used for spontaneous breathing, or time breathing to the learner giving positive pressure ventilation.
One or both of the blinking eyes are stuck open or closed.	Redirect the participant by having the ESP or the patient indicate that the condition is a normal state. Have the ESP discretely close eyes manually and have the patient state "I hope you don't mind if I close my eyes here while you do your work."
Other physical findings such as chest rise do not correlate with clinical interventions.	Have the ESP check and reassure normalcy.
Moulage problems such as wig or ulcer falls off.	Have the ESP discretely fix the error. If the learner notices before it gets fixed, state "Let me fix her wig—she gets embarrassed if it's not properly set."
Vocal cords do not close during the laryngospasm scenario.	Have an alternate scenario available to run on the fly, for example, bronchospasm. Discuss during debriefing.
Simulator Software and Programming Errors	
Scenario does not load or run as programmed.	Run scenario on the fly using your paper scenario flow diagram.
Software does not open or load.	Have the software available on backup computer. If available, use a different simulator. Run "low-technology" simulation by talking through the scenario with the participant to highlight educational goals and objectives.
Clinical Equipment Malfunction	
Anesthesia machine or ventilator alarms because pressure is too high or low.	Change the alarm limits on the equipment. Redirect participants by letting them know that a technician has been called, and they are working on the problem. Have a ESP play the role of a technician to resolve the problem.
Clinical equipment loses power or batteries need to be recharged.	If possible, plug in or replace battery. Add troubleshooting as part of scenario and discuss in debriefing.
Equipment is broken during the scenario.	Advise the participant that it was the only one available, and should proceed. If the equipment would have provided diagnostic value to move the scenario forward, give results to the participant.
Audiovisual Equipment Issues	
Debriefing room loses live audio/video feed in the middle of a scenario and participants cannot hear/see what is going on in the simulation.	Video-chat using videoconferencing unit, tablet, computer, or smartphone from the simulation room to debriefing room. Have participants observe and listen from inside the simulation room.
Audio connection is lost into simulation room and the patient cannot answer (speaker failure).	Have the ESP answer for the patient.
Audio is lost to ESP headphones (two-way communication between control room and simulation room fails).	Communicate with ESPs by passing notes, or by paging or texting. Step out of control room and let ESPs know of technical problem. Follow script exactly and have the ESPs come out if they are uncertain of actions.
Wireless Connectivity Issues	
Mannequin is not connecting.	Hardwire the mannequin to computer or router.
Internet-based digital audiovisual system is down.	Abandon video recording and bring everyone into the simulation room to view and participate.
Multimedia Integration Problems	
Integrating software or system is down and will not allow you to record or display audio/video in debriefing rooms.	When possible, go to basics and use camera without the integrated software. If not possible, see "Audiovisual equipment issues" above.
One of the integrated video, audio, or VGA inputs (i.e., vital signs) is experiencing delays and is not synced with the other feeds.	See "Audiovisual equipment issues" above.

are key to establishing a flow of information and resources to ensure smooth operations. Simulation is used for crisis management training for our learner participants. Those who work behind the scenes also need to practice what they preach. Teamwork and communication strategies from Crisis Resource Management and TeamSTEPPS tools should be fully utilized in the development and implementation of contingency plans (Agency for Healthcare Research and Quality, n.d.; Ostergaard et al., 2011).

Communication is absolutely critical for smooth operations and contingency planning. Implement a way to communicate between staff and educators—via paging, two-way radios, cell phone text, written notes, secret code signals, or gestures, or a combination of the above. After all the advance preparations, on the day of the session, having a huddle before each session and scenario can be a lifesaver. This allows last-minute changes to be shared and to take place on the basis of debriefing comments or other factors that only a few may be privy to. This is also a time to review with ESPs their cues, how the scenario should unfold, and what their contingency plans are if something goes off script. Situation monitoring by all staff is important to constantly assess for signs of derailing or potential pitfalls. Relaying this information in a timely manner will catch errors before they occur.

Establishing expectations with participants is also important. Learners appreciate having an orientation and simulation contract that delineates what the expectations of the day will be. Make sure that learners understand the channels of communication for relaying patient findings. For example, tell the learners during orientation that a embedded simulated nurse might provide information about skin changes because the simulator is not able to show a rash. If the rules of engagement are clear, learners will be able to engage appropriately.

A range of issues related to people is explored in Table 8.4.2. First, because this chapter focuses on behind the scenes, staff issues are discussed. The simulation program staff team is absolutely essential to a successful program. These are the people who coordinate scheduling, run the operations of the various simulators and technologies, and set up and clean up after each session. They support education in every respect. All staff should be thoroughly trained in their roles and responsibilities. More intense training will need to be given to those who will be in key positions. It should also be noted that staff may be absent, tardy, or need to be relieved for one reason or another. Backup staff should therefore be trained for each position. At the very least, instructions for each activity should be clearly delineated on a checklist so others can help when needed.

Training of personnel involved in simulation is absolutely critical. If trained, dedicated personnel are not available for each role because of funding and budget restrictions, then cross-training for the facilitator or operator is advised. All simulators and much of the audiovisual equipment, regardless of how much they are touted to be easy to use, are quite complex. This means that everything may be working correctly, but because of lack of training and familiarity with the equipment, problems could arise during a scenario. Many institutions hire simulation technicians or operators and just hope that the staff will eventually get the hang of it and learn things independently.

TABLE 8.4.2

People Problems and Contingencies

Example Problem	Contingency Plan
Your lead simulation technician calls in sick or your staff is stuck in traffic and the rooms are not set up yet.	Call in a backup technician. Set up a related task training station while you set up basic equipment or supplies needed for the first scenario.
Your staff is unprepared for the scenarios.	Give a quick overview of the scenario and explain how the scenario will unfold, its critical actions and events. Use cue cards.
The main educator has a personal emergency and is unable to teach.	Call a backup educator. Modify educational activity. Use low-technology simulation or other interactive exercises to illustrate the learning objectives.
The educator is using the mannequin as a prop to lecture with.	Pull the educator aside and let them know that learners can actually do hands-on procedures on the simulators. Orient new educators to capabilities and experiential learning theory. Ask for open reception to debrief after each teaching session. Redirect back to scenario by making the patient or ESP speak and stay in character.
The ESP is being too helpful and is revealing key points of the scenario.	Ask the ESP to step out of the room and advise them that they are being too helpful and that the participants need to identify key points on their own.
The ESP is overacting and is distracting from the scenario.	Tell the ESP that they are needed in the room next door and advise them appropriately. If they are still distracting, do not let them return to the scenario and talk to them after the session.
Participants are lost.	Provide a clear map and directions to the room. Place visible signs to direct them. Use a wireless headset to answer phones/inquires while you are setting up the rooms.
Participant is not buying into the scenario—says what he or she would do, but will not actually perform any of the tasks.	Have the ESP or patient redirect the participant by reminding them that he or she needs to perform the needed tasks.
An important visitor is brought by the administration for a personal tour during a high-stakes training event.	Have a prepared video or simulation recording that highlights trainings performed at your facility and training capabilities. Meet with the visitor after the scenario, or if appropriate invite the visitor to join in the facilitation and debriefing of scenario.

Although many operators do eventually learn on the job, this is not ideal as incorrect practices and shortcuts may be adapted. Training of simulation specialists can include vendor training, but should also include disassembly and reassembly of the equipment so they have complete understanding of each component. Also, it is critical that each person be expected to document any technical problem so that these are logged. The steps to resolving problems should also be noted so that they can serve as a reference for future problems.

Educators and facilitators are another group of people who need management and coordination. Clinicians are busy people who may not be adequately prepared to run simulations that they are asked to do infrequently. Staff support is crucial to help them with logistics, paperwork, directing the scenario, and assisting them in observing for key actions for later debriefing. More advanced educators can serve as directors of the scenario and observe learner actions simultaneously, but oftentimes, simulation operators can help by pointing out specific things that might be missed in the chaos of the scenario. Feedback to educators is a crucial aspect for quality assurance and program improvement.

Facilitating a debriefing session requires skill and practice. Not all educators are as well trained in this area, so providing cognitive aids to help them will make the session run smoothly. Approaches to debriefing should match the learning objectives and consider learner experiences and perspectives. In time-constrained sessions, a simple structure for debriefing using "plus/delta" (what went well?/what could be changed?) or the three-questions approach ("What went well? What could be improved? What will I do next time/how will I put this to practice?") may be easier to adapt or more appropriate compared to a more in-depth probing technique, whereas learning may require a deeper diagnosis of the reasons the learner performed an action versus coaching on the action itself. One example of this is the advocacy-inquiry method (Rudolph et al., 2007). Debriefing methods are evolving, and facilitation skills must be developed continuously and may be used together. Cognitive aids that provide sample questions to address both clinical management as well as teamwork skills offer educators a template for a more holistic debriefing.

Standardized patients are people who act in various roles. Embedded simulated persons are vital to scenario progression, especially in delivering specific cues needed to move a simulation training forward. For example, ESPs who play patients or patients' family members, a nurse, or a physician role could help push learners to action or redirect them if they go astray. Professional actors hired by the script are expensive, so most simulation programs use professional actors only for special occasions such as formal assessments. For formative simulation sessions, ESPs are played more commonly by simulation program staff or faculty to save on costs.

Embedded simulated persons help deliver critical information and allow for seamless transitions between simulated states. However, embedded simulated persons can sometimes derail the best-planned simulation scenario by inadvertently offering too much information, forgetting their lines, or simply introducing a negative tone to the simulation environment. Although these ESPs receive training to properly execute a scenario, sometimes inconsistencies or confusion make it necessary to create a contingency plan to rescue a scenario.

Learners might also provide unexpected consequences. Learners are often confused about what is simulated and what is real. Some have not accepted simulation as an immersive learning tool and remain on the sideline unable to get into character or see the simulator as anything other than a plastic dummy. Others have active imaginations, seeing or pretending to see things that are not really there. Still others get so immersed that they end up emotionally engaged and distraught when things go wrong. All of these possibilities are reasons to have for contingency plans.

The interplay of learners, faculty, staff, and ESPs make up the simulation performance. To minimize confusion, a proper orientation is necessary. This includes familiarizing participants with the simulated environment; the simulators, equipment, and supplies used in the scenarios; and the rules of engagement for what is real and what cannot be simulated. Create a "Fictional Contract" with the participants for simulation (Dieckmann, 2009).

It is also wise to use the "Rules of Improv." At the start of each scenario when learner participants enter the room, use the ESPs to orient them by stating the following:

1. Who you are (the learner): "Hi, Dr. Young, you're the intern on call today, right?"
2. Who I am (the ESP): "I'm the float nurse covering for another nurse who is on break."
3. Where we are: "Thanks so much for coming to the MICU."
4. What is happening: "I was just doing my usual assessments here with Mr. Johnson and he suddenly started having heart palpitations."

Because the learners are the main reason for running the simulation training, it is essential to redirect them if needed to optimize the learning opportunities. If ESPs stay in character, it is easier for participants to get into character. If educators lay out expectations at the beginning, participants will behave naturally and take advantage of the simulation experience.

Finally, people not involved with the education session can also interrupt an otherwise well-planned simulation session, not deliberately but as a matter of interest in simulation. The Dean could drop by for an unexpected tour with important potential donors. It would be inappropriate and unwise to ignore these important people, but at the same time, the educational session will suffer if you put it on pause. The best solution is to gauge the visitors' availability. If feasible, offer to have them observe and then give them a tour and talk to them after the scenario, or ask whether they would like to schedule an appointment so that you can spend dedicated time with them. If they do not have time and are just passing by, spend a few minutes to find out what they would like to know, then apologize and let them know you are about to run a simulation scenario. Get a staff member to assist. Provide them with a brochure and self-guided map/tour of the simulation program. Visitors should understand that these are educational sessions and will generally make concessions so that they do not disturb ongoing programs. A visitor policy should be in place, made visible, and enforced (Table 8.4.2).

THINGS BEYOND YOUR CONTROL

As much as facilitators try to take charge of and prevent all possible failures in the system, there are some things that are beyond control, such as:

1. Traffic
2. Facility issues: pipelines down, loss of pressure in pipelines, power loss
3. Renovation/construction noise
4. In situ or situated environments (Table 8.4.3)

DEVELOPING A CONTINGENCY PLAN

The chapter provides examples of possible breakdowns due to technology, people, and things beyond our control, along with some actionable solutions. However, there are many more possible problems and it is impossible to list every single one. As technology advances, new unanticipated

problems will arise. Therefore, more important than providing a litany of problems and solutions is to create and practice a systematic process for coming up with contingency plans to deal with problems.

Contingency planning can be broken down into several processes:

1. Assessment and Inventory of Needs and Risks ("What is going on? What could happen?")
2. Prevention Strategy ("What can we do ahead of time to prepare?")
3. Action Plan for Emergencies ("What are we going to do about it?")
4. Event Review, Reassessment, and Update ("How can we improve?")

The first step to contingency planning is to conduct a program assessment to determine what resources are available (equipment, people, time, and money) and what could go wrong. Consider the following while taking inventory of available assets and liabilities.

Dedicated Technicians

When it comes to technology, the best way to be prepared for the unexpected is to first and foremost know the equipment that will be used during the training session and do everything possible to prevent mechanical failure. For this reason, having dedicated technology-savvy simulation technicians or specialists who work with the equipment, day in and day out, can be beneficial and worth the investment. Dedicated personnel should be trained to operate, troubleshoot, and maintain clinical equipment and simulators in the simulation program and communicate with the team about known or potential problems with a specific piece of equipment that may affect a particular session. Creating a log of technical problems and their resolution is the beginning of contingency planning.

Many new programs purchase expensive equipment before they build their educational programs. Purchasing equipment before dedicated personnel have been identified to learn to use it is a disaster waiting to happen. If dedicated personnel are not available to help set up, maintain, repair, and run the simulators, it might be best to avoid spending money on highly complex simulators. Many simulators tout multiple advanced features when all that is really needed is the ability to display vital signs, palpate and auscultate, and defibrillate. There are creative low-budget ways to run simulation sessions without compromising the fidelity of the learning experience.

Dedicated Space

Having dedicated space can also reduce the amount of contingency planning and troubleshooting that needs to be done. If simulators and other equipment are in a set location and they do not need to be reconnected or plugged in every time a session is run, then there is less likelihood

TABLE 8.4.3

Other Problems and Contingencies

Example Case(s)	Contingency Plan
Traffic: Major freeway construction projects or accidents have your key educators delayed for up to an hour.	Play an educational game that complements the scheduled training. Prepare knowledge-based practice questions (Jeopardy) or use screen-based simulation or task trainers to fill time.
Facility issues: Pipeline is down.	Use E or H cylinders.
Renovation/construction: Construction in the building limits rooms to use.	Have a flexible schedule or add more in situ trainings.
Construction creates noise or noise is heard through walls in adjacent simulations.	During orientation, advise participants of the possibility of loud noise. Work with contractors to minimize noise during critical periods of time.
In situ: Patient care takes priority—a patient needs a room reserved for in situ simulation.	Have equipment and supplies ready to be transported to another room if one becomes available. Reschedule or move to the simulation program.
Participants have to leave to take care of patients before debriefing is over.	Prepare general debriefing notes that can be distributed to participants. Make sure that those who have to leave are followed up by one of the educators.

that something can get missed during the setup. Likewise, using a dedicated computer for the simulator controls can reduce problems with the simulators. Often simple things like changing a channel, com-port, or being connected to the wrong network (e.g., Internet vs. mannequin) are the source of many problems. Having the experience of relocating a simulation program three times in a period of 10 years highlights how frequent moves add headaches and contingencies. Constant movement causes confusion and parts can be easily misplaced. Trying to organize, label, and tag things together and maintain a general area for storage can help but inevitably something goes missing. Dedicated storage space and identified locations for equipment and supplies make setup and operations run much more efficiently.

Dedicated Audiovisual System and Communication Channels

The audiovisual component of a simulation program is another critical area where problems could occur. For instance, the live streaming of the simulation recording into a conference or debriefing room for observing participants is suddenly lost. It could be a wireless connectivity issue or a camera problem. By having a dedicated communication system in place, personnel will be able to identify, prioritize, and troubleshoot loose wires, misplaced parts, or incorrect connection figurations. Stepwise troubleshooting is easier if there is consistency in function and location. Should the wireless communication system fail for the staff and educators, a backup system such as using pagers and cell phones should take place.

The key to prevention of failures is vigilant adherence to systematic preparations and maintenance. It is easy to leave at the end of a long day and not put everything back in its place, checking to make sure equipment is ready at any time. However, factoring in that time to rebuild will save time in the long run. Documentation is crucial to preserve lessons learned by all parties involved in the process.

UPDATE YOUR CONTINGENCY PLANS

Contingency plans, once prepared, should not be treated as static documents. Rather, they should be regarded as dynamic documents that need to be regularly reviewed and updated with changing circumstances, educational programs, and technology. In reviewing and updating contingency plans, the following factors should be taken into account:

- New technology or space
- New scenarios that pose new challenges
- New staff/educators/learners
- Experiences, results from training or simulation exercises, and feedback

BEEN THERE, DONE THAT: HOW CAN I CONTINUE TO IMPROVE OR SUSTAIN WHAT I HAVE ACHIEVED?

A review and update of contingency plans should be done at minimum on an annual basis. This review should identify areas where plans need to be modified and further training is needed. There are several approaches to this review. In healthcare organizations, disaster drills are part of regular safety protocols. Most hospitals have annual simulations to increase awareness and prepare for anticipated emergencies (Bartley et al., 2006). With simulation contingencies, every session could be a drill. Continual assessment of how well each simulation program team member reacts to problems will provide insight for further training. Just as we use simulation for patient care practice, simulation exercises for testing and refining contingency plans can be very useful. These exercises also provide a means for building teamwork and professional development. Simulation exercises may be done purely as a paper exercise, through mock activities, or a combination of both approaches. Debriefing should follow immediately after the simulation exercise. This review can be done at an annual simulation retreat or time set aside for programming and development.

Another strategy to review what could improve a program is to prepare a Strengths, Weaknesses, Opportunities, and Threats (SWOT) analysis for the program, on the basis of institutional contingency planning operational manual. Questions to consider for SWOT analysis are listed in Table 8.4.4. As a team, make a diagram or list the simulation program's Strengths, Weaknesses, Opportunities, and Threats. Review lessons learned from other

TABLE 8.4.4

Questions to Consider for SWOT Analysis

Strengths	Weaknesses
1. What does your simulation program do well at?	1. What areas does your simulation program do poorly in?
2. Are your resources sufficient for your programmatic needs?	2. Are you constantly struggling with limited resources: educator recruitment and training, staff turnover, time and space constraints?
3. Are you reaching your market or target audience?	3. What problems frequently surface or could be avoided?
4. Is your personnel team well trained and talented?	4. Are your contingency plans effective?
Opportunities	**Threats**
1. What are the trends you see in usage?	1. Are there changes in leadership (political or economical)?
2. Are there new departments and areas for growth and development?	2. What are your competitors doing?
3. Do you have new simulation technologies?	3. What obstacles do you foresee?
4. Do you have a research and development team?	4. Is feedback reviewed and integrated?

high-tech systems that you foresee becoming integrated into simulation, such as electronic medical records. Advance planning for the future, opportunities to involve others including engineering and information technology, and developing own intranet for internal users are some examples of ways to continuously improve upon your operations. If there are plans for a build-out or expansion of the simulation center, get started on anticipating the needs and problems associated with renovation and new technology. The experience of moving several times over the past decade has highlighted many lessons to optimize operations in a single-suite simulation room as well as a multiroom facility. By examining the history and future goals, one is better able to anticipate what the next decade will look like. Being flexible and open to change is essential for evolving any simulation program.

Another way to prepare is to apply the Failure Mode and Effects Analysis (FMEA) model to gauge the adequacy of a contingency system (Duwe et al., 2005; Herzer et al., 2009). FMEA is a systematic, proactive method for evaluating a process to identify where and how it might fail and to assess the relative impact of different failures, to identify the parts of the process that are most in need of change. FMEA is different from a Root Cause Analysis, which reviews actions after the events have occurred. In FMEA, anticipated problems are reviewed and prevention and reaction strategies are identified. FMEA is used to examine processes for possible failures. By correcting the process, one can prevent failures from occurring rather than reacting to adverse events after failures have occurred. FMEA includes a team review of the following:

- Steps in the process
- Failure modes (What could go wrong?), the likelihood of occurrence and the ability to detect them
- Failure causes (Why would the failure happen?) and the strategies to fix them
- Failure effects (What would be the consequences of each failure?) and its severity

FMEA can also be instrumental for evaluating a new process before its implementation and to determine the impact of a proposed change to an existing process. A number of free Excel templates for FMEA can be found online.

SUMMARY

Simulation is a powerful educational tool, but with high reliance on technology, one can easily become encumbered by technical problems. Contingency planning for simulation is therefore critical to minimize disruptions to the educational experience. Contingency plans call for high integration of the talents of personnel, the advances of technology, and the experience and foresight to anticipate the future.

Contingency plan implementation involves a systematic approach of assessment, prevention, anticipation, reaction, review, and reassessment. Prevention is critical. All efforts should be made to prevent problems from occurring. This means checking and preparing any equipment or technology to be used the day before a session. Checklists and cognitive aids for scenario setup and equipment testing are strongly recommended for every educational activity.

If prevention requires skilled preparation, anticipation is an art of foresight. Anticipation of potential technical problems and anticipation of human interactions with the equipment are equally important. With experience, one can reasonably predict reactions and gauge how scenarios will unfold. Thinking ahead and planning for potential problems will help minimize surprise emergencies. Documenting these on a written contingency plan shows advanced foresight and preparedness.

When there are unexpected events occurring in the face of the best preparations, appropriate reactions make the difference between disaster and successful rescue so that those in the learner seats do not even notice that seamless smoothing was happening behind the scenes. The concepts of crisis resource management should be in practice:

1. React to the emergency in a calm and collected manner.
2. Call upon available resources.
3. Communicate clearly with all channels affected. Practice the teamwork and communication strategies that you teach in your simulation courses.

In conclusion, quality control is practiced when contingency plans are rehearsed, reviewed, and revised regularly. Contingency planning is essentially an evolving simulation scenario that all of us play a part in creating and reenacting. Having discussed the multitude of disaster possibilities and the strategies to overcome them before failures occur, we can ensure that we (as the behind-the-scenes team) get out alive and stress-free, but more importantly that our learners will leave with the best educational experience they could get with the resources we have.

REFERENCES

Agency for Healthcare Research and Quality. (n.d.). *TeamSTEPPS curriculum tools and materials*. Retrieved from http://teamstepps.ahrq.gov/abouttoolsmaterials.htm

Bartley, B. H., Stella, J. B., & Walsh, L. D. (2006). What a disaster?! Assessing utility of simulated disaster exercise and educational process for improving hospital preparedness. *Prehospital and Disaster Medicine, 21*(4), 249–255.

Dieckmann, P. (2009). Simulation settings for learning in acute medical care. In P. Dieckmann (Ed.), *Using simulations for education, training and research* (pp. 40–138). Lengerich, Germany: Pabst.

Dieckmann, P., Lippert, A., Glavin, R., & Rall, M. (2010). When things do not go as expected: Scenario life savers. *Simulation in Healthcare, 5*(4), 219–225.

Duwe, B., Fuchs, B. D., & Hansen-Flaschen, J. (2005). Failure mode and effects analysis application to critical care medicine. *Critical Care Clinics, 21*(1), 21–30, vii.

Herzer, K. R., Rodriguez-Paz, J. M., Doyle, P. A., Flint, P. W., Feller-Kopman, D. J., Herman, J., . . . Mark, L. J. (2009). A practical framework for patient care teams to prospectively identify and mitigate clinical hazards. *Joint Commission Journal on Quality and Patient Safety, 35*(2), 72–81.

Huang, Y. M., & Dongilli, T. (2008). Simulation center operations and administration. In R. Riley (Ed.), *A manual of simulation in healthcare* (pp. 11–24). London, England: Oxford University Press.

International Federation of Red Cross and Red Crescent Societies. (2012). *Contingency planning guide.* Geneva, Switzerland: Author. Retrieved from http://www.ifrc.org/PageFiles/40825/1220900-CPG%202012-EN-LR.pdf

Ostergaard, D., Dieckmann, P., & Lippert, A. (2011). Simulation and CRM. *Best Practice & Research Clinical Anaesthesiology, 25*(2), 239–249.

Rudolph, J. W., Simon, R., Rivard, P., Dufresne, R. L., & Raemer, D. B. (2007). Debriefing with good judgment: Combining rigorous feedback with genuine inquiry. *Anesthesiology Clinics, 25*(2), 361–376.

Stillsmoking, K. L., & Murray, W. B. (2008). Expect the unexpected: Managing a simulation session at a congress, away from home base. In R. R. Kyle & W. B. Murray (Eds.), *Clinical simulation: Operations, engineering, and management* (pp. 787–799). Burlington, MA: Academic Press.

CHAPTER 8.5

The Ethics of Simulation

Amy B. Smith, PhD, and Stephen E. Lammers, PhD

ABOUT THE AUTHORS

AMY B. SMITH started working with standardized patients (SPs) in the 1990s. She helped develop an SP program for medical students and has been involved in simulation at all levels of medical education from high-school students to senior healthcare providers. Dr. Smith understands the importance of ethical practice in teaching and assessment and is a champion for teaching ethics in medical education.

STEPHEN E. LAMMERS started working in clinical ethics in 1982. He helped develop the ethics program at Lehigh Valley Health Network. He is the coeditor of *On Moral Medicine: Theological Perspectives in Medical Ethics*. His recent research has focused on ethics education for medical students and medical residents.

ABSTRACT

Simulation begins in response to three ethical imperatives: keep patients, learners, and faculty safe; prevent errors; and facilitate engaged learning. This chapter reviews the central ethical issues involved in responding to those imperatives. Important is the safety, physical and psychological, of all participants; the careful use of resources; well-planned prebriefings and debriefings; and full explanations of the purpose of the planned simulations. If research is involved, a full consent of all participants is required. Many of the ethical issues that are found in healthcare in general are found as well in the practice of simulation.

CASE EXAMPLE

It is a Wednesday afternoon in the simulation center and learners are practicing their lumbar puncture skills on a partial task trainer. They practice and are checked off on a validated skill checklist and now feel confident to perform a lumbar puncture on a patient. A month after learning how to perform a lumbar puncture, a resident has his first opportunity on an actual patient. The resident cleans the site and prepares for the procedure. As he does, he notices that things feels different than what he remembered when he was in the learning session. The resident is uncertain about what to do. He is hesitant as he proceeds with the procedure.

What the learner did not know was that the task trainer he practiced with had been used many times, was old and worn out, but because of budget cuts and turnover in staff, the task trainer had not undergone routine maintenance. Is this an ethical concern?

INTRODUCTION AND BACKGROUND

Simulation begins with an important moral claim: we must do the best we can to keep patients safe while training the next generation of clinicians and retraining current clinicians so that they are kept up to date. If we can introduce clinicians to patients when these clinicians have more experience, we lessen the chances that vulnerable patients will be harmed. Ethics is not an add-on to simulation; an ethical claim drives the practice of simulation itself.

Thus, simulation is situated inside of healthcare, not alongside or outside of it. The practices of simulation in healthcare share many of the same ethical challenges and opportunities that are found in healthcare. As such, the ethics of simulation should be discussed within the context of the larger healthcare systems within which the practices of simulation are situated. Not only questions of informed consent and of research, but also issues of justice arise. These latter questions can be as broad as "Is this the wisest use of our limited resources?" or as focused as "Do our standardized patients have health insurance as part of their compensation?" (Taylor, 2011).

By now it should be clear that ethical questions run throughout most of the topics in this book. There are questions specific to management, education, research, the use of technology, and even the types of simulations. This chapter will focus on some of the general issues in ethics in and of simulation. As we proceed, we will point to questions that might be specific to a particular area of simulation. The effort here, however, is to introduce some general questions so that the simulation educator will be prepared for the specific questions that might arise. We hope to introduce a way of seeing what happens in simulation in light of the ethical imperatives that give rise to simulation in the first place. In this fashion, the educator is prepared to raise and address new questions that might arise, in whatever area of simulation the educator finds her/himself involved.

Questions of ethics are as much a matter of discovery as responding to well-rehearsed norms. Questions need to be appropriate to the matter at hand, and the search for answers should respect the dignity of all the participants. These are challenging tasks. In what follows, we will rely on the Society for Simulation in Healthcare's definition of simulation. They state that the purposes of simulation in healthcare are ". . . education, assessment, research, and health system integration in facilitating patient safety" (Society of Simulation in Healthcare, n.d.).

SIGNIFICANCE

Ethics—In the literature

Why do we need to talk about ethics in simulation? It is not simply that simulation begins with the imperatives mentioned above. It is also the fact that simulation raises ethical questions of its own. Clinicians will always have a first patient. What is at stake for that first patient and for that clinician? Training is critical in the preparation of clinicians prior to that first actual patient experience. That training is not simply technical. It is also a way to learn and practice collaboration through team training, interpersonal, interprofessional, and decision-making skills and not incidentally an opportunity for training in the ethics of the various healthcare professions.

Ziv et al. (2003) discuss the conflicting needs to ensure patient safety and to learn with actual patients. The questions of clinician competence and patient safety provide the context for the discussion of simulation. Because simulation is one method to train clinicians and to provide a level of competence prior to direct patient care, the question is, "Is it ethical *not* to use simulation in education and assessment?"

These same questions frame the discussion of the various issues within the practices of simulation. Keeping our attention on these questions keeps us from being distracted by other considerations that, while important, are not central to the matters at hand.

Healthcare Ethics

Ethical practices are grounded in the culture in which they are situated. For the purpose of this chapter, we will discuss ethics from an Anglo-American perspective. This is not to imply that these are the only ethical norms that exist.

Anglo-American healthcare ethics are marked by attention to questions of patient autonomy and choice. Other perspectives often raise questions of justice first and, in this chapter, we have tried to be sensitive to these perspectives. In the American context, questions of autonomy can become important, especially when research is being done. Simulation, however, more directly raises questions of beneficence (doing good for the patient) and nonmaleficence (preventing harm to the patient); (Beauchamp & Childress, 2013). These two concerns will be reiterated often in this chapter. It is also important to remember that when we seek to prevent harm, we do so not only to the patient but to all individuals involved with simulation, including staff, faculty, and standardized patients (SPs).

SIMULATION (INCLUDING TECHNOLOGY, STANDARDIZED PATIENTS, AND UNANNOUNCED STANDARDIZED PATIENTS)

Simulation in healthcare is delivered in many different ways: from low tech to high tech, from resource light to resource intense. Simulations can be delivered with high-technology equipment, human simulators, SPs, and virtual reality. The methods can also be combined to deliver hybrid simulations. Simulations also occur in various settings from large simulation programs, classrooms, the clinical environment, as well as the virtual environment. The ways simulation is delivered should be based on the goals and objectives of the program and the resources available.

What are the ethical considerations when developing a simulation activity? Patient safety and clinical needs come first. After that, the considerations include thinking of the resources, including the human resources (manpower) to conduct simulations. Human resources include those needed for planning, execution, and review. Just because a simulation program or institution has high-priced simulators, mannequins, and equipment does not mean that it is always the best or most effective way to provide learning and assessment. It is one way and there may be other more cost- or time-efficient methods to achieve the same goals.

Let us return to the Case Example. It has become standard practice to train clinicians using mannequins and partial task trainers. It has been shown that practice with simulation, deliberate practice with feedback and debriefing, improves performance. How close to reality are the experiences of practicing with mannequins and task trainers? Do learners have a false sense of confidence after they have simulated education? Can the mannequins and task trainers simulate the differences in the individual body composition of actual patients? There is always the possibility that technical issues may arise when using high-technology mannequins. These issues will have an impact on the realism, which will impact the learning. They key element is to stay focused on the learning objectives.

Technology (High, Low, and Midrange)

When developing educational and assessment activities, it is important to determine the learning objectives and outcomes and then determine whether simulation is the appropriate method to achieve the outcome. For example, it is usually not appropriate to place a novice learner in a high-technology simulation with many tasks. A novice learner needs to learn one task at a time before applying that learning in a high-technology simulation (Shemanko & Jones, 2008).

There are different levels of technology from high-cost, high-technology computer-controlled, lifelike mannequins to low-technology, inanimate mannequins and paper cases. High-technology simulations have a high degree of realism but it has to be asked whether this is always necessary? Resource questions persist at all levels. If a program has high-technology mannequins, do they have the resources to maintain the use of the mannequins, the human resources necessary to program and run the simulation, as well as the supplies and replacement skins needed for ongoing simulations (Rodgers, 2007; Shemanko & Jones, 2008)?

Standardized Patients

"Standardized patients (SPs) are individuals who are trained to portray a patient with a specific condition in a realistic, standardized, and repeatable way (where portrayal/presentation varies on the basis of learner performance only). SPs can be used for teaching and assessment of learners including but not limited to history/consultation, physical examination, and other clinical skills in simulated clinical environments. SPs can also be used to give feedback and evaluate student performance" (Association of Standardized Patient Educators, n.d.).

What are the ethical considerations when using SPs? There needs to be a thoughtful standard process in recruiting and hiring SPs. It is important to determine why an individual wants to work as an SP. Is it because they want to try to fix the healthcare system? Did they have a bad experience? Do the SPs have a history that might make them inappropriate for certain cases? It is the program's ethical responsibility to recruit appropriate individuals and assign them to appropriate cases. The organization has an ethical responsibility to ensure that these individuals come to know harm. A discussion of psychological harm to SPs and how to prevent this harm will be addressed later in this chapter.

Unannounced Standardized Patients

SPs who are trained to portray a patient, family member, or healthcare provider and enter the clinical environment unannounced to assess the provider's interaction with patients or the system are referred to in the literature as **unannounced standardized patients** (USPs), incognito standardized patients (ISPs), invisible patients, fake patients, secret shoppers, and mystery shoppers (Pott, 2008; Rethans et al., 2007; Siminoff et al., 2011). In this chapter, we will refer to these individuals as USPs, which avoids the potentially negative connotation associated with secret, mystery, or fake.

Why USPs? One of the central questions surrounding simulation is, "Does the training and assessment in a simulated setting transfer to actual patient care?" One way of assessing the transferability of skills is to employ USPs. Using USPs is the only choice for many to observe patient–clinician communication. There are ethical issues to consider when deciding to use USPs. Is using USPs deceptive? There are differing opinions.

There was objection by physicians when the Department of Health and Human Services wanted to use "mystery shoppers" to study the access to primary care (Rhodes, 2011). The Emergency Nurses Association and the American Academy of Emergency Medicine (2007) released a statement that they believe that using "mystery shoppers" in the Emergency Department is "not only dangerous and detrimental to quality care, but unnecessary since other more effective, less intrusive methods exist." Less intrusive methods include customer satisfaction surveys and direct observations. USPs are a way of testing two things: first, whether certain classes of persons have access to the system and second, what kind of care persons who do obtain access receive. However, those two matters do not have to be addressed in the same fashion. Research on access to care, as long as confidentiality is maintained, is relatively noninvasive, and the most reliable results come when persons are not informed that research is being done (Rhodes, 2011). The second practice—using USPs to determine the quality of care that patients receive—needs not only the protection of confidentiality but also the consent of the clinicians who are being observed. Siminoff et al. (2011) argue that using USPs is the only technique to observe how the clinician interacts with the patient in actual clinical settings and that this cannot be replicated with other methods. Observing clinicians with actual patients is valuable, but provides no standardization because each actual patient comes with their individual history and problems. Pott (2008) refers to the "invisible patient" to assess learners in the clinical environment without the learner knowing that the patient is actually an SP. He states that this type of assessment is worth the effort and resources.

Successful USP programs rely on flexibility and planning. Patient care always takes precedence and there are times when the unannounced activity needs to be postponed or rescheduled so as to not interfere with direct patient care. Planning an unannounced simulation involves discussions with stakeholders who may be involved regarding triage, registration, and medical records. It is important to decide whether a "dummy" medical record needs to be developed and how it will be implemented during the session and deleted after the encounter is over (Siminoff et al., 2011).

It is a challenge to notify providers in such a way as to not bias the results of the simulation. Consent is always an issue, however. At the end of a simulation in the Simulation Center or in another venue, learners can be told that within the next "n" months they will be visited by an USP in the clinical setting.

Will providing an USP program in the clinical setting improve practice habits? We believe that if there is effective feedback and debriefing after the session, practice habits will be improved. Miller (1990) created a four-level framework to assess clinical skills, competence, and performance. The pyramid begins with the knowledge base (knows), moving to knowing how to perform a skill (competence), followed by performing the skill in simulation (shows how), and ultimately doing the skill in practice (action). This method provides a way for clinicians to demonstrate the top of Miller's pyramid—the action or performing the skill in the clinical setting—and we can then measure whether what is performed and shown in simulation transfers to actual clinical performance (Miller, 1990). Providing actual benefit to patients provides support for the notion that using USP encounters is an ethical use of simulation.

SIMULATION CENTER VERSUS IN SITU

Simulation-based activities can be conducted in simulation centers or in the clinical environment (in situ). In situ simulation brings the simulation learning and training to the clinical environment in which the learners work versus taking the learners out of their work environment and taking them to a simulation center. In situ simulation is conducted in actual patient care areas using resources and actual members of the healthcare team (Wheeler et al., 2013).

The reason for selecting the location for the simulation activity should be based on the objective of the activity. Simulation centers provide training to students, new trainees, and healthcare providers where in situ simulation activities include practicing clinicians usually from different disciplines and professions. A systematic review by Rosen et al. (2012) found that in situ activities included multiple units, departments, and clinicians from different professions. Programs are using in situ simulation to identify latent safety threats, and results are showing that conducting in situ simulation with the purpose of identifying safety threats improves the safety climate in high-risk clinical settings (Patterson et al., 2013; Wheeler et al., 2013).

There are advantages and disadvantages with in situ simulation. Patterson et al. (2008) in *Advances in Patient*

Safety: New Directions and Alternative Approaches describe the challenges and benefits of in situ simulation.

Benefits

In situ simulation provides the opportunity to learn in context, for situated learning, and for training where you work. Benefits of in situ simulation include identifying systems issues within a particular context as well as knowledge gaps.

Systems integration is another potential benefit. Simulation-based activities can be used to test new facilities, equipment, and processes (Kobayashi et al., 2006; Patterson et al., 2008; Society for Simulation in Healthcare, n.d.).

Challenges

There are as many challenges as benefits to conducting in situ simulation. Being aware of the challenges and planning for them will provide the opportunity to conduct in situ simulation and reap the benefits of this type of training (LeBlanc, 2008).

Miller et al. (2012) studied in situ trauma simulations and observed an improvement in teamwork and communication during the simulation, but it was not sustained. In situ training requires resources including faculty time. Training needs to be ongoing.

Patterson et al. (2008) identify four areas of challenges in conducting in situ simulations: technical issues, logistics, cultural obstacles, and medical-legal concerns. As should be clear by now, we would add the use of resources. Technical issues include transportation, setup, and storage of simulators. If you use supplies on the unit, what is the cost and how do they get replaced?

Logistics

In situ simulation-based activities need to be made available to all shifts, including nights and weekends. Patients need to be kept safe 24/7. Questions to ask include "When are staff available? When is the equipment and space available?" One of the greatest challenges is finding time that is not too disruptive to patient care (Delac et al., 2013; Miller et al., 2012; Patterson et al., 2008).

Clinicians are concerned about taking time away from actual patient care and are concerned about what patients and families will think of this activity taking time from their care. They are concerned that this would be stressful for families. Cincinnati Children's Hospital Medical Center and the Children's Hospital of Philadelphia asked patients and families their perception of training in patient care areas. Responses included that the patients and families were glad that the clinicians were practicing and that the time waiting was not significant. If the simulation time is brief, the perception is that it is worth the wait (Patterson et al., 2008). Patients and families need to be told the why and what of the simulation. The explanation helps with the perception being positive, ongoing training versus a negative perception that their trusted providers make mistakes (Patterson et al., 2008). If patient safety is to continue to be a driving factor in simulation, in situ activities must always be considered, because those activities seem to have a higher probability of revealing problems in the delivery of patient care in today's healthcare environment.

RECORDING SIMULATIONS

There are always ethical concerns that need to be addressed when recording people. The most important questions to be asked are "What is the purpose of the recording? How are the recordings used? Are they being recorded for both formative and summative assessments? Are they for debriefing and for the learners to review or are they for research?" Learners cannot opt out of being recorded for educational purposes. They can opt out for research purposes.

How long and in what setting are the recordings stored? Recordings need to be kept in a secure location. Learners often worry that the recordings will show up on the Internet. Anyone being recorded needs to know why they are being recorded, how the recordings will be used, and how they will be stored.

When SP encounters are recorded, SPs should have the opportunity to view and reflect and be provided feedback on their performance. Recordings can also be used for training. All participants being recorded should sign a release or consent to be filmed. That release should include a date by which the recording will be destroyed. There is no standard best practice concerning the time frame to destroy the recordings. Some programs keep the recordings indefinitely and other programs destroy immediately after viewing the recording. The decision should be based on the purpose of the recording. If a clinician is being recorded for remediation purposes, this recording may need to be kept longer for legal and ethical issues versus a recording of a clinician in a formative learning encounter. The temptation will be to hold on to these recordings for as long as possible. Simulation center directors should resist these temptations. Given the changing pace of healthcare and the potential for negative consequences on those recorded, shorter rather than longer time frames should always be considered. Whatever time is chosen, steps should be put into place so that the destruction takes place as promised.

SIMULATION IN SUPPORT OF ETHICS

Simulation is not a set of practices that serves only the technical aspects of healthcare. Simulations can be used in the service of education in professionalism and ethics themselves. The imaginations of the simulation providers, the ethics and professionalism educators, and the availability of resources are the major constraints. For example, Vanlaere et al. (2012) designed a simulation exercise to foster empathy in nurses. Participants became elderly patients and were treated as such through such activities as bathing, feeding, being cared for, recreation, and so on. The second day of the exercise involved a debriefing of the patient participants as well as the simulated care providers. The goal was to see whether such exercises enhanced empathy in the providers who were patients for purposes of the exercise. Among the findings was the result that at least one experience during the simulation affected the learners in a profound way. How these findings become integrated into practice remains uncertain, for both the providers and the SPs.

Such an elaborate simulation exercise is only one example of how simulation can be at the service of professionalism and ethics. An SP being given bad news, an SP giving informed consent to an upcoming surgery, an SP expressing his fears about his rapidly approaching death, all of these scenarios can be used to help students (medical, nursing, allied health), residents (medical, nursing, pharmacy, pastoral care), as well as practicing clinicians develop the skills necessary to become excellent clinicians. Again, the issue is not whether simulation and ethics and professionalism can be of service to one another; the issue is how a particular simulation exercise serves a particular goal in the education of future clinicians.

PSYCHOLOGICAL SAFETY

What is **psychological safety**?

Gaba (2013) and Truog and Meyer (2013) state clearly that anyone who has a role in simulation needs to consider the psychological effects of simulation on learners and be responsible to ourselves, the learners, as well as patients and families. It is important to identify the needs of the learners, but also the needs of SPs, staff, and faculty.

Calhoun et al. (2013) describe a real case that illustrates the negative consequence of not speaking up. Members of a multidisciplinary team noticed that the physician ordered the wrong medication and no one spoke up, resulting in severe hypotension and bradycardia. It is the norm that clinicians work within a hierarchy and too often do not speak up to question the appropriateness of an action taken by someone in a more powerful position. This is commonplace throughout the workforce and deadly in healthcare. Training programs, such as the AHRQ Team-STEPPS program, are being developed around communication and speaking up. Clinicians need to be explicitly taught these skills needed for effective communication and be provided the time to practice the skills in a safe simulated setting.

The areas with the greatest concern for psychological safety include simulations around death and dying, and speaking up or challenging authority.

EXAMPLE AND COMMENTARY

Friday morning in the simulation center, an interdisciplinary team of clinicians comes together to participate in a patient safety simulation. One goal for the simulation is to assess how well the team can manage a trauma patient in shock. The case involves a critically ill patient that needs a number of immediate procedures for stabilization. The team provides IV fluids to the patient and moves on to the next procedure and assessment. No one is monitoring the patient's blood pressure and fail to notice that the patient needed blood products. A time-out is called at this point in the simulation. The patient would die if nothing further was done to treat the shock.

It is important to acknowledge what effect an action or inaction will have on the patient, family, and other clinicians. If the learners have the wrong diagnosis and the patient would die because of the wrong treatment, this needs to be discussed and identified. Many people argue that the SP should not die (Bruppacher et al., 2011). The alternative view is that learners need to understand that every action and inaction affects the life and death of those they are treating and need to experience this in a simulated environment (Rogers et al., 2011).

Psychological Harm to Learners

Simulations are stressful to learners. Learners experience physiological as well as psychological stress just thinking about having to perform in a simulation, talk with an SP, be videotaped, and receive feedback. Hulsman et al. (2010) studied the physiological and psychological stress of medical students communicating with SPs and found an increase in heart rate, mean arterial pressure, and cardiac output. Students in this study were presented two cases: history taking and delivering bad news. The students who delivered bad news first had a higher level of stress.

Simulation environments should be safe places to learn and make mistakes. Some stress is good, heightening the awareness of the situation and making an impact on the learner so that if they experience a similar situation, they can act effectively and efficiently. At the same time, it is imperative that learners are not placed in situations where the level of stress is too high and impacts their cognitive abilities.

There is discussion within the simulation community about allowing death of the simulated patient (e.g., the mannequin) to be a part of a case scenario (Bruppacher et al., 2011; Gaba, 2013; Truog & Meyer, 2013). As with all aspects of simulation, the developers need to consider the level of the learner and the objective of the scenario. The simulation environment needs to be one that promotes trust and safety. It is appropriate to allow the mannequin to die in certain situations if the appropriate treatment was not provided. This provides the teachable moment and a learning opportunity for learners to realize the impact of their actions or inaction. The vital component in these scenarios is the prebriefing and debriefing. Prebriefing is important for new learners or providers with little experience with these types of cases. Debriefing is critical to highlight and reinforce the correct action as well as to discuss the emotional issues surrounding the case. If possible, the schedule should allow enough time so that the case can be run a second time using what was learned so learners can leave with a positive outcome.

EXPERT'S CORNER

DEATH IN SIMULATION
Ignacio del Moral, MD, PhD
Founder and First President Elected, Spanish Society for Simulation in Healthcare

Sandra returned to the simulation center 3 years after her last training session. During the introduction to the course, she said, "I remember that room very well. Three years ago I was here and my patient died." That comment struck my attention, and I realized the impact death during simulated clinical scenarios has on our learners.

From the point of view of the educator, there are two types of scenarios in which death occur: (1) when the educator knows it in advance, regardless of the decisions of the learners and (2) when the scenario ends in death unexpectedly because of the learner's poor performance. The learner shares these same two points of view when it comes to death in a simulated scenario.

As clinical educators, we have a duty to address the issue of death in our curricula and also be aware of the impact it may have on our learners. Death in the simulation setting can have an impact in three different domains.

1. Impact on the learner's identity—"I'm not a good clinician, I am not worthy to work with patients."
2. Impact on the learning objectives—When death occurs, it can distract from other important learning objectives for the program.

3. Impact on the learner's psychological safety—"I feel sad and frustrated."

A deeper understanding of the impact death has on learners in simulated scenarios has led to personal insight into the matter. Because I always know if the scenario will end in death, I always let learners know in advance if death will be one of the topics of the day. Occasionally there is a situation where learner performance is poor and probably should result in death but, in this scenario, I choose to finish the case before death ensues. From my point of view, the risk of ending the scenario with an unexpected and unannounced death is that it will deflect attention away from the intended learning objectives. When I am concerned or frustrated about learner performance, I make it explicit during debriefing by discussing the issue, helping the learner understand the consequence of their actions, and supporting the learner to improve performance in the future.

Corvetto and Taekman (2013) reviewed the literature to examine the issue of allowing the mannequin to die. Should mannequins only be allowed to die if that was the objective of the simulation? Or should the mannequin be allowed to die unexpectedly? The biggest concern about allowing the mannequin to die is the psychological safety of the learners and their learning outcomes. Rogers et al. (2011) found in their work with medical students that the death of a "patient" provided an opportunity for the students to reflect about death and how that might transfer to the real clinical setting.

Clinicians receive little training or experience in dealing with death, dying, and end-of-life issues. Providing opportunities in a safe environment to experience these issues allows the learners to practice difficult skills that they may not otherwise encounter during training. Leavy et al. (2011) assessed student views on the benefits of participating in simulations when a patient dies and the effectiveness of the debriefing session in processing emotions. They state that students benefit in that they learn to process their anxieties and to develop coping skills.

Simulated death is an important and difficult teaching strategy for learners and faculty and "must be grounded in sound ethical principles that respect the teaching modality, promote a non-punitive culture around patient safety and interprofessional collaboration, and consider the well-being of learners" (Bruppacher et al., 2011, p. 317).

CASE EXAMPLE

Third-year medical students are coming to the Simulation Center for an end-of-the-year examination. One station is designed around giving bad news to a young woman who has a recurrence of breast cancer. The SP coordinator hired a number of women to portray this woman. One of the SPs playing this role fell out of character during the session. Only later did the coordinator learn that the SP's sister, who was 38 years old with two small children, recently died from breast cancer.

Psychological Harm to SPs

SPs are classified as another method or technique of simulation just like mannequins and virtual reality. SPs are human, however, and as humans they have emotions and feelings and take on the character of the person they are portraying. This method of training and assessment provides learners an opportunity to practice communication skills on actual people. Learners have an opportunity to practice how they would deliver bad news and review what worked and what was less than helpful for the patient and the family. The learner has a chance to receive feedback on how the news was presented and should have an opportunity to watch a recording of their performance and reflect on how it felt and what they did well and how they might communicate differently next time.

Depending on the scenario, the SP may react with denial, tears, anger, or even yelling and may receive the news over and over, allowing individual learners to present the same bad news. The SP needs to get back in character and take on the "burden" of this news for each new learner.

A key component of SP work is the preparation and support when portraying a difficult or emotionally charged patient or family member. Getting into character and staying in character can be exhausting. The SP often takes on the characteristics of the individual they are portraying and they need time after the case to come out of character. It is important for someone to check in with SPs after all performances, and it is most important when the SP is portraying someone receiving "bad" news, or is depressed, angry, and so on. There may be SPs that are unaware that they are holding the emotions until they debrief about the experience (Wallace, 2007, p. 257; see chapter 3.3).

What is an unexpected event when working with SPs? An example is the case with the SP who became emotional during a case about breast cancer that triggered emotions about her sister who died from breast cancer. All unexpected events cannot be avoided but to minimize the occurrence, SPs need to be screened for their case. When deciding which SPs should perform which cases, it is key to ask about history, comfort level, and confidence. Once an unexpected event occurs, it is the team's responsibility to deal with the event and provide support to the SP. Simulation cases have the potential to trigger emotions in anyone. This requires a plan and resources in place to deal with the emotions. The emotions should be discussed during debriefing.

Taylor (2011) discusses the moral commitment to avoid suffering and the aesthetic commitment to realistically portray it. SPs are an important part of training because they portray suffering of another (real vs. not real). When an SP portrays suffering, they cannot avoid suffering at some level. One reason to use SPs is to protect actual patients from risk and suffering, yet we place SPs in a situation where they take on the suffering of another and the SP may suffer as a result of this portrayal. A mechanism needs to be in place to protect and address physical and psychological safety of all individuals involved in simulation.

Psychological Harm to Faculty

Faculty have an important role in simulation. They are not only content experts but also role models. Faculty need to feel safe in the learning/teaching environment.

EXAMPLE AND COMMENTARY

Wednesday morning, the emergency medicine department sends an interdisciplinary team of learners, residents, and attending physicians to participate in Advanced Cardiac Life Support (ACLS) training. Dr. S. has not been involved with ACLS workshops since 2009 and was not aware of the guideline changes. The simulation team notices that Dr. S. is using an older version of the ACLS algorithm. There are two issues with this situation. First, the faculty member has not kept up to date with the current guidelines. Second, the resident has the potential problem of speaking up.

How can this be addressed without embarrassing the faculty, losing the credibility of that faculty member, and at the same time providing the most up-to-date information to everyone? Depending on when and who notices it, it should be noted that the algorithm has been updated and explain the updates. If possible, talking to the faculty member prior to the debriefing might provide a level of safety so they are prepared for the discussion. This having been said, it is an important issue to think through during the planning of an activity. In the real world, learners have to be willing to speak up if a faculty member's failure might compromise the patient.

Given the goal of simulation is patient safety, a key part of the learning is the debriefing session. Debriefing is a skill that takes practice. It is also a skill that needs to be exercised during every simulation exercise. It is not something to be done only if there is time before the next task in a busy schedule.

To make the most of a debriefing session, the environment needs to be one of safety in sharing what went well and what errors occurred. It must be clear that confidentiality will be maintained. If a faculty member makes an error, they need to have the skills to explain what they did and why. This illustrates to learners that everyone is human. This is a great opportunity for role-modeling—for taking ownership and displaying humility. This is especially important when the usual medical hierarchy comes into play and learners fear that their pointing out less-than-optimal faculty performance will have negative consequences for the learners. Simulations and debriefings should not be yet another series of places where a professional identity is formed that prizes silence over patient safety. One cannot emphasize enough that at critical junctures one has to remind oneself why one is doing the simulation in the first place and that is to enhance patient care.

EDUCATION VERSUS EDUCATION + RESEARCH

Not surprisingly, educators who use simulation spend the majority of their time planning and executing simulations of various kinds so that learners can begin and advance in their care of patients. What are the ethical issues that arise when the educators begin to think of contributing to the literature through research?

There is a large body of literature related to the ethics of research in medicine and anyone who wishes to do research should be familiar with it. Second, there are common practices and regulations associated with research that every healthcare provider should know. For example, if this is a case situated in the United States, has everyone on the research team been made aware of the responsibilities of researchers under the current Institutional Review Board (IRB) system? A wide variety of resources are available that serve as the foundation for ethics in US-based healthcare. The classic place to begin is with "**The Belmont Report**: Ethical Principles and Guidelines for the Protection of Human Subjects of Research" (U.S. Department of Health, Education, and Welfare, 1978). Beyond the

national requirements, are members of the team aware of the requirements of the IRB at their institution? Even if the research turns out to be exempt from full IRB review, members of the team need to learn what the practices of the local IRB are (see chapter 9.3).

Besides these general considerations, there are some specific questions that need to be asked by researchers in simulation. In particular, the setting of simulation lends itself to the possibility that learners, who are lower in status in power, will be subtly coerced into participating in a research project that grows out of a legitimate learning exercise. Learners need to be informed about what is expected of them and by continuing to participate, have given their consent to the learning exercise. Research participants need to give consent to the research component and, most importantly, need to be able to withdraw from the research. It may turn out that what this means in practice is that whatever data is collected around a particular participant will not be part of the data analyzed by the researcher. The possibility of nonparticipation as a research participant must be real. Even if the learner will be participating in whatever exercise is being investigated, they must always be able to insist that what they did does not "count" as part of the research.

Among other questions that would-be researchers need to address is what exactly is being pursued by the research. Some simulation research depends upon self-report by the learner. This type of research is not nearly as valuable as simulation research where there is some attempt to validate through some type of assessment, exactly how far the learner has progressed given the simulation intervention, or how the learner has been changed as a result of the intervention. The ultimate in research is to study the translation to patient outcomes over time (Hallenbeck, 2012).

Competency—Licensure/Certification

Simulation has become a method to assess competency. The American Heart Association has been using mannequins for certification of Basic Life Support (BLS) and ACLS.

The United States Medical Licensing Examination (USMLE) added computer-based case simulations in 1999, and in 2004 the Step 2 Clinical Skills (CS) was added (USMLE, 2007). There are three Steps of the USMLE that certifies that an individual has the minimum knowledge and clinical skills for the practice of medicine. Step 2 CS "uses standardized patients to test medical students and graduates on their ability to gather information from patients, perform physical examinations, and communicate their findings to patients and colleagues" (USMLE, 2013).

Levine et al. (2012) discuss the future of using simulation for licensure and certification. They state that the ethical benefits are significant. They believe that being trained and assessed using simulation prior to "real" patient encounters "reduces a patient's exposure to less-seasoned professionals."

THE HOW TO—NOVICE TO ADVANCED BEGINNER

Planning

Ensuring that simulations are conducted fairly and ethically starts with planning and preparation. The goals and objectives of the simulation need to be identified to determine what the best methodology is to achieve the stated outcome and to acknowledge when simulation is not the best method to achieve the outcome. During the planning phase, it is important to identify what resources are needed to ensure safe and effective simulations and develop a cost-benefit ratio.

Implementation

Preparation is key to a successful simulation experience. At the start of the simulation, it is important to set expectations with the learners, have them sign consent forms, and answer any questions. It is as important to provide time to debrief and be prepared for any unexpected responses during the simulation.

The simulation team should have a team huddle prior to the simulation to ensure that everything is in place prior to the learners' arrival. The simulation team should also debrief about the session and make notes about what worked and what changes should be addressed for future simulations.

A useful technique to capture what is working and what changes need to be addressed is by keeping a journal of events occurring during simulations.

BEEN THERE, DONE THAT: COMPETENT TO EXPERT

Interprofessional simulations, teamwork, and communication are vital components of patient safety. Healthcare is a team sport, yet traditionally we have trained in silos. Simulation is a methodology that encourages interprofessional training on teamwork and communication. The Interprofessional Education Collaborative Expert Panel (2011) developed core competencies for interprofessional collaborative practice and devoted one of the four domains to values/ethics for interprofessional practice. Communication and teamwork are factors in all that we do. Here again, the simulation team is a team and can model good teamwork and communication skills.

Scholarly activity includes evidence-based research, writing articles and books for publication, and sharing ideas in less peer-reviewed venues, blogs, listservs, and so on. Experienced simulation educators need to share what has worked, what has not worked, and what issues have been identified. Sharing can take place with colleagues at their own institution, at local, national, and international meetings, as well as writing and publishing.

Simulation educators have a responsibility to society to study simulation education to determine the methods and techniques that help learners understand and retain concepts, to identify whether the knowledge, behaviors, skills, and attitudes learned and practiced in the simulated environment translate to practice at the bedside. Rigorous research will influence future educational design, ultimately leading to better patient outcomes, safety, and public health (McGaghie, 2010; McGaghie et al., 2012). At the end of the day, it is the simulation educator's job to ask, answer, and share—"does this make a difference?"

SUMMARY

Simulation in healthcare provides a series of techniques to increase patient safety and provide better patient outcomes. It is our responsibility as everyone working in simulation—the learners and faculty, the patients and families and society—to be aware of the ethical considerations from the planning, to the implementation, to the debriefing, and to the sharing of information. Doing this will always be a work in progress. Ongoing reflection and practice in simulation will ultimately transfer to thoughtful practice in the clinical situation.

REFERENCES

Association of Standardized Patient Educators. (n.d.). *Terminology standards.* Retrieved from http://www.aspeducators.org/node/102

Beauchamp, T., & Childress, J. (2013). *Principles of biomedical ethics* (7th ed.). New York, NY: Oxford University Press.

Bruppacher, H., Chen, R., & Lachapelle, K. (2011). First, do no harm: Using simulated patient death to enhance learning? *Medical Education, 45*(3), 317–318. doi:10.1111/j.1365-2923.2010.03923.x

Calhoun, A., Boone, M., Miller, K., & Pian-Smith, M. (2013). Case and commentary: Using simulation to address hierarchy issues during medical crises. *Simulation in Healthcare: Journal of the Society for Simulation in Healthcare, 8*(1), 13–19. doi:10.1097/SIH.0b013e318280b202

Corvetto, M., & Taekman, J. (2013). To die or not to die? A review of simulated death. *Simulation in Healthcare: Journal of the Society for Simulation in Healthcare, 8*(1), 8–12. doi:10.1097/SIH.0b013e3182689aff

Delac, K., Blazier, D., Daniel, L., & N-Wilfong, D. (2013). Five alive: Using mock code simulation to improve responder performance during the first 5 minutes if a code. *Critical Care Nursing Quarterly, 36*(2), 244–250. doi:10.1097/CNQ.0b013e3182846f1a

Emergency Nurses Association & American Academy of Emergency Medicine. (2007, December). *Mystery shoppers' in emergency department statement.* Retrieved from http://www.ena.org/SiteCollectionDocuments/Position%20Statements/Mystery_Shoppers_in_the_Emergency_Department_-_ENAAAEM.pdf

Gaba, D. (2013). Simulations that are challenging to the psyche of participants: How much should we worry and about what? *Simulation in Healthcare: Journal of the Society for Simulation in Healthcare, 8*(1), 4–7. doi:10.1097/SIH.0b013e3182845a6f

Hallenbeck, V. (2012). Use of high-fidelity simulation for staff education/development: A systematic review of the literature. *Journal for Nurses in Staff Development: JNSD: Official Journal of the National Nursing Staff Development Organization, 28*(6), 260. doi:10.1097/NND.0b013e31827259c7

Hulsman, R., Pranger, S., Koot, S., Fabriek, M., Karemaker, J., & Smets, E. (2010). How stressful is doctor-patient communication? Physiological and psychological stress of medical students in simulated history taking and bad-news consultations. *International Journal of Psychophysiology:*

Official Journal of the International Organization of Psychophysiology, 77(1), 26–34. doi:10.1016/j.ijpsycho.2010.04.001

Interprofessional Education Collaborative Expert Panel. (2011). *Core competencies for interprofessional collaborative practice: Report of an expert panel.* Washington, DC: Interprofessional Education Collaborative.

Kobayashi, L., Shapiro, M., Sucov, A., Woolard, R., Boss, R., Dunbar, J., . . . Jay, G. (2006). Portable advanced medical simulation for new emergency department testing and orientation. *Academic Emergency Medicine: Official Journal of the Society for Academic Emergency Medicine, 13*(6), 691–695.

Leavy, J. D., Vanderhoff, C. J., & Ravert, P. K. (2011). Code simulations and death: Processing of emotional distress. *International Journal of Nursing Education Scholarship, 8*(1), 1–13.

LeBlanc, D. (2008). Situated simulation: Simulation to the clinicians. In R. Kyle & W. Murray (Eds.), *Clinical simulation: Operations, engineering and management* (pp. 553–557). New York, NY: Elsevier.

Levine, A., Schwartz, A., Bryson, E., & Demaria, S. (2012). Role of simulation in US physician licensure and certification. *The Mount Sinai Journal of Medicine, New York, 79*(1), 140–153. doi:10.1002/msj.21291

McGaghie, W. (2010). Medical education research as translational science. *Science Translational Medicine, 2*(19), 19cm8. doi:10.1126/scitranslmed.3000679

McGaghie, W., Issenberg, S., Cohen, E., Barsuk, J., & Wayne, D. (2012). Translational educational research: A necessity for effective health-care improvement. *Chest, 142*(5), 1097–1103. doi:10.1378/chest.12-0148

Miller, D., Crandall, C., Washington, C., & McLaughlin, S. (2012). Improving teamwork and communication in trauma care through in situ simulations. *Academic Emergency Medicine, 19*(5), 608–612. http://dx.doi.org/10.1111/j.1553-2712.2012.01354.x

Miller, G. (1990). The assessment of clinical skills/competence/performance. *Academic Medicine: Journal of the Association of American Medical Colleges, 65*(9 Suppl.), S63–S67.

Patterson, M. D., Blike, G. T., & Nadkarni, V. M. (2008). In situ simulation: Challenges and results. In K. Henriksen, J. B. Battles, M. A. Keyes, & M. L. Grady (Eds.), *Advances in patient safety: New directions and alternative approaches: Vol. 3. Performance and tools.* Rockville, MD: Agency for Healthcare Research and Quality Retrieved from http://www.ncbi.nlm.nih.gov/books/NBK43682/

Patterson, M. D., Geis, G. L., Falcone, R. A., LeMaster, T., & Wears, R. L. (2013). In situ simulation: Detection of safety threats and teamwork training in a high risk emergency department. *BMJ Quality & Safety, 22*, 468–477. doi:10.1136/bmjqs-2012-000942

Pott, L. (2008). The invisible standardized patient. In R. R. Kyle & W. Murray (Eds.), *Clinical simulation: Operations, engineering, and management* (pp. 379–383). New York, NY: Elsevier.

Rethans, J., Gorter, S., Bokken, L., & Morrison, L. (2007). Unannounced standardised patients in real practice: A systematic literature review. *Medical Education, 41*(6), 537–549. doi:10.111/j.365-2929.2006.02689.x

Rhodes, K. (2011). Taking the mystery out of "mystery shopper" studies. *The New England Journal of Medicine, 365*(6), 484–486.

Rodgers, D. L. (2007). *High-fidelity patient simulation: A descriptive white paper report.* Retrieved from http://sim-strategies.com/downloads/Simulation%20White%20Paper2.pdf

Rogers, G., de Rooy, N., & Bowe, P. (2011). Simulated death can be an appropriate training tool for medical students. *Medical Education, 45*(10), 1061. doi:10.1111/j.1365-2923.2011.04027.x

Rosen, M. A., Hunt, E. A., Provonost, P. J., Federowicz, M. A., & Weaver, S. J. (2012). In situ simulation in continuing education for the health care professions: A systematic review. *Journal of Continuing Education in the Health Professions, 32*(4), 243–254.

Shemanko, G. S. & Jones, L. (2008). To simulate or not to simulate: That is the question. In R. R. Kyle & W. Murray (Eds.), *Clinical simulation: Operations, engineering, and management* (pp. 77–84). New York, NY: Elsevier.

Siminoff, L., Rogers, H., Waller, A., Harris-Haywood, S., Epstein, R., Cario, F., . . . Longo, D. (2011). The advantages and challenges of unannounced standardized patient methodology to assess healthcare communication. *Patient Education and Counseling, 82*(3), 318–324. doi:10.1016/j.pec.2011.01.021

Society for Simulation in Healthcare. (n.d.). *What is simulation?* Retrieved from http://ssih.org/about-simulation

Taylor, J. (2011). The moral aesthetics of simulated suffering in standardized patient performances. *Culture, Medicine and Psychiatry, 35*(2), 134–162. doi:10.1007/s11013-011-9211-5

Truog, R., & Meyer, E. (2013). Deception and death in medical simulation. *Simulation in Healthcare: Journal of the Society for Simulation in Healthcare, 8*(1), 1–3. doi:10.1097/SIH.0b013e3182869fc2

U.S. Department of Health, Education, and Welfare. (1978). *The Belmont report: Ethical principles and guidelines for the protection of human subjects of research* (Publication No. (OS) 78-0012). Washington, DC: U.S. Government Printing Office.

United States Medical Licensing Examination. (2007). *United States medical licensing examination: Comprehensive review.* Retrieved from http://www.usmle.org/cru/updates/2007-08.html

United States Medical Licensing Examination. (2013). *United States medical licensing examination: Step 2 CS.* Retrieved from http://www.usmle.org/step-2-cs/

Vanlaere, L., Timmermann, M., Stevens, M., & Gastmans, C. (2012). An explorative study of experiences of healthcare providers posing as simulated care receivers in a "care-ethical" lab. *Nursing Ethics, 19*(1), 68–79. doi:10.1177/0969733011412103

Wallace, P. (2007). *Coaching standardized patients for use in the assessment of clinical competence.* New York, NY: Springer.

Wheeler, D. S., Geis, G., Mack, E. H., LeMaster, T., & Patterson, M. D. (2013). High-reliability emergency response teams in the hospital: Improving quality and safety using in situ simulation training. *BMJ Quality & Safety, 22*, 507–514. doi:10.1136/bmjqs-2012-000931

Ziv, A., Wolpe, P. R., Small, S. D., & Glick, S. (2003). Simulation-based medical education: An ethical imperative. *Academic Medicine, 78*(8), 783–788.

SECTION 9

Research

CHAPTER 9.1

Research in Healthcare Simulation

Marjorie Lee White, MD, MPPM, MA, and Dawn Taylor Peterson, PhD

ABOUT THE AUTHORS

MARJORIE LEE WHITE is an Associate Professor in the Department of Pediatrics, Division of Pediatric Emergency Medicine at the University of Alabama at Birmingham. She is also the Medical Codirector of the Pediatric Simulation Center at Children's of Alabama. She has been actively involved in simulation research for the past 7 years and is site coordinator for several multicenter simulation-based research studies.

DAWN TAYLOR PETERSON is the Director of Simulation Education & Research at the Pediatric Simulation Center at Children's of Alabama. She holds a PhD in Instructional Design, an Educational Specialist degree, and a Master of Arts in Education. Dr. Peterson is responsible for coordinating and tracking the Center's research projects including multisite and international studies.

ABSTRACT

This chapter serves to introduce the research process. It provides an overview of basic research concepts, strategies, and methods (i.e., quantitative, qualitative, and mixed methods), and provides examples of their use in the simulation field to date. High-quality research requires not only knowledge of the research process, but also appropriate attention to developing the structure to support the activity. This chapter is not intended to be comprehensive in nature but seeks to provide both a general framework as well as additional resources where one may develop more in-depth understanding.

CASE EXAMPLE

The new director of a simulation program is approached by his supervisor and asked about the research the program will be doing. The new director's boss suggests that he will need to report to the board about the scholarly productivity of the program. The board is interested in how the program is contributing to the literature about the impact of simulation and its educational effectiveness. One board member suggests that the only kind of research worth publishing is a randomized controlled trial, while another suggests that simulation activity might be best explored using qualitative methods. The new director wonders whether he has the time, resources, and ability to start doing research. He also wonders what sort of methods and resources are available to assist him in starting a research program.

THEMES

General Concepts of Simulation-Based Educational Research

Research is "the systematic investigation into and study of materials and sources in order to establish facts and reach new conclusions" (*Oxford English Dictionary*, 2013). Simulation-based educational research should follow accepted research methods. Research generally starts with a well-framed question, informed by a literature search, and clearly defined research proposal. It is in the development of the research question that the research methods can be appropriately chosen.

The purpose of this chapter is to provide an overview of common concepts often encountered in research as well as brief description of common methods used in research. No single chapter could provide all necessary information, as research is a multifaceted endeavor.

Recently, there have been efforts made to develop a framework to help education scholars conceptualize important research efforts. Cook et al. describe three classifications of studies by purpose: description, justification, and clarification. Descriptive studies do not contain statistical outcome data; rather they seek to provide explanatory information. Justification studies seek to answer questions about whether new interventions work. Clarification studies answer *how* and *why* questions and do so within conceptual frameworks (Cook et al., 2008).

Common Research Concepts: Hypotheses, Variables, Risk, Reliability, and Validity

Fundamentally, research involves the development of a **hypothesis** and measurement of variables to better understand specific situations and to reach conclusions. A hypothesis is a statement that summarizes the elements of the study including the sample, the **design**, and the predictor and outcome variables. The purpose of the hypothesis is to establish the basis for tests for significance or inference. The hypothesis is generally derived from the research question. A variable is a measurable characteristic of the subject being studied (American Educational Research Association et al., 1999). For instance, a variable that might be studied in simulation might be teamwork as measured by a teamwork scale. It is important for researchers to take into account confounding variables as well. A confounding is an extraneous variable in a statistical model that correlates (positively or negatively) with both the dependent variable and the independent variable. There are many possible confounding variables in the simulated setting. Examples might include the level of environmental fidelity or participants' past experiences.

Risk is a term used to describe the probability that an adverse outcome will occur during a specific period of time. Two major sources of statistical risk are important to address. Type I **errors** occur when a claim is made that is actually false. A Type I error corresponds to a "false-positive" test result. Type II errors occur when a claim is not made that should be made. A Type II error can be thought of as a "false-negative" test result. Early attention to questions of statistical importance including power analysis, sample size calculations, and the relationship between statistical and clinical/educational significance are best addressed with an expert in statistical analysis (McGahie et al., 2006; Yarris et al., 2012).

Reliability and validity are two concepts that are crucial to understand for those engaged in research. When measuring a particular variable, it is important to be sure that you are measuring what you think you are measuring. In this way, you are ensuring validity. A measure is considered reliable if it can be replicated. In describing both reliability and validity, one makes an argument to support these concepts and builds a case (Kazdin, 1995). There are three major types of reliability for instruments used in research: inter-rater, test–retest/intrarater, and internal consistency. Inter-rater reliability refers to the concept that multiple witnesses viewing the same event confer a similar score. There are statistical measures of agreement that are reported on the basis of the characteristics of the data (i.e., Cohen's kappa, Kendall's coefficient, and

intraclass correlation).Test–retest and intrarater reliability assesses the error related to individual changes over time and provides an estimate of stability. Internal consistency provides a measure of how well items fit together. One generally sees the reporting of a Cronbach's alpha or Kuder–Richardson values for internal consistency (Downing, 2004; Messick, 1989).

There are multiple types of validity that may need to be addressed when designing a study. It is impossible to make a valid argument before first establishing that you have reliable data. A new framework for providing sources or types of validity evidence describes content, internal structure, relations to other variables, and response to process and consequences. Researchers should develop a validity argument using a combination of different types of validity. Content validity can be addressed by expert review and use of published literature. Internal structure overlaps with reliability measures. Relations to other variables can be determined using correlation coefficients. Response process arguments address the reasoning and thought processes of learners. Addressing consequences can provide evidence to support validity or allow for detection of threats to validity (Downing, 2003; Kane, 2006; Messick, 1989). The application of these concepts to the simulated setting adds additional complexity. Tools used in educational research that are described as validated have not necessarily been validated in the setting in which new research will take place. Researchers may need to pay particular attention to the reliability and validity of the simulation itself.

Quantitative, Qualitative, and Mixed Methods

The purpose of research methods is to set out the rules by which data are collected, analyzed, and displayed in such a way that conclusions can be drawn. Qualitative and quantitative approaches represent a continuum. Often, **qualitative research** is seen as that which uses words and open-ended questions, whereas **quantitative research** focuses on closed-ended questions and numbers. **Mixed methods** research can be viewed as a combination of the two approaches and can be positioned between quantitative and qualitative methods on the spectrum. The next three sections provide a more in-depth discussion of quantitative, qualitative, and mixed methods research including examples from simulation-based educational research.

Quantitative Methods

Quantitative research is a means for testing hypotheses by examining the relationship among variables. This relationship is measured and analyzed using statistical procedures (Creswell, 2009). When researchers use quantitative methods, they often collect data on an instrument or test and use statistical analysis and interpretation to report this data. Hypotheses in quantitative methods are predictions that the researcher makes about what they expect the results to show. Variables are characteristics about individuals or organizations that can be measured or observed. More specifically, independent variables are those that cause, influence, or affect outcomes; dependent variables are those that are the outcome or result of the independent variables. Control variables are independent variables that researchers measure because of their potential to influence the dependent variables. Quantitative methods are used primarily in **experimental** and **nonexperimental research**. In experimental research, the researcher manipulates the independent variable and observes the effect. In nonexperimental research, there is no manipulation of the variable but an attempt is made to understand causal relationships or correlations.

There are numerous examples of using an experimental design in simulation research. In 2005, Wayne et al. published the results of their randomized trial with waitlist controls of internal medicine trainees who received training in Advanced Cardiac Life Support (ACLS) protocols in the simulated setting. In this research, all subjects had a baseline assessment and were randomized to an intervention (i.e., training sessions on the simulator) and then the waitlist crossed over to receive the intervention (Wayne et al., 2005). In 2009, Barsuk et al. reported their results of an observational cohort study of an educational intervention related to central venous catheter placement. Of note, members of this research team also applied quantitative research methods to multiple other clinical procedures including lumbar punctures, thoracentesis, paracentesis, hemodialysis catheter placement, and cardiopulmonary exam skills. In 2012, Schroedl et al. published their work demonstrating that simulation-based training improves patient care in the intensive care unit setting (Schroedl et al., 2012). Also in 2012, Seybert et al. reported the results of a randomized crossover study in which pharmacy students were randomized to receive either a problem-based learning curriculum or a simulation-based learning curriculum. Students were assessed for knowledge and clinical thinking (Seybert et al., 2012).

Significant problems have been reported with the use of randomized controlled trials in educational research (Krupat, 2010). Although randomization is a powerful tool for reducing bias, critics of randomized controlled trials in educational research point out that it is often difficult to tell whether the intervention is responsible for the effect or whether there is "contextual contamination" (Sullivan, 2011).

An example of nonexperimental, quantitative methods is found in the work of Shrader et al. This group sought to examine the relationship between interprofessional teamwork skills, attitudes, and clinical outcomes in the simulated setting. The research team administered a survey and rated performance using several checklists (Shrader et al., 2013).

Qualitative Methods

Qualitative research relies on the collection of qualitative data and follows a primarily exploratory scientific method.

Qualitative methods often use open-ended questions from interviews and observations. Practitioners analyze texts and images and develop **coding** schema for this data. The results are often themes and patterns of interpretation. Qualitative analysis is used when little is known about a topic or phenomenon and when the goal is to learn more about it (Creswell, 2009; Denzin & Lincoln, 1994; Strauss & Corbin, 1999).

Five specific types of qualitative research are commonly described: (1) ethnography, (2) case study research, (3) **grounded theory**, (4) phenomenology, and (5) narrative research (Johnson & Christensen, 2010). Grounded theory and narrative research are the most commonly used methods in educational research. It has been suggested that grounded theory is being used more frequently than before and is serving to meet a need for additional methods to explore important questions (Watling & Lingard, 2012).

An example of a recent qualitative analysis involved a group at the Center for Simulation, Advanced Education and Innovation, at The Children's Hospital of Philadelphia. This group sought to examine faculty motivation to teach in the simulated setting. The research team developed a scripted interview, performed the interview, developed a coding schema, and reported the major themes that emerged from the data (Deutsch et al., 2013).

Mixed Methods

In this arena, practitioners use both open- and closed-ended questions to develop multiple forms of data. Both statistical and text analysis can be used and information from both can be reported. Mixed method researchers use a combination of quantitative and qualitative concepts and approaches (Schifferdecker & Reed, 2009). The goal is to collect multiple sets of data using different research methods and approaches such that the result maximizes strengths and minimizes coinciding weaknesses (Lincol & Guba, 1985).

Educators at the Michener Institute for Applied Health Sciences performed a mixed methods evaluation that included survey assessments and qualitative focus groups to evaluate the simulation that was added into a new curriculum. They reported significant improvements in clinical preparedness (Bandali et al., 2012).

THE "HOW TO ..."

Huggett et al. describe the importance of collaboration in educational research and stress the importance of planning, implementation, and dissemination of outcomes (Huggett et al., 2011).

Preparation

Research starts with the identification of a topic that can be described in a short phrase. Experts suggest that drafting a working title early on can help to focus on the topic. Development of the research question is an additional early step. The PICOT mnemonic, which requires specification of the population, intervention, comparison intervention, outcomes of interest, and time can be used to help focus on a research question (Brian, 2006). In addition, Hulley et al. suggest that writing FINER MAPS (feasible, interesting, novel, ethical, relevant, manageable, appropriate, publishable, systematic) educational research questions may also help to set up a team for success (Hulley, 2007).

Successful programs of simulation-based educational research have often developed research teams with representation of various content expertise. Beginning researchers are well served to obtain assistance from those

---

EXPERT'S CORNER

RESEARCH IN HEALTHCARE SIMULATION
David M. Gaba, MD
Founding Editor-in-Chief, Simulation in Healthcare

First, I would like to reemphasize the notion identified first by me and mentioned in chapter 9.2 that research associated with simulation encompasses both research *about* simulation (e.g., its technology, its pedagogy, its impact, and outcomes) and research that *uses* simulation as a tool to study other key things (e.g., clinician performance and decision making, clinical processes, human factors of healthcare equipment).

Another point made in this chapter that should be reemphasized is that "scholarship" about or using simulation is broader than the typical conception of "research." Technological improvement, curricular innovation, and simulation application can be rigorous and meaningful but not necessarily be research. The dissemination vehicles for such activities may include modalities other than papers appearing in peer-reviewed indexed journals.

Having said that though, it remains true for the simulation community as for all healthcare communities of practice that the academic gold standard is publication of a research paper, systematic review, or significant new theoretical or conceptual piece in a peer-reviewed indexed journal. This is because such journals rely on careful review by external reviewers and by internal editors. Such a peer-review process allows both rigorous review against rising standards of scholarship, and flexibility to encompass innovative and novel conceptual, theoretical, or empirical work. For the journal that I edit, *Simulation in Healthcare* (*SiH*)—the official journal of the Society for Simulation in Healthcare—the process utilizes a review by the Editor-in-Chief (me) and nearly always also by one of nine Associate Editors. For manuscripts deemed worthy of further review, reviewers are chosen from a large pool of already vetted expertise within the community.

Despite roots that go back to the 1960s, 1970s, and 1980s for different aspects of simulation in healthcare, there has been a rapid growth in the last decade, which has yielded substantial innovation and scholarship. This has raised the standards for scholarly work. Activities that were novel 10 or 20 years ago are ordinary today. Studies of learning outcomes at the lowest Kirkpatrick levels—"reaction" of the learners, "self-efficacy," or "self-confidence"—and knowledge as measurable by simple tests (e.g., multiple-choice type) are no longer meaningful scholarship unless the application of simulation is extremely new and innovative. Studies without good control groups, or uncontrolled "before and after" paradigms are also unlikely to be considered with the same interest as they were years ago.

Thanks to William McGahie, PhD (originally from Northwestern University and now at Loyola University), and with additional contributions from me, the simulation field has adapted the "translational research" paradigm and nomenclature from biomedical science and clinical healthcare. The "T1" level means studies of clinical performance as measured during simulation. T2 is performance observed during actual clinical care. T3 is about whether patient outcomes are actually changed (and T3′ is about whether that change was cost-effective). I added additional levels discussed in "implementation science"—about how innovations get disseminated (T4) and adopted in the workplace (T5) to yield widespread changes in population health (T6). Much scholarship attempted today is at the T0 to T1 level. Only a little bit has been successfully attempted at the T2 and T3 levels—and most of that is about topics of very narrow clinical applications, where the complications are well-known; where we already conduct routine surveillance; and where the simulation intervention is also narrow. The poster child for such successful work is the T1/T2/T3/T3′ studies about simulation for central venous cannulation. But, "climbing the T ladder" is *very* difficult for any application. For many aspects of patient care, it may well be impossible to conduct robust studies of clinical performance or patient outcome. In an editorial in the February 2010 issue of *SiH*, I explained that such studies can be designed "on paper" but they would need to be so large, so long, so complex, and hence so expensive that they cannot be done in practice without a huge "deep pocket" with a long time horizon. For testing of medications, pharmaceutical companies can provide that deep pocket and horizon because when they hit a blockbuster drug, it can earn the company billions of dollars. There is no deep pocket for simulation research.

On the one hand, our community should seek to continue to raise the bar for good scholarship, while at the same time understanding, as well as educating our clinical and administrative counterparts in healthcare, about the realities of what can likely be proven with Level 1a evidence (i.e., multiple well-controlled randomized trials) and what can never be proven to that extent. I note that aviation (or nuclear power) has nothing like such "evidence-based" data showing that simulation saves lives, saves airplanes, or saves power plants, and they pretty much never will, as no one would volunteer to be in the "no-simulation" control group.

Hence, scholarship in our field can and should grow in rigor, in innovation, in novel applications and approaches. We should try harder to understand *how* simulation works and how it can be best conducted. We can also leverage simulation's power as a tool to study clinical processes and clinician performance. These approaches will just as likely make a major impact on healthcare delivery as would (possibly vain) attempts to prove unequivocally that simulation training saves hearts, brains, or lives.

with experience. A thorough literature search with the aid of a reference librarian can be an effective first step in the research process. The literature review should provide a framework for the importance of the study and can provide direction for the research questions and hypotheses. Maggio et al. (2011) have described 10 elements of an ideal literature search. Strong literature searches include searches of more than one database and are not limited to the databases of a single discipline. Theyw often use **Medical Subject Headings (MeSH terms)** and include the use of Boolean operators. Examples of databases to consider include MEDLINE via PubMed, ERIC, CINAHL, Web of Science, PsycINFO, ABI Inform, and SocINDEX.

After developing a research question and conducting a literature search, the next step is to develop a research protocol. A detailed, written research protocol can allow a research team to iron out conceptual differences and anticipate problems that may arise during data collection and analysis. A research protocol should include (1) Title, (2) Problem statement, (3) Purpose statement, (4) The research questions, hypotheses, or objectives, (5) The literature review, (6) The methods, and (7) Timeline. Once the protocol has been developed, the team can begin work after appropriate permissions and approvals have been obtained. (See chapter 9.3 for guidance on IRB-related activity.) There are multiple resources available to provide step-by-step assistance for research protocol development (Fraenkel & Wallen, 2000; Gall et al., 1996; Guyatt & Rennie, 2007; Hanson, 2006; Haynes et al., 2005; Linn & Gronlund, 2000).

Avoiding Pitfalls

Published articles have described flaws in simulation-based educational research that could be avoided with careful planning. McGaghie et al. (2006) point to inadequate literature searches (often limited to a single specialty), lack of awareness of research design, inadequate focus on reliability and power, and inconsistent statistical reporting characteristics. Authorship is an important discussion to have early on and to readdress when there are significant personnel changes. Most publications require certification that authors have participated sufficiently in the work, often in multiple phases, including conception and design, data analysis and interpretation, and manuscript drafting and revision.

Issues of intellectual property need to be addressed ideally before the research commences, but definitely at the stage of writing the final report. Some funded research might be carried out for agencies or organizations. Often, the results of the research and the report become the property of the commissioning organization and the report may have to be written in a particular format or for a particular audience, for example to support a government initiative. In addition, some funding organizations require listing the work with regulatory bodies (National Institutes of Health, n.d.).

Dissemination of Findings

There are many possible venues and formats for dissemination of simulation-based research. The major worldwide simulation societies including the Society for Simulation in Healthcare (SSH), the Association of Standardized Patient Educators (ASPE), the Association for Simulated Practice in Healthcare, the International Nursing Association for Clinical Simulation and Learning (INACSL), and the Society in Europe for Simulation Applied to Medicine (SESAM), to name a few, have meetings at which original research and innovations can be presented. In addition, general educational meetings such as the American Nurses Association's (ANA) Annual Quality Conference, the International Nursing Research Congress, and the American Association of Medical College's (AAMC) Research in Medical Education conference are possible venues for presenting original research. Many specialty societies have subgroups or meetings to which education-related research is welcomed. These subspecialty groups often have simulation interest groups from which research networks may grow. See Appendix A for a list of journals that may be interested in simulation education research findings. Kardong-Edgren et al. (2011) also provide a framework for acceptable inquiry.

EXPERT'S CORNER

GETTING STARTED IN SIMULATION-BASED RESEARCH
Joshua Hui, MD, MSCR, FACEP
Chair of Research Committee, Society for Simulation in Healthcare

After reviewing thousands of abstracts and defining selection criteria for scientific content of the International Meeting on Simulation in Healthcare (IMSH), I have a few common observations that I hope will be helpful to those embarking on the journey of simulation-based research.

First, simulation-based research should not be limited to educational-based inquiries. In fact, simulation modalities can be utilized as a valuable research tool to investigate questions that are difficult to answer in real settings because of safety or ethical concerns. For example, simulated scenarios are an excellent way to examine the differences in communication patterns between healthcare professionals of varying personalities, as long as the validity and the reliability of the scenarios and outcome measure are secure. Another example is a case series of root cause analyses through reenacted simulated scenarios for investigating errors in patient care delivery or poor patient outcomes. In fact, if the boundaries of simulation definition are pushed further, agent-based modeling and simulation could be considered to investigate factors that influence patient flow of an emergency department, which indeed has been done.

Second, because simulation research is often measuring educational outcomes, the usage of pre- and posttest study design is prevalent. Even so, simulation researchers should be diligent in considering the limitations of this study design and confounding variables. Some commonly overlooked areas of statistical analysis applicable to simulation studies include clustering effect and repeated measures. Furthermore, different linear and logistic modelings may be useful in addition to the commonly used pair-matched t-test, depending on the study design. For example, the odds ratio of being more "successful" in certain outcome measures after simulation can be calculated using logistic regression models.

Third, simulation-based research has matured beyond the use of simple survey data. Survey data in confidence levels that were very popular in the past are now recognized as a much less substantial form of evidence. These should not be used as sole evidence of the impact of simulation training. Meaningful outcome measures in both clinical and statistical senses must be sought.

Fourth, the value of a well-thought-out and thorough literature search in identifying knowledge gaps to support the merit of the study and its research question cannot be overemphasized. The importance of the literature search is further underscored by the recent growth of published simulation-based research. Remember that no study will ever be perfect in the eyes of reviewers, but lack of novelty is often noted even if the proposed study nears perfection.

Finally, researchers should consider the complexities of study design in correlation to the proposed research question to ensure the study does not exceed the capabilities of the simulation resources and/or scenarios. The fundamental concepts and importance of validity and reliability should receive even more attention and consideration given the limitations of simulation-based research.

BEEN THERE, DONE THAT: HOW CAN I CONTINUE TO IMPROVE OR SUSTAIN WHAT I HAVE ACHIEVED?

Institutions with successful programs and sustained records in publishing educational research have developed a cadre of faculty who have experience and are available to mentor a research team that includes specialists in research design, statistics, and educational theory. In addition, many institutions provide faculty with protected time for scholarly activity and have arranged local seed funding. In some institutions, education fellowships have fostered the conditions that allow for scholarly activity (Thomas et al., 2004).

Research Question Refinement

As suggested by Cook et al., starting with a well-framed question that seeks to answer more than a descriptive question is important. In addition, it will be important for advanced researchers to make sure that clarification studies are done before justification studies, if appropriate (Cook et al., 2008). In addition, recent work describing a new nomenclature for simulation research by Haji et al. might also be helpful when developing research questions. Work by this group supports further refinement of simulation-based medical education research into two subcategories: simulation-based education (SBET) and simulation-augmented education and training (SAET). In SBET, the learner experience occurs in the simulated environment and assessment of outcomes occurs in the simulated setting. In SAET, simulation is integrated with other educational opportunities and the outcomes can be assessed in multiple settings and can include behavior change and/or patient effects (Haji et al., 2013). Additional work has also focused efforts on the importance of evaluating cost of simulation-based research efforts, and a model for accounting and reporting costs has been proposed (Zendejas et al., 2013). Building cost information into future studies is an advanced feature. In addition, advanced researchers might also consider focusing on higher levels of translational science at the T2 or T3 level. T2 research would focus on translating patient level efforts to guidelines. T3 research would involve healthcare delivery or community engagement to produce improvements in the health of individuals and society (McGaghie et al., 2012).

Team Development

Successful research team members can be found outside the program or fostered within the organization. Looking both inside and outside the organization for discipline-specific expertise will likely broaden the pool of available resources. If team members cannot be found, there are training courses on educational research that are available both at simulation society meetings and nationally.

Securing Long-Term Support

It is known that the majority of healthcare educational research is not formally funded (Reed et al., 2005). In addition, the quality of published medical educational research is independently associated with funding ($p < .05$) (Reed et al., 2007). There are multiple possible sources of funding for simulation-based educational research. Often, local institutions will have mechanisms for supporting educational and/or innovative initiatives. In the United States, foundations such as the Josiah Macy, Jr. Foundation, the Kellogg Foundation, and the Robert Wood Johnson foundation have proven records in supporting clinical educational research. Federal funding, although limited, is also available. See Appendix B for suggestions of possible funding sources for simulation educational research.

SECTION 9 • Research

MultiCenter Collaboration

As has been the case in clinical research, the foundation of multicenter research networks will likely be a long-term solution to many of the methodological criticisms of simulation-based medical education. One example of a particularly active group is the INSPIRE—International Network for Simulation-based Pediatric Innovation, Research and Education (www.inspiresim.com). The members of research networks such as these can combine resources and assemble larger samples sizes to address some of the statistical limitations that have been present in research to date (Cheng et al., 2011).

SUMMARY

Case conclusion: The new director decides that he will start with a small mixed methods study. He recruits research partners from across the university including experts in instructional design, statistics, and research tool generation. He schedules weekly research meetings, starts idea generation and a literature search. He also applies for a local innovation grant to support his efforts and makes plans to attend the local research forum.

Research is a rigorous, multifaceted process. That simulation research seeks to measure human performance and technology adds additional complexity to the process. Attention to the statistics of measurement, research question, and hypothesis generation as well as team dynamics is crucial for success. Research in simulation-based education can utilize qualitative, quantitative, or mixed methods. There are myriad resources available to assist with these efforts. However, the basic principles of the research process remain unchanged, and opportunities to add to generalized knowledge are boundless.

REFERENCES

American Educational Research Association, American Psychological Association, & National Council on Measurement in Education. (1999). *Standards for educational and psychological testing.* Washington, DC: American Educational Research Association.

Bandali, K. S., Craig, R., & Ziv, A. (2012). Innovations in applied health: Evaluating a simulation-enhanced, interprofessional curriculum. *Medical Teacher, 34*(3), e176–e184.

Barsuk, J.H., Cohen E.R., Feinglass J., McGaghie W.C., Wayne, D.B. (2009). Use of simulation-based education to reduce catheter-related bloodstream infections. *Archives of Internal Medicine, 169,* 1420–1423.

Brian, H. R. (2006). Forming research questions. *Journal of Clinical Epidemiology, 59,* 881–886.

Cheng, A., Hunt, E. A., Donoghue, A., Nelson, K., Leflore, J., Anderson, J., … Nadkarni, V. (2011). EXPRESS—examining pediatric resuscitation education using simulation and scripting: The birth of an international pediatric simulation research collaborative—from concept to reality. *Simulation in Healthcare, 6,* 34–41.

Cook, D. A., Bordage, G., & Schmidt, H. G. (2008). Description, justification and clarification: A framework for classifying the purposes of research in medical education. *Medical Education, 42,* 128–133.

Creswell, J. W. (2009). *Educational research: Planning, conducting and evaluating quantitative and qualitative research* (3rd ed.). Upper Saddle River, NJ: Merrill.

Denzin, N., & Lincoln, Y. (1994). *Handbook of qualitative research.* Thousand Oaks, CA: SAGE.

Deutsch, E. S., Orioles, A., Kreicher, K., Malloy, K. M., & Rodgers, D. L. (2013). A qualitative analysis of faculty motivation to participate in otolaryngology simulation boot camps. *The Laryngoscope, 123*(4), 890–897.

Downing, S. M. (2003). Validity: On the meaningful interpretation of assessment data. *Medical Education, 37,* 830–837.

Downing, S. M. (2004). Reliability: On the reproducibility of assessment data. *Medical Education, 38,* 1006–1012.

Fraenkel, J. R., & Wallen, N. E. (2000). *How to design and evaluate research in education* (4th ed.). Boston, MA: McGraw Hill.

Gall, M. D., Borg, W. R., & Gall, J. P. (1996). *Educational research: An introduction* (6th ed.). White Plains, NY: Longman.

Guyatt, G., & Rennie, D. (2007). *User's guide to medical research: A manual for evidence-based clinical practice* (3rd ed.). Chicago, IL: AMA Press Printing.

Haji, F. A., Hoppe, D. J., Morin, M. P., Giannoulakis, K., Koh, J., Rojas, D., & Cheung, J. J. H. (2013). What we call what we do affects how we do it: A new nomenclature for simulation research in medical education. *Advances in Health Sciences Education, 19*(2), 273–280.

Hanson, B. P. (2006). Designing, conducting and reporting clinical research: a step-by-step approach. *Injury, 37*(7), 583–594.

Haynes, R. B., Sackett, D. L., Guyatt, G. H., & Tugwell, P. (2005). *Clinical epidemiology: How to do clinical practice research* (3rd ed.). New York, NY: Lippincott Williams & Wilkins.

Huggett, K. N., Gusic, M. E., Greenberg, R., & Ketterer, J. M. (2011). Twelve tips for conducting collaborative research in medical education. *Medical Teacher, 33*(9), 713–718.

Hulley, S. B. (2007). Conceiving the research question. In S. B. Hulley, S. R. Cummings, W. S. Browner, D. G. Grady, & T. B. Newman (Eds.), *Designing clinical research* (3rd ed.). Baltimore, MD: Williams & Wilkins.

Johnson, R. B., & Christensen, L. B. (2010). *Educational research: Quantitative, qualitative, and mixed approaches* (4th ed.). Thousand Oaks, CA: SAGE.

Kane, M. T. (2006). Validation. In R. L. Brennan (Ed.), *Educational measurement* (4th ed., pp. 17–64). Westport, CT: Praeger.

Kardong-Edgren, S., Gaba, D., Dieckman, P., & Cook, D. A. (2011). Reporting inquiry in simulation. *Simulation in Healthcare, 6*(7), S63–S66.

Kazdin, A. E. (1995). *Methodological issues and strategies in clinical research.* Washington, DC: American Psychological Association.

Krupat, E. (2010). A call for more RCTs (research that is conceptual and thoughtful). *Medical Education, 44*(9), 852–855.

Lincol, Y. S., & Guba, E. G. (1985). *Naturalistic inquiry.* Newbury Park, CA: SAGE.

Linn, R. L., & Gronlund, N. E. (2000). *Measurement and assessment in teaching* (8th ed.). Upper Saddle River, NY: Merrill, Prentice Hall.

Maggio, L. A., Tannery, N. H., & Kanter, S. L. (2011). Reproducibility of literature search reporting in medical education reviews. *Academic Medicine, 86,* 1049–1054.

McGaghie, W. C., Issenberg, S. B., Cohen, E. R., Barsuk, J. H., & Wayne, D. B. (2012). Translational educational research: A necessity for effective health-care improvement. *Chest, 142*(5), 1097–1103.

McGaghie, W. C., Issenberg, S. B., Petrusa, E. R., & Scalese, R. J. (2006). Effect of practice on standardized learning outcomes in simulation-based medical education. *Medical Education, 40*(8), 792–797.

Messick, S. (1989). Validity. In R. L. Linn (Ed.), *Educational measurement* (3rd ed., pp. 13–103). New York, NY: American Council on Education & Macmillan.

National Institutes of Health. (n.d.). *Public access policy.* Retrieved from http://publicaccess.nih.gov/citation_methods.htm

Oxford English Dictionary (Online ed.). (2013). Retrieved from http://oxforddictionaries.com/us/definition/american_english/research?q=research

Reed, D. A., Cook, D. A., Beckman, T. J., Levine, R. B., Kern, D. E., & Wright, S. M. (2007). Association between funding and quality of published medical education research. *Journal of the American Medical Association, 298*(9), 1002–1009.

Reed, D. A., Kern, D. E., Levine, R. B., & Wright, S. M. (2005). Costs and funding for published medical education research. *Journal of the American Medical Association, 294*(9), 1052–1057.

Schifferdecker, K. E., & Reed, V. A. (2009). Using mixed methods research in medical education: Basic guidelines for researchers. *Medical Education, 43*, 637–644.

Schroedl, C. J., Corbridge, T. C., Cohen, E. R., Fakhran, S. S., Schimmel, D., McGaghie, W. C., . . . Kane-Gill, S. L. (2012). Simulation-based learning versus problem-based learning in an acute care pharmacotherapy course. *Simulation in Healthcare, 7*(3), 162–165.

Seybert, J.A., & Weed, E. (2012). Benchmarking in Higher Education. In C. Secolsky (Ed.), *Measurement, assessment, and evaluation in higher education*. New York, NY: Routledge.

Shrader, S., Kern, D., Zoller, J., & Blue, A. (2013). Interprofessional teamwork skills as predictors of clinical outcomes in a simulated healthcare setting. *Journal of Allied Health, 42*(1), 1–6.

Strauss, A. L., & Corbin, J. M. (1999). *Basics of qualitative research: Grounded theory procedures and techniques*. Newberry Park, CA: SAGE.

Sullivan, G. M. (2011). Getting off the "gold standard": Randomized controlled trials and education research. *Journal of Graduate Medical Education, 3*(3), 285–289.

Thomas, P., Wright, S. M., & Kern, D. E. (2004). Education research at Johns Hopkins University School of Medicine: A grassroots development. *Academic Medicine, 79*(10), 975–980.

Watling, C. J., & Lingard, L. (2012). Grounded theory in medical education research: AMEE guide no. 70. *Medical Teacher, 34*, 850–861.

Wayne, D. B., Butter, J., Siddall, V. J., Fudala, M. J., Linquist, L. A., Feinglass, J., . . . McGaghie, W. C. (2005). Simulation-based training of internal medicine residents in advanced cardiac life support protocols: A randomized trial. *Teaching and Learning in Medicine, 17*(3), 210–216.

Yarris, L. M., Gruppen, L. D., Hamstra, S. J., Anders Ericsson, K., & Cook, D. A. (2012). Overcoming barriers to addressing education problems with research design: A panel discussion. *Academic Emergency Medicine, 19*(12), 1344–1349.

Zendejas, B., Wang, A. T., Brydges, R., Hamstra, S. J., & Cook, D. A. (2013). Cost: The missing outcome in simulation-based medical education research: A systematic review. *Surgery, 153*(2), 160–176.

APPENDIX A

Simulation, Teaching, and Subject-Specific Journals

Simulation Journals

The Journal for the Society of Simulation in Healthcare, http://journals.lww.com/simulationinhealthcare/pages/default.aspx

Clinical Simulation in Nursing, http://www.nursingsimulation.org

Teaching Journals

The following is a list of selected journals that accept submissions on educational research and innovations.

Academic Medicine, http://www.academicmedicine.org/

BMC Medical Education, http://www.biomedcentral.com/bmcmededuc/

Clinical Teacher, http://www.wiley.com/bw/submit.asp?ref=1743-4971&site=1

Education for Health: Change in Learning and Practice, www.educationforhealth.net

Journal of Continuing Education in the Health Professions, http://www.jcehp.com/

Journal of the International Association of Medical Science Educators, http://www.jiamse.org/

MedEdWorld, www.mededworld.org

MedEdPORTAL, http://services.aamc.org/30/mededportal/servlet/segment/mededportal/information/

Medical Education, http://www.mededuc.com/

Medical Education Online (MEO), http://www.med-ed-online.org/

Medical Teacher, http://www.medicalteacher.org/

Teaching and Learning in Medicine, http://www.siumed.edu/tlm/

Subject-Specific Journals

The following is a list of selected journals, listed by subject area, that frequently include articles on educational research and innovations in their respective discipline.

Anatomy: *The Anatomical Record: Advances in Integrative Anatomy and Evolutionary Biology,* http://www.wiley.com/WileyCDA/WileyTitle/productCd-AR.html

Clinical Anatomy, http://www.wiley.com/WileyCDA/WileyTitle/productCd-CA.html

Anesthesiology: *Anesthesiology,* http://journals.lww.com/anesthesiology/pages/default.aspx

Emergency Medicine: *Academic Emergency Medicine,* http://www.wiley.com/bw/journal.asp?ref=1069-6563

Family Medicine: *Family Medicine,* http://www.stfm.org/publications/familymedicine/index.cfm

Geriatrics and Gerontology: *Educational Gerontology,* http://www.tandf.co.uk/journals/authors/uedgauth.asp

Journal of the American Geriatrics Society, http://www.wiley.com/bw/journal.asp?ref=0002-8614&site=1

POGOe (Portal of Geriatric On-Line Education), http://www.pogoe.org

The Gerontologist, http://gerontologist.oxfordjournals.org/

Health Sciences: *Advances in Health Sciences Education,* http://www.springer.com/education/journal/10459?detailsPage=contentItemPage&CIPageCounter=138305

Internal Medicine: *American Journal of Medicine,* http://www.amjmed.com/

Annals of Internal Medicine, http://www.annals.org/

British Medical Journal, http://bmj.bmjjournals.com

Journal of the American Medical Association, http://pubs.ama-assn.org/

Journal of Evaluation in Clinical Practice, http://www.wiley.com/bw/journal.asp?ref=1356-1294

Journal of General Internal Medicine, http://www.springer.com/medicine/internal/journal/11606

Journal of the Royal Society of Medicine, http://jrsm.rsmjournals.com/

Lancet, http://www.thelancet.com

New England Journal of Medicine, http://authors.nejm.org/help/NewMs.asp

Southern Medical Journal, http://journals.lww.com/smajournalonline/pages/default.aspx

Medical Ethics: *Journal of Medical Ethics,* http://jme.bmj.com/

Medical Informatics: *Journal of the American Medical Informatics Association,* http://www.jamia.org/

Medical Informatics and the Internet in Medicine, http://www.ingentaconnect.com/content/14639238

Neurology: *Neurology,* http://www.neurology.org/

Nutrition: *American Journal of Clinical Nutrition,* http://www.ajcn.org/

OB-GYN: *American Journal of Obstetrics and Gynecology*, http://www.ajog.org/

Oncology: *Journal of Cancer Education*, http://www.informaworld.com/smpp/title~content=t775653660~db=all

Palliative Care: *American Journal of Hospice and Palliative Care*, http://ajh.sagepub.com/

Journal of Palliative Medicine, http://www.liebertpub.com/products/product.aspx?pid=41

Pediatrics: *Academic Pediatrics*, http://www.journals.elsevier.com/academic-pediatrics/

Pediatrics, http://pediatrics.aappublications.org/

Pharmacy: *Journal of Pharmacy Teaching*, [EBSCO; no public website]

Physiology: *Advances in Physiology Education*, http://advan.physiology.org/

Preventive Medicine: *American Journal of Preventive Medicine*, http://www.ajpm-online.net/

Primary Care: *Education for Primary Care*, http://www.radcliffe-oxford.com/journals/J02_Education_for_Primary_Care/

Psychiatry: *Academic Psychiatry*, http://ap.psychiatryonline.org/

Radiology: *Academic Radiology*, http://www.academicradiology.org/

Rehabilitation Medicine: *American Journal of Physical Medicine and Rehabilitation*, http://journals.lww.com/ajpmr/pages/default.aspx

Rheumatology: *Journal of Rheumatology*, http://www.jrheum.org/

Surgery: *American Journal of Surgery*, http://americanjournalofsurgery.com/

Journal of Surgical Research, http://www.journalofsurgicalresearch.com/

Urology: *Journal of Urology*, http://www.jurology.com/

Nursing Journals

Nurse Educator, http://journals.lww.com/nurseeducatoronline/pages/default.aspx

Journal of Nursing Education, http://www.healio.com/journals/JNE

Nursing Education in Practice, http://www.journals.elsevier.com/nurse-education-in-practice/

Nursing Education Perspectives, http://www.nlnjournal.org/

Journal for Nurses in Professional Development, http://journals.lww.com/jnsdonline/pages/default.aspx

Journal of Clinical Nursing, http://onlinelibrary.wiley.com/journal/10.1111/(ISSN)1365-2702

Journal of Forensic Nursing, http://journals.lww.com/forensicnursing/pages/default.aspx

Journal of Perinatal and Neonatal Nursing, http://journals.lww.com/jpnnjournal/pages/default.aspx

MedSurg Nursing, http://www.medsurgnursing.net/cgi-bin/WebObjects/MSNJournal.woa

Critical Care Nurse, http://ccn.aacnjournals.org/

Journal of Emergency Nursing, http://www.jenonline.org/

International Emergency Nursing, http://www.journals.elsevier.com/international-emergency-nursing/

Journal of Pediatric Nursing, http://www.pediatricnursing.org/

Journal of Gerontological Nursing, http://www.healio.com/journals/jgn

Miscellaneous Healthcare Education Journals

American Journal of Respiratory and Critical Care Medicine, http://www.atsjournals.org/journal/ajrccm

Canadian Journal of Respiratory Therapy, http://www.csrt.com/en/publications/journal.asp

Journal of Allied Health, http://www.ingentaconnect.com/content/asahp/jah

Journal of Interprofessional Care, http://informahealthcare.com/jic

Australian Journal of Physiotherapy, http://www.physiotherapy.asn.au/jop

Australian Occupational Therapy Journal, http://www.otaus.com.au/about/australian-occupational-therapy-journal

Social Work in Health Care, http://www.tandfonline.com/toc/wshc20/current

International Journal of Speach-Language Pathology, http://informahealthcare.com/journal/asl

Canadian Journal of Occupational Therapy, http://www.caot.ca/default.asp?pageid=6

Journal of Research in Interprofessional Practice and Education, http://www.jripe.org/index.php/journal/index

APPENDIX B

Possible Sources of Funding for Simulation-Based Research

Agency for Healthcare Research and Quality (AHRQ) Grants, http://www.ahrq.gov/fund/grantix.htm

Arnold P. Gold Foundation, http://humanism-in-medicine.org/index.php/programs_grants

Arthur Vining Davis Foundations, http://www.avdf.org/FoundationsPrograms/HealthCare.aspx

Association for Surgical Education Foundation (an arm of the Association for Surgical Education (ASE), which awards grants in its CESERT program—Center for Excellence in Surgical Education, Research and Training), http://www.surgicaleducation.com/mc/page.do?sitePageId=28551&orgId=ase

AstraZeneca Medical Education Research Grants, http://www.astrazenecagrants.com/

Fund for the Improvement of Postsecondary Education (FIPSE), http://www2.ed.gov/about/offices/list/ope/fipse/index.html

The Henry J. Kaiser Family Foundation, http://www.kff.org/

HRSA—U. S. Department of Health and Human Services, http://www.hrsa.gov/

National Institutes of Health, http://grants1.nih.gov/grants/index.cfm

NIH NCRR Science Education Partnership Award (SEPA) (R25), http://grants.nih.gov/grants/guide/pa-files/PAR-10-206.html

NBME Stemmler Medical Education Research Fund, http://www.nbme.org/research/stemmler.html

NSF Directorate for Education and Human Resources, http://www.nsf.gov/dir/index.jsp?org=EHR

The PEW Charitable Trust, http://www.pewtrusts.com/

Pfizer Medical Education Grants, http://www.pfizer.com/responsibility/grants_contributions/medical_education_grants.jsp

RSNA Foundation Radiology Education Grants, http://rsna.org

The Robert Wood Johnson Foundation, http://www.rwjf.org/index.jsp

Society for Academic Continuing Medical Education Research Grants in Continuing Medical Education, http://www.sacme.org/SACME_grants

CHAPTER 9.2

Simulation Research Considerations

Suzan E. Kardong-Edgren, PhD, RN, ANEF, CHSE, Peter Dieckmann, PhD, and James C. Phero, DMD

ABOUT THE AUTHORS

SUZAN E. KARDONG-EDGREN is a nurse researcher who concentrates on the use of technology to improve health professions education. Dr. Edgren is the Editor-in-Chief of *Clinical Simulation in Nursing.* Dr. Edgren cochaired the IMSH annual meeting in 2012 in Orlando. She currently holds the Jody De Meyer Endowed Chair in Nursing at Boise State University.

PETER DIECKMANN is a psychologist and head of research at the Danish Institute for Medical Simulation (DIMS), Copenhagen, Denmark. His research focuses on understanding simulation as a social practice, trying to optimize the interplay of concepts and technology. He also investigates human factors and organizational processes in simulation. He is the Past President of the Society in Europe for Simulation Applied to Medicine (SESAM) and cochaired the IMSH annual meeting in 2011 in New Orleans. Peter is an Associate Editor of the Journal *Simulation in Healthcare.*

JAMES C. PHERO serves as anesthesia attending faculty at The University of Cincinnati (UC) Medical Center. As Professor Emeritus of Anesthesiology, UC College of Medicine (UCCOM), he coordinates anesthesiology simulation and the Karl Storz Airway Center of Excellence. He is President of The International Federation of Dental Anesthesia Societies and Past President of The American Dental Society of Anesthesiology. Active on the SSH Research Committee, he cochaired the 2011 SSH Simulation Research Consensus Summit.

ABSTRACT

Drawing from seminal articles on the topic, this chapter provides researchers with a comprehensive overview of suggestions related to the use of simulation in health care. Ideas for research studies, theoretical models to help guide and strengthen research questions and concepts, building a research team, designing a study, recruiting subjects, interacting with Institutional Review Boards, resources for locating evaluation instruments with reliability and validity, and, finally, planning for publication of final results are presented. Novice researchers are more likely to produce a meaningful study if these ideas are addressed during the planning phase. Experienced researchers interested in developing a new program of research will find references and recommendations for entering the field.

CASE EXAMPLE

As new simulation faculty run multiple simulations, they begin to wonder about the best way to debrief participants to encourage maximum learning and retention. The faculty members involved in simulation activities search the literature and find some information, but many questions remain. At the same time, the school administrator is meeting with the Director of the Simulation Center and discussing her desire for the faculty to increase scholarly output and enhance the name and reputation of the simulation center. What to do? Are there activities that will contribute to addressing all of these issues? Perhaps there are. Conducting a high-quality research study and presenting findings at a conference is one way to meet this goal.

INTRODUCTION AND BACKGROUND

The capabilities and advantages of healthcare simulation are drawing the interest of both novice and experienced researchers to the field. Healthcare simulation is evolving rapidly, so there are many areas of research virtually untouched and crucial to further developing the science. The reviews of early simulation research and reporting indicate that the work was often not well done and would benefit from increased rigor (Cook et al., 2007; McGaghie et al., 2010).

Seeking to provide direction to individuals interested in conducting timely, high-quality simulation research studies, several seminal articles were produced. In 2008, "Simulation task force, the use of simulation in emergency medicine: A research agenda" was published in *Academic Emergency Medicine* (Gordon & Vozenilek, 2008). In 2011, "Setting a research agenda for simulation-based healthcare education: A synthesis of the outcome from an Utstein style meeting" was published in *Simulation in Healthcare* (Issenberg et al., 2011); and it provided a review of simulation science along with ideas for future research. In 2011, the Society for Simulation in Healthcare (SSH) held the first Research Consensus Summit on simulation in healthcare and published the results of that summit as a **monograph** in *Simulation in Healthcare* 2011. These articles help provide a blueprint for simulation researchers.

RESEARCH THE IDEA

Based on individual skills and interests, literature reviews, available resources, and experience, the research team will decide what study or series of studies is most reasonable to pursue. It is useful to get ideas of the "burning questions" of the day. There are a number of resources readily available that will provide ideas for the research team to consider. For example, in the 2011 SSH monograph on *Simulation Research*, Issenberg et al. (2011) provide a research agenda with proposed research questions grouped into three major themes: instructional design, translational research, and outcome studies. McGaghie et al. (2010) list research ideas and questions around 12 features and best practices of simulation. Additionally, the Society for Academic Medicine Simulation Task Force formulated research questions for consideration by all researchers (Bond et al., 2007).

Once the topic for research has been identified, the next step is completing a thorough literature review to assess the extent of what is known about this topic. Unfortunately, history has shown that "All too often the gap in knowledge that a study purports to close is actually the gap in the author's own knowledge base" (Gennaro, 2010). Searching the **grey literature** (defined by Polit and Beck, 2008, as "unpublished and less readily accessible research reports") may provide additional useful information. Search ProQuest for recently completed dissertations, journal databases, including CINAHL, ERIC, MEDLINE, PSYCHINFO, Science Direct, and simulation society websites. Consider expanding the literature search beyond a reliance on what may seem to be logical keywords. This will help in gathering all the citations that may be important to address the research question. To do this, scan the references of the articles you have already retrieved looking for other leads. Check the keywords listed with these articles for additional suggestions that you might not have been considered. Also, check simulation and topic related journals for their **in press articles**. These articles, typically listed on the journal's online website, are proofed and ready for publication when their turn in the queue arises. Abstract collections and proceedings of meetings can provide ideas about what work is in progress. Many of these abstracts will eventually appear in fully published formats. Finally, you can review monographs for discussions of needed research such as the SSH's Utstein monograph on research in simulation (Issenberg et al., 2011).

USE A THEORETICAL FRAMEWORK

Failing to use an identifiable theory to guide a research study is one of the most significant gaps in the science of simulation identified during the 2011 SSH Research Summit. Using a theoretical foundation "increases the cohesion of the research and builds a logical foundation for the discipline" (Nestel et al., 2011). It is possible to decide on a theoretical perspective and then build a program of research *around* this perspective; however, a simulation-focused research team has yet to report using this approach.

The following are among the more commonly used theoretical frameworks found in the simulation literature: Experiential Learning (Schön, 1983), "Thinking on Action" (Benner, 1984), "Thinking in Action" and "Novice to Expert" (Dewey & McDermott, 1973), Functional Psychology (Knowles, 1980), **Andragogy** (Vygotsky, 1962), Social Development and Cognition (Bandura, 1986; Schaefer et al., 2011, p. S32), Social Learning (Ericsson, 2004), Deliberate Practice for Expertise Development (Fitts & Posner, 1967), and Skill Learning, (Arthur et al., 1998; Schmidt & Lee, 2005). Other frameworks include Skills Decay and Retention (Kirschner, 2002), **Cognitive Load Theory** (Paas et al., 2003; van Merriënboer & Sweller, 2005), Situated Cognition (Onda, 2012; Paige & Daley, 2009) and Stress Inoculation (Meichenbaum, 1985).

An often-used framework for simulation-based education is the National League for Nursing—Jeffries Simulation Framework (Jeffries, 2005). An in-depth review of each of the Jeffries constructs in which further research needs were identified was completed in 2012 and published online in 2013 in *Clinical Simulation in Nursing*. As part of this project, Groom et al. (2014) provide research ideas for simulation design characteristics; Hallmark et al. (2014) provide research ideas in educational practices (see chapter 7.2 on Theory).

Each theory supplies an abundance of terms, definitions, and propositions around which to build a research study. Ensuring that all team members know, adopt, and use the same theoretical framework and terminology will help the team move forward in an efficient and effective manner. Seeking out and examining other studies that have used the same theory you have selected will often provide ideas and lessons that will be useful for your study.

CONSIDER THE DISTINCTION: RESEARCH *ON* SIMULATION OR RESEARCH *WITH* SIMULATION

Research and simulation may be linked in at least two different ways. The first way involves conducting research *on* simulation. The second involves conducting research with simulation. Research on simulation involves investigating simulation as a method. Such research *on* simulation makes simulation the object of the research. Research *with* simulation occurs when simulation is used as a method to investigate other research objects of interest (Dieckmann et al., 2011). In research on simulation, the aim is to refine the knowledge about simulation and its uses. One might say that simulation is the research object or dependent variable. In research with simulation, simulation is used to investigate another research object (e.g. actions of fatigued nurses). In this case, simulation is part of the research method or the independent variable. The assumption is made, however, when conducting research with simulation, that the research team knows enough about simulation to conduct simulation well.

Examples of research questions on simulation include:

- What are characteristics of effective debriefings (Raemer et al., 2011)?
- Which abilities should simulation facilitators have, when working with consultant-level participants?
- How can scenarios be best adapted to the various levels of learner abilities (Dieckmann et al., 2010)?

Examples of research questions using simulation as a method to investigate (research with simulation) include:

- Under what conditions would participants not execute an intention they formed earlier (Dieckmann et al., 2006)?
- How well do fatigued nurses follow the admission procedure of an emergency patient?
- Which pieces of patient information are prone to omission in handover situations (Manser, 2011)?

CONSIDER A HOT TOPIC—FOR EXAMPLE, TEAM TRAINING OR INTERPROFESSIONAL EDUCATION

Team training and interprofessional education using various simulation methodologies are emerging as important trends in the healthcare literature. (See chapter 2.4 for a more detailed discussion of Team Training). Emerging trends such as these provide opportunities for research. It is expected that published studies will be described well enough that another researcher could replicate the study to verify the results or apply the intervention to other populations or under different conditions. For example, there are papers that describe teamwork in ways that could be used to generate research ideas (Manser, 2011; Manser et al., 2009). These papers point to the importance of considering what is happening between the lines: what happens not only within the thoughts of people but also in the interactions between people. Members of different healthcare disciplines, often working in silos, will have different norms, values, and beliefs, which would need to be aligned, to some extent, to optimize the collaboration. Simulation could be used to analyze the variations of such norms, values, and beliefs or to explore how they might be influenced (Flin et al., 2013).

Other knowledge gaps related to team training and interprofessional education that could benefit from further research efforts include the optimal approach to assess the need for team training (Eppich et al., 2011), the most reliable and valid tools for team evaluations (Arnold et al., 2009; Okuyama et al., 2011; Sharma et al., 2011), understanding how in situ training compared with training at a simulation education center impacts educational and patient outcomes, and the effect of using clinicians versus nonclinicians as debriefers and facilitators.

THE RESEARCH TEAM APPROACH

A team-based approach often works well when novice researchers are developing a study. Planning and conducting a research study becomes more productive and fulfilling when using the team approach. Starting with individuals from several disciplines and then expanding the team as additional areas are identified provides synergy. Commonly, more ideas will be generated and a better research design results when a team is involved. This is especially true when the team manages to use the differences among its members to complement each other—for example, when the introverts keep on questioning the foundational thought behind the extroverts' actions, which, conversely, keeps the momentum moving forward. (See http://www.amazon.com/Quiet-Power-Introverts-World-Talking/dp/0307352153/)

Researchers at medical centers or larger health-related universities have access to individuals from a variety of disciplines, making the establishment of a multidisciplinary research team less challenging. Researchers based at smaller or stand-alone universities without multiple health professions programs will have to be creative to find other disciplines beneficial to their study design, for example: psychologists, human factors specialists, engineers, a methods consultant, social workers, physical therapists, pharmacists, communications experts, or exercise physiologists.

RESEARCH IN SIMULATION

Pamela R. Jeffries, PhD, RN, FAAN, ANEF
President, Society for Simulation in Healthcare (2014)

With the increased use of simulations in both academic and practice settings, there are extensive opportunities for research to be conducted in these healthcare arenas. Compared with the past, there are more evidence-based procedures using simulations being disseminated in the literature in addition to more descriptive studies on how to integrate clinical simulations into the healthcare curricula. Contemporary research topics include comparing or contrasting of different debriefing models, specific learning outcomes of a simulation activity, such as end-of-life care, discomfort of the learner, pain management, and various other concepts related to simulations. There continue to be many unexplored areas of research when using the simulation pedagogy that need to be studied, analyzed, and synthesized. Areas of further exploration could include evaluating the process, the learning outcomes, and the translational component regarding what is being learned in simulations that can make a difference in the quality of patient care and outcomes. To think about the research in simulations I have categorized research areas into *three categories* that can provide a few examples of underexplored areas.

PROCESS-BASED RESEARCH IN SIMULATIONS

Research questions focusing on the process of creating and implementing the simulations and debriefing may include a few of the following:

- Should learners have prework prior to coming to simulation lab/clinical so the time in simulations can be better utilized and a higher order of learning can take place? Having the preparation of content knowledge and skills, the focus could then be on the application and synthesis.
- Can virtual simulations be used as a prelearning methodology to foster a better learning and clinical performance opportunity when immersing learners and new graduates into the simulation environment?
- Do students learn from developing and creating their own clinical scenarios when information is provided? Is this an effective learning strategy?
- With the various types of debriefing methodologies, which one is the most effective? Does it matter which method is used?
- What are key criteria to establish to identify when a clinical event or activity would best be learned in a simulation environment?
- For which scenarios should we develop simulations—what are the key indicators?

LEARNING OUTCOMES FROM THE SIMULATION ACTIVITY

Research questions focusing on the learning outcomes of the simulation activity or event should be considered to ensure the activity is meeting the needs of the participant and used as the clinical educator intended. Research questions may include the following:

- When developing clinical simulations for a specific outcome, for example, effective communication, teamwork, or pain management, are the outcomes being achieved effectively and efficiently?
- Can we develop simulations to achieve more than one or two outcomes without creating too much complexity and overloading the participant(s)?
- How can the learning outcomes best be measured in a simulation?
- Is most of the learning occurring in the debriefing? How do we measure that?

TRANSLATION OF KNOWLEDGE, SKILLS, AND ATTITUDES TO THE CLINICAL ARENA IN OUR PATIENT CARE ENVIRONMENTS

Research questions focusing on the translation of knowledge, skills, and attitudes learned in simulation to the clinical arena are important considerations to add value to the simulation activities and the use of this pedagogy. Research questions may include the following:

- Are the knowledge, skills, and outcomes obtained in clinical simulation in the clinical lab and/or simulation center being transferred to the real clinical setting as the learner transitions to practice?
- When new graduates/practitioners learn a skill, behavior, or a plan of care in a simulation, are the skills, behaviors, and/or care model retained when practicing in the clinical environment?
- What are the best methods to measure the transference of knowledge, skills, and attitudes from the clinical simulation environment to real-world practice?
- How long are skills retained from a simulation before there is skill decay and a refresher is needed?
- Should the deliberative practice model be considered as the gold standard when teaching skills through simulations to novice practitioners and learners?
- What role do simulations play in practicing and retaining critical competencies of our healthcare providers? How often should skills be performed before decay occurs?

As one can see, there are numerous research questions that can be asked when studies are conducted to increase our evidence-base and contribution to the science of simulation pedagogy. Research studies need rigor, a strong theoretical foundation, and reliable, valid instruments to measure the outcomes and accomplishments of the simulation participants. Research studies should combine the focus interest of the researcher with the current state of the science. Creating research teams can enrich and expand the scientific studies in the area of simulations.

The role of the **principal investigator** (PI) is important and carries additional responsibility that cannot be delegated to others. Ultimately, the PI is responsible for the study design, the filing of all paperwork, reports, and manuscripts, the budget and its allocation, and the behavior of team members, including research assistants. If you are unclear about the responsibilities associated with the PI role or other roles, consult your local Office of Research or Institutional Review Board (IRB) for clarification.

It is wise to include an experienced statistician and/or methods consultant (qualitative or quantitative) from the beginning of study deliberations. The presence of an experienced statistician or methods person during the planning of a research design optimizes the quality of the research. These individuals will assist with data collection ideas the other members of the team might miss, and help prevent costly mistakes throughout the study process.

The optimal team size will vary depending on the specific research question, the research design, the experiences of each team member, and potential for schedule difficulties. The inclusion of undergraduate or graduate students can be a plus if the team has the time to mentor these student activities properly. Depending on the study design, consider adding a qualitative researcher to the team. There is limited qualitative work in simulation research currently, which makes this an important area for exploration (see chapter 9.1 for further information on qualitative research).

In addition to using a team approach, research groups frequently benefit from the use of experienced researchers from other institutions who serve as consultants. Consultants bring expertise in a subject area or in research methods. They can provide important perspectives and experiences to help season and support a relatively new research team. An experienced consultant researcher may save the team from inadvertently incorporating design flaws that can result in not receiving funding or in manuscript rejection.

In some cases, a researcher is alone with no one to help develop or implement a research project. In this situation, it is wise to access all the resources possible, including textbooks on study design. Being careful to adhere to standard research methodology and following the steps of the research process can produce a credible result. While there is nothing magical about conducting research, it is all too easy to miss key steps along the way while experience is being gained.

RESEARCH STUDY PLANNING: HOW TO BEGIN

After reading extensively to see what others have done on a chosen topic, it is time to sit down and plan. Form the research question, aims, purpose, and hypotheses on the basis of the literature review. When defining key terms, it is best to use well-accepted nomenclature and operational definitions. The use of standardized definitions such as those outlined by SSH or **INACSL** (INACSL Board of Directors, 2011) maximizes understanding and allows comparisons across studies. Once the team has decided on terminology, make sure to use the words and definitions consistently to minimize confusion.

An excellent website to assist with planning and reporting a study is http://www.equator-network.org/. Using the reporting guidelines found on this site, you can work backward to create a solid framework for building your study.

Some simulation researchers opt to start their research efforts with a descriptive study. According to Burns and Grove (2009, p. 237), descriptive studies are used to gain information about characteristics within a field, to identify problems within current practice, justify current practice, make judgments, or determine what others in similar situations are doing. In a descriptive study, variables are not manipulated, nor is there a specific treatment or intervention applied. Descriptive study designs can use either quantitative or qualitative methodologies or a combination of both. The term **triangulation** describes the use of multiple methods within a study in order to increase the credibility of the research by obtaining data from various perspectives (see chapter 9.1). The results from descriptive studies can provide fertile ground on which to build a series of studies.

Another starting point for a novice group of researchers is to duplicate a well-done study with a different group of participants or in a different environment. Schaefer et al. (2011) provided a list of well-designed experiments that might be duplicated. If you are considering replicating a study, it is important to check the stated limitations in the published report. The original researchers will often provide information about what they would do differently or what compromises they had to make in their study. These researchers may also provide advice about how to avoid their errors or how to improve the study. When well done, these studies can be used as roadmaps in designing your own well-planned study.

Many past studies in simulation have been underpowered, meaning the number of people or observations (also known as sample size) was insufficient to answer the research question(s). However, the means and standard deviations from their findings may permit you to determine the appropriate number of participants needed to achieve statistically meaningful results in a replication study. Repeating a previously published study as closely as possible may permit pooling the new findings with the prior study, thus creating a larger data set for more robust statistical analyses. Having the assistance of an appropriately qualified statistician is important for all research studies. Nowhere is it more important than when you are considering combining or comparing data sets across studies.

Determining an appropriate sample size for a specific research study is a statistical question. Acquiring an adequate sample is a logistical challenge. To achieve the requisite sample size, you may need to consider collaborating with another school or program. A secondary benefit of working with another center is that multisite studies are in favor with funding groups at present.

If you are dealing with a significant number of subjects, maintaining a log of activities can be problematic. You may want to consider using a tracking document similar to the one found on the Consolidated Standards of Reporting Trials (**CONSORT**) website (see http://www.consort-statement. org/consort-statement/flow-diagram). Tools such as these track how many participants were recruited and/or lost at each stage of the study and why. Another idea to jumpstart research in simulation is to consider using existing but previously unused archived materials. Scerbo et al. (2011) recommend feeding all the data collected into a retrievable and standardized system for potential use in other future research. The Medical University of South Carolina is saving all simulation in recorded digital files, in hopes that they will be usable in the future for doctoral students and their research (John Schaefer, personal communication). O'Shea et al. (2013) used archived student scenarios in obstetrics and pediatric rotations to evaluate communication. In an interesting twist, they included a graduate student from their department of communications in their data analysis team.

Do not be afraid to contact a study author. Authors are often flattered to be contacted for specific questions about repeating a study. It may also be possible to ask them to consult on a study design. The worst thing that can happen is that the researcher might say no. However, it is more likely that you will find an enthusiastic collaborator or consultant who will have the opportunity to build on their previous study through others.

What about doing a pilot study? Performing a pilot study helps verify design methodology and gather preliminary data. In addition, having pilot data often makes a study more competitive when competing for grant funding.

Randomization of subjects solves many problems in research design, as all participants have an equal chance of being assigned to the experimental or the control group. While this strengthens the results considerably, it is often impractical. Simulation research is often conducted on a floor of a hospital where the option of not training certain personnel is not possible or ethical. In academic research, the research team may have access only to convenience samples of readily available but preformed clinical groups.

The team should think carefully about where the study will be conducted and how the location might impact study design and results. Some projects are best done in situ, while some are better done in the simulation center (see chapter 2.2 for ideas on in situ simulation).

QUALITATIVE RESEARCH AND MIXED-METHODS STUDIES

Qualitative methodologies provide rich data that cannot be captured with quantitative research techniques. Qualitative rigor is derived from the philosophical stance used to determine the research questions, the data collection methods used, the thoroughness of the data collection (known as reaching saturation—the point where no new information is being uncovered), and, finally, the data analysis methods used. For a full explanation of all types of qualitative studies, see http://www.equator-network.org/resource-centre/library-of-health-research-reporting/reporting-guidelines/qualitative-research/. For examples of qualitative simulation research, see Reid-Searl et al. (2012) and Kelly and Fry (2013). When using qualitative methods, it is best to include a trained qualitative researcher on your team.

Mixed-methods studies use both quantitative and qualitative methods to answer research questions within the same study. Guidelines for reporting mixed-methods research can be found at http://www.equator-network.org/resource-centre/library-of-health-research-reporting/reporting-guidelines/mixed-methods-studies/. Pemberton

et al. (2013) provide an example of mixed-methods simulation research.

It may be beneficial to review the list provided by Schaefer et al. (2011) for ideas on design and models of well-designed studies. Review Cook and Campbell (1979) for quasi-experimental research designs, and use the strongest design possible. For example, a posttest only design is considered very weak. Unfortunately, in simulation research, posttest only design is fairly common. The strongest research design with posttests is frequently a Solomon 4-way, but it will require many participants and significant coordination.

Recruiting Subjects

Never underestimate the actual difficulty of recruiting participants for a research study. Long-term and repeated measures design studies are fraught with problems, for example, getting participants to come back on schedule for retesting. In simulation research, studies often involve gaining the cooperation of faculty members to build study participation into a course. The study must fit logically within the course objectives and parameters. The study can then use an **opt out** design. In this case, all students participate in the study activities, but students who opt out will not have their study data collected, or their study data will be deleted.

CONTROLLING VARIABLES

If the protocol involves conducting a study over multiple days, even a small change in how the room is laid out may affect how participants perceive the situation. If the same scenario is run multiple times, it is a plus to take a picture of the room setup and post it where the room monitors can be sure they are reproducing the same set of conditions for each person or team participating in a scenario. Depending on the study, it may also be important to report how much prior simulation experience the participants have received. Document the orientation given to all participants before entering the room to verify that they were given simulation objectives.

The actual training and calibration of the simulation teams and operators will affect your study findings. When documenting this, it is important to report the types of mannequins or Standardized Patients involved and the scenarios used, either commercially prepared or developed in-house. One might assume that commercially prepared scenarios have been vetted by outside groups, but this should be verified and documented. Home-grown scenarios also need to be tested for reliability and validity. At a minimum, multiple individuals familiar with the content should evaluate the scenarios to support its face validity. Statements about how the scenarios were validated should be included in the research findings. This is important as the team may be building in unusual regional or customary practices without knowing it.

Research Instruments

Tool development is a long, tedious, and specialized process with which few simulation research experts have experience. As such, it is best to use validated evaluation tools. However, this may be a problem if there are no tools to measure what the team has identified as the study's dependent variable or if existing tools around the topic were validated for a purpose different from the desired study. Boulet et al. (2011) suggest the work of Kane (1992, 2006) to help guide in tool development, should the team have to go this route. Kardong-Edgren et al. (2010) and Adamson et al. (2013) report over 20 evaluation instruments currently in use for simulation evaluation with more emerging every day. A scheduled and frequent literature scan may alert you to the perfect instrument for your study.

INSTITUTIONAL RESEARCH REVIEW

Many countries have requirements for formal institutional review of potential research studies. If you propose to conduct research in one of these countries, it is important that you meet with a representative of the Institutional Review Board early in the process. These individuals will provide you with the guidance you need to prepare required documents and complete required training. If you are in a country that does not require a formal review, make sure you determine what, if any, documentation you need to proceed. In addition, it is important that you get all communication from administration in writing. These documents may be required when you submit your research article for journal review. (For an in-depth discussion on the topic of working with an Institutional Review Board, see chapter 9.3).

Decide If Performing One Study or a Series of Studies

Spend some time with your research team discussing whether your research question can best be addressed in one study or whether a series of studies will be needed. Then map them out. A white board can be good for this, as it permits the group to erase, move, and connect lines multiple times over several hours before finalizing the research plan. For each study, consider the potential positive or negative results, plan the next logical step, and graph it out. This will save time in the long run, as the literature review will be more focused and research questions and terms will become clear to all early on.

INTERPRETING RESULTS

A statistician can provide depth, clarity, and a dose of reality to the study's research findings. Statisticians are cautious by nature and will help assure the team does not over- or understate the strength of the findings. They are invaluable with writing up the results section of the manuscript and getting the data into publishable tables. Discuss study results in light of what others who have done similar research have found. How similar or dissimilar are your results to previous work? Why might this be? What new or contradictory thoughts does the team have based on the study results?

The team must be forthcoming in discussing any study limitations. Think over the study and the limitations that were eventually discovered. Examples may include: one geographic location, only one unique type of student available, not enough subjects to obtain significant results. It is not always inappropriate or bad to have only a few subjects. Very good insights might come from *one* person.

REPORTING RESEARCH

The ultimate end point of simulation research is to change practice and improve patient care. Dissemination is the final, and, some may argue, the most important step in a research project. If well-done research is not reported, it might as well not have been done. It is arguably unethical to accept research funding and then not do the work to publish the findings. Note the emphasis on publishing; speaking at a conference is rewarding, but the audience is limited. Publishing your research findings reaches a much larger audience, and the article is archived where others can find the work. When publishing a research study, it is important to include enough detail that others can duplicate your work. Remember this when writing.

Before beginning to write up your study, select two potential journals for your work. Read several articles in both journals that match the type of reporting you are planning to use. Download the author guidelines for both journals, and write the manuscript based on your primary target journal. An excellent website to assist with reporting a study is http://www.equator-network.org/. Using guidelines such as these will lessen the risk that you forget something major. Often, researchers have worked on a study for so long, they assume readers know everything they do. Using these guidelines will minimize that risk.

Describe the procedures in your study in detail. For example, if debriefing was used in a study, explain the type of debriefing, and insert a copy of the debriefing script. Explain the training and experience level of the team's debriefers. If more than one individual was used for debriefing, document how standardized and calibrated their performance. If the mannequins were modified in any way, there should be a complete explanation included in the report.

Expect multiple revisions of a manuscript. Revise does *not* mean reject. Requested revisions mean that reviewers and an editor were interested enough to take the time to try to improve the work, for their readers. This is a gift. Accept it. Follow the author resubmission guidelines exactly. Read reviewer comments and answer every one, using a table format or a line-by-line reply to each reviewer.

State exactly how the comment was addressed in the revised manuscript. It is fine to disagree with a reviewer and to say so, in the reply to reviewers. State the reasons for your disagreement; the editor is the final arbiter in disagreements.

Once accepted, you can expect a delay in the actual publication of a manuscript. Publication delays can run more than a year for print journals, which often have a backlog of articles. A number of journals now place accepted articles in an "In press" or "Ahead of print" area on their websites. Many times, articles are cited ahead of print, as savvy researchers know where to look for the newest material.

BEEN THERE, DONE THAT: HOW CAN I CONTINUE TO IMPROVE OR SUSTAIN WHAT I HAVE ACHIEVED?

When listening to research report presentations at major conferences, one tends to feel that everything in these studies went flawlessly. In reality, it is almost *never* the case. Misunderstandings in protocol execution, problems with data collection, recruitment of participants, and squabbles over funding and authorship happen frequently. Dealing with unpredictable study participants, research partners, differences in equipment and faculty, simulation technicians, scenario facilitators, embedded actors, variations in presimulation orientation, and debriefing styles makes simulation research a very challenging undertaking, at the best of times. Expect the unexpected, and intervene early and often. The key to research is open communication and generating synergy to benefit the researchers and completion of the project.

SUMMARY

This chapter is a compilation of our years of research experience. It is meant as a short primer to assist a simulation center as it embarks on its first research study, which we hope would lead to a planned program of research. Carefully reviewing and thoughtfully using the ideas in this chapter should help novice researchers avoid many of the initial research mistakes others have made, and should lead to a high-quality research study and team.

REFERENCES

Adamson, K. A., Kardong-Edgren, S., & Willhaus, J. (2013). An updated review of published simulation evaluation instruments. *Clinical Simulation in Nursing, 9*(9), e327–e328. doi:10.1016/j.ecns.2012.09.004

Arnold, J. J., Johnson, L. M., Tucker, S. J., Malec, J. F., Henrickson, S. E., & Dunn, W. F. (2009). Evaluation tools in simulation learning: Performance and self-efficacy in emergency response. *Clinical Simulation in Nursing, 5*(1), e35–e43. doi:10.1016/j.ecns.2008.10.003

Arthur, W., Jr., Bennett, W., Jr., Stanush, P. L., & McNelly, T. L. (1998). Factors that influence skill decay and retention: A quantitative review and analysis. *Human Performance, 11*(1), 57.

Bandura, A. (1986). *Social foundations of thought and action: A social cognitive theory.* Englewood Cliffs, NJ: Prentice-Hall.

Benner, P. E. (1984). *From novice to expert: Excellence and power in clinical nursing practice.* Menlo Park, CA: Addison-Wesley.

Bond, W. F., Lammers, R. L., Spillane, L. L., Smith-Coggins, R., Fernandez, R., Reznek, M. A., ... Gordon, J. A. (2007). The use of simulation in emergency medicine: A research agenda. *Academic Emergency Medicine, 14*(4), 353–363. doi:10.1197/j.aem.2006.11.021

Boulet, J. R., Jeffries, P. R., Hatala, R. A., Korndorffer, J. R., Jr., Feinstein, D. M., & Roche, J. P. (2011). Research regarding methods of assessing learning outcomes. *Simulation in Healthcare: Journal of the Society for Simulation in Healthcare, 6(Suppl.)*, S48–S51. doi:10.1097/SIH.0b013e31822237d0

Burns, N., & Grove, S. K. (2009). *The practice of nursing research: Appraisal, synthesis, and generation of evidence* (6th ed.). St. Louis, MO: Saunders/Elsevier.

Cook, D. A., Beckman, T. J., & Bordage, G. (2007). Quality of reporting of experimental studies in medical education: A systematic review. *Medical Education, 41*(8), 737–745. doi:10.1111/j.1365-2923.2007.02777.x

Cook, T. D., & Campbell, D. T. (1979). *Quasi-experimentation: Design & analysis issues for field settings.* Boston, MA: Houghton Mifflin.

Dewey, J., & McDermott, J. J. (1973). *The philosophy of John Dewey.* New York, NY: Putnam Sons.

Dieckmann, P., Lippert, A., Glavin, R., & Rall, M. (2010). When things do not go as expected: Scenario life savers. *Simulation in Healthcare: Journal of the Society for Simulation in Healthcare, 5*(4), 219–225. doi:10.1097/SIH.0b013e77f74

Dieckmann, P., Phero, J. C., Issenberg, S. B., Kardong-Edgren, S., Ostergaard, D., & Ringsted, C. (2011). The first research consensus summit of the society for simulation in healthcare: Conduction and a synthesis of the results. *Simulation in Healthcare: Journal of the Society for Simulation in Healthcare, 6(Suppl.)*, S1–S9. doi:10.1097/SIH.0b013e31822238fc

Dieckmann, P., Reddersen, S., Wehner, T., & Rall, M. (2006). Prospective memory failures as an unexplored threat to patient safety: Results from a pilot study using patient simulators to investigate the missed execution of intentions. *Ergonomics, 49*(5–6), 526–543. doi:10.1080/00140130600568782

Eppich, W., Howard, V., Vozenilek, J., & Curran, I. (2011). Simulation-based team training in healthcare. *Simulation in Healthcare: Journal of the Society for Simulation in Healthcare, 6(Suppl.)*, S14–S19. doi:10.1097/SIH.0b013e318229f550

Ericsson, K. A. (2004). Deliberate practice and the acquisition and maintenance of expert performance in medicine and related domains. *Academic Medicine, 79(10 Suppl.)*, S70–S81.

Fitts, P. M., & Posner, M. I. (1967). *Human performance.* Belmont, CA: Brooks/Cole.

Flin, R., Bromiley, M., Buckle, P., & Reid, J. (2013). Changing behaviour with a human factors approach. *BMJ, 346*, f1416. doi:10.1136/bmj.f1416

Gennaro, S. (2010). Closing the gap. *Journal of Nursing Scholarship, 42*(4), 357. doi:10.1111/j.1547-5069.2010.01372.x

Gordon, J. A., & Vozenilek, J. A. (On behalf of the SAEM simulation task force and interest group, and the technology in medical education committee.) (2008). 2008 Academic medicine emergency consensus conference: The science of simulation in healthcare: Defining and developing clinical expertise. *Academic Emergency Medicine: Official Journal of the Society for Academic Emergency Medicine, 15*(11), 971–977.

Groom, J., Henderson, D., & Sittner, B. J. (2014). NLN/Jeffries simulation framework state of the science project: Simulation design characteristics. *Clinical Simulation in Nursing, 10*(7), 337–344.

Hallmark, B., Thomas, C., & Gantt, L. (2014). The education practices construct of the NLN/Jeffries simulation framework: State of the science. *Clinical Simulation in Nursing, 10*(7), 345–352.

The INACSL Board of Directors. (2011). Standard I: Terminology. *Clinical Simulation in Nursing, 7(4 Suppl.)*, S3–S7. doi:10.1016/j.ecns.2011.05.005

Issenberg, S. B., Ringsted, C., Ostergaard, D., & Dieckmann, P. (2011). Setting a research agenda for simulation-based healthcare education: A synthesis of the outcome from an utstein style meeting. *Simulation in Healthcare: Journal of the Society for Simulation in Healthcare, 6*(3), 155–167. doi:10.1097/SIH.0b013e3182207c24

Jeffries, P. R. (2005). A framework for designing, implementing, and evaluating simulations used as teaching strategies in nursing. *Nursing Education Perspectives, 26*(2), 96–103.

Kane, M. T. (1992). An argument-based approach to validity. *Psychological Bulletin, 112*(3), 527–535. doi:10.1037/0033-2909.112.3.527

Kane, M. T. (2006). Validation. In R. L. Brennan (Ed.), *Educational measurement* (4th ed., p. 17). Westport, CT: Praeger.

Kardong-Edgren, S., Adamson, K. A., & Fitzgerald, C. (2010). A review of currently published evaluation instruments for human patient simulation. *Clinical Simulation in Nursing, 6*(1), e25–e35. doi:10.1016/j.ecns.2009.08.004

Kelly, M. A., & Fry, M. (2013). Masters nursing students' perceptions of an innovative simulation education experience. *Clinical Simulation in Nursing, 9*(4), e127–e133. doi:10.1016/j.ecns.2011.11.004

Kirschner, P. A. (2002). Cognitive load theory: Implications of cognitive load theory on the design of learning. *Learning and Instruction, 12*(1), 1–10. doi:10.1016/S0959-4752(01)00014-7

Knowles, M. S. (1980). *The modern practice of adult education: From pedagogy to andragogy* (Rev. and updated ed.). Englewood Cliffs, NJ: Cambridge Adult Education.

Manser, T. (2011). Minding the gaps: Moving handover research forward. *European Journal of Anaesthesiology, 28*(9), 613–615. doi:10.1097/EJA.0b013e3283459292

Manser, T., Harrison, T. K., Gaba, D. M., & Howard, S. K. (2009). Coordination patterns related to high clinical performance in a simulated anesthetic crisis. *Anesthesia & Analgesia, 108*(5), 1606–1615. doi:10.1213/ane.0b013e3181981d36

McGahie, W. C., Issenberg, S. B., Petrusa, E. R., & Scalese, R. J. (2010). A critical review of simulation-based medical education research: 2003–2009. *Medical Education, 44*(1), 50–63. doi:10.1111/j.1365-2923.2009.03547.x

Meichenbaum, D. (1985). *Stress inoculation training.* New York, NY: Pergamon Press.

Nestel, D., Groom, J., Eikeland-Husebo, S., & O'Donnell, J. M. (2011). Simulation for learning and teaching procedural skills: The state of the science. *Simulation in Healthcare: Journal of the Society for Simulation in Healthcare, 6(Suppl.)*, S10–S13. doi:10.1097/SIH.0b013e318227ce96

Okuyama, A., Martowirono, K., & Bijnen, B. (2011). Assessing the patient safety competencies of healthcare professionals: A systematic review. *BMJ Quality & Safety, 20*(11), 991–1000. doi:10.1136/bmjqs-2011-000148

Onda, E. L. (2012). Situated cognition: Its relationship to simulation in nursing education. *Clinical Simulation in Nursing, 8*(7), e273–e280. doi:10.1016/j.ecns.2010.11.004

O'Shea, E. R., Pagano, M., Campbell, S. H., & Caso, G. (2013). A descriptive analysis of nursing student communication behaviors. *Clinical Simulation in Nursing, 9*(1), e5–e12. doi:10.1016/j.ecns.2011.05.013

Paas, F., Tuovinen, J. E., Tabbers, H., & Van Gerven, P. W. M. (2003). Cognitive load measurement as a means to advance cognitive load theory. *Educational Psychologist, 38*(1), 63–71.

Paige, J. B., & Daley, B. J. (2009). Situated cognition: A learning framework to support and guide high-fidelity simulation. *Clinical Simulation in Nursing, 5*(3), e97–e103. doi:10.1016/j.ecns.2009.03.120

Pemberton, J., Rambaran, M., & Cameron, B. H. (2013). Evaluating the long-term impact of the trauma team training course in Guyana: An explanatory mixed-methods approach. *American Journal of Surgery, 205*(2), 119–124. doi:10.1016/j.amjsurg.2012.08.004

Polit, D.F., & Beck, C.T. (2008). *Nursing research: Generating and assessing evidence for nursing practice.* New York, NY: Wolters Kluwer/Lippincott Williams & Wilkins.

Raemer, D., Anderson, M., Cheng, A., Fanning, R., Nadkarni, V., & Savoldelli, G. (2011). Research regarding debriefing as part of the learning process. *Simulation in Healthcare: Journal of the Society for Simulation in Healthcare, 6(Suppl.)*, S52–S57. doi:10.1097/SIH.0b013e31822724d0

Reid-Searl, K., Happell, B., Vieth, L., & Eaton, A. (2012). High fidelity patient silicone simulation: A qualitative evaluation of nursing students' experiences. *Collegian (Royal College of Nursing, Australia), 19*(2), 77–83.

Scerbo, M. W., Murray, W. B., Alinier, G., Antonius, T., Caird, J., Stricker, E., ... Kyle, R. (2011). A path to better healthcare simulation systems: Leveraging the integrated systems design approach. *Simulation in Healthcare: Journal of the Society for Simulation in Healthcare, 6(Suppl.)*, S20–S23. doi:10.1097/SIH.0b013e318227cf41

Schaefer, J. J., III, Vanderbilt, A. A., Cason, C. L., Bauman, E. B., Glavin, R. J., Lee, F. W., & Navedo, D. D. (2011). Literature review: Instructional design and pedagogy science in healthcare simulation. *Simulation in Healthcare: Journal of the Society for Simulation in Healthcare, 6(Suppl.)*, S30–S41. doi:10.1097/SIH.0b013e31822237b4

Schmidt, R. A., & Lee, T. D. (2005). *Motor control and learning: A behavioral emphasis* (4th ed.). Champaign, IL: Human Kinetics.

Schön, D. A. (1983). *The reflective practitioner: How professionals think in action.* New York, NY: Basic Books.

Sharma, B., Mishra, A., Aggarwal, R., & Grantcharov, T. P. (2011). Non-technical skills assessment in surgery. *Surgical Oncology, 20*(3), 169–177. doi:10.1016/j.suronc.2010.10.001

Society for Simulation in Healthcare. (2011). *Monographs from the first research consensus summit of the Society for Simulation in Healthcare 7.* New York, NY: Wolters Kluwer/Lippincott Williams & Wilkins.

Van Merriënboer, J. J. G., & Sweller, J. (2005). Cognitive load theory and complex learning: Recent developments and future directions. *Educational Psychology Review, 17*(2), 147–177.

Vygotsky, L. S. (1962). *Thought and language.* Cambridge, MA: MIT Press.

SECTION 9 • Research

CHAPTER 9.3

Institutional Review Board

Dawn Taylor Peterson, PhD, and Marjorie Lee White, MD, MPPM, MA

ABOUT THE AUTHORS

DAWN TAYLOR PETERSON is the Director of Simulation Education & Research at the Pediatric Simulation Center at Children's of Alabama. She holds a PhD in Instructional Design, an Educational Specialist degree, and a Master of Arts in Education. Dr. Peterson is responsible for coordinating and tracking the Center's research projects, including multisite and international studies. She coordinates scholarly activity for the Center's medical student research projects, resulting in significant Institutional Review Board–related activity.

MARJORIE LEE WHITE is an Associate Professor in the Department of Pediatrics, Division of Pediatric Emergency Medicine, at the University of Alabama at Birmingham. She is also Medical Co-Director of the Pediatric Simulation Center at Children's of Alabama and Director of Medical Student Simulation for the University of Alabama School of Medicine. She has been actively involved in simulation research for the past 8 years and is site coordinator for several multicenter simulation-based research studies.

ABSTRACT

Institutional Review Boards (IRBs) are designed for the purpose of reviewing and monitoring research efforts with the intent of protecting the rights of human subjects. This chapter will present a brief history of IRBs and human subject research along with the ethical considerations that must be considered when conducting educational research. The basic components of an IRB application will be discussed, and the three types of review categories will be explained. Electronic surveys and internet research will also be explored in regard to confidentiality and adherence to IRB standards. A section on International Ethics Committees is included as well as resources for those submitting to an IRB both in the United States and internationally. The end of the chapter contains a section geared toward simulation experts who have a fair amount of experience with IRBs. This section includes practical tips for managing large numbers of research studies and facilitating multisite research studies at the local level.

CASE EXAMPLE

The Simulation Coordinator at University Hospital Simulation Center has been asked by a nurse educator to develop a simulation course that will be used to reinforce concepts related to programming the intravenous pump. The nurse educator wants to collect data on the new simulation course and share the results at a regional nursing conference next year. The Simulation Coordinator explains that an Institutional Review Board (IRB) application must be completed and submitted for approval, but the unit educator insists that this type of research does not need IRB approval because it is an educational activity that would take place regardless of research. The Simulation Coordinator calls a colleague in the Southeastern Simulation Center across town to see how the situation would be handled in their center. The Director of Southeastern Simulation Center explains that they have a "blanket" IRB approval for all educational research and that they do not submit for individual educational research projects. The Simulation Coordinator then contacts a different colleague at the Northwest Regional Pediatric Simulation Center to inquire about their policies. The Director at Northwest Regional Pediatric Simulation Center says they do not typically submit for this type of research because the course would be required for staff whether it was considered "research" or not. Frustrated and confused, the Simulation Coordinator decides to contact a member of the local IRB to find an answer.

INTRODUCTION AND BACKGROUND: THE "WHY ..."

The use of high-technology simulation in clinical education has increased significantly over the past decade, resulting in large numbers of educational research studies being conducted in centers throughout the United States and around the globe (Kraus et al., 2012). Some clinical educators take the stance that submitting educational protocols to an IRB is not necessary for simulation centers because simulation has become standard in clinical education and will take place whether IRB approval is obtained or not. The key issue is whether the proposed educational research is considered **human subjects research** or a quality improvement project. Human subjects research is a systematic investigation whereby an investigator obtains information or data from a living individual through an intervention with the goal of developing or contributing to generalizable knowledge (Amdur & Bankert, 2011). Quality improvement projects are designed to identify and establish best practices within an organization, and participation in the educational initiative is at times required (Keune et al., 2013). The purpose of educational research projects in many simulation centers is to generalize the results to other learner populations and publish the findings, which indicates that the research is human subjects research and should be subject to ethical review.

Ethical issues are common in educational research although they do not seem as serious as those that exist in clinical research. Coercion and conflict of interest should both be considered by educational researchers as they design studies involving students, peers, and those they directly supervise. Because issues such as coercion and conflict of interest can be subtle, it is especially important for educational researchers to have a heightened sense of awareness of how these issues might be embedded in the procedures or methods of the study (Johnson & Christensen, 2010). Many educational researchers also have access to study populations that are convenient and readily available, and care should be taken to keep potential participants from feeling as if they are a captive population. Program directors must be particularly aware of hierarchical relationships that could impact participants' decisions to take part in a study (Keune et al., 2013).

Educational researchers must also ensure that studies are conducted with educational equivalency and equipoise (Egan & Mainous, 2012). Participants who are randomized to one intervention should receive equal educational benefits as those randomized to alternative interventions. Researchers should approach studies with an attitude of genuine exploration of which intervention is most effective for educating (i.e., equipoise). If one intervention is already known to be beneficial over another, then researchers should reconsider the study methods. An inherent conflict of interest is present when faculty and staff design studies for those whom they supervise with the anticipation that the project will yield publishable results. In light of this fact, investigators and research team members are not in a position to determine the ethical appropriateness of a study. It is best to look to an outside entity to review the study and protect the interests of participants (Moon & Khin-Maung-Gyi, 2009). The IRB was created primarily for this purpose.

While there are systems for the protection of human subjects in other countries, an IRB as described here is an American institution and is defined as a committee whose chief responsibility is to protect the rights and welfare of research participants and to assess the ethical acceptability of research proposals (Amdur & Bankert, 2011; Johnson & Christensen, 2010). Figure 9.3.1 briefly explains the list of events leading up to the creation of the IRB in the United States.

IRB members exist for the sole purpose of judging the ethical appropriateness of research studies and protecting participants from any type of risk or harm (Johnson & Christensen, 2010). While it seems difficult to imagine participants in educational research experiencing significant risk or harm, history is full of examples of individuals who were taken advantage of for the benefit of advancing science. In the context of simulation and educational research, it would be easy for investigators to coerce learners into participating in a study and then slightly alter data in order for the study to yield promising results (Johnson & Christensen, 2010). The attitudes of investigators and research team members who lead simulation can put additional pressure on participants to perform and give good feedback on evaluations. This perceived conflict of interest can also change the nature of the discussion during debriefing.

The literature is very clear on the necessity of submitting educational research proposals to an IRB (Amdur & Bankert, 2011; Cate, 2009; Egan & Mainous, 2012; Johnson & Christensen, 2010; Keune et al., 2013; Kraus et al., 2012; Moon & Khin-Maung-Gyi, 2009). But the question remains as to why some institutions and centers are still not doing it. A 2006 survey conducted by Dyrbye, Thomas, Papp, and Durning showed that only 60% of the clinician educators who responded to the survey had experience in submitting medical education protocols to an IRB. Fifty-one percent of those who responded to the survey said they would be more likely to submit an educational protocol if they knew more about the IRB's requirements regarding educational research. In an attempt to close the knowledge gap, the next section will focus on the IRB's requirements for submitting research protocols.

THE "HOW TO ..."

This section is intended to provide simulation educators and staff with basic information related to submitting an IRB application for educational research. The IRB application process, including the three types of IRB categories, will be explained after a brief discussion of IRB training

1948: The Nuremberg Code

The Nuremberg Code, which was a direct result of the Nuremberg trials, outlined the fundamental requirements for conducting human subject research. During World War II, Nazi physicians forced prisoners to endure horrific procedures for research purposes. The Nuremberg Code instituted the concept of informed consent, risk/benefit analysis, and the right to withdraw.

1955: The Wichita Jury Study

Social scientists from the University of Chicago audio taped jury deliberations in criminal trails that were being held in Wichita, Kansas. The purpose of the study was to explore the impact trail attorneys had on jury decision making. The jurors were not told they were being audio taped nor were they told the results would be discussed in academic forums. This event highlighted the issue of deception in research studies, and as a result, federal guidelines were created to protect individuals from exploitation.

1962: The Thalidomide Experience

Physicians commonly prescribed thalidomide to women in the 1950s to help ease symptoms related to pregnancy. However, women were not told that this was an investigatory drug. Several years after prescribing thalidomide to large numbers of women, it became evident that the medication caused severe birth defects in babies who were exposed to thalidomide in utero. The situation led to federal agency regulations requiring informed consent before treatment with any investigatory drug.

1964: The NIH Ethics Committee

The head of the National Institutes of Health (NIH), James Shannon, established a policy that required ethics committees to conduct a formal review of any research conducted by the Public Health Service.

1964: Declaration of Helsinki

This statement was developed by the World Medical Association in Helsinki, Finland in June 1964. It was built on the principles of the Nuremberg Code and describes the ethical standards involved in human subjects research. The Declaration of Helsinki has been amended six times since its creation in 1964. The most recent amendment was in 2008.

1966: *New England Journal of Medicine* - "Ethics of Clinical Research"

Henry Beecher, a physician from Harvard Medical School, published an article in the *New England Journal of Medicine* highlighting 22 research studies which compromised ethical standards such as informed consent and risk to participants. He challenged highly respected researchers to focus their attention on the ethical standards of conducting clinical research in the United States.

1973: Congressional Hearings on Health Care and Human Experimentation

Senator Edward Kennedy led a series of congressional hearings in 1973 as a result of public concern over the federally funded Tuskegee Syphilis Study that took place from 1932 to 1972. In this study, 300 uneducated sharecroppers living with syphilis in Macon County, Alabama were monitored to document the progression of the disease without treatment . The participants did not understand the nature of the study and were under the impression that they were receiving medical care. The study continued even after penicillin had been proven to be effective in the treatment of syphilis. The congressional hearings also investigated other clinical studies such as the Willowbrook Hepatitis Study (1950s) and the Jewish Chronic Disease Hospital Studies (1960s). In the Willowbrook study, health children living at an extended care facility for mental retardation were fed a solution containing the feces of children with active hepatitis. Parents of the healthy children were coerced into the study by being told that their child could not stay at the school unless they participated in the study. In the Jewish hospital studies, terminally ill and demented patients were injected with live cancer cells to study the spread of cancer among individuals with a weakened immune system. Informed consent was not obtained from the patients or from their families.

FIGURE 9.3.1   Events leading up to the creation of the Institutional Review Board.

The 1973 congressional hearings also investigated studies which resulted in ethical issues in the social sciences. In the 1960s Milgram studies, a psychologist named Stanley Milgram told participants that they were being recruited to help study the function of negative reinforcement in learning. The participants were asked to deliver electrical shocks to a person who was playing the role of the learner when they answered a question incorrectly. The participants were instructed to deliver stronger and stronger shocks as the study progressed which would have been potentially lethal. The participants were not told until after the study that they been deceived and the real purpose of the research was to explore the genocide of the Holocaust. Many of the participants admitted being emotionally distraught as a result of their involvement in the study and were upset to learn the real purpose of the research.

The Tearoom Trade Study in the early 1970s sought to investigate the behavior of homosexuals in public restrooms. Laud Humphries took license plate numbers of individuals who were frequenting a specific set of public restrooms to engage in anonymous homosexual behavior. He used this information to look up the names and addresses of the individuals and then visited them at their homes posing as an interviewer in order to collect information about the unknowing participant's family life and background. The individuals were not aware that they were being interviewed for a research study, nor did they know the findings of the study would be published with identifying information.

1974: National Research Act & the Creation of the IRB System
As a result of the congressional hearings led by Senator Kennedy in 1973, Congress passed the National Research Act which established the current IRB system. The intent of the IRB system was to provide regulatory oversight for all research involving human subjects. It is important to point out that Congress was not only concerned with the ethical standards involved in biomedical research but also those ethical standards that guide social science research. The Wichita Jury Study, the Milgram studies, and the Tearoom Trade study all highlighted a need for ethical guidelines in non-medical research involving human participants.

1979: The Belmont Report
The National Commission for Protection of Human Subjects of Biomedical and Behavioral Research convened in the Belmont Conference Center in Baltimore, Maryland to discuss research standards specifically related to vulnerable populations such as prisoners and children. The commission produced the Belmont Report which emphasized respect for persons, beneficence, and justice. The report serves as a guide for IRB members and researchers when evaluating the ethical nature of proposed research studies.

1981: Title 45, Part 46 of The Code of Federal Regulations (45 CFR 46)
The department of Health and Human Services along with the Food and Drug Administration created Title 45, Part 46 of the Code of Federal Regulations which is based on the Belmont Report. The regulations were revised as recently as 2009 and contain the department of Health and Human Services' guidelines for the protection of human research subjects.

1991: The Common Rule
Fifteen federal agencies adopted 45 CFR 46 as the basis for reviewing research involving human subjects. This federal policy or "Common Rule" was published in 1991 and governs any research taking place within the organizations who have adopted it.

(Amdur & Bankert, 2011; www.hhs.gov/ohrp)

FIGURE 9.3.1   *(continued)*

options. The process of **informed consent** will be reviewed as well as considerations related to special populations, electronic and internet research, and failure to comply.

IRB Training

Most **local IRB**s [i.e., IRBs that function as the oversight committee at an academic institution or other institution that conducts research (Moon & Khin-Maung-Gyi, 2009] require proof of ethics training for any individual who is listed on a protocol as a principal investigator, co-investigator, or other person involved in data collection or data analysis. Training requirements may vary slightly from institution to institution, but the majority of local IRBs will accept the Collaborative Institutional Training Initiative (CITI) module (https://www.citiprogram.org/irbpage.asp?language=english) or the National Institutes of Health (NIH) Protecting Human Research Participants module (http://phrp. nihtraining.com/users/login.php). Both courses are internet based and are free of charge. Topics covered include the history of ethical human subjects research, the research review process, and the concept of informed consent. Most local IRBs also require a yearly review course in addition to the initial IRB training by CITI or the NIH. The yearly update courses are typically designed and monitored by the local IRB office. Questions regarding required IRB training for investigators and other research personnel should be directed to the local IRB at the institution where the research will be taking place.

IRB Application Process

There are three research review categories that must be considered by investigators before submitting an application to an IRB. These categories are *exempt, expedited,* and *full review.* An **exempt study** is one that is determined by the IRB as not requiring initial or continuing review. The Code of Federal Regulations Title 45 Part 46 contains the parameters for studies that may be deemed exempt (Amdur & Bankert, 2011). Figure 9.3.2 is an example of an exempt study application that was submitted and approved by a local academic IRB.

This specific example involves collecting anonymous course evaluation data and analyzing learners' perceptions of the effectiveness of simulation (see Figure 9.3.3 for the course evaluation sheet used in this study). The investigators felt that the study involved no risk to participants. The IRB agreed and approved the study as exempt. However, the IRB still required that an information sheet be given to the participants to inform them of the study (see Figure 9.3.4 for an example of the information sheet used in this study). It is important to remember that the determination of exempt status is made by the IRB and not by the investigators. If an investigator submits an application for an exempt study, and the IRB does not feel the study is exempt, an expedited or full review protocol will be necessary.

Expedited and full review categories both require the investigator to fill out a human subjects protocol that is roughly a twenty-page application explaining the details of the study and the risks and benefits to the participants. While both of these categories require the same paperwork, the difference between the two categories is in the definition of the type of research and the number of IRB members required to approve the study. Expedited studies are those studies defined by the IRB as posing no more than minimal risk to the participants; minimal risk means that the research will cause no more harm or discomfort than that experienced in everyday life or in the context of the research environment (Amdur & Bankert, 2011). Expedited studies may be reviewed by one or more members of the approving IRB and must be reviewed on an annual basis (see Figure 9.3.5 for an example of an expedited human subjects protocol). The research study in Figure 9.3.5 was initially submitted as an exempt protocol. However, the IRB determined that the study involved minimal risk to the participants and an expedited protocol was required. (Note that much of the required information in the protocol related to human genes and biological specimens has been removed from this example to conserve space, and only the information pertinent to educational research has been included in the example; Figure 9.3.5.)

Research studies falling into the full review category are those studies that pose more than minimal risk to the participants and therefore require a full review by every member of the IRB (Amdur & Bankert, 2011). It is important to note that IRB committees meet at specific times throughout the year to conduct full reviews. Therefore, if an investigator believes a full review will be necessary, it is wise to submit the protocol in plenty of time for **full board review** and for any necessary revisions to be made. The length of time it takes to approve any research protocol depends on the number of protocols typically submitted throughout the year and the number of meetings the IRB schedules to review these protocols. Research studies submitted at large research institutions may take 3 to 6 months to be reviewed and approved if revisions are necessary. Investigators who submit at smaller institutions may be able to gain approval in 3 to 6 weeks. The turnaround time is highly variable across institutions, so it is best to check with the local IRB to determine their estimated operating timelines.

Typically, educational research involving simulation will fall into the exempt or expedited category because simulation centers are posing no more than minimal risk to the participants (Dyrbye et al., 2008). However, if a simulation center wishes to do educational research involving courses that include patients, patient families, or minors, it is likely that the IRB will require a full board review for this type of research. Examples of such research studies would be a Teen Trauma Prevention Program where simulation is used to show the dangers of unsafe driving to teen drivers or a course that uses simulation to educate families on asthma or diabetes maintenance prior to discharge. Both of these examples involve collecting data or studying the

Exempt Review Application

Indicate the type of review:

☒ **New**   ☐ **Continuing Review**   ☐ **Final Report**

1. Project Identification

a. Title of Project: **Learners' Perceptions of the Effectiveness of Simulation**

b. Principal Investigator (PI): **Donna Smith, PhD, RN**

2. Mark the category or categories below that describe the proposed research:

☒1. Research conducted in established or commonly accepted educational settings, involving normal educational practices, such as (i) research on regular and special education instructional strategies, or (ii) research on the effectiveness of or the comparison among instructional techniques, curricula, or classroom management methods. The research is not FDA regulated and does not involve prisoners as participants.

☐2. Research involving the use of educational tests (cognitive, diagnostic, aptitude, achievement), survey procedures, interview procedures or observation of public behavior, unless: (i) Information obtained is recorded in such a manner that human subjects can be identified, directly or through identifiers linked to the subjects; and (ii) any disclosure of the human subjects' responses outside the research could reasonably place the subjects at risk of criminal or civil liability or be damaging to the subjects' financial standing, employability, or reputation. Attach questionnaire(s) and/or surveys. If the research involves children as participants, the procedures are limited to educational tests and observation of public behavior where the investigators do not participate in the activities being observed. The research is not FDA regulated and does not involve prisoners as participants.

☐3. Research involving the use of educational tests (cognitive, diagnostic, aptitude, achievement), survey procedures, interview procedures, or observation of public behavior that is not exempt under category (2), if: (i) the human subjects are elected or appointed public officials or candidates for public office; or (ii) federal statute(s) require(s) without exception that the confidentiality of the personally identifiable information will be maintained throughout the research and thereafter. Attach to this application a copy of any questionnaire or survey to be used. The research is not FDA regulated and does not involve prisoners as participants.

☒4. Research involving the collection or study of existing data, documents, records, pathological specimens, or diagnostic specimens, if these sources are publicly available or if the information is recorded by the Investigator in such a manner that subjects cannot be identified, directly or through identifiers linked to the subjects. Attach a specimen release form if applicable. (*Specimens must be preexisting.*) The research is not FDA regulated and does not involve prisoners as participants.

☐5. Research and demonstration projects which are conducted by or subject to the approval of department or agency heads, and which are designed to study, evaluate, or otherwise examine: (i) public benefit or service programs; (ii) procedures for obtaining benefits or services under those programs;(iii) possible changes in or alternatives to those programs or procedures; or (iv) possible changes in methods or levels of payment for benefits or services under those programs. The protocol will be conducted pursuant to specific federal statutory authority; has no statutory requirement for IRB review; does not involve significant physical invasions or intrusions upon the privacy interests of the participant; has authorization or concurrent by the funding agency and does not involve prisoners as participants.

FIGURE 9.3.2   Example of Exempt Review Application.   *(continued)*

☐6. Taste and food quality evaluation and consumer acceptance studies, (i) if wholesome foods without additives are consumed or (ii) if a food is consumed that contains a food ingredient at or below the level and for a use found to be safe, or agricultural chemical or environmental contaminant at or below the level found to be safe, by the Food and Drug Administration or approved by the Environmental Protection Agency or the Food Safety and Inspection Service of the U.S. Department of Agriculture. The research does not involve prisoners as participants.

3. Briefly describe the proposed research: **Faculty and staff administer an anonymous course evaluation after every course that is taught in our simulation center. We would like to be able to present this anonymous data at conferences to show the learner's perceived effectiveness of simulation as a teaching tool.**

4. Describe how subjects/data/specimens will be selected. If applicable, include the sex, race, and ethnicity of the subject population: **Every learner, regardless of their discipline, completes an anonymous course evaluation after every simulation course. We would like to use the anonymous data from these evaluations to show the learner's perception of the effectiveness of simulation.**

5. Does the research involve deception? ☐Yes ☒No

6. Describe why none of the research procedures would cause a subject either physical or psychological discomfort or be perceived as harassment above and beyond what the person would experience in daily life: **None of the research would cause harm...the learner is always asked to complete a course evaluation after each simulation session. These evaluations are kept in a locked file cabinet in the simulation center.**

7. Describe the provisions to maintain confidentiality of data: **The course evaluations do not contain a place for the learner's name – they are strictly anonymous.**

8. Describe the provisions included in the research to protect the privacy interests of participants (e.g., others will not overhear your conversation with potential participants, individuals will not be publicly identified or embarrassed) **Course evaluations are a routine part of coming to the simulation center. Learners have completed evaluations after every course since the center's inception in 2008. This data is anonymous and is not discussed aloud.**

9. Will the research involve interacting with the subjects? ☒Yes ☐No
    If yes, describe the consent process and information to be presented to subjects, including:
    - That the activities involve research.
    - The procedures to be performed.
    - That participation is voluntary.
    - Name and contact information for the investigator.

When learners come to the simulation center, they are always given an anonymous evaluation form to complete after their course. We would provide a checkbox on the bottom of the course evaluation form so they can indicate that they do not wish their data to be used in any presentation or publication (see attached).

An information sheet will be shared after every course to inform the learners that their anonymous opinions may be shared unless they check the box at the bottom of the form (see attached).

Principal Investigator's Signature:_____ Date:_____

FIGURE 9.3.2 (continued)

SIMULATION PROGRAM EVALUATION

DATE _____   COURSE_____

I am a   ☐ MD   ☐ Resp Therapy   ☐ Other_____
          ☐ RN   ☐ Radiology Tech
          ☐ Chaplain   ☐ Med Student
          ☐ Pharmacist   ☐ Nursing Student

	Agree	Neutral	Disagree
Orientation to the simulation was appropriate.			
Length of time for simulation was appropriate.			
Length of time for debriefing was appropriate.			
This experience is applicable to my practice/profession.			
I found the simulations to be valuable learning experience.			
I found the debriefings to be valuable learning experience.			
This experience has increased my skill level in providing pediatric care.			
This experience has increased my confidence level in providing pediatric care.			
I would recommend this program to others.			

Two things I liked/learned today:

Two things I wish we had focused on or that could be improved:

Comment/Suggestions/Recommendations:

☐ **I do not wish for this anonymous information to be used in any presentation or publication.**

FIGURE 9.3.3   Course evaluation for exempt study in Figure 9.3.2.

effectiveness of simulation on patients or minors. Participants in a family education course may also be economically disadvantaged. The Code of Federal Regulations Title 45 Part 46 outlines specific populations such as children, prisoners, pregnant women, mentally disabled individuals, and educationally or economically disadvantaged persons as being vulnerable (Amdur & Bankert, 2011). If any of these special populations are involved in educational research, a full board review will be required.

Regardless of the type of participants who enroll in the study, investigators must obtain informed consent. Many educators think of informed consent as a signed document. However, informed consent is actually the process by which an investigator communicates the purpose,

procedures, risks, benefits, and confidentiality related to the study in such a way that the participant understands and agrees to participate (Amdur & Bankert, 2011; Johnson & Christensen, 2010). The **consent document** is the document signifying the participant's informed consent and is signed by the investigator, the participant, and a witness (Amdur & Bankert, 2011). Figure 9.3.6 shows the Informed Consent Document for the **expedited study** in Figure 9.3.5.

In certain very limited situations, the IRB may waive the requirement of informed consent. This type of waiver is granted only if the research cannot be practically conducted without the waiver and if the research involves no more than minimal risk to the participants. If a waiver of

<u>**Learners' Perceptions of the Effectiveness of Simulation**</u>

IRB Protocol # E125125125

Principal Investigator – Donna Smith - 222.526.6666
donna.smith@simulation.org

The purpose of this study is to investigate your perceptions of the effectiveness of simulation as a learning tool. After the simulation session, you will be asked to complete an anonymous evaluation form for this course just as you do for all scenarios in the Pediatric Simulation Center. Your total participation time will be less than one minute. If you do not wish to participate in this study, you may check the box at the bottom of the evaluation form that states you do not wish to have your anonymous information shared in any presentation or publication.

Participation in this research is voluntary and will in no way change your status as a resident or employee. If you are a student or employee, taking part in this research is not a part of your class work or duties. You can refuse to enroll, or withdraw after enrolling at any time before the study is over, with no effect on your class standing, grades, or job. You will not be offered or receive any special consideration if you take part in this research. All responses are anonymous.

If you have questions about this research, please contact the principal investigator, Donna Smith, at 222.526.6666 or donna.smith@simulation.org. If you have questions about your rights as a research participant, or concerns or complaints about the research, you may contact the Institutional Review Board at the University (222) 936-5555. Regular hours for the office of the IRB are 8:00 a.m. to 5:00 p.m. CT, Monday through Friday. You may also call this number in the event the research staff cannot be reached or you wish to talk to someone else.

FIGURE 9.3.4   Information sheet for exempt study in Figure 9.3.2.

informed consent is granted by IRB, there is usually the requirement of providing study information to the participants after they have participated in the study (Amdur & Bankert, 2011). It is more common in educational research studies for the IRB to grant a waiver of documentation of informed consent, which is different than a waiver of informed consent. When a waiver of documentation of informed consent is granted, the investigator still obtains verbal informed consent from the participant, but the participant's signature is not required. Investigators request this waiver when the only document linking the participant's name to the research is the consent document. Often in simulation education research, the participant's evaluations and test results are linked by a code known only to the participants. For this reason, many educational researchers will ask IRB for a waiver of documentation of informed consent, so there is no record of the names of those who participated in the study. Figure 9.3.7 shows an example of a waiver of informed consent documentation.

It is important to note that even in situations where documentation of informed consent is waived, the IRB may still require an information sheet that gives participants information on the purpose, procedures, risks, and benefits of the study. Contact information of the principal investigator and of the local IRB is typically provided on the information sheet as well (Refer back to Figure 9.3.4 for an example of an information sheet).

Electronic Surveys and Internet

Electronic surveys distributed via the internet have become popular tools in educational research due to the convenience of accessing participants. However, the use of electronic surveys and the internet adds a layer of complexity to the procedures of the study with regard to informed consent, privacy, and security. Informed consent indicates that the participant has been informed of the study and understands the details on the information sheet or consent

Human Subjects Protocol

Indicate the type of review you are applying for:

☐ Convened (Full) IRB *or*

☒ Expedited—See the <u>Expedited Category Review Sheet,</u> and indicate the category(ies) here:

☐1 ☐2 ☐3 ☐4 ☐5 ☐6 ☒7

IRB Protocol Title: <u>Medical Decision-Making Among Residents During a Simulated Patient Experience</u>

Investigator, Contacts, Supervisors

Name of Principal Investigator: <u>Lauren Nichols</u>

Describe the principal investigator's activities related to this protocol and provisions made by the PI to devote sufficient time to conduct the protocol:

<u>Dr. Nichols will organize the collection of data, the scheduling of resident time in the simulation center, and the debriefing sessions following each session. Her clinical time is exclusively with the General Inpatient Services, and she is already involved in resident education in that role. Research and education in the Simulation Center is a natural extension of her current duties.</u>

Describe the process that ensures that all persons assisting with the research are adequately informed about the protocol and their research-related duties and functions: <u>The team of persons who run and are involved with the Simulation Center meet weekly to discuss ongoing business. Discussion of this protocol will be on the agenda for discussion at these weekly meetings.</u>

Is this study funded? ☐Yes ☒No**If No,** specify that costs of the study will be covered by funds from the UAB department or other source named: <u>Costs of study will not exceed costs of resident education sessions which have already been occurring. Costs of printing paper for data analysis will be minor and will be absorbed by Simulation Center.</u>

Describe the facilities available for the conduct of the research. For research on UAB campus, include building names and room numbers: <u>The project will be conducted in the Simulation Center on the 3rd floor of Northwest Hospital.</u>

Purpose—in nontechnical, lay language

Summarize the purpose and objectives of this protocol, including any related projects, in one short paragraph.

<u>Our project has two phases, each with different purpose and objectives. In the first phase, we will use parallel simulated pediatric patient cases to evaluate whether residents show cognitive biases toward diagnostic error when presented with the incorrect diagnosis on a patient they are called to evaluate. We will evaluate residents' ability to recognize that the initial diagnosis was incorrect, make the correct diagnosis, and begin the appropriate therapy. We will evaluate the ability to demonstrate errors in diagnostic reasoning during a simulated patient encounter. We will use these simulated patient encounters to provide valuable resident education regarding teamwork and the pathophysiology of each illness. In the second phase of our project, we will provide post-session education to residents regarding causes and avoidance of diagnostic error in addition to the case-specific education they are receiving. We will repeat sessions with different simulated cases to evaluate the impact of the education on cognitive error and their ability to generalize and apply it to other situations.</u>

Background—in nontechnical, lay language

Summarize in 2-3 paragraphs past experimental and/or clinical findings leading to the formulation of this study. Include any relevant past or current research by the Principal Investigator. For drug and device studies summarize the previous results (i.e., Phase I/II or III studies).

<u>Pat Croskerry, an emergency medicine physician and expert in cognitive decision making theory, highlights an important disconnect between the importance of clinical judgment and diagnostic reasoning and the rate at which physicians fail in "this critical aspect of clinical performance (Croskerry, 2009)." Recently there has been a focus on diagnostic error as an important component of medical error. A subset of diagnostic error is in cognitive error, and in particular, the concept of premature closure. Premature closure is defined as the acceptance of a diagnosis before it has been fully verified (Croskerry, 2002).</u>

<u>The Northwest Hospital Committee for evaluation of Unplanned Transfers to a Higher Level of Care, on which Drs. Nichols and White serve, has documented repeatedly that premature closure is an all-too-frequent cause of mismanagement of patients admitted to the care of pediatric and other residents. There is significant literature both from the cognitive psychiatry domain and the medical education domain that can inform practitioners who access it (Ely, 2011; Mamede, 2010). In addition, there has been some work done in the simulated setting regarding the utility of this setting to teach metacognitive strategies (Bond, 2004 &2005). However, to date there have been no structured educational programs using simulation to educate pediatric residents on cognitive error.</u>

FIGURE 9.3.5   Example of Expedited Human Subjects protocol.

(continued)

Participants (Screening and Selection)

How many participants are to be enrolled at the university? **75-80 Interns and Residents**

If multi-center study, total number at all centers: _____

Describe the characteristics of anticipated or planned participants.

Participants will represent the demographics of residents (Pediatric and Medicine-Pediatrics) on their General Inpatient Pediatricsrotations. No one will be excluded. The current Pediatrics/Med-Peds residency program is approximately 30% male and 90% Caucasian.   Sex : **Male and Female**

Race/Ethnicity: **None targeted. No one will be excluded based on race/ethnicity.**

Age: **In general, residents are in their 20s and 30s; All participants will be older than 19 years of age.**

Health status: **None targeted or excluded. Most residents are healthy. Heath status will not affect participation in this study.**

From what population(s) will the participants be derived?

Participants will be residents (PGY 1 through PGY4) during their month-long rotations on the General Inpatient Pediatrics Service.Most residents and interns are from the Department of Pediatrics or are completing a combined Medicine/Pediatrics Residency. A few residents who participate will be from the Psychiatry, Family Medicine, and Anesthesia Residency Programs.

Describe your ability to obtain access to the proposed population that will allow recruitment of the necessary number of participants:

Drs. Nichols, Tindle, and White are attending physicians associated with the residency program. Dr. Tindle is Associate Pediatric Residency Program Director. Dr. Nichols is a former chief resident for the program. Residents are required to complete educational experiences in the simulation center as part of their educational experience on their General Inpatient rotations. All three faculty investigators are easily accessible by the house-staff.

Describe the inclusion/exclusion criteria:

All interns and residents will be eligible for inclusion in the study during their General Inpatient Pediatrics rotations. There are noexclusion criteria. Residents may opt out of the study by indicating they do not want to participate. Residents who choose not toparticipate will not miss out on the educational experience in the simulation center; we will simply not collect data from these sessions.

Indicate which, if any, of the special populations listed below will be involved in the protocol. Include the Special Populations ReviewForm (SPRF) if indicated.

☐ Pregnant Women: Attach SPRF—Pregnant Women, Fetuses, Neonates/Nonviable Neonates
☐ Fetuses: Attach SPRF—Pregnant Women, Fetuses, Neonates/Nonviable Neonates
☐ Neonates/Nonviable Neonates: SPRF—Pregnant Women, Fetuses, Neonates/Nonviable Neonates
☐ Prisoners: Attach SPRF—Prisoners
☐ Minors (<19 years old): Attach SPRF—Minors
☒ Employees or students at institution where research conducted
☐ Persons who are temporarily decisionally impaired
☐ Persons who are permanently decisionally impaired (e.g., mentally retarded)
☐ Non-English Speakers

For each box checked, describe why the group is included **and** the additional protections provided to protect the rights and welfare of these participants who are vulnerable to coercion: **This study is focusing on the process of diagnostic decision-making of residents at Northwest Hospital. Teams are comprised of residents and interns. Participation is voluntary and will in no way change the educational experience in the simulation center, status as a resident, or the resident's evaluation**.

List any persons other than those directly involved in the study who will be at risk. If none, enter "None": **None**

Describe the process (e.g., recruitment, chart review) that will be used to seek potential participants (e.g., individuals, records, specimens). Research recruitment by non-treating physicians/staff may require completion of Partial Waiver of Authorization for Recruitment/Screening. (See http://main.uab.edu/show.asp?durki=61981.)

Residents will be scheduled for sessions in the Simulation Center as part of their educational experience while on their General Inpatient Pediatrics rotations. When they arrive to the Sim Center, the study will be described to them by a member of the study team, and if they choose to participate, data will be collected on their performance. If they do not choose to participate in the study, they will still receive the educational experience of caring for simulated patients and no data will be collected.

FIGURE 9.3.5 (continued)

If you will use recruitment materials (e.g., advertisements, flyers, letters) to reach potential participants, attach a copy of each item. If not, identify the source (e.g., databases) from which you will recruit participants.
Participants will be recruited from the General Inpatient Pediatric teams (interns and residents).

Describe the procedures for screening potential participants.
A member of the investigation team will meet with the potential participants when they arrive for their simulated experience to describe the study and answer questions. Residents will be given information regarding the study and will choose whether or notthey would like to participate.

Protocol Procedures, Methods, and Duration of the Study—in nontechnical language
Describe the study methodology that will affect the participants—particularly in regard to any inconvenience, danger, or discomfort.**Participants will be residents who currently have a requirement for attending sessions in the Sim Center as part of their educational experience during their General Inpatient Pediatric rotation. Participating in the study will not change the experienceof simulation.**

Residents from General Inpatient Pediatric teams will come to the simulation center in teams of two. They will participate in two simulated cases chosen from a set of paired cases developed by the research team. They will be randomized to start a case with a stem that is misleading or with a control stem. For example, in the misleading case, a physician in the Emergency Department will ask the residents to come admit a patient in Room #303 with "asthma", and in the control scenario, the patient will be described as having "chief complaint of trouble breathing." The actual diagnosis in the example is congestive heart failure with respiratory symptoms. The remainder of the case is exactly the same; only the initial description the residents receive is different. Resident teams will do two cases; one of which has a misleading stem, and one of which does not (see below). We will test whether the misleading stem creates biases that lend toward errors in diagnostic reasoning by evaluating for delays in or lack of appropriate history-taking, physical exam, data collection, and therapy. Data will be collected about time to correct diagnosis for each of these simulations.

Sessions in the Simulation Center are routinely video-taped to allow for participants to view parts of their own simulation if helpful during their debriefing episodes. These tapes do not leave the Sim Center and are destroyed once they are no longer needed for this purpose.

Each simulated case experience is followed by a debriefing session led by one or two of the physicians on the Sim Center staff and this study protocol (Dr. Tindle Dr. White, or Dr. Nichols) The debriefing occurs as a team; both participants are present and discuss the case with the instructors. Confidentiality is preserved because the only people in the debriefing room are those who were directly involved in that simulated case. The remote location of the Simulation Center prevents debriefing sessions from being overheard. In past educational experience, residents respond very positively to these non-threatening, positive debriefing sessions.

In phase 1, debriefing sessions following the cases will focus on medical decision-making in general, and specifically on the pathophysiology of the illnesses of the simulated patients.
In phase 2, the research team will include instruction on cognitive forcing strategies and prevention of diagnostic error in the debriefing following simulation. Residents will return to the Sim Center, and we will continue our measurement to evaluate the effectiveness of this education and their ability to apply it to other simulated patient cases.

The educational content of Sim sessions is not optional. Only the data collection aspect is (Data Collection Instrument Included).

What is the probable length of time required for the entire study (i.e., recruitment through data analysis to study closure)?
24 months   What is the total amount of time each participant will be involved? **1-2 hours per academic year**

FIGURE 9.3.5   (continued)   (continued)

If different phases are involved, what is the duration of each phase in which the participants will be involved? If no phases are involved, enter "not applicable."

Phase 1: Approximately 6 months.   **Phase 2: Approximately 6 months-1 year.**

List the procedures, the length of time each will take, and the frequency of repetition, and indicate whether each is done solely for research or would already be performed for treatment or diagnostic purposes (routine care) for the population. *Insert additional table rows as needed.*

Procedure	Length of Time Required of Participants	Frequency of Repetition	Research (Res) –OR– Routine Care
Simulated Patient care	**1 hour**	**1-2**	☐Res ☒Routine
Data Collection: Demographics Sheet	**5 minutes**	**1-2**	☒Res ☐Routine

Will an interview script or questionnaire be used?   ☐Yes ☒No
   If Yes, attach a copy.

Will participants incur any costs as a result of their participation?   ☐Yes ☒No
If Yes, describe the reason for and amount of each foreseeable cost.

Will participants be compensated?   ☐Yes ☒No

Describe the potential benefits of the research.
Most research in diagnostic error has been done in Emergency Departments, areas where patient acuity, quantity, limitation of resources, and other factors increase cognitive load and the risk for cognitive mistakes. Education on strategies to prevent errors in these settings has been shown to be beneficial in decreasing their likelihood. There has been little to no research on the potential for cognitive errors in Pediatric Residents who also have risk factors for increased cognitive load. Residents' work hours are becoming even more restricted, adding the stress of feeling increasingly pressed for time to the risk factors of relative inexperience and high-levels of multitasking. Additionally, the number of hand-offs in patient care between care-givers seems to be exponentially increasing. Studying the risk factors involved in these hand-offs and the risk factors that cause failures in diagnostic reasoning will help to guide our educational efforts. Once we identify that they exist, we can begin to teach residents how to avoid them and improve patient care. The second part of our study will evaluate our effectiveness at just that.

Risks
List the known risks—physical, psychological, social, economic, and/or legal—that participants may encounter as a result of procedures required in this protocol. Do not list risks resulting from standard-of-care procedures. <u>Note.</u> *Risks included in this protocol document should be included in the written consent document.*
Participation in the study will not alter the residents' educational experience in the Simulation Center. The risks associated with simulation are no greater than the risks associated with their day-to-day activities. Risks of participation in this educational activity include potential emotional distress over being video-taped and watched by instructors along with embarrassment with performance. These are the risks of the educational experience, however, and are not increased by participation in this study.

Risks associated with study participation are the minimal risks of loss of data and/or confidentiality or of being overheard during participation during simulation.

Estimate the frequency, severity, and reversibility of each risk listed.
For this study, residents will participate for 1 hour each month they are on their General Inpatient Pediatrics (GIPS) rotation. PGY-1 and PGY-3 residents generally do two GIPS rotations per year, while PGY-2 and PGY-4 residents do one GIPS rotation per year. The risk of distress over being video-taped and the risk of embarrassment regarding poor performance are small. The residents are reassured that the videotapes are kept only in the Simulation Lab and then destroyed when they are no longer needed. No one except the participants in that particular scenario and the Simulation Center Staff will view the videos. The risk of embarrassment is greatly minimized by reassuring the participants that simulation is for their education, not evaluation or judgment. We start with the basic assumption that all participants are intelligent and capable and continue to work with participants with that assumption. Feedback they receive, though instructive, is positive, and focuses on playing up the areas of strength while working on the areas of weakness. The risk of loss of data and/or confidentiality is very unlikely given the measures described below. Similarly, the risk of being overheard during simulation is low due to the remote location of the Simulation Center.

FIGURE 9.3.5   *(continued)*

Is this a therapeutic study or intervention? ☐Yes ☒No

Do you foresee that participants might need additional medical or psychological resources as a result of the research procedures/interventions? ☐Yes ☒No

Do the benefits or knowledge to be gained outweigh the risks to participants? ☒Yes ☐No

☒Yes ☐No

Precautions/Minimization of Risks
Describe precautions that will be taken to avoid risks and the means for monitoring to detect risks.
All sessions will be performed in the Sim Center which is remote in location from other areas of the hospital, minimizing the chance of participants being overheard by others. The data collection forms will record performance information regarding each session. They will be kept in a locked cabinet in a locked office. Each form will be coded with a number corresponding to the individual participant. These numbers will be randomly assigned, and the key linking the participants' names and numbers will be kept separately from the documents themselves on a computer locked with a password. Evaluations will be turned into a basket anonymously. All data will be destroyed as soon as study and data collection are complete.

If hazards to an individual participant occur, describe (i) the criteria that will be used to decide whether that participant should be removed from the study; (ii) the procedure for removing such participants when necessary to protect their rights and welfare; and (iii) any special procedures, precautions, or follow-up that will be used to ensure the safety of other currently enrolled participants.
We do not anticipate participants incurring any hazards during this study. However, if an unforeseen hazard occurs, the investigative team will review the circumstances regarding the event and explore alternative approaches in order to avoid future hazards.

If hazards occur that might make the risks of participation outweigh the benefits for all participants, describe (i) the criteria that will be used to stop or end the entire study and (ii) any special procedures, precautions, or follow-up that will be used to ensure the safety of currently enrolled participants.
Participation in this study does not alter the residents' educational experience. We are collecting data regarding simulated patient experiences that will occur even without the study. Therefore, this study has minimal risks to participants. The investigative team currently meets weekly to discuss education and research ongoing in the Sim Center. We will use this opportunity to discuss any hazards that are occurring and solutions to prevent further hazards from occurring or potentially stopping the study if they cannot be prevented.

Informed Consent
Do you plan to obtain informed consent for this protocol? ☒Yes ☐No
If Yes, complete the items below.
If No, complete and include the Waiver of Informed Consent or Waiver of Authorization and Informed Consent, as applicable.

Do you plan to document informed consent for this protocol? ☒Yes ☐No
If Yes, complete the items below.
If No, complete the items below **and** include the Waiver of Informed Consent Documentation.

How will consent be obtained? **During the residents' initial presentation to the Simulation Center for their educational session, the study will be described. Residents will be given a copy of the Informed Consent document (included), and have the opportunity to ask and have their questions answered. They will indicate their consent to participate by singing the Informed Consent Document and filling out the Participant Demographics form.**

Who will conduct the consent interview? **A member of the investigative team.**

Who are the persons who will provide consent or permission? **The participants**

What steps will be taken to minimize the possibility of coercion or undue influence? **It will be explained clearly that they do not have to participate in the study. Participating or not will not change their educational experience.**

What language will the prospective participant or the legally authorized representative understand? **English**

What language will be used to obtain consent? **English**

FIGURE 9.3.5 *(continued)* *(continued)*

SECTION 9 • Research

If any potential participants will be, or will have been, in a stressful, painful, or drugged condition before or during the consent process, describe the precautions proposed to overcome the effect of the condition on the consent process. If not, enter "no such effect."
No such effect

How long will participants have between the time they are told about the study and the time they must decide whether to enroll? If not 24 hours or more, describe the proposed time interval and why the 24-hour minimum is neither feasible nor practical. **About 10 minutes, during their introduction to the Simulation Center. Risks to participation in the study are minimal and do not differ from risks of participation in simulated patient care without participation in the study. Residents are very busy during their General Inpatient Pediatrics Rotations. Requiring an hour of their time for the educational experience itself seems to some to be a stretch of the ever-increasing demands on their time. Because of its educational value, however, the Residency Program Directors have agreed in the importance of the simulation experience. Presenting the study to them during their regular scheduled session actually allows them time free from distractions to pay attention to what is described and carefully consider their participation. Any time more than 24 hours before participation is not practical, because they are often not reliably in one place for any length of time, and out of the Simulation Center will be burdened by distractions which may prevent careful thought regarding participation.**

Procedures to Protect Privacy
Describe the provisions included in the research to protect the privacy interests of participants (e.g., others will not overhear your conversation with potential participants, individuals will not be publicly identified or embarrassed).
Data obtained will be stored and evaluated in aggregate and coded fashion; no identifying information will be kept with it. The data collection forms will be coded with random numbers referring to the participant teams. A separate document will provide the key to be used for these numbers. The key will be stored in a locked file separately from the storage of the data collection sheets. Analysis of data regarding time to correct diagnosis and whether particular parts of the simulation were obtained (history, physical exam, and laboratory and radiology studies) will be done in aggregate such that data from no one participating team will be evaluated individually.

It is routine to obtain video during simulation sessions to be used for education. This is not unique to sessions involved in this study. Video obtained during these simulated experiences will be used for education only and destroyed after the educational session. Video cameras are installed in each of the Simulation Rooms and tape the mannequin, the participants, and the confederate nurse and confederate "parent" participants. They are used during the debriefing episode immediately following each simulated case scenario. Only the participants in that case and the instructors will view the videos. They are used only for educational purposes. After education, they are immediately destroyed. No one will view the videos in the future. No one will view the video of his/her peers.

Procedures to Maintain Confidentiality
Describe the manner and method for storing research data and maintaining confidentiality. If data will be stored electronically anywhere other than a server maintained centrally by UAB, identify the departmental and all computer systems used to store protocol-related data, and describe how access to that data will be limited to those with a need to know.
Data will be stored on a secure server within the Simulation Center. Only members of the Simulation team have access to this server.

FIGURE 9.3.5 (continued)

form. It is difficult to allow the participant to ask questions if an information sheet is provided electronically. One way to address this issue is to provide a FAQ (frequently asked question) sheet along with the information sheet. Investigators may also allow the participants to contact them via email with any questions they have about the study. This often leads to very specific contact information required by the local IRB. Another way to handle the situation is to provide participants with an electronic "debriefing" document after they have participated in the study. This document would review the purpose of the study, provide a brief description of the types of data collected, and would give more information on how the study was actually conducted (Johnson & Christensen, 2010). It is also important to request a waiver of documentation of consent from the IRB if an electronic information sheet is going to be used to inform participants and no signature will be required.

Privacy and security are both challenging issues when using electronic surveys and the internet to conduct educational research. Investigators must ensure that all participant information is transmitted securely and stored on a server that is protected from public access. Confidentiality can be maintained when using electronic surveys or the internet as long as the participants' information is available only to the IRB-approved investigators. It is extremely difficult to guarantee anonymity when using electronic surveys and the Internet. Anonymity indicates that the identity of the participants is being kept from everyone including the investigators. Surveys requiring demographic information cannot guarantee anonymity. Therefore investigators must be very thorough in describing the assurance of privacy and confidentiality to participants when electronic surveys and the internet are being used in educational research (Johnson & Christensen, 2010). It is also important to pay attention to the safety and security of electronic information that is collected for research purposes.

Failure to Comply

The Office of Human Research Protection's Division of Compliance Oversight (DCO) is responsible for handling situations in which investigators fail to comply with The Code of Federal Regulations Title 45 Part 46. The local IRB institution is responsible for reporting noncompliance issues to the DCO, and then the division determines what actions are necessary to protect human subjects. All letters of determination from the DCO are available beginning in the year 2000 and are posted on the DCO website. Letters of determination are listed in date order and are categorized by the institution who reported the incident of noncompliance. Some of the most common DCO determinations of noncompliance include the following: research conducted without IRB approval, inappropriate use of exempt categories of research, changes in research without IRB approval, failure to report unanticipated problems, and poorly maintained IRB files (Office of Human Research Protection, 2013a). It is always wise to ask the local

IRB when any types of questions arise related to educational research. Failure to do so could result in an ethics violation and a letter of determination publicly posted on the DCO website.

International Ethics Committees

Simulation is fairly well established as a teaching tool throughout North America, Europe, and Australia. But several countries in the Middle East such as Saudi Arabia, Qatar, the United Arab Emirates, and Israel have begun to see a huge growth in the use of simulation in clinical education. Simulation is also beginning to take root as a teaching tool in Africa, Asia, and South America (Davies & Alinier, 2011). As new simulation centers begin to open and grow, more educational research will naturally be conducted. For this reason, it is important to consider the ethical conduct of educational research in the international setting. Committees that review research to ensure human subjects' protection in countries other than the United States may be referred to as *ethics review committees* (ERCs), *research ethics committees* (RECs), *research ethics boards* (REBs), or possibly *internal review boards* (Amdur & Bankert, 2011).

The World Health Organization (WHO) Ethics Review Committee has developed a document for individuals and institutions involved in human subjects research, including biomedical, behavioral, social, and epidemiological research. This publication, entitled *Standards and Operational Guidance for Ethics Review of Health-Related Research with Human Participants*, is a collection of 10 research standards applicable to health-related research involving human participants. It is intended to serve as a benchmark for RECs to use when developing their own policies and procedures related to the ethical considerations of human subjects research. Any research project funded or supported by the WHO must be reviewed according to the standards in this publication (World Health Organization, 2013).

While social science research and protection for human subjects falls under the purview of the IRB in the United States, there are no universal international requirements for social science research with the exception of the aforementioned WHO publication. Many countries consider educational research as falling under the umbrella of the ethical review process for clinical research like the United States. However, some countries do not have an ethical review process for educational research. As recently as 2009, Dutch ethics committees considered educational projects and social science research as excused from ethical review (Cate, 2009). While more countries are beginning to consider social science and educational research as falling within the scope of ethical review guidelines, there is still much variation from country to country as to whether educational research is reviewed at the local level or at a central level. Some countries may have a central review board similar to **Central IRB**s in the United States that are not affiliated with any institution and are for-profit organizations

Informed Consent Document

TITLE OF RESEARCH: Medical Decision-Making Among Residents During a Simulated Patient Experience

IRB PROTOCOL NUMBER: X110611060

INVESTIGATOR: Lauren B, Nichols, MD
CO-INVESTIGATORS: Nancy M. Tindle, MD; Melanie Whitaker, MD; Lynn Zelnick RN; Amber Yasmin, RN

Explanation of Procedures

This research study is attempting to understand the process of medical decision-making by residents on the inpatient services. As part of your routine educational experience in the simulation center, teams of two (resident and intern pair) will be randomized to two scenarios which will be simulated cases of initial patient evaluations at the time of admission. In your teams, you will then evaluate and care for a simulated patient. Video will be made during each session to be used only for your education during the debriefing sessions after each case. This video will be destroyed after it is used for your debriefing session. Each two-case and debriefing session in the simulation center will last one hour. You are expected to attend one 1-hour session during each of your General Inpatient Pediatrics service months as part of your routine educational experience.

If you choose to participate in this research study, aspects of your performance will be timed and evaluated for appropriateness on medical decision-making. You will also be asked to complete a demographic sheet and a short evaluation of the experience as part of the research study.

Your participation in this research study is voluntary. You may choose to participate in the routine educational experience while choosing not to participate in the research component. If you choose not to participate in the research study, your experience will be the same; however, no data will be collected regarding your encounter.

Risks and Discomforts

The risks associated with simulation are no greater than the risks associated with your day-to-day activities. There is risk of loss of confidentiality. Measures such as coding, secure storage of data, destruction of video, and the remote location of the Simulation Center make this risk minimal.

Benefits

You may not benefit from participation in this research project. We hope that your clinical skills will be improved; however this cannot be guaranteed.

Alternatives

The alternative to this study is to decline to participate. This will in no way change your educational experience in the simulation center, your status as a resident, or your evaluation.

Confidentiality

Information obtained about you for this study will be kept confidential to the extent allowed by law. The following groups will have access to private information that identifies you by name: the Office for Human Research Protections (OHRP), and the Institutional Review Board (IRB). The results of this study may be published in the medical literature but no publication will contain information that will identify you.

Refusal or Withdrawal without Penalty

If you are a student or employee, taking part in this research is not a part of your class work or duties. You can refuse to enroll, or withdraw after enrolling at any time before the study is over, with no effect on your class standing, grades, or job. You will not be offered or receive any special consideration if you take part in this research.

FIGURE 9.3.6   Informed Consent Document for expedited study in Figure 9.3.5.

Cost of Participation

There will be no cost to you from taking part in this study.

Payment for Participation

There will be no payment for taking part in this study.

Questions

If you have any questions, concerns, or complaints about the research, please contact Dr. Lauren Nichols. She will be glad to answer any of your questions. Dr. Nichol's number is 255-212-2222. If you have questions about your rights as a research participant, or concerns or complaints about the research, you may contact the Director of the Office of the Institutional Review Board for Human Use (OIRB) at (255) 222-5555. Regular hours for the Office of the IRB are 8:00 a.m. to 5:00 p.m. CT, Monday through Friday. You may also call this number in the event the research staff cannot be reached or you wish to talk to someone else.

Signature of Participant	Date	Time

Signature of Witness	Date	Time

Signature of Person Obtaining Consent	Date	Time

FIGURE 9.3.6 (continued)

who typically receive payment for their services (Moon & Khin-Maung-Gyi, 2009).

The United States Department of Health and Human Services, Office of Human Research Protections has compiled a list of international human research standards including guidelines and organizations that govern human subjects research in 104 countries throughout the world. The compilation is intended for researchers, ethics committees, and sponsors of human subjects research in the international setting (Office of Human Research Protection, 2013b). Researchers wishing to conduct research abroad may consult this document for a list of resources if help from a local ethics committee is not available. The link for the compilation is listed in the resources section of this chapter.

The National Council on Ethics in Human Research (NCEHR) is an independent, Canadian organization dedicated to the protection of human volunteers as participants in research. The NCEHR does not restrict the protection of human participants to biomedical science but extends the protection of human participants to social science, education, and the humanities. In November of 2003, the NCEHR established a task force for developing an accreditation system for human subjects research protection (National Council on Ethics in Human Research, 2013).

International Training

In Canada, the Advisory Panel on Research Ethics offers free online courses to researchers and REBs. Their online course entitled *CORE* (Course on Research Ethics) is based on the guidelines contained in the Tri-Council Policy Statement: Ethical Conduct for Research Involving Humans (Panel on Research Ethics, 2013).

The European Network of Research Ethics Committees Network (EURECNET) is an association that promotes the collaboration of RECs and other comparable organizations across Europe. EURECNET also collaborates with national ethics councils on issues relating to human subjects research (European Network of Research Ethics Committees, 2013). EURECNET offers free online training modules, referred to as TRREE (Training and Resources in Research Ethics Evaluation), that include an introduction to research ethics, the roles and responsibilities of RECs, national regulations, and informed consent. The learning

Waiver of Informed Consent Documentation

- **Use this form** to request a waiver of the requirement
  - o   to obtain a signed consent document (cannot be used for FDA-regulated research) or
  - o   to give participants a signed copy of the document.
- **Do not use this form** to request a waiver of part or all of the informed consent process. Instead, use the Waiver of Consent or Waiver of Authorization and Informed Consent.

1. IRB Protocol Title: **The Use of High Fidelity Simulation in Genetic Counseling and Genetic Medical Education**

2. Principal Investigator: **Nancy Tindle, MD**

3. Choose one of the checkboxes below, indicating why the waiver of documentation is being requested for this research, and provide protocol-specific details as requested.

☐ Confidentiality Risk—Respond to Items a-c, below.
    a. Would the only record linking the subject and the research be the consent document?   ☐Yes ☐No
    b. Would the principal risk be the potential harm resulting from a breach in confidentiality?   ☐Yes ☐No
    c. Describe your plans to ask each subject whether he/she wants documentation linking his/her name with the research, and how each subject's wishes will govern (e.g., a document could be used for the informed consent process, subjects would be asked if they wanted a signed copy to document their consent, and those who did not would receive an unsigned copy)._____

☒ The research involves no greater than minimal risk and no procedures for which written consent is normally required outside the research context. Respond to Item a, below.
    a. Describe plans, if any, that you have for providing subjects with a written statement regarding the research. (*Note: The IRB may require that a written statement be given to the subject.*) **Participants will be provided an information letter as soon as they arrive for their regularly scheduled education session in the simulation center. This letter will inform them of the study.**

By signing this request for waiver of informed consent documentation, I certify the information included in it.

_____   _____
Principal Investigator's Signature   Date

FIGURE 9.3.7   Example of waiver of Informed Consent Documentation.

materials can be accessed at http://www.eurecnet.org/materials/index.html and are available in English, French, German, and Portuguese.

The Middle East Research Ethics Training Initiative (MERETI) is affiliated with the University of Maryland School of Medicine. Since 2005, more than fifty researchers have received certificates of training in research ethics. The majority of the researchers come from Egypt, Sudan, Jordan, Saudi Arabia, and Yemen. More information on the program and on training options can be found at http://medschool.umaryland.edu/mereti/.

BEEN THERE, DONE THAT: HOW CAN I CONTINUE TO IMPROVE OR SUSTAIN WHAT I HAVE ACHIEVED?

Many simulation centers have well-established research programs, and as a result, staff may have extensive experience submitting protocols and working regularly with IRB. This section is intended to offer practical advice for

centers with multiple educational research studies occurring throughout the year.

Organization and Storage

One of the most challenging issues in conducting multiple research projects is a safe and secure method of organizing and storing data and documents related to an IRB and to each individual study. A secure file server with automatic backup is a must. IRB documents such as the human subjects protocol, consent forms, demographic forms, surveys, posttests, approval letters, and so forth, can be housed in folders on a secure file server. Many IRBs are now returning approval letters and consent forms to the principal investigator in electronic formats, making the electronic storage of documents even easier. Any paper documents returned by the IRB can be scanned and stored with the electronic documents to prevent having both paper files and electronic files.

Organization of IRB documents and educational research materials is essential, especially in centers where numerous faculty and staff are involved in various research projects. Simulation centers at large academic institutions may have twenty to thirty IRB-approved research studies happening in any one period of time. Faculty and staff should be able to quickly and easily access consent forms and other IRB-related documents. Staff members should also have a convenient and secure location for data files to be stored and retrieved.

There are several different ways to organize files. They can be organized by course name, by principal investigator, or housed in one central folder titled *IRB*. Centers who already have established files for courses may find it easiest to create a new folder within an already existing course folder and title it *IRB*. All IRB-related documents, approval letters, and data files can be kept in this folder. Alternatively, if a large number of the principal investigators are not part of the simulation center staff, it may be easier to create a folder for each principal investigator. For instance, Dr. Smith has a folder on the server titled *Dr. Smith IRB*. Within that folder each of her studies have a folder—Respiratory Distress, Sharing Bad News, Chemotherapy Administration, and so forth—where consent forms, demographic surveys, and protocols are kept. If a simulation center is fortunate enough to have a research coordinator, it may make the most sense to have a single folder on the file server titled *IRB* where each individual study has its own folder for documents. Clearly, the most effective way of organizing IRB files will vary from center to center, depending on the staff and the number of people with access to the file server. The most important thing is that faculty and staff understand how documents are organized and can easily retrieve what they need in a timely manner.

Naming conventions are also helping when storing large numbers of files on a server. It is best to use shorter file names that make sense to the faculty and staff since most IRB protocol titles are lengthy (e.g., *IRB.Approval.Forensics. pdf* for a protocol titled *The Use of High-Fidelity Simulation in Teaching Residents How to Collect Forensic Evidence in the Emergency Department Setting*). It is also important to use dates in naming documents such as IRB amendments and renewals. Some educational research studies may last 3 or 4 years, and it is important to be able to locate specific protocol changes if needed (i.e., *March 2012 Amendment. Forensics.pdf*).

Another helpful tool in managing large numbers of research studies is the use of a tracking log. Figure 9.3.8 is an example of a tracking log that was created using tables in Word. Each research study can be easily reviewed, and important information such as renewals or protocol numbers can be found without having to search through multiple folders on a file server. The benefit of using tables in Word or of using an Excel spreadsheet is that the data can be sorted by renewal date, by protocol number, or by principal investigator. Storing the tracking log on a file server in the simulation center allows every faculty and staff member to have a quick glance at what research studies are approved

and whether or not data collection has begun. The file name of the log should reflect the most recent update of information on the log (e.g., *IRB.Tracking.Log. 3/15/13*).

Research Networks and Multisite Studies

Simulation centers that are involved in research networks or multisites studies will greatly benefit from having a research coordinator or a staff person who is assigned the responsibility of handling all of the IRB paperwork, including consent forms, protocol changes, and amendments. Multisite studies often result in several protocol changes in order to standardize the procedures of the study as much as possible. It is important to obtain IRB approval as early as possible when taking part in a multisite study so amendments can be submitted with plenty of time for approval before beginning data collection. Typically, the sponsoring institution will send out their IRB protocol for participating sites to use as an example for their local IRB application. Remember that local IRBs vary in their requirements, and some sites may accept another institution's IRB approval and allow for data collection. Other sites may have to begin a protocol from scratch and submit multiple amendments in order to obtain permission to begin the study. It is helpful to have a contact at the local site IRB that can be easily reached to get answers to questions.

Building a relationship with a person at the local IRB also allows insight into which protocols may be exempt and which may be expedited. It is extremely frustrating to complete a 23 page application for an expedited study only to find out the IRB would have accepted the 2-page application and allowed the study to be exempt. Briefly discussing the study with someone at the local IRB can give guidance in the right direction on which paperwork to fill out, including whether or not the study will be eligible for waiver of consent or waiver of documentation of consent. Many faculty and staff often find the IRB process to be frustrating and burdensome. However, having a contact at the local IRB with whom a relationship can be built can be invaluable in terms of time spent developing protocols, filling out amendments, and writing consent forms.

Conducting Research on Existing Courses

It is not uncommon for simulation faculty and staff to find themselves in a situation where they want to do educational research on a course that is already in existence and may or may not be required of certain populations of learners. Often, this type of research is considered exempt because the course is required and IRB approval is only required because the study involves analyzing anonymous data collected from students or employees. When submitting this type of protocol, it is necessary to highlight the required components of the course and compare those

Protocol Number	Study Title	Funding	Principal Investigator	Co-Investigators *Others on protocol	Approval Date	Status	Renewal Date	Contact
E121219003	Development of Interactive Simulation Video Cases for Medical Students in the Large Group Setting		Melanie Jones	Sam Smith	2/18/13	Data Collection Preparation	not required exempt protocol	MJ
X121011011	Counseling and Caring for Patients with Genetic Disorders: Simulated Cases for Pediatric Residents	Founders Fund	Samantha Carson	Nancy Tindle Lynn Zelnick	11/30/12	Data Collection in progress	11/30/13	Samantha
E120822005	Learners' Perceptions of the Effectiveness of Simulation		Donna Taylor	Marie Williams Amber Yasmin	9/5/12	Data Collection in progress	not required exempt protocol	Donna
X120711005	Treatment of Hyperkalemia in Patients with Renal Failure	Founders Fund	Nicki Selkirk	Nancy Tindle Kristin Dunston	8/3/12	Data Collection in progress	8/3/13	Nicki
X110311012	Medical Education Regarding Grandparent Caregivers and Pediatric Care	Donald W. Reynolds Foundation	Amanda Simpson	Hugh Elliott *Nancy Tindle *Lynn Zelnick *Amber Yasmin	5/30/12	Amendment approved May 30, 2012 Data Collection in progress	5/30/13	Amanda
E120419006	An Exploratory Study of Fatigue and Alertness Among Attending Physicians		Melanie Jones	Paul Stone Nancy Tindle Shawn Goodson Donna Taylor	5/17/12	Data Analysis	5/17/13	MJ
X110626010	Medical Decision-Making Among Residents During Simulated Patient Experience	Founders Fund	Lauren Neusome	Nancy Tindle Amber Yasmin Lynn Zelnick	8/31/11	Study Closed	8/31/12	Lauren

FIGURE 9.3.8 Example of a tracking log for IRB Activity.

with the research components of the course. This will help eliminate any confusion by the IRB member who is reviewing the protocol. The procedures section of the protocol should be very specific as in the following example: *Residents who come to the simulation center for the regularly scheduled required simulation course will be invited to participate in the study. The pretest, simulation, posttest, and course evaluation are required of every student regardless of whether or not they choose to participate in the study as these components are part of the third year medical student clerkship curriculum. The research component of the course includes a short demographic form. After informed consent, students who fill out the demographic form are indicating their willingness to participate in the study and to allow their tests and evaluation data to be analyzed and linked with their demographic information. All pretests, posttests, evaluations, and demographic forms will be correlated with a unique code developed by the student (e.g., year of birth followed by last three letters of middle name) and students' data will remain anonymous and reported in aggregate form.* Of course, some research on existing courses may be much more complex, and it is advisable to contact a local IRB member prior to beginning the IRB application to discuss the study and determine the type of application needed.

SUMMARY

All healthcare-related education research, whether simulation is involved or not, should be submitted to an IRB for review (Kraus et al., 2012). Investigators involved in multisite research have reported remarkable differences in IRB expectations among institutions (Dyrbye et al., 2008). Therefore, it is best to consult the local IRB at the institution where the research will take place if investigators have any questions as to the category of research or the requirements of informed consent. International ethics committees exist in most countries and at some academic institutions abroad. As with IRBs in the United States, educational researchers should view them as a resource and as an objective means to protect all human subjects who are involved in educational research.

RESOURCES

Resources within the United States

The local IRB at the institution where the research will take place is the best resource for answering questions related to simulation education research or human subjects research. The list below contains additional information related to human research guidelines and policies within the United States.

Office for Human Research Protections (OHRP)
Home Page
www.hhs.gov/ohrp

Office for Human Research Protections (OHRP)
Guidebook
www.hhs.gov/ohrp/irb/irb_guidebook.htm

Office for Human Research Protections (OHRP)
Guidance Topics by Subject
www.hhs.gov/ohrp/policy/index.html#topics

Office for Human Research Protections (OHRP)
OHRP Compliance Oversight: Determination Letters
www.hhs.gov/ohrp/compliance/letters/index.html

Office or Research Integrity
Home Page
www.ori.dhhs.gov

OHRP Archived Materials
Nuremberg Code
Belmont Report
Children in Research
Conflicts of Interest
http://www.hhs.gov/ohrp/archive/index2.html

Protection of Human Subjects
45 Code of Federal Regulations Part 46
www.hhs.gov/ohrp/humansubjects/guidance/45cfr46.html
Western Institutional Review Board (WIRB)
Home Page
http://www.wirb.com/Pages/default.aspx

International Resources

Canadian National Guidance Document
Tri-Council Policy Statement—Ethical Conduct for Research Involving Humans
http://www.pre.ethics.gc.ca/pdf/eng/tcps2/TCPS_2_FINAL_Web.pdf

Community Research and Development Information Service (a division of the European Commission)
Guidance Note for Researchers and Evaluators of Social Sciences and Humanities Research
http://ec.europa.eu/research/participants/data/ref/fp7/89867/social-sciences-humanities_en.pdf

Council for International Organizations of Medical Sciences
International Ethical Guidelines for Biomedical Research
http://www.cioms.ch/publications/layout_guide2002.pdf

Middle East Research Ethics Training Initiative
(sponsored by the University of Maryland School of Medicine)

MERETI brochure and network blog
http://medschool.umaryland.edu/mereti/

The United Nations Educational, Scientific and Cultural Organization (UNESCO)
International Bioethics Committee (IBC)
http://www.unesco.org/new/en/social-and-human-sciences/themes/bioethics/international-bioethics-committee/

United States Department of Health and Human Services
The International Compilation of Human Research Standards
http://www.hhs.gov/ohrp/international/intlcompilation/intlcomp2013.pdf.pdf

World Health Organization
Standards and Operational Guidance for Ethics Review of Health-Related Research with Human Participants
http://whqlibdoc.who.int/publications/2011/9789241502948_eng.pdf

REFERENCES

Amdur, R., & Bankert, E. A. (2011). *Institutional review board member handbook* (3rd ed.). Sudbury, MA: Jones and Bartlett.

Cate, O. T. (2009). Why the ethics of medical education research differs from that of medical research. *Medical Education, 43*(7), 608–610. doi:10.1111/j.1365-2923.2009.03385x

Davies, J., & Alinier, G. (2011). The growing trend of simulation as a form of clinical education: a global perspective. *International Paramedic Practice, 1*(2), 58–62.

Dyrbye, L. N., Thomas, N. R., Papp, K. K., & Durning, S. J. (2008). Clinician educators' experiences with institutional review boards: Results of a national survey. *Academic Medicine, 83*(6), 590–595.

Egan, M., & Mainous, A. G. (2012). The tension between educational equivalency and equipoise in medical education research. *Family Medicine, 44*(1), 5–6.

European Network of Research Ethics Committees. (2013). *Welcome to EUREC.* Retrieved from http://www.eurecnet.org/index.html

Johnson, R. B., & Christensen, L. B. (2010). *Educational research: Quantitative, qualitative, and mixed approaches* (4th ed.). Thousand Oaks, CA: SAGE.

Keune, J. D., Brunsvold, M. E., Hohmann, E., Korndorffer, J. R., Jr., Weinstein, D. F., & Smink, D. S. (2013). The ethics of conducting graduate medical education research on residents. *Academic Medicine, 88*(4), 1–5. doi:10.1097/ACM.0b013e3182854bef

Kraus, C. K., Guth, T., Richardson, D., Kane, B., & Marco, C. A. (2012). Ethical considerations in education research in emergency medicine. *Academic Emergency Medicine, 19*(12), 1328–1332. doi:10.1111/acem.12019

Moon, M. R., & Khin-Maung-Gyi, F. (2009). The history and role of institutional review boards. *Virtual Mentor: American Medical Association Journal of Ethics, 11*(4), 311–321.

National Council on Ethics in Human Research. (2013). *Welcome to the National Council on Ethics in Human Research.* Retrieved from http://www.ncehr-cnerh.org/

Office of Human Research Protection. (2013a). *Compliance oversight.* Retrieved from http://www.hhs.gov/ohrp/compliance/

Office of Human Research Protection. (2013b). *International compilation of Human Research Standards.* Retrieved from http://www.hhs.gov/ohrp/international/intlcompilation/intlcompilation.html

Panel on Research Ethics. (2013). *The TCPS 2 tutorial course on research ethics (CORE).* Retrieved from http://ethics.gc.ca/eng/education/tutorial-didacticiel/

World Health Organization. (2013). *Ethics and health.* Retrieved from http://www.who.int/ethics/publications/research_standards_9789241502948/en/index.html

Resources

10.1 Resources

CHAPTER 10.1

Resources*

Alicia Gill Rossiter, MSN, ARNP, FNP, PNP-BC, Susan Garbutt, DNP, RN, CIC, CNE, and Rita F. D'Aoust, PhD, ACNP, ANP-BC, CNE, FAANP, FNAP

ABOUT THE AUTHORS

ALICIA GILL ROSSITER is Coordinator of Graduate Nursing Simulation at the University of South Florida (USF) College of Nursing. She is responsible for coordination and implementation of graduate nursing simulation and interprofessional education activities at multiple locations within the USF Health interdisciplinary simulation consortium. She is also a Lieutenant Colonel in the United States Air Force Reserves, serving as adjunct faculty at the Uniformed Services University of the Health Sciences in Bethesda, Maryland.

SUSAN GARBUTT is the Simulation Coordinator/Lecturer in Nursing at the University of Tampa, where she collaborates with graduate and undergraduate nursing faculty to develop and implement simulation scenarios across the curriculum. An early adopter of simulation, Dr. Garbutt has been using clinical simulation to teach nursing students and health care professionals since 2003. Dr. Garbutt has presented at national and international conferences on patient safety, evidence-based practice, and clinical simulation.

RITA F. D'AOUST is the Associate Dean for Academic Affairs and the Director for Interprofessional Initiatives at the University of South Florida College of Nursing. Dr. D'Aoust has a long history in developing innovative undergraduate and graduate curriculum and an extensive background in simulation, including development of a simulation center and the integration of simulation into undergraduate, graduate, and interprofessional curricula. She is the primary investigator of a HRSA grant—Integrating Technology into Nursing Education and Practice—a Web-based training module to educate faculty on incorporation of informatics, simulation, and telehealth into nursing curriculum.

ABSTRACT

A comprehensive reference for evidence-based current simulation resources is critical to the success of any simulation education program. This chapter provides a comprehensive resource for evidence-based simulation education resources. All of the resources from this textbook are compiled in this chapter to serve as a quick reference guide for simulation educators who work with simulation in academic, practice, and/or community settings.

CASE EXAMPLE

You are the Simulation Program Director responsible for managing all aspects of the simulation program at a large university Simulation Program. Your Simulation Program is interdisciplinary and serves medical students, nursing students, physical therapy students, and pharmacy students. In addition, you have a cooperative agreement with the largest hospital in your area, and provide simulation experiences to validate competencies for the licensed healthcare providers on their staff. You are a certified simulation educator, and committed to using the best evidence-based resources to support your simulation program.

---

*Resources in this chapter are also available online at http://www.ssih.org/News/Defining-Excellence

INTRODUCTION AND BACKGROUND

Simulation educators are busy, and must excel at multi-tasking. When key stakeholders approach the simulation educator/simulation director with a new idea for program innovation or expansion, the simulation educator needs a ready reference to locate the most current information on the best evidence-based resources for simulation education. The purpose of this chapter is to serve as a comprehensive quick reference guide to simulation resources. This chapter compiles all of the resources in the chapters in this text, in an easy-to-use quick reference guide format. Links are also available online at http://www.ssih.org/News/Defining-Excellence

1. Simulation Standards
   a. 1.1 SSH Accreditation Standards
      Society for Simulation in Healthcare
         http://www.ssih.org/Accreditation
   b. 1.2 The INACSL Standards of Best Practice
      International Nursing Association of Clinical Simulation and Learning (INACSL)
         www.inacsl.org
   c. 1.3 Simulation Center Program Metrics
      Society for Simulation in Healthcare (SSH)
         http://ssih.org/committees/accreditation
      The American College of Surgery, Accredited Education Institutes (ACS-AEI)
         http://www.facs.org/education/accreditationprogram/
      The American Society of Anesthesiology (ASA)
         https://simapps.asahq.org/
      The American College of Obstetrics and Gynecology (ACOG)
         http://www.acog.org/
      Programmatic requirements for Accreditation Council for Graduate Medical Education (ACGME)
         http://www.acgme.org/acgmeweb/GraduateMedicalEducation/AccreditedProgramsandSponsorSearch.aspx
      IMSH
         http://www.ssih.org/Events/IMSH-2015
      Vanderbilt's Center for Experiential Learning and Assessment
         https://medschool.vanderbilt.edu/cela/
      Peter M. Winter Institute for Simulation Education and Research (WISER)
         http://www.upmc.com/about/why-upmc/quality/Pages/wiser.aspx
      SimPORTAL
         http://www.simportal.umn.edu
      University of Washington (UW)
         http://isis.washington.edu
      The Vanderbilt Program in Interprofessional Learning (VPIL)
         https://medschool.vanderbilt.edu/vpil/
   d. 1.4 Development of the SSH Certified Healthcare Simulation Educator (CHSE) Program: Design of Valid, Defensible and Cost Effective Program
      Society for Simulation in Healthcare (SSH)
         https://ssih.org/certification/chse-examination
      SSH Healthcare Simulation Educator Certification Program
         http://www.ssih.org/Certification
      Australian Society for Simulation in Healthcare (ASSH)
         http://www.simulationaustralia.org.au/divisions/about-assh
      The International Nursing Association for Clinical Simulation & Learning (INACSL)
         http://www.inacsl.org
      The London Deanery
         http://www.londondeanery.ac.uk/
      National League for Nursing (NLN)
         http://www.nln.org/
      Society in Europe for Simulation Applied to Medicine (SESAM)
         http://www.sesam-web.org/
   e. 1.5 Quality Improvement
      National Patient Safety Foundation (NPSF)
         http://www.npsf.org
      Institute of Medicine (IOM)
         http://iom.edu/
      Institute for Healthcare Improvement
         IHI.org
      National Quality Forum (NQF)
         http://www.qualityforum.org/Home.aspx
      Statistical Method from the Viewpoint of Quality Control by Walter A. Shewhart
         https://openlibrary.org/books/OL2723003M/Statistical_method_from_the_viewpoint_of_quality_control
      Six Sigma
         http://sixsigmaonline.org/index.html
      Lean
         http://www.ihi.org/resources/pages/ihiwhitepapers/goingleaninhealthcare.aspx
         http://www.qualitymeasures.ahrq.gov/expert/expert-commentary.aspx?id=32943
         http://www.iom.edu/Global/Perspectives/2012/LeanApproach.aspx
2. Types of Simulation Programs
   a. 2.1 Creating the Infrastructure for a Successful Simulation Program
      Northern New England Simulation Education and Research Consortium (NNESERC)
         www.nneserc.org
      Community Health Education and Simulation Center (CHESC)
         http://nwhospital.org/chesc/welcome.asp
      Institute for Simulation and Interprofessional Studies (ISIS)
         http://isis.washington.edu/

ResearchResearch
    http://www.researchresearch.com/
h. 4.8 Working with Vendors
none
5. Management
  a. 5.1 Business Needs and Asset Assessment
     Stakeholder Map
         http://www.stakeholdermap.com
  b. 5.1.1 CASE STUDY—Group Purchasing
     none
  c. 5.1.2 Business Expansion for Providing Mainte-
     nance of Certification Course none
  d. 5.2 Policies and Procedures : SSH Policy and
     Procedure Manual Template at http://www.ssih.
     org/Portals/48/Docs/Resource%20Library/
     SSH_Policy_Manual.pdf
  e. 5.3 Writing and Implementing a Strategic Plan
     Society for Simulation in Healthcare's Accredi-
     tation Standards
         http://ssih.org/Portals/48/
         Accreditation/14_A_Standards.pdf
  f. 5.4 Developing a Systematic Evaluation Plan
     none
  g. 5.5 Management of Standardized Patient
     Centers
     The Association for Standardized Patient Educa-
     tors GTA/MUTA special interest group
         http://www.aspeducators.org/
     ASPE SP Trainer List-serve
         http://depts.washington.edu/hsasf/clinical/
         learnmoreSP.html
     Association of Standardized Patient Educators
     (ASPE)
         http://aspeducators.org/core-curriculum.
         php
  h. 5.6 Simulation Alliances, Networks, and
     Collaborations
     Healthy Simulation
         http://healthysimulation.com/
     Agency for Healthcare Research and Quality
         http://www.ahrq.gov
     Bay Area Simulation Collaborative (BASC)
         www.cinhc.org › Programs › California
         Simulation Alliance
     California Simulation Alliance (CSA)
         www.californiasimulationalliance.org
     Rural Northern Area Simulation Collaborative
     (RNASC)
         www.cinhc.org › Programs › California
         Simulation Alliance
     Capital Area Simulation Collaborative
     (CASC)
         https://www.californiasimulationalliance.
         org/CSACollaboratives.aspx
     Central Valley Simulation Collaborative
     (CVSC)
         http://www.cinhc.org

Southern California Simulation Collaborative
(SCSC)
    www.cinhc.org › Programs › California
    Simulation Alliance
San Diego Simulation Collaborative (SDSC)
    www.cinhc.org › Programs › California
    Simulation Alliance
Oregon Simulation Alliance (OSA)
    http://oregonsimulation.com/about/
Southeast Indiana Health Care Consortium
    www.eiahec.org/sei-sim.html
Tennessee Simulation Alliance
    www.tnsim.org/
Hawaii Statewide Simulation Collaborative
    thssc.nursing.hawaii.edu/content/meet-staff
Florida Healthcare Simulation Alliance
    http://www.floridahealthsimalliance.org/
    About/WhatistheFHSA.aspx
    Victorian Simulation Alliance (VSA)
    http://www.vicsim.org/index.
    php?option=com_content&view=article&id=
    1&Itemid=2
6. Environmental Design
  a. 6.1 Building a Simulation Center: Key Design
     Strategies and Considerations
     none
  b. 6.2 Space: Potential Locations to Conduct Full-
     scale Simulation-based Education
     none
  c. 6.3 Technical Infrastructure
     none
  d. 6.4 Transitioning to a New Center
     none
7. Educational Development
  a. 7.1 Assessing Learning Needs
     none
  b. 7.2 Common Theories in Healthcare Simulation
     Pamela Jeffries' Simulation Model
         http://www.aacn.nche.edu/membership/
         members-only/presentations/2012/12bacc/
         Richardson-Goldsamt-Jeffries.pdf
         http://livingbooks.nln.org/hits/chapter_03/
         Jeffries_article_NEP.pdf
     The International Nursing Association for Clini-
     cal Simulation and Learning (INACSL)
         https://www.inacsl.org/
  c. 7.3 Assessment in Healthcare Simulation
     none
  d. 7.4 Continuing Medical Education (CME)
     Alliance for Continuing Education in the
     Health Professions (ACEHP)
         www.acehp.org/
     Accreditation Council for Continuing Medical
     Education (ACCME)
         http://www.accme.org
     American Nurses Credentialing Center (ANCC)
         www.nursecredentialing.org/

8. Faculty Development
    a. 8.1 Educator Training Simulation Methodology Courses
       SSH Committee for Certification of Healthcare Simulation Educators
          ssih.org/certification
    b. 8.2 Debriefing
       National Aeronautics and Space Administration
          http://www.nasa.gov
       Objective Structured Assessment of Debriefing (OSAD)
          http://www1.imperial.ac.uk/cpssq/cpssq_publications/resources_tools/osad/
       Debriefing Assessment for Simulation in Healthcare (DASH)
          http://www.harvardmedsim.org/debriefing-assesment-simulation-healthcare.php
    c. 8.3 Realism and Moulage
       FEMA
          Moulage Kit. Retrieved from https://hseep.dhs.gov/hseep_vols/viewResults.aspx?qsearch='moulage'
    d. 8.4 Expecting the Unexpected: Contingency Planning for Healthcare Simulation
       TeamSTEPPS
          http://teamstepps.ahrq.gov/abouttoolsmaterials.htm
       Failure Mode and Effects Analysis (FMEA) model
          http://www.isixsigma.com/tools-templates/fmea/quick-guide-failure-mode-and-effects-analysis/
       International Federation of Red Cross and Red Crescent Societies—Contingency planning guide
          http://www.ifrc.org/PageFiles/40825/1220900-CPG%202012-EN-LR.pdf
    e. 8.5 The Ethics of Simulation
       TeamSTEPPS
          http://teamstepps.ahrq.gov
       Belmont Report: Ethical Principles and Guidelines for the Protection of Human Subjects of Research
          http://www.hhs.gov/ohrp/humansubjects/guidance/belmont.html
9. Research
    a. 9.1 Research in Healthcare Simulation
       Society for Simulation in Healthcare (SSH)
          www.ssih.org/
       Association of Standardized Patient Educators (ASPE)
          www.aspeducators.org/
       Association for Simulated Practice in Healthcare
          www.aspih.org.uk/
       International Nursing Association for Clinical Simulation and Learning (INACSL)
          https://www.inacsl.org/
       Society in Europe for Simulation Applied to Medicine (SESAM)
          www.sesam-web.org/
       American Nurses Association (ANA)'s Annual Quality Conference
          www.nursingworld.org/
       International Nursing Research Congress
          congress.nursingsociety.org/
       Association of American Medical Colleges (AAMC)'s Research in Medical Education
          https://www.aamc.org/
       International Network for Simulation-based Pediatric Innovation, Research and Education (INSPIRE)
          www.inspiresim.com
    b. 9.2 Simulation Research Considerations
       Society in Europe for Simulation Applied to Medicine (SESAM)
          www.sesam-web.org/
       Society for Academic Emergency Medicine
          http://www.saem.org
       INACSL
          https://www.inacsl.org/
    c. 9.3 Institutional Review Board
       Collaborative Institutional Training Initiative (CITI)
          https://www.citiprogram.org/irbpage.asp?language=english
       National Institutes of Health (NIH) Protecting Human Research
          Participants module. Retrieved from http://phrp.nihtraining.com/users/login.php
       The Office of Human Research Protection's Division of Compliance Oversight (DCO)
          http://www.hhs.gov/ohrp/compliance/
       The World Health Organization (WHO) Ethics Review Committee
          http://www.who.int/ethics/en/
       The United States Department of Health and Human Services, Office of Human Research
          http://www.hhs.gov/ohrp/humansubjects/
       The National Council on Ethics in Human Research (NCEHR)
          www.ncehr-cnerh.org/
       Advisory Panel on Research Ethics (Cananda) (*CORE*—Course on Research Ethics)
          http://www.pre.ethics.gc.ca/eng/education/tutorial-didacticiel/
       The European Network of Research Ethics Committees Network (EURECNET) (Training and Resources in Research Ethics Evaluation—TRREE)
          http://www.eurecnet.org/materials/index.html
       The Middle East Research Ethics Training Initiative (MERETI)
          http://medschool.umaryland.edu/mereti/

Office for Human Research Protections (OHRP)
  www.hhs.gov/ohrp
Office for Human Research Protections (OHRP)
  www.hhs.gov/ohrp/irb/irb_guidebook.htm
Office for Human Research Protections (OHRP)
  www.hhs.gov/ohrp/policy/index.html#topics
Office for Human Research Protections (OHRP)
  www.hhs.gov/ohrp/compliance/letters/index.html
Office of Research Integrity
  www.ori.dhhs.gov
OHRP Archived Materials
  http://www.hhs.gov/ohrp/archive/index2.html
Protection of Human Subjects
  www.hhs.gov/ohrp/humansubjects/guidance/45cfr46.html
Western Institutional Review Board (WIRB)
  http://www.wirb.com/Pages/default.aspx
Canadian National Guidance Document
  http://www.pre.ethics.gc.ca/pdf/eng/tcps2/TCPS_2_FINAL_Web.pdf

Community Research and Development Information Service (a division of the European Commission)
  ftp://ftp.cordis.europa.eu/pub/fp7/docs/ethical-guidelines-in-ssh-research_en.pdf
Council for International Organizations of Medical Sciences
  http://www.cioms.ch/publications/layout_guide2002.pdf
Middle East Research Ethics Training Initiative (sponsored by the University of Maryland School of Medicine)
  http://medschool.umaryland.edu/mereti/
The United Nations Educational, Scientific and Cultural Organization (UNESCO)
  http://www.unesco.org/new/en/social-and-human-sciences/themes/bioethics/international-bioethics-committee/
United States Department of Health and Human Services
  http://www.hhs.gov/ohrp/international/intlcompilation/intlcomp2013.pdf.pdf
World Health Organization
  http://whqlibdoc.who.int/publications/2011/9789241502948_eng.pdf

INDEX

Page numbers followed by "*f*" and "*t*" denote figures and tables, respectively.